Encyclopedia of TOXICOLOGY

Volume 2 F–P

Encyclopedia of TOXICOLOGY

Volume 2 F–P

Editor-in-Chief

Philip Wexler

Toxicology and Environmental Health Information Program
National Library of Medicine
National Institutes of Health
Bethesda, Maryland

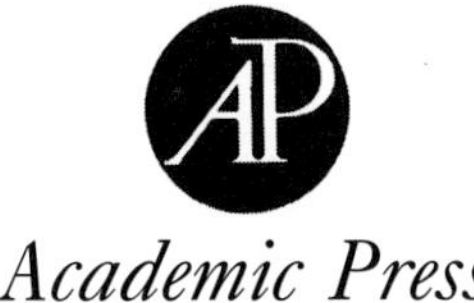

Academic Press

San Diego London Boston New York Sydney Tokyo Toronto

The following articles are U. S. government works in the public domain:

Carbamate Pesticides
Combustion Toxicology
Medical Surveillance
Nerve Gases
Nitrogen Mustards
Organotins
Risk Assessment, Ecological
Sarin
Soman
Sulfur Mustard
Tabun
VX

This book is printed on acid-free paper. ∞

Academic Press
a division of Harcourt Brace & Company
525 B Street, Suite 1900, San Diego, California 92101-4495, USA
http://www.apnet.com

Academic Press Limited
24-28 Oval Road, London NW1 7DX, UK
http://www.hbuk.co.uk/ap/

Library of Congress Card Catalog Number: 98-84114

International Standard Book Number: 0-12-227220-X (set)
International Standard Book Number: 0-12-227221-8 (volume 1)
International Standard Book Number: 0-12-227222-6 (volume 2)
International Standard Book Number: 0-12-227223-4 (volume 3)

PRINTED IN THE UNITED STATES OF AMERICA
98 99 00 01 02 03 MM 9 8 7 6 5 4 3 2 1

Contents

Volume 2

F

Federal Insecticide, Fungicide and Rodenticide Act 1
Fentanyl 2
Fentanyl Derivatives, Illicit 3
Fenthion 4
Fenvalerate 5
Fluorine 6
Fluoxetine 7
Folic Acid 8
Folpet 9
Food Additives 10
Food and Agriculture Organization of the United Nations 20
Food and Drug Administration 25
Food, Drug, and Cosmetic Act 27
Forensic Toxicology 28
Formaldehyde 33
Formamide 34
Formic Acid 35
Foxglove 36
Freons 37
Furan 39
Furfural 40

G

Gallium (Ga) 43
Gastrointestinal System 44
Generally Recognized As Safe (GRAS) 51
Ginger Jake 52
Ginseng 52
Glutathione 53
Glutethimide 54
Glyceraldehyde 55
Glycerol 56
Glycol Ethers 57
Glyphosate 60
Gold (Au) 61
Good Laboratory Practices 61
Guaifenesin 65

H

Hazard Identification 67
Hazardous Waste 70
Helium 73
Hemlock, Poison 73
Hemlock, Water 74
Heparin 74
Heptachlor 76
Heptane 77
Heptanone 78

Heroin 79
Hexachlorobutadiene 81
Hexachlorocyclopentadiene 82
Hexachlorophene 83
Hexane 85
Holly 88
Hormesis 88
Host-Mediated Assay 92
Hydrangea 94
Hydrazine 95
Hydrobromic Acid 96
Hydrochloric Acid 97
Hydrocodone 98
Hydrofluoric Acid 100
Hydrogen Peroxide 101
Hydrogen Sulfide 102
Hydroiodic Acid 105
Hydromorphone 105
Hydroperoxides, Organic 107
Hydroxylamine 107
Hymenoptera 108
Hypersensitivity, Delayed-Type 109
Hypoglycemics, Oral 110

I

Ibuprofen 113
Immune System 114
Indole 139
Indoor Air Pollution 140
Information Resources in Toxicology 148
International Agency for Research on Cancer 170
International Life Sciences Institute—North America 173
International Programme on Chemical Safety 173
International Register of Potentially Toxic Chemicals 177
International Union of Toxicology 180
Investigative New Drug Application 182
In Vitro Test 183
In Vivo Test 184
Iodine 186
Iron (Fe) 187
Isocyanates 189
Isoniazid 189
Isoprene 190
Isopropanol 191

J

Jequirity Bean 195
Jimsonweed 196

K

Kerosene 197
Kidney 198

L

LD_{50}/LC_{50} 227
Lead (Pb) 230
Levels of Effect in Toxicological Assessment 233
Levothyroxine 234
Lidocaine 235
Life Cycle Assessment 237
Lily of the Valley 244
Limonene 245
Lindane 245
Liothyronine 246
Lipid Peroxidation 247
Lithium (Li) 253
Liver 253
Loperamide 262
Loxapine 262
LSD 264
Lye 265
Lyme Disease 266

M

Malathion 269
Mancozeb 270
Manganese (Mn) 271
Marijuana 272
Maximum Allowable Concentration 274
Maximum Tolerated Dose 274
Mechanisms of Toxicity 275
Medical Surveillance 279
Meperidine 283
Meprobamate 285
Mercaptoethanol, 2- 286
Mercapturic Acid 287
Mercury (Hg) 288
Mescaline 289
Metallothionein 290
Metals 291
Methadone 292
Methamidophos 293
Methane 294
Methanol 295
Methaqualone 297
Methomyl 298
Methoprene 299
Methoxychlor 299
Methoxyethanol 301
Methoxypsoralen 302
Methyl Acrylate 302
Methylamine 303
Methyl Bromide 304
Methylcholanthrene, 3- 305
Methyl Disulfide 306
Methyldopa 307
Methylene Chloride 308
Methyl Ethyl Ketone 310
Methylenedioxymethamphetamine 311
Methyl Isobutyl Ketone 312
Methylmercury 314
Methylnitrosourea 316
Methyl Parathion 317
Methyl *t*-Butyl Ether 318
Methyprylon 319
Metronidazole 320
Mevinphos 321
Microtox 322
Minoxidil 324
Mistletoe 325
Mitomycin C 326
Mixtures 326
Modifying Factors of Toxicity 327
Molecular Toxicology—Recombinant DNA Technology 335
Molybdenum (Mo) 343
Monoamine Oxidase Inhibitors 344
Monosodium Glutamate 345
Morning Glory 346
Morphine 347
Mouse Lymphoma Assay 348
Mouthwash 350
Multiple Chemical Sensitivities 351
Mushrooms, Coprine 354
Mushrooms, Cyclopeptide 355
Mushrooms, Ibotenic Acid 357
Mushrooms, Monomethylhydrazine 358
Mushrooms, Muscarine 359
Mushrooms, Psilocybin 360
Mustard Gas 362
Mutagenesis 363
Mycotoxins 369

N

Naphthalene 371
Naphthylisothiocyanate, 1- 373
National Center for Toxicological Research 373
National Environmental Policy Act 374
National Institute for Occupational Safety and Health 375

National Institute of Environmental Health Sciences 376
National Institutes of Health 377
National Library of Medicine/TEHIP 378
National Toxicology Program 378
Nematocides 380
Nerve Gases 380
Neurotoxicity, Delayed 385
Neurotoxicology: Central and Peripheral 389
Niacin 414
Nickel (Ni) 415
Nicotine 417
Nitric Oxide 418
Nitrite Inhalants 419
Nitrites 420
Nitrobenzene 421
Nitroethane 423
Nitrogen Mustards 424
Nitrogen Tetraoxide 426
Nitromethane 427
Nitrosamines 428
N-Nitrosodimethylamine 429
Nitrous Oxide 430
Noise: Ototraumatic Effects 431
Norbormide 438
Nutmeg 439

O

Occupational Safety and Health Act 441
Occupational Safety and Health Administration 442
Occupational Toxicology 442
Octane 450
Oil, Crude 451
Oil, Lubricating 453
Oleander 454
Opium 455
Organisation for Economic Co-operation and Development 456
Organochlorine Insecticides 464
Organophosphate Poisoning, Intermediate Syndrome 465
Organophosphates 467
Organotins 471
Oxygen 472
Ozone 473

P

Paraquat 475
Parathion 476
Paregoric 478
Penicillin 478
Pentachloronitrobenzene 479
Pentachlorophenol 480
Pentane 481
Pentazocine 482
Perchloric Acid 483
Periodic Acid 484
Permethrin 484
Permissible Exposure Limit 485
Peroxisome Proliferators 486
Pesticides 494
Petroleum Distillates 495
Petroleum Ether 496
Petroleum Hydrocarbons 497
Peyote 500
Pharmacokinetic Models 501
Pharmacokinetics/Toxicokinetics 503
Phenanthrene 512
Phencyclidine 512
Phenol 514
Phenothiazines 515
Phenylmercuric Acetate 516
Phenylpropanolamine 518
Phenytoin 519
Phorbol Esters 520
Phosgene 522
Phosphoric Acid 523

Photoallergens 523
Photochemical Oxidants 528
Phthalate Esters Plasticizers 529
Picloram 530
Picric Acid 531
Piperonyl Butoxide 532
Platinum (Pt) 533
Poinsettia 534
Poisoning Emergencies in Humans 534
Pokeweed 550
Pollution, Air 551
Pollution Prevention Act 559
Pollution, Soil 560
Pollution, Water 566
Polybrominated Biphenyls 573
Polychlorinated Biphenyls 574
Polycyclic Aromatic Amines 576
Polycyclic Aromatic Hydrocarbons 577
Polyethylene Glycol 577
Polymers 578
Population Density 580
Potassium (K) 584
Primidone 585
Procainamide 586
Prometryn 588
Propachlor 588
Propane 589
Propanil 590
Propargite 591
Propazine 591
Propene 592
Propionic Acid 593
Proposition 65 594
Propoxur 594
Propoxyphene 595
Prostaglandins 596
Prunus Species 597
Pseudophedrine 598
Psychological Indices of Toxicity 599
Pyrethrin/Pyrethroids 610
Pyridine 611
Pyridoxine 612
Pyriminil 613

Volume 3

Q

Quartz 1
Quinidine 2
Quinine 3

R

Radiation Toxicology 5
Radon 19
Ranitidine 20
Red Dye No. 2 21
Red Tide 22
Reproductive System, Female 23
Reproductive System, Male 38
Reserpine 49
Resistance to Toxicants 50
Resource Conservation and Recovery Act 51
Respiratory Tract 52
Rhododendron Genus 86
Rhubarb 87
Riboflavin 87
Rifampin 88
Risk Assessment, Ecological 89
Risk Assessment, Human Health 103
Risk Characterization 109
Risk Communication 110
Risk Management 113
Rotenone 114

S

Saccharin 117
Safe Drinking Water Act 118
Salicylates 118
Salmonella 120
Sarin 121
Saxitoxin 124
Scombroid 125
Scorpions 126
Selenium (Se) 127
Sensitivity Analysis 128
Sensory Organs 130
Sertraline Hydrochloride 135
Shampoo 136
Shellfish Poisoning, Paralytic 137
Shigella 138
Short-Term Exposure Limit 138
Sick Building Syndrome 139
Silver (Ag) 144
Sister Chromatid Exchanges 144
Skeletal System 146
Skin 151
Snake, Crotalidae 179
Snake, Elapidae 180
Society of Environmental Toxicology and Chemistry 182
Society of Toxicology 183
Sodium (Na) 185
Sodium Fluoroacetate 186
Sodium Sulfite 187
Solanum Genus 188
Soman 189
Speed 192
Spider, Black Widow 193
Spider, Brown Recluse 194
Staphylococcus aureus 196
State Regulation of Consumer Products 197
Structure–Activity Relationships 198
Strychnine 201
Styrene 202
Sudan Grass 203
Sulfites 205
Sulfur Dioxide 205
Sulfur Mustard 206
Surfactants, Anionic and Nonionic 209

T

2,4,5-T 211
Tabun 213
TCDD 215
Tellurium (Te) 216
Terbutaline 217
Terfenadine 218
Tetrachloroethane 219
Tetrachloroethylene 220
Tetrachlorophenoxyacetic Acid 222
Tetrahydrofuran 222
Tetranitromethane 224
Tetrodotoxin 225
Thalidomide 226
Thallium (Tl) 227
Theophylline 228
Thiamine 230
Thiazide Diuretics 230
Thioacetamide 232
Thioxanthenes 232
Thiram 234
Threshold Limit Value 235
Thyroid Extract 236
Tin (Sn) 237
Tissue Repair 238
Titanium (Ti) 244
Tobacco 245
Tobacco Smoke 247
Toluene 248
Toluene Diisocyanate 250
Toluidine 251
Toxicity, Acute 252

Toxicity, Chronic 259
Toxicity, Subchronic 264
Toxicity Testing, Alternatives 269
Toxicity Testing, Aquatic 273
Toxicity Testing, Behavioral 282
Toxicity Testing, Carcinogenesis 289
Toxicity Testing, Dermal 293
Toxicity Testing, Developmental 305
Toxicity Testing, Inhalation 319
Toxicity Testing, Reproductive 328
Toxicology 338
Toxicology, Education and Careers 341
Toxicology, History of 347
Toxic Substances Control Act 354
Toxic Torts 356
Triadimefon 371
Trichloroethanes 372
Trichloroethylene 372
Tricyclic Antidepressants 375
Trihalomethanes 376
Trinitrotoluene 377

U

Uncertainty Analysis 379
Uranium (U) 381
Urethane 382

V

Valproic Acid 385
Vanadium 386
Vanillin 387
Veterinary Toxicology 388
Vinyl Chloride 403
Vitamin A 404
Vitamin D 405
Vitamin E 406
VX 407

W

Warfarin 411
Wisteria 412

X

Xylene 415

Y

Yew 419
Yohimbine 420

Z

Zinc (Zn) 423

Glossary of Key Terms *425*
Contributors *433*
Index *441*

Volume 1

Guide to Encyclopedia *xix*
Foreword *xxiii*
Preface *xxxv*

A

Absorption 1
Academy of Toxicological Sciences 7
ACE Inhibitors 7
Acenaphthene 9
Acetaldehyde 10
Acetaminophen 11
Acetic Acid 13
Acetone 14
Acetonitrile 16
Acetylaminofluorene 17

Acetylcholine 18
Acetylene 20
Acetylsalicylic Acid 21
Acids 22
Aconitum Species 23
Acrolein 24
Acrylamide 25
Acrylic Acid 26
Acrylonitrile 27
Adiponitrile 28
Aerosols 30
A-esterase 30
Aflatoxin 33
Agency for Toxic Substances and Disease Registry 34
Alachlor 35
Alar 36
Albuterol 37
Aldicarb 38
Aldrin 39
Algae 40
Alkalies 41
Alkyl Halides 42
α-Methylfentanyl 44
α-Naphthyl Thiourea 45
Aluminum (Al) 46
Aluminum Phosphide 48
Amdro 49
American Academy of Clinical Toxicology 50
American Association of Poison Control Centers 50
American Board of Toxicology 51
American College of Medical Toxicology 53
American College of Toxicology 53
American Conference of Governmental Industrial Hygienists 55
Ames Test 56
Aminoglycosides 58
Amiodarone 59
Ammonia 60
Ammonium Nitrate 61
Ammonium Perchlorate 62
Amphetamine 63
Amphibians 64
Amyl Nitrate 65
Analytical Toxicology 66
Androgens 69
Animal Models 70
Anthracene 73
Anticholinergics 74
Antimony (Sb) 76
Anxiolytics 77
Aramite 79
Arsenic (As) 80
Arum 82
Asbestos 82
Ascorbic Acid 84
Aspartame 85
Astemizole 86
Atrazine 87
Atropine 87
Avermectin 89
Azinphos-Methyl 90

B

Bacillus cereus 93
BAL 93
Baneberry 94
Barbiturates, Long-Acting 95
Barbiturates, Short-Acting 97
Barium (Ba) 99
Baygon 100
BCNU 101
Behavioral Toxicology 102
Belladonna Alkaloids 128
Benadryl 130
Benomyl 131

Benz[a]anthracene 132
Benzene 133
Benzene Hexachloride 134
Benzidine 136
Benzo[a]pyrene 137
Benzodiazepines 139
Benzyl Alcohol 141
Benzyl Benzoate 143
Beryllium (Be) 144
Beta Blockers 145
Biguanides 146
Bioaccumulation 148
Bioconcentration 151
Biomagnification 152
Biomarkers, Environmental 153
Biomarkers, Human Health 154
Biotransformation 159
Bismuth (Bi) 174
Bleach 174
Blood 176
Boric Acid 182
Boron (B) 183
Botulinum Toxin 184
Brodifacoum 185
Bromine 187
Bromobenzene 188
Bromoform 189
Buckthorn 190
Butadiene, 1,3- 191
Butane 192
Butter Yellow 193
Butyl Ether 194
Butyl Ethyl Ether 195
Butyl Methyl Ether 196
Butyl Nitrite 196
Butylamines 197
Butylated Hydroxyanisole 198
Butylated Hydroxytoluene 199
Butyraldehyde, *n*- 201
Butyric Acid 202
Butyronitrile 203
Butyrophenones 203

C

Cadmium (Cd) 207
Caffeine 209
Calcium Channel Blockers 211
Calomel 212
Camphor 213
Captafol 214
Captan 215
Carbamate Pesticides 216
Carbamazepine 218
Carbaryl 219
Carbofuran 221
Carbon Dioxide 222
Carbon Disulfide 223
Carbon Monoxide 224
Carbon Tetrabromide 226
Carbon Tetrachloride 227
Carbonyl Sulfide 228
Carboxylesterases 229
Carboxylic Acids 232
Carcinogen Classification Schemes 232
Carcinogen–DNA Adduct Formation and DNA Repair 237
Carcinogenesis 246
Cardiovascular System 268
Castor Bean 288
Catecholamines 288
Cell Proliferation 290
Centipedes 295
Cephalosporins 295
Charcoal 296
Chemical Industry Institute of Toxicology 297
Chloral Hydrate 298
Chloramphenicol 299

Chlorbenzilate 300
Chlordane 301
Chlordecone 303
Chlordimeform 304
Chlorine 306
Chlorine Dioxide 307
Chlorobenzene 308
Chloroform 310
Chloromethyl Ether, bis- 311
Chlorophenols 312
Chlorophenoxy Herbicides 313
Chloropicrin 315
Chloroquine 316
Chlorothalonil 317
Chlorpheniramine 318
Chlorpromazine 319
Chlorpyrifos 322
Chlorzoxazone 324
Cholesterol 325
Choline 325
Cholinesterase Inhibition 326
Chromium (Cr) 340
Chromosome Aberrations 342
Chrysene 344
Ciguatoxin 346
Cimetidine 346
Cisplatin 347
Clean Air Act 349
Clean Water Act 350
Clofibrate 351
Clonidine 352
Clostridium perfringens 353
Cobalt (Co) 353
Cocaine 355
Codeine 356
Coke Oven Emissions 357
Colchicine 358
Combustion Toxicology 360
Comprehensive Environmental Response, Compensation, and Liability Act 374
Coniine 375
Consumer Product Safety Commission 376
Copper (Cu) 376
Corrosives 378
Corticosteroids 379
Cosmetics 380
Cotinine 382
Coumarins 383
Creosote 384
Cromolyn 385
Cyanamide 386
Cyanide 387
Cyclodienes 389
Cyclohexane 390
Cyclohexene 391
Cyclophosphamide 392
Cypermethrin 393
Cysteine 395

D

2,4-D 397
Dalapon 398
DDT 399
Decane 400
DEET 401
DEF 402
Deferoxamine 403
DEHP 404
Delaney Clause 405
Deltamethrin 405
Deodorants 406
Detergent 407
Developmental Toxicology 408
Dextromethorphan 453
Diazinon 454
Diazoxide 455
Dibenz[a,h]anthracene 456
Dibenzofuran 457
Dibromochloropropane 458
Dibutyl Phthalate 459
Dicamba 460

Dichlone 461
Dicholorobenzene 461
Dichloroethanes 462
Dichloroethylene, 1,1- 463
Dichloroethylene, 1,2- 465
Dichloropropene, 1,3- 467
Dichlorvos 468
Dieldrin 469
Diesel Exhaust 470
Diesel Fuel 471
Diethyl Ether 474
Diethylamine 475
Diethylene Glycol 475
Diethylstilbestrol 477
Diflubenzuron 478
Difluoroethylene, 1,1- 478
Digitalis Glycosides 479
Dimethoate 481
Dimethyl Sulfoxide 483
Dinitroanilines 484
Dinitrophenols 485
Dinitrotoluene 487
Dinoseb 489
Dioctylphthalate 490
Dioxane, 1,4- 492
Dioxins 494
Diphenhydramine 496
Diphenoxylate 497
Diphenylhydrazine 498
Disc Batteries 499
Distribution 500
Disulfiram 503
Dithiocarbamates 504
Diuron 506
Dominant Lethal Tests 506
Dose–Response Relationship 508

E

E. coli 515
Ecological Toxicology 515
Ecological Toxicology, Experimental Methods 516
EDTA 520
Effluent Biomonitoring 521
Emergency Response 527
Endocrine System 531
Endrin 535
Environmental Hormone Disruptors 536
Environmental Processes 538
Environmental Protection Agency, National Health and Environmental Effects Research Laboratory 540
Environmental Toxicology 541
Eosinophilia–Myalgia Syndrome 541
Epichlorohydrin 554
Epidemiology 555
Ergot 560
Erythromycin 561
Ethane 562
Ethanol 563
Ethanolamine 565
Ethchlorvynol 566
Ethene 567
Ethyl Acetate 568
Ethyl Acrylate 569
Ethylamine 570
Ethylbenzene 571
Ethyl Bromide 572
Ethylene Glycol 573
Ethylene Glycol Monoethyl Ether 575
Ethylene Glycol Mono-*n*-butyl Ether 576
Ethylene Imine 577
Ethylene Oxide 578
European Commission 579
European Society of Toxicology 584
Excretion 585
Exposure 588
Exposure Assessment 592
Exposure Criteria 594
Eye Irritancy Testing 598

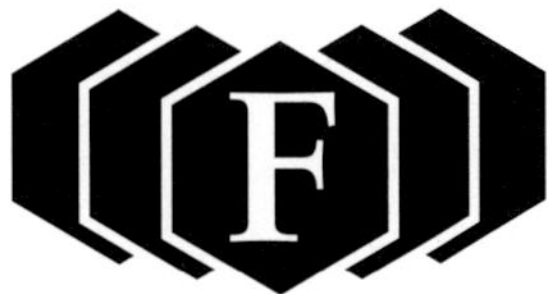

Federal Insecticide, Fungicide and Rodenticide Act

The Federal Insecticide, Fungicide and Rodenticide Act (FIFRA) is the main statute under which all pesticides are distributed and sold in the United States. Federal regulation of pesticides started with the Insecticide Act of 1910, which was directed primarily toward protecting consumers from fraudulent pesticide products; it remained the major law governing pesticide products for 37 years. The Insecticide Act was essentially a labeling statute and did not require registration of products or establish any significant safety standards.

The Insecticide Act was replaced by FIFRA in 1947. FIFRA required that pesticides be registered by the secretary of agriculture before being distributed or sold in interstate or foreign commerce and required label warnings and instructions for safe use for highly toxic products. Since that time, there have been numerous amendments to FIFRA to bring the statute to its current form, and these have been linked with other major federal reorganizational changes. In particular, on December 2, 1970, President Nixon created the U.S. EPA. EPA assumed the pesticide regulatory functions of USDA and with the 1972, 1975, 1978, 1980, 1988, and 1990 amendments, FIFRA has become an increasingly complex statute with greatly increased authority to regulate pesticide products. The regulations governing pesticides are administered by EPA's Office of Pesticide Programs.

FIFRA requires that every pesticide to be sold or distributed in interstate and intrastate commerce be registered. A registration is equivalent to a license to sell or distribute a pesticide in commerce. Registration is based on submission to EPA, by the registrant, data "demonstrating that the pesticide will not cause unreasonable adverse effects on human health or the environment when it is used according to approved label directions"; FIFRA is a risk-balancing statute that does not state that pesticides must be free of all potential risk. It also considers economic and social costs and benefits. A pesticide must also be registered with the appropriate agency in each state in which it is to be used and, in some states such as California, pesticide registration requirements may be even more stringent than those of EPA.

An application for an EPA pesticide registration must be accompanied by data establishing that it is efficacious and can be used without causing unreasonable adverse effects. In registering new products, pesticide manufacturers have the responsibility of providing the data necessary to demonstrate that a material will not present unreasonable risks to humans or the environment. This requires the manufacturer to conduct a comprehensive battery of tests to determine acute and chronic mammalian toxicity, potential adverse effects on other nontarget species (birds and fish), environmental fate and transport, and other factors. The likelihood that the material will leave residues in food crops or might leach into groundwater is also evaluated. The tests required to get a single new pesticide product on the market may cost as much as $40 million and the process may take from 6 to 8 years.

Toxicology data are among the most time-consuming and costly to generate. They are designed to establish the potential adverse effects of the pesticide by different routes of exposure (oral, inhalation, and dermal) and include a complete series of acute, subchronic, and chronic animal studies; metabolism and pharmacokinetic studies; and a battery of tests to determine potential mutagenic activity. While certain exemptions for specific uses may be granted, the tests typically required under FIFRA include acute oral, dermal, and inhalation toxicity; skin and eye irritation; skin sensitization; subchronic (90-day feeding); developmental (teratology); and two-generation reproductive and chronic oncogenicity. Several of these, such as the developmental toxicity and oncogenicity studies, are usually conducted with two different species. The primary objective of toxicology testing under FIFRA is to establish no-observed-effect levels (NOELs) or lowest-observed-effect levels for noncarcinogenic endpoints and cancer potency factors ($q1^*$ values) for materials classified as carcinogens. The NOEL values are used to calculate a reference dose (RfD) (once termed the acceptable daily intake). The RfD is considered to be the daily dose of the pesticide that could be consumed by humans each day, for a lifetime, without causing any adverse effects. The RfD is obtained by applying a "safety factor" or "uncertainty factor" to the NOEL. The uncertainty factor reflects the degree of uncertainty in the data; if the data are good, the factor may be relatively small (perhaps 10) but if the toxicology data are uncertain, it may be as great as 1000. A typical safety factor is about 100, a factor of 10 being used to express uncertainty in extrapolating from animals to humans and an additional factor of 10 to cover possible differences in susceptibility in the human population.

All tests required for FIFRA must be conducted according to FIFRA Good Laboratory Practices (GLP) that specify the minimum practices and procedures that must be followed to ensure the quality and integrity of the data submitted in support of a pesticide registration. GLP regulations were initially promulgated in 1983. Compliance with GLP standards are monitored through a program of laboratory inspections and study audits coordinated through the EPA.

If, after a pesticide product has been registered and in commerce for some time, new data become available that suggest that criteria for determining unreasonable adverse effects have been exceeded, a special review (formally called a Rebuttable Presumption Against Registration) can be initiated. The special review may result in no change in the registration status of the pesticide (if the criteria for unreasonable risk are found not to have been exceeded) or may lead to restrictions in the use of a pesticide or the complete suspension or cancellation of the registration.

—Chris F. Wilkinson

Related Topics

Delaney Clause
Food, Drug, and Cosmetic Act
Good Laboratory Practices
Levels of Effect in Toxicological Assessment
Pesticides
Pharmacokinetics/Toxicokinetics
Risk Assessment, Ecological
Risk Assessment, Human Health
Risk Characterization
Toxicity Testing
Uncertainty Analysis

Fentanyl

- CAS: 437-38-7
- SYNONYMS: Phentanyl; Sublimaze; Duragesic
- PHARMACEUTICAL CLASS: Synthetic opioid analgesic
- CHEMICAL STRUCTURE:

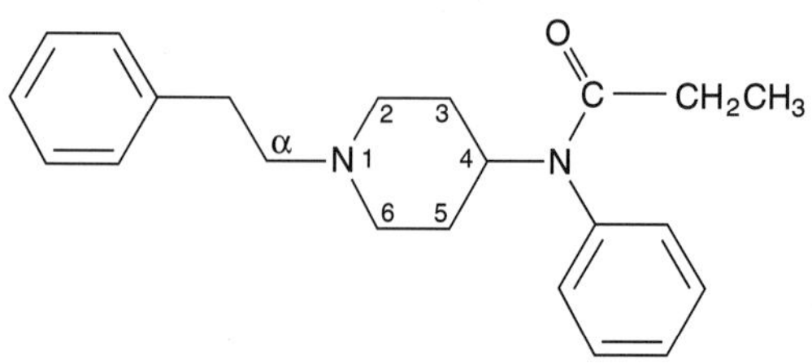

Uses

Intravenous fentanyl is an analgesic supplement. Intramuscular fentanyl is a potent analgesic and presurgery medication. Transdermal fentanyl is utilized to manage chronic pain. Fentanyl and its derivatives have high-dependence liability (see Fentanyl Derivatives, Illicit).

Exposure Pathways

Exposure may occur through the parenteral, oral, and dermal routes.

Toxicokinetics

Parenteral fentanyl is rapidly absorbed and effects are observed in minutes. Transdermal absorption differs. Absorption is temperature dependent. The dermal area under the patch absorbs medication and becomes a depot of fentanyl. This delivery system is designed to deliver a constant amount of drug over hourly intervals. Absorption is accomplished by the mechanism of a gradient difference between the saturated drug in the patch and skin layers. The drug is metabolized by the liver. Metabolism occurs by N-dealkylation to norfentanyl and inactive metabolites. Fentanyl is highly protein bound (80–86%). The average volume of distribution is 6 liters/kg. Up to 85% of the drug is eliminated in the urine in 3 or 4 days. The half-life of fentanyl is 3–12 hr. The half-life increases in persons with hepatic failure and in the geriatric population. The half-life of transdermal fentanyl is different. After removal of the patch, there is continued absorption from the skin depot. The serum concentration falls 50% in an average of 17 hr.

Mechanism of Toxicity

Fentanyl stimulates μ-opioid receptors in the central nervous system (CNS). It binds at the receptor site causing changes in response to pain. The precise sites and mechanism are not understood. It is believed that fentanyl alters the release of different neurotransmitters from the nerves sensitive to pain. Opioid receptors are postulated to have many different binding sites. The ability of fentanyl to produce its effect may be related to its degree of agonist effect on the opioid receptor sites. It can produce profound CNS and respiratory depression through mechanisms common to other opioids.

Human Toxicity

The toxic effects of fentanyl include respiratory and CNS depression, bradycardia, hypotension, miosis, decreased gastrointestinal motility, and feelings of euphoria. High doses produce marked muscular rigidity.

Clinical Management

Basic and advanced life-support measures should be performed as needed. Activated charcoal may be utilized to adsorb fentanyl if it has been ingested (as in the ingestion of a fentanyl patch). Whole bowel irrigation should be considered if a fentanyl patch has been ingested. Naloxone is the specific pharmacologic antagonist for fentanyl.

Animal Toxicity

Fentanyl exhibits an excitatory effect on cats and horses. Its effect on dogs is similar to the human response. Naloxone can be used on animals.

—Denise A. Kuspis

Fentanyl Derivatives, Illicit

- Synonyms: 3-Methyl-fentanyl (3MF); China white; synthetic heroin; designer fentanyl; street fentanyl; α-methylfentanyl (see separate entry for α-Methylfentanyl)
- Pharmaceutical Class: Synthetic opioid
- Chemical Structure:

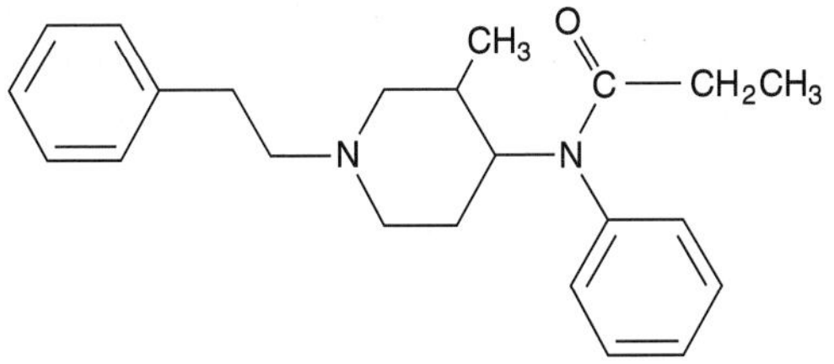

3-Methyl-fentanyl

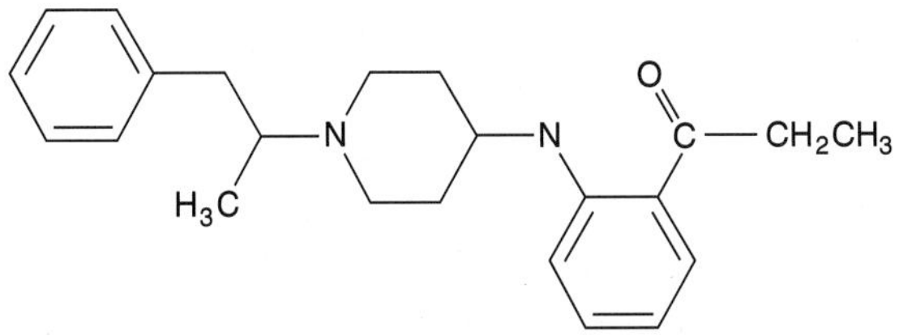

-Methyl-fentanyl

Uses
Illicit fentanyl is synthesized in clandestine laboratories solely for substance abuse.

Exposure Pathways
Illicit fentanyl may be nasally insufflated as powder or solubilized and injected intravenously.

Toxicokinetics
Little is known about the toxicokinetics of illicit fentanyls. Kinetics may change with each manufactured product. Street fentanyl is rapidly absorbed. Addicts report the onset of action or "rush" within 90 sec. Fatal overdose victims have been found with the intravenous needle still in the vein. It is believed that street fentanyl is metabolized by the liver.

Mechanism of Toxicity
Illicit fentanyl's action is one of opioid receptor agonist. The exact opioid receptor sites are not known but appear similar to those of fentanyl.

Human Toxicity
The toxic effects of street fentanyl include rapid onset of respiratory and central nervous system depression. Euphoria is prevalent. Bradycardia, hypotension, miosis, and decreased gastrointestinal motility also occur.

Clinical Management
Basic and advanced life-support measures should be initiated immediately. Activated charcoal may be utilized to adsorb street fentanyl in patients who have ingested it. Naloxone (Narcan) is the specific antidote for this drug. Higher than traditional dosages of naloxone may be required to counteract the opioid effects.

—*Denise A. Kuspis*

Fenthion

- CAS: 55-38-9
- SYNONYMS: *O*,*O*-dimethyl *O*-(4-methylmercapto-3-methylphenyl) thiophosphate; DMTP; Baycid; Baytex; Entex; Lebaycid; Mercaptophos; Queletox; Spotton; Tiguvon; code designations include BAY-29493 and S-1752
- CHEMICAL CLASS: Organophosphorothionate pesticide
- CHEMICAL STRUCTURE:

CH_3O, CH_3O, S, P, O, SCH_3, CH_3

Uses
Fenthion is an effective stomach and contact insecticide against fruit flies, leafhoppers, and cereal bugs. It is available in varying concentrations in wettable powders, fogging agents, emulsifiable concentrates, ultralow-volume sprays, dusts, and granules.

Exposure Pathways
Dermal exposure is most common, but other exposure routes are possible.

Toxicokinetics
Fenthion is well absorbed through the skin and the gastrointestinal tract. Unlike most other phosphorothionates, toxicity from fenthion develops slowly and persists for several days, with the persistence being relatively independent of the route of exposure. It appears that a significant amount of fenthion is converted to the sulfoxide and sulfone before the parent compound undergoes oxidative desulfuration. After dermal application in cows, fenthion and various metabolites were found in the fatty tissues. There is no evidence of *S*-methyl isomerization, and cleavage of the O-methyl ester is a minor reaction.

With a dermal exposure of radiolabeled fenthion, 45–55% of the radioactivity was recovered in the urine in the form of water-soluble hydrolysis products. Approximately 2% each was recovered in the feces and urine. In steers, fenthion and its metabolites, fenthion sulfoxide, fenoxon, and fenthion sulfone, were found in the fat 3 days after a dermal application. Fenthion and metabolites (except fenthion sulfone) were found in the feces as long as 10 days after application.

Mechanism of Toxicity
Fenthion exerts toxicity through indirect inhibition of acetylcholinesterase, i.e., following matabolic activa-

tion to the oxon. Following extensive acetylcholinesterase inhibition, acetylcholine accumulates in synaptic regions and disrupts cholinergic transmission in the central and peripheral nervous systems (see Cholinesterase Inhibition).

Human Toxicity

In the majority of documented cases of exposure to fenthion, a delay in severe toxic effects occurs. The typical clinical signs from organophosphate poisoning are present (e.g., salivation, lacrimation, urination, and diarrhea). Respiratory depression and pulmonary edema may also occur. Possible symptoms of toxicity from chronic fenthion exposure are tingling and numbness in the limbs, back pain, numbness, and generalized muscle weakness. Fenthion appears to be capable of inducing the intermediate syndrome (see Organophosphate Poisoning, Intermediate Syndrome) but does not induce delayed neurotoxicity.

Clinical Management

For exposure to eyes, eyelids should be held open and the eyes flushed with copious amounts of water for 15 min. For exposure to skin, affected areas should be washed immediately with soap and water. The victim should receive medical attention if irritation develops and persists.

For exposure through inhalation, the victim should be removed to fresh air and, if not breathing, given artificial ventilation. The victim should receive medical attention as soon as possible.

First aid for ingestion victims would be to induce vomiting, keeping in mind the possibility of aspiration of solvents. Gastric decontamination should be performed within 30 min of ingestion to be most effective. Initial management of acute toxicity is establishment and maintenance of adequate airway and ventilation. Atropine sulfate in conjunction with 2-PAM can be administered as an antidote. Atropine by intravenous injection is the primary antidote in severe cases. Test injections of atropine (1 mg in adults and 0.15 mg/kg in children) are initially administered, followed by 2–4 mg (in adults) or 0.015–0.05 mg/kg (in children) every 10–15 min until cholinergic signs (e.g., diarrhea, salivation, bronchial and secretions) decrease. High doses of atropine over several injections may be necessary for effective control of cholinergic signs. If lavage is performed, endotracheal and/or esophageal control is suggested. At first signs of pulmonary edema, the patient should be placed in an oxygen tent and treated symptomatically.

Animal Toxicity

Oral LD_{50} values in rodents range from about 150 to 250 mg/kg. Dermal toxicity values are somewhat higher (LD_{50} about 500 mg/kg). Fenthion does not appear to be a teratogen in experimental studies. Several epidemiological and experimental studies suggest that fenthion exposure may have long-lasting effects on the visual system.

—Thuc Pham

Related Topics

Cholinesterase Inhibition
Organophosphate Poisoning, Intermediate Syndrome
Organophosphates
Pesticides

Fenvalerate

- CAS: 51630-58-1
- SYNONYMS: Sumicidin; Pydrin; Phenvalerate; cyano(3-phenoxyphenyl)methyl 4-chloro-α-(1-methylethyl)benzeneacetate
- CHEMICAL CLASS: Type II synthetic pyrethroid insecticide
- CHEMICAL STRUCTURE:

Uses
Fenvalerate is a restricted-use pesticide for insects on cotton, peanuts, soybeans, sugarcane, and sunflowers.

Exposure Pathways
Dermal contact is the main route of exposure, but fenvalerate is sometimes accidentally inhaled or ingested.

Toxicokinetics
Fenvalerate is absorbed readily following ingestion, dermal exposure, or inhalation. Plasma levels of pyrethroids are not clinically useful. Fenvalerate undergoes ester cleavage to alcohol followed by rapid hydroxylation. Fenvalerate is distributed to lipid-rich tissues including the brain. Elimination from fatty tissues is slow, with a half-life of 2–7 days. Fenvalerate is eliminated through urine.

Mechanism of Toxicity
Fenvalerate has low toxicity in mammals due to its rapid metabolic breakdown. It acts directly on nerve axons by prolonging sodium channel opening. In small animals, type II pyrethroids cause salivation, chewing, burrowing, choreoathetosis, and seizures. They also cause lower action potential amplitude, marked membrane depolarization, and eventual total neural activity blockade.

Human Toxicity: Acute
Oral ingestion commonly results in headaches, dizziness, weakness, nausea, and vomiting. The solvent appears to markedly affect toxicity. A more concentrated dose may cause seizures and coma. Common adverse effects of inhalation are runny nose and scratchy throat. Hypersensitivity reactions that may be noted include wheezing, sneezing, shortness of breath, pneumonitis, pulmonary edema, bronchiospasm, and chest pain. Eyes exposed to fenvalerate may develop mild to severe corneal damage. Dermal exposures cause tingling and burning sensations and numbness of the skin. Excitability, tremors, incoordination, numbness, seizures, and coma may result from massive exposure.

Human Toxicity: Chronic
Fenvalerate does not pose significant chronic hazard potential.

The ACGIH TLV-TWA is 5 mg/m^3. The minimal lethal dose is probably in the range of 10–100 g.

Clinical Management
Prevention of absorption may be accomplished by gastric lavage followed by activated charcoal. Basic and advanced life-support measures should be used as necessary. Treatment is primarily supportive and should monitor the development of respiratory distress, seizures, and hypersensitivity reactions. Dermal and ocular exposures should be irrigated with large amounts of water, and other adverse reactions should be treated symptomatically.

Animal Toxicity
Fenvalerate is a powerful paralytic toxin in insects causing "quick knockdown." Fish are extremely sensitive to fenvalerate, but birds are resistant. Dermal and inhalation toxicities in experimental animals are low, and mutagenicity and teratogenicity tests have been negative. Demyelination in peripheral nerves has been reported in experimental animals.

The oral LD_{50} values vary among species. The reference dose is 2.5E-2 mg/kg/day. The no-observed-effect level is 125 ppm.

—Carey Pope and Janice Reeves

Related Topics

Neurotoxicology: Central and Peripheral
Pyrethrin/Pyrethroids

Fluorine

- CAS: 7782-41-4
- Chemical Class: Halogen
- Chemical Symbol: F

Uses
Fluorine is combined either directly or indirectly with other elements to form flourides, and it is used in hydroflouric acid and fluoropolymers and refrigerating agents.

Exposure Pathways

Dermal exposure, inhalation, or ingestion are possible routes of exposure.

Toxicokinetics

Chronic ingestion of flourides causes exaggerated buildup on teeth, bones, and ligaments. Exposure to skin, eyes, and mucous membranes has a corrosive effect.

Mechanisms of Toxicity

Fluoride interferes with metabolism of cells and enzymes. It is a cross-linking agent (does not occur in elemental state in nature.) It is a metabolic inhibitor, interfering with calcium metabolism and electron transport.

Human Toxicity

Chronic overabsorption can cause hardening of bones, calcification of ligaments, and buildup on teeth. Fluoride can cause irritation or corrosion to eyes, skin, and nasal membranes. Inhalation may be fatal. The ACGIH TLV for fluorine is 1 ppm.

Clinical Management

Skin or mucousal burns should be washed for 15–60 min under running water. Burns should be coated with a water-based magnesium dioxide ointment with at least 20% glycerin, no oil. Affected eyes should be washed in running water for 15 min then irrigated with saline solution for 30–60 min. If ingested, soluble calcium should be administered. Milk or cream should be consumed every 4 hr to relieve gastric upset.

—*Shayne C. Gad and Jayne E. Ash*

Fluoxetine

- CAS: 54910-89-3
- Synonyms: *N*-methyl-3-phenyl-3-[(a,a,a-trifluoro-*p*-tolyl)oxy]propylamine hydrochloride; Prozac
- Pharmaceutical Class: Selective serotonin reuptake inhibitor; bicyclic antidepressant unrelated to tricyclic or tetracyclic compounds
- Molecular Formula: $C_{17}H_{18}F_3O$
- Chemical Structure:

F_3C–(C₆H₄)–O–$CHCH_2CH_2NHCH_3$ (with phenyl on CH)

Uses

Fluoxetine is used to treat depression, anorexia, bulemia, obesity, obsessive–compulsive disorder, premenstrual syndrome, panic attacks, narcolepsy, kleptomania, and diabetic neuropathy.

Exposure Pathways

Fluoxetine is available orally as capsules or liquid. Ingestion is the most common route of exposure.

Toxicokinetics

Fluoxetine is rapidly and completely absorbed orally, reaching a peak in 6–8 hr. Food does not affect absorption. Fluoxetine is N-demethylated in the liver to an active metabolite, norfluoxetine, and many other minor inactive metabolites. Both fluoxetine and norfluoxetine are then conjugated prior to excretion. Protein binding is 94%. The volume of distribution is estimated to be 11–88.4 liters/kg. Approximately 2.5% of the drug is renally excreted unchanged and 10% as the norfluoxetine metabolite. A total of 65% of radiolabeled fluoxetine is recovered in the urine after 35 days and 15% is recovered in the feces. The elimination half-life of fluoxetine is 48–72 hr, averaging almost 70 hr. The half-life of norfluoxetine is 7–9 days. The elimination half-life for both is prolonged in patients with hepatic disease.

Mechanism of Toxicity

Fluoxetine has been found to cause selective central nervous system (CNS) neuronal uptake inhibition of serotonin. While fluoxetine may bind to adrenergic, muscarinic, and histaminic receptors, it has not been shown to have the profound effects on catecholamine that are common to tricyclic antidepressant overdose patients.

Human Toxicity

The therapeutic dose of fluoxetine ranges from 20 to 60 mg/day. At therapeutic levels, the most commonly reported adverse effects are headache, nervousness, insomnia, drowsiness, tremor, nausea, anorexia, and diarrhea. Patients reported to have overdosed with fluoxetine have had a benign course with very little neurologic or cardiovascular toxicity. A decreased level of consciousness is the most common effect noted in overdose patients. Reported neurologic clinical symptoms include tremor, confusion, ataxia, insomnia, and coma. Seizures have been rarely reported following either therapeutic dosing or overdose. Cardiovascular symptoms seldom occur. The most common cardiovascular effects include mild tachycardia, bradycardia, and hypertension. No consistent EKG changes have been noted. Other symptoms reported are a flu-like syndrome, nausea, vomiting, and diarrhea. The estimated lethal dose is 1200–2000 mg. However, most fluoxetine-related fatalities occur in patients who have taken a concurrent tricyclic antidepressant overdose. It has been disputed that therapeutic dosing of fluoxetine has been associated with the development of mania, psychosis, and suicidal ideation. Fluoxetine use may be associated with serotonin syndrome following both therapeutic use and overdose, primarily in combination with other serotonergic agents.

Clinical Management

All basic and advanced life-support measures should be implemented. Gastric decontamination should be performed. Fluoxetine is readily adsorbed by activated charcoal. Aggressive supportive care should be instituted. There is no specific antidote for fluoxetine overdose. Hemoperfusion and hemodialysis are ineffective.

Animal Toxicity

Six dogs were given intentional overdoses of oral fluoxetine during preclinical testing. Five of the six dogs had grand-mal seizures. All recovered with standard veterinary doses of intravenous diazepam. Chronic administration of fluoxetine has led to increased phospholipids in mice, rats, and dogs; this increase was reversed when the drug was discontinued.

—Douglas J. Borys

Folic Acid

- CAS: 59-30-3
- SYNONYMS: Vitamin B_9; folacin; folate; pteroylmonoglutamic acid; glutamic acid; *N*-(*p*-(((2-amino-4-hydroxy-6-rteridinyl) methyl)amino)benzoyl)-,l
- PHARMACEUTICAL CLASS: Water-soluble vitamin
- MOLECULAR FORMULA: $C_{19}H_{19}N_7O_6$
- CHEMICAL STRUCTURE:

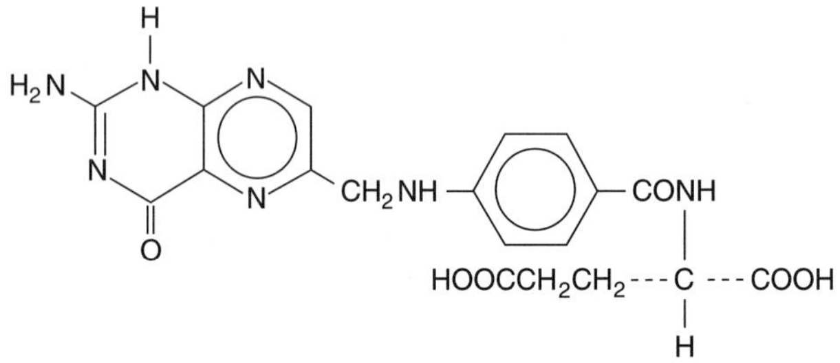

Uses

Folic acid is a nutritional supplement used during deficiency (sprue). Folic acid needs increase during chronic diseases, such as malabsorption liver disease, alcoholism, and during pregnancy and lactation.

Exposure Pathways

Routes of exposure are oral, intravenous, intramuscular, and subcutaneous. Dietary sources of folic acid are green leafy vegetables, some fruits, legumes, eggs, yeast, whole grain cereals, lean beef, veal, liver, and kidneys. Heat destroys folic acid in cooked foods.

Toxicokinetics

Folic acid is almost completely absorbed from the gastrointestinal tract, mostly in the upper duodenum. Peak serum levels occur within 30–60 min. Folic acid is converted in the liver to tetrahydrofolic acid in the presence of ascorbic acid by dihydrofolate reductase. Tetrahydrofolic acid and its derivatives are distributed into all body tissues with approximately half of it in the liver. It is excreted renally almost entirely as metabolite. Excessive amounts of folic acid (beyond the daily needs) are excreted unchanged in the urine.

Mechanism of Toxicity

Unknown

Human Toxicity: Acute

Toxicity is unlikely even after acute ingestions of 100 times the recommended daily allowance. Allergic reactions have been reported.

Human Toxicity: Chronic

Chronic large doses may interfere with sleep patterns and cause malaise, irritability, and gastrointestinal symptoms such as anorexia, nausea, bloating, flatulence, and bad taste. Seizure threshold may be lowered in epileptics and progression of neurologic injury in pernicious anemia has also been reported.

Clinical Management

Acute ingestions seldom require treatment. In cases of chronic excessive use, the patient should be instructed to discontinue the supplement. Any toxic symptoms should be treated symptomatically.

Animal Toxicity

Acute toxicity is not expected and it would be unlikely for animals to be given chronic folic acid overdoses.

—Denise L. Kurta

Related Topic

Developmental Toxicology

Folpet

- CAS: 133-07-3
- Synonyms: Acryptan; Faltan; Faltex; Folnit; Folpan; Folpel; Folpex; Ftalan; Fungitrol II; Intercide TMP; Phaltan; Phaltane; Spolacid; Thiophal; Vinicoll; ENT 26539; SHA 081601
- Chemical Class: *N*-[(trichloromethyl)thio] phthalimide fungicide
- Chemical Structure:

O, C, C, O, $NSCCl_3$

Uses

Folpet is a broad-spectrum contact fungicide used on various fruits, vegetables, berries, flowers, and ornamentals. It is also used on seeds, plant beds, and structural surfaces and is added to some paints and plastics for antifungal purposes. Folpet is useful only for prevention of fungal growth and not for treatment of an existing infection.

Exposure Pathways

Folpet is available as dustable or wettable powders or as a suspension concentrate. Eye and skin or respiratory exposure may occur during production or application of folpet. Ingestion of contaminated food products is also a potential route of exposure.

Toxicokinetics

Folpet is readily absorbed following oral administration in rats. Metabolites of folpet in rats are tetrahydrophthalimide and phthalimide, which may be further metabolized to phthalic acid and ammonia. Studies indicate folpet does not require enzymatic activation and may be detoxified by glutathione conjugation.

Mechanism of Toxicity

In target organisms, folpet acts by blocking fungal growth. Toxicity in nontarget organisms is probably due to multiple mechanisms. Glyceraldehyde-3-phosphate dehydrogenase activity and O-demethylase activity in liver microsomes are inhibited by folpet. Folpet has been shown to uncouple oxidative phosphorylation and may act as a hapten, stimulating the immune system to produce allergic responses against folpet and other structurally similar compounds.

Human Toxicity: Acute

Local irritation can result following dermal, ocular, or respiratory contact with folpet. Ingestion of folpet may cause vomiting and diarrhea leading to dehydration and electrolyte depletion. Exposure to folpet has been linked to contact dermatitis. In rats, folpet and the related fungicides captan and captafol have been shown to decrease cytochrome P450 activity and increase serum enzymes suggesting hepatotoxicity.

Human Toxicity: Chronic

Folpet is classified as a probable human carcinogen (B2). It has induced neoplastic growth in the duodenum of several strains of mice and has tested positive for mutagenicity in multiple *in vitro* assays. Researchers have thoroughly examined the possible teratogenic effect of folpet due to its structural similarity to the known human teratogen thalidomide. All test results for teratogenicity were negative.

Clinical Management

For eye contact, the eyes should be flushed immediately with generous amounts of water. For dermal exposure, contaminated clothing should be removed and the skin should be washed thoroughly with soap and water. A physician should be contacted promptly if irritation does not subside. In fully conscious patients, emesis with syrup of ipecac should be used for substantial ingestion of folpet. After emesis, activated charcoal with sorbitol should be administered, unless diarrhea is already present, in which case only the charcoal should be given. If the patient is not fully conscious, an endotracheal tube should be inserted and the gastric contents removed. Gastric lavage should be performed with activated charcoal containing sorbitol. Some charcoal should remain in the stomach upon removal of the endotracheal tube. Severe dehydration and electrolyte depletion can be treated with intravenous infusion of glucose and normal saline Ringer's solution or Ringer's lactate.

Animal Toxicity

Reported LD_{50} values vary greatly depending on the route of exposure. Folpet is slightly toxic via oral and dermal routes with reported oral LD_{50} values >10,000 mg/kg in rats and dermal LD_{50} values >22,600 mg/kg in rabbits. In contrast, intraperitoneal LD_{50} values of 40 and 68 mg/kg have been reported in rats. The large differences in LD_{50} values between oral and intraperitoneal routes are most likely due to route-dependent differences in absorption.

—*Paul R. Harp*

Related Topic

Pesticides

Food Additives

Introduction

The issue of food safety is a highly emotional and often nonexact science that routinely has been viewed differently by the public and regulatory agencies responsible for enforcing a diverse group of rules and regulations. To complicate matters, various international governments and agencies have approached the problem with different degrees of concern and legislation, and thus certain compounds that have explicit approval for incorporation into foods in some countries are totally banned elsewhere. For example, in the United States, the number of compounds that can legally be added to food approaches 3000, whereas in Europe, the number permitted is approximately 1/10 this number. This in turn tends to frustrate some consumers into concluding that their government does not have their health and safety as high priorities.

Through the years, most consumers have naturally concluded that compounds intentionally added, with government approval, to their food supply are the key threats to their health, whereas from a practical standpoint, potential microbiological problems have a far greater impact on their health and well-being. Also, through the years, some compounds approved for food use have eventually been banned, further lowering consumer confidence.

Another concern that can also be frustrating to the public is the role of diet and its supplementation on health. The trends toward diets lower in total fat and salt or high in fiber are some simplistic examples that have in some instances resulted in the approval and use of additional additives in the manufacture of formulated foods. The role of diet and cancer is also of major concern, and some consumers believe that food additives can cause cancer.

The extreme over consumption of almost any compound can lead to death due to toxicity. However, equally as important is the prolonged consumption of sublethal levels of naturally occurring compounds. A primary example of this latter scenario is the intentional elevated consumption of the compound selenium. Thus, responsible agencies not only have to be concerned about the addition of compounds that are not naturally occurring but also be concerned about naturally occurring compounds that can be toxic if consumed at elevated levels.

Also of potential concern is the presence of various agricultural chemicals used in the production, processing, and distribution of our food supply. These chemicals have been referred to as unintentional food additives and include compounds such as insecticides and pesticides. Uncertainty about their benefits and safety has led to a rise in organically grown foods, which are loosely defined as foods grown without the use of agricultural chemicals.

Most consumers lack a practical definition of a food additive. In actuality, a food additive can be a single approved compound or a mixture of compounds that can find their way either intentionally or unintentionally into any aspect of food production, storage, processing, packaging, distribution, and consumption. Using this accepted legal definition, most consumers are surprised to discover that compounds such as salt and sugar are food additives. Thus, various food additives have been used for centuries and should not be considered to be exclusively a group of nontraditional compounds concocted in the laboratory.

Most consumers also do not realize that a compound, whether it is or is not naturally occurring, cannot be automatically incorporated into their food supply. There is a distinct protocol for obtaining legal permission for such use, and a key checkpoint centers around toxicological concerns. However, human toxicity data may be difficult to obtain for obvious reasons. Thus, for numerous compounds, laboratory animal toxicity data are extrapolated to humans, a sometimes controversial technique.

The fact that the United States has the most reasonably priced, diverse, and safe food supply in the world can be directly attributed to the appropriate use of food additives. For example, the use of chemical preservatives as antimicrobial agents in various foods dramatically minimizes the role of various types of food-borne problems. Also, the use of certain antioxidants minimizes essential fatty acid degradation during processing and prolonged storage of lipid-containing foods, thereby preserving their nutritional significance. The intentional addition of nutrients normally degraded during processing and storage is another example of food additives improving the nutritional quality of our food supply.

Historical Significance

Without question, through the centuries, food adulteration has been an ongoing concern. Early examples included the addition of sawdust to ground spices and the addition of water to milk and wine. One could argue that these abuses did not compromise food safety but were purely immoral acts for economic gain. Thus, in the modern world, most countries have in place detailed legislation and inspection procedures governing food abuses that could have direct bearing on the quality and safety of their food supply. One could argue that in most societies, food quality and subsequent safety are controlled by competition, but the introduction of new foods and the use of food additives need to be government directed to protect the public from potentially immediate (toxic) and long-term health and safety issues.

In the United States, uniform federal legislation directed toward food was sparked by the publication of *The Jungle*, a book by Upton Sinclair, in which he detailed abuses that were apparently common occurrences in the processing of certain foods. This resulted in the passage of the Pure Food and Drug Act in 1906. Later, in 1938, the manufacture of cosmetics was also included under the federal Food, Drug and Cosmetic Act.

Food additives were specifically addressed with the passage of the 1958 Food Additives Amendment, while color additives were defined in the 1960 Color Additives Amendment. Of continued ongoing interest was the Delaney Clause associated with the 1958 amendment. It rather simply stated that any compound that can be demonstrated to be a carcinogen could not be used in food. This concept not only covered existing food additives but also was assumed to apply to any food itself. Since no usage levels were specified for the compound or food in question, one could probably demonstrate that most foods and additives could effectively be banned from our food supply. This concept can be further clouded if one presupposses mutagenicity to be a precursor for carcinogenicity. For example, most foods when heated can be demonstrated to possess mutagenic properties via the microbial Ames test. As a result, the Delaney Clause has been the rallying point against the use of food additives.

Historically, the use of numerous agricultural chemicals was covered under the Federal Insecticide, Fungicide and Rodenticide Act. This act, along with the 1958 act, was modified by the 1996 Food Quality Protection Act, which stated that the Delaney Clause now does not apply to pesticide residues in food. The new law also changed and expanded various pesticide regulations, turning the focus to health-based-standard approach and to pesticide residue safety.

Although most of the previously mentioned legislation has been in effect for decades, groups still express concern over the safety of our food supply relative to food additives. Two of the main areas of contention are the concept of zero tolerance and benefits-to-risk ratio. With zero tolerance, a residue level of zero is permitted for certain compounds in a food at the time of consumption. However, as more sensitive analytical techniques are developed, some residues that had been measured as zero are now measurable at a greater than zero level, thereby banning the food containing them for human consumption. The benefits-to-risk concept usually represents a somewhat educated estimate as to, at a certain usage level, what would be the projected number of adverse incidences attributable to the compound in question. The key question becomes "What will be the potential total consumption within a population over time?" As with any toxicological concern, consumption versus body weight, especially for infants and children, is a key factor to be considered. Since the benefits-to-risk ratio is part of the preapproval process, proven data are typically not available and thus opponents of food additives are concerned that the public will eventually become the "test subjects" for new food additive usage.

Another concept that concerns food additive components is the government generally recognized as safe (GRAS) list. A large number of the currently approved food additives in the United States are on this list. Historically, the GRAS list served as the "Grandfather" clause for food additive use. Simply stated, it permits the continued use of compounds that have been in use for long periods of time for which no adverse effects have been demonstrated to date. Invariably, compounds from this list are removed for approved use when subsequent research identifies concerns with the compound. Opponents insist that all compounds on the GRAS list should unequivocally be tested to ensure their safety.

The FDA is charged with ensuring the safety of the United States food supply; however, in actuality, they rely on private enterprise to demonstrate the safety of food additives before they are officially approved by the FDA. Opponents question this approach since they feel that not all data will be presented to the FDA for review.

Key Classes of Additives

The Federal Food, Drug and Cosmetic Act of 1938 along with its subsequent amendments which are administered by the FDA are central to the U.S. food safety. These laws recognize five broad categories of compounds associated with the U.S. food supply. They include intentional food additives, color additives, prohibited substances, GRAS compounds, and unavoidable constituents. Compounds on most of these lists are continually changing, with new compounds being added and others removed or their use restricted to certain foods or levels.

Relative to intentional additives, a key issue that has to be addressed before a compound is approved is its functional merit. Therefore, one of the simplest ways of classifying food additives is by their function in foods. The following sections provide a brief listing and description of the most important categories of intentional food additives based on function.

Antibrowning Agents

Foods such as fresh-cut fruits and vegetables along with dried versions of these products can darken during processing and storage due to a process that is commonly called enzymatic browning. When these products are exposed to air, the enzyme polyphenol oxidase can react with naturally occurring substrates, such as catechol and caffeic acid, to produce discoloration. The rate of enzymatic browning can be controlled either by eliminating one of the three required reactants—enzyme, air, or substrate—or by chemical means. Compounds such as citric and ascorbic acids can be used to adjust pH to a point where enzymatic activity is decreased or, more commonly, sulfites are used to retard the reaction.

The use of sulfiting agents in products such as wines and in salad bar items has potential cause for concern, especially with asthmatics. Therefore, current law requires that a special notation be placed on the product label or in a conspicuous location when sulfiting agents are added to food systems.

Sulfites can degrade important nutrients, such as thiamin, methionine, and tryptophan, as well as induce lipid oxidation. In animal studies, diets containing up to 8% sulfites resulted in reduced growth due to thiamin deficiency, glandular hyperplasia, hemorrhaging, ulceration, necrosis, and stomach inflammation. The acute intraperitoneal LD_{50} for sodium bisulfite in various test animals is in the 300–600 mg/kg body weight range.

Anticaking Agents

These compounds have the unique ability to preferentially bind moisture, thereby maintaining the free-flow properties of such products as salt, powdered sugar, and finely ground spices, especially after these products are opened in moist climates. A typical compound in this category is calcium stearate, which in addition to its anticaking properties can also be a source of calcium in the diet. Compounds such as tricalcium phosphate can also be used as anticaking agents. The compound is ground into a fine powder, which is then mixed with salt crystals for example. The powder coats the salt granules and prevents them from sticking together, thereby resulting in a free-flowing salt.

Antimicrobial Agents

Through the centuries, various forms of food preservation have been practiced. These include drying, heating, freezing, and the use of high concentrations of chemicals such as salt, sugar, and wood smoke. In recent times, additional chemicals have been identified that can retard or prevent the growth of various forms of microorganisms such as bacteria, yeast, and molds. Obviously, microbial growth in various foods can dramatically lower aesthetic quality and, in some cases, present serious health concerns.

Some of the most commonly used chemical preservatives in the United States include benzoates, propionates, and sorbates. Benzoic acid, usually in the sodium salt form, is very effective in controlling bacteria and yeast growth, especially in acidic foods. Interestingly, benzoic acid has been found to be naturally occurring in cranberries, certain types of plums, and various spices including cinnamon and cloves. Propionic acid is usually marketed as its sodium or calcium salt and is very effective against mold growth and, thus is commonly used in combination with benzoic acid to retard all types of microbial activity in various foods. In addition, it has found widespread application in baked goods, in which mold growth is the primary form of microbial activity. Another major application for propionic acid is as a surface dip to retard mold growth in packaged cheese. Sorbic acid, which is usually marketed as its potassium salt, in turn, is quite effective against yeast and molds but somewhat less effective against bacteria. It is effective in food systems having a pH of up to 6.5 and, thus, is commonly used in a wider variety of foods than benzoates and propionates. Other less commonly used but approved chemical preservatives include acetic acid and various acetates.

Food additive opponents question the use of chemical preservatives in general by noting that they can serve as an easy and inexpensive alternative to other forms of preservation, thereby discouraging good manufacturing practices and proper storage conditions. On the other hand, it can be argued that the use of chemical preservatives in conjunction with other forms of food preservation has greatly expanded the availability and shelf life of numerous foods in the United States.

Antioxidants

Traditionally, compounds in this category have been used to control lipid oxidation in fat-containing foods. This type of oxidation occurs in several stages. The first stage involves the reaction of residual oxygen attacking the unsaturated double bonds in a fatty acid chain. This next results in the formation of lipid peroxides, and then there is an actual fatty acid chain cleavage resulting in short-chain aldehydes. These short-chain aldehydes, such as pentanal, have a characteristic odor that is commonly referred to as rancid. A rancid fat, or oil or food containing a rancid fat source, dramatically decreases food acceptability.

Compounds that have antioxidant properties have the ability to preferentially bind oxygen before it can attack fatty acids. There are obviously other ways to prevent oxygen attack in lipid systems, with the most simple being the purging of oxygen from the system via techniques such as nitrogen flushing or vacuum packaging. However, once the package is opened, oxygen will be naturally reintroduced and, with storage, rancidity can develop.

The origins of antioxidants can either be naturally occurring or synthetic. Examples of naturally occurring antioxidants include lecithin, cephalin, carotene, and tocopherol. However, in general, tocopherol and related naturally occurring antioxidants are usually not as effective as synthetic antioxidants and are less stable to heat processing. Some of the most widely used synthetic antioxidants include butylated hydroxyanisole (BHA), butylated hydroxytoluene (BHT), and propyl gallate. Relative to synthetic antioxidants, BHA and BHT are usually used in combination since they display synergism. Their maximum permitted usage level in most foods is 0.02% based on the fat content of the food. However, levels up to 0.1% are permitted in other food systems such as chewing gum.

Certain antioxidants, including BHA and BHT, are permitted in food packaging materials such as the paper or plastic liners normally found in cereal boxes. They are applied to the inner surface during liner manufacture and volatilize into the dry cereal when the package liner is sealed.

The average LD_{50} in test animals for BHA and BHT is from 2000 to 3000 mg/kg body weight, whereas the estimated average consumption of these compounds in the American diet is 0.04 mg/kg body weight.

Coloring Agents

Food appearance is one of the primary factors that govern food acceptability. In turn, one of the ways to influence food appearance is by the addition of coloring agents. Normally, food color can be influenced by heat processing and exposure to light during prolonged storage. For example, the color in nonheated processed fruits and vegetables can be quite attractive but fading usually occurs when these products are heat processed to extend their shelf life. Ready-to-eat cereal-based foods are major users of coloring agents.

These compounds can either be naturally occurring, such as anthocyanin-based grape skin extract and beet juice powder, or synthetic. Normally, the synthetic compounds are more effective at a given concentration and possess greater stability to factors such as heat processing, pH, and exposure to light.

Through the years, synthetic colorants have come under a great deal of scrutiny and, as a result, some that were previously approved have been banned or their use has been limited to specific foods. A classic example was the use of F-D-&-C Red No. 2, which for quite some time was the major red synthetic colorant used in the American food supply. However, its use is now banned in the United States since it was subsequently shown to be carcinogenic in animals. It has been replaced by F-D-&-C Red No. 40.

Red No. 2 was originally approved for food use in the United States in 1929. However, research published in 1966 demonstrated that when fed to dogs at a level of 1% over a period of 7 years, chronic follicular cystitis of the bladder, hemosiderotic focal lesions of the liver, and atrophy of the adrenal zona glomerulosa were observed. Interestingly, Red No. 2 was not banned in the United States until 1976.

All synthetic colorants have to be certified and come in two forms, namely dyes and lakes. Dyes function by actually dissolving in a food system, while lakes are insoluble pigments that color by dispersion.

One synthetic colorant that has been shown to cause adverse reactions to sensitive individuals is the compound tartrazine (F-D-&-C Yellow No. 5). As a result, if it is used as a coloring agent in a food, it must be listed as a separate ingredient instead of being grouped under the term "artificial color(s)" on the ingredient statement.

Yellow No. 5 has been reported to initiate allergic reactions in certain individuals, such as asthmatics. Symptoms include itching, hives, tissue swelling, asthma, and rhinitis. Chronic urticaria has also been associated with tartrazine ingestion.

Curing Agents

Compounds such as sodium nitrite are commonly used as part of the cure mixture for various processed meats such as ham and frankfurters. These products normally have a characteristic pink color. Nitrite decomposes to nitrous oxide, which in turn reacts with naturally occurring meat pigments to produce the pink colored compound nitrosomyoglobin. In addition to serving as a color precursor, nitrite has antimicrobial properties.

Due to the fact the nitrite can react with amino acids during heat processing to produce carcinogenic nitrosamines, the amount of nitrite that legally can be added is strictly limited. However, intentionally added nitrite is not the only potential source of nitrosamines in our diet. For example, nitrates can be microbially converted to nitrites. Thus, foods and water supplies that contain high nitrate levels due to excessive fertilization can undergo significant microbial activity before processing. Nitrosamines also can result from poor oral hygiene when microbes convert food residues containing high levels of nitrate to nitrites. These nitrites in turn can react in the gut with amino acid residues to produce nitrosamines.

Dough Conditioners

Dough conditioners represent a wide variety of both inorganic compounds, such as phosphates, and organic compounds, such as enzymes, that have the physical and chemical abilities to modify the protein and/or starch components in cereal-based flours. By modifying or standardizing flour structure, subsequent dough mixing time can be reduced and baked loaf volume can be increased. Since mixing time and loaf volume can vary among flour batches, the use of these additives permits the production of more uniform bakery items.

Drying Agents

The function of these compounds is similar to that of anticaking agents in that they can preferentially absorb moisture from other food ingredients to keep them from becoming soggy. For example, nut pieces included in a bakery dry mix can be precoated with corn starch. The corn starch in turn absorbs moisture before it can enter the nut, thereby keeping the remainder crisp.

These compounds can also absorb moisture that may migrate through flexible packaging material, thereby maintaining low water activity in the packaged dried food. Low water activity in turn discourages microbial activity and extends product shelf life.

Emulsifiers

Compounds of this type have the ability to promote the formation of suspensions in liquid or semiliquid food systems that normally are not miscible. A simple example would be the manufacture of a salad dressing that has large amounts of water and oil as its major ingredients.

These compounds are normally charged and thus have the ability to orientate themselves in such a fashion that they lower the surface tension among ingredients, thereby permitting an emulsion to form. Lecithin is a classical example of a naturally occurring emulsifying agent, while mono- and diglycerides are examples of modified naturally occurring compounds.

Enzymes

Enzymes are naturally occurring protein-based compounds that have the unique ability to react with specific food components such as lipids, proteins, and carbohydrates.

Numerous food items are routinely made by the action of specific carbohydrases on simple (sugar) to complex (starch) substrates. For example, invert sugar can be made by the action of invertase on sucrose, while enzymatic starch degradation can produce products such as corn syrup and high fructose corn syrup (HFCS).

Residual pectin, which is a carbohydrate derivative naturally present in various fruit juices, can produce a cloudy juice. However, by adding pectinase, the pectin is degraded and thus cloud formation is eliminated.

Protease can be used to modify meat protein structure, thereby resulting in tenderization, while protease added to beer prevents cloud formation due to low levels of protein that are normally present. Proteases are also quite critical to the manufacture of products such as soy sauce and certain types of cheese.

A major nonfood use for enzymes is in various detergents and stain removers. These are usually mixed-enzyme preparations that specifically attack protein and/or fat-containing stains on clothing.

Firming Agents

Traditional heat processing of various fruits and vegetables usually results in a significant loss of firmness, thereby resulting in a product whose textural properties are significantly different than the fresh form of the product in question. Specific examples of compounds that function by maintaining firmness or crispness would be the use of alum in pickles and the use of calcium salts in canned whole tomatoes.

Flavor Enhancers

Compounds in this category are also commonly known as intensifiers or potentiators; they have the unique ability to increase the flavor properties in certain foods. They work especially well in meat and vegetable-based foods but apparently do not function effectively in dairy and cereal-based foods.

Throughout this century, a limited number of naturally occurring compounds have been shown to possess potentiation properties. Without question, the most widely known flavor potentiator is monosodium glutamate (MSG). It is naturally present in many foods but is present at relatively high concentrations in certain seafoods, cheeses, condiments such as soy sauce, and in concentrated tomato products. It can also be thermally and enzymatically produced.

Its intentional addition to food has led to concern among certain individuals who claim to experience adverse reactions to MSG. This is commonly referred to as "Chinese Restaurant Syndrome," which has been characterized as producing overall weakness, palpitation, and numbness in the neck. Severe asthmatics have also reported adverse reactions that appear to be dose related. As a result, the U.S. government is currently considering the mandatory listing of the amount of MSG present in foods.

A major reason for ongoing concern relative to the addition of MSG to food is that a series of early studies reported significant physiological changes in various test animals, such as retina degeneration, brain lesions, convulsions, vomiting, adulthood obesity, and diabetes. However, subsequent studies clearly demonstrated that these specific reactions relative to added MSG ingestion were species specific.

Other commonly used potentiators include inosine monophosphate and guanosine monophosphate, which are commonly called 5′ nucleotides. They function at lower concentrations than MSG but since all three compounds display synergism, they are commonly used in combination if intentionally added to food. All three compounds are also synergistic to salt.

Aside from adding the pure forms of these compounds to food systems, some food processors add ingredients that can result in their formation during heating. Others add ingredients that contain high levels of these compounds. This includes ingredients such as soy sauce and hydrolyzed protein sources, which are produced by either acidic or enzymatic hydrolysis of a protein source in the presence of salt. Using this process, released glutamic acid, which is the predominant amino acid in most protein sources, is converted to MSG.

Flavor Adjutants

These can be used in the manufacture of both liquid and dry flavoring ingredients. In the case of liquid flavorants, they represent a solvent that aids in flavor compound solubility and dispersibility. Typical compounds in this category include ethanol (vanilla extract) and propylene glycol. In the case of dry flavoring agents, these can include various starches and gums that first aid in converting a liquid flavoring to its dry form through a process which is commonly known as encapsulation, which in turn protects the active flavor ingredients against oxidation and also aids in dispersing/dissolving the flavorant when incorporated into a food system.

Flavoring Agents

Flavoring agents represent the largest number of individual compounds approved as food additives in the United States and thus include approximately 1800 diverse compounds coming from both natural and synthetic (imitation) sources. Although there are many compounds in this category, their combined usage level is rather low since most are used at minimal concentrations due to their potency.

The flavor of most foods is due to the presence of numerous flavor-related compounds. Therefore, in order to duplicate an accurate flavor, many compounds are required. Compounds possessing unique flavor properties range from relatively simple acids to esters, aldehydes, lactones, and numerous forms of heterocyclics.

A vast majority of the compounds approved as flavor additives were first identified as naturally occurring flavor components. Once their structures are elucidated, in most cases they can be synthesized in the organic chemistry laboratory or via biosynthesis. Current regulations define biosynthesized compounds as being "natural," whereas those synthesized in the laboratory are classified as "imitation" despite the fact that they are structurally identical. In some instances, approved flavoring agents are purely synthetic and have not been identified to date as naturally occurring.

Interestingly, there are numerous examples in the world of naturally occurring flavoring agents (vanilla being one) where usage far exceeds supply. This has resulted in the synthetic production to augment the natural counterpart. Also, the flavor intensity and complexity of naturally occurring flavoring agents can vary from year to year because they are derived from natural sources, and thus one theoretical advantage of imitation flavors is that they can be formulated to be more uniform over time.

Flour-Treating Agents

These are compounds similar to dough conditioners that result in modified flour properties. Perhaps the best example of compounds in this category would be bleaching agents for flour. Bleach not only modifies flour color from gray to white, therefore improving product acceptability, but also can modify protein structure, thereby decreasing dough mixing time and also producing a more tender product.

Formulation Aids

These compounds improve the efficiency of mixing and processing ingredients. For example, during the weighing and blending of dry spice ingredients or during the grinding of spices, a great deal of dust can be produced, which can present a health and dust explosion hazard. In these situations, antidusting compounds can be added to minimize dust formation. Another example would be the addition of antifoaming agents to certain juices and liquid products. This aids in the rapid filling of containers.

Fumigants

Almost all agricultural products at harvest contain live insects or eggs deposited by aphids. These forms of insect life can then be present during processing and subsequent storage. If these products are minimally processed, they may even be present at time of consumption. Therefore, fumigation represents a very effective way of ensuring that insects in any form of their life cycle are not present in the final product. Cereals destined for long-term storage before milling, along with various spices, are routinely fumigated to control insect contamination. However, there are increasing heath concerns with the use of fumigants, especially for the workers using them; thus lower usage levels and the elimination of certain approved fumigants is a certainty in the future. In addition, environmental concerns exist with the release of fumigants into the atmosphere.

A logical alternative to fumigation, especially for spices, is irradiation. Certain countries, including the United States, do permit the irradiation of certain foods, but the widespread use of irradiation to control insect growth as well as a preservation technique still faces many hurdles.

Humectants

Certain foods and/or ingredients expected to have a semimoist consistency have a tendency to dry out over time. Examples of such foods include shredded coconut, raisins, and marshmallows. Therefore, compounds can be added to maintain moisture content. In the case of shredded coconut, propylene glycol is added.

Leavening Agents

Two forms of cereal-based baked goods are available. In the case of yeast leavened products, the carbon dioxide produced via yeast as a by-product is the means by which a product expands. The other type is chemically leavened products in which carbon dioxide is released from the incorporation of baking powder or soda. This latter category is typified by inorganic compounds normally added to produce products such as muffins and pancakes.

Lubricants

These compounds aid in food processing itself or are used in conjunction with food processing equipment. For example, pipe sections are usually connected with the aid of gaskets and clamps. The gaskets in turn are usually coated with a food-grade jell to minimize leakage. Another example would be the spraying of bread and muffin pans so that the respective products can easily and quickly be removed after baking. These compounds are usually food-grade lipids, oils, or jells. Another equipment use application would be the lubrication of agitators in food processing vessels.

Nonnutritive Sweeteners

Traditional sweeteners, such as sugar and honey, aside from their sweetening properties are also a source of calories and thus are considered to possess nutritional properties. In turn, there are various natural and synthetic compounds that have sweetening properties ranging from several hundred to several thousand times that of sucrose. Therefore, to obtain the same sweetening level from one of these compounds compared to sucrose, a very small amount of compound is required, and thus its caloric contribution is almost nonexistent. Therefore, the use of these compounds in place of sugar can reduce overall caloric intake, which is a key factor relative to weight reduction. In addition, there are certain individuals who for medical reasons cannot tolerate significant amounts of traditional sweeteners, and thus the use of nonnutritive sweeteners provides them the opportunity to consume sweet-tasting foods without compromising their health. Another potential advantage of nonnutritive sweeteners is that they possess anticariogenic properties.

Interestingly, most of the naturally occurring nonnutritive sweeteners have limited potential since they are usually present at relatively low concentrations, which in turn makes their extraction and purification economically limiting. In addition, most of them are structurally protein based and thus are not stable to heat processing or suitable for long-term storage in certain food systems. On the other hand, most of the synthesized compounds are more stable.

Through the years, various approved nonnutritive sweeteners have been banned or their use has been curtailed due to unforeseen health concerns. The most classical example was cyclamate, which had been used in the United States for decades. Another such compound was saccharin. Although it is still permitted in our food supply, a warning label regarding its use is required. A similar compound is Aspartame or Nutrisweet, which also requires a warning label concerning the fact that people lacking the ability to metabolize phenylalanine should restrict their use since the compound is composed of the two amino acids aspartic acid and phenylalanine. Also, during its approved use, both new and reoccurring concerns have surfaced that are currently being further investigated. Other nonnutritive sweeteners have been approved both internationally and in the United States with food approval being given on a food item by food item basis.

Nutritive Sweeteners

These compounds are sweeter than sucrose but, based on the amount required to equal the sweetening power of sucrose, they contribute to caloric intake. Common compounds in this category are corn syrup and HFCS. HFCS has found its largest application as a replacement for sucrose in various carbonated and noncarbonated drinks. Since it is sweeter than sucrose on an equal weight basis, less HFCS is required in formulating such products. In addition to its sweetening properties, HFCS can add thickness or viscosity to liquid drinks, thereby improving their acceptability. HFCS can also function as a humectant in certain foods due to its ability to bind water and thus lower water activity in semimoist foods.

Nutrient Additives

This represents another major category of food additives based on the total weight consumed. Typical common compounds include vitamins and minerals as well as amino acids. In most cases, these represent compounds that can be lost or diminished via various forms of food processing. As a result, opponents suggest that these compounds would not have to be added to our food supply if our foods were not so overprocessed. However, this group usually fails to realize that in many cases heat processing, for example, actually improves the overall nutritional quality of certain foods via inactivation of certain naturally occurring antinutritional components such as urease and trypsin inhibitors.

Another useful function of these compounds is that they can be added to certain foods at levels higher than normally present to make the food in question more nutritionally sound or to actually expand the individual nutrient profile normally found in the food of question.

The U.S. government has historically been a strong proponent of nutrient addition to the food supply. Two very typical and practical examples are the nationwide availability of iodized salt and enriched wheat flour. Currently, the U.S. government is considering expanding the added nutrient profile to enriched flour through the addition of biotin.

pH Control Agents

There are numerous instances in food processing in which the use of acidifying agents, alkalies, buffers, and neutralizing agents is very beneficial to the process as well as the resulting product. Numerous vegetables, especially tomato-based products, are routinely acidified with citric acid prior to canning. Reducing pH shortens the heat processing time required to ensure commercial sterility. In turn, if heat processing time is reduced, nutrient retention along with flavor, color, and textural properties are improved.

In the manufacture of soy protein isolate, both acidic (food-grade HCL) and basic (food-grade NAOH) are used. HCL is used to lower the soy protein to its isoelectric point where the protein precipitates out. Once this fraction is recovered, the pH is adjusted upward with NAOH to resolublize the protein.

Processing Aids

This group represents a wide variety of compounds that assist in making various food processing operations simpler and faster. This includes the uses of alkali to chemically remove the peel from products like potatoes and using various floculants and filter aids to remove various solids. Another example is the use of immobilized enzyme technology to remove undesirable protein from a liquid or semiliquid product on a continuous basis.

Propellants and Gases

These are approved food-grade gases such as nitrogen for use in pressurized cans such as for whipped toppings and CO_2 for use in carbonated beverages.

Sequestrants

The presence of significant amounts of free metals such as iron and copper can produce unwanted color changes in certain foods as well as catalyzing off-flavor development such as rancidity. Sequestrants such as ethylenediaminetetraacetic acid (EDTA) have the unique ability to bind these reactive metals before they can react during processing or storage.

Solvents

These compounds are used in processing to effectively extract certain compounds or classes of compounds from various foods. Typical examples would be the solvent extraction of caffeine from coffee, the production of a liquid oleoresin extract from spices, and the selective extraction of oil from soybeans. In most cases, after the initial extraction, the mixture is usually heated under partial vacuum to selectively recover the solvent for reuse. Hexane, ethanol, and methylene chloride are typical solvents used with food systems.

Stabilizers/Thickeners

This class of compounds is usually composed of natural and chemically modified starches as well as plant, animal, microbial, and seaweed-derived hydrocolloids. They all have the ability to immobilize all or a portion of a liquid in liquid or semiliquid systems. By varying the type and amount of additive, a liquid product can be slightly thickened or completely jelled. They can also be used to suspend solids, like spices, in products such as salad dressings.

Surface Active Agents

These compounds have the ability to quickly and completely disperse or dissolve solids in liquid systems. They permit the rapid and complete wetting and rehydration of dry components added to liquid systems such as cocoa powder into liquid milk.

An example of a naturally occurring surface active agent is lecithin, while examples of synthetic compounds include dioctyl sodium sulfosuccinate and sorbitan esters.

Surface Finishing Agents

Common compounds in this category include edible food-grade waxes, shines, and protective coatings that can be applied to fruits such as apples and vegetables such as cucumbers to enhance attractiveness and prevent product moisture loss.

Conclusion

In conclusion, from this brief presentation, it should be appreciated that there are numerous functional uses for many naturally occurring as well as synthetic compounds in our food supply. In turn, the use of these compounds permits the production of a diverse variety of foods at an economical price. It is conceded that approved additives have on occasion been removed from our food supply when direct evidence has been presented to question the safety of such compounds.

It can be appreciated from the previous discussion that structurally, approved food additives can range from simple to very complex. Also, considering the large number of compounds involved, it is quite impressive that through the years, only a small number of such compounds have been banned, with the remainder demonstrating no adverse physiological or toxicological properties. One should remember that the overconsumption of any compound (e.g., salt) or food can result in distress which may require immediate medical attention. Detailed toxicological properties of specific food additives can be found in the references listed under Further Reading and elsewhere in the encylopedia.

Further Reading

Ayres, J., and Kirschman, J. (Eds.) (1981). *Impact of Toxicology on Food Processing*. AVI, Westport, CT.
Furia, T. E. (Ed.) (1975). *Handbook of Food Additives*, 2nd ed. CRC Press, Cleveland, OH.
Maga, J., and Tu, A. (Eds.) (1995). *Food Additive Toxicology*. Dekker, New York.
Taylor, S., and Scanlan, R. (Eds.) (1989). *Food Toxicology*. Dekker, New York.
Tu, A. (Ed.) (1980). *Survey of Contemporary Toxicology*, Vol. 1. Wiley, New York.

—Joseph A. Maga

Related Topics

Food and Agriculture Organization of the United Nations
Food and Drug Administration

Food and Agriculture Organization of the United Nations

The Food and Agriculture Organization of the United Nations (FAO) was established on October 16, 1945, with the goal to promote global sustainable development of agriculture, fisheries, forestry, and food production and security, quality, and safety as well as the related socioeconomic issues in the member countries. There are 174 member countries in the organization (1995). The headquarters of FAO is located in Rome and is organizationally divided into eight departments, with five regional, five subregional, five liaison, and more than 100 country offices with functions dealing with regional and in-country activities and projects. Five specialized offices within FAO headquarters assist the director-general in directing and managing this, the largest specialized agency of the United Nations system.

Within FAO headquarters there are two departments with responsibilities which include toxicology-related activities. They are the Economic and Social Department (ES) and the Agriculture Department.

The Economic and Social Department, within its Food and Nutrition Division (ESN), houses the Secretariat of the Joint FAO/WHO Food Standards Program established in 1962 and implemented through the Codex Alimentarius Commission (CAC). CAC is an intergovernmental body that meets alternately in Rome and Geneva at the headquarters of the two parent organizations, FAO and World Health Organization (WHO), every odd number of years. The aims of CAC are to protect the health of the consumer and facilitate international trade through the harmonization of national legislation and regulations through establishing international codes of practice, general standards for food additives and contaminants, food commodity standards, maximum limits for residues of pesticides and residues of veterinary drugs in foods, food labeling standards, methods of analysis, etc. The preparatory work for these activities is accomplished by the CAC subsidiary bodies, the Codex General Subject and Commodity Committees (27). Three of these Codex committees are especially important in this connection: the Codex Committee on Food Additives and Contaminants (CCFAC), the Codex Committee on Residues of Veterinary Drugs in Foods (CCRVDF), and the Codex Committee on Pesticide Residues (CCPR).

The Food and Nutrition Division also provides the FAO Secretariat of the Joint FAO/WHO Expert Committee on Food Additives (JECFA). The JECFA was established in the mid-1950s by FAO and WHO to assess chemical additives in food on an international basis. The first meeting was held in 1956 in response to recommendations made in 1955 at a FAO/WHO Conference on Food Additives meeting in Geneva.

When the CAC was formed it decided to utilize the expert scientific advice provided by JECFA on matters relating to the toxicological and specifications activities of food additives. A system was established whereby the Codex Committee on Food Additives, a general subject committee, identified food additives that should receive priority attention, which were then referred to JECFA for assessment before being considered for inclusion in Codex Food Standards.

Over the years, JECFA responsibilities have been expanded to include evaluation/assessment of food contaminants and residues of veterinary drugs in food. JECFA's advice and evaluations are used by the currently existing CCFAC and CCRVDF. JECFA also provides scientific advice directly to FAO, WHO, and their member states. Requests for assessment may come directly from them. JECFA cooperates very closely with Codex but is not a component of the CAC.

Specialists invited to serve as members of JECFA are independent scientists who serve in their individual capacities as experts and not as representatives of their governments or employers. They also understand that the discussions at the meetings are confidential. The goal is to establish safe levels of intake and to develop specifications for identity and purity for food additives or maximum residue limits when veterinary drugs are used in accordance with good practice in the use of veterinary drugs.

As of 1997, a total of 49 meetings of JECFA have been held and over 1000 food additives including 240 flavoring agents, 31 contaminants, and 77 veterinary drugs evaluated. The reports are published in the WHO Technical Report Series. The toxicological evaluations, which summarize the data that serve as the basis for the safety assessments, are published in the WHO Food Additives Series. The specifications and residue evaluations are published in the FAO Food and Nutrition Paper Series.

JECFA meetings are convened twice a year, with one session devoted to the evaluation of food additives and contaminants and the other to the evaluation of residues of veterinary drugs in foods. The meetings are open only to the invited experts and the Joint Secretariat. JECFA can hold hearings during the meeting in which those who have submitted data for evaluation are invited to answer specific questions by the committee to clarify the submission. The JECFA procedures do not permit the committee to discuss the substances under review when the nonmembers are present during these hearings.

JECFA is one body. The discussions are held and decisions made in plenary sessions. The drafting, however, is done in separate groups. In the case of food additives, the FAO experts are responsible for proposing specifications of identity and purity for food additives. The three main objectives of the specifications prepared by the committee are to identify the substance that has been subjected to biological testing, to ensure that the substance is of the quality required for safe use in foods, and to reflect and encourage good manufacturing practice.

To familiarize the reader with the JECFA food additive specifications, those of ammonium polyphosphate are provided in Fig. F-1, as extracted from the Food and Nutrition Paper No. 52, Addendum No. 2 (FAO, 1993).

FAO experts also prepare data sheets for the substances on the agenda to provide the committee with the information on the physical and chemical characteristics of the additive, on the raw material(s) used in commercial production of the additive, and on methods of manufacture by which the raw material(s) is converted into a finished commercial food additive. It is acknowledged that some of these data may be trade secrets. Therefore, such data are held in strict confidence. Furthermore, the data sheets include information on impurities including intermediates, functional use(s) with the technological purpose for using the additive and the levels of use on a commodity basis, estimate(s) of daily intake by humans, reactions and fate in food, and effects on nutrients. In the case of contaminants, FAO experts are responsible for gathering information on human intakes and methods of analysis in food.

Acceptable daily intakes (ADI) for food additives and residues of veterinary drugs and provisional tolerable weekly intakes (PTWI) for contaminants are prepared by the WHO experts.

In JECFA meetings dedicated to the evaluation of veterinary drug residues, the FAO experts are responsible for proposing maximum residue limits (MRLs) for foods of animal origin based on pharmacokinetic and metabolism studies in experimental animals, target animals, and in humans when available; radiolabeled residue depletion studies in target animals from zero withdrawal time to periods beyond the recommended

SYNONYM	INS No. 452(v)
DEFINITION	
Chemical name	Ammonium polyphosphate
C.A.S. number	6833-79-9
Chemical formula	Heterogeneous mixture of ammonium salts of linear condensed polyphosphoric acids of general formula $H_{n+2}P_nO_{3n+1}$
Assay	Content not less than 55.0% and not more than 75.0% on an anhydrous basis, calculated as P_2O_5
DESCRIPTION	Aqueous solution
FUNCTIONAL USES	Sequestrant, emulsifier
CHARACTERISTICS	
IDENTIFICATION TESTS	
A. Solubility	Freely soluble in water
B. pH	4.0–9.0 (1% solution)
C. Positive test for ammonia[a]	Passes test
D. Positive test for phosphates[a]	Mix 0.5 g of sample with 10 ml of nitric acid and 50 ml of water, boil for 30 min, and cool. Test the resulting solution.
PURITY TESTS	
Cyclic phosphate[a]	Not more than 8% calculated as P_2O_5 content
Fluoride[a]	Not more than 10 mg/kg
Arsenic[a]	Not more than 3 mg/kg (Method II)
Lead[a]	Not more than 5 mg/kg Dilute 2 g of the sample to 20 ml with water, neutralise with strong ammonia or dilute acetic acid using phenolphthalein TS as the indicator. Test this solution as directed in the Limit Test, using 10 μg of lead ion (Pb) in the control.
Heavy metals[b]	Not more than 20 mg/kg Test 1 g of the sample as directed in Method I under the Limit Test.
METHOD OF ASSAY	Determine the content calculated as P_2O_5 according to the General Method* "Phosphate Determination as P_2O_5", Method I.

* These specifications were prepared at the 41st session of JECFA (1993) superseding earlier specifications published in the Compendium of Food Additive Specifications (1992).

[a] See General Methods (Guide to JECFA Specifications), FNP 5/Rev.2 (1991).

[b] See General Methods (Guide to JECFA Specifications), FNP 5/Rev.2 (1991).

FIGURE F-1. Food additive specifications for ammonium polyphosphate

withdrawal time (these studies should provide information on total residues, including free and bound residues, and major residue components in order to select a marker residue and target tissue); unlabeled drug depletion studies for analysis of marker residue in target animals including muscle, liver, kidney, fat, eggs, milk, and honey as applicable (this should include studies with appropriate formulations, routes of application, and species using up to maximum recommended doses); methods for routine analysis that may be used by authorities for the detection of residues in target tissue; and the acceptable daily intake proposed by the WHO experts and the standard food intake of 300 g of muscle, 100 g of liver, 50 g of kidney, 50 g of fat, 100 g of eggs, and 1.5 L of milk. Other assumptions and variables may also be involved in determining MRLs, including safety factors used in establishing ADIs, withdrawal times, the contribution of bound residues, and the bioavailability of residues.

In this terminology a veterinary drug is any substance applied or administered to any food-producing animal, such as meat or milk-producing animals, poultry, fish or bees, whether used for therapeutic, prophylactic, or diagnostic purposes or for modification of physiological functions or behavior.

MRL is the maximum concentration of residue resulting from the use of a veterinary drug, expressed in mg/kg or μg/kg on a fresh weight basis. It is based on the type and amount of residue considered to be without toxicological hazard for human health as expressed by the ADI. Consideration is also given to residues of the compound that occur in food of plant origin and/or environment (the same active ingredient may be used as a veterinary drug and pesticide).

Metabolic studies identify and quantify the residues. These studies should simulate the conditions of use of the drug in animal husbandry as closely as practicable. The pharmacokinetics (distribution and elimination) of the residues should be examined between the time of administration of the drug and the time the animals enter the human food supply.

The withdrawal time after administration of a drug is the time during which animals or animal products should not be harvested by fishing, milking, slaughtering, egg collection, etc. for human consumption.

The total residues of a drug in animal-derived food consist of the parent drug, together with all the metabolites and drug-based products that remain in the food after the administration of the drug to food-producing animals. The amount of total residues is generally determined by means of a study using the radiolabeled drug and is expressed as the parent drug equivalents in mg/kg or μg/kg of the food.

The use of veterinary drugs in food-producing animals can result in residues that are neither extractable from tissues nor readily characterized (bound residues). The extractable residues are the residues extracted from tissues or biological fluids by means of aqueous acidic or basic media, organic solvents, and/or hydrolysis with enzymes (e.g., sulfatase or glucuronidase) to hydrolyze conjugates. The nonextractable residues are obtained by subtracting the extractable residues from the total residues and comprise residues of the drug incorporated through normal metabolic pathways into endogenous compounds (e.g., amino acids, proteins, and nucleic acids) or chemically bound residues derived by interaction of residues of the parent drug or its metabolites with macromolecules. These residues may be of toxicological concern. The bioavailable residues are the residues that can be shown, by means of an appropriate method, to be absorbed when fed to experimental (laboratory) animals. In the absence of relevant residue data, it should be assumed that all of the residue is bioavailable and that its potency is equal to that of the most toxic component of the residue.

A marker residue is a residue whose level decreases in a known relationship to the level of total residues in tissues, eggs, or milk. In other words, a marker residue is, or is representative of, the residue of toxicological concern in the target tissue and/or milk/eggs. Identification of a marker residue is important because it is the substance determined for control purposes in the enforcement of MRLs by the national authorities and other parties concerned.

A target tissue is defined within JECFA as the edible animal tissue (muscle, liver kidney, or fat) for which the MRL is recommended and that may be analyzed for purposes of the enforcement of the MRL.

In assessing the safety of veterinary drug residues, the Expert Committee determines the MRL expressed in terms of a named marker residue for target tissues of interest of individually specified animal species. The committee identifies at least two target tissues whenever possible, with one being muscle or fat and the other liver or kidney. Selection of an appropriate target tissue permits regulation of the MRL in international trade in meat (liver and kidney not available) as well as in national control programs.

In summary, when an ADI is established, consideration of the estimated intakes of the relevant foods by human beings allows an assessment to be made of a safe and acceptable residue level for the relevant animal tissue(s). If the levels of residues estimated from supervised trials, when the drug is administered according to good practices in the use of veterinary drugs (only the amount which is necessary to obtain the desired effect is used), are below those considered toxicologically acceptable, then the levels determined by good practice will dictate the acceptable residue level, provided that practical analytical methods are available at that level for routine residue analysis. The committee is reluctant to establish MRLs lower than a level twice that of the limit of quantitation of the previous analytical method.

If the levels of residues found in practice exceed those determined to be acceptable from the toxicological evaluation and consumption data, then drug use in the food-producing animals may need to be modified to reduce residue concentrations in edible tissues to acceptable levels. Possible modifications include extending the withdrawal periods and changing the drug dosage, formulation, or method of application.

When it has been determined that an ADI is unnecessary because the compound of interest is produced endogenously in human beings and animals, then the establishment of an acceptable residue limit is also unnecessary. At the other extreme, when an ADI has not been allocated because, on toxicological grounds, the safety of the compound cannot be assured, then no acceptable residue limit should be established.

The principles outlined here apply to the evaluation of residues of all veterinary drugs. For the establishment of tolerance limits for residues of certain chemotherapeutic agents, however, the antimicrobial properties of the residues must also be taken into account. Antimicrobial properties will become the determining factor in safety evaluation when the toxicity of the substances to be considered is so low that their residues in food could, from the toxicological viewpoint, be tolerated even at the height of therapeutically effective tissue concentrations. At the microbial level, concern for food safety is centered on the question of whether or not residues of antimicrobial agents ingested via food of animal origin pose a danger to human health by exerting a selective pressure on the intestinal flora and thus favoring the growth of microorganisms with natural or acquired resistance.

With regard to withdrawal times, the committee does not attempt to derive, from the residue kinetics, the appropriate withdrawal times to be observed in order to ensure that the concentration of residues in food will be below the established MRL. Residue kinetics and withdrawal times depend on various parameters strictly linked to a given veterinary drug including, but not limited to, the pharmaceutical formulation, the concentration of the active ingredient, the dosage, and the route of administration. The determination of the appropriate withdrawal time for a given veterinary drug in order to comply with an assigned MRL is the responsibility of the appropriate national authority. Nevertheless, when determining MRLs, the committee verifies that those that it recommends can be achieved through realistic withdrawal times and established good practices in the use of veterinary drugs.

To demonstrate how the ADI and MRLs are linked together and how the maximum ingested residue of parent drug and its equivalents is calculated, the following information is presented as extracted from the Food and Nutrition Paper No. 41/6 (FAO, 1994) and the Technical Report Series No. 851 (WHO, 1995).

Based on the ADI of 0–6 μg/kg of body weight for levamisole (parent drug) established by the committee, the permitted daily intake of parent drug and/or its equivalents is 360 μg for a 60-kg person.

The following factors were considered in estimating the MRLs: the ADI; the parent drug is a suitable residue marker and is 2.4% of the total residues; all the residues in muscle and fat are equivalent to parent drug; 50% of the residues in liver are bound and 15% of these bound residues are bioavailable; the residues in kidney are qualitatively similar to those in liver; it is assumed that all bioavailable residues in liver and kidney are equivalent to parent drug; and the residues are similar in cattle, sheep, and pigs.

The committee recommends MRLs of 10 μg/kg for muscle, kidney, and fat and 100 μg/kg for liver of cattle, sheep, poultry, and swine expressed as parent drug. Because residues in eggs at recommended dose level, at 1 day withdrawal, are approximately 1000 μg/kg, the committee considered that levamisole should not be used in laying hens.

The previous assumptions can be used to calculate maximum theoretical daily intake of levamisole equivalents if a consumer ate the standard meat diet containing concentrations of levamisole at the proposed MRLs. The maximum ingested residue of parent drug and its equivalents is 397 μg per day, which consists of 14 μg/day of parent drug and 383 μg/day of levamisole equivalents. The calculation is shown in Table F-1.

Considering the inherent uncertainty of the total levamisole equivalents based on levamisole as the marker residue and considering that only a small proportion of the total residues are used to estimate the total levamisole equivalents (397 μg), the committee considered this value to be equivalent to the maximum ADI.

Depending on the subject of the meeting, the outcome of the JECFA meetings will be the ADIs for food additives or veterinary drug residues, PTWIs for food contaminants, MRLs for residues of veterinary drugs, or specifications for identity and purity of food additives. The MRLs and specifications are then discussed by the CCRVDF and CCFAC, respectively, and if found

TABLE F-1
Calculation of Maximum Ingested Residue of Levamisole (Parent Drug) and Its Equivalents

Tissue	*Standard intake (kg)*	*MRL (μg/kg)*	*UD (μg)*[a]	*EQ (μg)*[a] *Free*	*EQ (μg)*[a] *Bound*	*Total (μg)*
Muscle	0.300	10	3	125	0	125
Liver	0.100	100	10	208	31	239
Kidney	0.050	10	0.5	10	2	12
Fat	0.050	10	0.5	21	0	21
Total	0.500	—	14	364	33	397

[a] UD, unchanged drug; EQ, parent drug equivalents.

acceptable, forwarded to the CAC for adoption as Codex Maximum Residue Limits and Codex Specifications. The ADIs for food additives and PTWIs for contaminants are used by the CCFAC in the preparation of general standards for food additives and contaminants and in recommending of maximum-use levels of food additives or guideline levels of food contaminants in food. Aside from the Codex committees, the outcomes of the JECFA evaluations are freely available to all parties concerned.

The Agriculture Department, within its Plant Production and Protection Division, includes the FAO Secretariat of the Joint Meeting of the FAO Panel of Experts on Pesticide Residues in Food and the Environment and the WHO Toxicological and Environmental Core Assessment Groups, otherwise known as the Joint FAO/WHO Meeting on Pesticide Residues (JMPR). JMPR was established following the resolution of the FAO Conference in 1962 by the Codex Alimentarius Commission to recommend maximum residue limits for pesticide residues and environmental contaminants in specific food products, including methods of sampling and analysis to ensure safety of food containing residues.

The JMPR meetings are closed to nonmember participation and are held annually in September, alternately in Rome and Geneva. WHO-invited members are responsible for proposing ADIs for the substances on the agenda. FAO-invited members draft maximum residue limits for substances under evaluation based on findings in supervised field trials conducted in various countries worldwide. The ADI and MRL proposals are discussed, examined, and the decisions made in the plenary when all the committee members are present. The report of the meeting and the *Evaluations, Part I–Residues* are published in the FAO Plant Production and Protection Paper Series and the *Evaluations, Part II–Toxicology* as a WHO/IPCS publication.

The cooperation between the JMPR and the Codex Committee on Pesticide Residues is close. CCPR identifies those substances which require priority evaluation. After the JMPR evaluation, CCPR discusses the recommended MRLs and forwards them, if they are acceptable, to the Codex Alimentarius Commission for adoption as Codex Maximum Residue Limits.

—*Juhani Paakkanen*

This entry was prepared by J. Paakkanen, Nutrition Officer, Food and Nutrition Division of the Food and Agriculture Organization of the United Nations and is reproduced here by permission of that organization.

Related Topics

Food Additives
Food and Drug Administration
Information Resources in Toxicology
International Life Sciences Institute–North America
International Programme on Chemical Safety
International Register of Potentially Toxic Chemicals
Pharmacokinetics/Toxicokinetics

Food and Drug Administration

The name "Food and Drug Administration" was first provided by the Agriculture Appropriation Act of 1931 (46 Stat. 392), although similar law enforcement functions had been in existence under different organizational titles since January 1, 1907, when the Food and Drug Act of 1906 (21 U.S.C. 1-15) became effective.

The United States Food and Drug Administration's (FDA) activities are directed toward protecting the health of the nation against impure and unsafe foods, drugs and cosmetics, and other potential hazards.

Office of Operations

The Office of Operations advises and assists the commissioner and other key officials on compliance-oriented matters; develops and administers all agency field operations and provides direction and counsel to regional Food and Drug directors; administers regulation of biological products under the biological product control provisions of the Public Health Service Act and applicable provisions of Federal Food, Drug, and Cosmetic Act; works to develop an acquired immunodeficiency syndrome (AIDS) vaccine and AIDS diagnostic tests and conducts other AIDS-related activities; develops and administers programs with regard to the safety, composition, quality (including nutrition), and labeling of foods, food additives, colors, and cosmetics; develops and administers programs for controlling unnecessary exposure of humans to, and ensures the safe and efficacious use of, ionizing and nonionizing radiation-emitting electronic products; develops and administers programs with regard to the safety, effectiveness, and labeling of medical devices for human use; and develops and administers programs with regard to the safety and effectiveness of animal drugs, feeds, feed additives, veterinary medical devices (medical devices for animal use), and other veterinary medical products.

The Office of Operations includes the Office of Regulatory Affairs, the regional field offices, the Center for Biologics Evaluation and Research, the Center for Drug Evaluation and Research, the Center for Food Safety and Applied Nutrition, the Center for Devices and Radiological Health, the Center for Veterinary Medicine, the National Center for Toxicological Research, the Office of AIDS Coordination, the Office of Orphan Products Development, and the Office of Biotechnology.

Center for Drug Evaluation and Research

The Center for Drug Evaluation and Research develops FDA policy with regard to the safety, effectiveness, and labeling of all drug products for human use and reviews and evaluates new drug applications and investigative new drug applications for human use. It develops and implements standards for the safety and effectiveness of all over-the-counter drugs and monitors the quality of marketed drug products through product testing, surveillance, and compliance programs.

The center coordinates with the Center for Biologics Evaluation and Research regarding activities for biological drug product, including research, compliance, and product review and approval, and develops and promulgates guidelines on current Good Manufacturing Practices for use by the drug industry. It develops and disseminates information and educational material dealing with drug products to the medical community and the public in coordination with the Office of the Commissioner. It conducts research and develops scientific standards on the composition, quality, safety, and effectiveness of human drugs; collects and evaluates information on the effects and use trends of marketed drug products; monitors prescription drug advertising and promotional labeling to ensure their accuracy and integrity; and analyzes data on accidental poisonings and disseminates toxicity and treatment information on household products and medicines.

In carrying out these functions, the center cooperates with other components of the FDA, other Public Health Service organizations, governmental and international agencies, volunteer health organizations, universities, individual scientists, nongovernmental laboratories, and manufacturers of drug products.

Center for Biologics Evaluation and Research

The Center for Biologics Evaluation and Research administers regulation of biological products under the biological product control provisions of the Public Health Service Act and applicable provisions of the Federal Food, Drug, and Cosmetic Act. It provides dominant focus in the FDA for coordination of the AIDS program, works to develop an AIDS vaccine and AIDS diagnostic tests, and conducts other AIDS-related activities. It inspects manufacturers' facilities for compliance with standards, tests products submitted for release, establishes written and physical standards, and approves licensing of manufacturers to produce biological products.

The center plans and conducts research related to the development, manufacture, testing, and use of both new and old biological products to develop a scientific base for establishing standards designed to ensure the continued safety, purity, potency, and efficacy of biological products and coordinates with the Center for Drug Evaluation and Research regarding activities for biological drug products, including research, compliance, and product review and approval.

The center plans and conducts research on the preparation, preservation, and safety of blood and blood products; the methods of testing safety, purity, potency, and efficacy of such products for therapeutic use; and the immunological problems concerned with products, testing, and use of diagnostic reagents employed in grouping and typing blood.

Center for Food Safety and Applied Nutrition

The Center for Food Safety and Applied Nutrition conducts research and develops standards on the composition, quality, nutrition, and safety of food and food additives, colors, and cosmetics. It conducts research designed to improve the detection, prevention, and control of contamination that may be responsible for illness or injury conveyed by foods, colors, and cosmetics and coordinates and evaluates the FDA's surveillance and compliance programs relating to foods, colors, and cosmetics.

The center also reviews industry petitions and develops regulations for food standards to permit the safe use of color additives and food additives; collects and interprets data on nutrition, food additives, and environmental factors affecting the total chemical result posed by food additives; and maintains a nutritional data bank.

Center for Veterinary Medicine

The Center for Veterinary Medicine develops and conducts programs with respect to the safety and efficacy of veterinary preparations and devices; evaluates proposed use of veterinary preparations for animal safety and efficacy; and evaluates the FDA's surveillance and compliance programs relating to veterinary drugs and other veterinary medical matters.

Center for Devices and Radiological Health

The Center for Devices and Radiological Health develops and carries out a national program designed to control unnecessary exposure of humans to, and ensure the safe and efficacious use of, potentially hazardous ionizing and nonionizing radiation. It develops policy and priorities regarding FDA programs relating to the safety, effectiveness, and labeling of medical devices for human use and conducts an electronic product radiation control program, including the development and administration of performance standards.

The center plans, conducts, and supports research and testing relating to medical devices and to the health effects of radiation exposure and reviews and evaluates medical device premarket approval applications, product development protocols, and exemption requests for investigational devices. It develops, promulgates, and enforces performance standards for appropriate categories of medical devices and Good Manufacturing Practice regulations for manufacturers. It also provides technical and other nonfinancial assistance to small manufacturers of medical devices.

The center develops regulations, standards, and criteria and recommends changes in FDA legislative authority necessary to protect the public health; provides scientific and technical support to other components within the FDA and other agencies on matters relating to radiological health and medical devices; and maintains appropriate liaison with other federal, state, and international agencies, with industry, and with consumer and professional organizations.

For more information, contact the Food and Drug Administration, 5600 Fishers Lane, Rockville, MD 20857. Telephone: (301) 594-6740.

—David M. Krentz and Harihara M. Mehendale

(Adapted from information supplied by FDA)

Related Topics

Food Additives
Food and Agriculture Organization of the United Nations
Food, Drug, and Cosmetic Act
Information Resources in Toxicology
Investigative New Drug Application

Food, Drug, and Cosmetic Act

- Title: FDCA
- Agency: U.S. FDA

- YEAR PASSED: 1938; subsequently amended multiple times
- GROUPS REGULATED: Pharmaceutical, food, cosmetics, and biologics companies

Synopsis of Law

The federal Food, Drug, and Cosmetic Act (FDCA) is administered by the U.S. FDA and controls the introduction of human and animal drugs, direct food additives, indirect food additives (such as packaging materials), and components of cosmetics. In the case of new human or animal drugs, safety and efficacy must be established before approval for marketing by the U.S. FDA. The approval process is lengthy. For the investigational new drug phase, industry is required to file with the U.S. FDA certain toxicity data at a stage when the investigation of the potential therapeutic usefulness of a chemical in a limited number of humans or animals is desired. As the efficacy of the drug in the treatment of a particular disease is established through clinical trials, these data, together with additional animal toxicity testing data, are filed as part of a new drug application or new animal drug application for review of safety and efficacy by U.S. FDA. Ultimately, as a consequence of the U.S. FDA review, the new drug application is either approved or deficiencies in the data are cited.

While informal guidelines do exist for what the FDA considers to be adequate toxicity testing for certain stages in human clinical investigation, it has not proposed guidelines for the conduct of particular animal toxicity studies. The FDA has, however, issued regulations governing Good Laboratory Practices in the conduct of animal toxicity studies.

Under the same act, industry must show that a chemical intended for direct addition to food, such as a preservative or flavoring agent, or a new polymer having indirect contact with food, such as in a packaging material or can coating material, is safe for its intended use. Results of animal toxicity tests are submitted to the U.S. FDA for review as part of a food additive petition. If the data demonstrate the safety of the chemical to the U.S. FDA, a regulation is published in the *Federal Register* allowing the chemical to be used for a particular purpose in food or in contact with food. U.S. FDA has issued guidelines for the type of toxicity studies that should be conducted in support of a food additive petition (these guidelines are commonly referred to as the Red-book); however, U.S. FDA has not given any guidelines on methodology. The Red-book has been revised and currently is under review.

Currently, there are no requirements for the U.S. FDA to review cosmetic formulations for safety prior to marketing. While the FDCA only requires that cosmetics be free of any "poisonous and deleterious" substances, responsible suppliers of ingredients for use in cosmetics and manufacturers of the final product have conducted relevant toxicity studies where appropriate.

—*Shayne C. Gad*

Related Topics

Delaney Clause
Food Additives
Food and Agriculture Organization of the United Nations
Food and Drug Administration
Generally Recognized as Safe (GRAS)
Good Laboratory Practices
Investigative New Drug Application
State Regulation of Consumer Products
Toxic Torts

Forensic Toxicology

Forensic toxicology is the branch of medical science that applies the principles and knowledge of toxicology to issues and problems in the field of law. To achieve this, the discipline of forensic toxicology combines techniques of analytical chemistry with essential principles of toxicology to address medicolegal issues relating to the effects of toxic substances on humans. Analytical chemistry deals with the techniques and methods for determining the identity and relative amounts of unknown components in a sample of matter. Toxicology has been defined as the study of poisons. A frequently used definition of a poison is one provided by the physician–alchemist, Paracelsus (1493–1541). He noted that "All substances are poisons; there is none which is not a poison. The right dose differentiates a poison from a remedy." For this reason, forensic toxicology involves the use of proper chemical or analytical techniques to identify potentially any chemical substances in biological systems and examining the effects of these substances on humans. In assisting the judicial system in deciding whether a chemical substance could have a medicolegal impact on the outcome of a legal matter, the forensic toxicologist must first establish the presence and exact identity of that chemical substance (prescription or illicit drug or poison) in an individual and establish a relationship between exposure to that chemical and the occurrence of an injurious effect or death.

Poisoning is usually an act contrived of evil intentions. The poisoner seeking the death of another individual is often very discreet about the manner in which a poison is introduced into the body of a victim. Great precaution is often taken to conceal the steps leading to the completion of this activity. Therefore, establishing that the cause of death of an individual is due to poisoning, whether by accident, suicide, or homicide, is a difficult task requiring the application of a vast amount of knowledge. For the forensic toxicologist, this may involve knowledge of a number of factors and reliance on the expertise of other professionals. The forensic toxicologist must have an inquisitive mind, be familiar with a wide variety of chemicals and poisons, and be conversant with current knowledge regarding the "drug culture," including the flow, distribution, and patterns of use of illicit drugs. In the normal course of their duties, forensic toxicologists work closely with other professionals. For example, when called upon to assist in establishing the cause of a sudden death, the forensic toxicologist would probably work with a medical examiner, a team of scientists, nurses, police officers, and other law enforcement personnel. The knowledge and information provided by each of these professionals may either collectively or individually assist the forensic toxicologist in resolving the mysteries surrounding the death.

A typical forensic toxicological investigation to determine a cause of death or to determine the presence or absence of a drug or poison in an individual begins with the collection of an appropriate biological specimen. The biological specimens usually collected from living individuals are peripheral blood and urine. Blood is of particular usefulness to the forensic toxicologists because the presence of a drug or poison in blood indicates that absorption has taken place. Additionally, good correlation exists between the blood levels of most drugs and poisons and the pharmacological and/or behavioral effects exerted on humans. Urine drug levels, on the other hand, only indicate that a subject had been exposed to the drug in question without definitive information as to the exact time of exposure or possible physiological effects. Nevertheless, the acquisition of a urine sample from an individual provides a noninvasive method of gaining valuable information regarding the presence or absence of a drug in the body of an individual. Occasionally, gastric contents, saliva, and hair samples may also be collected from living individuals. The case is reported of an arresting police officer who saw a man suspected of possessing and distributing a white powder believed to be cocaine. However, before an arrest could be made the suspect stuffed the white powder and its plastic wrapper into his mouth and swallowed the crucial evidence. Upon finally arresting the man, part of the forensic investigation involved toxicological analysis of available body fluids. In this instance, acquisition of gastric or stomach contents from the suspect is indicated and despite the risks involved, a gastric lavage must be performed. The forensic toxicologist should request and analyze the gastric contents from this living individual as part of the battery of tests to be performed. By analyzing a sample of the stomach contents the toxicologist may be able to answer questions about the chemical identity of the white powder.

For deceased subjects, specimens should be collected before embalming the body. Embalming may cause a dilution, destruction, or false indication of the presence of a drug or chemical in the decedent's body. The specimens collected from a decedent will include samples of other body fluids and organs since drugs and other chemicals distribute themselves in body fluids and organs with varying affinities. Whenever possible, a portion of the liver and whole kidneys should be obtained from deceased persons suspected of dying from a drug overdose or chemical toxicity. The liver is the organ primarily responsible for the detoxification of foreign substances such as drugs and chemicals in the body and tends to sequester most of them in high concentrations. Kidneys are the major organs responsible for the excretion of most drugs and poisons, particularly heavy metals, and are also expected to contain high concentrations of these poisons. Additionally, depending on the case history presented, the forensic toxicologist should request and analyze samples from specific tissues and organs collected from a decedent. For instance, the eye fluid or vitreous humor may be the preferred specimen to be analyzed for the presence of alcohol in the driver of a fatal accident whose blood or other bodily fluids become contaminated by stomach alcohol as a result of injuries received. Because the vitreous humor is anatomically well isolated from the stomach and is well protected from microbiological degradation, it may be the preferred specimen to be analyzed for the presence of alcohol in motor vehicle fatalities when blood or other bodily fluids become contaminated by stomach alcohol as a result of injuries received. Certain toxicants, such as the organometallic compounds (methylmercury and trimethyltin), and drugs, such as the anticancer drug doxorubicin, have great affinities for the nervous system. For example, when called upon to investigate the cause of a sudden death of a cancer patient being treated with doxorubicin, in addition to analyzing the usual biological specimens, the toxicologist should also analyze a sample of the brain tissue for the presence and concentration of the drug since the drug is selectively toxic to brain cells and tissues. If doxorubicin is found to be present in high concentrations in the brain, the forensic toxicologist may be able to ascribe the cause of death to doxorubicin toxicity with a high degree of certainty and not necessarily to the effects of the cancer as it might appear superficially.

The specimens should be collected by qualified personnel and each container into which a specimen is placed must bear a label with the name of the subject, the type of specimen in the container, date and time of the collection of the specimens, and the signature of the person collecting the specimen. Forms and labels are usually developed to take inventory of the specimens collected and to document the activities at the collection site. Frequently, a police officer is at the scene of the collection of the specimen and that officer should also append his or her signature on the labels and form. The specimens collected should be properly packaged with the proper documentation and case history if available and transferred to a forensic laboratory for analysis. From a legal perspective, the specimens are part of the evidence that can be introduced in legal proceedings, as is any analysis to be performed by a forensic toxicologist. For this reason, the processes involved in the transfer of the specimens from the collection site to the forensic laboratory must be carefully documented to establish a "chain of custody." The chain of custody ensures that only authorized personnel handle the specimens and thereby ensure their integrity.

Once in the laboratory, the types of toxicological analyses to be performed on the specimens will depend on several factors. In fact, the types of drugs or poisons to which any population of people are exposed will vary with the prevailing social, political, economic, and religious climate. Sometimes a specimen may arrive in a toxicology laboratory with a request for the analysis of a specific type of drug or poison. Other times, however, the type of analysis to be performed will be determined largely by the case history or other factors associated with the specimen. For example, the analysis performed on biological specimens taken from the driver of a vehicle involved in a traffic accident may involve first and foremost the determination of the presence or absence of alcohol and/or other commonly abused drugs such as marijuana or cocaine, primarily because of the overwhelming involvement of these drugs in traffic fatalities. However, the type of analysis to be performed on a decomposed body may involve searching for drugs and poisons other than alcohol. During decomposition, certain drugs initially present at death may be destroyed and others produced either by virtue of bacterial activity or by changes in the ambient environment.

To the untrained individual, determining both the presence and amount of an unknown drug or poison in an individual is a daunting task. However, systematic and well-standardized methods aimed at detecting the largest possible number of commonly encountered toxic substances have been developed over the years to assist the forensic toxicologist. Generally these methods have focused on the type of biological matrix being analyzed and the chemical class to which a drug or poison belongs. Thus, the method used in analyzing for a poison such as arsenic in hair will be different from that used in analyzing for alcohol in blood. Today, the forensic toxicologist has available to him or her all the modern techniques of analytical chemistry and is able to rely on a wide variety of methods to determine the presence of many poisons in a biological sample.

A classification scheme that is commonly employed involves placing poisons in the following groups: corrosive agents, gases and volatile agents, metallic poisons, nonvolatile organic agents, and miscellaneous poisons. The corrosive agents include the mineral acids and bases. This group of poisons also consists of a number of household products which are formulated with caustic compounds. This group of poisons can be analyzed using basic chemical and clinical techniques which take advantage of physical properties, such as solubility, acidity, or basicity, and observable color changes of the poisons. Gaseous and volatile poisons include several compounds, such as acetone, acetaldehyde, isopropanol, toluene ethanol, methanol, and several other organic solvents. This class of poisons can generally be determined using gas-liquid chromatography techniques. Metallic poisons include arsenic, mercury, lead, and other heavy metals. The method of choice in analyzing for metallic poisons is atomic absorption spectrometry. The nonvolatile organic group contains by far the largest number of prescription and illicit drugs. Drugs such as the antipsychotic agents, antidepressants, amphetamines, central nervous system stimulants, and hallucinogens belong to this group. Extraction techniques which take advantage of the acidic, basic, neutral, or amphoteric nature of these drugs are combined with appropriate instrumental methods to analyze for these compounds. Miscellaneous poisons will include agents such as plant and animal toxins and any other chemical substance whose detection from biological specimens will involve the application of some or all of the techniques described including immunoassay techniques.

Regardless of the type of toxicological analysis eventually performed on a biological specimen, it is essential to follow specific and well-established scientific and good laboratory procedures. A clean laboratory environment should be maintained and only chemicals of the highest grade and purity should be used for analysis. Instruments and equipment should be properly calibrated and maintained in proper working condition. The forensic toxicologist must be aware of the constraints and demands imposed by the judicial system and ensure that the techniques and procedures used in the laboratory are based on firm, well-established, and generally accepted scientific foundation as well as satisfying the criteria of admissibility established by the courts. Historically, in the United States, most courts deferred to the landmark ruling of Frye vs United States Of America in 1923 as a criterion for judging whether a scientific principle or method is "generally accepted" by those expected to be familiar with its use. Recently, the "Frye test" has undergone a change in U.S. federal courts in order to allow the introduction of valid scientific data or information gathered from rapidly advancing scientific techniques or novel tests into evidence. A variety of scientifically valid analytic procedures and instruments are used in forensic toxicology laboratories to analyze biological specimens. The type of procedure or instrument used for the detection of a particular drug or analyte will depend on the type of analyte or drug sought. Usually, however, the first line of tests performed are nonspecific screening tests designed to determine the presence or absence of a class or group of drugs. If a positive result is obtained with these tests, a second test using a different procedure based on physicochemical principles different from the first is performed to identify and confirm the particular drug. Some of the instruments that are currently used for the unequivocal identity of most drugs or chemicals are gas chromatography/mass spectrometry, atomic absorption spectrometry, and high-performance liquid chromatography

The relevance and importance of the toxicological analysis to the overall forensic investigation resides in the correct interpretation of the test results. To this end, the forensic toxicologist must bring his or her knowledge of human anatomy, biochemistry, physiology, pharmacology, pathology, and concepts in other basic sciences to bear on the test results. Following the analysis, a written report detailing the outcome of the test is sent out to the agency or party submitting the specimens for analysis. Usually this report will conclude any further involvement of the toxicologist in the issues surrounding the specimen. For example, a test result of "0.18 g of ethanol per 100 milliliters of blood" which is reported following the analysis of a blood specimen obtained from a motorist suspected of operating a vehicle under the influence of alcohol may be all that is needed by the arresting agency to sustain a charge of "operating under the influence of alcohol" against the motorist because in most countries it is unlawful to operate a motor vehicle while having a bodily alcohol content that is $\geq$0.10 g of ethanol per 100 milliliters of blood. However, instances arise when the forensic toxicologist will have to provide detailed interpretation of the result of the analysis.

Should the presence of the metabolite or biotransformation product of a drug be detected in the body of an accused individual, the forensic toxicologist will have to rely on several factors such as age, weight, gender, and health status of the accused as well as relevant concepts in toxicology to aid in the interpretation of that result. A 45-year-old female was charged with operating her vehicle under the influence of drugs, causing the death of another individual. The accused reportedly failed to obey a traffic signal and drove her vehicle through a red light into an oncoming vehicle, killing its occupant. She fled the scene of the accident but was later apprehended. In her defense, she stated that she was being treated by her physician for depression and had consumed her medication after the accident but prior to her arrest. Toxicological analysis showed the presence of the prescribed drug in addition to two major metabolites of the parent drug. In this case, simply sending out a toxicology report without interpretation or a summary of what the results mean is unlikely to assist the court in adjudicating the matter fairly. Because there is an admission by the defendant in this case to the consumption of the drug, it is in answering the question of whether the presence of the drug may have been responsible for the defendant's behavior at the time of operating her vehicle that the toxicologist's expert knowledge can assist the court in an impartial ruling on this case. If the prescribed medication is a short- or long-acting drug, the toxicologist may be able to use information on the relative half-life (time required to break down half of the original dose) of the medication and amount of metabolite detected upon analysis to ascertain the approximate time of drug intake. The toxicologist should be ready to provide this type of information to assist in the resolution of the matter.

A forensic toxicologist may be subpoenaed as a witness to offer testimony pertaining to the results of the analysis performed. Two distinct types of testimony may be offered by the toxicologist. First, he or she may testify only to the results of the analysis performed. This type of testimony is known as objective testimony and involves furnishing the court with information such as the identification and description of the specimen analyzed, the manner in which the specimen arrived in the laboratory, the location of the laboratory, a description of the methods used for analysis, and education and training which qualify the toxicologist to perform the tests used. The second type of testimony offered by the toxicologist is known as expert testimony. For this type of testimony, the toxicologist is presented as an expert witness and can offer interpretive opinions on his or her own results as well as those obtained by other scientists. To be accepted by the court as an expert witness, the toxicologist must be qualified, usually in the presence of a jury. In testifying as an expert witness, the forensic toxicologist must be very familiar with current scientific knowledge on the topic at hand. All conclusions must be based on sound scientific knowledge and the information presented to the court with impartiality, integrity, and honesty. It is only by providing the court with scientific knowledge in this manner that the forensic toxicologist truly functions in his or her role as one who applies the principles and knowledge of toxicology to the resolution of problems in the field of law.

The role of the forensic toxicologist continues to be pivotal to society, particularly when it comes to the administration of justice. The findings from a forensic toxicological analysis can be combined with those from a medical examiner or forensic pathologist to establish the cause or causes of death. Because many drugs, chemicals, or poisons do not produce characteristic and clinically observable tissue or organ damage to the medical examiner, the contribution by a forensic toxicologist is invaluable if a cause of death is probably due to a drug or poison. It is a truism that the administration of justice has become a multidisciplinary mosaic of law, science, and modern technology. As long as society continues to strive to ensure that justice is properly is carried out for all and sundry, reliance on the activities of the forensic toxicologist in cases involving human exposure to chemicals and their possible role in causing injury or death will be expected to continue. A society in which the unfortunate reliance on drugs (prescription and illicit) has become a way of life for some is bound to have its share of sudden unexplained deaths, traffic accidents, and other serious outcomes of drug exposure and toxicity. The forensic toxicologist will continue to contribute to the overall knowledge gained about drugs as society continues to grapple with the identity and toxicity of new drugs, particularly "designer drugs" and their analogs.

Further Reading

Cravey, R. H., and Baselt, R. C. (1981). *The Science of Forensic Toxicology. Introduction to Forensic Toxicology.* Biomedical Publications, Davis, CA.

DiMaio, D. J., and DiMaio, V. J. M. (1993). *Forensic Pathology.* CRC Press, Boca Raton, FL.

Eckert, W. G. (Ed.) (1997). *Introduction to Forensic Sciences*, 2nd ed. CRC Press, Boca Raton, FL.

Frye vs. United States (1923). 54 App. D.C. 46, 293 Fed 1013.

Garriot, J. C. (Ed.) (1996). *Medicolegal Aspects of Alcohol Determination in Biological Specimens,* 3rd ed. Lawyers & Judges Publishing, Tucson, AZ.

Gossel, T. A., and Bricker, J. D. (1990). *Principles of Clinical Toxicology*, 2nd ed. Raven Press, New York.

Klaassen, C. D. (Ed.) (1996). *Casarett & Doull's Toxicology: The Basic Science of Poisons*. McGraw-Hill, New York.
Matson, J. V. (1994). *Effective Expert Witnessing*, 2nd ed. Lewis, Boca Raton, FL.
Skoog, D. A., and West, D. M. (1982). *Fundamentals of Analytical Chemistry*. CBS College Publishing.

—Felix Adatsi

Related Topics

Analytical Toxicology
Toxic Torts
Toxicology, Education and Careers

Formaldehyde

- CAS: 50-00-0
- SYNONYMS: Formalin; formic aldehyde; formal; methaldehyde; methanal; methyl aldehyde methylene oxide; oxomethane; oxymethylene
- CHEMICAL CLASS: Aldehyde
- CHEMICAL STRUCTURE:

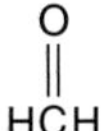

Uses

Formaldehyde has several commercial, industrial, and medical uses. It is utilized in the production of urea formaldehyde foam, paint pigments, and in the processes responsible for generating wrinkle-free, crease-resistant fabrics. In medicine, it has been used as a disinfectant, antiseptic, deodorant, and a tissue fixative. It is also an embalming agent.

Exposure Pathways

Formaldehyde is classified as a hazardous substance that may be absorbed through the skin, inhaled, and ingested. As a contaminant of smoke and photochemical smog, formaldehyde is ubiquitous in the environment.

Toxicokinetics

Formaldehyde will undergo reactions characteristic to all aldehydes. Metabolically it can undergo oxidation to an acid (formic acid), reduction to an alcohol (methanol), and conjugation with glutathione (*S*-acyl glutathione). The conjugation product forms rapidly and is the direct substrate for oxidation reactions that may follow.

Mechanism of Toxicity

Metabolic products will contribute to the toxicity of formaldehyde. The formation of formic acid will result in general acidosis, corrosion of the gastrointestinal tract, and other systematic effects. Formaldehyde also serves as an allergen due to its ability to combine with protein in the epidermis. This combination results in a hapten–protein complex that sensitizes T lymphocytes. Exposure can result in sensitization and contact dermatitis upon subsequent exposures.

Human Toxicity

Toxicity of formaldehyde is related to metabolic products and, as a result, individual variability will determine toxic outcomes. Human ingestion of 4 oz of formaldehyde has resulted in both death and survival. Systemic acidosis may appear upon ingestion along with corrosion and hemorrhaging of the digestive tract. Allergic sensitization may occur after exposure. This may lead to contact dermatitus with subsequent skin exposure, as well as asthmatic attack upon inhalation exposure. Inhalation may also result in irritation of the respiratory tract and pulmonary edema. Formaldehyde is an animal carcinogen and a mutagen.

Clinical Management

There is no specific antidote for formaldehyde exposure. Contact with skin should be followed by a soap and water wash for a minimum of 15 min. For inhalation exposure, the victim should be moved to fresh air and, if not breathing, given artificial respiration. If breathing difficulties are apparent, oxygen may be administered. After ingestion, decontamination with milk or water should be followed with a bolus of charcoal (1 g/kg) and a mild saline cathartic. Dialysis may be started if severe acidosis or deteriorating vital signs are apparent. Electrolytes and blood methanol levels should be monitored.

Animal Toxicity

In rats, the oral LD_{50} ranges from 0.2 to 0.8 g/kg, the subcutaneous LD_{50} is 0.42 g/kg, and the inhalation LC_{50} is 250 ppm/4 hr and 815 ppm/0.5 hr.

—*Kathryn Kehoe*

Related Topics

Indoor Air Pollution
Respiratory Tract
Sensory Organs
Skin

Formamide

- CAS: 75-12-7
- SYNONYMS: Carbamaldehyde; methanamide; formimidic acid
- CHEMICAL CLASS: Amide, aliphatic
- MOLECULAR FORMULA: $HCONH_2$

Uses

Formamide is widely used as a solvent in the manufacture and processing of plastics. It is used as a solvent for glue, as a softener in paper manufacturing, and as a solubilizer in latex paints. It is frequently used on a smaller scale in research laboratories in the preparation of formamide denaturing polyacryamide and agarose gels. It is a component used in hybridization of nucleic acids and during *in situ* hybridization of human chromosomes.

Exposure Pathways

Formamide may be swallowed, inhaled, or absorbed through the skin. It is classified as an irritant. Inhalation represents the most common route of exposure industrially and in a research setting.

Toxicokinetics

Literature regarding the metabolism and distribution of formamide is lacking. Formamide was once reported to be a metabolic breakdown product of dimethylformamide, but this is now considered controversial. The toxicokinetics of the better studied dimethylformamide is described as complicated and also remains unclear.

Mechanism of Toxicity

The toxicity of formamide is considered to be identical to that of its analog, dimethylformamide. However, the target organ for dimethylformamide is the liver, while that of formamide is the kidney.

Human Toxicity

While the liver is not affected by repeated formamide exposure, nephrotoxicity has been reported. After chronic exposure, renal tubular cells displayed necrosis and regeneration. Thrombocytopenia and lymphopenia were also indicated. Formamide is also described as a fetotoxin and teratogen. Exposure to the pregnant female may cause embryonic deformity.

Clinical Management

Exposed persons should be removed from the source of exposure and treated symptomatically. Inhalation exposure may involve central nervous system effects and results in liver function impairment. Changes in leukocyte and platelet counts have been noted in rats. Artificial respiration should be performed if the victim is not breathing.

After dermal exposure, the affected area should be washed with mild soap or detergent for 15–20 min. Symptoms of irritation and dermatitis should be treated.

For ingestion, gastric lavage or emesis should be performed. Oxygen should be given if respiration is depressed. Because there is no antidote, it is important to treat symptoms as they occur.

Animal Toxicity

Prolonged exposure to formamide has caused reduced organ weight and polycythemia in rats. Liver and kidney damage has also been noted. Rabbits repeatedly exposed to formamide during pregnancy showed adverse fertility effects and fetal developmental abnormalities.

The oral LD_{50} is 5577 mg/kg in rats and 3150 mg/kg in mice. The dermal LD_{Lo} in rabbits is 6 gm/kg; the intravenous LD_{Lo} in dogs is 1500 mg/kg; and the inhalation TC_{Lo} in rats is 1500 ppm/6H/2W-I.

—*Kathryn Kehoe*

Formic Acid

- CAS: 64-18-6
- SYNONYMS: Aminic acid; formylic acid; methanoic acid; myrmicyl
- CHEMICAL CLASS: Organic acid
- MOLECULAR FORMULA: CH_2O_2
- CHEMICAL STRUCTURE:

HCOOH

Uses

Formic acid is added to silage to improve its nutritional value. It is an animal feed additive, food preservative, and constituent of flavor enhancer formulations. In the manufacturing industry, it is used as an acidulating agent in dyeing and finishing textiles; in leather tanning; wool dyeing; preparation of organic esters; pesticide manufacturing; electroplating; as an antiseptic in wine and beer brewing; and as a coagulating agent for rubber latex.

Exposure Pathways

In industry, exposure to formic acid can occur through the oral, dermal, and inhalation routes. Formic acid can also be produced in the mouth and stomach from ingested formaldehyde. Formic acid can also be produced in the liver and other organs from the metabolism of methanol and formaldehyde (see Methanol and Formaldehyde).

Toxicokinetics

Formic acid can be readily absorbed from the digestive tract and the respiratory system. Systemic absorption of formic acid produces acidosis, neuropathy, and visual and mental disturbances. Acidosis can also be produced when formic acid is produced by liver aldehyde dehydrogenase from formaldehyde. Formaldehyde in turn can be produced metabolically by alcohol dehydrogenase from methanol. Formic acid is oxidized to carbon dioxide by the folate-dependent pathway. Some formic acid is excreted unchanged in the urine.

Mechanism of Toxicity

Exposure to formic acid may produce irritation and acid burns at the site of contact. Oral exposure may produce salivation, vomiting, diarrhea, gastritis, and pain. Dermal contact produces dermal irritation, dermatitis, and ulceration of membranes. Accidental splash in the eyes may result in irritation, lacrimation, and pain. Inhalation of vapors, mists, or aerosols may result in increased nasal discharge, cough, throat discomfort, and pulmonary edema. Systemic absorption of large doses of formic acid may result in damage to the liver, kidneys, and eyes.

Human Toxicity

The main target organs for formic acid poisonings are the respiratory and gastrointestinal systems, skin, eyes, liver, and kidneys. Symptoms include severe acidosis, severe osmolar gap, hypotension, renal failure, apnea, ocular damage, circulatory collapse, and death.

Clinical Management

If ingested, alert victims may be given milk or water to dilute the formic acid. Careful gastric aspiration with a nasogastric tube may be attempted to limit systemic absorption. The goal of the clinical management is to correct the acidosis. Acidosis may be treated with sodium bicarbonate or by hemodialysis. Immediate hemodialysis may remove formic acid from systemic circulation. Acid-base balance, electrolytes, and kidney function should be monitored closely.

Animal Toxicity

Formic acid is slightly toxic by the inhalation route. The LC_{50} has been estimated to be 15 g/m^3/15 min in rats and 6.2 g/m^3/15 min in mice. Rats consuming a diet containing 0.5–1.0% formic acid for 6 weeks experienced a reduced organ and total body weight compared with controls. The same response was noted when rats were given formic acid in their drinking water at a concentration of 0.5–1.0%. The oral LD_{50} has been reported to be 1076 mg/kg in mice and 1830 mg/kg in rats.

—*Heriberto Robles*

Related Topics

Acids
Alkalies

Foxglove

- SYNONYMS: *Digitalis purpurea, Digitalis obsura, Digitalis ferruginea*—Scrophulariaceae family; digitalis; fairy bells; fairycap; fairy glove; fairy thimbles; rabbit flower; lady's thimbles; lion's mouth; throatwort; witch's thimbles; folks glove; willow-leaves foxglove; revebjelle
- DESCRIPTION: Foxglove is an erect biennial herb with simple toothed leaves and a central stalk of pink, purple, yellow, or white tubular, bell-shaped pendent flowers about 3 in. long and numerous. This herb grows up to 4 ft high. Foxglove is a cultivated plant in the western United States and Hawaii; it is native to Britain and Europe. It is found in open land, roadsides, and waste areas and is commonly grown in gardens.

Uses

Foxglove contains approximately a dozen different cardiac glycosides, the most prominent being digitoxin. An extract of foxglove, digitalis, has been used medicinally for decades (see Digitalis Glycosides).

Exposure Pathways

The most common route of exposure is ingestion of any part of the plant or of any material or drug derived from the plant.

Toxicokinetics

Limited useful data are available for plants containing glycosides; however, reference will be made in relationship to the toxicokinetics of digitoxin.

Digitoxin is readily and completely absorbed (90–100%) from the gastrointestinal tract. Peak absorption occurs between 4 and 12 hr postingestion, but in overdose, peak amounts can be delayed. Absorption of digitalis glycosides from plant debris may be slower than from medicinals. Digoxin is a by-product of digitoxin metabolism (80%). After a single ingestion, the major serum and urine metabolite formed is digoxin. Plasma protein binding is extensive (97%) and there is a relatively small apparent volume of distribution (0.6 liters/kg). Digitoxin is metabolized by the liver by removing sugar (digitoxose) to form epidigitoxigenin, which is then conjugated to an inactive metabolite.

The elimination half-life is very long, approximately 100 hr or 4–6 days. It is slowly eliminated, with 60–80% of the dose appearing as metabolites in the urine.

Mechanism of Toxicity

Foxglove contains approximately a dozen cardiac glycosides, most prominently digitoxin. There are also other physiologically active chemical constituents including digitonin, digitalin, antirhinic acid, digitalosmin, and digitoflavone. The toxins are cardiac or steroid glycosides. A combination of an aglycone or genin and one to four sugar molecules is in each cardiac glycoside. The aglycones are derivatives of cyclopentenophenanthrene, and the sugars are unusual methyl pentoses. These influence the heart in two ways: stronger cardiac contractions and slower contractions through vagal stimulation, prolonging diastole. There is also a significant interference of the sodium–potassium pump mechanism mediated by adenosine triphosphatase. With the decrease in intracellular potassium, electrical conduction is impaired and progressive electrical changes occur. The normal resting membrane potential is reduced with a decreased ability of the myocardial cells to act as pacemakers and eventually there is complete loss of myocardial electrical function with asystole.

Human Toxicity: Acute

Foxglove plant poisoning is fairly uncommon. Many ingestions have been from foxglove tea. Some references state as little as two or three leaves can produce serious toxicity. Foxglove toxicity resembles oleander and digitoxin poisoning. Gastrointestinal symptoms develop within several hours and may include mouth and throat pain, nausea, vomiting, cramping, abdominal pain, and diarrhea. This is followed by central nervous system changes (e.g., severe headache, drowsiness, vision disturbances, confusion, hallucinations, tremors, and convulsions), hyperkalemia, dysrhythmias, and heart block. Yellow haloes are classic symptoms of digitalis leaf poisoning but usually are not seen with commercial digoxin poisoning. Severe overdose results in hyperkalemia and loss of excitability of cardiac tissue. There is often marked difficulty in managing these cases due to the inactivity of the myocardial muscle. The myocardium may even lose its ability to respond to electrical pacing. Foxglove tea poisoning has been associated with ventricular tachycardia, junctional rhythms, and atrial fibrillation with high-grade atrioventricular block requiring 6 days to revert to normal. One report described a patient suffering from confusion and visual disturbances lasting 5 days and EKG changes until 10 days. Elevated digitoxin levels confirm toxicity (in the absence of simultaneous consumption of digitalis preparations).

Therapeutic digitoxin levels range from 18 to 22 ng/ml (23–28.18 nmol/liter). Toxicity in most patients is above 25 ng/ml (32 nmol/liter). Levels, however, do not guide management due to cross-reactivity.

Human Toxicity: Chronic

Chronic toxicity may develop following the use of herbal products or teas that contain foxglove. The development of toxicity is unpredictable since the digitalis glycoside content of these products is not standardized.

Clinical Management

Basic and advanced life-support measures should be utilized as necessary. Gastrointestinal decontamination can include syrup of ipecac if it is administered within 30 min after ingestion and the patient is asymptomatic. However, the decision to induce emesis is controversial and must be considered carefully since emesis may produce vagal effects. Gastric lavage is also useful followed by activated charcoal. Multiple-dose activated charcoal (every 2–6 hr) may be effective in adsorbing digitalis glycosides from plant debris. Furthermore, digitoxin is enterohepatically circulated and multiple-dose activated charcoal may enhance elimination by preventing reabsorption of digitoxin. Treatment with digitoxin immune Fab should be considered in those with severe symptomatology who fail to respond to conventional therapy. Atropine is useful in treating varying degrees of heart block and bradycardia induced by digitalis. Phenytoin and lidocaine are useful for ventricular dysrhythmias (premature ventricular contractions, ventricular tachycardia, and bigeminy), with phenytoin improving conduction through the atrioventricular node. Magnesium has been reported to reverse arrhythmias from digoxin. Amiodarone was successfully used for ventricular fibrillation refractory to cardioversion. Bretylium can also be used if other antiarrhythmics are unsuccessful. Pacemaker insertion should be considered in patients with severe bradycardia and/or slow ventricular rate due to second-degree atrioventricular block who fail to respond to atropine and/or phenytoin and conventional therapy.

There is marked variability in response to ingestion of cardiac-glycoside-containing plant parts (e.g., leaves and stems) depending on various factors (e.g., the season, age of plant, and humidity). Therefore, all patients with a history of ingestion should have decontamination, a baseline EKG, and electrolyte monitoring and replacement (if necessary) and should be observed for 4–6 hr. Patients presenting with any signs of toxicity should be admitted to a monitored setting for a least a 24-hr observation.

Animal Toxicity

Signs and symptoms of toxicity in animals and livestock would be similar to those in humans. Livestock symptoms include diarrhea, bloody stools, anorexia, weakness, urge to urinate, and arrhythmias. Treatment should consist of symptomatic and supportive care.

—*Lanita B. Myers*

Related Topic

Cardiovascular System

Freons

- CAS: The CAS registry number is dependent on the specific freon compound.

- PREFERRED NAME: Chlorofluorocarbons (CFCs)
- SYNONYMS: Halons; halocarbons; freon 12; freon 13; freon 22; freon 113; freon 114; CFC-12; CFC-13; CFC-22; CFC-113; CFC-114
- CHEMICAL CLASS: Halogenated solvent
- MOLECULAR FORMULA:

Freon 12: CCl_2F_2

Freon 113: $C_2Cl_3F_3$

Freon 22: $CHClF_2$

Uses

Freons are commonly used as refrigerants and propellants in many types of aerosols. They are also used as selective solvents for degreasing.

Exposure Pathways

Inhalation (pulmonary route) is the main source of toxic exposures to chlorofluorocarbons. Dermal exposure may also occur. Ingestion would be intentional.

Toxicokinetics

Chlorofluorocarbons have low dermal absorption characteristics. Absorption by the lungs is slow based on data collected from animal studies. The main factor affecting the fate of chlorofluorocarbons is the amount of body fat. Chlorofluorocarbons are concentrated in the body fat and are slowly released into the blood at concentrations that do not present a risk of cardiac sensitization.

Loss of CFC-113 from tissues is rapid during the postexposure period with virtually 100% clearance within 24 hr of exposure. Chlorofluorocarbons compounds partition preferentially into lipid-rich tissues and are poorly metabolized. Significant accumulation occurs in brain, liver, and lung tissues compared to blood levels.

Chlorofluorocarbon compounds are cardiac sensitizing agents.

Mechanism of Toxicity

The exact mechanism of central nervous system (CNS) depression has not been determined, but the most plausible hypothesis is change in membrane fluidity that alters the neural transmission. No significant histological damage has been noted in the brains of animals exposed to lethal concentrations.

Chronic skin irritation occurs as a result of defatting of the skin. Ventricular fibrillation is due to the direct sensitization of the myocardium to endogenous catecholamines.

Human Toxicity

Eye and skin irritation has been observed following exposure to chlorofluorocarbons. No corneal opacity has been noted as a result of exposure to chlorofluorocarbons.

Chlorofluorocarbons are very toxic when inhaled at high concentrations and/or for extended periods of time. Lower concentrations or brief periods of exposure result in transient eye, nose, and throat irritation. Chlorofluorocarbons are acutely toxic but do not appear to induce chronic toxicity. Temporary CNS depression, dizziness, headache, confusion, and incoordination are associated with exposure to high concentrations (>2500 ppm in air). Gross overexposure may lead to abnormal liver function or fatality. Intentional sniffing of aerosols has resulted in sudden death. There is significant individual variability in response to chlorofluorocarbons.

Pulmonary edema, bronchial constriction, and lung irritation may also occur following inhalation exposure to high chlorofluorocarbon concentrations.

Clinical Management

Oral exposures to liquid chlorofluorocarbons has not been described, probably due to rare occurrence of exposure by this route. Due to low toxicity, emesis would probably not be necessary.

Following inhalation overexposure, a quiet, calm atmosphere should be provided to prevent an adrenaline surge if cardiac arrhythmias have not yet occurred. Minimum physical exertion is also recommended. Administration of Dilantin usually improves atrioventricular conduction.

Exposure of the eyes to liquid chlorofluorocarbons or significant air concentrations should be treated by irrigating the eyes with tepid water for at least 15 min.

Animal Toxicity

The chief effects observed in animals following exposure to chlorofluorocarbons are CNS depression, respiratory tract irritation, and mild liver effects. Cardiac dysrhythmias and mild chemical conjunctivitis have also been noted.

Chlorofluorocarbons are more acutely toxic to rabbits than to mice via the oral route of exposure. Dogs have demonstrated vomiting, lethargy, nervousness, and tremors following inhalation exposure to chlorofluorocarbons. High-concentration exposures to dogs, monkeys, and rats resulted in cardiac arrhythmias. A 2-year inhalation exposure to rats did not demonstrate any hepatotoxic effects.

Animal testing indicates no carcinogenic, mutagenic, embryotoxic, or reproductive effects. Generally, no changes in offspring were noted when doses of chlorofluorocarbons were below those associated with maternal toxicity (both oral and inhalation exposures).

—Kathryn A. Wurzel

Furan

- CAS: 110-00-9
- SYNONYMS: Axole; divinylene oxide; 1,4-epoxy-1,3-butadiene; furfuran; oxacyclopentadiene; oxole; tetrole
- CHEMICAL CLASS: Five-membered aromatic heterocyclics

Uses

Furan is a solvent used in the organic synthesis of pyrrole, tetrahydrofuran, and thiophene. It is also used as a solvent for resins and in the production of lacquers.

Exposure Pathways

The most significant route of exposure for furan is via inhalation. However, oral and dermal exposure may also occur.

Toxicokinetics

Animal studies suggest that furan is readily absorbed via all routes of exposure. Furan is oxidized by the cytochrome P450 enzymes in the liver and other tissues and may form epoxide intermediates; however, the precise intermediates have not yet been identified. Other intermediates of furan include enedials and dialdehydes, which are metabolized to CO_2 and eliminated. Examination of urinary output following furan administration in animals revealed a complex mixture of mercapturate metabolites of furan.

Mechanism of Toxicity

Furan is metabolized by the cytochrome P450 enzymes in the liver and other tissues. The furan ring undergoes oxidative cleavage and forms highly reactive furan radical cations or epoxides, which react directly with cellular necleophiles. These reactive metabolites may react directly with DNA or with cellular proteins to produce disruption of cellular functions and cell death. There is some evidence to suggest that the reactive metabolites of furan may induce mutations in cellular genes.

Human Toxicity

Inhalation of furan vapors may produce central nervous system (CNS) depressant effects including headache, nausea, dizziness, drowsiness, and confusion. Acute exposure to high concentrations may produce unconsciousness and/or death. Direct contact with vapors or liquid will irritate or burn skin and eyes. Oral ingestion may be associated with CNS depressant effects similar to those following inhalation exposure.

Very little information is available concerning the chronic toxicity of exposure to furan. Industrial use of furan is confined to closed systems due to the volatility of the compound; therefore, the potential for direct exposure to furan is limited. The public exposure to commercial furan is minimal. Many natural foods contain the furan ring structure and substituted furans may be formed through cooking of simple carbohydrates.

Clinical Management

If inhalation exposure occurs, the source of contamination should be removed or the victim should be moved to fresh air. Artificial respiration should be administered or, if the heart has stopped, cardiopulmonary resuscitation should be administered if necessary. If dermal contact has occurred contaminated clothing should be removed and the affected area washed with water and soap for at least 5 min or until the chemical is removed. Contaminated eyes should be flushed with lukewarm, gently flowing water for 5 min or until the chemical is removed. If ingestion occurs, vomiting should not be induced. Water should be given to dilute the compound. If vomiting occurs naturally, have victim lean forward to reduce risk of aspiration. Aspiration of compound into the lungs may produce chemical pneumonitis, requiring antibiotic treatment and administration of oxygen and expiratory pressure.

Animal Toxicity

Furan has been shown to be cytotoxic in animal models and may cause cell damage in tissues and organs which show cytochrome P450 oxidase activity. Furan was evaluated for carcinogenicity in rats and mice in a 2-year study by the National Toxicology Program. The primary toxic effects of furan were observed in the liver of treated animals. Cholangiocarcinogma of the liver was observed in all dosed rats and was detected as early as 9 months into the study. The incidence of combined liver carcinomas and adenomas in male rats showed a significant dose-related increase. A significant increase in liver adenomas was observed in treated females. The incidences of combined liver adenomas and carcinomas were also increased for all treated groups of mice. Several types of nonneoplastic liver lesions were observed in treated mice and rats. Toxic hepatitis of dose-related severity was noted in all dosed rats, in male mice at doses $\geq$8 mg/kg, and in female mice at doses $\geq$15 mg/kg. Doses of 2 and 4 mg/kg/day did not produce hepatitis.

Repeated exposure to furan vapors at various concentrations resulted in histopathological liver changes and structural or functional changes in the trachea or bronchi.

The inhalation LC_{50} in mice was reported as 120 mg/m^3 (acute pulmonary edema). The oral LD_{Lo} (lowest published lethal dose) in dogs has been reported as 234 and 140 mg/kg (convulsions or effect on seizure threshold). The inhalation TC_{Lo} (lowest published toxic concentration) in rats has been reported as 200 mg/m^3/4 hr, 500 mg/m^3, and 5 mg/m^3/4 hr (CNS disturbance).

—*Linda Larsen*

*Furfural**

- CAS: 98-01-1
- SYNONYMS: 2-Furancarboxaldehyde; 2-furanaldehyde; 2-formylfuran; 2-furfural
- CHEMICAL CLASS: Five-membered heterocyclic aldehyde

Uses

Furfural is an insecticide, fungicide, and germicide. It has multiple industrial uses, including production of durite, solvent refining of petroleum oils, acceleration of vulcanization, and a component of rubber cements. It is used in the extractive distillation of butadiene. It is a colorless or reddish-brown oily liquid having an almond-like odor and a caramel-like taste. It is only slightly volatile, having a boiling point of 162°C, and its vapor density is about three times that of air. Odor is detectable at levels as low as 24 μg per cubic meter.

Exposure Pathways

Inhalation of furfural vapor and dermal contact with liquid furfural are the most common routes of exposure.

Toxicokinetics

Furfural is rapidly absorbed from the gut and lungs and is also absorbed percutaneously following dermal exposure. Metabolism is rapid. The aldehyde group is oxidized to form furoic acid, the majority of which is conjugated with glycine to produce furoylglycine. A small portion of the acid is decarboxylated to form CO_2 or condensed with acetic acid to form furanacrylic acid, which is excreted as furanacryluric acid.

Furfural has been shown to be distributed throughout the tissues and organs in rats. At 72 hr following oral administration, the concentration of labeled furfural and its metabolites was highest in the liver and kidneys and lowest in the brain.

The major route of elimination is via the kidneys as the glycine conjugates, with more than 60% excreted

* Information Source: Hazardous Substance Data Bank, Bethesda, MD, July 1996.

as furoylglycine within the first 24 hr after oral administration. Only 3–7% is excreted in the feces and less than 1% is excreted in expired air. The half-life of an oral dose is approximately 2–2.5 hr.

Mechanism of Toxicity

Little is known about the mechanism of action in humans, but some information is available from animal studies. Inhalation exposure in rats is associated with pulmonary irritation, parenchymal injury, and the regenerative proliferation of type II pneumocytes. The activity of acid and alkaline phosphatases and glutamic–pyruvate transaminase is increased, whereas that of arginase and succinate dehydrogenase is decreased. The concentration of lactic acid in the lungs is increased. The activity of glutathione-*S*-transferase is also increased concurrently with a decrease in the concentration of glutathione. After single oral doses given to rats and mice, the effects on the liver are transient and involve scattered eosinophilic globular formation and increased mitotic figures without zonal or massive necrosis. Repeated oral administration results in cirrhotic changes including bridging necrosis and hydropic degeneration of hepatocytes in the parenchyma. Daily intraperitoneal administration to rats caused a time-reversible decrease of respiratory enzyme activity. This results in a degeneration of the processes of reverse resorption in the nephron and may be the cause of the observed functional insufficiency of the kidneys.

Human Toxicity

Furfural vapors are a strong irritant to the skin and mucous membranes of the eyes and respiratory tract. Acute exposure to high concentrations has caused severe lung congestion. Chronically exposed workers have complained of headache, fatigue, itching of the throat, lacrimation, loss of the sense of taste, numbness of the tongue, tremor, and possibly chronic bronchitis. Furfural is also a strong skin irritant and chronic contact can result in irritant dermatitis which may become eczematous. Skin sensitization has been reported and furfural is a photosensitizer. Workers with preexisting respiratory and/or skin disorders may be more susceptible to the effects of furfural exposure. Exposed workers have been reported to show increased levels of sister chromatid exchanges. Evidence for carcinogenicity of furfural is inadequate in humans and limited in experimental animals. It is not classifiable in terms of human carcinogenicity.

Animal Toxicity

Furfural has a high acute toxicity. Inhalation of 260 ppm was fatal to rats but caused no death in mice or rabbits. Pigs exposed 6 hr/day for 4 weeks at 130 ppm suffered liver damage, but at 63 ppm no ill effects were noted. Central nervous system depression with brain lesions has been reported in animals. Brain biochemical changes have also been reported.

Ingested furfural has produced liver cirrhosis in rats. Rabbits exposed to vapors for several hours a day manifested hepatic and renal lesions and hematologic changes. Administration of a single lethal dose produced a pronounced inhibitory effect on the medullary vegetative centers and brain nuclei with signs of congestion in liver, kidneys, and brain, with degenerative lesions in liver and kidneys.

The inhalation exposure of cats to very high levels of furfural (2800 ppm) for 30 min resulted in death due to pulmonary edema. The oral LD_{50} in rats is between 50 and 100 mg/kg and the intraperitoneal injection LD_{50} is between 20 and 50 mg/kg. The symptoms appear to be weakness, ataxia, and unconsciousness. Inhalation exposures (220 mg/m^3, 5 hr/day, six times/week for 12 weeks) caused changes in the hypothalamic–hypophyseal–adrenal system of rats which affected bodily adaptation processes. Decreases in brain noradrenaline levels and adrenal gland adrenaline content occurred. Brain acetylcholinesterase concentration increased and urinary 17-hydroxycorticosteroid and 17-ketosteroid excretion decreased. Subchronic inhalation of furfural by Syrian golden hamsters resulted in atrophy and hyperplasia of olfactory epithelium in the nasal cavity, and cats exposed at higher levels demonstrated pulmonary edema.

—*A. J. Nordone, D. E. Sharp, and R. A. Parent*

Related Topics

Pesticides
Sister Chromatid Exchanges

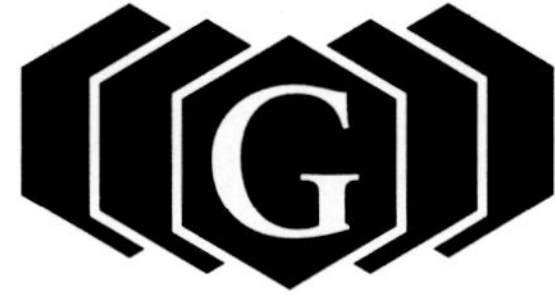

Gallium (Ga)

- CAS: 7440-55-3
- Selected Compounds: Gallium arsenide (GaAs; CAS: 1303-00-0); gallium phosphide (GaP; CAS: 12063-98-8)
- Chemical Class: Metals

Uses

Medicinally, radioactive gallium has been used to locate bone lesions, and nonradioactive gallium has been used as an antitumor agent. Gallium has been used experimentally as an adjunct to *cis*-platinum cancer chemotherapy. It has also been used to treat hypercalcemia. Industrially, gallium is used in special high-temperature thermometers, in place of mercury in arc lamps, and as a component of metal alloys. Gallium arsenide and gallium phosphide are used in semiconductors for light-emitting diodes.

Exposure Pathways

The most common route of exposure to gallium is parenteral injection. There are not any reported cases of gallium toxicity from occupational exposure. Gallium is relatively rare; it is obtained as a by-product of copper, zinc, lead, and aluminum refining.

Toxicokinetics

Gallium is not readily absorbed orally, but when administered parenterally it is easily taken up by various tissues. Once absorbed, gallium concentrates in the bone (where it appears to be quite stable). Gallium also concentrates in the liver, kidneys, and spleen but is soon released and excreted in the urine.

There is no information on the effects of gallium on enzymes, either as an agonist or as an antagonist.

Mechanism of Toxicity

Gallium can interfere with the structural integrity of transferrin, the iron-binding protein that transports iron in the serum. Gallium is believed to bind in the protein methionine. In microorganisms like *Escherichia coli*, gallium suppresses the synthesis of low-molecular-weight polypeptides. It also concentrates on the surface of the cell envelope.

Human Toxicity

When used as a diagnostic tool, gallium has produced dermatitis in some patients. Gallium can also lead to gastrointestinal distress. Reported bone marrow depression may result from radioactivity and not from gallium itself.

Clinical Management

Experimentally, deferoxamine mesylate has been effective in treating gallium toxicity. Ethylenediaminetetraacetic acid and meso-2,3-dimercaptosuccinic acid have not been effective.

Animal Toxicity

In different species of animals, gallium was responsible for renal damage, blindness, and paralysis. Gallium concentrates in tumors in experimental animals.

—Arthur Furst and Shirley B. Radding

Related Topics

Metals
Radiation
Radioactivity

Gastrointestinal System

Introduction

The gastrointestinal (GI) system or tract begins with the mouth and ends in the anus. The primary function of the GI system is the digestion and absorption of food, including solids and liquids, and the provision of a barrier to many potentially harmful ingested substances. Digestion is the breakdown or hydrolysis of food into smaller molecules in preparation for absorption into the body. Absorption is the transport of nutrients across the intestinal cell. The GI system also includes the exocrine pancreas which secretes proteolytic digestive enzymes into the duodenum, which facilitates the digestion of sugars, protein, and fats. The endocrine functions of the pancreas are considered in the entry titled Endocrine System. Bile salts produced by the liver also play a critical role in the absorption of fats and fat-soluble vitamins and the effects of xenobiotics on bile metabolism.

The GI tract provides the second largest surface area for direct contact of xenobiotics after the lung. Agents can contact the GI tract directly after oral ingestion and through the swallowing of particles that have been cleared from the respiratory tract by mucociliary clearance. Other potential routes of contact include direct introduction into the rectum, which is a route of administration for certain drugs. Agents metabolized by the liver and excreted in bile come into direct contact with the small intestine and can be continually recirculated because of enterohepatic circulation, which is described under Liver.

From a toxicological perspective, the GI tract is an important organ system since it is the initial site of contact of many environmental agents including food contaminants which have the potential to produce a broad array of toxicological effects. The GI tract is the target organ for a significant number of poisonings due to either inadvertent ingestion of medications, household products, and other items by children or intentional ingestion of poisons by adults during suicide attempts. GI symptoms are also common manifestations of systemic toxicity from a wide variety of toxic agents. Knowledge and recognition of such symptoms can be essential in identifying a toxic condition.

This entry provides an overview of the anatomy and physiology of the GI system and later describes the type of toxic effects that can be observed with different classes of agents.

Anatomy and Physiology

The GI tract is composed of several segments that have specialized functions with respect to digestion and absorption but share common anatomical and histological features. The GI tract can be considered as a tube composed of several layers. The tube consists of (1) an inner mucosal layer that contains mucous and the specialized cells; (2) a submucous layer that consists of loose connective tissue containing blood and lymphatic vessels, inflammatory cells, and nerve fibers; (3) a muscular layer containing many smooth muscles that is responsible for peristalsis; and (4) a serosal layer or covering. The specialized cell types vary in each GI tract segment and reflect the specialized function of each GI segment with respect to digestion and absorption. The individual segments are discussed below.

Oral Cavity and Pharynx

This segment of the GI tract includes the mouth and tongue, the pharynx, and oropharynx. The primary functions of the oral cavity are (1) as a storage place for food to enable chewing and mixing of food with salivary enzymes, and (2) as a passage for transport to the esophagus. Salivary amylase helps break down starch. The oral cavity is lined by stratified squamous columnar epithelium, which is keratinized in areas subject to a high degree of mechanical friction such as the tongue and palate. The mucosa also contains mucous glands. The pharynx is also lined by stratified squamous columnar epithelium, but unlike the oral cavity it has striated muscle that is not under voluntary control. The connective tissue surrounding the cavity is loose and highly vascularized. When presented with antigenic stimuli, this tissue can become edematous quickly and lead to obstruction of the airway, a potentially life-threatening condition.

Esophagus

The esophagus is a musculomembranous conduit that extends from the pharynx to the stomach and is approximately 23–25 cm in length in an adult. It is lined by stratified squamous columnar epithelium and surrounded by a muscular layer composed of longitudinally arranged smooth muscle bundles. The submucosa contains many nerve fibers. It also contains submucous glands, which are mainly present in the lower and upper portions of the esophagus and are thought to be continuations of the minor salivary glands in the oropharynx.

The primary functions of the esophagus are the transport of solid and liquids into the stomach and the prevention of retrograde flow or reflux of gastric contents. Aspiration of gastric contents into the lung can produce serious lung injury. These functions require coordinated esophageal motor activity. Manometric pressure studies have revealed that the esophagus has two areas of increased pressure, or sphincters, that function to prevent reflux. An upper sphincter at the level of the cricopharyngeal muscle remains closed most of the time due to its elastic properties and the tonic contraction of the cricopharyngeal and inferior pharyngeal muscles. A lower esophageal sphincter just proximal to the gastroesophageal junction also remains closed much of the time. Both sphincters must relax in response to a peristaltic wave and later increase in pressure to prevent gastric reflux.

The control mechanisms for the lower esophageal sphincter are complex and not well understood. The sphincter is innervated by preganglionic parasympathetic fibers of the vagus nerve and postganglionic inhibitory and excitatory neurons of the symptomatic nervous system. However, vagotomy or surgical cutting of the vagus nerve does not abolish sphincter tone. Many agents can decrease lower esophageal tone such as cholinergic muscarinic agonists, gastrin, and α-adrenergic agonists. Other substances, such as nicotine, β-adrenergic agents, nitric oxide, and dopamine, cause a decrease in the sphincter tone. It is not clear whether these agents play a role in the normal functioning of the tone of the lower esophagus or whether the effects are pharmacological. Smoking and high-fat meals lead to a decrease of tone and can produce symptoms of heartburn, which is due to reflux of gastric contents into the esophagus.

Stomach

The key function of the stomach, a bag-like widening of the digestive tract, is to secrete gastric acid and pepsin (an enzyme to digest food); however, very little absorption of food takes place in the stomach, except for some lipid-soluble substances such as alcohol. In humans, the stomach is composed of four main segments: the cardia, the fundus, the body, and the antrum (Fig. G-1). The cardia, a narrow portion just distal to the gastroesophageal junction, is primarily lined with mucous secreting cells. The fundus is the proximal portion that lies above the gastroesophageal junction and is largely composed of cells that secrete mucous and hydrochloric acid. The body is the part that lies proximal to the angle above the lesser curvature and contains similar cells. The antrum is located distal to the angle of the lesser curvature and is demarcated from the duodenum by the pyloric sphincter. The stomach also contains a muscular layer which facilitates mixing of the stomach contents with hydrochloric acid and pepsin. The surface of the stomach has coarse rugae, which are infoldings of the submucosa and mucosa that provide a larger area for digestion.

The stomach is lined with a mucosal surface that is punctuated by gastric pits leading to gastric glands. Foveolar cells, which secrete mucin, line the surface of

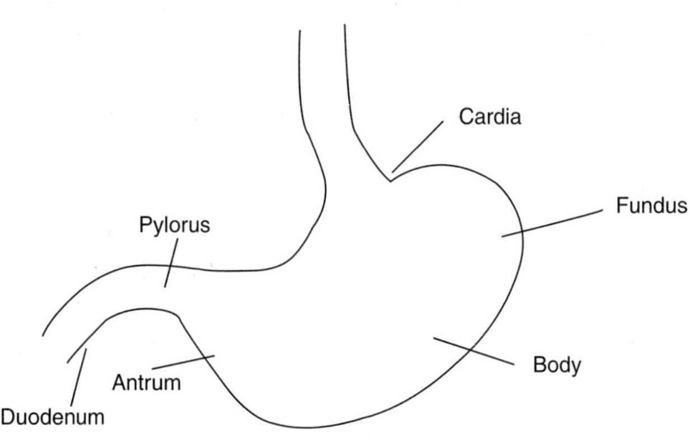

FIGURE G-1 The stomach.

the stomach and the gastric. These are tall and columnar cells that contain clear mucin-containing granules. Neck cells are located in the gastric pits, which are probably progenitor foveolar cells. Various glands empty into the gastric pits, including cardiac glands in the cardia stomach section, which mainly secrete mucous; gastric glands in the body and fundus, which contain large numbers of parietal cells; and pyloric or antral glands in the antral stomach, which contain large numbers of mucous secretory cells.

The individual cell types reflect specialized gastric digestive functions. The stomach secretes hydrochloric acid and pepsinogen, which digest food but can also damage gastric tissues which must be protected from these factors. Hydrochloric acid is secreted by approximately 1 billion parietal cells located in the fundus and body of the stomach secrete. The cells are interspersed along the course of mucous glands and secrete hydrochloric acid at a concentration that is approximately 3 million times that found in blood. Parietal cells contain large numbers of intracellular tubulovesicular structures derived from endoplasmic reticulum. The endoplasmic reticular membranes contain a hydrogen–potassium ATPase that pumps hydrogen ion across a membrane in exchange for potassium.

Proteolytic proenzymes pepsinogen 1 and 11 are released by chief cells which are located at the base of gastric glands found also in the body and fundus of the stomach. Chief cells have morphological features of cells that synthesize protein and are characterized by an extensive endoplasmic reticulum and numerous apical secretory granules. Pepsinogen is activated by the stomach's low pH environment and is inactivated by the high pH (>6) in the duodenum.

Mast cells and enterochromaffin-like cells found in the interstitium and among parietal cells contain histamine, which acts on parietal cell receptors to stimulate the release of hydrochloric acid. The histamine receptor on parietal cells is designated as H2 and is blocked by H2 blockers such as cimetidine which are widely used to treat peptic ulcers.

The factors associated with the regulation of gastric acid secretion are complex and involve chemical, neural, and hormonal influences. The stomach and small intestine contain several endocrine cells that affect the release of gastric acid. The most important factor that stimulates the release of hydrochloric acid is gastrin, a hormone that is released into circulation by G cells which are located in the epithelial lining of the pyloric glands in the antrum of the stomach, duodenum, and proximal jejunum. Gastrin is released in response to food in the stomach and small intestine. Stimulation of the vagus nerve results in the release of acid via the muscarinic cholinergic receptors located on the parietal cells. Vagal stimulation is also thought to stimulate the release of gastrin into the circulation and lower the parietal threshold for releasing gastrin into the circulation.

Gastric acid secretion can be inhibited by several mechanisms including acid in the stomach (pH 3 inhibits gastrin release), acid in the duodenum, the presence of fat in the pancreas, and hypertonic fluids or hyperglycemia. Somatostatin, a hormone produced by antral mucosal endocrine cells (D cells), inhibits the release of gastrin by directly inhibiting the parietal cells. Somatostatin is also present in other gastrointestinal tissue and the pancreas. C cells, endocrine cells in the proximal small intestine, secrete secretin in response to mucosal acidification, which also decreases gastric secretion.

The stomach has several protective mechanisms against hydrochloric acid and pepsinogen. The primary defense is the presence of gastric mucous, a large polymeric glycoprotein that is secreted by mucous glands throughout the stomach. Gastric mucous exists in two phases: (1) an insoluble mucous gel layer that coats the stomach and has a low diffusion coefficient for H^+ and (2) in gastric juice as a soluble phase. Mucous secretion is enhanced by cholinergic stimulation of muscarinic receptors and occurs in response to mechanical and chemical irritation of the stomach. Other protective mechanisms exist, including the secretion of bicarbonate by nonparietal cells via carbonic anhydrase, and are present in foveolar and parietal cells. Gel thickness increases in response to secretion of E series prostaglandins and is decreased by nonsteroidal, antiinflammatory medications. The other protective mechanism is tight cell junctions between surface epithelial cells, which are almost impermeable, to back diffusion of hydrochloric acid or pepsin. Prostaglandins of the E series which are in the gastric mucosa are thought to play a role by stimulating the secretion of gastric acid mucous and bicarbonate and by maintaining blood flow to the gastric mucosa which is necessary to maintain the integrity of cell surfaces and promote the epithelial renewal.

Small Intestine

The primary functions of the small intestine are digestion and absorption of food. The adult small intestine is approximately 6 m in length and is composed of the duodenum, ileum, and jejunum. Digestion occurs primarily in the upper small intestine and requires the action of pancreatic enzymes such as amylase, lipase, and trypsin, which are released from the pancreas into the duodenum, and bile salts from the biliary system. Absorption largely takes place in lower portions of the small intestine.

The mucosa or lining of the small intestine is enormous. A characteristic feature of the small intestine is the mucosal lining, which is principally composed of enterocytes that contain numerous villi that serve as absorptive areas. The villi extend into the lumen and appear as finger-like projections covered with epithelial cells. The villi also contain microvilli, which are also composed of microfilaments that form a brush border. Absorption of nutrients is also enhanced by motility of the small intestine, which places food in proximity to capillaries and lymphatic lacteals that serve as absorptive channels, and by the direct movement of villi.

Several types of absorptive mechanisms exist for nutrients including active transport, passive diffusion, facilitated diffusion, and endocytosis. Endocytosis occurs when the outer plasma membrane surrounds soluble or particulate nutrients in the gastrointestinal tract and engulfs the contents. This process is similar to phagocytosis.

Carbohydrates, or starches, which are complex polysaccharides, are hydrolyzed to oligosaccharides and disaccharides by the action of pancreatic amylase. Disaccharides, including lactase, sucrase, and maltase, are enzymatically split by enzymes contained in the microvilli of enterocytes. Glucose and other monosaccharides are absorbed by an active transport mechanism and this action is coupled to energy derived from a sodium pump mechanism.

Proteins are initially broken down in the stomach by pepsins, but completion of digestion occurs in the duodenum by the action of pancreatic trypsin and chymotrypsin. This results in the formation of oligopeptide, dipeptides, and amino acids. Dipeptides are broken down by dipeptidases located on the microvilli and the cell cytoplasm. Amino acids are absorbed rapidly in the duodenum and jejunum by active transport mechanisms, including the generation of sodium ions.

Most dietary fat is composed of long-chain triglycerides, which contain saturated and unsaturated fats. The stomach's churning action acts to reduce the particle size of fats. In the duodenum, hydrolysis of triglycerides occurs through the action of pancreatic lipase, colipase, and bile salts, which form a ternary complex. Bile salts, which are synthesized by the liver, have detergent properties and enable the formation of micelles, which are emulsions of triglycerides or fats with bile salts. The micelles enable pancreatic lipase enzyme to access the water–fat-insoluble phase. Colipase, a pancreatic enzyme, acts to place the pancreatic lipase in close proximity to the surface of a triglyceride droplet and is necessary for the action of lipase. Lipase hydrolyzes the triglyceride to form 2-monoglycerides and fatty acids. Monoglycerides are released from micelles and come into contact with the cell surface, where they are absorbed by diffusion. Once inside the cell, the fate of fatty acid is dependent on chain length. Long-chain fatty acids are esterified to triglycerides by enzymes in the endoplasmic reticulum and interact with cholesterol phospholipids and apoproteins to form chylomicrons and very low-density lipoproteins. Medium-chain fatty acids are not reesterfied and enter the portal venous system, where they are transported and bound by albumen. Other nutrients absorbed in the small intestine include fat-soluble vitamins, iron, calcium, water, and sodium.

Bile salts are absorbed from the ileum or terminal portion of the small intestine and are recirculated via portal vein. If the ileum is diseased as in Crohn's disease, bile salts may not be absorbed, and fat absorption, including absorption of fat-soluble vitamins, may be impaired.

Endocrine cells are scattered among walls of the small intestine including the villi and crypts The cells can release a large array of secretory products into the bloodstream. The hormones play a key role in the digestive process and exert actions through neurocrine and paracrine mechanisms. Products released in the small intestine include gastrin, somatostatin, secretin, cholecystokinin, motilin, neurotensin, enteroglucagon, vasoactive intestinal polypeptide, gastrointestinal polypeptide, and other agents.

The small intestine in addition to other portions of the mucosa and submucosa of the alimentary tract contain a large number of individual T and B cells, macrophages, and plasma cells. This lymphoid tissue becomes confluent in the ileum and forms unencapsulated nodules, which are macroscopically visible and known as Peyer's patches. The M (membrane) cells are present in the epithelial tissue overlaying the GI tract and can transcytase antigenic macromolecules from the intestine to intact lymphocytes. The tissue with lymphocyte tissue in the appendix and mesenteric lymph nodes constitute the mucosa-associated lymphoid tissue. This system forms part of the afferent link of the intestinal immune system and is involved in the secretion of IgA, which serves as a defense mechanism against external pathogens. Other mucosal epithelial surfaces in the body (e.g., respiratory tract and genitourinary tract) contain similar populations of lymphocytes that serve to protect pathogenic organisms.

Large Intestine

The large intestine or colon is approximately 1.5 m in length. The principal function of the colon is to reabsorb water and electrolytes that are present inside a liquid luminal stream. In contrast to the small intestinal mucosa, the lining of the colon is composed of columnar absorptive cells that have shorter, flat, and no villi and microvilli. The mucosa is punctuated by tubular crypts that extend to the mucosal layer and contain goblet cells, which secrete mucous; Paneth cells, which secrete lysozyme; endocrine cells; and undifferentiated goblet cells. Cellular proliferation is confined to the crypts and cells differentiate and migrate to the surface to replace superficial epithelial cells lost to surface abrasion or degeneration Lymphoid tissue is found in the mucosa and submucosa.

Cellular Replication

The GI tract has one of the highest rates of cell turnover of mitosis of any organ system. The highest rate of mitosis is in the small intestine, where between 60 and 75% of cells are turned over on a daily basis. Over 50% of the cells in the stomach pylorus are turned over daily and 10% of the cells of the colon are replaced. Agents that are known to interfere with cellular replication, such as alkylating agents or antimetabolites used in cancer chemotherapy, can have potential effects on the GI tract by interfering with normal regeneration of the cells the are undergoing rapid replacement.

Intestinal Flora

The GI tract is not sterile and bacteria are continually swallowed to the stomach with food. Hydrochloric acid limits the concentration of bacteria in the stomach. In contrast, the large and small intestine contain numerous bacteria. Intestinal bacteria may contain several enzymes including β-glucosidase, β-galactosidase, and β-glucuronidase. These enzymes may play a role in transforming medications to their active form or affecting their excretion. Administration of ampicillin leads to an increase in the excretion of conjugated estrogens. Diets rich in meat, which has been identified as a risk factor for cancer of the colon, also increase β-glucuronidase activity in fecal bacteria. Gastrointestinal bacteria also play a role in metabolizing some compounds into more toxic forms such as reducing azo dyes, which are used in some food additives. Some bacteria, like *Lactobacilli,* may serve to decrease the risk of cancer.

Exocrine Pancreas

The pancreas contains cells that have endocrine and exocrine functions. The gland is largely formed of acinar cells, which secrete digestive enzymes or their precursor into the duodenum. Exocrine function is subject to hormonal and neural regulation. Islets of Langerhans contain strands of cells including B and A cells that secrete insulin and glucagon respectively and form the endocrine portion of the gland.

Toxicant Effects on the GI System

Toxic effects can be mediated in the gastrointestinal system by several mechanisms, which are discussed in the following sections.

Direct Mucosal or Cellular Injury

Xenobiotics that contact the mucosal or other cells of the GI tract produce irritation characterized by inflammation, degeneration, and/or proliferation. The type of toxic effect that is manifest is dependent on several factors including chemical characteristics of the agent, dose or magnitude of exposure, and type of tissue involved.

Erosions or a superficial ulceration of the mucosa can occur focally or diffusely. Erosions are due to focal necrosis of the epithelium and associated stroma and are restricted to the superficial layers. Diffuse irritation accompanied by an inflammatory reaction is called enteritis. Ulcers, in contrast, are deeper lesions extending beyond the mucosa and penetrating into the adjacent tissue layers. Chronic irritation can produce proliferative lesions including dysplasia, which potentially could become malignant.

Ingestion of strong alkali and acids has the potential to produce severe tissue destruction or liquefaction necrosis. Alkali with a pH of >11.5–12 and acids with a pH <2 can produce significant corrosive injury. Other substances such as phenol may not be highly alkaline but can still produce corrosive injury. Alkali are found in many commercial products, such as household and industrial cleaners, dishwasher soaps and drain openers, and low-phosphate detergents. Factors affecting the degree of tissue injury or destruction include the amount ingested, the duration of contact with tissue, concentration, pH, physical form, titratable alkaline, and acid reserve.

This liquefaction process has four distinct phases:

1. Inflammatory phase: This phase lasts 1 or 2 days and consists of marked fibroblastic proliferation. In this stage, perforations may occur.

2. Necrotic phase: This phase occurs 1–4 days after injury. Cells die from coagulation of intracellular protein. Vascular thrombosis and bacterial invasion may worsen the underlying injury. The esophagus is especially vulnerable to perforation during this phase.

3. Granulation phase: This phase begins 3–5 days postinjury when necrotic tissue sloughs. Granulation tissue begins to fill in tissue defects and connective tissue begins to form in 10–12 days.

4. Constriction phase: This phase occurs 2.5–3 weeks following injury and is related to the formation of collagen in the healing lesion. Marked narrowing of the esophageal lumen may occur as the collagen fibers begin to contract.

The most frequent injury following alkali ingestion is esophageal burns. Diffuse circumferential esophageal burns are more common in patients ingesting liquid forms of concentrated alkaline corrosives; granular forms tend to produce more oral burns and esophageal burns that are in patches or streaks. Gastric injuries may also be more common in patients ingesting liquid alkaline corrosives or solids that have been placed in capsules. Intestinal burns, mostly duodenal, have been reported but are much less frequent. Severe duodenal injury may be more common with suicidal ingestions. From a clinical perspective, the absence of visible oral burns does not reliably exclude the presence of esophageal burns. Symptoms of stridor, vomiting, and drooling can indicate serious esophageal injury.

Sequelae associated with ingestions of caustics include a tracheoesophageal and aortoesophageal fistulae; strictures of the mouth, esophagus, and stomach; and esophageal carcinoma. In severe cases, gastrointestinal bleeding or perforated viscus with mediastinitis or peritonitis may develop. Strictures are more likely to develop after second- or third-degree or circumferential burns.

Several other agents produce GI tract irritation by interfering. Gastric ulcers have been associated with the use of antiinflammatory medications including aspirin and nonsteroidal antiinflammatory medications. The mechanism is thought to be the inhibition of cyclooxygenase, which is required for prostaglandin secretion. Prostaglandins play a key role in maintaining mucosal defenses of the stomach. Other agents that can cause severe injury to the GI tract include salicylates, heavy metals, and iron.

Several agents have been associated with producing acute pancreatitis or inflammation of the pancreas. The main causes are alcohol and a disturbance of the bile duct, which account for approximately 50% of cases. Drugs with a clear association include sulfonamides, thiazide diuretics, tetracycline, azathioprine, estrogens, and valproic acid. The mechanism for the underlying injury is not well understood. Possible associations have been reported with other medications including methyldopa, procainamide, and L-asparaginase. A relationship between corticosteriods has not been established. Chronic pancreatitis is primarily due to alcohol.

Interaction with Receptors of the GI Tract

Gastrointestinal function can be affected by interaction with cellular receptors. Stimulation of cholinergic muscarinic receptors by agents such as cholinesterase inhibitors (organophosphate pesticides and carbamates)and nicotine and opioid withdrawal can lead to an increase in motility and secretions of the GI tract. This process can lead to symptoms of abdominal pain, cramps, and diarrhea. Similarly, the administration of drugs that block with cholinergic muscarinic receptors functioning (e.g., atropine, tricyclic antidepressants, opiates, and sedative hypnotic medications) can slow motility and lead to constipation.

Indirect Effect

Vomiting can occur as a consequence of the interaction of a chemical with the central chemoreceptor zone or vomiting center in the forth ventricle of the brain. This results in GI symptoms caused by an indirect effect. Glycosides, opiates, nicotine, and possibly carbon monoxide may act in this manner. Vomiting can also occur as a consequence of local gastrointestinal tract stimulation from a wide array of agents including soaps, detergents, solvents, metals (including arsenic and thallium), and toxins associated with several types of food poisonings.

Allergic Reactions

The GI tract can be a site of hypersensitivity reactions. Angioedema of the mouth including the pharynx can occur following use of several medications including ACE inhibitors. The reaction is mediated via IgE.

Carcinogenesis

Cancers of the gastrointestinal tract represent a large proportion of malignancies in the United States. Colorectal cancer is the second most common malignancy in the United States. There is strong evidence that gastrointestinal cancers are affected by environmental factors since there are considerable geographical differences between cancer incidence of the same organ and migration studies have demonstrated that migrants who move to new countries over time will experience the same risks or cancer rate as the people in the host country.

Oral cavity cancers have been associated with cigarettes, alcohol, and chewing tobacco or snuff. Cancer of the oral cavity is not common in the Western world but frequently found in some developing countries including India, where it accounts for approximately 80% of all malignancies. Risk factors associated with oral cancers include excessive alcohol consumption, although the effects of alcohol are sometimes hard to differentiate from tobacco use since persons commonly smoke and drink. Chewing of tobacco has been identified as a principal risk factor. Other factors include a history of ionizing radiation exposure and nutritional deficiencies including iron in association with Plummer–Vinson syndrome.

Esophageal cancer has been related to the use of alcohol and nitrosamines. Other risk factors include a history of ingestion of alkaline corrosive agents, including lye. Nutritional deficiencies have also been linked to this type of malignancy.

Gastric neoplasms were among the most frequent malignancies at the turn of the century, but the incidence has decreased in the past 50 years even though there have been no major advances in diagnosis or treatment. Factors that have been linked to gastric cancer include nitrate ingestion as well as other dietary factors. Persons with atrophic gastritis who have hypochlorhydria or a relative lack of stomach acid are at greater risk. This may be secondary to the presence of bacteria, which are normally killed in an acid gastric environment and that transform nitrates to nitrites, which can eventually form carcinogenic nitrosamines.

Colon cancer has been associated with several factors including radiation exposure, limited physical activity, dietary fat intake, high meat intake, and nitrosamines. Fats may increase the risk of cancer by changing the intestinal flora or increasing the concentration of bile acids or because of a secondary effect on metabolism of xenobiotics. Negative associations have been associated with intake of fresh vegetables and meats. Other risk factors include family polyposis, chronic ulcerative colitis, and family cancer syndrome.

Further Reading

Cotran, R. S., Kumar, V., and Robbins, S. L. (1994). *Robbins Pathologic Basis of Disease*, 5th ed. Saunders, Philadelphia.

—*M. Joseph Fedoruk*

Related Topics

Absorption
Acids

Alkalies
Carbamate Pesticides
Carcinogenesis
Corrosives
Endocrine System
Liver
Metals
Organophosphates
Poisoning Emergencies in Humans

Generally Recognized As Safe (GRAS)

- Title: Part of amendments to 1958 Amendment to Food, Drug and Cosmetic Act (FD&C Act)
- Agency: U.S. FDA
- Year Passed: 1958
- Groups Regulated: Food processors and industry

Synopsis of Law

When Congress enacted the 1958 food additive amendments to the Food, Drug and Cosmetic Act (FD&C Act), certain food ingredients that had long been in use were exempted from the premarketing testing and approval processes introduced for food additives. An ingredient in use prior to January 1, 1958, could be classified as "generally recognized as safe" (GRAS) based on a demonstration that it had a common use in food. A substance could also be classified as GRAS based on documentation that it is "generally recognized, among experts qualified by scientific training and experience to evaluate its safety, as having been adequately shown through scientific procedures (. . . or experience based on common use in food) to be safe under the conditions of its intended use."

U.S. Congress developed the GRAS concept because it did not consider it either wise or practical to subject substances such as baking soda, pepper, salt, and vinegar to the new requirements it had imposed on food additives. There are currently approximately 2000 GRAS substances.

The FD&C Act defines a food additive as:

> Any substance the intended use of which results or may reasonably be expected to result, directly or indirectly, in its becoming a component of or otherwise affecting the characteristics of any food (including any substance intended for use in producing, manufacturing, packing, processing, preparing, treating, packaging, transporting, or holding food; and including any source of radiation intended for any such use). [FDCA, Title 21, *Code of Federal Regulations*(CFR)]

It is clear from this language that intention is a key criterion by which food additive status is to be judged. It is also clear that the intended use of a substance is not limited to its direct addition to food, but includes any use that "results or may reasonably be expected to result" in the introduction of some substance into food that would not otherwise be present. The important distinctions among so-called direct and indirect additives will be further discussed.

The FD&C Act creates further distinctions. In particular, the law goes on to exclude several groups of intentionally added substances from the legal category of food additives. Thus, the FD&C Act recognizes as distinct substances GRAS despite the fact that the FD&C Act and the regulations (e.g., 21 CFR 170.3) scrupulously avoid defining food, except in an exception sense—"food means articles used for food or drink by man or other animals . . . (and includes) chewing gum . . . articles used for components of any such article"—it regards foods as GRAS when they are added to other food, for example, green beans in vegetable soup. It also regards a number of food ingredients as GRAS; these ingredients are listed under 21 CFR 182, 184, and 186. However, it is important to note that not all substances recorded by the U.S. FDA as GRAS are listed as such. The language used in 21 CFR 182.1(a) acknowledges that there are substances the U.S. FDA regards as GRAS which are not listed in the CFR. This accomplishes the following: (1) It leaves the door open for additional nonlisted substances to be affirmed as GRAS by the agency, and (2) it reinforces the concept that substances can be deemed GRAS whether or not they are listed by the U.S. FDA or listed on a publicly available list. It is important to note that GRAS substances, although used like food additives, are not regulated food additives because the act states in section 201(s): "The term 'food additive' means any substance the intended use of which results . . . in its becoming a component . . . of any food . . . if such substance is not generally recognized . . . to be safe."

Therefore, to be GRAS is not to be a regulated food additive. Although GRAS listings technically apply only to ingredients used in foods, such listings are also considered for ingredients used in cosmetics, drugs, and devices.

—Shayne C. Gad

Related Topics

Food Additives
Food and Drug Administration
Food Drug and Cosmetic Act

Ginger Jake

- REPRESENTATIVE COMPOUND: Triorthocresnyl phosphate (TOCP)
- CHEMICAL CLASS: Organic phosphate compounds

Uses

During Prohibition in the 1930s, ginger (contaminated with organophosphates such as TOCP) was added to alcohol for taste. Ginger Jake syndrome resulted from consuming bootleg liquor or ginger beer.

Exposure Pathways

Ingestion is the primary route of exposure; dermal contact and inhalation are also possible routes.

Toxicokinetics

Ginger Jake is primarily absorbed from gastrointestinal tract; but it may be absorbed from the skin, eyes, and lungs as well. It is detoxified in liver by P450 monoxygenases.

Mechanism of Toxicity

Organophosphate-induced delayed neurotoxicity is caused by Ginger Jake. The key toxin is the *ortho* isomer of tritolylphosphate. It inhibits production of neuropathic target esterase, which prompts degeneration of axons of large diameter and myelmic sheaths. Seventy-percent inhibition of this esterase is the threshold trigger for organophosphate-induced ascending neuropathy (OPIAN).

Human Toxicity

Exposure leads to OPIAN or "Ginger Jake" walk. The onset is identified by muscle weakness, chest tightness, gastrointestinal cramps, irregular rhythms, diarrhea, urination, miosis, emesis, lacrimation, and salivation. This leads to a second stage of hyperactivated reflexes and spasms. The condition can lead to long-term damage in the lower extremities.

Clinical Management

Respiratory symptoms should be treated with PO_2. For heart and liver, atropine and then PAM should be administered and the patient monitored for at least 48 hr. If ingested, emetic and activated charcoal should be administered within 4–6 hr of ingestion. Exposed skin should be washed with mild soap and water. Direct contact should be avoided.

Animal Toxicity

Toxicity in animals differs with species. In laboratory testing, hens and cats are most susceptible to OPIAN. The classic test to determine the potential for an organophosphate to induce the syndrome is termed the old "hen" test.

More recently, the levels of neurotoxic esterase (NTE) have been measured.

—Jayne E. Ash and Shayne C. Gad

Related Topics

Neurotoxicity, Delayed
Neurotoxicology: Central and Peripheral
Organophosphate Poisoning, Intermediate Syndrome of
Organophosphates

Ginseng

- SYNONYMS: *Panax quinquefolium*; American ginseng

- ◆ DESCRIPTION: Ginseng is a long-stemmed herb with palmate leaves. Flowers are yellowish green and bloom in groups of two to four. Red drupe berries appear in clusters. This herb is native to the Orient but widely cultivated in the United States for export.

Uses

Ginseng is used for many medicinal and rejuvenating reasons domestically and abroad. Traditional Chinese medicine values ginseng as a nerve and cardiac stimulant, a treatment for impotence, to promote metabolism, and to moderate blood pressure and blood sugar levels. Two or three grams is considered therapeutic. Fifty grams has been prescribed but has resulted in adverse side effects.

Exposure Pathways

Exposures occur via ingestion (e.g., teas and soups). Ginseng cigarettes are also available. A topical preparation is used to approximate wound edges. In the United States, it is widely accepted as an effective demulcent.

Mechanism of Toxicity

All plant parts contain 13 capon glycosides. Two of these agents have a prolonged antiinflammatoray action similar to that of nonsteroidal antiinflammatory medications. Another component is thought to affect corticosteroid secretion in the central nervous system. The fusiform roots are recognized for their vitamin and mineral content.

Human Toxicity

In large therapeutic doses, patients may suffer insomnia, depression, and nervous behavior. When used in chronically excessive doses, patients may suffer from hypertension, insomnia, dermal blemishes, and morning diarrhea. Hypertension and depression may result from abrupt withdrawal after chronic use.

Clinical Management

Supportive care may be indicated. Discontinue use of the herbal preparation.

—*Regina Wiechelt*

Glutathione

Glutathione, also referred to as GSH, is an endogenous component of cellular metabolism, a tripeptide composed of glycine, cysteine, and glutamic acid. It normally is present in the liver at a concentration of 10 m*M*. It is an integral part of the biotransformation of xenobiotic substances.

Unlike amino acids, glutathione conjugation involves electrophilic substrates or those which can easily convert to electrophiles. Some of this is done nonenzymatically. Glutathione *S*-transferases, or ligandin, aids the enzymatic conjugation by catalyzing the reaction, converting GSH to GS^-. Glutathione *S*-transferases comprise about 10% of total cellular protein.

Glutathione can conjugate with xenobiotics in many ways. It may displace an electron withdrawing group, putting GS^- in its place. It may add itself (GSH) to the substrate. It may also respond to a substrate formed from earlier metabolism. A xenobiotic may stereoselectively conjugate, removing one or more of the peptides.

Glutathione conjugation helps contribute to detoxification by binding electrophiles that could otherwise bind to proteins or nucleic acids, resulting in cellular damage and genetic mutations. Exaggerated presence of glutathione *S*-transferase may indicate resistance to chemical toxicity. Different glutathione *S*-transferase responses to different chemicals between species may indicate susceptibility to toxic effects.

On the other hand, glutathione conjugation may activate the toxic moiety within a xenobiotic. Activation mechanisms involving glutathione include:

- Toxic metabolites released from conjugation with haloalkanes, organic thiocyanates, and nitrosoguanides
- Electrophilic sulfur mustards formed from conjugation with vicinal dihaloalkanes
- Conjugates of halogenated alkenes activated by β lyase in the kidney
- Toxic metabolites produced from γ-glutamyltranspeptidase degradation of quinones, quinoneimines. and isothiocyanates

A classic example of glutathione-related toxicity is acetaminophen. Phase 1 metabolism of acetaminophen by P450 results in a toxic metabolite. Glutathione conjugation breaks down and detoxifies the metabolite and excretes it as mercapturic acid. Sufficient glutathione is a key player in this protective biotransformation. If as much as 70% of endogenous glutathione is already consumed, the toxic activation may take place. It takes only 15.8 g of acetaminophen to reduce glutathione levels to the point where hepotoxicity may occur.

Glutathione conjugates have two routes of excretion—via bile or via urine. Conjugates eliminated in the urine are first converted to mercapturic acids in the kidney. Mercapturic acid is defined as N-acetylated, S-substituted cysteine conjugates arising from conjugation of a xenobiotic with glutathione. Its biosynthesis involves conjugation of the GSH itself. Glycine and glutamic acid are removed; then cysteine is conjugated further by interaction with *N*-acetyltransferase. This last step converts the substance to mercapturic acid.

Conjugation with mercapturic acid may also activate hepatoxins. It may cleave with γ-glutamyltranspeptidase, an enzyme implicated in the degradation quinones, quinoneimines, and isothiocyanates. Acetaminophen also increases the urinary excretion of mercapturic acid and cysteine conjugates, enabling the formation of its own hepatoxic metabolites. Treatment with mercaptamine, a synthetic mercapturic acid, can reduce acetaminophen intoxication.

—*Shayne C. Gad and Jayne E. Ash*

Related Topics

Biotransformation
Kidney
Liver
Metallothionein

Glutethimide

- CAS: 77-21-4
- Synonyms: Doriden; Dorimide; 2-ethyl-2-phenylglutarimide; 3-ethyl-3-phenyl-2,6-piperidinedione
- Chemical Class: Piperidinedione derivative
- Molecular Formula: $C_{13}H_{15}NO_2$
- Chemical Structure:

C_2H_5 5 3 1 O N O H

Uses

Glutethimide was once used as a sedative–hypnotic agent. Its use has generally been abandoned because of its acute and chronic toxicity, abuse potential, and the availability of more favorable alternatives.

Exposure Pathways

Ingestion is the most common route of both accidental and intentional exposure to glutethimide. It is available as 500-mg tablets.

Toxicokinetics

Glutethimide is slowly and erratically absorbed from the gastrointestinal tract. Peak serum concentrations occur within 1–6 hr following a therapeutic dose. Glutethimide is metabolized by the liver to conjugated and unconjugated metabolites, two of which are active. These active metabolites, 4-hydroxy-2-ethyl-2-phenylglutarimide (4-HG) and α-phenyl-γ-butyrolactone, accumulate in overdose patients and contribute to the toxic effects of glutethimide. 4-HG has been found to be twice as potent as the parent compound.

Protein binding is 50%. The volume of distribution is 1.7 liters/kg. Glutethimide is highly lipid soluble and accumulates in the brain and adipose tissue. The elimination half-life for glutethimide is approximately 10–12 hr but is prolonged in overdose.

Mechanism of Toxicity

Glutethimide depresses the central and autonomic nervous systems. The pharmacologic mechanism of glutethimide is not well understood. It produces effects comparable to those of phenobarbital. In addition, it possesses marked anticholinergic activity.

Human Toxicity: Acute

Ingestion of a single 500-mg tablet is likely to produce toxicity in a child. The potentially toxic and lethal doses of glutethimide in adults are generally accepted to be

3 and 10 g, respectively. Acute overdose with glutethimide results in central nervous system (CNS) depression ranging from lethargy to profound coma. Prolonged and fluctuating coma may occur due to redistribution of active metabolites from adipose stores and from enterohepatic recirculation. Hypotension and respiratory depression may develop. Anticholinergic manifestations, such as mydriasis, thick bronchial secretions, urinary retention, and hyperthermia, may complicate the clinical course. Pulmonary and cerebral edema, cardiovascular shock, and seizures may develop in severe cases.

Human Toxicity: Chronic

Chronic use of high doses of glutethimide may produce psychologic and physical dependence. Abrupt discontinuation of therapy may result in withdrawal signs and symptoms such as nausea, vomiting, tremulousness, tachycardia, fever, delirium, hallucinations, and seizures. Unlike opioid withdrawal, glutethimide withdrawal can be life-threatening.

Clinical Management

Basic and advanced life-support measures should be implemented as necessary. Gastrointestinal decontamination procedures should be used as appropriate based on the patient's level of consciousness and history of ingestion. Activated charcoal can be used to adsorb glutethimide. The patient's level of consciousness and vital signs should be monitored closely. Obtunded patients with reduced gag reflex should be intubated. Respiratory support including oxygen and ventilation should be provided as needed. There is no antidote for glutethimide. If hypotension occurs it should be treated with standard measures including intravenous fluids, Trendelenburg positioning, and dopamine hydrochloride by intravenous infusion. Standard measures for the management of seizures and cerebral edema should be employed. Hemodialysis and hemoperfusion may be effective for the active removal of glutethimide but should be reserved for severe cases when standard supportive measures are inadequate. The occurrence of withdrawal signs and symptoms indicates the need to reinstitute glutethimide therapy and gradually reduce the dose until discontinued. A barbiturate such as phenobarbital or a benzodiazepine may be substituted for glutethimide.

—Gregory P. Wedin

Glyceraldehyde

- CAS: 367-47-5
- SYNONYMS: DL-glyceraldehyde; 2,3-dihydroxypropanal; α,β-dihydroxypropionaldehyde; glyceric aldehyde; glycerose; 2,3-dihydroxypropionaldehyde
- CHEMICAL CLASS: Aldose

Uses

Glyceraldehyde is a naturally occurring chemical in living organisms, including humans. To obtain energy from food, animals must convert simple carbohydrates derived from plants, or sugars, to carbon dioxide and water. Glyceraldehyde is an intermediate in the conversion of the carbohydrate fructose, which is in turn a constituent of sucrose, or table sugar (sucrose is a disaccharide consisting of glucose and fructose).

Glyceraldehyde is used in biochemical research and nutrition; in the preparation of polyesters and adhesives; as a cellulose modifier; and in the tanning of leather.

Glyceraldehyde can exist as two different isomers, D-glyceraldehyde and L-glyceraldehyde, so named because these isomers are "mirror images" (i.e., they cannot be superimposed upon each other). A good analogy for this is the left and right hand of an individual: Both are virtually identical in structure and function, but they can never be matched or superimposed on each other because they are mirror images. D- and L-glyceraldehyde are also mirror images of each other (as are other sugars) and are used as "reference" chemicals because each is one of the simplest molecules to compare other molecules (such as sugars and amino acids) against. Thus, the conformation of the alcohol and aldehyde group around the center carbon of D-glyceraldeyde helps scientists to evaluate the structure and nomenclature (identity) of other simple sugars, such as glucose. This makes glyceraldehyde an important tool and reference standard for the biochemist.

Exposure Pathways

Only persons involved in the manufacture and production of glyceraldehyde would be expected to be exposed to significant concentrations of glyceraldehyde. Because it is a solid at room temperature, exposure would be anticipated to occur only through contact with the skin or by inhalation of airborne dust. Liquids are generally present as an aqueous solution (40%).

Toxicokinetics

Glyceraldehyde is an intermediate in the metabolism of fructose. In the liver, fructose is converted to fructose-1-phosphate by the enzyme fructokinase. Fructose-1-phosphate is then converted to glyceraldehyde and dihydroxyacetone phosphate by the enzyme fructose-1-phosphate aldolase. Glyceraldehyde is then converted to glyceraldehyde-3-phosphate by the enzyme glyceraldehyde kinase. Glyceraldehyde-3-phosphate is a high-energy intermediate that may now move into the glycolysis cycle, which allows the body to extract energy to make ATP, which can then be used to run other metabolic functions (like muscle contraction).

Human Toxicity

Because glyceraldehyde is a normal metabolic intermediate, this chemical cannot be readily categorized as a "toxic" chemical: Given a large enough exposure or dose, any chemical can result in toxic injury. As with any aldehyde/alcohol, very high air concentrations or accidental ingestion of large amounts would be expected to overwhelm the body's natural defenses and produce an adverse effect (e.g., eye, nose, lung irritation from airborne dust; and stomach ache/nausea following ingestion).

Clinical Management

Persons who have been overcome by high concentrations or doses of glyceraldehyde should be removed from the area of high exposure. Medical attention should be sought. Treatment should be similar to first aid followed for any high-level exposure: irrigation of eyes with copious amount of water, washing of exposed skin with soap and water, and supportive therapy following ingestion.

Animal Toxicity

The median lethal dose (LD_{50}) for glyceraldehyde in rats is 2 g/kg, which, generally speaking, places it in the category of slightly to moderately toxic. The chemical is also slightly toxic by the intraperitoneal route. No other data are available on animal toxicity.

—Stephen Clough

Glycerol

- CAS: 56-81-5
- SYNONYMS: Glycerin; 1,2,3-propanetriol; 1,2,3-trihydroxypropane; glyceritol; glycyl alcohol
- MOLECULAR FORMULA: $C_3H_8O_3$

Uses

Glycerol is used as a solvent for flavors and food colors. It is also used as a humectant, plasticizer, emollient, and sweetener. It is used in the manufacture of dynamite (nitroglycerol), cosmetics, liquid soaps, liqueurs, printing and copying inks, lubricants, pharmaceuticals (toothpaste, laxatives, and drugs), antifreeze in automobiles, and gas meters.

Exposure Pathways

Inhalation, dermal contact, ocular contact, and ingestion are the exposure pathways for glycerol.

Toxicokinetics

Oral exposure results in rapid absorption through the gastrointestinal tract with rapid distribution in the blood. Most glycerol is incorporated into the body fat. Seven to 14% is excreted unchanged in the urine within 2.5 hr of ingestion with approximately 80% of metabolism occurring in the liver and 10–20% occurring in the kidneys. Glycerol metabolism in the liver is initiated by glycerokinase, with glycerol further metabolized to carbon dioxide and water or utilized in glucose or glycogen synthesis. Some glycerol may combine with free fatty acid to form triglycerides.

Mechanism of Toxicity

The medicinal action of glycerol as a laxative is a result of an increase in water absorption and irritation effects which cause evacuation of the bowel.

Human Toxicity

Toxicity following acute ingestion of excessive amounts of glycerol-based laxatives is generally minimal and limited to the gastrointestinal tract. Aspiration may result in pneumonitis. Adverse effects following oral administration include mild headache, dizziness, nausea, vomiting, thirst, and diarrhea. Repeated application of 100% glycerin to the surface of the eye causes extensive changes in the endothelium but most of these changes disappear within 90 min after cessation of exposure. Severe dehydration, cardiac arrhythmias, and hyperosmolar nonketoic coma may be fatal. Hemolysis, hemoglobinuria, and renal failure may occur.

Clinical Management

Due to the generally low toxicity of glycerol and potential aspiration hazard, emesis is not generally recommended following ingestion. Activated charcoal should only be used in the event of very large ingestions due to the potential for induction of vomiting. Dehydration, electrolyte imbalance, hyperglycemia, and acidosis or alkalosis require management by the clinician. Excessive diarrhea should be treated with high fluid intake and monitoring of fluid and electrolyte status.

Animal Toxicity

Rhabdomyolysis in experimental animals may cause death by an unknown mechanism. It has been determined that the effect is not a result of free radical formation or blood endotoxins. Intramuscular injection in rabbits results in necrosis of muscle fibers and disruption in cell plasma membrane. Extensive regeneration is apparent 7–14 days following exposure: Changes are similar to muscular dystrophy. The glycol myopathy may be a good model for pathophysiological studies of Duchennes muscular dystrophy.

Current data are not sufficient to determine the carcinogenicity of glycerol.

—*Kathryn A. Wurzel*

Glycol Ethers

- Structures and Synonyms: This is a large and diverse group of compounds that can be divided into two general classes, the ethylene glycol ethers and the propylene glycol ethers. Names, structures, synonyms, and CAS numbers for commonly used glycol ethers are presented in Table G-1.

Uses

Glycol ethers are extensively used in industrial applications as solvents for the manufacture of lacquers, varnishes, resins, printing inks, and textile dyes; as anti-icing additives in brake fluids; and as gasoline additives. In addition, they are used in consumer products such as latex paints and cleaners.

Exposure Pathways

Dermal contact and inhalation of vapor/aerosol/mist are the primary routes of exposure. Although the oral route of exposure would not be expected during proper use of the material, there is the potential for accidental ingestion to occur.

Toxicokinetics

Glycol ethers are absorbed readily after oral, dermal, or inhalation exposure. In addition, for the ethylene series, the ratio of the oral LD_{50} to the dermal LD_{50} is approximately 1, indicating that an equivalent amount of material can be absorbed by either route. The differences in toxicity between the ethylene series and the propylene series appears to be due the metabolites produced. The ethylene glycol ethers are metabolized via the alkoxyacetaldehyde to the respective alkoxyacetic acid. For example, ethylene glycol monomethyl ether (EGME) is metabolized to methoxyacetic acid, which has been shown to produce the same biological effects as the parent compound, EGME. However, in the propylene glycol ether series, propylene glycol monomethyl ether (PGME) is metabolized to propylene glycol, which is further metabolized to carbon dioxide.

Mechanism of Toxicity

The testes, bone marrow, and embryo contain large numbers of rapidly dividing and differentiating cells, and it is possible that one or more processes of cell division and differentiation are affected. The difference between the toxicity of the ethylene glycol ethers and the propylene glycol ethers may be due to the formation of a toxic metabolite, the alkoxyacetic acid, while the propylene glycol ethers are metabolized to a non-toxic metabolite.

TABLE G-1
Names, Structures, and Abbreviations of Some Commonly Used Glycol Ethers

Ethylene glycol ethers[a]	$R{-}O{-}CH_2{-}CH_2{-}OH_2$	
R = CH_3	EGME:	ethylene glycol monomethyl ether (CAS 109-86-4) Synonym: 2-methoxyethanol
R = $CH_3{-}CH_2$	EGEE:	ethylene glycol monoethyl ether (CAS 110-80-5) Synonym: 2-ethoxyethanol
R = $CH_3{-}CH_2{-}CH_2$	EGnPE:	ethylene glycol monopropyl ether (CAS 2807-30-9) Synonym: *n*-propoxyethanol
R = $CH_3\,CH\begin{smallmatrix}CH_3\\CH_3\end{smallmatrix}$	EGiPE:	ethylene glycol isopropyl ether (CAS 109-59-1) Synonym: 2-isopropoxyethanol
R = $CH_3{-}CH_2{-}CH_2{-}CH_2$	EGBE:	ethylene glycol monobutyl ether (CAS 111-76-2) Synonym: 2-butoxyethanol
R = C_6H_5	EGPhE:	ethylene glycol phenyl ether (CAS 122-99-6) Synonym: 2-phenoxylethanol
Propylene glycol ethers[b]	$R{-}O{-}CH_2{-}CH(CH_3){-}OH$	
R = CH_3	2PG1ME[c]	2-propylene glycol 1-methyl ether (CAS 107-98-2) Synonym: 1 methoxy-2-propanol
R = CH_3	1PG2ME[c]	1-propylene glycol 2-methyl ether (CAS 1589-47-5) Synonyms: 2-methoxy-1-propanol
R = $CH_2{-}CH_3$	2PG1EE	2-propylene glycol 1-methyl etheryl ether (CAS 1569-02-4) Synonyms: 1-ethoxy-2-propanol

[a] The class of ethylene glycol ethers also includes the acetate derivatives of EGME, EGEE, EGnPE, EGBE; the ethylene glycol diakyl ethers; diethylene glycol ethers; and triethylene glycol ethers.
[b] The acetate derivatives of 2PG1ME and 1PG2ME, dipropylene glycol alkyl ethers, and tripropylene glycol ethers are also included in the class of propylene glycol ethers.
[c] 2PG1ME and 1PG2ME are isomers and are generally referred to collectively as PGME.

Human Toxicity

Acute effects of overexposure include central nervous system (CNS) changes (depression, ataxia, dysarthria, somnolence, tremor, personality change, and blurred vision); irritation of the eyes, nose, and throat; renal failure (including albuminuria, hematuria, and oxaluria); hemorrhagic gastritis; metabolic acidosis; and macrocytic anemia. An oral dose reported to cause lethality was 3 g/kg. There have been a number of reports in which workers were exposed to glycol ethers in the workplace. Fatigue, weakness, lethargy, anemia, bone marrow hypoplasia, and other abnormalities of hematological parameters (immaturity of neutrophils with some abnormal cells and low platelet concentration) have been reported in workers at exposure concentrations ranging from approximately 60 to 4000 ppm. There does not appear to be an association between exposure to glycol ethers and adverse effects on human testes.

Workplace exposure limits have been established for several of the compounds (Table G-2); however, OSHA is considering applying an additional uncertainty factor to glycol ethers, which would lower the current limits.

Clinical Management

If ingestion has occurred, emesis or gastric lavage may be useful if initiated within 30 min. If acidosis is present, it can be treated with intravenous sodium bicarbonate (1 or 2 mEq/kg for adults and 1 mEq/kg for children) every 1 or 2 hr as needed. Hemodialysis may be indicated in cases of severe acid-base and/or fluid-

TABLE G-2
Threshold Limit Values[a]

Compound	*TWA (ppm)*	*TWA (mg/m³)*
EGME	5	16
EGEE	5	18
PGME	100	369
EGMEA[b]	5	24
EGEEA[c]	5	27

[a] Adopted by the American Conference of Industrial Hygienists (ACGIH).
[b] EGMEA, ethylene glycol monomethyl ether acetate.
[c] EGEEA, ethylene glycol monoethyl ether acetate.

electrolyte abnormalities or in cases of renal failure. Animal data suggest that ethanol therapy may inhibit the formation of toxic metabolites: Administer a loading dose of 7.6–10 ml/kg of 10% ethanol in D5W intravenously over a 30-min period to achieve a blood ethanol concentration of 100–130 mg/dl. The oral loading dose is 0.8–1.0 ml/kg of 95% ethanol in 6 oz of orange juice over a 30-min period. Follow the loading dose with a maintenance dose of 1.39 ml/kg/hr of 10% ethanol in D5W by intravenous infusion (if dialysis is also being used, the maintenance dose may have to be increased to compensate for the loss of ethanol). For children, the loading and maintenance dose are the same with the target blood level of 100 ml/dl.

Animal Toxicity

Glycol ethers as a class are not acutely toxic by the oral route. Inhalation exposure to high concentrations of compounds in the ethylene series can cause lethality. However, exposure to compounds in the propylene series was not lethal to rodents even at nearly saturated concentrations.

The monoalkyl ethylene glycol ethers have been shown to possess a wide spectrum of biological activity, with some variation in the range of effects and potency among the individual compounds (Table G-3). For example, laboratory animals treated with EGME were observed to develop testicular atrophy, bone marrow hypoplasia (pancytopenia) with secondary effects on red blood cell and white blood cell indices, and was teratogenic and embryotoxic/fetotoxic in pregnant animals. EGEE produced a similar pattern of toxicity, while EGnPE and EGBE caused hemolysis and embryotoxicity/fetotoxicity without causing teratogenicity or effects on the bone marrow and testes. Therefore, it appears that the testicular and bone marrow effects decrease with increasing size of the alkoxy group, with the maximal effects observed for EGME. EGnPE and EGBE cause hemolysis without affecting the bone marrow; in general, the hemolytic effects appear to increase with the size of the alkoxy group. In addition, the hemolytic effects are more pronounced in mice, rats, and rabbits compared to dogs and man, which are less affected. The testicular effects have been observed in mice, rats, rabbits, and dogs, and the hematological effects have been observed in mice, rats, rabbits, cats, dogs, and man. However, PGME and other propylene glycol ethers do not cause the testicular or hematological effects and are not teratogenic, although fetotoxicity has been reported in some studies at concentrations which also produced maternal toxicity. There are also reports that EGEE and EGBE cause kidney enlargement without functional impairment. EGME has been reported to affect conditioned avoidance behavior in trained rats, and PGME has been reported to cause CNS depression. In general, the acetates derived from the glycol ethers have the same toxicological activity as the parent glycol ether. However, the acetate of PGME does appear to have teratogenic potential in rabbits, in contrast to the parent compound PGME. A

TABLE G-3

Summary of Effects in Laboratory Animals from Some Commonly Evaluated Glycol Ethers

Compound	*Fetus*[a]	*Testes*[b]	*Blood*[c]	*Bone marrow*[d]	*Kidney*[e]	*Nervous system*[f]	*Overall NOEL (ppm)*
EGME	+ (T)(F)(B)	+	+	+	NR	+	10
EGEE	+ (T)(F)(B)	+	±	+	+	−	10
EGnPE	+ (F)	−	+	−	NR	NR	100
EGiPE	NR	−	+	−	NR	NR	
EGBE	+ (F)	−	+	−	+	−	50
PGME	+ (F)	−	−	−	NR	+	1500

Note. +, Exposure to the compound produced one or more of the effects listed for the respective organ system in one or more species; −, exposure did not cause an effect in this organ system; ±, exposure to the compound produced a slight or equivocal response; NR, not reported.

[a] Effects include teratogenicity (T), fetal toxicity/embryo toxicity (F), and alterations in behavioral performance of pups (B).

[b] Effects include testicular atrophy and testicular edema.

[c] Effects include hemolysis, anemia, and decreased white blood cell count.

[d] Effects include bone marrow hypoplasia.

[e] Effects include kidney enlargement without functional impairment.

[f] Effects include inhibition of the secondary conditioned–avoidance response and central nervous system depression.

number of the glycol ethers have been evaluated with respect to potential mutagenicity and, in general, they were not mutagenic in a variety of test systems. The overall or lowest no-observed-effect levels (NOELs) for several of the commonly studied compounds are presented in Table G-3 and range from 10 ppm for EGME and EGEE to 1500 ppm for PGME. However, additional information continues to be developed for this class of compounds and could change the NOELs. Therefore, the NOELs presented in Table G-3 should only be used as a general indicator of relative compound potency.

—Linda A. Malley and David M. Krentz

Glyphosate

- CAS: 1071-83-6
- SYNONYMS: *N*-phosphonomethyl glycine; Roundup (41%); Honcho; Weedoff; Rattler; Jury; Glifinox; Glycel
- CHEMICAL CLASS: Organic phosphate herbicide
- CHEMICAL STRUCTURE:

$$HO-\overset{\displaystyle O}{\overset{\|}{C}}-CH_2-NH-CH_2-\overset{\displaystyle O}{\overset{\|}{\underset{\displaystyle OH}{\underset{|}{P}}}}-OH$$

Uses

Glyphosate is the active ingredient in several commercial herbicides for nonselective weed control.

Exposure Pathways

The primary route of exposure to glyphosate is through accidental or intentional ingestion. Dermal exposure is not typically associated with systemic effects.

Toxicokinetics

Glyphosate is rapidly absorbed following oral ingestion. Dermal absorption is very low. Glyphosate is metabolized to aminomethyl phosphonic acid. High concentrations have been found in the kidneys, liver, brain, and blood following intentional oral ingestion. Glyphosate is rapidly excreted in the urine in large amounts. Usually within 24–48 hr, glyphosate is undetectable in the urine.

Mechanism of Toxicity

Several mechanisms have been proposed for glyphosate, such as uncoupling of mitochondrial oxidative phosphorylation, inhibition of aryl hydrocarbon hydroxylase activity, and inhibition of cytochrome P450 activity. However, surfactants present in many commercial preparations (i.e., Roundup), are considered to be responsible, in part, for the observed toxicity. In contrast to organophosphate insecticides, glyphosate is not a significant inhibitor of acetylcholinesterase.

Human Toxicity: Acute

The primary effects following ingestion include mucous membrane irritation, abdominal pain, vomiting, diarrhea, hypotension, oliguria, and anuria. Esophageal and gastric erosions have occurred after ingestion of concentrated solutions (41% glyphosate). In fatal cases, hypovolemic shock, cardiac arrhythmias, metabolic acidosis, and pulmonary edema have been reported. However, glyphosate has relatively low toxicity, with mortality rates of only 17% in suicidal cases. Ingestions of 150 ml or less have not resulted in deaths.

Human Toxicity: Chronic

Dermatitis resembling sunburn has been reported following prolonged skin exposure. There is no evidence of carcinogenicity in humans and only one tumorigenic response has been observed in experimental animals.

Clinical Management

Due to the possibility of esophageal erosion, emesis is not recommended. Activated charcoal and a cathartic should be administered following ingestion of large amounts of glyphosate. Oral irrigation and dilution may be sufficient for smaller ingestions. In severe cases, basic life support, such as fluid replacement for hypovolemic shock, should be provided. Hemodialysis is indicated in patients with renal failure.

Animal Toxicity

Glyphosate is a compound of low mammalian toxicity. Oral LD_{50} values for laboratory rodents are >4 g/kg. The dermal LD_{50} value in rabbits is about 5 g/kg.

—Kevin N. Baer

Related Topic

Pesticides

Gold (Au)

- CAS: 7440-57-5
- REPRESENTATIVE COMPOUNDS: Gold salts; sodium gold chloride
- CHEMICAL CLASS: Metal

Uses

Gold has found many industrial uses because of its excellent electrical and thermal conductivity properties. It is used for plating other metals and as an alloying metal. It is used in the manufacture of jewelry, dental inlays, art, currency, and electronic components. Gold has also found use in medicine in the treatment of certain cancers, rheumatoid arthritis, discoid lupus (a rare skin disease), and in specialized surgical procedures.

Exposure Pathways

The most common exposure pathway is through dermal contact. Inhalation and oral exposure to gold dust may occur in occupational settings.

Toxicokinetics

Gold dust and gold salts are poorly absorbed from the gastrointestinal tract.

Mechanism of Toxicity

The main mechanisms believed to be responsible for gold salt toxicity is the formation of gold–protein complexes that elicit immune reactions. That is, gold salts may act as a hapten with subsequent antibody production against the gold–protein complex. The gold–protein–antibody complexes may in turn accumulate in the glomerular subepithelium. A second possible mechanism of gold salt toxicity is that antibodies may be formed against kidney tubular cells damaged by gold.

Human Toxicity

Oral administration of excessive amounts of gold salts have been found to produce pancytopenia in certain individuals. In addition, therapeutic doses of gold salts given for the treatment of rheumatic disease may produce adverse side effects such as dermatitis, immune complex hypersensitivity, nephrotoxicity, and peripheral neuropathy.

Clinical Management

Further exposure to gold or gold salts should be prevented. A physician should be consulted if gold is being used as a therapeutic agent. Supportive treatment should be provided.

Animal Toxicity

Animal experiments have shown that gold dust is not carcinogenic to rats. However, subcutaneous implantation of gold sheets was able to induce tumors.

—Heriberto Robles

Related Topic

Metals

Good Laboratory Practices

In 1976 the U.S. FDA first proposed Good Laboratory Practices (GLPs) in an attempt to ensure the integrity of data generated during nonclinical laboratory studies. The regulations came in the wake of a realization that certain basic laboratory practices were not routinely followed by all laboratories performing safety assessment studies. In many cases, personnel involved in the conduct of a study were no longer employed by the laboratory, and the data collected were insufficient for determining what had happened during the study. The essence of the GLPs require that a well-defined, organizational structure exists and that a paper trail be established, through which the course of events for a study can be reconstructed. Personnel not directly involved in the conduct of a study must monitor each study to ensure the testing facility management and regulatory agencies that the facilities, equipment, personnel, methods, practices, records, and controls do, in fact, conform to the requirements of the GLPs.

The FDA GLPs were revised and the final rule was adopted on September 4, 1987. On August 17, 1989, the U.S. EPA issued two final rules for its Good Laboratory Practice Standards. One rule addressed studies conducted to meet pesticide registration requirements under the Federal Insecticide, Fungicide, and Rodenticide Act (FIFRA), and the other rule addressed studies required for industrial chemicals under the Toxic Substances Control Act (TSCA).

In other countries, similar regulations were adopted. During the early 1980s, use of GLPs were adopted for regulatory studies by the Organisation for Economic Cooperation and Development and the following Japanese regulatory agencies: the Ministry of Health and Welfare; the Ministry of International Trade and Industry; and the Ministry of Agriculture, Forestry and Fisheries. While the GLPs for the various agencies differ slightly, they are essentially the same.

As with most legal documents, the GLPs are open to a fair degree of interpretation. Sponsors (the study initiator or supporter) maintain or contract quality assurance personnel to evaluate a laboratory's compliance with the GLPs. Laboratories must have personnel who are not involved in the study review study procedures and data to ensure GLP compliance. Thus, an entire profession has evolved around the interpretation and application of the GLPs. Many circumstances do not fit neatly into the letter of the law. The views and interpretations presented in this discussion of the GLPs represent those of the author and are based on practical application, scientific validity, and the underlying essence of the GLPs to ensure that study data are collected in such a way that the integrity of the data is preserved and that the course of events for a study can be reconstructed.

The beginning of the paper trail for studies performed in accordance with the GLPs is the study protocol. All studies must have a protocol. The protocol indicates the scope of the work to be performed and the parties involved. The protocol must be approved by the study sponsor and signed and dated by the study director. Any changes to the protocol must include the reason for the change and be signed and dated by the study director.

The study director is the individual charged with the overall responsibility for technical conduct of the study and with ensuring that all GLPs are followed. The study director must have the training, education, and experience necessary to serve as the single point of control for the study. The study director has the ultimate responsibility for the implementation, documentation, and interpretation of the study. All events that could compromise the outcome of a study must be acknowledged by the study director.

The study director is designated by the management of the laboratory performing the study. The role of the study director becomes increasingly complicated when several laboratories are involved in study conduct. How does the study director oversee functions at other laboratories? How can the study director ensure GLP compliance at other laboratories? Often a representative of the sponsor coordinates the activities of the various laboratories. Should this individual be the study director? In this case, which laboratory's management designates the study director?

This dilemma is probably best rectified by recognition of a main testing facility, that being the facility managing the administration or application of the material being tested. The study director, appointed by the main testing facility's management, must be aware of the aspects of the GLPs that may be compromised by conducting studies at more one facility. The GLP issues should first be addressed in the protocol by specifying the laboratories involved, the scope of work they are to perform, record retention and reporting requirements for each of the laboratories, and quality assurance responsibilities for each of the laboratories. In the GLP compliance statement, which is discussed later, the study director should indicate the role that each laboratory assumed in meeting the requirements of the GLPs.

In addition to appointing a study director, the testing facility management must ensure that a sufficient number of trained personnel and adequate resources are available to complete a study in a timely manner. The management establishes and approves the practices and procedures necessary to conduct the studies in a manner that ensures the quality and integrity of the data. The practices and procedures must be formalized in written documents called standard operating procedures (SOPs).

The GLPs indicate some specific procedures that require SOPs, such as observations of the test systems (test organisms), collection and identification of specimens, and maintenance and calibration of equipment. SOPs must be readily available in the study area so that personnel can easily consult them, if necessary, while performing a procedure. Revisions to SOPs must be documented in such a way that identification of the version of an SOP in use at any given time is possible.

The GLPs are not specific when it comes to the contents of SOPs, except for the maintenance and calibration of equipment. Equipment SOPs must indicate the frequency and procedures for testing, calibrating, or standardizing equipment as well as the personnel responsible for these functions. The GLPs require that detailed records be kept for all equipment inspections, maintenance, testing, calibration, and standardizing operations. Records of both routine and nonroutine maintenance must be kept for all pieces of equipment used in the generation, measurement, or assessment of data and for facility environmental control equipment. Routine maintenance records must indicate whether or not the maintenance procedures followed SOPs. Nonroutine maintenance records must include information regarding the nature of the problem and how the problem was discovered.

For certain pieces of equipment, the advantages of keeping detailed maintenance records are clear. The records can be used to support, after the fact, that a piece of equipment was functioning properly at its time of use. For example, with a piece of equipment such as a balance, a log of calibrations or verifications using standard weights can provide reasonable assurance that weights recorded during a study were accurate. On the other hand, is a record necessary for the routine cleaning of a microscope or the nonroutine replacement of a microscope's ocular? Would these maintenance records add in any way to the validity of histopathological findings? Clearly, if a malfunction in a piece of equipment would not compromise study integrity, an SOP should not be needed.

Another critical aspect of the GLPs is the integrity of the chemicals used in a study. Chemicals can be broadly classified as standard reagents or study-specific compounds. The GLPs require that reagents and solutions be labeled as to their identity, titer or concentration, storage requirements, and expiration date. Additional requirements are imposed on study-specific compounds.

Study-specific compounds, referred to as substances or articles, depending on the version of the GLPs, can be placed in one of two or three categories, again depending on the version of the GLPs. The FDA GLPs recognize two categories: test articles and control articles. The EPA GLPs (both FIFRA and TSCA) recognize three categories—test substances, control substances, and reference substances—but include control substance in parentheses after reference substance, implying that they are the same. The three Japanese GLPs refer only to test and control articles or substances. None of this would be much of a problem, except that test, control, and reference substances or articles must be characterized prior to use in a study. Therefore, one must know whether a material is considered a test, control, or reference substance or article.

The test article or substance is the compound, mixture, or device, etc. under study, which is regulated by, for which a permit is sought, etc. Control substance, as defined in the FIFRA GLPs means

> Any chemical substance or mixture, or any other material other than a test substance, feed, or water, that is administered to the test system for the purpose of establishing a basis for comparison with the test substance for known chemical or biological measurements.

Is a vehicle, defined in the FIFRA GLPs as "any agent which facilitates the mixture, dispersion, or solubility of a test substance with a carrier," or a carrier, defined in the FIFRA GLPs as "any material, including but not limited to feed, water, soil, nutrient media, with which the test substance is combined for administration to a test system," a control substance if one compares the response of organisms receiving the test substance with organisms receiving only the vehicle or carrier? Frequently, corn oil is used as a carrier for oral administrations, and the control group receives the corn oil without the test substance. Should the corn oil also be classified as a control substance and be characterized? (Interestingly, various TSCA testing guidelines define the term carrier to be synonymous with the GLP term vehicle, and therefore not synonymous with the GLP term carrier.)

A key part of the definition of control substance is "for the purpose of establishing a basis for comparison." A vehicle or carrier is not administered for the purpose of establishing a comparison, but it is necessary for the administration of the test substance. The purpose of administering a vehicle or carrier to a control group is to ensure that any effects seen in groups receiving the test substance are not attributable to the vehicle or carrier. Classically, materials that are administered to establish a basis for comparison have been called positive controls. Positive control substances are used in testing because they are known to elicit an effect that may be suspected with the test substance. Only substances clearly administered as a positive control should be considered "control substances" and be subjected to characterization requirements.

To further sink in the mire of substance definition, reference substance is defined in the FIFRA GLPs as

> Any chemical substance or mixture, or analytical standard, or material other than a test substance, feed, or water, that is administered to or used in analyzing the test system in the course of a study for the purposes of establishing a basis for comparison with the test substance for known chemical or biological measurements.

So the only difference between a control substance and a reference substance is the inclusion of analytical standards.

As stated earlier, test, control, and reference substances need to be characterized. Characterization typically includes determining the identity, purity, and composition. Determining purity requires an analytical standard for comparison. The analytical standard also needs to be characterized; this includes purity determination.

There are other requirements for test, control, and reference substances. The stability of the test, control, or reference substance must be determined, but it may be determined during the course of the study. If, however, a substance is determined to be unstable, then the integrity of the study may be compromised. Stability under conditions of storage at the test site must also be known. Storage stability is often known prior to the study in vague terms, such as ambient temperature storage or frozen storage. Again, if a substance is not stable under the exact storage conditions at the testing facility, a study may be compromised.

Solubility, if pertinent to study conduct, is another parameter that must be determined prior to beginning the experimental portion of a study. Solubility can be affected by many factors, such as temperature; ideal solubility and the solubility obtainable during a study may differ considerably. For an aquatic toxicology study, in which solubility is a crucial parameter, mixing times are usually scent compared to the amount of time a chemist may allow for solubility determinations at a bench. Does determination of ideal solubility add to study integrity?

Labeling requirements for test, control, or reference substances include name, chemical abstract service registry number or code number, batch number, expiration date, and storage conditions. If the study has an experimental duration of more than 4 weeks, then a reserve sample must be collected and retained.

The GLPs require that the receipt of distribution of each batch of test, control, or reference substance is documented. The accountability of test substance may be critical in reconstructing study events. If results suggest that an improper dose or concentration level was used, records showing the amounts used for formulations may be able to support the presupposition.

Facilities must be adequate to ensure that test, control, or reference substances are stored properly and are not contaminated. Standard operating procedures that address the receipt, identification, storage, handling, mixing, and method of sampling for test, control, or reference substances are required. Handling practices must be sufficient to prevent cross-contamination among various substances.

Mixtures of a test, control, or reference substance with a carrier that are used for administration to a test system must be analyzed for uniformity or homogeneity, concentration, stability, and, if relevant, solubility. These analyses ensure that the specified amount of a test, control, or reference substance is being administered to the test system. Normally acceptable parameters for these analyses, such as all homogeneity analyses being within 10% of the target concentration, should be specified in an SOP but must also be left open to the discretion of the study director. Of course, these analyses do not ensure that a test system actually receives the proper amount of a test, control, or reference substance, but only that the proper amount is in the mixture with the carrier.

A testing laboratory must have adequate facilities for the housing and care of the test systems. Test systems are any animal, plant, microorganism, or chemical or physical matrix to which the test, control, or reference substance is applied or administered for study. Separation of test systems must be sufficient for the isolation of individual projects. Separation can be accomplished through the use of different rooms or protective barriers. Additionally, there must be sufficient space for the storage of supplies for the care and maintenance of the test systems.

All studies are concluded by the issuance of a final report. Many requirements for the final report are listed in the GLPs. The final report must be signed and dated by the study director. The final report, all raw data and supporting documentation, protocols, and specimens must be retained, with the exception of various samples that may not afford further evaluation. Archiving facilities must be adequate to prevent deterioration and allow for orderly storage and expedient retrieval. Materials must be retained for as long as a sponsor holds a permit for research or marketing to which the study is applicable—at least 5 years following submission in support of a research or marketing permit or 2 years if the study is not submitted in support of an application, whichever is longer.

All applications of toxicological safety assessment studies in support of a research or marketing permit must include a compliance statement that is signed by the sponsor, study director, and, in the case of FIFRA submissions, the applicant. The compliance statement must indicate that all requirements of the GLPs were followed, must state any aspects of the GLPs that were not followed, or must state that the person was not a study sponsor, did not conduct the study, and has no knowledge as to whether the GLPs were followed.

Submission of a false compliance statement is a criminal offense. Therefore, the various ambiguities in the GLPs and their interpretations have legal implications. Study directors, laboratory management, and study sponsors should be aware of these gray areas and, if in doubt, should so indicate in the compliance statement.

—Shayne C. Gad

Further Reading

Chengelis, C. P., Gad, S. C., and Holson, J. (1995). *Regulatory Toxicology*. Raven Press, New York.

Gad, S. C., and Errico, P. (1996). *Handbook of Data Recording, Maintenance and Management for the Biomedical Sciences*. Raven Press, Boca Raton, FL.

Related Topics

Analytical Toxicology
Effluent Biomonitoring
Federal Insecticide, Fungicide, and Rodenticide Act
Food and Drug Administration
Organisation for Economic Cooperation and Development
Toxic Substances Control Act

Guaifenesin

- CAS: 93-14-1
- SYNONYMS: Glyceryl guaiacolate; α-glyceryl guaiacol ether; guaianesin; Robitussin
- CHEMICAL STRUCTURE:

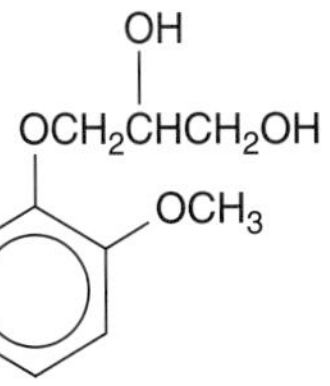

OH
OCH_2CHCH_2OH
OCH_3

Uses

Guaifenesin is used as a respiratory tract expectorant.

Exposure Pathways

Guaifenesin is available in liquid or capsule form for oral dosing. Accidental or intentional exposure occurs most commonly by ingestion.

Toxicokinetics

Guaifenesin is well absorbed from the gastrointestinal tract, specifically from the intestine. It is hydrolyzed 60% in the blood within 7 hr. Following hydrolysis, urinary metabolites include β-(4-hydroxy-2-methoxyphenoxy)lactic acid, β-(2-methoxyphenoxy)lactic acid, and guaiacol glyceryl ether. The metabolites are excreted via the kidneys. Following oral administration, no unchanged drug is detected in the urine.

Mechanism of Toxicity

Guaifenesin lacks specific toxicity. It stimulates respiratory tract secretions by irritating the gastric mucosa. It facilitates the evacuation of secretions from the respiratory tract by decreasing sputum viscosity, thus relieving difficulty in expectoration. Unlike antitussives, it does not inhibit or suppress cough. Toxicity associated with guaifenesin will generally result from the presence of antihistamines, decongestants, analgesics, cough suppressants, and/or alcohol in preparations containing a combination of ingredients.

Human Toxicity

Guaifenesin is of low order of toxicity. Adverse effects are primarily minor gastrointestinal complaints. Doses larger than those required for expectorant action may produce vomiting, but gastrointestinal upset is rare at ordinary dosage levels.

Clinical Management

Basic and advanced life-support measures should be instituted as indicated. When guaifenesin is the sole substance ingested, treatment of the exposure is rarely necessary. In situations of overdose, in which guaifenesin is ingested in multisymptom products containing antihistamines, decongestants, and/or cough suppressants, treatment is directed toward that which is appropriate to the coingestant(s). Consideration should be given to the alcohol content of liquid preparations of guaifenesin and combination products.

—Carole Wezorek

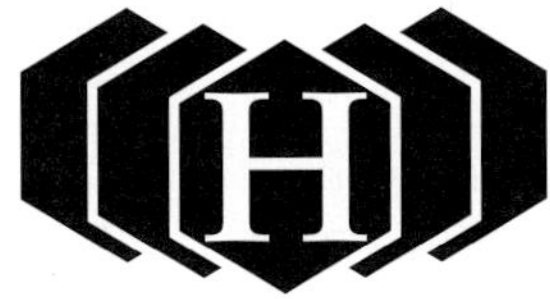

Hazard Identification

Hazard identification is the first step in the risk assessment process and addresses two questions: (1) Does a given material present a potential hazard, and (2) What type of adverse health effect(s) is it likely to cause? Is it, for example, a neurotoxicant, a developmental toxicant, or a potential carcinogen?

Hazard identification depends on a careful scientific evaluation of several different types of information:

- Physical characteristics (e.g., corrosivity, flammability, and reactivity with other substances)
- Results of *in vivo* animal testing studies
- Results of *in vitro* laboratory tests (e.g., cell cultures or isolated tissues)
- Results of epidemiological studies with human populations
- Structure–activity analysis (i.e., comparisons with the known toxicity of structurally similar chemicals)

In Vivo Animal Studies

The most commonly used information in hazard identification is obtained from animal bioassays. Although the use of animals in toxicity testing has become a highly controversial topic in recent years, responsible studies with a variety of species of laboratory animals (mainly rats, mice, guinea pigs, rabbits, dogs, and occasionally primates) frequently represent our only source of information on which to judge the potential adverse effects of a chemical on humans. While always associated with a good deal of uncertainty, the use of animals in toxicology testing rests on the premise that the results observed in animals are applicable to humans.

Chemicals usually can cause multiple effects and the outcome of an exposure is likely to depend on the length of time over which an exposure occurs, the primary route of exposure, the sensitivity of the individual or species, and the resulting dose. Effects can occur as a result of exposure at the point of contact (e.g., skin, eyes, gastrointestinal tract, and respiratory tract) or any internal or systemic target. Animal bioassays are often placed in one of three major groups based primarily on the duration of exposure period; these groups are acute, subacute and subchronic, and chronic.

Acute Studies

Acute studies are designed to evaluate the possible adverse effects that may occur after short-term exposure (e.g., 24 hr or less to about 1 week). Exposure may occur from one or possibly a few exposures to the test substance over the time period. In humans, such exposures might result from one-time accidents or other unusual incidents. Acute effects may occur in any system and can range from mild irritation of the eyes, skin, and respiratory tract to comma and death.

Subacute and Subchronic Studies

Subacute studies occur over time periods that are greater than a week up to several months. Subchronic studies address exposures that occur for period of about 90 days. Both subacute and subchronic studies involve repeated, usually daily, exposures to the test substance. These studies have been used to reflect effects that might result from continual occupational exposures that can occur over a period of several weeks or months. Subchronic studies in rodents (lifetime of 2 years) have been used as the basis for exposure criteria that is intended to protect against the occurrence of adverse effects in humans for exposures that are anticipated to occur over 1–7 years. Animals are observed daily throughout the course of the study and observations made with respect to clinical signs of toxicity (e.g., loss of body weight, incoordination, and loss of balance), general appearance, and/or unusual behavioral patterns. At the end of the study, all animals are sacrificed and a gross and microscopic pathological examination of selected tissues is conducted. Included with subchronic and subacute studies are special developmental toxicity studies in which pregnant animals are exposed daily to the test chemical throughout the critical stages (organogenesis) of fetal development. It should be noted that some chemicals (e.g., thalidomide) exert their adverse effects at very specific points in fetal development so that even single acute exposures during that critical period can cause an effect.

Chronic Studies

Chronic studies are typically conducted for periods >90 days and usually as close as possible to the length of the lifetime of the test animal. In some cases, as with bioassays for carcinogenesis, the animals are exposed daily for the lifetime (usually 18 months in mice and 2 years in rats). Chronic studies focus on identifying effects (e.g., such as cancer or certain reproductive effects) that might occur following continuous exposure over several generations.

The results of animal bioassays for toxicity form the basis of risk assessment and risk management under most regulatory statutes at the federal, state, and international levels. To obtain consistency and to ensure that the studies are designed, conducted, and analyzed in a sound scientific manner, experimental protocols for animal studies are required to meet various U.S. federal statutes. Requirements are all carefully described in the *Code of Federal Regulations*. The study guidelines consist of a series of Standard Evaluation Procedures that clearly specify factors like the number of animals per test group, the number of treatment groups, methods of chemical administration, types of observations that must be made and detailed procedures, and endpoints for clinical, hematological, ophthalmoscopic, and histopathologic evaluation. A study that does not follow the appropriate guidelines may not be acceptable to the regulatory agency. Currently, attempts are being made to standardize (harmonize) the test guideline requirements in different countries (e.g., United States, Canada, and the Europe Union) that are often somewhat different from one another.

Depending on the physicochemical nature of the chemical and the route of exposure of particular concern or relevance to expected human exposures, the test materials may be administered orally [by incorporation in food or water or by gavage (feeding tube) directly into the stomach], dermally (application to the skin), or by inhalation in the form of a gas or aerosol. In most cases, the test chemical is administered in a substance that is believed to be a toxicologically inert vehicle (such as saline or corn oil) and the observations in the treated animals are compared with those in control animals receiving only the vehicle. The tests are usually conducted with groups of control animals and three or more groups receiving different doses of the test material; groups of each sex are employed. The number of animals in a treatment group varies depending on the nature of the test, ranging from about 6–20 animals for acute and subchronic studies to 50–60 animals in chronic cancer bioassays.

In Vitro Tests in Hazard Identification

In vitro tests are tests in which chemical interactions with any of a wide variety of organs, tissue preparations, cell cultures, enzymes, receptors, etc. are studied "in the test tube." Such studies have always been considered important tools in studying the effects of toxic chemicals and identifying the mechanisms through which toxicity occurs and usually complement *in vivo* studies with intact animals. Indeed, with growing concern over the use of animals in laboratory research, there has been a concerted effort in recent years to develop a number of *in vitro* tests that might serve as alternatives for some *in vivo* tests; despite some success, there remains a strong consensus that both types of testing will continue to be required.

The intact animal in a toxicity study is equivalent to a black box. It is possible to make gross observations on toxic signs, symptomology, and clinical effects but these seldom provide the details required to understand the precise mechanisms of toxicity or the primary cause of the adverse effects occurring at the subcellular level. The use of *in vitro* systems allows, for example, measurements of the ability of a neurotoxicant to inhibit cholinesterase, identifies potentially reactive metabolites formed in the liver, or demonstrates the ability of a compound to bind to a macromolecular receptor like DNA. *In vitro* studies are also extremely important in metabolic studies and the identification of reactive intermediates. The use of specific intact organs or a variety of cell or tissue cultures of human, animal, plant, or microbial origin often provides useful laboratory models for studying the potential of a compound to penetrate skin or damage the cornea of the eye or otherwise interact with living tissues. Adverse effects may be indicated through changes in cell turnover, membrane permeability, or damage to cell organelles (e.g., mitochondria).

The results of *in vitro* studies to determine genetic toxicity have become an important component in assessing the carcinogenic potential of a chemical. Thus, an important part of the routine testing of all chemicals now involves a battery of *in vitro* tests to determine each chemical's potential mutagenicity or clastogenicity (DNA damage). These tests include the well-known Ames mutagenicity test with various strains of Salmonella, cytogenetic, and unscheduled DNA synthesis assays employing various cell cultures including those of human cells. A positive result with these types of tests suggests genotoxic or mutagenic potential that is taken into account in the total weight of evidence evaluation of carcinogenicity.

Epidemiology in Hazard Identification

Since epidemiology relates directly to the incidence of illness or toxicity in humans (see Epidemiology), the existence of positive epidemiological data is most relevant to assessing potential human hazard or risk. The major advantages of epidemiological studies are that they are usually based on large numbers of humans exposed to "real-world" levels of the chemical. Any effects observed are directly relevant to humans and do not require the type of extrapolations used to related animal studies to humans.

Unfortunately, epidemiological data can only be obtained retrospectively after a chemical has been on the market for a number of years and, obviously, cannot play a role in the prospective hazard evaluation of a new chemical.

Structure–Activity Relationships

In the absence of any other information, the analysis of possible structure–activity relationships (SARs) is often useful as a first attempt at hazard identification. SAR analysis involves a comparison of the structural, physical, and chemical properties of a chemical with unknown hazards with those of similar chemicals having known toxic effects. In some cases, SAR analysis may simply provide a qualitative indicator of a specific type of activity (i.e., if it is a polycyclic aromatic hydrocarbon it is likely to be treated as a suspected carcinogen in the absence of any toxicity data). In other cases, SAR relationships can actually be used to obtain a quantitative estimate of an effect (e.g., with homologous series of compounds or organophosphorus cholinesterase inhibitors). SAR analysis is frequently used by regulatory agencies to develop a series of triggers of concern. Thus, when faced with a new chemical that has never been tested, the presence of certain functional groups may represent indicators of possible toxicological concern.

It is important to recognize, however, that SAR analysis can be misleading and must be used cautiously. With some chemicals, the requirements for exerting an adverse effect are very specific, and small, seemingly insignificant changes in structure (e.g., the *ortho*, *meta*, or *para* position of an aromatic substituent) can make an enormous change in biological activity.

—*Chris F. Wilkinson*

Related Topics

Ames Test
Analytical Toxicology
Animal Models
Biomarkers, Human Health

Epidemiology
Good Laboratory Practices
In Vitro Test
In Vivo Test
Risk Assessment, Human Health
Structure–Activity Relationships
Toxicity, Acute
Toxicity, Chronic
Toxicity, Subchronic
Toxicity Testing

Hazardous Waste

There are two definitions of hazardous waste. The first definition was written into legislation by the U.S. Congress, and the second, which has its basis in the first, was written into regulation by the U.S. EPA. In 1976, U.S. Congress defined the term "hazardous waste" in the Resource Conservation and Recovery Act (RCRA), an amendment to the Solid Waste Disposal Act of 1965, as

> A solid waste, or combination of solid waste, which because of its quantity, concentration, or physical, chemical, or infectious characteristics may—(A) cause, or significantly contribute to an increase in mortality or an increase in serious irreversible, or incapacitating reversible, illness; or (B) pose a substantial present or potential hazard to human health or the environment when improperly treated, stored, transported, or disposed of, or otherwise managed. (42 USC 6903(5))

In Subtitle C of RCRA, Congress created the framework for the "cradle-to-grave" management of hazardous waste. The broad, subjective statutory definition of hazardous waste, however, did not specify which wastes would be subject to Subtitle C and its accompanying regulatory scheme. A more precise definition of hazardous waste was needed in order to determine exactly which wastes would be subject to RCRA Subtitle C regulation. Therefore, the U.S. Congress directed U.S. EPA to promulgate regulations identifying the characteristics of hazardous waste and listing particular hazardous wastes, "taking into account toxicity, persistence, and degradability in nature, potential for accumulation in tissue, and other related factors such as flammability, corrosiveness, and other hazardous characteristics" (42 USC 6921(a)). In 1980, U.S. EPA fulfilled this statutory mandate by promulgating 40 CFR Part 261, which is titled *Identification and Listing of Hazardous Waste*. Since then, U.S. EPA modified Part 261 to reflect Congressional intent and trends in waste generation.

In the regulatory sense, hazardous waste identification relies not so much on a definition as on a series of steps that involve checking against lists of waste exclusions and inclusions. The three steps of the hazardous waste identification process are codified at 40 CFR 262.11.

The first step of hazardous waste identification is determining whether a material is a solid waste. A solid waste is any material that is discarded. (The modifier "solid" is not indicative of the physical state of the material. That is, a solid waste may be in the liquid or gaseous phases as well as the solid phase.) A material is considered discarded when it is abandoned, recycled, or inherently waste-like. Abandonment occurs when a material is disposed of; burned/incinerated; or accumulated, stored, or treated before, or in lieu of, abandonment. Recycling occurs when a material is used in a manner that resembles disposal (e.g., placed on the ground); burned to recover its energy; reclaimed to recover a usable product; or accumulated speculatively. In addition, a few specific materials have been designated inherently waste-like (e.g., certain dioxin-containing wastes) and are considered solid wastes when recycled in any manner. However, a number of materials do not meet the definition of solid waste when discarded because the materials qualify for one of several statutory or regulatory exclusions from the definition of solid waste. For example, in order to avoid duplicative regulations, materials regulated and managed under the Clean Water Act or the Atomic Energy Act are exempt from the definition of solid waste (40 CFR 261.4(a)(2) and 261.4(a)(4), respectively).

The second step in the hazardous waste identification process is determining whether a solid waste qualifies for one of the statutory or regulatory exclusions from the definition of hazardous waste. Several exclusions from the definition of hazardous waste appearing in the regulations have their origins in the statute. For instance, U.S. EPA incorporated Congress' Subtitle C exclusion for cement kiln dust into the regulations at

40 CFR 261.4(b)(8). In addition, U.S. EPA has promulgated a number of exclusions independently of Congress, all of which are codified in 40 CFR 261.4(b). For example, U.S. EPA exempted all solid wastes routinely generated in residences from the definition of hazardous waste (40 CFR 261.4(b)(1)). Waste-specific exclusions may also be obtained on a site-by-site basis by petitioning U.S. EPA.

The third step of hazardous waste identification is determining whether a solid waste that is not specifically excluded is a hazardous waste. There are two broad categories of hazardous waste: listed and characteristic. The hazardous waste determination process in 40 CFR 262.11 states that the listings are reviewed first. If a solid waste does not meet any of the listing descriptions, then the characteristics are checked. The listings are intended to regulate common hazardous wastestreams by specifically listing them by name or by description. The characteristics, on the other hand, are written as broad descriptions, each of which may capture an unspecified number of solid wastes within hazardous waste regulation. All hazardous wastes are assigned a waste code consisting of an initial letter and a number. Listed waste codes begin with an "F," "K," "P," or "U," while all characteristic waste codes begin with the letter "D."

A waste is listed by U.S. EPA if it meets one of the three criteria codified in 40 CFR 261.11. First, a waste can be promulgated as a listed waste if it exhibits any of the four characteristics (a detailed discussion of the characteristics follows). Although a waste may be listed because it exhibits a characteristic, it is not defined in the regulations in terms of its characteristic(s). Rather, U.S. EPA defines such wastes in terms of the process by which it is generated or by its chemical name. For example, K044 is listed because it exhibits a characteristic, but its listing description reads, "wastewater treatment sludges from the manufacturing and processing of explosives," without reference to the characteristic.

Second, a waste can be listed because it contains any of the toxic constituents listed in 40 CFR Part 261 Appendix VIII, provided the concentration of the constituent in the waste, the persistence of the constituent, any toxic degradation products of the constituent, as well as other factors are taken into account. Hazardous constituents are listed in Appendix VIII if the constituents have been shown in scientific studies to have toxic, carcinogenic, mutagenic, or teratogenic effects on humans or other life forms. The majority of listed wastes have been listed in this manner.

Finally, a waste can be listed if it has been found to be fatal to humans in low doses or, in the absence of data on human toxicity, it has been shown in studies to

- Have an oral LD_{50} toxicity (rat) <50 mg/kg, or
- Have an inhalation LC_{50} toxicity (rat) <2 mg/liter, or
- Have a dermal LD_{50} toxicity (rabbit) <200 mg/kg, or
- Be otherwise capable of causing or significantly contributing to an increase in serious, irreversible, or incapacitating reversible illness.

Wastes listed in this manner are classified as acute hazardous wastes which become subject to full hazardous waste regulation in smaller quantities than those for other hazardous wastes. An example of an acute listed hazardous waste is P042, a discarded, unused solution of pure epinephrine.

Based on the first three criteria, U.S. EPA has promulgated several hundred listed wastes, dividing the listed wastes into three groupings: wastes from nonspecific sources ("F wastes"), wastes from specific sources ("K wastes"), and (two types of) commercial chemical products ("P or U wastes").

Before a characteristic of hazardous waste can be promulgated it must be assessed against two criteria that are codified in 40 CFR 261.10. The first criterion is that a waste exhibiting the characteristic in question must meet the broad statutory definition of hazardous waste. The second criterion is that the characteristic must be able to be measured using standardized test methods or detected through knowledge of the waste. Based on these criteria, U.S. EPA has identified four characteristics of hazardous waste: ignitibility, corrosivity, reactivity, and toxicity. For each characteristic, U.S. EPA has promulgated at least two distinct properties. A solid waste need only exhibit one property of one characteristic to be subject to regulation as a characteristic hazardous waste.

EPA has identified four properties of ignitibility. One of the four properties pertains to liquids that are not aqueous solutions containing less than 24% alcohol by volume. A liquid meeting this description that has a flash point $<60°C$ (140°F), as determined by a specified closed cup test, is one example of an ignitible hazardous waste that carries the waste code D001.

Two properties of corrosivity have been identified by EPA, either of which can render a solid waste a hazardous waste, identified by the waste code D002. An aqueous solid waste that has a pH ≤ 2 or ≥ 12.5, as measured by a specified test, is a corrosive hazardous waste. Likewise, a liquid solid waste that corrodes steel at a rate >6.35 mm/year at 55°C, as measured by a specified test, is also a corrosive hazardous waste.

A solid waste is hazardous for reactivity if it displays any one of eight separate properties that U.S. EPA has specified. Unlike the other three characteristics of hazardous waste, several of the properties of reactivity rely on subjective criteria rather than scientifically measured properties. In such cases a generator of a solid waste must make a judgment about the regulatory status of the waste based on his/her knowledge of the nature of the waste. For example, a solid waste that forms potentially explosive mixtures with water, or a waste that is normally unstable and readily undergoes violent change without detonating, is a D003 reactive waste.

The final characteristic, toxicity, is defined by the concentration levels of 40 hazardous constituents—26 organics, 8 metals, and 6 pesticides—in an extract of a representative sample of waste. The extract is obtained by subjecting a sample to the Toxicity Characteristic Leaching Procedure, a test designed to estimate the ability of the contaminant to leach if the waste containing it were placed in a landfill. The concentration levels of hazardous constituents measured in a waste extract are compared to maximum allowable concentrations limits established in the regulations. If any of the regulatory concentration limits are equaled or exceeded, the wastestream (not just the extract) is a characteristic hazardous waste for toxicity. Each of the 40 toxicity characteristic (TC) waste codes, D004–D043, corresponds to a different hazardous constituent (e.g., a waste exceeding the regulatory limit for lead is D008 and for mercury it is D009).

It is important to note that the same chemical or compound can be regulated as different listed wastes based on the manner in which it is generated. For example, American Petroleum Institute (API) separator sludge from the petroleum refining industry is identified by the waste code K051. Separator sludge generated in a unit other than an API separator would not be K051 because it does not meet the listing description which, as a K listing, specifies the source of the sludge. The same waste generated in another type of separator would most likely be captured by either F037 or F038, neither of which, as F-listed wastes, specifies the source of the wastestream. In addition, if neither listing applies, the sludge could be regulated as a characteristic hazardous waste with the waste code D018 if it meets or exceeds the regulatory limit of the toxicity characteristic for benzene.

According to 40 CFR 262.11, the person(s) who produces a waste (generator) is responsible for carrying out the hazardous waste identification process. First, the generator must review all hazardous waste listings. Only if no listings apply is the generator required to check for characteristics, using testing and/or process knowledge. Although it is not necessary for hazardous waste identification purposes to determine whether a listed waste is also characteristic, it may be necessary to take the added step of identifying characteristics to determine the appropriate treatment for the waste. If a solid waste does not meet a listing description and it does not exhibit any of the four characteristics, it is not a hazardous waste as defined by the federal regulations.

Hazardous waste identification is the first step in determining how a waste must be managed. Wastes that meet the definition of hazardous waste are subject to comprehensive federal regulations (40 CFR 262-279) that govern the generation, transportation, storage, treatment, disposal, and recycling of hazardous waste. The level of regulation varies based on criteria such as the amount of waste generated at a site on a monthly basis, the nature of the waste, and, in some cases, whether the waste is recycled. All hazardous waste regulations are similar in that they are intended to ensure the safe management of hazardous waste from cradle to grave.

—Kristin M. Fitzgerald and Cynthia Hess

Related Topics

Clean Water Act
Environmental Toxicology
Resource Conservation and Recovery Act

Helium

- CAS: 7440-59-7
- SYNONYMS: Helium, compressed; helium, refrigerated liquid (cryogenic liquid)
- CHEMICAL CLASS: Nonflammable gas; simple asphyxiant
- MOLECULAR FORMULA: He

Uses

Liquid helium is used to produce low temperatures. The inert, nonflammable gas is used in balloons and in scientific studies (e.g., meteorological). It is also used in inert gas shielding for arc welding, in filling light bulbs, as a carrier gas in chromatography, and as a substitute for nitrogen in air supplies for deep diving.

Exposure Pathways

Exposure is possible through inhalation of the gas or dermal contact with liquid helium.

Toxicokinetics

Helium is an inert gas that acts in the lungs as an asphyxiant by keeping oxygen from reaching the blood.

Mechanism of Toxicity

Helium may displace oxygen, leading to oxygen deficiency.

Human Toxicity

Helium is nontoxic at normal temperature and pressure. The primary concern is its ability to displace oxygen in the air. Oxygen content must remain above 19% by volume in order to prevent symptoms of oxygen deficiency. Skin contact with liquid helium can cause frostbite.

Clinical Management

Rescue workers must wear a self-contained breathing apparatus before entering areas of oxygen deficiency. If a victim is unconscious or does not respond, the victim should be moved to fresh air. If breathing has stopped, trained personnel should begin artificial respiration or, if the heart has stopped, cardiopulmonary resuscitation. Oxygen may be administered by a person trained in its use.

Animal Toxicity

Studies in animals indicate that helium acts as a simple asphyxiant.

—Mary Lee Hultin

Related Topic

Respiratory Tract (Asphyxiant)

Hemlock, Poison

- SYNONYMS: *Conium maculatum*, Umbelliferae family; spotted hemlock; deadly hemlock; poison parsley; poison stinkweed

Exposure Pathways

Ingestion of plant parts is the route of exposure.

Mechanism of Toxicity

Coniine (piperidine alkaloid), *N*-methyl coniine, conhydrine, λ-coniceine, and pseudconhydrine are the toxins identified. Coniine has a number of pharmacological activities resembling nicotine (see Coniine). It is capable of producing stimulation followed by depression of autonomic ganglia. An intracellular mechanism appears to be responsible for a myoneuro-blocking effect.

Human Toxicity

Poison hemlock toxicity has effects similar to those of nicotine (see Nicotine). The alkaloid content varies significantly between species, plant parts, and geographic location. The alkaloid concentration increases in all parts as the plant matures but remains the highest in the roots. Initial central nervous system (CNS) stimulation, nausea, vomiting, and sore throat are followed by cardiorespiratory depression and ascending paralysis.

Clinical Management

Standard decontamination should be employed including lavage and administration of activated charcoal and a cathartic. Symptomatic and supportive care should follow.

Animal Toxicity

All animal species (except certain small birds) appear to be affected similarly with muscle tremors, salivation, dyspnea, vomiting, polyuria, CNS depression, and death.

—Rita Mrvos

Related Topics

Toxicology, History of

Hemlock, Water

- Synonyms: *Cicuta maculata*, Apiaceae (carrot) family, Cicuta species; Cowbane; snakeweed; wild carrot; poison parsnip; spotted hemlock; masquash root; beaver poison; false parsley; fever root; wild parsnip

Exposure Pathways

Exposure occurs via ingestion of any plant part (especially the root).

Mechanism of Toxicity

The major toxicity results from the central nervous system (CNS) stimulant properties of cicutoxin. Cicutoxin is concentrated in the roots but also may be found in aboveground parts. A mouthful of the root may be sufficient to kill an adult. Death results from status epilepticus, possibly caused by excessive stimulation of cholinergic receptors in the basal ganglia or brain stem.

Human Toxicity

All parts of the plant are considered toxic with the root being the most toxic portion. In a typical case of water hemlock poisoning, severe nausea, vomiting, and abdominal pain begin within 15–90 min postingestion. These symptoms are rapidly followed by seizures and profound CNS depression. Excess salivation, diaphoresis, flushing, and dizziness are also commonly seen. The major toxicity is related to CNS stimulation. Death usually results from status epilepticus and respiratory failure.

Clinical Management

A patient exposed to water hemlock may convulse suddenly and without warning; therefore, it is important to establish intravenous access immediately. Decontamination with gastric lavage is preferred. Syrup of ipecac should never be used to induce emesis. Activated charcoal and a cathartic should be administered. Seizures respond to diazepam followed by phenytoin. Hemodialysis or hemoperfusion may be attempted in severe cases although it is not clear if these procedures will be beneficial. Further care should be symptomatic and supportive.

Survivors may experience long-term effects including changes in sensorium with impaired intellectual function and acute anxiety reactions.

Animal Toxicity

All species of animals are at potential risk for poisoning with symptoms similar to those found in humans.

—Rita Mrvos

Heparin

- Synonyms: Heparin sodium (CAS: 9041-08-1); heparin calcium (CAS: 37270-89-6)
- Pharmaceutical Class: Anticoagulant
- Chemical Structure:

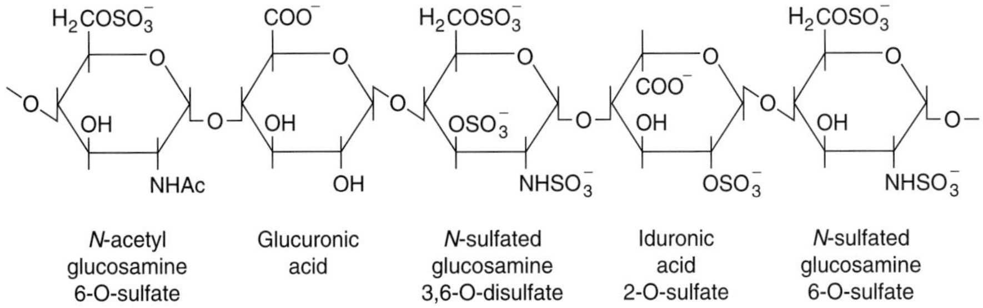

N-acetyl glucosamine 6-O-sulfate — Glucuronic acid — *N*-sulfated glucosamine 3,6-O-disulfate — Iduronic acid 2-O-sulfate — *N*-sulfated glucosamine 6-O-sulfate

Uses

Heparin is a heterogenous mixture of anionic sulfated glycosaminoglycans of 5000–30,000 Da molecular weight commercially derived from bovine lung or porcine intestinal mucosa. It is used as an anticoagulant for the prevention and treatment of thromboembolic disease. It is also used during extracorporeal circulation and hemodialysis and to maintain patency of indwelling vascular catheters.

Exposure Pathways

Heparin is not absorbed orally. It is administered parenterally. It is available as heparin calcium (porcine intestinal mucosa) or heparin sodium (bovine lung or porcine intestine).

Toxicokinetics

Subcutaneous administration has a delayed onset of anticoagulant effect of 20–60 min. Intravenous administration has an immediate onset. Heparin binds to a number of plasma proteins. The volume of distribution is 40–60 ml/kg in adults. The pharmacokinetics of heparin is complex and incompletely understood. Clearance consists of a more rapid but saturable mechanism involving the reticuloendothelial system and a slower phase that includes renal excretion. Heparin is partially depolymerized and desulfated by the reticuloendothelial system. Larger molecular weight heparin moieties are cleared more rapidly than smaller. The half-life of heparin is dose dependent and both the half-life and the anticoagulant effect increase disproportionately with increasing dose. At a dose of 400 U/kg the half-life is 150 min and at 800 U/kg it is 6 hr. Heparin metabolites and a small amount of unchanged heparin are excreted into the urine.

Mechanism of Toxicity

Heparin serves as a catalyst for antithrombin III (AT III), a plasma protein that inactivates activated serine proteases of the coagulation cascade, most importantly activated factors II (thrombin) and X. Only the larger heparin species (standard heparin) are capable of inactivation of factor II. (Heparin also catalyzes the inactivation of factor II by heparin cofactor II, a more minor pathway.) These effects result in systemic anticoagulation. Heparin possesses platelet aggregating properties. Heparin also may induce the production of platelet aggregating antibodies. Heparin interferes with aldosterone synthesis and by an unknown mechanism has led to osteoporosis during longer term use.

Human Toxicity: Acute

Bleeding is the major complication of heparin therapy. The risk of bleeding is related to the dose administered. Bleeding can occur virtually anywhere and may be minor or catastrophic. Adrenal hemorrhage with subsequent adrenal insufficiency has been reported.

Two forms of heparin associated thrombocytopenia (HAT) have been observed. Transient, mild, and benign thrombocytopenia seen soon after initiation of heparin therapy is felt to be due to the platelet aggregating properties of heparin. A second, more severe form of HAT, typically seen later, is believed to be due to heparin-dependent platelet aggregating antibodies. The risk of the more severe form of HAT has been estimated to be less than 3% to up to 10%. The onset is generally 5–8 days post initiation of heparin therapy but may occur sooner with reexposure. HAT may occur with any dose of heparin but the frequency is greater with higher therapeutic dosing schedules. HAT is complicated by thrombosis in 10–20% of cases. These thrombi form predominately in the arterial circulation and are associated with significant morbidity and mortality. Thrombotic complications include arterial thrombosis, myocardial infarction, stroke, gangrene, and death. Hyperkalemia may be seen with heparin therapy due to aldosterone synthesis inhibition.

Human Toxicity: Chronic

Bone pain, osteopenia, rib fractures, and vertebral fractures have been reported with long-term use. Heparin does not cross the placenta and some authorities consider its use safe in pregnancy. Comorbid conditions may account for the increased rates of prematurity and fetal mortality reported in some studies.

Clinical Management

The anticoagulant effect of heparin is best monitored by the activated partial thromboplastin time. If an excessive dose of heparin has been administered, careful monitoring for signs of bleeding or hemodynamic compromise are indicated. If there is no clinical evidence of bleeding, or bleeding is minor, discontinuation of heparin may be all that is necessary. With massive overdoses or with clinical evidence of serious hemorrhage, the use of protamine sulfate should be considered. Protamine sulfate is a specific antidote for heparin. When rapid neutralization of heparin is necessary, protamine is administered at a dose of approximately 1 mg per 100 units heparin. Considerable variation exists and treatment should be individualized with careful monitoring. Complications of protamine include hypotension, anaphylaxis, and pulmonary vasoconstriction. If a declining platelet count is observed, platelets should be monitored more frequently. If thrombocytopenia develops, heparin therapy should be discontinued as soon as an alternate form of therapy is instituted (e.g., vena caval ligation and warfarin). If the platelet count is less than 20,000/μl or a thrombotic complication occurs, heparin should be discontinued immediately. Thrombolytic therapy or embolectomy may be necessary with thrombosis. Antiplatelet agents such as aspirin may also be beneficial in this situation.

—Michael J. Hodgman

Related Topics

Blood
Cardiovascular System

Heptachlor

- CAS: 76-44-8
- SYNONYMS: 1,4,5,6,7,8,8-Heptachloro-3a,4,7,7a-tetrahydro-4,7-methanoindane; Drinox; Heptagran; Heptamul
- CHEMICAL CLASS: Synthetic organochlorine insecticide
- CHEMICAL STRUCTURE:

H H Cl Cl H Cl-C-Cl Cl H Cl H Cl

Uses

Heptachlor is used as an insecticide.

Exposure Pathways

Exposure to heptachlor may occur via ingestion, inhalation, or dermal contact.

Toxicokinetics

The absorption of heptachlor through the skin is very efficient. Heptachlor is also absorbed very effectively via the respiratory and gastrointestinal tracts. As with other organochlorine insecticides, fiber and fat content in the diet affects the absorption rates; a lack of these generally favors increased absorption through the gastrointestinal tract.

Heptachlor is metabolized primarily by liver microsomal enzymes to the epoxide form (which is more toxic than the parent compound) and to less toxic and more easily excreted products including 1-chloro-3-hydroxychlordene, 1-hydroxychlordene, and 1-hydroxy-2,3-epoxychlordene.

Heptachlor tends to sequester in adipose tissue and organs with high fat content. The epoxide is the primary storage form. Metabolites of heptachlor are primarily excreted in the urine.

Mechanism of Toxicity

The activity of γ-aminobutyric acid, that of inducing uptake of Cl^- ions by neurons, is blocked. This results in only a partial repolarization of activated neurons leading to an uncontrolled excited condition. Additionally, both Ca^{2+}, Mg^{2+}-adenosine triphosphatase (ATPase) and Na^+,K^+-ATPase functions are inhibited by heptachlor. This leads to increased intracellular-free calcium concentration in neurons and the release of neurotransmitters. These neurotransmitters potentiate depolarization of adjacent neurons in a chain-reaction fashion, propagating stimuli through the central nervous system (CNS).

Human Toxicity

The toxic effects of heptachlor are the same as those of chlordane. Generally, nausea, vomiting, and dizziness precede CNS symptomatology. Convulsions usually follow these symptoms, although convulsions have been reported in the absence of other warning symptoms. Convulsions usually manifest themselves within 0.5–3 hr after ingestion or dermal exposure and are often accompanied by confusion, incoordination, excitability, or coma (in some cases). Respiratory arrest may result from acute exposure to high doses (see Chlordane).

Clinical Management

Treatment is symptomatic. Anticonvulsive treatment with diazepam or phenobarbital is usually effective for control of convulsions. Cholestyramine treatment has increased elimination of heptachlor.

Animal Toxicity

The toxic effects of heptachlor in animals are the same as those of chlordane. Chlordane toxicity in animals is similar to that of other organochlorine insecticides except tremor is absent. CNS involvement produces hyperexcitability and convulsions. Immunosuppression has been reported in mice prenatally exposed to chlordane. The incidence of hepatomas is increased in mice, but not in rats, fed chlordane.

—Benny L. Blaylock

Related Topics

Neurotoxicology: Central and Peripheral
Organochlorine Insecticides
Pesticides

Heptane

- CAS: 142-82-5
- Synonyms: *n*-Heptane; dipropyl methane; Gettysolve-C; heptyl hydride; heptan (Polish); eptani (Italian); heptanen (Dutch); UN1206, DOT
- Chemical Class: Aliphatic hydrocarbon (C7)
- Molecular Formula: C_7H_{16}

Uses

n-Heptane is a colorless, flammable liquid that is lighter than, but insoluble in, water. It has a definite petroleum odor that is easily detected at air concentrations of 200 ppm or greater. It is used as the knock-testing "standard" for octane rating measurements. Triptane, or 2,2,3-trimethyl butane, is used in aviation fuel. All isomers are used in organic synthesis and are ingredients of gasoline, rubber solvent naphtha, and other petroleum mixtures that are utilized as fuels or solvents. Naturally occurring heptane is isolated from natural gas, crude oil, or pine extracts.

Exposure Pathways

Although heptane exists at room temperature as a liquid, the most adverse effects observed in people or animals exposed to this solvent are via inhalation. The most common exposure routes in industry (in order of decreasing importance) are inhalation, dermal contact, and ingestion.

Toxicokinetics

Heptane is converted to hydroxy derivatives (e.g., alcohol) by cytochrome P450 mixed function oxidase system before being converted to keto forms. It may then be conjugated to the glucuronide and subsequently excreted.

Mechanism of Toxicity

Most of the current toxicological information available in the literature suggests that heptane is, physiologically speaking, more neurotoxic than other aliphatic hydrocarbons such as pentane, hexane, and octane. Debilitating peripheral neuropathy, such as that seen upon chronic exposure to *n*-hexane, has not been observed in animals or humans. Some cases of polyneuritis, observed in the absence of hexane exposure, might be attributed to the presence of heptane in a solvent mixture. In any event, no one to date has discerned a true toxic mechanism for *n*-heptane. To be safe, NIOSH recommends a workplace environmental limit (TWA) of 85 ppm for heptane, with a 15-min ceiling of 440 ppm. On a weight/volume scale, this is the same limit imposed for pentane, hexane, and octane and is most likely designated to prevent polyneuropathy found following hexane exposure.

Human Toxicity

Heptane is considerably toxic to the human nervous system (neurotoxic). Acute exposure symptoms include distorted perception and mild hallucinations. Humans exposed to 0.1% (1000 ppm) heptane exhibited dizziness in 6 min; higher concentrations caused marked vertigo and incoordination. Humans accidentally exposed to high concentrations showed similar symptoms, as well as mucous membrane irritation, nausea, and lassitude. All these symptoms will pass quickly upon recovery in fresh air, but the recovery period is still longer than that for pentane or hexane.

Finally, several authors have noted signs of polyneuropathy or polyneuritis in groups of people exposed to mixtures of solvents that contain significant quantities of heptane. Heptane is also very flammable and is therefore an explosion and/or fire hazard (lower and upper explosive limits are 1.05 and 6.7% by volume, respectively).

Clinical Management

Persons who are exposed to high concentrations should vacate or be removed from the source of the vapor and seek fresh air. Care should be taken to keep areas of high concentration free from ignition sources, such as sparks from static electricity and use of explosion-proof apparatus.

Animal Toxicity

Rats exposed to heptane showed neurologic signs that are very similar to those seen following exposure to technical-grade hexane. Righting reflexes in mice are affected at a concentration of 40 mg/liter (approximately 0.96%), while 70 mg/liter (approximately 1.7%) was lethal. Narcosis has also been shown in mice exposed to air concentrations of 1–1.5% for 3–50 min. Other permutations of concentration and exposure period caused convulsions, tetany, respiratory arrest, and death.

—Stephen Clough

Related Topic

Neurotoxicity: Central and Peripheral

Heptanone

- CAS: 106-35-4
- Preferred Name: 3-Heptanone
- Synonyms: Butyl ethyl ketone; ethyl butyl ketone; heptan-3-one
- Chemical Class: Ketone
- Molecular Formula: $C_7H_{14}O$

Uses

Heptanone is used as a synthetic flavoring agent and as a solvent for lacquers, finishes, and resins.

Exposure Pathways

Exposure may occur through oral, dermal, or inhalation routes, although ingestion of 3-heptanone is rare.

Toxicokinetics

Ketones are absorbed into the bloodstream after ingestion, inhalation, or dermal exposure. 3-Heptanone is metabolized to the neurotoxins 6-hydroxy-3-heptanone and 2,5-heptanedione. Conjugation with glucuronic acid, sulfuric acid, or glutathione also occurs prior to excretion in the urine, with glucuronic acid conjugation being the prominent pathway. 3-Heptanone has been identified in the urine of humans who have not been exposed.

Mechanism of Toxicity

3-Heptanone is metabolized to neurotoxic diketones. Central nervous system (CNS) depression is due to anatomic and morphological nerve degeneration characterized by large multifocal axonal swellings ("giant" axonal neuropathy) in the CNS and the peripheral nervous system. Myelin damage is a secondary effect. The peripheral nervous system is more severely affected than the CNS. Inhalation exposures have failed to produce sufficient neurotoxic metabolites to result in neuropathy.

Human Toxicity

3-Heptanone may cause mild skin irritation after a single exposure. Repeated skin contact may result in dermatitis. Systemic effects from exposure include CNS depression, headache, nausea, vertigo, incoordination, narcosis, coma, and cardiorespiratory failure. Ketones may potentiate the hepatotoxicity of halogenated hydrocarbons and inhibit aromatic hydrocarbon metabolism.

Clinical Management

Victims should be removed immediately to fresh air after inhalation. Copious dilution is appropriate after ingestion, dermal exposures, or eye exposures. Patients should be treated symptomatically. Plasma ketone levels are generally not clinically useful.

Animal Toxicity

Mild irritation results from dermal exposure of rabbit skin and eyes. The LD_{50} for dermal exposure in the rabbit was reported to be >20 ml/kg for 24 hr. Inhalation exposures in rats have resulted in ataxia, prostration, CNS depression, and death at high concentrations. The inhalation LC_{50} is 2000 ppm for 4 hr in rats. Inhalation of 500 ppm for 10 days resulted in piloerection, vasodilation, and lacrimation but did not cause pathological lesions in the lungs, liver, or kidneys in rats. Longer term inhalation studies at 700 ppm did not result in clinical signs of neurotoxicity, although a decrease in total white blood cells was reported. The toxicity of 3-heptanone is low by the oral route. The oral LD_{50} has been reported to be 2760 mg/kg in rats. Chronic feeding studies have resulted in neurotoxicity and neuropathological lesions only at high doses.

—*Janice M. McKee*

Related Topic

Neurotoxicology: Central and Peripheral

Heroin

- CAS: 561-27-3 (diamorphine)
- Synonyms: Acetomorphine; diacetylmorphine hydrochloride; diamorphine hydrochloride; heroin hydrochloride
- Pharmaceutical Class: Opioid analgesic
- Chemical Structure:

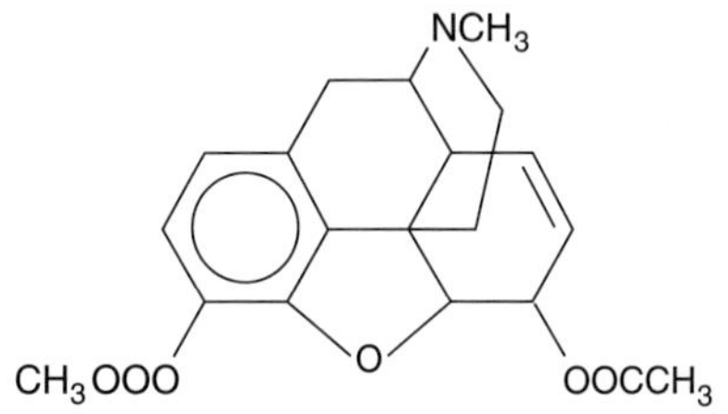

Uses

Heroin has been used as an analgesic for moderate to severe pain. In the United States, it is a schedule I substance and, therefore, does not have a medicinal use. It is a drug of abuse.

Exposure Pathways

Administration can be parenteral, sublinqual, oral, rectal, or by nasal insufflation. As a common drug of abuse, heroin is usually present in the street product at concentrations of 2–7%; purer forms of up to 90% are occasionally available.

Toxicokinetics

Heroin is rapidly absorbed from all sites of administration. It has a high lipid membrane solubility, thus leading to rapid absorption from the blood and the blood–brain barrier. Heroin undergoes complete presystemic metabolism to morphine following oral administration. Peak morphine serum levels have occurred

30 min after ingestion. With parenteral administration, peak levels have occurred in 10–15 min (heroin and 6-acetylmorphine, 10 min; morphine, 15 min).

Heroin in rapidly hydrolyzed in whole blood to 6-monoacetylmorphine (6-MAM). The liver then converts most of the 6-MAM to morphine. These two metabolites are the primary contributors to pain relief. It is widely distributed in tissues. Protein binding is 40%. The volume of distribution approximates 25 liters/kg. The half-life of heroin in blood is less than 20 min, approximately 3 min after parenteral administration. The elimination half-life is 60–90 min. Urine yields primarily morphine in the free or conjugated form.

Mechanism of Toxicity

Heroin's primary toxic principle is its profound ability to depress the central nervous system (CNS). Opioid analgesics bind with stereospecific receptors at many sites within the CNS. Heroin, similar to other opioids, exerts its pharmacologic effect by acting at μ, κ, and δ receptors in the brain. Although the precise sites and mechanisms of action have not been fully determined, alterations in the release of various neurotransmitters from afferent nerves sensitive to painful stimuli may be partially responsible for the analgesic effect. Activities associated with the stimulation of opiate receptors are analgesia, euphoria, respiratory depression, miosis, and reduced gastrointestinal motility.

Human Toxicity: Acute

Toxicity occurs when heroin's pharmacologic effects are exaggerated (as in an overdose). Any amount of heroin can be potentially toxic, especially when the purity of this illicit drug is not known. Heroin depresses the CNS, thereby producing coma and cessation of respirations. Pulmonary edema is one of the most frequent complications of heroin overdose. Respiratory arrest may occur. Miosis is often present but may be absent in the presence of hypoxia or mixed drug overdoses. With depression of the CNS, there is also a decrease in sympathetic tone and an increase in parasympathetic tone. This yields bradycardia and hypotension. Hypothermia may also occur as a result of peripheral vasodilation. Urine can be screened for heroin metabolic products. Blood heroin levels are not clinically useful but can be detected for up to 36 hr. 6-MAM has a short half-life in serum, but it can be detected by gas chromatography and by mass spectrometry in the urine.

Human Toxicity: Chronic

Chronic users of heroin may develop tolerance to some of its effects, thereby necessitating larger doses to develop the characteristic "high." Cessation of use can result in withdrawal. Classic symptoms are restlessness, insomnia, hypertension, tachypnea, tachycardia, vomiting, and diarrhea.

Clinical Management

Basic life-support measures should be instituted as necessary. Intensive support therapy may be required to correct respiratory failure and shock. Respirations must be supported and monitored until all symptoms disappear. Pulmonary edema should be managed with appropriate ventilatory support. If taken orally, gastrointestinal decontamination should be based on the patient's level of consciousness or decrease in gag reflex. Activated charcoal may be used to adsorb the heroin. A cathartic may be given to aid elimination of the activated charcoal–heroin complex. Heroin is often smuggled via "body packing," whereby an individual swallows receptacles (often condoms) containing heroin to evade customs officials. Whole bowel irrigation may be a useful way to enhance their elimination from the gastrointestinal tract.

The specific antagonist naloxone hydrochloide is used to counteract respiratory depression and coma. A dose of 0.4–2.0 mg is given intravenously and can be repeated at intervals of 2 or 3 min if necessary. The therapeutic effect of naloxone may be of shorter duration than that of the opiate activity; therefore, a naloxone continuous infusion may be of benefit. Arterial blood gases, vital signs, and level of consciousness should be monitored continuously until cessation of symptoms.

Animal Toxicity

Dogs respond similarly to humans exposed to heroin. Symptoms may include drowsiness, ataxia, vomiting, respiratory depression, miosis, coma, and hypotension. Opiates and their derivatives have an excitatory effect on the CNS of cats and horses. Naloxone may be used at 0.02 mg/kg if needed.

—*Lisa Scheuring-Mroz*

Related Topics

Neurotoxicology: Central and Peripheral
Poisoning Emergencies in Humans

Hexachlorobutadiene

- CAS: 87-68-3
- SYNONYMS: Hexachloro-1,3-butadiene; hexachlorobuta-1,3-diene (HCBD); perchlorobutadiene
- CHEMICAL CLASS: Chlorinated hydrocarbon
- CHEMICAL STRUCTURE:

$$CCl_2{=}CCl{-}CCl{=}CCl_2$$

Uses

Hexachlorobutadiene is used as a pesticide and is an industrial by-product.

Exposure Pathways

Hexachlorobutadiene may be toxic by inhalation, ingestion, and dermal exposure.

Toxicokinetics

In rabbits, hexachlorobutadiene is absorbed through the skin. Two major pathways of metabolism have been suggested which call for mediation either by cytochrome P450 or by glutathione conjugation. In rats, hexachlorobutadiene was found in lungs, blood, liver, brain, kidneys (proximal section of the nephron), spleen, and mesentery after a single injection (unspecified). Following oral administration of a nephrotoxic dose (200 mg/kg) of hexachloro-1,3-butadiene to male rats, the principal route of excretion was biliary, with 17–20% of the dose being eliminated on each of the first 2 days. Fecal excretion was <5% of the dose per day, suggesting enterohepatic recirculation of biliary metabolites. Urinary excretion was small, not exceeding 3.5% of the dose during any 24-hr period.

Mechanism of Toxicity

Increased toxicity is due to glutathione conjugation, renal processing of the glutathione-*S*-conjugate, and formation of reactive intermediates by β-lyase.

Human Toxicity

Hexachlorobutadiene is on the NIOSH list of suspected carcinogens because it has the potential to cause kidney and lung cancer. The ACGIH TLV is 0.02 ppm. A group of 205 vineyard workers who were exposed seasonally to hexachlorobutadiene (0.8–30 mg/m^3 in air over the fumigated zones) showed multiple toxic effects contributing to the development of hypotension, cardiac disease, chronic bronchitis, disturbances of nervous function, and chronic hepatitis.

The following combination of tests may be useful for detecting renal dysfunction in occupationally exposed workers: examination of urine with reagent strips for the presence of glucosuria and proteinuria and quantitative determination of at least two proteins, one of the high molecular weight for glomerular function and one of the low molecular weight for tubular function. Some value has also come from the determination of the lysosomal enzyme *N*-acetyl-β-D-glucosaminidase in urine.

Clinical Management

No specific treatment is available. Patients acutely and chronically exposed should be monitored for renal, hepatic, and pulmonary damage. At least some of the renal toxicity appears to be reversible, so supportive care is indicated. Emesis may be indicated and is most effective if initiated within 30 min of ingestion. Charcoal slurry, aqueous or mixed with saline cathartic or sorbitol, should be administered. A saline cathartic should be administered, unless sorbitol–charcoal slurry is used.

In cases of inhalation exposure, the victim should be moved to fresh air and monitored for respiratory distress. If cough or difficulty in breathing develops, the victim should be evaluated for respiratory tract irritation, bronchitis, or pneumonitis. Supplemental oxygen (100% humidified) should be administered with assisted ventilation as required.

Exposed eyes should be irrigated with generous amounts of tepid water for at least 15 min. If irritation, pain, swelling, lacrimation, or photophobia persist, the patient should see a doctor. Exposed areas should be washed extremely thoroughly with soap and water. A physician may need to examine the area if irritation or pain persists.

Animal Toxicity

The oral LD_{50} (single dose) is 90 mg/kg in guinea pigs, 87–116 mg/kg in mice, and 200–350 mg/kg in rats. The dermal LD_{50} at 7 hr was 126 mg/kg in rabbits.

Hexachlorobutadiene causes lung, liver, and renal injury (renal proximal tubular dysfunction) in animals. Eye and nose irritation have been reported in animals exposed to 250 ppm for 4 hr and 110 ppm for 6 hr.

In a 30-day study in rats, 30, 65, and 100 mg/kg/day resulted in renal toxicity, increased kidney : body weight ratio and renal tubular degeneration, necrosis, and regeneration; 100 mg/kg/day resulted in decreased food consumption and body weight and minimal hepatocellular swelling at 100 mg/kg; and 10, 30, 65, and 100 mg/kg/day resulted in hemoconcentration. A statistically significant increase of kidney tumors was observed in male and female rats fed diets containing hexachlorobutadiene (99% pure) at 20 mg/kg body weight/day for 22 months.

At dosages high enough to cause maternal toxicity (decreased weight gain) and slight fetal toxicity (decreased fetal weight) hexachlorobutadiene was not teratogenic.

Unscheduled DNA synthesis has occurred in experimental animals. Mutations have been produced in *Salmonella typhimurium* and sister chromatid exchange has occurred in the hamster ovary cell.

—*Robin Guy*

Related Topics

Glutathione
Pesticides
Sister Chromatid Exchange

*Hexachlorocyclopentadiene**

- CAS: 77-47-4
- SYNONYMS: 1,2,3,4,5,5-Hexachloro-1,3-cyclopentadiene; hexachloropentadiene; perchlorocyclopentadiene; HCCP
- CHEMICAL CLASS: Chlorinated cyclic hydrocarbon

Uses

Hexachlorocyclopentadiene is used as a chemical intermediate for many insecticides, polymer resins, flame retardants, resins, dyes, and pharmaceuticals. It is also used to make shock-proof plastics, acids, esters, ketones, and fluorocarbons. Hexachlorocyclopentadiene is a yellow-green dense oily liquid, and its vapor has a density approximately nine times that of air. Its odor is detectable at approximately 1.5 mg/m^3 of air.

Exposure Pathways

Although occupational exposure appears to be the main source of human contact, certain segments of the population may be exposed through ingestion of contaminated drinking water or contaminated fish. People living in the vicinity of hazardous waste disposal sites containing this compound may be exposed by inhalation of contaminated air. Workers involved in the manufacture or handling of this compound or treatment of wastes containing this compound could potentially be exposed by inhalation or dermal exposure.

Toxicokinetics

Hexachlorocyclopentadiene can be absorbed orally, dermally, and by inhalation. Following oral exposure in rats dosed in diet, 70% of the labeled dose appeared in feces while 15% appeared in urine, an indication that most of the compound was not absorbed. Of that absorbed, accumulation in the kidneys, liver, ovaries, and fat was reported. Inhalation of hexachlorocyclopentadiene by rats was reported to result in

* Information Source: Hazardous Substance Data Bank, National Library of Medicine, Bethesda, MD, July 1996

84% retention with some accumulation in trachea and lungs.

Degradation apparently occurs in the gut since little of the analyzed fecal material was of an apolar nature.

Rats given 6 mg/kg of hexachlorocyclopentadiene orally excreted 33% in urine and 10% in feces in 7 days. Most excretion occurred during the first 24-hr period following dosing. The kidneys retained 0.5% of the compound, while the liver retained ≥0.5%.

Mechanism of Toxicity

Hexachlorocyclopentadiene's mechanism of toxicity is not well described; however, because of its characteristics as a chlorinated hydrocarbon, it would be expected to stimulate liver enzyme activity.

Human Toxicity

Eye and throat irritation has been reported in humans. Independent of the exposure route, the lung appears to be a major target organ resulting in cough, dyspnea, and chest pains. Headache and nausea are common after exposure. Exposed workers have developed reversible subclinical elevations of liver function tests and reversible proteinuria. Skin irritation and blistering may occur from direct contact with liquid hexachlorocyclopentadiene, and skin contact with vapor has been reported to result in skin irritation. Reported human cases have generally been mild.

The acceptable daily intake for hexachlorocyclopentadiene is 0.00462 mg/day. The OSHA 8-hr TWA is 0.01 ppm. Hexachlorocyclopentadiene is not classifiable in terms of carcinogenicity in either humans or animals.

Animal Toxicity

Approximate lethal doses for rats and rabbits by single oral administration were between 420 and 620 mg/kg. The animals showed diarrhea, lethargy, and decreased respiration. Rabbits were reported to show diffuse degenerative changes in the brain, heart, liver, and adrenal glands; necrosis of the epithelium of renal tubules; and severe hyperemia and edema of the lungs by skin absorption.

Acute range-finding (14-day) and subchronic (90-day) inhalation studies were conducted with Sprague–Dawley rats and subchronic (90-day) inhalation studies were conducted with monkeys. The studies with rats showed steep dose–response curves with male rats being more sensitive than females. The threshold for toxic effects was <0.5 ppm hexachlorocyclopentadiene. Observation of lesions in the olfactory and bronchiolar epithelium as well as inflammatory exudate in the lumen of the respiratory tract was consistent with observed impaired respiratory function, confirming the lungs as the main target organ. Lacrimation, salivation, tremors, and degenerative changes in the brain, heart, liver, adrenal glands, and kidneys have been observed in animal inhalation studies. Hexachlorocyclopentadiene is reported to be noncarcinogenic based on inhalation studies in rats and mice.

F344 rats and B6C3F1 mice were exposed to hexachlorocyclopentadiene by gavage at 0–150 and 0–300 mg/kg, respectively, and all high-dose mice died on study. Liver : brain weight ratios were significantly increased in the exposed groups of female rats. Kidney:brain weight ratios in females significantly increased after 75 and 150 mg/kg exposure. In female mice, the kidney : brain weight ratios significantly increased at all doses, and the lung : brain weight increased after exposure at 300 mg/kg dose.

Pregnant mice and rabbits were administered up to 75 mg/kg/day of hexachlorocyclopentadiene by gavage during active oogenesis. Teratogenic effects have not been observed; however, nephrosis and acute tubular necrosis were seen in the dams.

Hexachlorocyclopentadiene has shown negative findings in the *Salmonella typhimurium* assay for mutagenesis with and without activation and in *Escherichia coli.*

—R. A. Parent, T. R. Kline, and D. E. Sharp

Hexachlorophene

- CAS: 70-30-4
- SYNONYMS: 2,2′-Methylenebis(3,4,6-trichlorophenol); 2,2′-dihydroxy-3,3′,5,5′,6,6′-

hexachlorodiphenylmethane; bis(3,5,6-trichloro-2-hydroxyphenyl)methane; hexachlorophane

- CHEMICAL STRUCTURE:

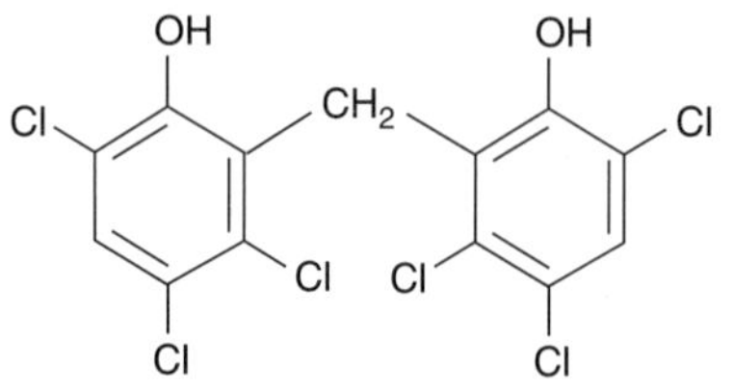

Uses

Hexachlorophene is used as an agricultural chemical, detergent, therapeutic agent, and wood preservative. It is used as a topical antiinfective, fungicide, germicide, bactericide, and disinfectant.

Exposure Pathways

Hexachlorophene exposure is usually dermal as a bactericide. It is sometimes used as a topical treatment for acne vulgaris to suppress associated staphylococci.

Toxicokinetics

Hexachlorophene is well absorbed orally and dermally and through mucosal surfaces. In rats, up to 55% of dermally applied hexachlorophene is absorbed in 24 hr. Dermal absorption is enhanced by dimethylsulfoxide and dermatitis or skin abrasions. Placental transfer has been demonstrated in rats. Hexachlorophene is converted to hexachlorophene-β-D-glucuronide in the rat and rabbit. Some hexachlorophene has been found in the blood and adipose tissue. Hexachlorophene was administered intraperitoneally to rats and rabbits; excretion was slow; most (48–83%) was excreted unchanged in the feces. Hepatic function is important determinant in removal of hexachlorophene. In a rat study, within 3 hr after administration, 50% was excreted in the bile. Rats given intraperitoneal doses excreted about 5% of the dose in the urine and none as CO_2; more than 70% of the material was excreted in feces.

Mechanism of Toxicity

Following skin absorption, hexachlorophene enters the nervous system and results in intramyelinic edema, splitting the intraperiod line of myelin in both the central nervous system (CNS) and the peripheral nervous system. Experimental studies with erythrocyte membranes show that hexachlorophene binds tightly to cell membranes, resulting in osmotic swelling of erythrocyte membranes by altering their permeability to sodium and potassium. Hexachlorophene uncouples oxidative phosphorylation.

Human Toxicity

The estimated lethal dose in humans is 1–10 g. Dermal application, especially in neonates or on damaged skin, of highly concentrated (≥3%) preparations on several occasions or repeated applications of less concentrated preparations may result in significant toxicity or death. An erythematous desquamative rash may occur following repeated dermal application, especially in neonates or in high concentrations (≥3%). Cutaneous hypersensitivity may occur.

Acute ingestion of large amounts (≥30–60 m for an adult) or repeated ingestion of small amounts may also cause significant toxicity or death. Dermal, gastrointestinal, and neurologic effects are the most common toxic manifestations. Cardiorespiratory arrest may occur most notably following acute ingestion of large amounts. Lethargy frequently occurs as an early manifestation of toxicity.

Blindness has occurred after repeated ingestion.

Clinical Management

Plasma hexachlorophene levels have not been demonstrated to correlate well with clinical effects. Hexachlorophene may cause seizures. The risk of seizures during emesis may preclude the use of ipecac syrup. Charcoal slurry, aqueous or mixed with saline cathartic or sorbitol, should be administered. The usual charcoal dose is 30–100 g in adults and 15–30 grams in children (1 or 2 g/kg in infants). If seizures cannot be controlled with diazepam or they recur, phenytoin or phenobarbital should be administered. The patient should be checked for cerebral edema. Exposed eyes should be irrigated with copious amounts of tepid water for at least 15 min. Vigorous washing with soap and water should be followed by washing with 70% isopropanol or olive oil or castor oil, followed by a second vigorous soap and water cleansing, may increase removal of hexachlorophene.

Animal Toxicity

Rats fed 500 ppm (25 mg/kg/day) showed weakness in their hindquarters, which progressed to paralysis.

Microscopic examination of the brain and spinal cord revealed a particular edema of white matter resembling spongy degeneration of white matter in infants. When the animals were removed from the hexachlorophene diet, they recovered gradually over a period of weeks; similar signs were noted in the monkey.

Oral administration of hexachlorophene to rats causes degeneration of spermatogenic cells. In sheep, 2500 mg/kg followed 2 days later by a dose of 50 mg/kg also caused extensive damage to spermatogonia; after 21 days there was neither sperm in epididymis nor spermatogenesis.

Oral LD_{50}s in rats were 187 and 67 mg/kg; 56 mg/kg in the female rat; 120 mg/kg in the rat weanling; 9 mg/kg in the rat suckling (10 days old); 63–87 mg/kg in the female Wistar rat; and 58–87 mg/kg in the male Wistar rat.

—*Robin Guy*

Related Topic

Neurotoxicology: Central and Peripheral

Hexane

- CAS: 110-54-3
- Preferred Name: *n*-Hexane
- Synonyms: Dipropyl; Esani; Heksan; AI3-24253; hexanen; hexyl hydride; NCI-C60571; HSDB 91; Skellysolve B
- Chemical Class: Aliphatic hydrocarbon
- Chemical Structure:

$$CH_3CH_2CH_2CH_2CH_2CH_3$$

Uses

n-Hexane is used for determining the refractive index of minerals, for calibrations, as a paint diluent, and in thermometers. It is also used as a solvent in the extraction of soybean oil, cottonseed oil, flaxseed oil, safflower seed oil, and other oil seeds. It is used as a denaturant for alcohol, and as a cleaning agent in the textile, furniture, and leather industries. *n*-Hexane is a common laboratory reagent and a component of many products associated with the petroleum and gasoline industries.

Exposure Pathways

Humans can be exposed to *n*-hexane via inhalation, ingestion, or dermal contact.

Toxicokinetics

Acute exposure usually occurs by inhalation. *n*-Hexane may be absorbed orally or percutaneously. *n*-Hexane has a vapor density of 2.97 and it is heavier than air. *n*-Hexane is believed to be metabolized through cytochrome P450 system and phenobarbital pretreatment of liver microsomes induced 2- and 3-hydroxylation of *n*-hexane sixfold. 3,4-Benzpyrene suppresses 2-hydroxylation and stimulates 3-hydroxylation of *n*-hexane. For humans, 2, 3-hydroxy hexane is responsible for various toxicities. In environment, *n*-hexane does not absorb UV light in the environmentally significant range (>290 nm); therefore, it will not undergo hydorlyiss or direct photolysis.

Mechanism of Toxicity

n-Hexane is biotransformed to 2-hexanol and further to 2,5-hexanediol by cytochrome P450 mixed function oxidases by Ω^{-1}oxidation. 2,5-Hexanediol may be further oxidized to 2,5-hexanedione, the major metabolite of *n*-hexane in humans. Identification of 2,5-hexanedione as the major neurotoxic metabolite of *n*-hexane proceeded rapidly after its discovery as a urinary metabolite. 2,5-Hexanedione has been found to produce a polyneuropathy indistinguishable from *n*-hexane. 2,5-Hexanedione is many times more potent than *n*-hexane, a parent compound in causing neurotoxicity in experimental animals. It appears that the neurotoxicity of 2,5-hexanedione resides in its γ-diketone structure since 2,3-, 2,4-hexanedione and 2,6-heptanedione are not neurotoxic, while 2,5-heptanedione and 3,6-octanedione and other γ-diketones are neurotoxic.

Human Toxicity

An estimated 2.5 million workers are occupational exposed to *n*-hexane. This commonly used solvent was not regarded as industrial hazard until the discovery of its neurotoxic potential since its acute toxicity is quite low. Vapor concentrations of many hundreds of parts per million are tolerated for several minutes without causing discomfort among workers. In recognition of the neurotoxic property of *n*-hexane, the ACGIH has recommended a TLV of 50 ppm, expressed as an 8-hr TWA. There are a number of epidemiology studies reported for *n*-hexane.

Acute exposure to hexane causes central nervous system (CNS) depression. Chronic exposure to an average air concentration of 450–650 ppm for as little as 2 months may result in peripheral neuropathy, characterized by muscular weakness, loss of sensation, and impaired gait. Hexane has been reported to be the most highly toxic member of the alkanes. When *n*-hexane is ingested, it causes nausea, vertigo, bronchial irritation, general intestinal irritation, and CNS effects. It poses an acute aspiration hazard. It has been reported that about 50 g of *n*-hexane may be fatal to humans. An exposure of 880 ppm for 15 min can cause eye and upper respiratory tract irritation in humans. Blurred vision has been mentioned in association with *n*-hexane polyneuropathy. It was concluded that *n*-hexane vapor levels of less than 100 ppm for 8 hr per day were not likely to produce a clinical neuropathy, but mild subclinical changes in muscle strength and nerve conduction velocity may occur.

In humans, 2000 ppm of *n*-hexane for 10 min resulted in no effects. However, 5000 ppm caused dizziness, giddiness, slight nausea, headache, and eye and throat irritation. Three women had motor polyneuropathy following industrial exposure to an adhesive agent containing 80.4% *n*-hexane. In the nerves, there were polymorphous changes in the myelin sheaths and axons of large diameter fibers. Muscles showed denervation changes, with lymphocytic infilatrates and phagocytosis. Three cases of *n*-hexane neuropathy in the shoe industry were reported. In the most severe cases, symptoms consisted of dysarthria, disproportionate ataxia of gait, blurred vision, and sometimes after recovery of peripheral neuropathy, appearance of leg spasticity.

Out of 1662 workers exposed to organic solvents, which consisted mainly of *n*-hexane and a small amount of toluene, 53 were found to have sensory polyneuropathy, 32 had sensorimotor polyneuropathy, and 8 had sensorimotor polyneuropathy with amyotrophy. Cranial nerve involvements, such as visual disorders and facial numbness, were observed. About 50% showed denervation and reinnervation of the nerves. Among 93 cases of *n*-hexane polyneuropathy during a large outbreak in 1968, 44 were studied. Over a few years, most of the cases were completely recovered (except for a few with mild sensory impairment) after establishing 100 ppm as the maximal allowable concentration of *n*-hexane and providing well-equipped ventilation systems in individual houses. During rescreening in 1981, 21 cases with mild *n*-hexane polyneuropathy were observed, revealing mostly the same features as in the previous outbreak in 1968. It may be suggested from this data that, despite <50 ppm of *n*-hexane concentration in a room, sandal workers have suffered from neurotoxicity from this organic solvent.

In a cross-sectional study, nerve conduction velocities were determined in 59 workers employed in press proofing factories in Taipei. Workers were divided into exposure categories on the basis of air concentrations of *n*-hexane (>100, 50–99, and <50 ppm) and *n*-hexane concentrations in the cleaning solvent used (>50, 49–10, and $<10\%$). Fifteen members (25%) of the study group were found to have polyneuropathy. In one factory where all 6 employees developed polyneuropathy, the air concentration of *n*-hexane was determined to be 190 ppm. In other factories, workers exposed to *n*-hexane at levels of <100 ppm showed a significant decrease in motor nerve conduction velocities.

n-Hexane is currently under review for its carcinogenicity; however, it is not classified as a carcinogen at the present time. A reference concentration of 2E-1 mg/m^3 is considered based on an epidemiological inhalation study with an uncertainty factor of 300. Critical effects were reported to be neurotoxicity and electrophysiologial alterations.

Clinical Management

Oral Exposure

In general, gastric emptying is not indicated except in selected cases in which a history of a large ingestion is obtained. An activated charcoal slurry, aqueous or mixed with saline cathartic or sorbitol, can be administered for oral exposure. The U.S. FDA suggests 240 ml of dilutent per 30 grams of charcoal. The usual charcoal dose is 30–100 g in adults and 15–30 g in children. In symptomatic patients (e.g., coughing, choking, and tachypnea), blood gases should be monitored to ensure adequate ventilation and a baseline chest X-ray should be obtained. Ventilation and oxygenation should be maintained for pulmonary edema with close arterial blood gas monitoring. Early use of positive end expiratory pressure and mechanical ventilation may be needed to maintain oxygen pressure (PO_2) >50 mm Hg with FIO_2 less than 60%.

Inhalation Exposure

The victim should be moved to fresh air to decontaminate. The person should also be monitored for respiratory distress. If cough or difficulty in breathing develops, respiratory tract irritation, bronchitis, or pneumonitis should be evaluated. Supplemental oxygen (100% humidified) should be administered with assisted ventilation as required.

Eye Exposure

Exposed eyes should be irrigated with copious amount of tepid water for at least 15 min. If irritation, pain, swelling, lacrimation, or photophobia persist, the patient should be seen in health care facility.

Dermal Exposure

The exposed area should be washed thoroughly with soap and water to decontaminate. A physician may need to examine the area if irritation or pain persists.

Animal Toxicity

Hexane has been reported to be three times as acutely toxic to mice as is pentane. A concentration of 30,000 ppm produced CNS depression within 3060 min. Concentrations ranging from 35,000 to 40,000 ppm produced convulsions and death. When mice were exposed to an atmosphere containing 2.5–3% of *n*-hexane for 4 days, liver growth was observed after 24 hr. Mice were exposed to commercial hexane (65–70% *n*-hexane) for 24 hr a day, 6 days a week for 1 year. Exposure levels ranged from 100 to 2000 ppm. Atrophy and degeneration of hindleg muscle fibers were present in animals exposed to 1000 and 2000 ppm of *n*-hexane.

Pregnant Fischer 344 rats were exposed to 1000 ppm *n*-hexane for 6 hr per day on Days 8–12 of gestation. Postnatal growth of pups born to dams exposed to 1000 ppm on Days 8–16 of gestation was significantly depressed compared to controls. New Zealand rabbits exposed in inhalation chambers to 3000 ppm *n*-hexane 8 hr per day for 8 days showed changes in the lungs, emphysema, necrotic phenomena in bronchiolar epithelium, and athelectasis. Epicutaneous administration of *n*-hexane to guinea pigs caused progressing nuclear pyknosis and junctional separation between the basement membrane and the basal cells of the skin.

Male rats were exposed by inhalation to several concentrations of hexane, administered continuously or intermittently. In rats exposed to 1000 ppm hexane 24 hr per day, 5 days per week for 11 weeks, the fifth component of the brain stem auditory-evoked response included increase in latency and decrease in amplitude, reflecting a brain stem dysfunction. Latency returned to normal within 5 weeks after termination of exposures, but amplitude did not. Latency of the compound action potential of the ventral caudal nerve of the tail of these rats was also increased and this effect was still present 22 weeks after termination of the exposure.

Adult rats were exposed to hexane at different concentrations of *n*-hexane. Lung tissue was then examined. The direct toxic effect to pneumocytes could be demonstrated as definite regressive alterations, such as fatty generation and change of lamellar bodies of type II pneumocytes as well as increased detachment of cells. After chronic inhalation of solvents, conspicuous aggregation of lamellar discharge material of type II pneumocytes can be seen and, probably as a result of an irritated fat metabolism, there were large lysosome-like bodies with densely packed lipid material in type I pneumocytes.

New Zealand rabbits exposed in inhalation chambers to 3000 ppm *n*-hexane 8 hr per day for 8 days showed changes in lungs, emphysema, necrotic phenomena in bronchiolar epithelium, and atelectasis. The injection of hexane in rabbits caused edema and hemorrhaging of the lungs and tissue, with polymorphonuclear leukocytic reactions. In rabbits, dermal application of 2–5 mg/kg for 4 hr has resulted in ataxia and restlessness. No deaths occurred at 2 mg/kg; however, some occurred at 5 mg/kg.

Hexane was found to be negative when tested for mutagenicity using the Salmonella microsome preincubation assay, following the standard protocol approved by the National Toxicology Program. Hexane was tested in as many as five *Salmonella typhimurium* strains (TA1535, TA1537, TA97, TA98, and TA100) in the presence and absence of rat and hamster liver S9 at doses of 0.001, 0.0033, 0.010, 0.033, 0.100, and 0.333 mg/plate. Some cultures exhibited slight clearing of the background bacterial lawn at the two highest doses tested.

—Leyna Mulholland

Related Topics

Neurotoxicology: Central and Peripheral
Pollution, Water

Holly

◆ SYNONYMS: Aquifoliaceae family, Ilex species; *Ilex aquifolium*—Prick holly, sparked holly, Christmas holly, crocodile holly, English holly, European holly, Oregon holly; *Ilex vomitoria*—emetic holly, deer holly, yaupon, Indian black drink, Appalachian tea, Carolina tea, evergreen cassena, cassena; *Ilex opaca*—American holly

Exposure Pathways

Exposure occurs via ingestion of plant material (i.e., leaves and berries).

Mechanism of Toxicity

It is believed the saponins may be responsible for gastrointestinal effects, although the exact mechanism of action is unknown. The toxins involved include ilicin, tannic acid, ilexanthin, ilicic acid, and (in *I. aquifolium*) cyanogenic glycosides. These toxins may be found in the leaves and fruit (berries) of the plant.

Human Toxicity

Although symptoms will vary with different types of holly, the predominant toxic effect appears to be gastrointestinal irritation. Ingestion of small amounts of plant material may result in mild to moderate gastritis resulting in nausea, vomiting, abdominal pain, and diarrhea. Mild central nervous system (CNS) depression may be evident. Ingestion of the thorny leaf can cause mechanical irritation. Larger amounts have the potential to cause more severe gastrointestinal irritation along with varying degrees of CNS depression.

Clinical Management

The main goal of therapy for holly ingestions is fluid replacement and supportive care. There is no specific antidote available. Initial management should consist of gastric emptying if the ingestion is discovered soon after exposure. Syrup of ipecac may be used for this purpose. Activated charcoal may be given as well as intravenous fluid replacement if oral liquids cannot be tolerated.

Animal Toxicity

Gastrointestinal irritation may be seen along with CNS depression. Death in animals is rare.

—*Rita Mrvos*

Hormesis

Introduction

Hormesis is commonly defined as a beneficial or stimulatory effect caused by exposure to low doses of an agent known to be toxic at higher doses. Conceptually, this represents a dose–threshold model for toxicity where hormetic effects become smaller (after a maximum) with increasing dose up to a threshold, after which toxicity increases with dose (Fig. H-1A). Not surprisingly, proponents of hormesis are frequently at odds with other scientists, particularly those who favor a no threshold, linear dose–response curve (Fig. H-1B) or a "hockey stick" dose–response curve (Fig. H-1C). The beneficial effects that have been attributed to exposure to low doses of toxic agents in laboratory animals include increased life span, improved rates of growth and development, decreased tumor incidence, and increased resistance to infection and tolerance to radiation. Some of these effects have been reported to occur commonly after exposure to low doses of a wide variety of physical and chemical agents.

Radiation Hormesis

The most intensively studied area of hormesis research has been exposure to low-level ionizing radiation

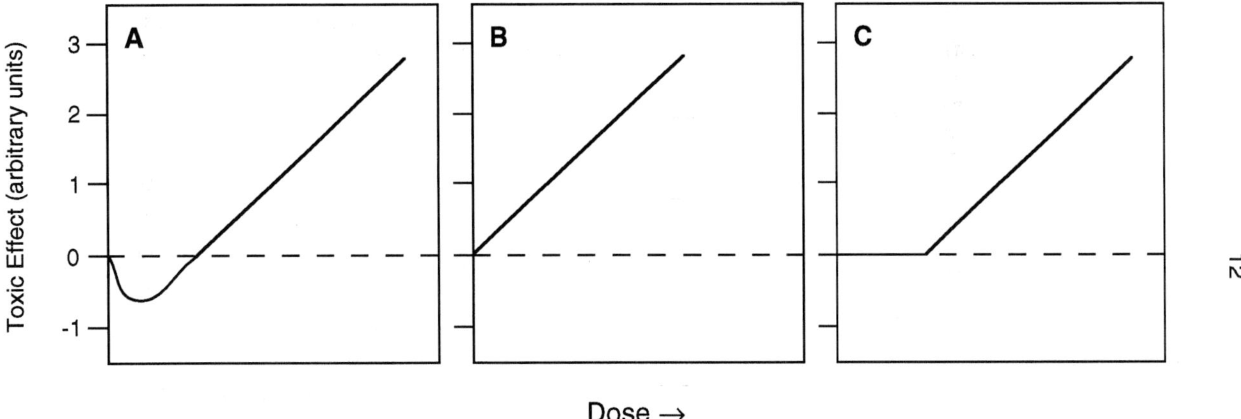

FIGURE H-1. Idealized dose–response curves for the (A) hormesis, (B) linear, and (C) threshold hypotheses. A "positive" toxic effect is regarded as detrimental, whereas a "negative" toxic effect is beneficial (hormetic).

(LLIR). The concept that LLIR can produce beneficial effects in biological systems challenges the conventional radiation paradigm which asserts that (1) radiation exposure is harmful at all dose levels (i.e., there is no threshold); and (2) there are no effects at low doses that cannot be predicted from effects observed at high dose levels (i.e., linear or near-linear dose–response curve). As an indication of the controversial nature of this area of research, several investigators have vigorously defended their belief in the potential beneficial effects of LLIR, with some even suggesting that LLIR exposure is essential for "maximum evolutionary fitness" (Parsons, 1990). In this context it must be remembered that background radiation is ubiquitous and that the level can vary markedly from locale to locale.

There is no doubt that biological systems can respond to exposure to toxic physical and chemical agents in a manner that often reduces the severity of the insult. Frequently, these responses are a result of altered gene expression, such as the increased synthesis of heat shock or stress proteins following exposure to thermal or oxidant stress. Such protective effects have also been demonstrated experimentally following exposure to low-level radiation when discrete, sensitive cellular and/or biochemical endpoints are measured. For example, the level of oxygen free radical scavengers, which protect against the toxic effects of radiation, was shown to increase in bone marrow cells of mice after whole body exposure to as little as 0.1 gray (Gy) of cesium-137 gamma irradiation (Feinendegen *et al.*, 1987) (The Gy is a unit of dose absorbed by a material and is equivalent to 1 J per kilogram.) Temporary suspension of DNA synthesis was also observed after 0.01 Gy exposure, which might result in the formation of fewer free radical-mediated DNA lesions during the exposure and facilitate the repair of lesions caused by free radical attack. If a higher concentration of radical scavengers or antioxidants were produced or released than required for neutralization of the excess free radicals produced by irradiation treatment of the mice, this would be viewed as radiation hormesis, the case made by Feinendegen and co-workers. The "excess" radical scavengers available might produce a beneficial effect by protecting against the damage caused by background radiation, by subsequent free radical challenges induced by radiation exposure, or, alternatively, by normal cellular metabolism.

Wolff and colleagues believe they have evidence for a hormetic response of human lymphocytes to LLIR (Shadley and Wolff, 1987; Wiencke *et al.*, 1986). Growth of lymphocytes in the presence of 0.01–0.10 μCi/ml of [^{3}H]thymidine or very low (.005–0.01 Gy) doses of X-rays, while not producing deleterious effects, appears to confer resistance to chromosomal breakage upon subsequent exposure to 1.5 Gy of X-rays. [The curie (Ci) is a unit of radioactive source activity and is equivalent to 3.70×10^{10} disintegrations per second.) The low-dose radiation-associated decrease in DNA damage could be eliminated by the addition of 3-aminobenzamide, an inhibitor of poly(ADP-ribose) polymerase when added after the high-dose exposure. This indirect evidence suggests that the LLIR exposure induces a DNA repair mechanism involving this enzyme. Critics of these studies have suggested that the small doses of LLIR employed would result in only very small, transient increases above the normal steady-state concentration of intracellular free radicals and thus would be an unlikely trigger to activate repair mechanisms.

Investigations with the protozoan *Paramecium tetraurelia* and the cyanobacterium *Synechococcus lividus* have provided evidence for hormesis using cell growth parameters as a biological endpoint (Planel *et al.*, 1987). The growth rate of either organism within chambers shielded from normal background radiation was depressed up to 50% when compared with growth in unshielded chambers. Critical to the hormesis concept, the growth rate in shielded chambers could be restored to unshielded values when the organisms were subjected to LLIR exposure at doses comparable or slightly greater than normal background levels (7–20 mGy/year). This LLIR stimulatory effect disappeared at dose rates >50 mGy/year. The authors interpreted these data to suggest that LLIR stimulates proliferation of these single-cell organisms, although an exact mechanism(s) was not demonstrated.

Epidemiological studies involving large populations remain the best means available for the study of potential hormetic effects in humans. A study of atomic bomb survivors from Nagasaki suggested that significantly lower (65% of control) mortality rates from noncancerous diseases exist in males exposed to 50–149 cGy of bomb-related radiation versus unexposed, age-matched controls (Mine *et al.*, 1990). However, these data conflict with those of other studies that have failed to produce significant evidence for beneficial effects among atomic bomb survivors exposed to low levels of radiation (Bloom *et al.*, 1987; Kato *et al.*, 1987). Some proponents of radiation hormesis have suggested that the lack of hormetic effects among atomic bomb survivors is because the data set represents the effects of acute exposure to radiation and is, therefore, not a valid comparison to the chronic, LLIR exposure ideally associated with hormesis.

The relationship of the annual cancer incidence rate in various cities and states of India to the intensity of background radiation has been reported by Nambi and collaborators (Nambi and Soman, 1987). The annual age-adjusted mortality rate from all cancers in five major Indian cities was found to decrease at a rate of 0.3 per millirem/year increase in the external background radiation dose from a hypothetical incidence level of 79 per 100,000 corresponding to a hypothetical "zero environmental radiation" level. (The rem is a unit of the biological effects of radiation and is equivalent to the dose absorbed × a quality factor specific for individual types of radiation.) A similar study (Wang *et al.*, 1990) from the Guangdong province of China examined two similar population groups of 60,000 people living in adjacent areas but whose exposure to background radiation was 330 and 114 mrem/year, respectively. An analysis of total cancer mortality from 1970 to 1986 failed to show a significant beneficial (hormetic) effect in the high background group. When nonleukemic cancers of inhabitants aged 40–70 years from 1970 to 1986 or all cancers within the entire population from 1975 to 1978 were considered separately, however, a significant 14.6% lower cancer mortality rate in the high background group was found. Interpretations of these studies are controversial and have been criticized primarily with respect to the problems associated with the limited time spans evaluated, lack of an accurate assessment of radiation exposures, and confounding factors such as smoking, diet, and lifestyle.

Thus, even though some of the data collected to date suggest that low-dose radiation may protect against subsequent environmentally mediated carcinogenesis, it is apparent that the hormetic response remains very difficult to validate unequivocally.

Chemical Hormesis

Numerous reports of chemical-mediated hormesis in response to exposure of plants or animals to a wide variety of compounds appear in the literature. Chemical hormesis is characterized by a biphasic or U-shaped dose–response curve (Fig. H-1A), where very low doses of toxicant have a beneficial or stimulatory effect, relative to control exposures, and moderate to high doses are obviously toxic. The concept of chemical hormesis also challenges the linear, no threshold dose–response model (Fig. H-1B) or the hockey stick model (Fig. H-1C), especially with respect to carcinogens. Metals, in particular, have received much attention with respect to possible hormetic effects. Administration of 22 mg/kg of tetramethyl lead, a known central nervous system (CNS) toxicant, for 60 days to pregnant rats, and subsequently to their offspring, was reported to produce an increase in weight gain in the absence of deleterious effects on brain weight or morphology (Cragg and Rees, 1984). The authors have presumed this represents a stimulatory effect of low levels of lead on body growth, although it could also result from stimulation of appetite.

Preexposure of the tidal fish *Fundulus heteroclitus* to 0.05 mg/liter concentrations of cadmium prior to partial amputation of the caudal fin resulted in a 5–15% faster rate of regeneration in water containing 0.1 mg/liter cadmium compared with unexposed fish allowed to regenerate in "clean water" assumed to be cadmium free (Weis and Weis, 1986). This effect, however, was observed in only two of three experiments conducted. While the mechanism for this effect was not clear, the increased rate of regeneration was hypothesized to be due to an overcompensation of homeostatic regulation resulting in accelerated growth.

Low concentrations of carcinogenic polycyclic aromatic hydrocarbons (PAHs) have also been evaluated for a potential hormetic effect. Exposure of grunion embryos (*Leuresthes tenuis*; a freshwater teleost) to 7 ppb of benzo[*a*]pyrene resulted in significantly increased respiration rates compared with unexposed controls (Hose and Puffer, 1984), whereas at higher concentrations of 24.2, 361, or 868.8 ppb, respiration rates were not significantly different from control. Although no benefit of the increased respiration rate is obvious, it may be that this or similar metabolic responses to low-level PAH exposure represent an overcompensatory response typical of hormesis. It might be argued, however, that an adaptive biological response to low toxicant exposure in the absence of a clearly demonstrated benefit, preferably at the molecular mechanism level, does not constitute hormesis.

Hormesis studies in humans have been performed using populations exposed occupationally to toxic chemicals. Chronic exposure to low levels (5–40 ppm) of the hepatotoxicant, trichloroethylene (TCE), was recently associated with changes in cholesterol metabolism rather than causing hepatic cell damage (Nagaya *et al.*, 1993). In particular, elevated levels of serum high-density lipoprotein associated cholesterol (HDL-C) were noted, while levels of the serum enzymes aspartate aminotransferase, alanine aminotransferase, and γ-glutamyl transpeptidase were unaffected. Because HDL-C is thought to be protective against coronary heart disease and to improve longevity, elevated serum levels may have a beneficial effect. However, the significance of the trend for HDL-C to increase with the dose of low-level exposure was only marginal ($p = 0.08$). Furthermore, evidence for decreased incidence of heart disease and/or increased longevity was not part of this epidemiological study; perhaps a follow-up investigation is possible. What we are left with is the demonstration of a biological change that is apparently associated with low-level occupational exposure to TCE and that may be beneficial. However, further epidemiological studies employing definitive biological endpoints, with careful controls for lifestyle and other variables, are required to definitively demonstrate that chemical hormesis is a common beneficial mechanism resulting from low-level exposure to toxic chemicals in humans.

Conclusions

Many reports of hormesis occur in the scientific literature. In their comprehensive reviews, Luckey (1980) and Stebbing (1982) have collected more than 1000 published articles relating to the effects of radiation and chemicals on biological systems. As stated previously, adaptations based on changes in gene expression and/or posttranslational protein modification are common (Sorger, 1991; Nebert *et al.*, 1990). Whether or not such alterations are beneficial to the organism, an essential component of hormesis, is very difficult to determine, particularly from studies designed for other purposes. While many of the studies that purport to show hormesis suffer from flaws in experimental design and an unimpressive response (the difference between biological significance and statistical significance is relevant here), the volume of published research material alone suggests that further clarification is necessary! Important aspects that must be evaluated include the dose–response relationship and the specific mechanism or mechanisms of the "hormetic effect." Additional work should entail both reevaluation of data sets from previous studies in which appropriate endpoints have been evaluated or additional data can be obtained from archived material and carefully designed new experiments. Recently, Calabrese and Baldwin (1993) reexamined the data from a previous chemical toxicity study and identified numerous examples of possible chemical hormesis for a variety of endpoints studied.

In closing, it must be emphasized that chronic exposure of organisms to physical or chemical stressors can result in changes in gene regulation that confer a protective (detoxication) effect against the stressor in the exposed organism. The issue remains, however, whether chronic exposure to low concentrations of toxic chemicals or radiation can infer long-term beneficial effects to the organism and whether this is a general protective response.

Further Reading

Bloom, E. T., Akiyama, M., Kusunoki, Y., and Makinodan, T. (1987). Delayed effects of low-dose radiation on cellular immunity in atomic bomb survivors residing in the United States. *Health Phys.* 52, 585–591.

Calabrese, E. J., and Baldwin, L. A. (1993). Possible examples of chemical hormesis in a previously published study. *J. Appl. Toxicol.* 13, 169–172.

Cragg, B., and Rees, S. (1984). Increased body : brain weight ratio in developing rats after low exposure to organic lead. *Exp. Neurol.* 86, 113–121.

Feinendegen, L. E., Muhlensiepen, H., Bond, V. P., and Sondhaus, C. A. (1987). Intracellular stimulation of biochemical control mechanisms by low-dose, low-LET irradiation. *Health Phys.* **52,** 663–669.

Hose, J. E., and Puffer, H. W. (1984). Oxygen consumption rates of grunion (*Leuresthes tenius*) embryos exposed to the petroleum hydrocarbon, benzo[*a*]pyrene. *Environ. Res.* 35, 413–420.

Kato, H., Schull, W. J., Awa, A., Akiyama, M., and Otake, M. (1987). Dose–response analyses among atomic bomb survivors exposed to low-level radiation. *Health Phys.* 52, 645–652.

Koppenol, W. H., and Bounds, P. L. (1989). Hormesis [comment]. *Science 245*, 311.

Luckey, T. D. (1980). *Hormesis with Ionizing Radiation.* CRC Press, Boca Raton, FL.

Macklis, R. M., and Beresford, B. (191). Radiation hormesis. *J. Nucl. Med.* 32, 350–358.

Mine, M., Okumura, Y., Ichimaru, M., Nakamura, T., and Kondo, S. (1990). Apparently beneficial effect of low to intermediate doses of A-bomb radiation on human lifespan. *Int. J. Radiat. Biol.* 58, 1035–1043.

Nagaya, T., Ishikawa, N., Hata, H., and Otobe, T. (1993). Subclinical and reversible hepatic effects of occupational exposure to trichloroethylene. *Int. Arch. Occup. Environ. Health* **64,** 561–563.

Nambi, K. S. V., and Soman, S. D. (1987). Environmental radiation and cancer in India. *Health Phys.* 52, 653–657.

Nebert, D. W., Petersen, D. D., and Fornace, A. J. (1990). Cellular responses to oxidative stress: The [Ah] gene battery as a paradigm. *Environ. Health Perspect.* **88,** 13–25.

Parsons, P. A. (1990). Radiation hormesis: An evolutionary expectation and the evidence. *Int. J. Radiat. Appl. Instrum. A* **41,** 857–860.

Planel, H., Soleilhavoup, J. P., Tixador, R., Richoilley, G., Conter, A., Croute, F., Caratero, C., and Gaubin, Y. (1987). Influence on cell proliferation of background radiation or exposure to very low, chronic g radiation. *Health Phys.* **52,** 571–578

Shadley, J. D., and Wolff, S. (1987). Very low doses of X-rays can cause human lymphocytes to become less susceptible to ionizing radiation. *Mutagenesis* **2,** 95–96.

Sorger, P. K. (1991). Heat shock factor and the heat shock response. *Cell* **65,** 363–366.

Stebbing, A. R. D. (1982). Hormesis—The stimulation of growth by low levels of inhibitors. *Sci. Total Environ.* **22,** 213–234.

Wang, Z., Boice, J. D., Jr., Wei, L., Beebe, G. W., Zha, Y., Kaplan, M. M., Tao, Z., Maxon, H. R., III, Zhang, S., Schneider, A. B., Tan, B., Wesseler, T. A., Chen, D., Ershow, A. G., Kleinerman, R. A., Littlefield, L. G., and Preston, D. (1990). Thyroid nodularity and chromosome aberrations among women in areas of high background radiation in China. *J. Natl. Cancer Inst.* **82,** 478–485.

Weis, P., and Weis, J. S. (1986). Cadmium accumulation and hormesis in *Fundulus heteroclitus* during fin regeneration. *Environ. Res.* **39,** 356–363.

Wiencke, J. K., Afzal, V., Olivieri, G., and Wolff, S. (1986). Evidence that the [^{3}H]thymidine-induced adaptive response of human lymphocytes to subsequent doses of X-rays involves the induction of a chromosomal repair mechanism. *Mutagenesis* **1,** 375–380.

—Christopher J. Sinal and John R. Bend

Related Topics

Dose–Response Relationship
Radiation

Host-Mediated Assay

The host-mediated assay (HMA), developed in the late 1960s by Gabridge and Legator, is an approach for providing the *in vivo* metabolism of a whole animal (the host) for assessing effects on indicator cells that are placed in the host during chemical exposure and then removed for *in vitro* measurements of mutagenicity. As shown by James and Elizabeth Miller of the University of Wisconsin, due to the limited metabolic capacity of most bacterial and mammalian target cells used in *in vitro* genetic toxicology, a number of chemicals found mutagenic and carcinogenic in whole animals are without genetic effects *in vitro* in the absence of a provision for *in vivo* metabolism to convert the chemicals to electrophiles capable of interacting with nucleic acids and proteins.

The HMA is of historical significance to the field of genetic toxicology testing because its development preceded that of the now widely used addition of exogenous liver homogenates (e.g., the 9000*g* supernatant fraction, termed S9) to approximate *in vivo* metabolic pathways in *in vitro* test systems and because, in the early 1970s, the HMA was one of three original screening tests recommended (together with the dominant lethal test and the *in vivo* cytogenetic assay) for evaluating the mutagenic effects of chemicals. However, the concept of growing cells in an *in vivo* environment predates the HMA. In 1887, cells were grown in a tube obtained from reeds and implanted in a host animal, and applications which continued into the first half of the twentieth century included maintaining cell lines in animals before the development of chemically defined culture medium.

In the host-mediated mutagenicity assay as initially defined, a microbial indicator organism in which mutation frequencies can be measured is injected into the peritoneal cavity of the host, and the host is treated with a potential chemical mutagen. Subsequently, the microorganisms are withdrawn from the host, and the induction of mutants is assessed following growth of the microorganism *in vitro*. Application of the HMA was then expanded to include additional sites of inoculation and recovery of the indicator cells (blood, intestinal tract, liver, spleen, lungs, and testes) and the use of other than bacterial indicator cells, including *Neurospora*, yeast, and various types of mammalian cells. It is of some historical interest that the L5178Y

$$tk^{+/-} \longrightarrow tk^{-/-}$$

mouse lymphoma cell mutation assay was initially developed with descendants of cells which had been passaged as ascites cultures in mice, before the definition of culture medium; hence, it was thought that the L5178Y cells would be ideally suited for use in the HMA.

Since its definition, the HMA has been used to evaluate several hundred chemicals, with the measured genetic effects including forward and reverse mutations, recessive lethal mutations, mitotic gene conversion, mitotic recombination, differential DNA repair, sister chromatid exchanges, chromosome deletions and aberrations, and alterations in cellular and colony morphology. However, the HMA was not universally successful, in part because in the early 1970s it was initially coupled with mutagenesis systems that had been insufficiently defined and validated. However, other problems included a failure to allow for animal-to-animal variability, contamination of bacterial indicator cells with intestinal flora, and difficulties in differentiating between mammalian indicator cells and cells from the host.

Thus, the HMA was no longer recommended for mutagenicity testing for regulatory submissions when the technically more straightforward and less expensive use of S9 metabolic activation became available and it was found that, because subcellular systems contain predominantly activating enzymes, few, if any, chemicals were found positive in the HMA that were not also positive for mutagenicity with S9. Since a goal of initial mutagenicity testing, particularly for regulatory submissions, is to identify chemicals for subsequent evaluations of potential hazard to humans, an approach that tips the balance of metabolic reactions in favor of activation reduces the risk of overlooking potentially hazardous chemicals.

It must be remembered, however, that *in vitro* S9 metabolic activation systems cannot address *in vivo* fate processes such as absorption, storage and excretion, hormonal influence, and specific tissue biochemistry, including hydrolysis and preferential enzymatic detoxification. In addition, a number of apparently false-positive responses obtained for rodent noncarcinogens in *in vitro* assays may to be associated with chemicals that possess innate genotoxic activity that is unexpressed *in vivo*.

Although after a decade of use HMA mutagenicity testing was essentially abandoned, today, a number of problems initially encountered with the HMA have been resolved or are capable of resolution. *In vitro* mutagenesis systems have now been extensively defined and evaluated; animal-to-animal variability can be minimized by using a sufficient number of animals per dose; and both contamination of indicator cells and difficulties in differentiating between cells from the host and mammalian indicator cells are precluded when the target cells are contained within devices such as diffusion chambers (consisting of two circular semipermeable membranes, about the size of a dime, attached to a narrow Teflon ring) which are then surgically implanted in the host.

Diffusion chambers, coupled with the HMA approach, have also been used for organ culture, hematopoietic research, and in pharmacodynamic studies to assess the effects of various chemotherapeutic agents on human tumor cells and, recently, to maintain genetically engineered cells *in vivo* for utilization of their specialized cellular products for human gene therapy. Thus, the host-mediated assay approach may be of future utility in toxicology research not only to examine the basis for a lack of concordance between *in vitro* and *in vivo* test results but also to evaluate the efficacy and potential risks of developed approaches for human genetic therapy.

—*Ann D. Mitchell*

Related Topics

Ames Test
Analytical Toxicology
Carcinogenesis
Chromosome Aberrations
Developmental Toxicology
Dominant Lethal Tests
In Vitro Testing
In Vivo Testing
Molecular Toxicology
Mouse Lymphoma Assay
Mutagenesis
Sister Chromatid Exchanges
Toxicity Testing, Alternatives
Toxicity Testing, Aquatic
Toxicity Testing, Behavioral
Toxicity Testing, Carcinogenesis
Toxicity Testing, Dermal
Toxicity Testing, Developmental
Toxicity Testing, Inhalation

Hydrangea

- SYNONYMS: *Hydrangea arborescens*; *Hydrangea macrophylla*; *Hydrangea paniculata*; seven bark; wild hydrangea
- PHARMACEUTICAL CLASS: Cyanogenic glycosides

Uses

There are no known uses for hydrangea.

Exposure Pathways

Exposure occurs via dermal contact and ingestion.

Toxicokinetics

Small doses of cyanide are converted to thiocyanate by an enzymatic reaction catalyzed by rhodanese. The rhodanese system can detoxify large amounts of cyanide but may not respond quickly enough to prevent fatalities.

Mechanism of Toxicity

The leaves and buds contain hydrangin, which has the potential to produce cyanide (see Cyanide). When the plant material is ingested, it reacts slowly in the acid pH of the stomach. Once transportation into the alkaline medium of the duodenum occurs, the process is hastened. Hydrocyanic acid is produced forming a stable complex with the ferric iron and cytochrome oxidase, thereby inhibiting the activity of the enzyme and aerobic metabolism. Cells containing cytochrome oxidase become hypoxic because they are unable to utilize available oxygen.

Human Toxicity

Cyanide toxicity due to accidental exposure is rare. Sudden severe vomiting and epigastric pain are usually the first symptoms present. Respirations are rapid at first and then become slow and labored. Acidosis is usually present as a result of the Kussmaul respiration. Syncope, progressive loss of consciousness, and seizures ensue after gastrointestinal symptoms. Allergic contact dermatitis due to the sensitizer hydrangenol has been reported.

Clinical Management

In asymptomatic patients, gastric lavage and/or activated charcoal and observation are all that is necessary. Induction of emesis following large ingestions is contraindicated due to the potential rapid development of symptoms. In symptomatic patients, ignore gastric decontamination procedures until life-support measures have been instituted. Cyanide antidote kit administration may be necessary.

Animal Toxicity

Toxicity associated with hydrangins is not known in animals, but ruminal microorganisms have the ability to degrade cyanogenic glycosides causing the release of hydrogen cyanide.

—*Brenda Swanson Biearman*

Hydrazine

- CAS: 302-01-2
- SYNONYMS: Diamine; hydrazine anhydrous
- CHEMICAL CLASS: Miscellaneous nitrogen compounds
- MOLECULAR FORMULA: H_4N_2

Uses

Hydrazine is a chemical intermediate for explosives, heat stabilizers, textiles, agricultural chemicals, dyes, and pharmaceuticals (antituberculants and sickle cell anemia). It is a reducing agent for many transition metals.

Exposure Pathways

Inhalation, dermal contact, and ingestion are the possible exposure pathways for hydrazine.

Toxicokinetics

Hydrazines are absorbed by all routes of administration. In dogs, absorption of hydrazine through the skin is rapid with hydrazine detected in blood within 30 sec. Hydrazine is acetylated very rapidly in most mammalian species and excreted in the urine as the diacetyl metabolite. Hydrazine is possibly degraded to ammonia. The excretion of hydrazine in the urine has been determined through intravenous or subcutaneous administration. Dogs receiving high doses of hydrazine (approximately twice the LD_{50}) excreted 5–11% of the dose within 4 hr. The rate of appearance in the blood is dependent on whether the exposed individual is a fast or slow acetylator.

Hydrazine is distributed rapidly to most tissues with the highest levels appearing in the kidneys. Loss from all tissues was extensive by 24 hr; within the first 2 hr approximately 20% of the dose was expired.

Mechanism of Toxicity

Under the effect of hydrazine, single carbon compounds are incorporated to yield O^6-methylguanine and a 7-methylguanine in DNA. The methyl group stems from metabolism of *S*-adenosylmethionine. This activity stimulates guanylate cyclase which catalyzes production of guanosine monophosphate, which has been implicated in malignant transformation. Adrenal hormones may be partly responsible for the mechanism by which hydrazine exerts effects on the liver.

Human Toxicity

Hydrazine is a violent poison with strong caustic action on the skin and mucous membranes. Skin contact may cause severe dermatitis. Skin contact with anhydrous hydrazine can result in caustic-like burns and dissolved hair. Hydrazine can cause injury to the blood and liver. Hydrazine is classified as a local irritant, convulsant, hepatotoxin, and hemolytic agent. Exposure can result in anorexia, vomiting, cardiac depression, and hypotension. Acute respiratory exposure to low concentrations can cause delayed death (days) and produce bronchial mucous destruction and pulmonary edema.

Hydrazine vapors may cause eye irritation, while contact with liquids may result in severe eye damage. Delayed eye irritation is also an effect of hydrazine exposure. Facial edema, conjunctivitis, and salivation have occurred following exposure.

Clinical Management

Lavage, with the airway protected, is recommended rather than emesis following ingestion. Emesis to remove hydrazines may be severely limited by their irritancy and their tendency to produce convulsions and coma. Pyridoxine (vitamin B_6) may be antidotal. Administration of diazepam is indicated if convulsions occur.

Overexposure via inhalation should be treated first by moving the individual to an area of fresh air and monitoring for respiratory distress. Skin should be washed thoroughly with soap and water following direct dermal contact.

Animal Toxicity

Inhalation exposure in guinea pigs and dogs resulted in rapid weakness, significant liver damage, and lesser damage to kidneys and lungs. Muscular tremors have been noted in dogs following inhalation exposure.

The extent of the effect on the blood system of rats became more severe with increase in animal age.

Exposure of pregnant toads to hydrazine during the neurulation stage of development resulted in teratogenic effects. Pregnant rats exposed to hydrazine had dose-related embryolethality and maternal toxicity.

There is insufficient data in humans but sufficient data in laboratory animals to classify hydrazine as a possible human carcinogen [increased tumor incidence in mouse (pulmonary tumors), rats (liver tumors), and hamsters (liver tumors)]. Hydrazine also reduces the latency period associated with the development of tumors in exposed rats. Hydrazine has been shown to be mutagenic in bacteria, viruses, and mammalian cell assays.

—*Kathryn A. Wurzel*

Hydrobromic Acid

- CAS: 10035-10-6
- Synonyms: Hydrogen bromide; hydrogen bromide, anhydrous; anhydrous hydrobromic acid
- Chemical Class: Inorganic acid; corrosive
- Chemical Structure: H-Br

Uses

Hydrobromic acid is used in the manufacture of inorganic bromides for use in photography, pharmaceuticals, industrial drying, textile finishing, engraving, lithography, and in fire retardants. It is also used as a reagent in analytical chemistry.

Exposure Pathways

Exposure may occur by the oral, inhalation, dermal, or ocular routes.

Toxicokinetics

No information is available regarding the toxicokinetics of hydrogen bromide in humans or animals.

Mechanism of Toxicity

The primary mechanism by which hydrogen bromide exerts its toxic effects is via irritation upon contact with tissues. Hydrogen bromide is a potent irritant of the tissues of the mouth, nose, eyes, and respiratory tract.

Human Toxicity

Subjective responses of six human volunteers exposed to levels ranging from 2 to 6 ppm for several minutes were reported as follows: exposure to 5 or 6 ppm resulted in nasal irritation in all volunteers and throat irritation in one volunteer. Eye irritation was not reported at any of the tested concentrations. One individual noted nasal or throat irritation at the 3 ppm level. Odor was detectable at all concentrations tested. Higher levels of inhalation exposure can produce pulmonary edema. If a solution is splashed on the skin or eyes, it will cause a burn. Ingestion can cause burns of the stomach. The OSHA PEL is 3 ppm (10 mg/m^3) as an 8-hr, time-weighted average. ACGIH and NIOSH recommend 3 ppm as a ceiling concentration. The IDLH level is 50 ppm.

Clinical Management

Personnel not wearing personal protective equipment should be restricted from areas of spills or leaks until cleanup has been completed. In the case of exposure to the eyes or skin from hydrogen bromide solutions, contaminated skin or eyes should be flushed with copious amounts of water for at least 15 min. If an individual inhales large amounts of hydrogen bromide, this person should be moved to fresh air at once. Artificial respiration should be performed if breathing has stopped. In the event of ingestion of hydrogen bromide solution, large quantities of water or milk should be given immediately, provided the individual is conscious. Vomiting should not be induced.

Animal Toxicity

In a comparative toxicity study, hydrogen bromide caused more severe burns to the skin than hydrogen chloride or hydrogen iodide. In another study comparing the acute toxic effects of hydrogen fluoride, hydrogen bromide, and hydrogen chloride, rats were exposed to 1300 ppm hydrogen bromide for 30 min. Rats were separated in two groups. The first group consisted of ordinary mouth-breathing rats and the second group consisted of rats fitted with an apparatus to simulate nose breathing. More than twice as many rats in the pseudo-mouth-breathing group died as in the nose-only group and none died in the control group. The location of the lesion was found in the nasal passages of the nose-breathing group and in the trachea of the pseudo-mouth-breathing group. The inhalation (LC_{50}) in rats is 2858 ppm for 1 hr. The inhalation LC_{50} in mice is 814 ppm for 1 hr.

—*Mary Lee Hultin*

Related Topics

Acids
Corrosives

Hydrochloric Acid

- CAS: 7647-01-0
- SYNONYMS: Aqueous hydrogen chloride; hydrogen chloride; HCl; muriatic acid; spirits of salt; chlorohydric acid; hydrochloride
- CHEMICAL CLASS: Inorganic acid; corrosive
- CHEMICAL STRUCTURE: Cl-H

Uses

Uses of hydrochloric acid include neutralization of alkaline products, ore reduction, metal pickling, and cleaning. Hydrogen chloride is used in the manufacture of alkyl chlorides via hydrochlorination, polymerization, alkylation, and nitration reactions. Hydrochloric acid is also used in the treatment of oil and gas wells and in removal of scale from boilers and heat exchange equipment. Hydrochloric acid use is also reported in food processing and in therapeutics as an acidifying agent.

Exposure Pathways

Exposure may occur via dermal or ocular contact, ingestion, or inhalation.

Toxicokinetics

Hydrochloric acid is highly water soluble and, when inhaled, reacts with the surface components of the upper respiratory tract; therefore, it is generally retained or deposited at this site. Highly concentrated hydrochloric acid can overwhelm the scrubbing capacity of the upper respiratory tract and penetration to the bronchioles and alveoli may result.

Mechanism of Toxicity

Hydrogen chloride is an irritant. With acid burns, loss of cell membrane integrity and cellular death/necrosis are preceded by erythema and edema. Edema of the cornea and conjunctiva, skin, surface mucosa, and deep respiratory tissues occurs with substantial exposure. Changes in permeability and liquid transport across cell membranes are associated with alveolar damage.

Human Toxicity

Concentrated solutions may cause severe burns. Exposure to hydrogen chloride gas or solutions of hydrogen chloride may cause eye irritation and permanent damage with loss of sight. Inhalation immediately causes severe irritation with cough and choking sensation. Inflammation and ulceration of the upper respiratory tract occurs, and pulmonary edema can occur if hydrogen chloride gas is inhaled deeply. Excessive exposures (e.g., 1000–2000 ppm) for a few minutes can cause life-threatening pulmonary edema. Severe breathing difficulties may be delayed in onset. In workers, exposure to 50–100 ppm for 1 hr was barely tolerable. Short exposure to 35 ppm caused irritation of the throat; 10 ppm was considered the maximal concentration allowable for prolonged exposure. Occupational ceiling exposure limits are 5 ppm to 7 mg/m^3. Human asthmatics exposed to 0.8 or 1.8 ppm hydrogen chloride for 45 min did not exhibit exposure-related alterations in pulmonary function tests performed immediately after exposure.

Ingestion may cause corrosion of the mucous membranes, esophagus, and stomach with dysphagia, nausea, vomiting, intense thirst, and diarrhea. Circulatory collapse and death may occur. Chronic exposure to hydrogen chloride may cause erosion of the teeth, bronchitis, and gastritis. Repeated exposure of the skin to dilute solutions of hydrogen chloride may cause a rash.

Clinical Management

If solutions of hydrogen chloride or strong concentrations of hydrogen chloride gas get into the eyes, the eyes should be washed immediately with large amounts of water, lifting the lids occasionally. If skin exposure occurs, contaminated clothing should be removed and the exposed areas flushed with water. In the event of exposure to high concentrations, the exposed person should be moved to fresh air. Artificial respiration should be performed if breathing has stopped. In the case of accidental ingestion, a conscious person should be given large amounts (8–16 oz) of water to drink. Vomiting should not be induced.

Animal Toxicity

Rabbits and guinea pigs were studied for acute effects. When exposed to 4350 ppm hydrogen chloride for 30 min, all animals died. A level of 650 ppm for 2–6 hr was fatal to all animals. Most deaths were due to respiratory effects, although some animals died as a result of liver damage. Inhalation exposure to 65 ppm for 6 hr on each of 5 days produced the following reactions: pulmonary changes, mucous membrane irritation, lymph node hyperplasia, and reversible weight loss. A 90-day inhalation study in mice and rats using 10, 20, or 50 ppm exposures found slight weight gain decreases in the high-exposure groups of both species and rhinitis in rats. However, there were no changes in hematology, clinical chemistry, or urinalysis. Macrophage accumulation in peripheral tissues was noted in the high-dose mice, and all groups of mice developed eosinophilic globules in the nasal epithelium. In another 30-min inhalation study using guinea pigs, both pulmonary and sensory irritation were found. Doses of 320–1380 ppm produced sensory irritation in 1–6 min. Evidence of sensory irritation included decreased respiratory rate and lengthening of the expiratory phase due to stimulation of the trigeminal nerve. Baboons exposed to 500, 5000, or 10,000 ppm hydrogen chloride for 15 min were observed for 3 months following exposure. Respiratory rates and minute volumes were increased following exposure and the higher doses caused reversible decrease in arterial PO_2. However, 16,570 and 17,290 ppm doses administered to baboons for 5 min produced severe dyspnea and death after 18 and 76 days, respectively. The RD_{50} (concentration eliciting a 50% decrease in respiratory rate) in the mouse was 309 ppm. One chronic inhalation study used 10 ppm exposures to rats for their lifetimes. More treated animals than controls exhibited hyperplasia in the nasal mucosa. There was an increased incidence of laryngeal–tracheal hyperplasia compared to the controls. The U.S. EPA used this chronic data as a basis for development of an inhalation reference concentration (or acceptable daily exposure) of 0.02 mg/m^3.

The inhalation LC_{50} (1-hr duration) was 3124 ppm in rats and 1108 ppm in mice. The oral LD_{50} in rabbits was 900 mg/kg.

—Mary Lee Hultin

Related Topics

Acids
Corrosives
Pollution, Air

Hydrocodone

- CAS: 125-29-1
- Synonyms: Calmodid; curadol; dihydrocodeinone acid tartrate; dihydrocodeinonum bitartaricum; duodin; hydrocodonhydrogentartrat;

hydrocodoni; hydrocodonum; hydrocodonium; hydroconi; hydroconum; kolikodal; orthoxycol; procodal

- PHARMACEUTICAL CLASS: Opioid analgesic
- CHEMICAL STRUCTURE:

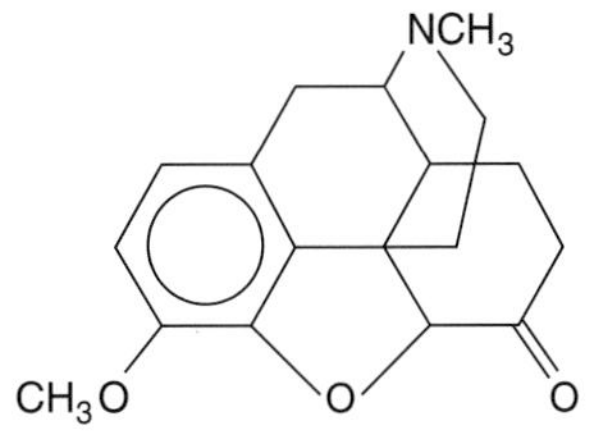

NCH_3 CH_3O O O

Uses

Hydrocodone is used as an analgesic and as an antitussive. It can be a drug of abuse.

Exposure Pathways

Ingestion is the most common route of exposure to hydrocodone. It is available in tablets and syrup.

Toxicokinetics

Hydrocodone is well absorbed from the gastrointestinal tract with peak serum levels occurring approximately 1 hr after ingestion. Peak analgesia generally occurs 2 hr after dose. Extended release products can provide up to 12 hr of antitussive effects. Hydrocodone is metabolized in the liver by O-demethylation, N-dealkylation, and 6-keto-reduction. The primary metabolites of hydrocodone are norcodeine, hydromorphone, 6-β-hydrocodol, 6-α-hydrocodol, 6-β-hydromorphal, and 6-α-hydromorphol. All metabolites are active with pharmacologic activity. Distribution sites and the volume of distribution have not been well defined. The kidneys are the main site of excretion. Unchanged drug (approximately 12%) and metabolites are excreted in the urine. The elimination half-life is approximately 3.8 hr.

Mechanism of Toxicity

Hydrocodone is a semisynthetic, centrally acting narcotic analgesic and antitussive agent. It is postulated that the drug's antitussive effects come from its direct depression of the medulla. Analgesic effects are related to the stimulation of opiate receptors in the central nervous system (CNS). Interaction with the opioid receptors mimics the actions of endogenous enkephlins and endorphins. These actions result in the therapeutic effects of analgesia, sedation, euphoria, and decreased gastrointestinal motility.

Human Toxicity: Acute

Toxicity occurs when the pharmacologic effects are increased, as can occur in an overdose. The depression of the CNS yields the primary symptoms. The typical overdose patient may present with extreme somnolence and skeletal muscle flaccidity. This can then progress to stupor or coma. Miosis is usually present unless the individual is acidotic or hypoxic. Life-threatening depression of respiration occurs, which may produce apnea or respiratory arrest. Pulmonary edema is often a complication. Bradycardia and hypotension may occur if there is an increase in parasympathetic tone. Hypothermia may also occur as a result peripheral vasodilation. A toxic dose has not been established but can be very close to a therapeutic dose—especially in children. Hydrocodone is often combined in products with acetaminophen; therefore, patients should also be evaluated for hepatotoxicity secondary to acetaminophen overdosage. Hydrocodone can be qualitatively detected in urine by EMIT homogenous enzyme immunoassays. Peak serum levels are 0.024 mg/liter; toxic levels may reach 0.1–1.3 μg/ml but are of little prognostic or therapeutic value.

Human Toxicity: Chronic

Opiates have a high potential for abuse. Chronic users may develop tolerance, thus necessitating larger doses for the desired effect. Toxic effects in chronic abuse can yield a decrease in immunity leading to frequent infections and possible AIDS. Abrupt cessation can cause withdrawal, yielding restlessness, insomnia, hypertension, tachypnea, tachycardia, vomiting, and diarrhea.

Clinical Management

Basic life-support measures should be instituted as necessary. Intensive support therapy may be required to correct respiratory failure and shock. Respiration must be supported and monitored until all symptoms disappear. Pulmonary edema should be managed with appropriate ventilatory support. If taken orally, gastrointestinal decontamination should be based on the patient's level of consciousness or decrease in gag reflex.

Activated charcoal may be used to adsorb the hydrocodone. A cathartic may be given to aid peristalsis. The specific antagonist naloxone hydrochloride is used to counteract very rapidly respiratory depression and coma. A dose of 0.4–2.0 mg is given intravenously and can be repeated at intervals of 2 or 3 min if necessary. The therapeutic effect of naloxone may be of shorter duration than that of the opiate activity; therefore, a naloxone continuous infusion may then be of benefit. Arterial blood gases, vital signs, and level of consciousness should be monitored continuously until cessation of symptoms. *N*-acetylcysteine therapy may be necessary if toxic acetaminophen levels are present.

Animal Toxicity

Dogs respond similarly to humans; symptoms may include drowsiness, ataxia, vomiting, respiratory depression, miosis, coma, and hypotension. Opiates and their derivatives have an excitatory effect on the CNS of cats and horses. Naloxone may be used at 0.02 mg/kg if needed.

—*Lisa Scheuring-Mroz*

Hydrofluoric Acid

- CAS: 7664-39-3
- SYNONYMS: Hydrogen fluoride; hydrofluoride
- CHEMICAL STRUCTURE: HF

Uses

Hydrogen fluoride is used in fluorocarbons, fluoropolymers, aluminum production, stainless steel pickling, uranium processing, glass etching, oil well acidizing, and gasoline production.

Exposure Pathways

Accidental dermal exposure is the most common route for humans.

Toxicokinetics

Hydrofluoric acid rapidly corrodes and penetrates the skin and/or mucous membranes. Fluoride ions are then readily absorbed but are rapidly almost completely bound to available calcium and magnesium ions. The resulting salts are excreted.

Mechanisms of Toxicity

Hydrogen fluoride is toxic by ingestion, inhalation, and (most commonly) by dermal exposure. It is highly corrosive to the skin and mucous membranes with very short (5 sec or less) exposures at concentrations of 0.003% and above. It causes a liquefying necrosis at the site of contact. Absorption of fluoride ions leads to systemic fluoride poisoning, in turn leading to hypokalemia and hypomagnesemia potentially resulting in neuromuscular paralysis and cardiac arthemyias.

Human Toxicity

The ACGIH TLV ceiling for inhalation exposure is 3 ppm. Hydrofluoric acid is highly corrosive and can cause systemic fluoride poisoning with neuromuscular paralysis (tetany).

Clinical Management

If the exposure is to the skin, all clothing should be removed from the affected region. The region should be copiously irrigated with water and then treated with a calcium gluconate paste. For exposure by any route, a 10% solution of calcium gluconate should be slowly infused (intravenously) to a total of 0.5 ml/kg.

Animal Toxicity

The inhalation LC_{50} is 1276 ppm in rats and 342 ppm in mice. The intraperitoneal LD_{Lo} in rats is 25 mg/kg. It is very corrosive to the skin, mucous membranes, and eyes.

—*Shayne C. Gad*

Related Topics

Acids
Corrosives

Hydrogen Peroxide

- CAS: 7722-84-1
- SYNONYMS: Albone; carbamide peroxide; hydrogen dioxide; hydroperite; hydroperoxide; inhibine; perhydrol; peroxan; urea hydrogen peroxide; urea peroxide
- PHARMACEUTICAL CLASS: Antiinfective, topical antiseptic, cleansing agent
- MOLECULAR FORMULA: H_2O_2

Uses

Dilute concentrations of hydrogen peroxide are used as an antiseptic. It is also effective in loosening cerumen that occludes the auditory canal. Industrial-strength (35%) food-grade hydrogen peroxide is being sold and promoted by health food outlets for use in "hyperoxygenation therapy."

Exposure Pathways

Ingestion is the most common route of exposure. Hydrogen peroxide is absorbed orally and via inhalation, dermal, or ocular contact or instillation into body cavities.

Toxicokinetics

Following exposure, absorption is rapid.

Mechanism of Toxicity

Hydrogen peroxide is an oxidizing agent that liberates oxygen upon application to tissue. The effects last only as long as the oxygen is being released and are of short duration. For each volume of 3% solution, 10 volumes of oxygen are released. The major toxic effect of ingestion of concentrated hydrogen peroxide is rupture of the colon secondary to liberation of oxygen. Corneal exposure to industrial-strength (>10%) solution can result in delayed corneal ulcerations. Delayed pulmonary edema has occurred after inhalation of concentrated formulations.

Human Toxicity

Household Strength (3%)

Ingestion of small amounts may cause mild irritation to mucosal tissue causing spontaneous vomiting. However, most exposures are not associated with any adverse sequelae. Gastric distention and possible rupture of the colon secondary to the release of oxygen are possible but rare. Eye exposure results in immediate pain but severe eye injury is rare. Dermal exposure causes a white discoloration to the skin lasting 2 or 3 hr. Ulcerative colitis has occurred after administration of dilute hydrogen peroxide enemas.

Industrial Strength (>10%)

Exposures are corrosive causing burns to the mouth, throat, esophagus, stomach, cornea, and skin. Ingestions of even small amounts of solutions containing >30% hydrogen peroxide have resulted in death. Complications include seizures, ruptured colon, gas embolization, and respiratory failure. Death can occur rapidly from apnea resulting from mechanical asphyxia.

Inhalation of large amounts of hydrogen peroxide causes pulmonary irritation and has resulted in respiratory arrest.

Chronic Toxicity

Interstitial lung disease was associated with chronic exposure to aerosol hydrogen peroxide concentrations of 41 mg/m^3 (the upper regulatory limit is 1.5 mg/m^3 in the workplace). Chronic use of hydrogen peroxide as a mouthwash may cause hypertrophy of the papillae of the tongue.

Clinical Management

Ingestion

Following exposure to dilute hydrogen peroxide, dilution or irrigation with water is usually the only treatment necessary. Exposure to concentrated solutions (>10%) requires rapid and extensive treatment. Dilute with 8 oz of fluid in adults and 4 oz in children. Excessive fluid intake may cause vomiting. Syrup of ipecac should be avoided due to the potential for burns and/or seizures. Transportation to a medical facility is mandatory. The patient should be monitored for dyspnea or seizures. Diazepam, phenytoin, or phenobarbital can be used for seizures. An initial ear–nose–throat exam is necessary with a follow-up esophagoscopy within the first 24 hr. The use of hyperbaric oxygen has been used in cases of severe gas emboli in patients with respiratory compromise or central nervous system symptoms.

Inhalation

The patient should be moved to fresh air and monitored for respiratory distress. Humidified supplemental oxygen (100%) should be administered with assisted ventilation if dictated by symptoms.

Eye Exposure

The eye(s) should be irrigated with copious amounts of tepid water for at least 15 min. If symptoms persist an ophthalmology exam is indicated.

Dermal Exposure

The exposed area should be irrigated with tepid water for at least 15 min. This area should be washed with soap and water. If irritation or pain persists a medical exam is necessary.

Animal Toxicity

Small amounts of hydrogen peroxide (3% solution) may be used to induce vomiting in companion animals (such as dogs) that have ingested poisons and need gastric decontamination.

—*C. Lynn Humbertson*

Hydrogen Sulfide

- CAS: 7783-06-4
- SYNONYMS: Sulfur hydride; dihydrogen sulfide; hydrosulfuric acid; stink damp; sewer gas
- MOLECULAR FORMULA: H_2S
- CHEMICAL STRUCTURE:

H : S : H

Uses

Hydrogen sulfide is formed naturally and is commonly found in petroleum deposits, volcanic gases, natural sulfur springs, natural gas deposits, and anywhere organic matter is decaying (e.g., manure and sewage). It may be produced when sulfide or sulfuric acid is used in mixtures or in tanning, glue making, metal recovery, and rubber vulcanizing. It may be released to the environment during leather production and production of heavy water for nuclear reactors. Hydrogen sulfide is used as a reagent in analytical chemistry.

Exposure Pathways

Hydrogen sulfide is a colorless gas and most human exposures occur via inhalation. However, exposure may also occur via ingestion or skin contact. It may be released in the body after ingestion of soluble inorganic sulfide salts. Soluble salts have been used experimentally to evaluate exposure to hydrogen sulfide and have been administered by injection in laboratory animals.

Average ambient air background levels are low and range from 0.001 to 0.092 mg/m^3 in the locations that have been studied.

Toxicokinetics

Hydrogen sulfide gas is quickly absorbed through the lungs. Absorption through the skin is limited, but does occur. Sulfides may be oxidized by nonenzymatic or enzymatic mechanisms. Hydrogen sulfide may spontaneously oxidize to the sulfate of thiosulfate once in the body. Thiosulfate can bind methemoglobin and form sulfmethemoglobin, which autooxidizes. Hydrogen sulfide may also be metabolized by reacting with disulfide and/or metal containing proteins or reacting with oxygen to produce sulfate. The liver and kidneys contain a sulfide oxidizing system.

Most hydrogen sulfide is eliminated from the body in the urine as sulfate after oral exposure. Some may be excreted in the volatile form through the lung. The amount excreted by a particular route (e.g., in the urine and through the lung) is influenced by the route through which exposure occurred.

Mechanism of Toxicity

Systemic effects are caused by changes that occur at the cellular level. Hydrogen sulfide inhibits cellular (mitochondrial) respiration. It binds proteins that are important to mitochondrial electron transport (cytochrome aa and cytochrome oxidase) and inhibits the conversion of molecular oxygen to water and the generation of adenosine triphosphate (ATP). ATP provides the energy required for many cellular functions. The mechanism of toxicity is similar to that of cyanide (see Cyanide).

Inhibition of respiration on the cellular level inhibits cellular function. Systems in the body with the highest oxygen demand are most vulnerable to its effects. These include the central nervous system, particularly the area that controls breathing, and the heart. High-level acute exposure may cause death due to a depressant effect on the respiratory center in the brain (which controls breathing).

Chemoreceptors in the carotid body (small body of vascular tissue that is sensitive to changes in the concentration of oxygen in the blood) are believed to be responsive to sulfide in the blood and react to cause changes in breathing (rapid and/or deep breathing), respiratory depression, and apnea (transient cessation of breathing).

Human Toxicity

Hydrogen sulfide is a highly toxic gas. Adverse effects may occur at the site of contact (e.g., lungs, eyes, and skin) or systemically. It is a local irritant at low concentrations and may be irritating to all contact surfaces (eyes, skin, and respiratory tract). Contact with the vapor may cause irritation and /or conjunctivitis to the eyes (gas eye). Prolonged or high-level exposure may cause more serious local effects (e.g., pulmonary edema).

Systemic effects are serious and can be life threatening. Signs and symptoms of exposure also may include headaches, fatigue, dizziness, confusion, cardiac effects (e.g., tachycardia and bradycardia), cough, respiratory depression, nausea, cyanosis, and shortness of breath. Symptoms may progress to include pulmonary edema, apnea, seizures, coma, and death.

The likelihood of adverse effects due to exposure to hydrogen sulfide depends on (1) the concentration in the air, (2) how long the individual is exposed, and (3) the individual's sensitivity to the effects of the chemical. For example, an individual with lung disease (e.g., emphysema or asthma) may exhibit certain symptoms before a healthy individual. Certain effects have been observed after exposure to hydrogen sulfide at different ranges of concentrations. Generally, the shorter the duration of exposure, the higher the concentration associated with effects.

Exposure to high concentrations (1000–2000 ppm or greater; "knockdown concentration") paralyzes the respiratory center; breathing may stop and collapse and death can occur within seconds. Exposure to 700 ppm can be rapidly fatal. Pulmonary edema can occur after short-term exposure to 250–600 ppm. Prolonged exposure to 50 ppm has also been associated with pulmonary edema. Eye and respiratory tract irritation has been observed after exposure to a wide range of concentrations (50–500 ppm).

The sense of smell may be lost shortly after exposure to atmospheres ranging from 50 to 150 ppm. Exposure to 14–25 ppm may cause burning eyes, headache, loss of appetite, weight loss, and dizziness. Conjunctivitis (eye irritation) has been reported after exposure to atmospheres containing 10–14 ppm hydrogen sulfide.

Hydrogen sulfide from an industrial source was released intermittently in the City of Terre Haute, Indiana, over a period of 2 months. Ambient air concentrations were reported to range from 0.002 to 8 ppm. During that time, residents (total of 27) complained of nausea, headache, shortness of breath, sleep disturbance, and throat and eye irritation.

Hydrogen sulfide has a strong odor resembling rotten eggs. There is a wide range in the reported odor thresholds in air. ACGIH reported a geometric mean as 0.0045 ppm and an accepted value range from 0.001 to 0.13 ppm for those studies it had reviewed. Odor does not provide a reliable warning of overexposure. The sense of smell becomes rapidly fatigued and cannot be relied on to warn of the continuous presence of hydrogen sulfide. Loss of sense of smell has been observed to occur after exposure to atmospheres containing between 50 and 150 ppm hydrogen sulfide.

Different agencies have developed exposure criteria for hydrogen sulfide (summarized in Table H-1). Criteria is usually developed based on prevention of an effect that occurs at low doses which should then prevent the occurrence of other more serious effects known to occur at higher doses. U.S. EPA's chronic reference concentration of 9E-4 mg/m^3 (0.645 ppb) was set to prevent inflammation of the nasal mucosa in the general population over a lifetime exposure. The OSHA PEL Ceiling of 20 ppm with a 50 ppm for a maximum of 10 min was set to protect workers against risk of "eye irritation and conjunctivitis." The ACGIH TLV is 14 mg/m^3, with a STEL of 21 mg/m^3.

Clinical Management

The victim should be removed to fresh air and away from the source of exposure. Caution should be exercised by the rescuers as high concentrations of hydrogen sulfide can kill within seconds. Oxygen should be provided if there is respiratory distress. Providing life sup-

TABLE H-1
Summary of Exposure Criteria Commonly Used for Hydrogen Sulfide

Agency	*Criteria (ppm)*		*Averaging time*
U.S. EPA	RfC	0.006, 45	24 hr a day for a lifetime
OSHA	Ceiling	20	NA
OSHA	Maximum peak	50	10-min maximum peak
NIOSH	Ceiling	10	10 min
NIOSH	IDLH	100	NA
ACGIH	TLV TWA	10	8 hr over a lifetime of work
ACGIH	STEL	15	15 min
ACGIH	EPRG 1	100	1 hr
ACGIH	EPRG 2	30	1 hr
ACGIH	EPRG 3	0.1	1 hr
NRC	EEGL	50	10 min
NRC	EEGL	10	24 hr
NRC	CEGL	1	90 days

Abbreviations used; NA, not applicable or not available; U.S. EPA, United States Environmental Protection Agency; RfC, reference concentration; NIOSH, National Institute for Occupational Safety and Health; OSHA, Occupational Safety and Health Act; ACGIH, American Congress of Governmental Industrial Hygienists; IDLH, Immediately Dangerous to Life and Health; EPRGs, Emergency Planning Response Guidelines; NRC, National Research Council; EEGL, Emergency and Continuous Guideline Levels; CEGL, Continuous Exposure Guidelines Levels.

port quickly may be critical to patient survival in certain cases. Administration of naloxone and dextrose may be indicated. For irritation, contaminated clothing should be removed and contaminated skin washed. Medical attention should be sought immediately for all symptomatic exposures. Patients who have had significant exposures should be closely monitored in the hospital.

Symptoms resemble those observed in cyanide poisoning and cyanide antidote kits may be useful for emergency treatment. Amyl nitrate by inhalation and intravenous sodium nitrite may be appropriate for certain patients.

In laboratory animals, inducing methemoglobinemia with nitrates provides protection (even antidotal properties) against sulfide poisoning because the hydrosulfied anion (HS-) can bind methemoglobin and form sulfmethemoglobin. This treatment has been used in some instances in humans.

Animal Toxicity

There is a fairly large body of animal data characterizing the toxicity of hydrogen sulfide. Studies have been conducted in monkeys, dogs, rabbits, mice, rats, and guinea pigs in which animals have been exposed via both inhalation and dermal contact. Inhalation studies have documented responses at different atmospheric concentrations over varying periods of time. Both local and systemic effects have been observed.

Monkeys exposed via inhalation to hydrogen sulfide at 504 ppm for various time periods exhibited eye irritation, changes in gray matter (brain tissue), necrosis in certain areas of the brain, moderate changes in the liver, hyperemia, ataxia, anorexia, sudden loss of consciousness, and cardiac arrest. Exposure to 20 ppm for 90 days was associated with weight loss and an increase of amylase and alkaline phosphatase in the blood.

Rats and mice exposed via inhalation to hydrogen sulfide at concentrations varying from 0.01 to 101 ppm for various time periods exhibited irritation of the respiratory tract, anorexia, reduced weight gain, weight loss, changes in the lung, nerve cell abnormalities, changes in certain blood cells (increase in reticulocytes and changes in the mean corpuscular volume), and death.

Rabbits exposed via inhalation to hydrogen sulfide at 72 ppm exhibited disturbed liver, brain, kidney metabolism, serum protein, enzyme and mineral changes, decreased myocardial enzymes, cardiac irregularities, and unconsciousness. Dermal exposure resulted in changes in blood chemistry.

Dogs exposed via inhalation to a range of concentrations of hydrogen sulfide from 100 to 1800 ppm exhibited effects ranging from local irritation to respiratory paralysis and immediate death.

—Betty J. Locey

Related Topics

Respiratory Tract
Sensory Organs

Hydroiodic Acid

- CAS: 10034-85-2
- SYNONYMS: Anhydrous hydroiodic acid; hydrogen iodide; hydrogen monoiodide
- CHEMICAL CLASS: Inorganic acid; corrosive
- CHEMICAL STRUCTURE:

H—I

Uses

Hydroiodic acid was formerly used as an expectorant in chronic bronchitis and bronchial asthma. It is used in the manufacture of disinfectants. It is also used for analytical purposes (e.g., as a chemical intermediate for inorganic iodides and organic synthesis.)

Exposure Pathways

Exposure may occur via ingestion, dermal or ocular contact, or inhalation.

Mechanism of Toxicity

Hydroiodic acid is a strong irritant. When used as an expectorant, hydroiodic acid is believed to act by irritating the gastric mucosa, which then stimulates respiratory tract secretion.

Human Toxicity

Inhalation of hydrogen iodide can cause irritation of the upper respiratory tract. A concentration of 35 ppm has been shown to cause irritation of the throat after short exposure. More severe exposures may result in pulmonary edema and laryngeal spasms. As with other acids, oral ingestion may produce oral and esophageal burns with more severe burns occurring in the stomach. Initial signs and symptoms may not reliably predict the extent of injury to the gastrointestinal tract. Tachycardia, hypotension, and circulatory collapse may occur as a result of the ingestion of concentrated corrosive iodine solutions. Severe burns may occur with dermal exposure. Systemic toxicity could result in acute hepatic injury. Repeated exposures to fumes may cause erosion of the teeth.

Clinical Management

In the case of inhalation exposure, the victim should be moved to fresh air. Trained personnel may administer oxygen and monitor the patient for signs of respiratory distress. Contaminated clothing and shoes should be removed and isolated. In the case of skin or eye contact, the skin or eyes should be flushed with running water for at least 15 min. Contact lenses should not be worn when working with this chemical. In the case of accidental ingestion, vomiting should not be induced. Bicarbonate should not be given to neutralize. From 4 to 8 oz of water or milk should be given to adults (2–4 oz to children) for dilution. The victim should be kept quiet and normal body temperature maintained.

Animal Toxicity

A toxicity study compared the toxicity to rat skin of hydrogen iodide, hydrogen bromide, and hydrogen chloride. Hydrogen bromide caused the most severe burns in the rats. No data are available on animal studies examining effects from inhalation or ingestion.

—Mary Lee Hultin

Related Topics

Acids
Corrosives

Hydromorphone

- CAS: 466-99-9
- SYNONYMS: 7,8-Dihydromorphinone; dihydromorphinone; 6-deoxy-7, 8-dihydro-6-oxomorphine; Dilaudid
- PHARMACEUTICAL CLASS: Semisynthetic opiate agonist
- CHEMICAL STRUCTURE:

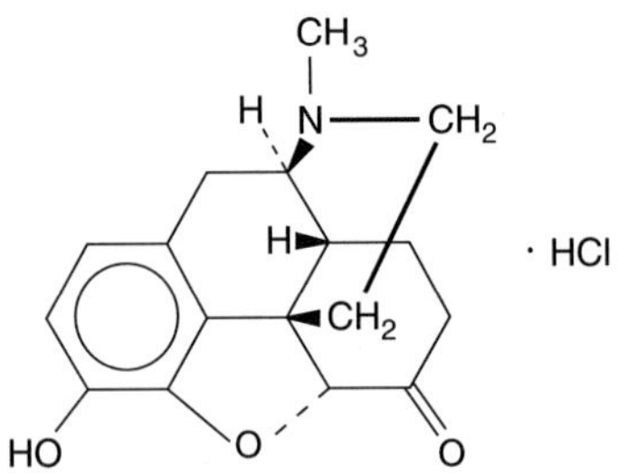

Uses

Hydromorphone is used as an analgesic for moderate to severe pain and as an antitussive. It is also a drug of abuse.

Exposure Pathways

Hydromorphone is available commercially as hydrochloride salt. It is available in oral, parenteral, and rectal forms.

Toxicokinetics

Hydromorphone is well absorbed following oral, rectal, and parenteral administration. It is incompletely absorbed from the gastrointestinal tract with a 62% bioavailability compared to intravenous administration. Peak plasma levels occur within 1.5–2 hr after oral administration and within 0.5–1 hr after intramuscular administration. The duration of action is approximately 4 or 5 hr. Hydromorphone is metabolized primarily in the liver, where it undergoes conjugation with glucuronic acid. Identified metabolites are conjugated hydromorphone, conjugated 6-α-hydroxyhydromorphone, and conjugated 6-β-hydroxyhydromorphone. The volume of distribution following intravenous administration is 1.22 liters/kg. After intravenous administration, hydromorphone has biphasic distribution: an α phase of 1.27 min followed by a β distribution phase life of 14.7 min. Hydromorphone is excreted primarily in the urine as the glucuronide conjugate. The elimination half-life of the parent compound is 1.5–4 hr.

Mechanism of Toxicity

Hydromorphone is a morphine derivative and approximately seven or eight times as potent as morphine on a milligram-to-milligram basis. As an opiate agonist, it exerts its effects by acting centrally on the central nervous system (CNS). Hydromorphone's interaction with opiate receptors causes the majority of its effects. The three main types of receptors are μ, κ, and δ. Stimulation of these receptors yields respiratory depression, miosis, reduced gastrointestinal motility, analgesia, euphoria, and sedation.

Human Toxicity: Acute

The incidence of adverse effects from hydromorphone is greater than that of other opiate agonists such as morphine, methadone, and codeine. Symptoms can occur with therapeutic use and with abuse. A typical overdose victim presents with extreme somnolence and skeletal muscle flaccidity. This can then progress to stupor or coma. Miosis is usually present unless the individual is acidotic or hypoxic. Life-threatening respiratory depression occurs, which can progress to apnea or respiratory arrest. Pulmonary edema may be a complication. Bradycardia and hypotension may occur if there is a decrease in sympathetic tone. Hypothermia may also occur as a result of peripheral vasodilation. Hydromorphone levels are not clinically useful but can confirm usage. A radioimmunoassay of hydromorphone in human plasma is available. It can quantify hydromorphone in the 2.5–20 ng/ml range with minimum sensitivity at 1.0 ng/ml. Hydromorphone can be qualitatively detected in the urine.

Human Toxicity: Chronic

Opiates have a high potential for abuse. Chronic users may develop tolerance, thus necessitating larger doses for the desired effect. Toxic effects in chronic abuse can yield a decrease in immunity leading to frequent infections and possibly AIDS. Abrupt cessation can cause withdrawal with such symptoms as restlessness, insomnia, hypertension, tachypnea, tachycardia, vomiting, and diarrhea.

Clinical Management

Basic life-support measures should be instituted as necessary. Intensive support therapy may be required to correct respiratory failure and shock. Respirations must be supported and monitored until all symptoms disappear. Pulmonary edema should be managed with appropriate ventilatory support. If taken orally, gastrointestinal decontamination should be based on the patient's level of consciousness or decrease in gag reflex. Activated charcoal may be used to adsorb the hydromorphone. A cathartic may be given to enhance elimination of the activated charcoal–hydromorphone complex. The specific antagonist naloxone is used to counteract respiratory depression and coma. A dose of 0.4–2.0 mg is given intravenously and can be repeated at intervals of 2 or 3 min. The therapeutic effect of naloxone may be of shorter duration than that of the opiate activity; therefore, a naloxone continuous infusion may then be of benefit. Arterial blood gases, vital signs, and level of consciousness should be monitored continuously until cessation of symptoms.

Animal Toxicity

Dogs act similarly to humans—symptoms may include drowsiness, ataxia, vomiting, respiratory depression, miosis, coma, and hypotension. Opiates and their derivatives have an excitatory effect on the CNS of cats and horses. Naloxone may be used at 0.02 mg/kg if needed.

—*Lisa Scheuring-Mroz*

Hydroperoxides, Organic

- Representative Compound: *tert*-Butyl hydroperoxide (CAS: 75-91-2)
- Synonyms: 2-Hydroperoxy-2-methylpropane; 1,1-dimethylethyl; TBH
- Chemical Class: Peroxides
- Chemical Structure:

```
       H   H
HO—O—C—C—CH3
       H   H
```

Uses

tert-Butyl hydroperoxide is used as a polymerization initiators.

Exposure Pathways

Dermal contact and inhalation are routes of exposure.

Toxicokinetics

tert-Butyl hydroperoxide oxidizes human erythrocyte glutathione with a half-life of 4.5 sec at 37°C.

Mechanism of Toxicity

tert-Butyl hydroperoxide is soluble in water, ethanol, ether, and chloroform. It accelerates oxidation of glutathione and decreases the metabolism of sodium hexabarbitol in rat livers.

Human Toxicity

tert-Butyl hydroperoxide is a mutagen and irritant. It causes eye and skin irritations.

Clinical Management

Respiratory therapy should be administered to exposed individuals. Contaminated clothing should be removed. Exposed skin should be washed with soap and water. Exposed eyes should be flushed with water for at least 15 min.

Animal Toxicity

tert-Butyl hydroperoxide is a mutagen and teratogen. It produced lethal birth defects and TBH-positive offspring. In rabbits, it produced sever skin irritation at 500 mg and eye irritation with a 150-mg rinse.

—*Shayne C. Gad and Jayne E. Ash*

Hydroxylamine

- CAS: 7803-49-8
- Synonym: Oxammonium
- Chemical Class: Reducing agent
- Molecular Formula: NH_2OH
- Chemical Structure:

H—NH—OH

Uses
Hydroxylamine is used as a reducing agent in photography and industrial chemistry. Salts are used in the production of nylon and in other industrial chemical synthesis.

Exposure Pathways
Routes of exposure include dermal contact, inhalation, and (potentially) ingestion. Most extensive exposure is occupational, in industry.

Mechanism of Toxicity
Hydroxylamine acts as a reducing agent when absorbed systemically, producing methemoglobin and the formation of Heinz bodies in the blood. It can induce hemolytic anemia. It inhibits platelet aggregation and is a "nitric oxide" vasodilator.

Human Toxicity
Hydroxylamine produces methemoglobin when systemically absorbed, potentially resulting in cyanosis, convulsions, hypotension, and coma. It is a marked irritant to skin and mucous membranes. Long-term exposures at lower levels can induce hemolytic anemia. It is a dermal and pulmonary sensitizer.

Clinical Management
Treatment consists of administration of methylene blue (1% solution), 0.1 ml/kg intravenously over a 10-min period.

Animal Toxicity
Hydroxylamine is a positive dermal sensitizer in guinea pigs and mice. The intraperitoneal LD_{50} is 60 mg/kg in mice and 59 mg/kg in rats. Hydroxylamine is a strong dermal and ocular irritant. It is reported to be a teratogen in rabbits but not in rats. It is an *in vitro* mutagen in most test systems.

—*Shayne C. Gad*

Hymenoptera

◆ SYNONYMS: Bees; wasps; ants

Exposure Pathways
Hymenoptera envenomation results from the subcutaneous injection of venom via a stinging or biting apparatus.

Mechanism of Toxicity
Hymenoptera venom components differ among bees, wasps, and ants. Honeybee venom includes phospholipase A, hyaluronidase, and various other allergens. Local skin reactions occur as a result of endogenous inflammatory response to the injected foreign proteins and enzymes. Multiple stings or bites can result in a generalized systemic reaction. Following multiple stings, large amounts of injected venom may cause the release of vasoactive substances, which can lead to hypotension and shock. Allergic (anaphylactic) reactions occur as a result of antibody production from a previous sensitization (bite or sting). The resulting IgE-mediated reaction triggers the release of such vasoactive substances as histamine and leukotrienes.

Human Toxicity
Clinical manifestations following a bite or sting can be classified into three groups. The first and most common reaction is a mild local tissue reaction characterized by slight swelling, redness, itching, and pain at the site of the bite or sting. The second involves a systemic reaction resulting from multiple bites or stings (typically ≥50–100). Symptoms may include nausea, vomiting, headache, and loss of consciousness. Renal failure and seizures are rare but have been documented. Lastly, allergic reactions may develop as a result of an individual's sensitization from a prior sting. This may range from a simple urticarial reaction to anaphylaxis. The latter is characterized by laryngeal edema, bronchospasm, difficulty breathing, wheezing, hypotension, cardiovascular collapse, and death. Anaphylactic reactions may occur within 15 to 30 minutes of a sting. Although unrelated to toxicity, any bite or sting may result in local infection.

Clinical Management

Basic and advanced clinical life support may be required for those individuals exhibiting anaphylactic reactions following a bite or sting. Honeybees possess barbed stingers which remain imbedded in the skin along with the venom sac. Following a bee sting, the stinger should be removed using a stiff card (e.g., credit card) scraped across the skin at an angle. Do not grasp the stinger since doing so will contract the attached venom sac and force more venom into the skin. Nonallergic local reactions following small numbers of bites or stings can generally be managed outside of the hospital setting. The home remedy of applying meat tenderizer to the sting site is not effective. The enzyme, papain, is not absorbed into the skin and, therefore, cannot inactivate the venom. Best results are obtained by washing the site well with soap and water, applying an iodine- or alcohol-based disinfectant locally, and using a cold compress to decrease swelling and pain. Antihistamines may help relieve itching and swelling. Stings to the throat have occurred during the process of accidentally swallowing a bee or wasp that had fallen into a soft drink. Swelling of the oropharynx occurred and impaired breathing. These cases represent a medical emergency and should be managed in a health care facility. Patients with multiple stings (50–100), those with a history of anaphylaxis, and those exhibiting an allergic reaction to a sting should be managed in an emergency department setting. Patients with multiple stings should be observed. Only supportive care and observation is required. Urticarial reactions may be managed with antihistamines with or without subcutaneous epinephrine depending on the severity of the reaction. Anaphylaxis must be treated promptly and aggressively. Intravenous fluids should be started immediately. Evaluate respiratory status and establish an airway with supplemental oxygen, if necessary. Subcutaneous epinephrine 1:1000 should be administered immediately. Intravenous diphenhydramine may be used but it is of secondary importance. A vasopressor is occasionally required in addition to intravenous fluids to manage hypotension.

—*Gary W. Everson*

Related Topics

Poisoning Emergencies in Humans
Scorpions
Snake, Crotalidae
Snake, Elapidae
Spider, Black Widow
Spider, Brown Recluse

Hypersensitivity, Delayed-Type

The immune response of lymphocytes *in vivo* to antigens can cause inflammatory reactions. Inflammation produced at 24–48 hr after challenge with antigen is called delayed-type hypersensitivity (DTH) and is a result of the immune response of T lymphocytes to antigen. Although antibody plays no role in DTH, antibody is responsible for inflammatory reactions produced immediately (anaphylactic) or within a few hours (Arthus) after an antigen challenge. In the skin, DTH reactions are characterized grossly by induration (hardening) and erythema and microscopically by the accumulation of large numbers of macrophages and lymphocytes. However, DTH reactions can occur in all tissues in the body where immune and inflammatory cells are present. The DTH inflammation is caused by the *in vivo* production and release of lymphokines by T lymphocytes stimulated by contact with antigen. Examples of lymphokines important in DTH are macrophage activating factor, interleukin-1, interleukin-2, tumor necrosis factor, and interferon. These lymphokines cause the accumulation and activation of large numbers of lymphocytes and monocytes–macrophages at the site of antigen exposure. Because only a small number of antigen-specific lymphocytes are present at any site (e.g., skin) at the time of antigen exposure, the accumulation and activation of a significant number of macrophages at the site is gradual and requires 1 or more days.

DTH is produced mainly to infectious agents (e.g., tuberculosis, leprosy, leishmaniasis, and fungal infections). Although the cellular immunity causing DTH can be protective, frequently the enzymes and mediators produced by macrophages in DTH immunity damage infected tissues without removal of the infectious agent. The tissue damage is apparently caused by chronic antigenic exposure from the persistence of these infectious agents. Clinically, skin tests are used to measure DTH to infectious agents that cause disease. For example, in tuberculosis, immunity to the tubercle bacillus can be tested by an intradermal injection of tuberculin or purified protein derivative.

In addition to infectious agents, DTH can also be produced to chemicals, foods, and other sensitizing agents. Contact dermatitis can be induced by topically applied drugs (e.g., neomycin, diphenhydramine, chloramphenicol, benzocaine, and sulfonamides) and other chemicals (e.g., nickel and dinitrochlorobenzene). Poison ivy, poison oak, and primula are examples of plant materials that cause DTH reactions. The small molecular weights of these sensitizing agents allow them to penetrate the skin, where they bind proteins either covalently or noncovalently as haptens. These hapten–protein conjugates then sensitize, and reexposure results in DTH.

Further Reading

Gallin, J. I. (1993). Inflammation. In *Fundamental Immunology* (W. E. Paul, Ed.), pp. 1015–1032. Raven Press, New York.

Plaut, M., and Zimmerman, M. (1993). Allergy and mechanisms of hypersensitivity. In *Fundamental Immunology* (W. E. Paul, Ed.), pp. 1399–1425. Raven Press, New York.

Roitt, I. M., Brostoff, J., and Male, D. K. (1985). Hypersensitivity–Type IV. In *Immunology*, pp. 22.1–22.10. Mosby, St. Louis.

Turk, J. L. (1980). Delayed hypersensitivity. In *Research Monographs in Immunology*. Elsevier/North Holland, Amsterdam.

—*David E. Bice*

Related Topics

Immune System
Skin

Hypoglycemics, Oral

- Preferred Name: Sulfonylureas
- Synonyms:

First-generation sulfonylureas—acetohexamide, Dylmelor (CAS: 968-81-0); chlorpropamide, Diadenese (CAS: 94-20-2), Orinase (CAS: 64-77-7); tolazamide, Tolynase (CAS: 1156-19-0); tolbutamide

Second-generation sulfonylureas—glipizide, Glucotrol (CAS: 29094-61-9); glyburide (glibenclamide), Diabeta (CAS: 10238-21-8)

- Pharmaceutical Class: All sulfonylureas are arylsulfonylureas, with substitutions on the benzene and the urea groups producing the different drugs.
- Chemical Structure:

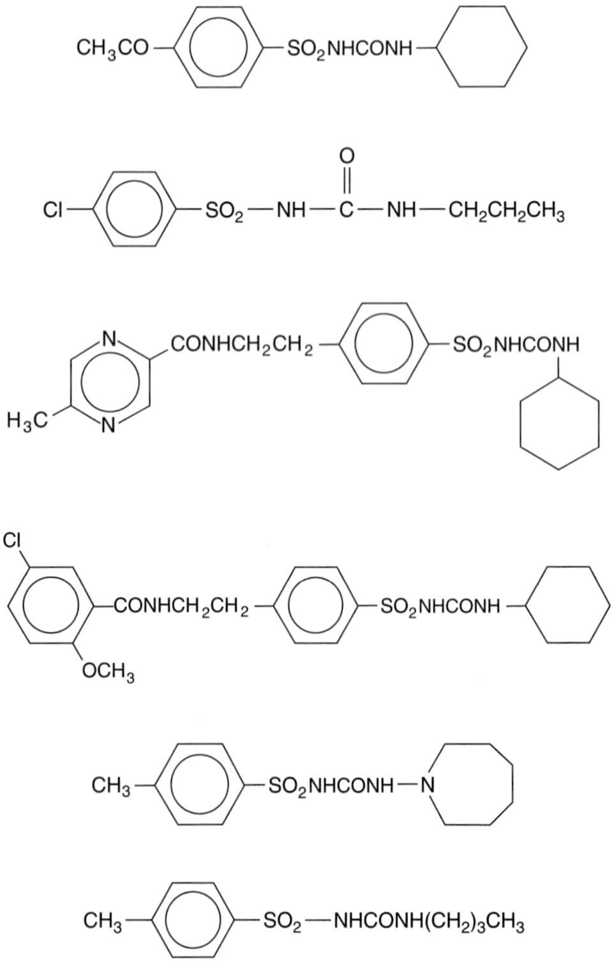

CH_3CO—(benzene)—$SO_2NHCONH$—(cyclohexane)

Cl—(benzene)—SO_2—NH—C(=O)—NH—$CH_2CH_2CH_3$

H_3C—(pyrazine)—$CONHCH_2CH_2$—(benzene)—$SO_2NHCONH$—(cyclohexane)

Cl, OCH_3—(benzene)—$CONHCH_2CH_2$—(benzene)—$SO_2NHCONH$—(cyclohexane)

CH_3—(benzene)—$SO_2NHCONH$—N(azepane)

CH_3—(benzene)—SO_2—$NHCONH(CH_2)_3CH_3$

Uses

Sulfonylureas are used in the treatment of non-insulin-dependent diabetes mellitus.

Exposure Pathways

All sulfonylureas are available as tablets only, with the exception of tolbutamide, which is available as tablets and a sterile solution for injection.

Toxicokinetics

Sulfonylureas are readily absorbed from the gastrointestinal tract with the exception of tolazemide, which is absorbed somewhat more slowly. Oral bioavailability of all sulfonylureas is complete. Peak plasma levels occur within a range of 1–8 hr. However, in overdose the duration of effect is a more important factor than onset of action. There is extensive biotransformation of sulfonylureas by the liver. Those with active metabolites are acetohexamide and chlorpropamide. Sulfonylureas are highly protein bound, from 92 to 99%, except for acetohexamide, which is 65–90%. Glyburide may accumulate in deep body compartments, allowing for later redistribution after withdrawal of the drug. Sulfonylureas are cleared primarily in the urine as metabolites. Glyburide is also cleared to a significant amount as the parent drug in the feces via biliary secretion. The half-lives of sulfonylureas are generally less important clinically than durations of action, which range from 8 to 72 hr.

Mechanism of Toxicity

Sulfonylureas cause a depolarization of the cell membrane of the β cells of the pancreatic islets by increasing calcium influx and increasing membrane permeability to potassium. This causes a release of preformed insulin into circulation.

Human Toxicity

The cascade of symptoms from sulfonylurea overdose reflect the patient's hypoglycemic state. Initially the patient may present with restlessness, diaphoresis, altered mental status, combative behavior, tremors, or confusion. An infant or small child may be difficult to feed. Nausea, vomiting, or abdominal pain may also occur. This will be followed by increasing central nervous system depression, seizures, and coma if the patient's blood glucose continues to fall. Most other effects reflect persistent hypoglycemia. In small children and poorly nourished patients, the onset of hypoglycemia may be sudden. In severe cases hypotension, tachycardia, and eventually cardiac arrest may occur. Hypokalemia may occur as serum potassium is shifted intracellularly along with glucose, during the persistent hyperinsulinemic state. Metabolic acidosis may also occur. A disulfiram-like reaction may occur with concomitant ethanol and sulfonylurea use.

Clinical Management

Basic and advanced life-support measures should be utilized as necessary. Gastrointestinal decontamination procedures should be used as deemed appropriate to the patient's level of consciousness and the history of the ingestion. Activated charcoal effectively binds sulfonylureas. The cornerstone of therapy is glucose replacement. Continuous intravenous 10% glucose in water via a peripheral line is usually sufficient. However, patients may require additional boluses of D50W to maintain an adequate blood glucose. Frequent blood glucose monitoring is recommended due to the prolonged effect of most sulfonylureas. Patients are at greatest risk during or after periods of fasting, such as sleep. Glucose therapy should be titrated to the patient's serial blood glucose measurements. Additional oral glucose via frequent snacks and meals will be helpful but usually not sufficient by themselves. In cases of persistent hypoglycemia unresponsive to glucose therapy, diazoxide may be helpful by altering calcium influx in the beta cell and, therefore, reducing insulin secretion. In adults, octreotide, a somatostatin analog, may be used at a rate of 30 ng/kg/min.

Animal Toxicity

Sulfonylureas are not routinely used in animals. Hypoglycemia, lethargy, and seizures can occur.

—Henry A. Spiller

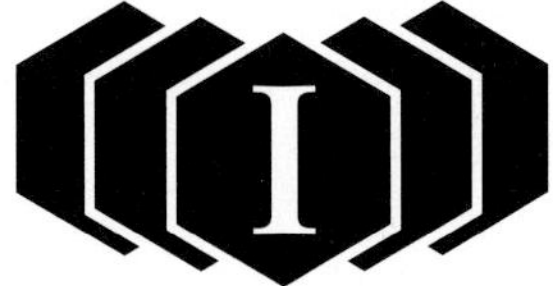

Ibuprofen

- CAS: 15687-27-1
- Synonyms: 2(4-Isobutylphenyl) propionic acid; 2-(*p*-isobutylphenyl) propionic acid; Motrin; Rufen; Midol 200; Motrin-IB; Advil; Nuprin; Medipren; Pamprin IB; Haltran; Profen
- Pharmaceutical Class: A substituted phenylalkanoic acid nonsteroidal antiinflammatory and analgesic agent
- Chemical Structure:

$(CH_3)_2CHCH_2-C_6H_4-CH(CH_3)COOH$

Uses

Ibuprofen is used for analgesic, antipyretic, and antiinflammatory purposes.

Exposure Pathways

Ibuprofen is available in tablet and liquid dosage forms. Ingestion is the most common route of both accidental and intentional exposure to ibuprofen.

Toxicokinetics

Ibuprofen is rapidly absorbed after ingestion, and peak concentrations in plasma are observed after 1 or 2 hr. The absorption half-life in plasma is approximately 2 hr. Ibuprofen is extensively metabolized, yielding four urinary metabolites formed by hydroxylation and by further oxidation of the primary alcohol to a carboxyl group. Ibuprofen is highly bound (99%) to plasma proteins. However, the drug occupies only a fraction of the total drug binding sites during therapeutic use. The volume of distribution approximates 0.11–0.19 liters/kg. Ibuprofen passes slowly into synovial spaces and may remain there in higher concentration as the concentrations in plasma decline. Ibuprofen has been demonstrated to pass easily across the placenta. The excretion of ibuprofen is rapid and complete. Approximately 90% of an ingested dose is excreted in the urine as metabolites or their conjugates, and 10% is eliminated as free drug. A single oral dose is completely excreted over 24 hr as the major metabolites, which are the hydroxylated and carboxylated compound.

Mechanism of Toxicity

The mechanism of ibuprofen-induced toxicity is obscure. Acute renal failure is postulated to result from decreased production of intrarenal prostaglandins. In turn, this will decrease the renal blood flow and glomerular filtration rate.

Human Toxicity: Acute

Ibuprofen overdoses generally do not appear to cause serious toxicity. Acutely, ibuprofen overdosage does not prolong the elimination half-life. Adults and children have ingested overdoses of ibuprofen that have resulted in blood concentrations 20 or more times greater than therapeutic levels with few adverse effects. In a 2-year survey undertaken to document ibuprofen-induced toxicity, 17 of 19 children (89%) ingesting up to 2.4 g of the drug remained asymptomatic and 13 of 23 adults (56%) ingesting 1.4–24 g were asymptomatic. Abdominal pain, nausea, vomiting, lethargy, and drowsiness are the most frequently reported symptoms. In rare instances of massive acute overdose, apnea, seizures, metabolic acidosis, renal failure, and coma have occurred.

Human Toxicity: Chronic

The chronic ingestion of excessive amounts of ibuprofen may produce similar toxicity but in a more insidious fashion.

Clinical Management

Treatment of acute overdoses of ibuprofen should consist of basic poison management and symptomatic supportive care. Ingestions of <100 mg/kg may be diluted with small quantities of milk or water to minimize gastrointestinal upset. Larger volumes of diluent may result in enhanced absorption of ibuprofen. Pediatric ingestions of 100–200 mg/kg require gastrointestinal decontamination via syrup of ipecac-induced emesis or activated charcoal as deemed appropriate by the child's level of consciousness and the history of the ingestion. Ingestions >200 mg/kg may require hospital evaluation and treatment. Children ingesting >400 mg/kg have the greatest risk for serious toxicity and require referral to a health care facility for assessment. Activated charcoal may be used to adsorb ibuprofen or concomitant ingestants. Serum ibuprofen levels are not readily available and do not influence patient management. The primary utility of the ibuprofen nomogram is to predict which initially asymptomatic patients are likely to remain so.

Animal Toxicity

Ibuprofen is not recommended for use in animals. Dogs appear to be exquisitely sensitive to the propionic acid group of nonsteroidal antiinflammatory drugs and easily develop gastric ulcers and renal failure.

—Bonnie S. Dean

Immune System

Introduction

The role of the immune system may be stated succinctly as the preservation of integrity. This system is charged with identifying that which is "self" and that which is "nonself." Examples of self are all the tissues, organs, and cells of the body. Examples of nonself are a variety of opportunistic pathogens, including bacteria and viruses, and transformed cells or tissues (i.e., tumors). The great complexity of the mammalian immune system is an indication of the importance, as well as the difficulty, of this task. If the immune system fails to recognize as nonself an infectious entity or the neoantigens expressed by a newly arisen tumor, then the host is in danger of rapidly succumbing to the unopposed invasion. This aspect of immunocompetence is the reason why the immune system is often made synonymous with "host defense." Alternatively, if some integral bodily tissue is not identified as self, then the immune system is capable of turning its considerable defensive capabilities against that tissue, and an autoimmune disease may be the end result. This aspect of immunocompetence emphasizes the tremendous destructive potential which is associated with the host defense mechanisms of the immune system. The cost to the host of these mistakes, made in either direction, may be quite high. The fact that mistakes can occur in either direction is discussed below as a continuum. Because the cost of mistakes in immunocompetence can be so high, and because of the tremendous diversity involved in the identification of self versus nonself, a complex array of organs, cells, soluble factors, and their interactions has evolved to regulate this system and minimize the frequency of errors in either direction.

Definition of Immunotoxicology

Studies in animals and humans have indicated that the immune system, like most organs, is a potential target organ, and that damage to this system can be associated with morbidity and even mortality. These studies coupled with tremendous advances in the science of immunology have caused an almost exponential growth in our understanding of immunotoxicology during the past 10 years. Immunotoxicology can be most simply defined as the study of adverse effects on the immune system resulting from occupational, inadvertent, or therapeutic exposure to drugs, environmental chemicals, and, in some instances, biological materials. Collectively, these agents are frequently referred to as xenobiotics, where "xeno-" means foreign and "-biotic" means anything affecting biology.

Adverse Effects

A critical component of this definition is the term "adverse." The need to determine whether an effect is adverse is what differentiates toxicology from other branches of biomedical science. Consequently, immunotoxicology is not merely the demonstration of treatment-related changes in a component of the immune system. Not all treatment-related changes are adverse. Some changes may be beneficial, some may be indifferent, and some are of unknown or uncertain consequence. It is inappropriate to declare an effect to be adverse simply because an adverse consequence cannot be ruled out. The long-term credibility of any scientific discipline depends on involved scientists being forthcoming when there is uncertainty, or when the effects have no known adverse consequence. Some have attempted to classify as adverse any effect which is undesired or unwanted. This definition of adverse effect is social or cultural in nature and has little scientific utility because social definitions may vary as a matter of individual preferences. The term adverse has been defined in classical toxicology as the undesired side effects of a drug, which are deleterious. This definition of an adverse effect differentiates between undesired (unwanted) effects that are deleterious and those that are not, thereby avoiding the quagmire associated with social definitions.

The evolution of immunotoxicology has been based in large part on the design and validation of critical experimental approaches to most clearly answer the question, Is an observed effect adverse or is it not? For the purposes of this entry, an adverse effect in immunotoxicology will be defined as a xenobiotic-induced change in the ability to perform an immune function. A suppression in immune functional ability would obviously be deleterious if the host were to encounter an opportunistic pathogen. As noted previously, an exaggerated immune response can also be deleterious. The utility of this definition is that it focuses attention on a specific functional ability. This definition does not explicitly address the issue of a xenobiotic-induced change in a structural component of the immune system, i.e., such as a change in the weight of an immune organ or a histopathological change in an immune organ. This omission is a deliberate one because a structural change without a concomitant change in a functional component would fall into the category of a treatment-related effect of unknown or uncertain consequence. As such, the demonstration of a treatment-related structural change in itself cannot be considered an adverse immunotoxicological effect.

Immunotoxicology as a Continuum

Because the primary role of the immune system is the discrimination of self versus nonself, immunotoxic effects can occur in either direction. As such, immunotoxicology can be thought of as a continuum, which is depicted as the solid dark vertical arrow in Fig. I-1. A xenobiotic-induced change in immunocompetence

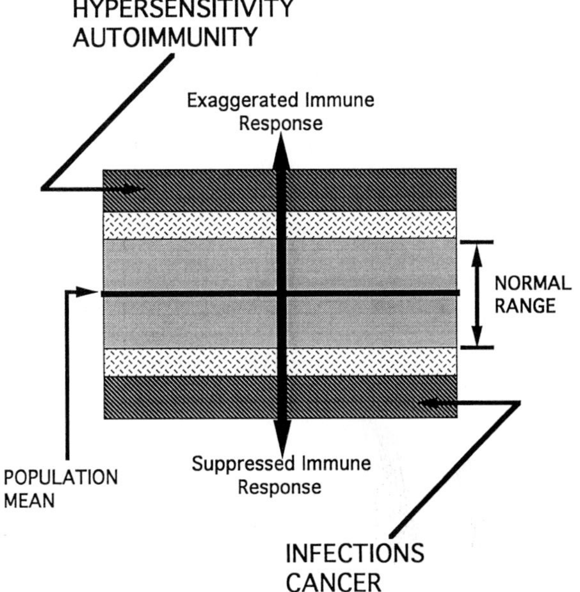

FIGURE I-1. Immunotoxicology is a continuum. There are adverse consequences associated with both suppressed and exaggerated immune responses.

from the normal range, which is manifest as an underactive immune system, is shown as a "suppressed immune response," while a xenobiotic-induced change manifested as an overactive immune system is shown as an "exaggerated immune response." The adverse (i.e., deleterious) consequences of suppressed immune function would reflect an inability to recognize nonself and are depicted as infections and cancer. The adverse consequences of exaggerated immune function would reflect an inability to recognize self and are depicted as hypersensitivity and autoimmunity. A hypersensitivity response is most simply defined as an acquired immune response which occurs in an exaggerated or inappropriate form, causing tissue damage. Autoimmune disease occurs when the reactions of the immune system are directed against the body's own tissues.

Treatment-related effects which are not clearly manifested as adverse are depicted in Fig. I-1 as the lightly shaded areas both above and below the normal range. The consequences of immunotoxicology are also described in greater detail in later sections of this entry. It is also important to emphasize that whether a treatment-related effect on the immune system is manifest as adverse or not in a given individual is dependent on where that individual is positioned in relationship to the normal range and the population mean. For example, an individual with a suppressed immune system, such as someone with the acquired immunodeficiency syndrome (AIDS) or any of a number of congenital immune deficiencies, could benefit by being exposed to a drug or chemical which causes immunostimulation. Similarly, an individual with an autoimmune disease can be treated therapeutically with an immunosuppressive drug. It is also important to note that it is routine to treat an individual scheduled for an organ/tissue transplant with an immunosuppressive drug. The goal of this therapy is to purposefully lower that individual's capacity to identify self versus nonself in order to decrease the chances that the transplant (i.e., an example of nonself) will be rejected. However, there are consequences associated with this treatment which are consistent with the continuum depicted in Fig. I-1.

Organization of the Immune System

The mammalian immune system is a complex system which is dependent on the integration of, and orchestrated cooperatively between, several organs, cells, and soluble factors. Components of the immune system are distributed throughout the body. An appreciation of the organization of the various components of the immune system is essential to understanding immunotoxicology. By knowing the role played by a given component of the immune system in host defense mechanisms, one can begin to understand the consequences of a xenobiotic-induced change in the function of that component.

Organs of the Immune System

The organs of the body which comprise the immune system and/or contribute to immune function include the bone marrow, spleen, thymus, lymph nodes, a network of lymphoid tissue along secretory surfaces (i.e., the so-called mucosa-associated lymphoid tissue or MALT), and the skin. Lymphoid organs can be classified in two ways. The first classification is based on the role that organs play in the development of the immune system and/or its ability to elicit a response.

Primary and Secondary Lymphoid Organs

Primary lymphoid organs are those organs in which the production of the cells of the immune system takes place. For example, bone marrow is a primary organ and contains a pluripotent stem cell which serves as the precursor to red blood cells (i.e., erythrocytes) and myeloid progenitors (which ultimately differentiate into granulocytes, mast cells, monocytes, and platelets), in addition to lymphoid progenitors (which ultimately differentiate into the various types of lymphocytes). Hematopoiesis is a general term used to refer to the production of the cells of the blood, and it can be subdivided into erythropoiesis, myelopoiesis, and lymphopoiesis, respectively, based on the cell lineages described previously. Lymphoid progenitors will emerge from the bone marrow and travel to other primary lymphoid organs where the final stages of lymphocyte maturation take place. As described later, mature lymphocytes play a major role in discriminating between self and nonself because they are endowed with surface receptors characterized by tremendous specificity. Lymphoid progenitors which receive their final education in the thymus are called thymus-derived lymphocytes or T cells. The other major subtype of lymphocyte is the B cell, so named because it was originally characterized in the chicken as a lymphoid progenitor which receives its final education in a primary lymphoid organ called the Bursa of Fabricious, an outpocketing of gastrointestinal epithelium. Although there is no Bursa in mammals, fetal liver, spleen, and adult bone marrow are considered the "bursal equivalents" and function as the primary lymphoid organs for the production of B cells. The process of lymphopoiesis takes place within specific regions of the thymus and bursal equivalents called microenvironments and is regulated by specialized cells (bone marrow stromal cells and thymic epithelial cells) and their soluble factors (including the interleukins IL-3, IL-7, IL-9, and IL-12; see Table I-1), which comprise the microenvironments. The stages of lymphopoiesis are generally believed to be antigen independent, where antigen is defined as any substance which can stimulate a specific immunological reaction. The surface receptors of lymphocytes, mentioned previously, are directed toward "antigen." Although lymphopoiesis is neither antigen dependent nor antigen driven, a role for antigen cannot be excluded because factors secreted during an antigen-specific reaction in the periphery can promote various forms of hematopoiesis in the bone marrow. Moreover, although antigen is not a driving force for lymphocyte development, the antigen receptors on the surface of lymphocytes play a critical role. Many immature lymphocytes have the potential to respond to self products and therefore pose a threat. During development, immature B cells in the bone marrow and immature T cells in the thymus will have an opportunity to interact with neighboring cells which express surface proteins indicative of self. These self proteins are encoded for by the major histocompatibility complex (MHC). If the antigen receptor on any lymphocyte binds too effectively to these MHC-derived proteins, then that cell will be eliminated. This process of negative selection is thought to be mediated by one of two possible mechanisms. Either this inappropriate recognition of self proteins triggers apoptosis, which is programmed cell death, and the lymphocytes are eliminated, or these cells become anergic, which is an induced lack of responsiveness to antigenic stimulation. This process of negative selection is not limited to self proteins obviously associated with the microenvironments of the bone marrow and thymus. Self proteins from different parts of the body are actually transported to these primary lymphoid organs to probe lymphocytes for reactivity against distant tissues.

Secondary lymphoid organs are those organs in which the antigen-dependent proliferation and differentiation of specific lymphocytes takes place. These organs are responsible for the dissemination of an antigen-specific immune response and include lymph nodes, spleen, and the various types of MALT, which are further defined below. An appreciation for the role that secondary lymphoid organs play in the immune system can be derived from the fact that swollen lymph nodes (i.e., as a consequence of the antigen-specific lymphoproliferation) are a hallmark indicator of certain types of infections.

Internal and External Lymphoid Organs

The second classification of lymphoid organs is based on their location, with some being classified as internal organs and others being classified as external organs. The internal lymphoid organs include the bone marrow, thymus, spleen, and some lymph nodes. The external lymphoid organs include all the components of MALT as well as the lymph nodes draining MALT. As indicated previously, MALT is defined as lymphoid tissue associated with mucosa. This tissue can be subdivided into more specific regions based on the anatomical location, and includes gut-associated lymphoid tissue (including Peyer's patches and the appendix) and bronchus-associated lymphoid tissue. The skin is another example of an external organ for which the contribution to the immune system is sometimes underappreciated. Although the skin does not contain organized lymphoid tissue, there are immune components associated with the skin that are interconnected with other immune organs, leading to the concept of the so-called skin-associated lymphoid tissue. An appreciation for the important role that skin plays as a "first line of defense" in the immune system can be derived from the fact that when this barrier is breached, as occurs following an abrasion and especially so after a severe burn, a serious consequence is an increase in the incidence and severity of infections.

The importance of this second classification of lymphoid organs is that the two locations behave somewhat independently in host defense. An immune response mediated primarily by internal lymphoid organs is generally referred to as a systemic immune reaction or systemic immunity, while an immune response mediated primarily by external lymphoid organs is generally

TABLE I-1
Cytokine Network

Cytokine	*Other names*	*Cell source*	*Cell target and actions*
Interferon-α (IFN-α)		Leukocytes	B cells: proliferation and differentiation NK cells: stimulates cytolytic activity T_C cells: increases generation APCs: increases MHC I and II expression Others: increases MHC I and FcR expression; induces antiviral state
IFN-β		Fibroblasts	Similar to IFN-α
IFN-γ		T_H cells	B cells: stimulates IgG2a synthesis and inhibits IL-4-induced IgE/IgG1 synthesis APCs: increases MHC I and II expression Macrophages (macs): activates cytolytic activity NK cells: stimulates cytolytic activity Others: increases MHC I expression; induces antiviral state
Interleukin 1 (IL-1)	Endogenous pyrogen	Monocytes/macs	T_H cells: stimulates production of lymphokines, especially IL-2 and expression of IL-2R B cells: proliferation and differentiation Macs: stimulates production of cytokines, IL-1, IL-6, and tumor necrosis factor-α (TNF-α) Brain: fever response
IL-2	T cell growth factor (GF)	T_H cells	T_H cells: stimulates proliferation and release of lymphokines (especially T_{H1} cells) B cells: proliferation and differentiation NK cells: activates
IL-3	Multicolony stimulating factor (CSF)	T_H cells	Bone marrow (BM): promotes growth of stem cells to granulocytes, macs, and mast cells
IL-4	BCGF; B cell stimulating factor (BSF)	T_H cells (B cells)	B cells: stimulates IgE and IgG1 production and increases MHC II expression T_H cells: promotes generation; synergizes with IL-2
IL-5	T cell replacing factor (TRF); BCGF II	T_H cells	B cells: proliferation and differentiation; stimulates IgA production
IL-6	IFN-β_2	T_H cells Monocytes Endothelial cells Fibroblasts	T cells: proliferation and differentiation B cells: proliferation and differentiation Others: similar profile of activity to IL-1; synergizes with IL-1
IL-7	Lymphopoietin	BM stroma	T cells: induces growth of immature cells B cells: induces growth of immature cells
IL-8	Neutrophil-activating factor (NAF)	Monocytes	Neutrophils: chemotaxis; granular exocytosis; respiratory burst
IL-9		T_H cells	BM: stimulates growth of erythroid and megakaryocyte precursors Others: promotes mast cell growth B cells: acts synergistically with IL-4 in production of IgE and IgG1
IL-10		T_H cells (B cells)	T_{H1} cells: inhibits lymphokine synthesis T_{H2} cells: promotes generation Monocytes: inhibits cytokine synthesis T_C cells: stimulates IL-2-dependent growth Mast cells: stimulates growth
IL-11		Fibroblasts BM stroma	BM: stimulates hematopoietic cell growth Others: stimulates T-dependent antibody response; resembles IL-6
IL-12	NK cell stimulatory factor (NKSF)	Monocytes/macs B cells	NK cells: activates cytotoxicity T_{H1} cells: stimulates proliferation and lymphokines production, especially IFN-γ T_{H2} cells: inhibits generation (negative feedback) T_C cells: activates; synergizes with IL-2

(*continues*)

TABLE I-1 (*Continued*)

Cytokine	*Other names*	*Cell source*	*Cell target and actions*
Lymphotoxin	Tumor necrosis factor-β (TNF-β)	T cells	Target cells: kills
Macrophage activating factor	MAF	T_D cells	Macs: activates cytotoxicity and proinflammatory actions
Macrophage inhibiting factor	MIF	T_D cells	Macs: inhibits migration
Transforming growth factor-β	TGF-β	Lymphocytes Macs	B cells: suppresses growth; inhibits IgM and IgG production; decreases MHC II expression T cells: suppresses growth Monocytes: inhibits TNF production; chemotaxis; induces IL-1 and IL-6 expression
Tumor necrosis factor-α	Cachectin (TNF-α)	Monocytes/macs	Tumor cells: cytotoxicity Others: similar profile of activity of IL-1; promotes antiviral state

referred to as a local immune reaction or local immunity. As will be described in greater detail, there are also differences in the specific effector functions associated with systemic and local immunity.

Cells of the Immune System

The most obvious example of a cellular component of the immune system is the lymphocyte and includes all the various subtypes of T and B cells. As indicated previously, the fundamental distinction of T cells versus B cells is based on the specific primary lymphoid organ in which the final stages of lymphopoiesis takes place. As described below, these cell types can also be distinguished based on their respective functions within the immune system as well as by phenotypic characteristics. For the purposes of this entry, a phenotype will be defined as a marker expressed on the surface of a cell which is genetically determined and which is frequently associated with the specific function of that cell. Other important examples of cellular components of the immune system include monocytes, macrophages, granulocytes, mast cells, and natural killer cells (NK cells). As with the lymphocytes, the specific functions of these cells as they relate to the immune system will be described in greater detail. Some of these cells are oftentimes found circulating in the blood. Examples of circulating cells include monocytes, granulocytes, and NK cells. Other cells important to the immune system are typically tissue bound and include mast cells and macrophages. Macrophages present in tissue constitute the mononuclear phagocytic system, which was formerly known as the reticuloendothelial system. Macrophages located in specific anatomical regions have been frequently given distinct names, including Kupffer cells (liver), Langerhan cells (skin), microglia (brain), osteoclasts (bone), follicular dendritic cells (B cell regions of lymphoid tissue), and interdigitiating dendritic cells (T cell regions of lymphoid tissue). The issue of whether a lymphocyte is circulating or noncirculating is a bit more complex than for most of the other cellular components of the immune system. The blood circulation contains only a minor part of the body's total lymphocyte count (estimated at about 1%), which is a relatively select population, the so-called recirculating lymphocyte pool. As such, an assessment of only the blood lymphocyte pool provides an incomplete inventory of the body's immune system as it relates to lymphocytes because it ignores the activities of the nonrecirculating cells. In general, the recirculating lymphocyte pool does not include cells that are in a state of activation, proliferation, or differentiation. As indicated previously, the dissemination of an antigen-specific reaction takes place in secondary lymphoid organs, especially lymph nodes. The lymphatic system represents a second circulatory system of conducting vessels (i.e., lymphatic capillaries and/or lymphatics), loose aggregates of lymphoid tissues (i.e., nodules), and more highly organized and structured organs (i.e., lymph nodes). Through this system passes lymph, a collection of tissue fluids rich in globulins and lymphocytes. As lymph passes through draining lymph nodes, it becomes progressively more enriched with lymphocytes. Lymphocytes within lymph can empty back into the blood circulation via the thoracic duct. After entry into the blood, these lymphocytes will eventually find their way into a lymph node, at which point they may either remain in the circulating blood or reenter the lymphatic circulation. Therefore, lymphocytes and their products are transported between lymphoid organs and throughout the body via the blood and the lymph. However, it is again important to emphasize that the percentage of the total lymphocyte count in the blood is normally very small.

Soluble Products of the Immune System

Soluble products also play an important role in the immune system and are oftentimes the primary mediator of a given effector function by the immune system. Some soluble products of the immune system are secreted by lymphocytes. For example, immunoglobulins (Igs) are secreted by B cells. It is important to emphasize that an antibody is an immunoglobulin molecule secreted by a B cell during an immune response that specifically reacts with the antigen. Therefore, "immunoglobulin" and "antibody" are distinct terms that are often used somewhat interchangeably as they pertain to effector functions by the immune system. A second example of a lymphocyte-derived soluble product is the variety of substances secreted by T cells called lymphokines. Although lymphokines have been described as being hormone-like, they are probably more analogous to neurotransmitters because of their very localized sites of action and because of the signal transduction pathways they trigger in responsive cells. Specific examples of lymphokines, including the interleukins, will be provided and are summarized in Table I-1. It is important to emphasize that lymphokines are a subgroup of a larger family of soluble factors secreted by a variety of cells, called cytokines, which can modulate immune function, and that both lymphokines and cytokines can affect cells, organs, and tissues outside of the immune system. Some soluble products are secreted by cells of the immune system other than lymphocytes. For example, monocytes/macrophages are also capable of secreting cytokines, which are sometimes referred to as monokines and which include some interleukins, such as IL-1, IL-6, IL-8, and IL-12, and other factors, such as tumor necrosis factor (TNF). Some soluble products with important roles in the immune system originate outside of the immune system. One example is interferon, which is actually a heterogenous family of proteins of two types. Type I or viral interferons are induced by infection and consists of interferon-α (IFN-α) and -IFN-β, which are secreted by leukocytes, and fibroblasts or epithelial cells, respectively. Type II or immune interferon, consists of IFN-γ, which is secreted by T cells (therefore, IFN-γ can be classified as a lymphokine) in response to specific antigens. A second example of a soluble product which originates outside of the immune system is complement, which is primarily produced in the liver. Complement is actually a group of about 20 proteins, including several proteases, that activate and split each other in sequential order. The specific functional roles played by complement and the other soluble products of the immune system will be discussed later

Immune Response

Innate versus Acquired Immunity

Foreign substances, including the various examples of nonself indicated in the introduction, can provoke two basic types of immune responses, innate (also called nonspecific) immunity and acquired (also called specific) immunity. One of the easiest ways to present and understand the functions of the various cells and soluble products of the immune system is in the context of these two types of immune responses, which each make significant contributions to host defense capability. The principal difference between these two types of immunity is the role of the antigen, which was defined previously as any substance which can trigger a specific immunological reaction. In this context, it is important to note that an antigenic determinant on the surface of a microbe or tumor cell is usually about 10 amino acids in size and can be made up of polypeptides, carbohydrates, or lipids, and that a given type of microbe or tumor cell can express several different types of antigens as well as multiple copies of a given antigen. Innate immunity is considered to be antigen independent and occurs without prior exposure to antigens. Acquired immunity is considered to be antigen dependent and comprises all of the specific immunological reactions alluded to in the definition of antigen. Acquired immunity can be subdivided into humoral immunity and cell-mediated immunity, which are described in greater detail later.

Because innate immunity can be triggered upon the initial encounter with a foreign substance, its components are oftentimes called the first lines of defense. As such, it is appropriate to consider the skin as a component of innate immunity. Similarly, the following bodily functions contribute to host defense and should be considered parts of innate immunity: the lysosomal enzymes found in salivary, lacrimal, and vaginal secretions, which have bacteriastatic properties; the cough reflex, which is an important mechanism to clear the bronchial passages of irritants and potential infectious microbes; and the fever response, which is an important reaction to an infection because of the limited temperature range for the growth of most bacteria.

More traditional components of the innate immune defense system include phagocytic cells such as neutrophils and macrophages, NK cells, and the soluble products, type I interferon and complement. Neutrophils and macrophages are the primary cells involved in inflammatory responses. Their contribution to innate immunity is based on their abilities to phagocytize (i.e., to engulf; literally the foreign particle becomes enclosed by the cell membrane of the phagocyte into a phagosome) and to kill bacteria. The latter mechanism is carried out either by the extracellular release of lysosomal enzymes, oxygen radicals, bactericidal proteins, and proteinases or by the intracellular fusion of phagosomes containing the microbes and lysosomes containing these destructive mediators. Phagocytic cells are attracted to the site of infection or inflammation, a process known as chemotaxis, by a number of factors including some complement components and some cytokines, which are discussed later. Moreover, microbial cells and other foreign particles are also capable of attracting the attention of phagocytic cells directly because of unique properties. For example, bacteria produce peptides with an unusual chemical structure beginning with formyl-methionine sequences that are produced in very small amounts by mammalian host tissue. Therefore, large amounts of formyl-mehtionine peptides will stimulate neutrophil chemotaxis and phagocytosis. A second example has been identified in macrophages which have receptors for sugars typically found on many microbial organisms, i.e., mannose, L-fructose, and galactose. The destructive capabilities of both macrophages and neutrophils can also be modulated by cytokines, primarily lymphokines produced by antigen-specific T cells, as discussed later

NK cells are leukocytes of lymphoid or myeloid origin with the ability to kill target cells without prior sensitization. NK cells require intimate contact with target cells before lysis can take place. One postulated mechanism for cytolysis involves the production and secretion of a cytolytic protein, perforin, which functions to produce transmembrane channels in the target cell and ultimately leads to porous membrane lesions and cell death. The mechanism for attachment by NK cells to their target cells is accomplished through an as yet poorly understood chemical means by which these cells seem to recognize certain viral or tumor-associated markers. As with the macrophage, the killing capability of NK cells can be modulated by T cell-derived lymphokines, most notably IFN-γ.

In addition to their ability to produce and release destructive inflammatory mediators, neutrophils and monocytes/macrophages can contribute to the innate immune response by the production and release of cytokines. The cell sources, targets, and actions for a number of cytokines are summarized in Table I-1. IL-1 has been the most studied interleukin because it was the first one to be discovered and because it triggers a wide variety of activities in several organ systems. For the purposes of this entry, the discussion will be limited to actions of IL-1 associated with the innate immune response which include the activation of neutrophils, macrophages, and NK cells; cytostatic and cytotoxic actions for some tumor cells; the induction of the fever response in the brain (IL-1 has been identified as the "endogenous pyrogen"); and the stimulation of some acute phase reactive proteins by the liver. IL-6 is produced by a number of different cell types and possesses a profile of activity similar to IL-1, including the following actions: an increase in the synthesis of the major acute phase reactive proteins by the liver and pyrogenic activity in the brain. IL-1 and IL-6 are known to act synergistically. IL-8 is produced by activated monocytes and macrophages and acts on neutrophils as a chemotactic factor and as a stimulus for enzyme release and an oxidative burst. IL-12 is also synthesized by monocytes/macrophages in response to bacteria or other parasites and acts on NK cells to activate them. TNF is produced predominantly by activated macrophages and it draws its name from the fact that it was originally isolated as a factor which was capable of triggering a hemorrhagic lesion in transplanted tumors.

However, the effects of TNF are now known to extend well beyond that original definition. For example, TNF produces many of the same actions that were identified for IL-1, and these two cytokines can act synergistically. TNF is also known as cachectin because of its association with the wasting syndrome (cachexia) characteristic of chronic diseases, including some malignancies. It is important to emphasize that IL-1, IL-6, IL-12, and TNF also have actions on lymphocytes, and these immunoregulating properties are discussed later. The fact that certain cytokines can contribute to both innate and acquired immunity is an indication of their interdependency. The fact that certain soluble products and cells contribute to multiple components of the immune system is also an indication of the overlapping nature of host defense capabilities, a concept which is sometimes referred to as the redundancy of the immune system.

As noted previously, interferon exists as two types, and it is the type I or viral interferons IFN-α and IFN-β, which are produced in an antigen-independent fashion, that contribute to the innate immune response. As with the phagocytic cells, the trigger for the production of type I interferon is a unique feature of the genetic makeup of viruses. Viruses make much greater quantities of double-stranded RNA than do mammalian cells, and the presence of large amounts of double-stranded RNA stimulates the production of viral interferon. Although the sources of IFN-α and IFN-β are different (i.e., leucocytes and fibroblasts or epithelial cells, respectively), their effector functions are similar and include the following actions: stimulation of NK cells, induction of antiviral activity, and cytostasis for some tumor cells.

Complement is not a single soluble factor but a carefully regulated system of about 20 functionally linked proteins. The linkage is provided by the facts that many complement proteins have protease activity, and that they interact in an ordered cascade, the so-called complement cascade. With several steps in the cascade, there is the cleavage of small-molecular-weight peptides, which possess most of the biological activities attributed to the complement system. A detailed description of this obviously complicated system is beyond the scope of this entry. Instead, two points will be emphasized, the mechanisms for activating the complement cascade and the biological activities of some of the products of the complement system. The latter point will be discussed as it relates to the relative contributions of innate versus acquired immunity to host defense. The classical activation of the complement cascade is triggered by immunoglobulin complexes with antigen and will be discussed in the following section. The alternative pathway of the complement cascade is triggered by nonimmune specific activators, most notably polysaccharides associated with the surface of some microbes. Although these two activational schemes differ in the way that nonself triggers the complement cascade, there are common mediators in the two pathways and the biological consequences of the complement components are similar. There are receptors for various components of complement (usually designated CR) located on both neutrophils and macrophages. Some complement peptides (most notably, activated C3b, C5a fragment, and the activated complex of C567) function as chemotactic factors for these inflammatory cells. Other complement peptides (most notably, activated C3b) will attach to the microbe and facilitate the adherence and subsequent phagocytosis of the microbe by neutrophils and macrophages, a process known as opsonization. Finally, the terminal product of the complement cascade, the activated complex of C6789, can form a lytic unit which can attack the cell membrane and directly kill the microorganisms by punching holes in their cell membrane. It is thought that most cells of the host are equipped with surface proteases that inactivate complement and protect them from cytolysis.

Humoral versus Cell-Mediated Immunity

Acquired immunity is antigen dependent and comprises all the specific immunological reactions associated with lymphocytes. In light of the existence of an antigen-specific defense system, a legitimate question becomes why we have such an elaborate nonspecific immune system. One of the primary reasons may be that an acquired immune response takes time. For example, 5 days are needed to generate a primary antibody response, and the body must rely on the innate immune system to hold the infection in check during this time. As noted previously, acquired immunity can be subdivided into two effector arms, humoral immunity and cell-mediated immunity. The "humor" (i.e., a bodily fluid) associated with humoral immunity is the secreted form of immunoglobulin in the blood. The "cells" associated with cell-mediated immunity are the various subpopulations of T cells.

Because immunoglobulin is the primary effector for humoral immunity, this component of the immune system is associated with the activities of antigen-specific B cells. The steps involved in an acquired immune response by B cells and the regulation of B cell activity are depicted in Fig. I-2 and described later. In this section, the emphasis will be on the specific contributions that immunoglobulin makes to the function of the immune system. The basic structure of the immunoglobulin or antibody molecule consists of four protein chains of two types—i.e., two identical light chains and two identical heavy chains. These protein subunits are linked in a fixed and precise orientation to form a "Y"-shaped molecule. The "forked" end of the antibody molecule contains two variable regions and is the site which recognizes and binds the specific antigen. To accommodate the many antigens that exist, these variable regions differ from antibody molecule to antibody molecule. Each type of antibody molecule is synthesized by a clone or family of identical antigen-specific B cells. The "closed" end of the antibody molecule is nearly identical among all antibodies and is called the constant region. Although the constant region of the antibody molecule is not involved in the specific binding of antigen, this component of the molecule is critical to the effector functions of immunoglobulin, as described later. The remaining feature of the immunoglobulin molecular structure that needs to be emphasized is that the heavy chains can vary in type, which gives rise to the various major classes of immunoglobulin, namely, IgM, IgG (there are four subclasses of IgG), IgE, IgA (there are two subclasses of IgA), and IgD. The existence of multiple types of Ig adds to the repertoire with which the humoral arm of acquired immunity can add to host defense, as discussed later. The different types of Ig also provide insights into the complexities associated with B cell biology. Surface Ig is the hallmark feature of the B cell and is one of the principal phenotypic markers used to identify and enumerate B cells. Surface Ig is also a "receptor" in the truest sense of the term. The ligand for this receptor is the antigen, and because of the molecular structure of Ig, this ligand–receptor (i.e., antigen–antibody) interaction is the driving force for the tremendous specificity associated with humoral immunity. It is important to emphasize that the cytoplasmic region of surface Ig contains only three amino acid residues, which makes it difficult, if not impossible, to ascribe signal transduc-

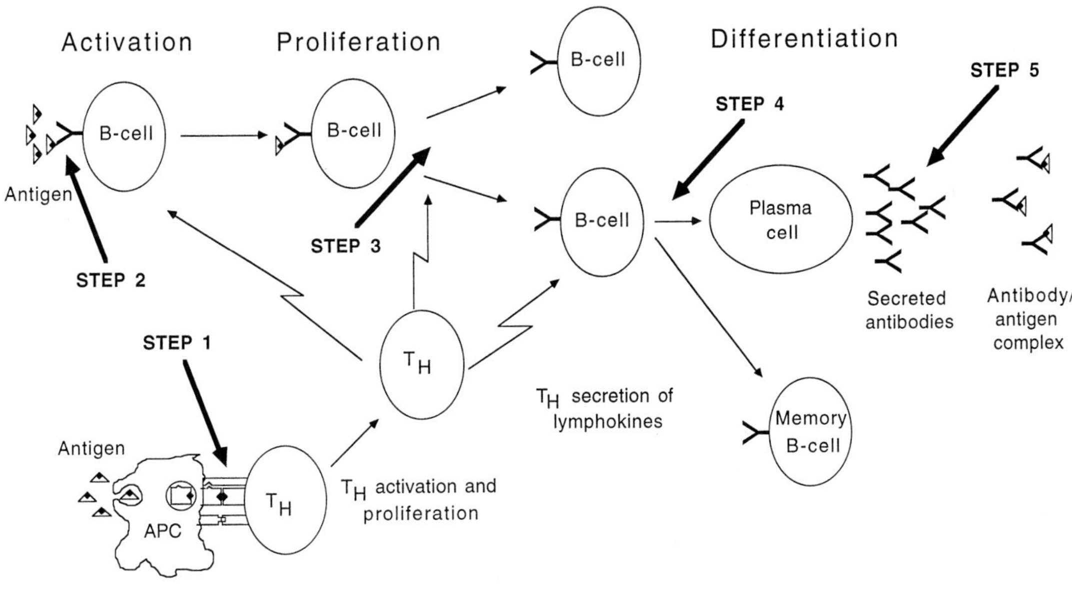

FIGURE I-2. Generation of an antibody response. An antibody response is an example of an acquired immune response and is characterized by a five-step process. The production of memory cells is also depicted.

tion as being mediated via this domain. However, it has been shown that surface Ig can associate with type I transmembrane glycoproteins to form a B cell receptor (BCR) complex, which can generate the necessary signal transduction pathways to trigger activation and proliferation in B cells in the presence of the appropriate ligand (antigen). Virgin B cells express either IgM or IgD or both on their surface. The function of IgD is limited to its role as a receptor on B cells, and it cannot mediate any of the effector functions associated with the other classes of Ig. IgM is the first class of Ig to be released by the B cell after antigen challenge during a primary antibody response. In the serum, IgM exists as a pentamer. Depending on the nature of the antigen, B cells can undergo a process known as class switching, which results in the generation of IgG, IgA, or IgE. As described later, the T cell plays a critical role in class switching through the release of a variety of lymphokines. Antigens triggering this type of interaction between B and T cells are therefore called T-dependent antigens. Some antigens can trigger an antibody response in a T-independent fashion and are generally limited to the production of IgM.

Once released, the various forms of Ig possess a number of effector functions to engage the antigen. It is important to emphasize that a given microbe, tumor cell, or foreign protein can express several types of antigens and multiple copies of these antigens. If the antigen to which an antibody is directed is associated with the toxic portion of a molecule, then the antibody can neutralize the toxin. The production of neutralizing antibodies is frequently a problem in the therapeutic application of recombinant proteins generated through biotechnology. This problem can become a rate-limiting step in the preclinical testing of human-derived proteins in animal models because they are perceived as nonself by their hosts. Another example of the ability of antibodies to neutralize occurs when the antibody is directed against an antigen on the surface of an infectious particle which serves as the cellular adhesion site. In the presence of the antibody, the infectious particle cannot attach to the cellular target to initiate infection. Although the neutralizing capabilities of antibodies are known, in actuality, they play a relatively minor role in the effector functions associated with humoral immunity in host defense. In particular, it is important to emphasize that antibody can only bind to an antigen and, in itself, cannot destroy anything.

Most of the effector functions of humoral immunity are mediated by processes activated by antibody. Moreover, the effector processes activated by antibody have already been described as key participants in innate immunity. For example, the classical activation of the complement cascade is triggered by antigen–antibody complexes and is specifically mediated by the constant region of the Ig molecule. Both IgM and IgG can activate the complement system in this manner, which results in all of the biologically active components identified previously, including the lytic unit, the chemotactic factors, and the complement peptides which opsonize the microbe to facilitate its phagocytosis. IgM and IgG can function to opsonize some microbes independent of complement activation in an antigen-dependent fashion because macrophages and neutrophils have receptors on their surface which recognize the constant region of Ig (Fc receptors; FcR). Fc receptors also play a major role in the ability of IgG to participate in a process known as antibody-dependent cellular cytotoxicity, whereby antigen-specific antibody attaches via FcR to certain types of cells, including NK cells, enabling these cells to attach intimately to the target cell and trigger cell death. Finally, Fc receptors are also the primary effector mechanism for IgE, which is the principal immune defense against certain types of parasitic infections (most notably, helminths) and is produced primarily by the external immune system along secretory surfaces. IgE binds to Fc receptors on the surfaces of mast cells and basophilic granulocytes. Once bound to FcR, IgE can serve as an antigen-specific receptor on the surface of these inflammatory cells to trigger the release of a variety of proinflammatory factors, including the vasoactive amines (histamine) and products of the arachidonic cascade (leucotrienes and prostaglandins).

IgA is the principal antibody present in a number of secretions and is the major antibody associated with the external immune system. IgA lacks the effector functions identified previously and acts mainly in immune exclusion (prevention of entry of potentially infectious entities into the body). As noted previously, there are differences in the immune effector mechanisms associated with the internal immune system or systemic immunity and the external immune system or local immunity. Systemic immunity is mediated by IgM and IgG, the latter of which is the major form of Ig found in the blood. Local immunity is mediated primarily by IgA and IgE. The contribution by the external immune system should not be underestimated because about half of the body's lymphocytes are associated with this system, and its capacity for Ig synthesis is about 1.5 times that of the internal immune system.

The other arm of the acquired immune system is cell-mediated immunity, for which antigen-specific T cells play the primary effector role. The antibody associated with humoral immunity is particularly effective against extracellular pathogens and it is a major constituent of serum. However, immunoglobulins are water-soluble proteins which cannot venture across the lipid membranes of cells. Therefore, cell-mediated immunity is needed to defend against intracellular pathogens such as protozoans, fungi (*Candida*), viruses, and certain bacteria (*Mycobacteria* and *Listeria*). Cells infected with these types of intracellular microbes are able to signal the body that they are infected by expressing pieces of the microbe on their surface. Cell-mediated immunity is also an important defense against certain types of malignancies. Central to this component of immune function, which is sometimes referred to as immunosurveillance, is the concept that tumor cells express antigens on their surface that are not found on normal tissue counterparts, so-called tumor-specific antigens.

As with the B cell, the antigen specificity of T cells is derived from a surface receptor. For T cells, the antigen receptor is a heterodimeric molecule (either the α,β heterodimer or the γ,δ heterodimer) which has a constant and a variable region, similar to that previously described for the Ig molecule. Moreover, as with surface Ig, the T cell receptor (TCR) cannot in itself mediate transmembrane signal transduction, and it is coupled on the cell surface with the CD3 molecule, where "CD" stands for cluster of differentiation, which has become the standard nomenclature to refer to a multitude of surface markers. CD3 consists of at least four invariant polypeptide chains and is thought to mediate the signal transduction associated with binding of the TCR to antigen. The expression of CD3 has become the hallmark feature of the T cell and is the principal phenotypic marker used to identify and enumerate T cells. Although there are similarities, there are also major differences between the TCR and its counterpart in the B cell. First, it is clear that there are structural differences between the TCR and BCR, and that T cells recognize different antigenic determinants than those recognized by B cells. Second, the TCR complex includes a number of different accessory molecules, namely CD4 and CD8, which play essential roles in the recognition of antigen by T cells. CD4 and CD8 also serve as important phenotypic markers for distinct subpopulations of T cells, T helper cells (T_H; Note: as indicated below, some $CD4^+$ cells are classified as T_D cells by virtue of their primary role in mediating a delayed hypersensitivity response) and T suppressor/T cytotoxic cells (T_S/T_C), respectively. The importance of these various subpopulations is described in greater detail below. Finally, unlike the B cell, in which the secreted form of Ig becomes the primary effector for humoral immunity, neither the TCR nor any component of its complex are secreted for effector function. Antigen-specific T cells contribute to host defense capabilities by two basic mechanisms. One type of T cell, which is usually designated T_D and expresses the CD4 phenotype, orchestrates an inflammatory response called a delayed hypersensitivity response through the release of a variety of lymphokines. Some T_D-derived lymphokines are capable of causing cell lysis independently of a direct attachment between effector and target cell and are called lymphotoxins. As with the ability of antibody to activate effector functions in humoral immunity, other T_D-derived lymphokines act to markedly stimulate the destructive capabilities of inflammatory cells associated with innate immunity and include macrophage-activating factor, macrophage-inhibiting factor (inhibits the directed movement or chemotaxis of macrophages at the site of infection), and IFN-γ, which stimulates both macrophages and NK cells. The second type of T cell is designated T_C for T cytotoxic and expresses the CD8 phenotype. As the name implies, T_Cs are capable of killing target cells in an antigen-specific fashion through intimate contact. These T cells are thought to play the major role in the rejection of a foreign tissue graft or transplant. Although T_Cs and NK cells have many similarities, including the enhanced activity in response to IFN-γ and the postulated role for cytolytic proteins such as perforin, they recognize their targets differently. Only T_Cs are antigen driven and require initial exposure to antigen to become active. Interestingly, T_C cells have been recently shown to be capable of producing a protein which interacts with perforin and renders it lytically inactive, thereby providing these cells with some resistance to their killing capability.

Regulation of an Acquired Immune Response

As emphasized throughout this entry, antigen plays the critical role in providing the driving force and the specificity of an acquired immune response. This type of response can be regulated by several general mechanisms including cellular cooperativity, the cytokine network, and genetically determined regulation. Cellular cooperativity can be mediated by both direct cell-to-cell contact and the release of soluble factors, especially the lymphokines. The "cytokine network" is a relatively recent term used to emphasize the fact that cytokines can both up- and downregulate lymphocyte activity. Genetically determined regulation is mediated by two major types of proteins encoded for by the MHC. In humans, MHC-derived proteins are called human lymphocyte antigens. MHC class I proteins are expressed on all cells of a given host and are critically involved in the designation of self versus nonself. These surface markers determine tissue compatibility and are the primary targets (i.e., antigens) in allograft or transplant rejection. MHC class II proteins are expressed only on certain types of immune cells and play a central role in the control of cellular interactions during an immune response.

All three of these mechanisms will be highlighted in the discussion of the five basic steps of an acquired immune response, which are illustrated below and which are depicted in Fig. I-2 for the generation of an antibody response. It is important to emphasize that these same five steps are involved in the generation of a cell-mediated immune response:

Step 1: antigen recognition and presentation

Step 2: lymphocyte activation

Step 3: lymphocyte proliferation

Step 4: lymphocyte differentiation

Step 5: effector function

Step 1: Antigen Recognition and Presentation

Thus far, antigen has been depicted as the structures associated with a foreign substance that allow it to be recognized as nonself and to therefore provide the driving force for an acquired immune response. It has also been emphasized that both B and T cells are equipped with surface molecules that effectively function as the receptors for antigen, allowing these cells to recognize antigen in a highly specific manner. Generally speaking, the form of the antigen as it appears on the foreign substance when it is introduced into the host is not the form of the antigen which is recognized by the "antigen receptors" on the surface of lymphocytes. The antigen must be taken up by specialized cells and "processed" so that the most immunogenic components can be "presented" to the lymphocytes. As depicted in Fig. I-3, cells carrying out this step of an acquired immune system are called antigen presenting cells (APCs). In order to present antigen to T cells, the immunogenic components must be presented in the context of MHC molecules, i.e., a T cell can only recognize antigen if the APC and the T cell share the same MHC type and antigen recognition by T cells is said to be MHC restricted. The role of MHC in antigen processing and presentation is shown in Fig. I-3. During antigen processing, the microbe or foreign particle is internalized within a vesicle and broken down. The most immunogenic components become associated with MHC-derived proteins, which are produced by the endoplasmic reticulum, and the antigen–MHC protein complex is returned to the surface of the APC. T_H cells, which express CD4 on their surface, can only recognize antigen in the context of MHC class II molecules, and all APCs which can present antigen to T_H cells must express MHC class II molecules. As noted previously, CD4 molecules play an accessory role in the recognition of antigen by T_H cells, and it is the CD4 molecule which recognizes the MHC class II antigens. Some examples include macrophages in the spleen, dendritic cells in lymph nodes, and Langerhan cells in the skin. While it is true that many APCs can also be classified as phagocytic cells, antigen processing and presentation and phagocytosis are two distinct functions. This point can be readily appreciated by the fact that B cells are recognized as efficient APCs under conditions of low antigen concentration. The participation of B cells in antigen processing and presentation occurs by virtue of their ability to complex with antigen via their surface immunoglobulin and by the fact that B cells can express MHC class II molecules on their surface. Moreover, because B cells are able to recognize antigen via surface immunoglobulin, antigen presentation to B cells is not MHC restricted. Antigen presentation to T_S/T_C cells is also known to be MHC restricted. Because these cells express CD8 on their surface as an accessory molecule to the TCR complex, recognition of antigen can only take place in the context of MHC class I antigens. As noted previously, most cells of the body express MHC class I proteins. When a cell becomes infected, it alerts

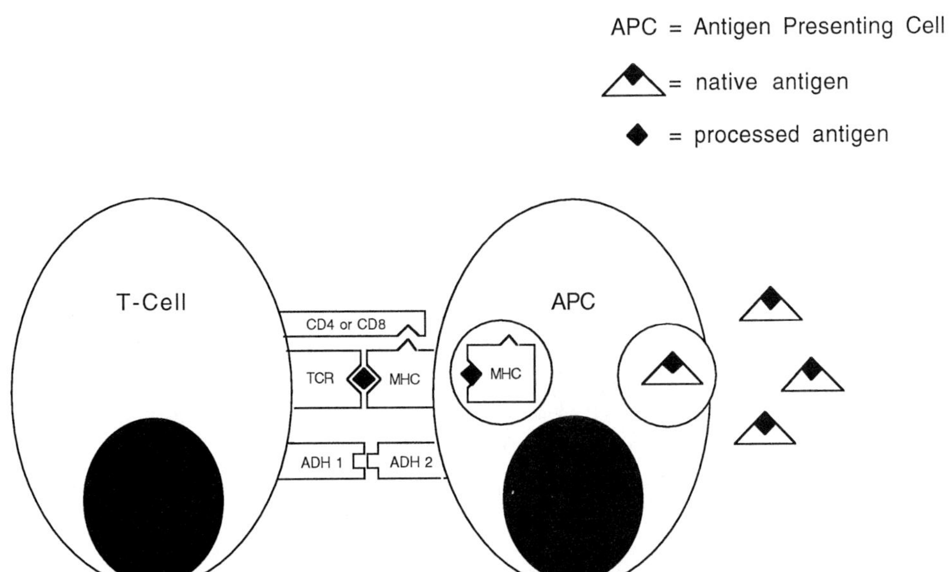

FIGURE I-3. Antigen presentation to T cells. The roles of antigen processing and of MHC-derived proteins in antigen presentation, the first step in the five-step process to generate an acquired immune response, are depicted.

T cells of the infection by coexpressing some antigenic determinant of the microbe in a complex with MHC class I proteins. This situation makes sense when one considers that T_C cells are $CD8^+$ and are the primary effector cells to engage certain types of virally infected cells and tumors (i.e., those tumors which express tumor-specific antigens) as well as allografts (i.e., a transplant of nonself, with different MHC class I proteins expressed). One final point about MHC proteins which needs to be emphasized is that their expression can be upregulated by certain cytokines, most notably the interferons, as summarized in Table I-1. One final point that needs to be emphasized about the process of antigen presentation is that other cell surface molecules, depicted in Fig. I-3 as adhesion molecules, play important roles in the cell-to-cell contact.

Step 2: Lymphocyte Activation

Because both the BCR and TCR are effectively the receptors for the ligand, which is antigen, once an antigen has been processed and presented to a specific B or T cell in the proper confirmation, it can trigger a number of second messenger systems which ultimately initiate transcription. The cell becomes activated and begins to move into the cell cycle toward mitosis and cell division. An important part of this process is the upregulation of surface receptors for cytokines which facilitate the movement of these cells through the cell cycle to proliferate and subsequently to differentiate. Because these receptors are generally expressed in very low levels in a resting cell, only the antigen-activated cells become responsive. In general, as shown in Fig. I-2, antigen-specific T_H cells are the primary source of these lymphokines. The ability of B cells to respond to the majority of antigens is critically dependent on these T_H cell-derived lymphokines, and these antigens are called T-dependent antigens. Other antigens, usually large polymeric molecules with repeating antigenic determinants, are able to trigger B cell responses without requiring T_H cell-derived lymphokines, and these antigens are called T-independent antigens.

Step 3: Lymphocyte Proliferation

The third step in an acquired immune response is the proliferation by antigen-specific lymphocytes. This step is often referred to as "clonal expansion," where a clone is a family of cells having an identical antigenic specificity. Therefore, a "polyclonal activator" is a substance which can trigger the proliferation of several clones, generally not in an antigen-specific fashion. Mitogens, substances which can cause lymphocytes to enter mitosis, are examples of polyclonal activators. A "monoclonal antibody" is a genetically engineered antibody which has a single antigenic specificity because it is produced by a homogenous clone of cells.

As depicted in Fig. I-2 and described previously, the movement of antigen-activated lymphocytes into proliferation is regulated by lymphokines produced predominately by antigen-specific T_H cells. The characteristics of many of these lymphokines are summarized in Table I-1. IL-2, which was previously known as T cell growth factor, is of particular importance to T cells, including T_C and T_H cells. In the latter cell type, this lymphokine functions as an autocrine growth factor (i.e., a factor which can stimulate proliferation in the same cells where it is produced). IL-2 can also promote the proliferation of B cells, as can the following T_H cell-derived lymphokines: IL-4, IL-5, IL-6, and IL-1, a cytokine produced by macrophages/monocytes. As indicated in Table I-1, some cytokines act as negative regulators of cell growth. Of particular importance to both B and T cells is transforming growth factor-β (TGF-β).

Step 4: Lymphocyte Differentiation

The proliferation in step 3 can be repeated several times (i.e., "clonal expansion"). Eventually, the lymphocytes will stop proliferating and will begin to differentiate into antigen-specific effector cells. As with proliferation, this step in an acquired immune response is under the control of lymphokines produced primarily by T_H cells. One of the critical steps in the differentiation of B cells is the "switch" to the specific type of immunoglobulin molecule that will ultimately be secreted. As indicated in Table I-1, IFN-γ stimulates the production of IgG2-α, IL-4 stimulates the production of IgE and IgG1, IL-5 stimulates the production of IgA, and IL-9 can act synergistically with IL-4 to stimulate IgE and IgG. A fully mature antibody-secreting B cell is called a plasma cell. A number of cytokines can also increase the generation of T_C cells including all types of interferon, IL-2, IL-4 (this action is synergistic with IL-2), IL-10, and IL-12.

Step 5: Effector Function

The basis for the effector function by antigen-specific lymphocytes—especially antibody-secreting B cells, T_D cells, and T_C cells—and the participation of other cellular components of the immune system in acquired immunity—including NK cells, macrophages, and neutrophils—have already been emphasized in other sections of this volume. It has also been emphasized that T_H cells play an important effector role in acquired immunity as regulators in the growth and differentiation of B cells and T_C cells. In this regard, it is important to note that both populations of T cells whose participation in an acquired immune response is mediated by the secretion of lymphokines, i.e., T_H and T_D cells, are characterized by the expression of CD4.

Recent evidence has suggested that there are at least two subpopulations of T_H cells, designated T_{H1} and T_{H2}. To date, the distinction between these two populations has been operationally defined and is based on the respective profiles of lymphokines which are produced: whereas both T_{H1} and T_{H2} cells produce IL-3 and GM-CSF; only T_{H1} cells produce IL-2 and IFN-γ, and only T_{H2} cells produce IL-4, IL-5, IL-6, and IL-10. The importance of this phenomenon can be derived from the discussion of the primary effects of these lymphokines. By virtue of the production of IL-2 and IFN-γ, T_{H1} cells will facilitate the generation of a cell-mediated immune response. In contrast, T_{H2} cells will facilitate the generation of a humoral immune response by virtue of producing lymphokines which support B cell function. Moreover, as indicated in Table I-1, T_{H1} cells can downregulate the activity of T_{H2} cells via the production of IFN-γ, and T_{H2} cells can downregulate the activity of T_{H1} cells via the production of IL-4 and IL-10. The basis for this "cross talk" between the two types of T_H cells has been called the cytokine network. An important outcome of this cytokine network is that under certain conditions, a cell type traditionally characterized as a "helper" cell can actually "suppress" an immune functional component (i.e., T_{H1} cells can suppress T_{H2} cells via IFN-γ, and T_{H2} cells can suppress T_{H1} cells via IL-4 and IL-10).

Certain types of T cells expressing CD8 are known to function as antigen-specific T_S cells. T_S cells are activated under conditions designed to induce immunological tolerance, previously referred to as a state of anergy, and their importance can be confirmed in cell transfer experiments. The mode of action of T_S cells is uncertain and may involve the secretion of soluble factors as described for T_H cells. T cell-derived suppressor factors have been shown to be associated with APCs, such as macrophages. The action of T_S cells is also thought to be capable of being directed toward T_H cells and B cells in an antigen-specific fashion. Therefore, it becomes obvious that the relative balance between T_H cells and T_S cells can exert tremendous influence over the magnitude of a given immune response and can even dictate if an immune response occurs.

Memory Cells: the Goal of Vaccinations/Immunizations

One final point about acquired immunity needs to be emphasized. During the five steps of an acquired immune response, some of the antigen-specific and activated lymphocytes will undergo proliferation but will not be stimulated to differentiate and become effector cells, which have a relatively short half-life during a primary immune response. As shown in Fig. I-2, these cells will instead be programmed with the same antigenic specificity and will be returned to the blood and/or lymph circulation as long-lived memory cells. Upon reinfection with the same microbe, the secondary immune response, which is initiated by these memory cells, will occur quicker and with greater intensity. In the case of a humoral immunity, whereas IgM is the predominate Ig released during a primary immune response, IgG is the predominate Ig released during a secondary immune response. The generation of memory cells is the goal of vaccinations and immunizations where the host is injected with nonpathogenic (i.e., inactivated or attenuated) forms of infectious microbes. As children, we are vaccinated to several infectious organisms, including measles, mumps, diphtheria, tuberculosis, rubella, and poliomyelitis. Just prior to the winter months throughout a good portion of the United States, many people elect to receive the latest influenza vaccines, the so-called "flu shots." These are all examples of vaccinations and the objective is to clonally expand antigen-specific memory cells. Often, the responses to childhood vaccines, sometimes called "recall antigens," are checked as an assessment of human immunocompetence.

Consequences of Immunotoxicity

Having established an appreciation of the immune system, with an emphasis on its functional organization and capabilities, it is now possible to begin to discuss the consequences of immunotoxicity beyond the generalized concept of a continuum, as depicted in Fig, I-1. However, prior to discussing more specific consequences of immunotoxicity, especially the immunosuppressive part of the continuum, the concepts of redundancy and immunological reserve need to be emphasized. While the immune system can be divided into innate and acquired immunity, it is important to emphasize that this classification is based on the role that antigen plays in triggering a response. As described in previous sections, the immune system often has several overlapping mechanisms to cope with a given opportunistic pathogen, regardless of how the response is triggered. Moreover, the same effector mechanisms that are involved in innate host defense capabilities are activated in acquired immunity, and the progression from innate to acquired immunity is generally associated with greater intensity (i.e., greater destructive capability). The concept of overlapping effector function is often called the redundancy of the immune system. For example, phagocytic inflammatory cells, complement-derived peptides, and antibodies are all involved in the defense against bacterial infections. The first two effectors are prime players in innate immunity and are markedly activated by antigen-specific antibody in acquired immunity. Similarly, macrophages, NK cells, interferons, T_C cells, and T_D cell-derived inflammatory lymphokines are all involved in the defense against viral infections. Again, the first two effectors are prime players in innate immunity and are markedly activated by antigen-specific T cells in acquired immunity. The importance of redundancy is that the consequences of suppression of a given component of the host defense capabilities are sometimes minimized because of these overlapping systems. This phenomenon is sometimes referred to as immunological reserve. The redundancy and reserve of the immune system is thought to have evolved because of the diverse nature of pathogens with which it must cope to protect self. Moreover, a point about opportunistic pathogens, which is too often ignored, is that they are generally not passive players in their assault on the host. It is a characteristic of most successful infectious organisms that they can elicit different mechanisms to evade detection and/or to minimize the full effects of the host's defense capabilities. Moreover, microbes also evolve rapidly, enabling them to devise new means to evade the inherited defenses of species that evolve much more slowly. Therefore, even if the manifestation of the suppression of a given functional component is not clearly associated with disease, this immunotoxic effect should still be considered adverse because it does represent a loss in functional capabilities.

When the immune system is suppressed, the most severe consequences will be an increase in the incidence and severity of infections and/or an increase in the incidence and progression of malignancies or cancer. The specific types of infections which are increased can provide some clues as to the specific components of the immune system which were suppressed. For example, suppression of humoral immunity (i.e., antibody production) and/or its associated effector systems, such as phagocytic cells (i.e., macrophages and neutrophils) and the complement cascade, will be characterized by infections mediated by extracellular pathogens, including some bacteria and parasites. In contrast, suppression of cell-mediated immunity and/or its associated effector systems, such as NK cells and the interferons, will be characterized by infections mediated by intracellular pathogens, including protozoans, viruses, and some bacteria, as well as by increased tumor formation. That these are consequences of immunosuppression in man cannot be argued based on a multitude of studies in individuals with congenital or acquired immune deficiencies or in patients undergoing long-term treatment with immunosuppressive drugs subsequent to organ or tissue transplantation. That these are consequences of exposure to suspected immunotoxic (i.e., immunosuppressive) xenobiotics in animal models also cannot be argued, primarily because extensive dose–response characterizations can be conducted under well-controlled experimental conditions and because changes in various immune functional parameters can be correlated with changes in host resistance models. However, this is not the case in humans, where there are few clear-cut examples of, or convincing evidence for, xenobiotic-induced immunosuppression outside of a therapeutic context. What becomes clear (even in the animals studies) is that the effects of immunotoxic drugs and chemicals are generally much more subtle than either the immune dysfunctions associated with congenital conditions or those produced by drugs used for immunosuppressive therapy.

As indicated in Fig. I-1, the other side of the immunotoxicity continuum is manifested either as a hypersensitivity response or as an autoimmune disease. A hypersensitivity response is an acquired immune response (i.e., by definition, it is manifested on second contact with a particular antigen) which occurs in an exaggerated or inappropriate form to cause tissue damage and which is a characteristic of the individual (i.e., there is a genetic predisposition).

Autoimmune disease occurs when the reactions of the immune system are directed against the body's own tissues and is also characterized by a genetic susceptibility. Examples of autoimmune diseases include myasthenia gravis, in which cholinergic receptors, especially those associated with neuromuscular junctions, are targeted; multiple sclerosis, in which myelin is targeted; and rheumatoid arthritis, in which connective tissue, especially the synovial lining of joints, is targeted. The terms "hypersensitivity" and "autoimmunity" are often confused and are certainly interrelated. Based on their definitions, a hypersensitivity response can be a mechanism by which an autoimmune disease is produced. In contrast to the situation regarding suppression, in which the immune system is by and large a passive target for xenobiotic-induced changes, exaggerated immune responses can be mediated by two entirely different types of interactions by the immune system with drugs and chemicals. First, the immune system can again be a passive target for the enhancing effects of drugs and chemicals, such as occurs when a xenobiotic mimics or causes the aberrant production of immunomodulatory cytokines or when a xenobiotic disrupts the regulatory mechanisms which serve to protect self (i.e., suppress a suppressor). Another way that xenobiotics can enhance immune function is by acting as an adjuvant, which is defined as any substance which nonspecifically enhances the immune response to an antigen. The classic adjuvant is complete Freund's adjuvant (CFA), which is a water-in-oil emulsion containing killed mycobacteria. The effectiveness of adjuvants in enhancing immune responses can be demonstrating by the fact that animals are often injected with CFA to increase the production of antigen-specific antibodies and by the desire to develop an adjuvant that is safe in man (i.e., CFA produces severe side effects) which could be used in conjunction with vaccines or immunotherapy. The specific mechanism(s) for the actions of an adjuvant, including CFA, is not known. Moreover, the existence of environmental adjuvants is controversial and/or poorly studied. Therefore, adjuvants will not be further discussed in this entry.

In the second type of interaction, the components of the immune system are active participants in that the xenobiotic or some fraction of a xenobiotic is recognized as nonself and therefore provides the driving force for the response. Drugs and chemicals which are capable of triggering an immune response are generally low-molecular-weight substances some inherent reactivity. For the most part, the xenobiotic cannot be considered an antigen, simply because in itself it is not capable of stimulating an immune response. Instead, these substances are called haptens, which are defined as small molecules that can act as antigenic determinants but which cannot stimulate an immune response by themselves. The immune response is triggered when the hapten binds to some tissue of the host, the so-called carrier. This property is called the sensitizing potential of the hapten and is associated with its inherent reactivity. Hapten-specific immune responses are therefore triggered only in the presence of the hapten–carrier complex and can be mediated either by humoral immunity (i.e., antibody), as in an allergic response, or by cell-mediated immunity (i.e., specifically a delayed hypersensitivity response), as in contact dermatitis. The damage associated with either type of hypersensitivity response can be directed against the tissue which is bound by the hapten. Therefore, the morbidity associated with hypersensitivity responses can be manifested in a number of ways depicting the target tissues, including contact dermatitis, rhinitis, allergy, and anaphylaxis. Animal models have been developed which can clearly demonstrate the sensitizing potential of xenobiotics. Moreover, hypersensitivity disease has become an important human health problem in industrialized societies. One striking example of the consequences of hypersensitivity disease in humans is occupational asthma, which is one of the most common occupational ailments in the Western world. However, it is important to emphasize that the establishment of a cause and effect relationship is more straightforward in the case of hypersensitivity than immune suppression. The onset of hypersensitivity is always a consequence of exposure to an exogenous agent. On the other hand, the repercussions of immune suppression following exposure to a xenobiotic, especially one that produces only modest changes in immunocompetence, in most cases will be subtle. These consequences will likely be manifested as a slightly greater susceptibility to common opportunistic infections, such as those responsible for the common cold or the flu.

The situation with autoimmunity is much more complex than hypersensitivity responses. Animal models exist for many autoimmune conditions, and autoimmunity has been clearly demonstrated in humans, although it is a relatively infrequent occurrence. Therefore, the existence of autoimmune disease and the expected consequences cannot be denied. However, the ability of drugs and chemicals to exacerbate or trigger autoimmune disease in either animal models or humans is poorly understood. In fact, of all the possible consequences of immunotoxicity, autoimmunity is unquestionably the least understood. Primarily because of the strong genetic component in the susceptibility to autoimmunity, deciphering the exact role of xenobiotics in the induction of these conditions has proven to be very difficult.

Mechanisms of Immunotoxicity

As described previously, the immune system is a complex, widely distributed and tightly regulated series of overlapping effector functions designed to allow the discrimination between self and nonself. As such, the immune system is characterized by a number of features that make it vulnerable to being targeted by exposure to xenobiotics. Several of these features are briefly highlighted below.

Immune System Features Associated with Vulnerability to Xenobiotics

- Many of the effector functions of the immune system are dependent on a multitude of cell types, which all share a common precursor, the pluripotent stem cell. Therefore, any damage to the stem cell would be expected to have devastating consequences, several of which would extend beyond the immune system, most notably involving the red blood cell. Fortunately, the stem cell has proven to be refractory to xenobiotic-induced perturbation and is only affected by high doses of radiation. However, the subsequent steps of hematopoiesis have been shown to be affected by exposure to chemicals, with benzene being a classic example. Acute toxicity to benzene is associated with pancytopenia, aplastic anemia, and, at high doses, immunosuppression and leukemia.
- The generation of mature lymphocytes with the capability of being programmed to respond against nonself in an antigen-specific manner but without the risk of responding to self is

dependent on a complex maturational process that takes place in primary lymphoid organs, such as the bone marrow and thymus. Therefore, xenobiotic-induced damage to these microenvironments can contribute to immunosuppression as well as problems with immune regulatory functions.

- Proliferation (i.e., the clonal expansion of reactive lymphoid cells) is a critical step in any acquired immune response. Therefore, any drug or chemical with antiproliferative properties has the potential to be immunosuppressive. Many types of immunosuppressive drugs are in fact antiproliferative, including cyclophosphamide, methotrexate, and azathioprine. Moreover, many types of anticancer drugs which target highly proliferating cells exhibit immunosuppression as an important side effect. An aspect centered around proliferation, which is rarely considered in immunotoxicology, is the malignant processes of immunocompetent cells. Leukemias and lymphomas are characterized by uncontrolled proliferation of T cells, B cells, or monocytes. However, because these cells are arrested in a specific stage of maturation or differentiation, even though there is tremendous proliferation, these conditions are generally associated with decreased functional capabilities and are manifested as a profile of activity comparable to that associated with exposure to antiproliferative drugs or chemicals (i.e., immunosuppression). As noted previously, benzene is an example of a chemical which can trigger leukemias, and ethylene oxide is an example of a chemical which has been associated with the development of lymphomas. Because these conditions are most appropriately categorized as types of cancers, they will not be further discussed in this entry.
- Virtually all aspects of immunity are dependent on recognition of surface structures and can be regulated by a multitude of soluble products. Therefore, any drug or chemical that affects protein synthesis, gene expression, and/or receptor expression has the potential to disrupt immune function.
- The immune system is characterized by a unique distribution, and many of its components are located close to the principal sites of absorption, including the gastrointestinal tract, the pulmonary tract, and the skin. Therefore, the immune system is in a position to be exposed to potentially high concentrations of drugs and chemicals. This phenomenon is especially important in hypersensitivity responses where the primary portal of entry of the hapten can determine the specific site of the reaction.
- Some components of the immune system have metabolic capability including some forms of the cytochrome P450 system. Therefore, some chemicals, which are inert in their parent form but can be metabolized to reactive intermediates, can be activated by the immune system. However, it is important to emphasize that the metabolic capability of the immune system is minor when compared to other organ systems, most notably the liver, and that it possesses only a small repertoire of metabolizing enzymes. This point is discussed below as a major type of indirect mechanism of immunosuppression.
- The immune system is not only regulated by its own products but also exquisitely sensitive to products generated by other systems. Two examples, that will be discussed below as major types of indirect mechanisms of immunosuppression, are changes in neuroendocrine status and liver damage.

Direct and Indirect Effects of Xenobiotics

The remaining discussion of the mechanisms of immunotoxicity will be presented from the perspective of the following three general consequences of immunotoxicity: immunosuppression, hypersensitivity, and autoimmunity.

One of the critical features of any discussion of the mechanisms of immunosuppression must be the appreciation that robust changes in immune function can be mediated by either direct or indirect effects (or both) of a xenobiotic. Direct effects can be associated with distinct types of cells. Perhaps the best example is cyclosporin A and related immunosuppressive drugs, such as rapamycin and FK-506, which specifically target T cells via an interaction with cytosolic and/or nuclear proteins to disrupt antigen-induced activation of transcription. To date, despite the tremendous evolution of the discipline of immunotoxicology, no other xenobiotic associated with occupational or environmental exposure has been as well characterized from a mechanistic perspective as cyclosporin A. Nonetheless, a few examples are worthy of mention. Cannabinoids, the active ingredients of marijuana, have been demonstrated to somewhat selectively suppress T cell function. The mechanism of action appears to be mediated by a specific cannabinoid receptor that is located in the plasma membrane and that is associated with a G-protein coupled signal transduction pathway. Binding of cannabinoid ligands, such as δ-9-tetrahydrocannabinol, to cannabinoid receptors results in the inhibition of adenylate cyclase, the enzyme that converts ATP to AMP. Some chemicals have been shown to selectively affect macrophage function, including asbestos. The effects on macrophage function are frequently manifested as a deficit in antigen-presenting capabilities. The mechanism of action of asbestos is mediated by the fact that the asbestos fibers are phagocytized by the macrophages to the point where they appear to become engorged. Perhaps the most studied environmental chemical for effects on the immune system has been 2,3,7,8-tetrachlorodibenzo-I-dioxin, which is also know as TCDD or dioxin. While it appears that dioxin may affect multiple cell types, it is apparent that the B cell is an especially sensitive target. The mechanism of action for the immunotoxic effects of dioxin is unknown. Although many of the actions by dioxin are mediated by a specific cytosolic receptor with a profile of activity similar to steroid receptors (i.e., the ligand–receptor complex can act as a transcription factor), to date there is no definitive evidence implicating a specific target gene or genes, or transcription in general, in the immunotoxicity by dioxin. Recent results from a number of laboratories have suggested that the actions of TCDD on immunocompetent cells, including the B cell, may be mediated by an aberrant activation of a kinase system, which is triggered in part by a change in intracellular calcium. Another chemical which has been shown to affect multiple cell types is the semiconductor, gallium arsenide. Arsenic has been identified as the primary immunosuppressive component and both macrophages and T cells have been identified as targets. In macrophages, antigen processing and presentation was identified as a functional target. The effect on T cells was manifested as an antiproliferative effect mediated through a decreased expression of surface molecules and could be reversed by the exogenous addition of IL-2, IL-5, and IL-6. Finally, a group of chemicals which have been widely studied for effects on the immune system are the polyaromatic hydrocarbons (PAHs), such as benzo(*a*)pyrene [B(*a*)P] and 7,12-dimethylbenzanthracene (DMBA). PAHs represent a prototypical class of carcinogens, and this action is mediated by the generation of a reactive intermediate, which is capable of binding directly to macromolecules like DNA. The mechanism of immunotoxicity also appears to be dependent on the generation of the reactive intermediates, and the available evidence suggests that certain types of immunocompetent cells, most notably the macrophage, have enough metabolic capability to activate PAHs such as B(*a*)P and DMBA. The specific macromolecular target which is responsible for the immunosuppression is not known, although it appears that these chemicals can affect multiple cellular targets. Interestingly, there are reports that exposure to PAHs can disrupt the production of immunomodulatory cytokines. Specifically, B(*a*)P has been reported to decrease the production of IL-1, and the suppression by DMBA can be reversed by the exogenous addition of IL-2.

A number of chemicals with demonstrable suppression of immune function have been determined to produce this action via indirect effects. By and large, the approach which has been most frequently used to support an indirect mechanism of action is to show immunosuppression after *in vivo* exposure but no immunosuppression after *in vitro* exposure to relevant concentrations. One of the most often cited mechanisms for an indirect action is centered around the limited metabolic capabilities of immunocompetent cells and tissues. A number of chemicals have caused immunosuppression when administered to animals but were essentially devoid of any potency when added directly to suspensions of lymphocytes and macrophages. Many of these chemicals have been demonstrated to be capable of being metabolized to reactive metabolites, including dimethylnitrosamine, aflatoxin B_1, and carbon tetrachloride. Interestingly, a similar profile of activity (i.e., suppression after *in vivo* exposure but no activity after *in vitro* exposure) has been demonstrated with the potent immunosuppressive drug cyclophosphamide. With the exception of the PAHs, few chemicals have been demonstrated to be metabolized when added directly to immunocompetent cells in culture. A primary role for a reactive intermediate in the immunosuppression by dimethylnitrosamine, aflatoxin B_1, carbon tetrachloride, and cyclophosphamide has been confirmed in studies in which these xenobiotics were incubated with suspensions of immunocompetent cells in the presence of metabolic activation systems (MASs). Examples of MASs include primary hepatocytes, liver microsomes, and liver homogenates. In most cases, confirmation for a primary role by a reactive metabolite has been provided by *in vivo* studies in which the metabolic capability was either enhanced or suppressed by the administration of an enzyme inducer or a metabolic inhibitor, respectively.

While the demonstration that the immunosuppression by a given chemical is mediated by a metabolite, and not the parent compound, is an important observation, it does not in itself account for the mechanism of action. One indirect mechanism of action, which is consistent with a role by metabolism, involves a primary consequence of the generation of many reactive intermediates, i.e., liver damage. Among many different types of adaptive responses, the liver is capable of secreting a number of soluble factors. Some of these soluble factors have been demonstrated to be capable of affecting immune responses. Most notably, as pointed out in Table I-1, TGF-β has been previously described as being capable of suppressing both T and B cell effector functions. Both carbon tetrachloride and cocaine have each been shown to cause immunosuppression and liver damage over a comparable dose range. Support for a role by a serum factor was obtained by studies in which serum from either carbon tetrachloride-treated or cocaine-treated mice suppressed the function of immunocompetent cells from untreated mice. Confirmation for a role by TGF-β was obtained by demonstrating its presence in the serum of treated mice and by showing that the suppression by the serum could be reversed by a neutralizing antibody against TGF-β.

The liver damage associated with exposure to cocaine is a relatively minor component of its profile of activity. Cocaine is an abused substance which has been studied most extensively for its effects on the brain and on behavior. Cocaine is capable of triggering robust changes in a number of neuroendocrine factors, some of which have been demonstrated to suppress immune function. In particular, it has been proposed that cocaine is able to cause immunosuppression at least in part through an elevation in plasma corticosterone as a consequence of the stimulation of the hypothalamic–pituitary–adrenal neuraxis. Ethanol (i.e., at least after acute exposure) and morphine are two other examples of xenobiotics which are suspected of producing their primary actions on the immune system via neuroendocrine effects. In most cases, the evidence is based on a measurable increase in serum coriticosterone at doses capable of causing immunosuppression and on the ability of the glucocorticoid antagonist, RU-486, to reverse the suppression.

Hypersensitivity Reactions

Three points about hypersensitivity reactions have already been emphasized. First, the ability of a drug or chemical to trigger a hypersensitivity reaction is due to an inherent property of the xenobiotic (i.e., hapten), its sensitizing potential. Second, in a hypersensitivity reaction, the immune system plays an active role in mediating the response against the hapten. Third, both antigen-specific antibody (i.e., humoral immunity) and antigen-specific T cells (i.e., cell-mediated immunity) can be the effectors which are responsible for the tissue damage associated with hypersensitivity reactions. Traditionally, different types of hypersensitivity have been classified by a scheme originally proposed in 1963. Although the Coombs and Gell classification scheme is still widely used today, it is important to emphasize that the different types of hypersensitivity reactions rarely appear individually and are most often seen as mixed components. Nonetheless, this classification still represents one of the easiest ways to appreciate how the immune system is involved with the tissue damage-associated hypersensitivity reactions. The first three types of hypersensitivity reactions (I–III) are mediated by antigen-specific antibody, while the fourth type of hypersensitivity reaction (IV) is mediated by antigen-specific T cells.

Type I

A type I hypersensitivity reaction is the classic example of an allergic reaction and is also called an immediate hypersensitivity reaction because of its rapid appearance upon challenge in a sensitized individual. The primary mediator for a type I reaction is IgE, which is produced by antigen (hapten)-specific B cells in a T cell-dependent fashion and which binds by its constant region to the Fc receptors on the surface of mast cells and basophils. As such, hapten-specific IgE can rightfully be considered a true biomarker for exposure in sensitized individuals. Therefore, in the absence of antigen-specific IgE, it is inappropriate to label a condition as an allergic reaction. This situation is true for occupational allergy, where only the presence of antigen-specific IgE should be accepted as a criteria for exposure to a suspected respiratory sensitizer. Upon a second contact with the hapten, the mast cells and basophils will be stimulated to degranulate and release a variety of vasoactive substances, which are the mediators of the inflammatory response and the accompanying tissue damage. The target organs for a type I reaction include the gastrointestinal tract, skin, lungs, and vasculature. Anaphylaxis is a systemic type I reaction which can be life threatening. As noted previously, many hypersensitivity reactions have a genetic component, and atopy is a term used to describe a genetic predisposition toward the development of IgE-mediated reactions against common environmental antigens, such as pollen and dust.

In the section on the effector functions of antibody, it was emphasized that IgE was a primary player in the host defense against a variety of parasites. Therefore, it could be easily argued that individuals endowed with an ability to mount a robust IgE response possessed a distinct survival advantage over individuals without such a defense mechanism against parasitic infections. However, in most developed nations, parasitic infections have been all but eliminated. Interestingly, in most developing nations, while parasitic infections are still a problem, the incidence of allergy or chemically induced hypersensitivity reactions is very low. Taken together, these two observations have prompted the speculation that the incidence of allergy and chemically induced hypersensitivity reactions in industrialized societies is due, at least in part, to the fact that the components of the immune system associated with the production of IgE, in the absence of parasites, are now free to react to other nonparasitic substances in a counterproductive way.

Type II

A type II hypersensitivity reaction is also called a cytolytic reaction because the damage is mediated by hapten-specific antibodies which are capable of triggering cytotoxicity in the target cell. The antibodies involved in a type II reaction are both IgM and IgG, with the latter type predominating. The specific effectors which are responsible for the cell damage include both the complement system and phagocytic cells, and these effectors are activated exactly as described in the section on humoral immunity. The target organs for type II reactions include many cell types circulating in the blood. Examples of type II reactions include xenobiotic-induced hemolytic anemia or agranulocytosis.

Type III

A type III hypersensitivity reaction is also called immune complex disease. Examples of type III reactions include the Arthus reaction and serum sickness. The damage associated with type III reactions is mediated by the generation of hapten-specific antibody, primarily IgG. The basis for the damage associated with type III reactions is that soluble antigen–antibody complexes are deposited in key anatomical locations, such as small capillary beds in the skin or the glomerular regions of the kidney. As described in the section on humoral immunity, the classical activation of the complement cascade is mediated by antigen–antibody complexes. Therefore, the deposition of immune complexes can cause a very localized activation of the complement cascade resulting in the generation of chemotactic peptides as well as the lytic unit. The target organs for type III reactions include blood vessels in the skin, joints, and lungs and the glomerular regions of the kidney.

Type IV

A type IV hypersensitivity reaction is also called a delayed hypersensitivity reaction because of its delayed appearance (i.e., after 24–48 hr) following challenge in a sensitized individual. This is the only type of hypersensitivity reaction which is not mediated by antibody and is instead dependent on the generation of hapten-specific T cells, specifically the T_D cells, which contribute to the inflammation and the accompanying tissue damage by the generation and release of a variety of lymphokines. Classic examples of type IV reactions include the response that some individuals have to poison ivy (i.e., again emphasizing the genetic component to hypersensitivity reactions) and contact dermatitis. Target organs besides the skin include the lungs (i.e., the target organ for the well-studied tuberculin reaction), CNS, thyroid, and other organs.

Recent studies to characterize the basis for chemically induced hypersensitivity have uncovered an important interplay between type I hypersensitivity reactions, manifested primarily as respiratory sensitization, and type IV hypersensitivity reactions, manifested primarily as contact sensitization. The most important observation came from studies which showed that a predominantly respiratory sensitizer would still trigger an IgE response when applied topically. The basis for this observation can be accounted for by the cytokine network model which was described previously as an important cross talk between humoral immunity and cell-mediated immunity. Basically, a chemical with the capability of being a respiratory sensitizer will trigger an IgE response regardless of its route of exposure because it "selects" or supports the development of a T_{H2}-dependent response, with the associated cytokine profile, IL-4, IL-5, and IL-10. In contrast, a chemical which lacks the capability of being a respiratory sensitizer; but which can still trigger contact dermititis, will select or support a T_{H1}-dependent response, with the associated cytokine profile, IL-2 and IFN-γ.

Autoimmune Responses

If increased incidence and/or severity of infections represents the critical consequence of a suppressed immune response, then autoimmunity represents the antithesis for an exaggerated immune response. As noted previously, the characterization of the onset and progression of autoimmune conditions has been complicated by the critically important role that genetics plays in this process. While the exact association to drugs and chemicals as factors is poorly understood, several potential mechanisms have been proposed to account for this association. By definition, autoimmunity is the harmful consequences associated with an immune response which is mediated against self. Therefore, most of the mechanisms which have been proposed are centered around either a xenobiotic-induced change in the antigens associated with self or a xenobiotic-induced change in the recognition of self. Autoimmune responses that are driven by the first mechanism are associated with several possibilities which are identified as follows:

- Immune responses can be directed toward a foreign (i.e., nonself) antigen which has a similar chemical structure to an antigen which characterizes self.
- Immune responses can be directed toward a new nonself antigen that has become nonspecifically absorbed to a cell membrane. This mechanism is essentially the description of the sensitizing potential of a hapten and is one of the reasons why there is some overlap between hypersensitivity reactions and autoimmune conditions.
- Immune responses can be directed against a self antigen which is normally shielded or hidden but which becomes available or expressed following exposure to a xenobiotic or during a disease process. Again, this is a potential area of overlap between hypersensitivity reactions and autoimmune disease. As described previously, hypersensitivity reactions can be mediated by the activation of immune effector processes which possess considerable destructive capability. Therefore, it is possible that one of the consequences of the tissue damage caused by a hypersensitivity reaction could be the expression of hidden antigens, which then sets the stage for the initiation of an autoimmune condition.

The second mechanism for autoimmunity is a change in the way that self is recognized. As described previously, the repertoire of antigen-specific immune effector mechanisms must develop with the capability of recognizing a tremendous number of nonself antigens while preserving the ability to recognize an equally vast number of self determinants. There are several regulatory mechanisms which are involved in this critical process that could be targeted to contribute to the onset and/or progression of autoimmune disease. First, T_S cells can play an important regulatory role in preventing an exaggerated immune response. Therefore, the suppression of T_S cells could result in an inappropriate recognition of self antigens. Second, an important step in the maturation of both T and B cells is negative selection, whereby these cells are probed for their recognition of self determinants. Lymphocytes with antigen receptors that can recognize self determinants are either destroyed via the stimulation of apoptosis or these cells are rendered anergic. An important part of the probing process is centered around the transfer and presentation of self determinants of organs or tissues distal to the microenvironments of the thymus or bone marrow. Recent evidence has suggested that this process may be one of the more sensitive targets for triggering an autoimmune mechanism. As such, any xenobiotic-induced changes in the movement of self determinants to the primary lymphopoietic organs and/or any xenobiotic-induced changes in the primary lymphopoietic organs themselves can be a mechanism for autoimmunity.

Autoimmune diseases may be tissue specific, where the damage is associated with a specific type of tissue or a specific organ, or tissue nonspecific, where the signs and symptoms are associated with several organs and tissues. The targets from the perspective of the primary sites of tissue damage in autoimmune disease are many and varied. The following organs, cells, and organelles have all been determined to be the site of autoimmune reactions: nuclei (specifically histones and/or single-stranded DNA—one of the hallmark indicators of certain types of autoimmune disease is the expression of anti-nuclear antibodies), red blood cells, lymphocytes, neutrophils, platelets, immunoglobulins (primarily IgG), striated muscle (cholinergic receptors), smooth muscle, mitochondria, skin (basement membranes), thyroid (thyoglobulin), kidney (glomerular and tubular basement membrane), central nervous system (myelin), connective tissue (synovial lining of joints), lung, and liver. Both cell-mediated immunity and humoral immunity can be involved as effector mechanisms in causing the damage in autoimmune conditions.

Multiple Chemical Sensitivity

Although the issue of hypersensitivity disease is perhaps much more complex than originally suspected, all four types of hypersensitivity reactions and several types of autoimmune conditions are well established and recognized by both the scientific and the clinical communities. In contrast, there are a number of conditions which have little or no clinical definition and which are not currently recognized by the scientific community as being immune-mediated conditions. The most prevalent of these conditions is most frequently called multiple chemical sensitivity (MCS), although it has other names including idiopathic environmentalintolerances, chemical hypersensitivity syndrome, and twentieth-century disease. MCS usually refers to a constellation of varied symptoms that some people believe are caused by exposure to low-molecular-weight chemicals at trace levels normally considered to be safe. Not only has there been no evidence brought forth to establish any kind of a link to an immune-mediated disease or reaction but also few, if any, of the rules of causality have been met for any given chemical. This condition is being championed by so-called clinical ecology laboratories, which have generally based their claims for immune damage on very subtle changes in the expression of surface markers on lymphocytes which have not been validated. Specifically, the functional consequences (if any) associated with these subtle changes are rarely known; the regulatory mechanisms responsible for controlling the expression of these surface markers are not known; and there is next to no database available on xenobiotic-induced changes in these surface markers. Despite the absence of a legitimate scientific basis, MCS and similar conditions will have a tremendous impact on human health in the years ahead. These conditions are driving a good share of toxic torte litigation at tremendous cost to society. MCS is clearly not without its proponents, and the impact is already being felt in different parts of the country. For example, in Marin County, California, an ecology house, an 11-unit, federally funded housing project designed to provide an odor-free environment for low-income people who are "disabled" by the smells and odors of everyday living, has been constructed at a cost of \$1.8 million. The basis for the ecology house is that individuals with MCS are eligible for disability, and the funds used to construct the ecology house were from Housing and Urban Development which had been earmarked for low-income disabled persons. The design of the ecology house prohibits all carpeting, paints, pesticides, fluorescent lighting, and natural gas lines. Moreover, individuals who live in the ecology house cannot wear any perfumes, colognes, or deodorants or use any other scented products, including detergents. Advocates of MCS are now calling for the construction and implementation of odor-free zones and entrances in all public buildings. All these activities will occur at tremendous expense to society as a whole and are directed at a condition, MCS, which has been described as "a name in search of a disease." Most experts agree that there is no immunological basis for MCS and suggest that treatments of MCS should target underlying psychological problems in individual sufferers, not the elimination of environmental odors.

Approaches to Immunotoxicology

The situation with MCS emphasizes that the discipline of immunotoxicology will continue to evolve as a meaningful and interpretable subdiscipline of toxicology only if the best scientific approaches are applied. One of the key issues facing immunotoxicology which has scientific, political, and societal implications is the approach to immunotoxicity testing for regulatory purposes. Several U.S. government agencies with regulatory responsibilities, including the FDA and the EPA, have drafted recommendations for guidelines for immunotoxicity testing strategies. All testing strategies to date recognize the complexity of the immune system as a target organ and recognize that no single immune parameter can be used with sufficient confidence to test for the hazard of immunotoxicity. Therefore, historically, immunotoxicity has been assessed by a battery of assays usually structured in a multitiered approach. However, recent validation studies, most notably studies conducted by the National Toxicology Program, have indicated that immunotoxicity can be assessed with a finite number of assays. Several concepts that have had an impact on the evolution of a testing strategy are highlighted as follows:.

- Although the concept of required immunotoxicity testing is a relatively recent development, the toxicity of the immune system has been an important part of routine toxicity testing for some time. The endpoints have included weights and histological evaluation of key immunocompetent organs, including the spleen and thymus, leukocyte counts and differentials, and some parameters in clinical chemistry, including globulin measurements. However, while it is acknowledged that these standard toxicology endpoints are important and can provide some indication of immunotoxicity, it is generally recognized that they are not sufficient as a predictor of immunotoxicity hazard. It has been estimated that as many as 30% of known immunotoxic chemicals would be missed if only these endpoints were used. Moreover, while it is accepted that these endpoints become better predictors when chemicals are assessed at high doses (i.e., at or above the maximum tolerated dose), it is recognized that these types of exposures will also increase the likelihood that indirect mechanisms of immunotoxicity (i.e., such as neuroendocrine changes, liver damage, or effects on other organ systems) will be involved.
- Most experts in the field of immunotoxicology recognize that immunotoxicity can only be measured if the immune system is asked to perform its function. Therefore, a specific functional parameter is now recognized as a critically important component of the first tier of a testing strategy. One of the most sensitive indicators of immunosuppression in most animal models has been the primary response to an antigen. An especially sensitive parameter has proven to be the antibody response to a T cell-dependent antigen. The sensitivity of this type of assay is consistent with the description of this response as being dependent on the cooperativity of multiple cell types, including the B cell as the primary effector cell, T cells as important regulatory cells, and APCs. Regardless of the specific immune parameters included in a testing strategy, the interpretation for immunotoxicity can only be made in the context of a well-designed study from the perspective of the dose–response relationship.
- Because an increase in the incidence and/or severity of infection has been consistently identified as one of the hallmark indicators of immunosuppression, a great deal of effort has been put forth into the design and characterization of host resistance models. One of the key features of these characterizations has been the correlation of changes in various host resistance models with changes in specific immune parameters. These results have consistently indicated that changes in specific immune functional parameters are associated with the predicted/anticipated changes in host resistance models. It is now generally accepted that host resistance models are not a feasible choice as an initial predictor of immunotoxicity because of their complexity and cost and that these models are best positioned in the second tier of a testing strategy.
- Because immunotoxicity exists in a continuum, it is important to measure xenobiotic-induced

changes in immune function in both directions. By and large, more effort has been invested in the validation of studies to address the immunosuppressive part of the continuum. However, recent validation studies have been conducted to address the sensitizing potential of chemicals, including a major effort by the National Toxicology Program.

- One of the obvious and most important goals of an experimental immunotoxicity testing strategy is to enable the best extrapolations between the results generated in the animal models and the potential risk of immunotoxicity in humans. One of the recent fallouts of this goal has been the recognition that the historic approaches that have been used in clinical immunology may not have much use in human immunotoxicology. While these endpoints are sufficient to detect immunodeficiencies associated with either congenital disorders or immunosuppressive drug therapy, they do not possess the necessary sensitivity to detect the more subtle consequences of xenobiotic-induced immunotoxicity. Specifically, many of these endpoints, including mitogen-induced lymphoproliferation, the analysis of lymphocyte surface markers, and the response to recall antigens, have been demonstrated to lack appreciable sensitivity in most animal studies. As a result, several recent proposals have been put forth to reevaluate the way that we measure immune function in humans. Most of these testing strategies have incorporated plans to measure the primary response to a new antigen, and several of these testing strategies have recommended using newly developed vaccines as the new antigen.

The immune system has unquestionably been identified as a potential target organ for drugs and chemicals. Therefore, the hazard exists. The assessment of the risk associated with xenobiotic-induced immunotoxicity represents one of the key challenges for this discipline in the immediate future.

Further Reading

Burrell, G. R., Dean, J. H., and Munson, A. E. (Eds.) (1995). *Methods in Immunology,* 2-vol. set. Wiley-Liss, New York.

Burrell, R., Flaherty, D. K., and Sauers, L. J. (Eds.) (1992). *Toxicology of the Immune System—A Human Approach.* Van Nostrand Reinhold, New York.

Paul, W. E. (Ed.) (1993). *Fundamental Immunology*, 3rd ed. Raven Press, New York.

Roitt, I. M., Brostoff, J., and Male, D. K. (Eds.) (1989). *Immunology*, 2nd ed. Gower Medical, New York.

Smialowicz, R. J., and Holsapple, M. P. (Eds.) (1995). *Experimental Immunotoxicology.* CRC Press, Boca Raton, FL.

Subcommittee on Immunotoxicology and the Committee on Biologic Markers (Eds.) (1992). *Biologic Markers in Immunotoxicology.* National Academy Press, Washington, DC.

Michael P. Holsapple and Norbert E. Kaminski

Related Topics

Biomarkers, Human Health
Blood
Delayed-Type Hypersensitivity
Molecular Toxicology
Multiple Chemical Sensitivities
Polyaromatic Hydrocarbons
Psychological Indices of Toxicity
Resistance to Toxicants
Sensitivity Analysis
Skin

Indole

- CAS: 120-72-9
- SYNONYMS: 2,3-Benzopyrrole; 1-benzopyrrole; 1-azaindene
- CHEMICAL CLASS: Organic dye; originally a coal tar dye and essential oil constituent
- MOLECULAR FORMULA: C_8H_7N

Uses

Indole is used as a chemical reagent and in the preparation of perfumes.

Exposure Pathways

Dermal contact, inhalation, and ingestion are all possible routes of exposure.

Human Toxicity

Indole is a possible human carcinogen.

Animal Toxicity

Indole is a possible carcinogen. The oral LD_{50} in rats is 1 g/kg. The oral LD_{Lo} in mice is 1070 mg/kg. The intraperitoneal LD_{50} in mice is 117 mg/kg. The dermal LD_{50} in rabbits is 790 mg/kg.

—*Shayne C. Gad*

Indoor Air Pollution

Introduction

Most people are concerned about the quality of the air that they breathe when outdoors, but until recently they were much less aware that the indoor air environment may contain some of the same pollutants found outdoors and quite a number of different ones. However, indoor air pollution is, in fact, not a new problem. When early humans discovered fire and used it to heat their shelters, they must have found that one of its undesirable side effects was production of and exposure to smoke. Attempts to provide adequate ventilation may have been made, but success was only partial in that mummified human lungs from the preindustrial age show considerable carbonaceous pigmentation.

It has become increasingly evident that the indoor environment is a significant source of personal exposure to various air contaminants, some of which can reach fairly high concentrations. However, any health effects from exposure to indoor air pollutants are a function of the total exposure, which is the relationship between air concentration and exposure duration. Thus, even when indoor concentrations are low, exposures may be of long duration and the total, or cumulative, dose can be quite high. This reflects the fact that people can spend upwards of 90% of their time indoors, be it at home, at the office, or in shopping malls. In many instances, indoor sources actually provide the bulk of personal exposure to certain airborne toxicants and the only source of exposure to others. Furthermore, the population exposed largely indoors is much more diverse than that exposed in occupational environments or even in ambient outdoor air; in addition to healthy adults, it includes infants, children, and people with medical conditions, all of whom may be especially vulnerable to certain toxicants.

For a long time, remaining indoors was considered to afford protection from air pollution, and early studies of indoor air quality were generally concerned with examining the ratios of indoor to outdoor concentrations of various contaminants since it was felt that indoor contaminant levels were controlled primarily by outdoor concentrations. Outdoor pollutants can indeed infiltrate indoors through cracks and other openings in buildings and through ventilation systems, or they be carried indoors on building occupants. However, the relative amount of an outdoor pollutant found indoors depends largely on its physicochemical properties. For example, highly reactive gases and large particles may be removed from the air prior to entering an indoor environment, and resulting indoor concentrations would be much lower than those found outdoors. On the other hand, very small particles or less reactive gases may occur indoors at levels that approach 80% of those found outdoors.

It is now very clear that indoor air contaminants are not totally derived from outdoor sources, but that numerous contaminants can be directly released into the indoor environment from local sources, such as cooking over an open flame, from smoking, from heating systems, from modern synthetic building and furnishing materials, from consumer products, and even from natural sources, including the normal biological activities of building occupants. Many of these contaminants have been found to occur in increasing levels over recent years due to the attempt to make homes, and other buildings, more airtight for energy conservation. This reduces the rate of air exchange between the outside (fresh air) and inside environments. For example, older homes may have air exchange rates which are 2–10 times greater than those found in newer houses. The result is that levels of many indoor contaminants can be many times higher than the concentration of these same materials in the outdoor environment, if they occur outdoors at all.

Buildings are not the only sources for exposure to indoor air contaminants. Many people spend a significant portion, often up to 5%, of their day in transit, and transportation provides additional opportunities for exposure to various toxicants. Although the air exchange rate in most forms of transportation is generally higher than in buildings, in many cases the number of occupants per unit volume of air is much greater. A good example of this is modern aircraft, which also may recirculate as much as 50% of the interior air, leading to the accumulation of contaminants such as ozone and cigarette smoke.

The major sources of air pollutants found in buildings are described below. However, the mere presence of a potential contaminant source does not necessarily mean that exposure will ensue. This is because the extent of exposure, if any, often depends on the physical nature of a source or the manner in which it is used; an example of this is asbestos, as will be discussed later. Furthermore, the health significance of exposure to indoor pollutants may not always be clear. While many of these toxicants may have adverse effects under exposure conditions found in occupational and other environments, often much less is known about biological responses with prolonged exposures at concentrations common in indoor environments.

Sources of Indoor Air Contaminants

Combustion By-Products

One very common source of indoor air pollutants is the combustion of biomass or fossil fuels, such as in gas ranges (including pilot lights), wood burning stoves and fireplaces, and gas and kerosene space heaters. These emit both particles and gases. The former consist of carbon soot, various mineral constituents of the fuels, and organic compounds, while the latter include carbon monoxide, carbon dioxide, nitrogen dioxide, nitric oxide, and, depending on the fuel used, sulfur dioxide and various organics. The amounts of specific contaminants emitted vary depending on the fuel type, the combustion process used, and the nature of the appliance. For example, properly operated gas ranges emit little if any particulate matter, while wood burning stoves emit much greater amounts. When properly used and vented, many potential contaminants from combustion sources do not remain within the indoor environment, thus becoming outdoor pollutants. However, because combustion activities tend to be episodic, short-term indoor concentrations can be quite high for unvented or improperly vented systems.

About half of all homes in the United States use natural gas for cooking, a typical example of unvented combustion and a major source of indoor nitrogen dioxide and carbon monoxide, especially in kitchen areas. Other generally unvented combustion sources are gas and kerosene space heaters, found in about 10% of homes in the United States. Emissions from the latter are similar to those from gas-fueled devices, but particles from kerosene heaters consist of carbon onto which may be adsorbed organic chemicals (e.g., hydrocarbons), many of which show significant mutagenic activity. Wood stoves are also used for home heating in many areas, and while they are generally vented outdoors, improper venting or lack of proper seals can also result in significant indoor contamination by organic-coated carbon particles. The actual exposure to contaminants from any of these combustion sources depends on the degree of venting used while the appliance is in operation and the extent and pattern of its use, but indoor concentrations of nitrogen dioxide and carbon monoxide are generally higher than those outdoors when significant sources are present, especially in the winter when interior ventilation tends to be reduced.

Nitrogen Dioxide

Any high-temperature combustion process in air initially generates nitric oxide and some nitrogen dioxide, but the former becomes rapidly oxidized to the latter. Combustion processes may produce other forms of nitrogen oxides, such as nitric acid vapor; however, the toxicological significance of these is not certain.

When natural gas ranges are in operation for home cooking, indoor nitrogen dioxide levels are generally higher than those found outdoors and are always above those found in homes using electric ranges. The average daily concentration in homes using gas for cooking purposes can range from 0.05 to 0.5 ppm, but short-term peaks of 1 ppm are not uncommon. The result is that personal exposures to nitrogen dioxide are primarily driven by indoor sources in homes using gas appliances.

Nitrogen dioxide is an upper respiratory tract irritant and has, in some cases, been linked to an increased incidence of acute respiratory infection in children residing in homes using gas for cooking. There is also some suggestion that nitrogen dioxide, at concentrations found indoors, may increase asthmatic symptoms. However, controlled laboratory and epidemiological studies have not as yet resulted in a consistent pattern of responses that allow an unequivocal conclusion as to the potential health effects of indoor exposure.

Carbon Monoxide

Carbon monoxide is produced during the incomplete combustion of carbon-containing fuels, such as natural gas, kerosene, and wood. Its production rate by gas ranges is actually greater than that for nitrogen dioxide, and indoor levels can be several times greater than those found outdoors. Concentrations ranging from 2 to 15 ppm have been found in homes using gas for cooking. In some cases, indoor levels are enhanced by carbon monoxide derived from automobiles housed in garages attached to residences or in office buildings.

Carbon monoxide binds very strongly to hemoglobin in red blood cells, resulting in the production of carboxyhemoglobin (COHb); this can actually be used as a marker for exposure to carbon monoxide. The presence of COHb impairs the normal transport of oxygen within the blood and can result in adverse effects on tissues, such as those in the cardiovascular and nervous systems which have high oxygen needs.

Symptoms of acute carbon monoxide poisoning range from headache to death. Prolonged exposure can affect the body due to oxygen deprivation, a condition known as tissue hypoxia. Levels of carbon monoxide encountered indoors have been found to result in disorientation in exposed individuals and can exacerbate symptoms in people with cardiovascular disease, perhaps increasing mortality. The effects of prolonged exposures to indoor concentrations on the health of normal individuals are, however, not certain.

Wood Smoke

The use of wood for space heating in homes has increased during the past 25 years in a number of areas in the United States. Wood smoke is a complex mixture of gases and particles, including carbon monoxide, nitrogen dioxide, sulfur dioxide, and various organic compounds. The amount of each produced depends on burn rate, the type and quantity of wood used, and its moisture content. Wood stoves are generally vented outdoors, and the newer ones even operate under negative pressure and should contribute little contamination to the indoor air environment. However, some indoor pollution may occur from faulty venting, leakage, or during non-airtight conditions such as during start-up, stoking, and reloading. There has not, however, been adequate characterization of the influence of wood combustion on indoor air quality. Furthermore, while individual constituents of wood smoke are irritants and carcinogens, any health hazard due to indoor exposure is not known, although there is some evidence that it may increase chronic respiratory symptoms, such as cough and wheeze, in children.

Environmental Tobacco Smoke

One indoor air pollutant of recent concern in terms of potential effects on public health is tobacco smoke, which contains over 4000 different chemical compounds emitted as particles or gases and is the largest single source of air contamination in many indoor environments. Environmental tobacco smoke is the term used to describe the smoke found indoors and which consists of a combination of that emitted into air from the burning end of a cigarette, cigar, or pipe (sidestream smoke) plus the smoke that is actively inhaled from the mouth end (mainstream smoke) and subsequently exhaled. Generally half of a cigarette is consumed by active smoking and the other half by smoldering.

The combustion conditions differ when a cigarette is puffed compared to when it smolders, so the actual ratios of chemical constituents in sidestream and mainstream smoke also differ, although qualitatively the materials are similar. Because mainstream smoke becomes diluted by inhalation and subsequent exhalation, the bulk of environmental tobacco smoke actually consists of sidestream smoke, which has higher concentrations of a number of toxic and carcinogenic chemicals than found in mainstream smoke. While the amount of these inhaled by the nonsmoker compared to the active smoker is reduced by dilution in room air, environmental tobacco smoke is the source of numerous toxic and carcinogenic contaminants in indoor environments; some of the major ones are listed in Table I-2. Particulate levels in the smoking areas of some build-

TABLE I-2
Major Indoor Air Contaminants Derived from Environmental Tobacco Smoke

In vapor/gas phase	*In particulate phase*
Acetone	Aniline
Acrolein	Benzo(*a*)pyrene
Ammonia	Carbon
Carbon dioxide	Nicotine
Carbon monoxide	Metals (nickel, arsenic, cadmium)
Formaldehyde	Phenol
Hydrogen cyanide	
Nitrogen oxides	
Pyridine	

ings can be up to 25 times greater than those in nonsmoking areas, reaching concentrations above 300 $\mu g/m^3$. Nitrogen dioxide and benzene have also been found to be significantly elevated in the homes of smokers compared to those of nonsmokers.

Passive smoking, or involuntary smoking, is the term used to describe the inhalation of environmental tobacco smoke by nonsmokers. The amount of smoke to which any individual is exposed is quite variable, depending on the number of sources (i.e., active smokers), the degree of building ventilation which affects dilution, and the presence of any air cleaning devices. Personal exposures to passive smoking can be assessed using biological markers in body fluids, such as saliva, blood, or urine. The most sensitive and specific of these markers are nicotine and its major metabolite, cotinine. Following smoke exposure, the latter remains longer in the body than does the former and is therefore a better monitor of chronic exposure. Its assessment clearly indicates that passive smoking is a significant source of exposure to cigarette smoke, with cotinine levels in nonsmokers approaching 10% of those found in active smokers.

Exposure to environmental tobacco smoke has been linked to various diseases and symptoms, particularly in children of smoking parents. Within this group, responses include increased acute respiratory infection, such as bronchitis and pneumonia, especially in infants; increased frequency of chronic respiratory symptoms (i.e., cough, phlegm, and wheezing) and middle ear infections; and reduced lung function and rate of lung growth. Effects in adult nonsmokers are not as conclusive in terms of alterations in lung function, but irritation of the eyes and of the upper and lower respiratory tract do occur, and environmental tobacco smoke may increase the risk of developing cardiovascular disease. Exposure may affect adults with concurrent cardiovascular or pulmonary disease to a greater extent than healthy individuals. Exacerbation of symptoms in asthmatics, especially children, also occurs, and smoke exposure may actually be a risk factor for new cases of asthma. Effects on birth weight of babies when the mother is exposed have been reported in some instances.

Environmental tobacco smoke is a significant risk factor for lung cancer in nonsmokers, and it has been classified as a respiratory carcinogen by IARC. The increased individual risk can be 30–50% depending on the extent of exposure, and exposure to environmental tobacco smoke is estimated to be responsible for lung cancer deaths among nonsmokers in the United States.

Volatile and Semivolatile Organic Compounds

Volatile organic compounds (VOCs) consist of various classes of carbon-containing chemicals that are gases at room temperature. They are found in essentially all indoor locations, released by offgassing from numerous sources, such as construction and decorating materials, pesticides, consumer products, paints, paint removers, furnishings, carpets, and from combustion of wood, kerosene, and tobacco. While more than 500 volatile organic compounds have been identified in indoor air, about 50 occur most commonly. The major sources for many of these are listed in Table I-3. In older homes, the total concentration of all volatile organics can range from 0.02 to 1.7 mg/m^3, while in newer homes, levels of 0.5–19 mg/m^3 have been found. Such indoor exposure to organic compounds is much greater than that which occurs outdoors, with indoor concentrations of some materials being 10 times higher than those outdoors and with short-term peaks reaching 1000 times higher.

Semivolatile organic compounds, which are solids or liquids at room temperature, are also found in indoor air, derived from pesticides, wood preservatives, floor waxes and polishes, and from combustion sources. These have, however, not been as extensively categorized indoors as have the volatile chemicals.

TABLE I-3
Common Indoor Sources of Volatile Organic Compounds

Chemical class	*Examples*	*Typical sources*
Aldehydes	Formaldehyde	See Table I-4
Hydrocarbons		
Aliphatic	Propane, butane, undecane, pentane	Cooking and heating fuel, aerosol propellants, lubricants, perfume, glues
Aromatic	Benzene, styrene, toluene, xylene	Paint, varnish, glue, cleaners, lacquers, combustion sources
Halogenated	Chloroform, 1,1,1-trichloroethane, trichloroethylene, methylene chloride, *p*-dichlorobenzene	Pesticides, dry-cleaning solvents, aerosol propellants, degreasing agents, paint strippers
Alcohols	Methanol, hexanol	Window cleaners, paint, adhesives, cosmetics
Ketones	Acetone	Lacquers, polish removers, adhesives
Terpenes	α-Pinene, limonene	Air fresheners, polishes, fabric softeners

Many volatile organic compounds are known or suspected human carcinogens (e.g., benzene, vinyl chloride, chloroform, and *p*-dicholorobenzene) and many more are respiratory tract irritants or can affect the central nervous system (e.g., toluene and xylene). Furthermore, many organic chemicals have distinct odors, which can act as stressor agents affecting response. Exposure to volatile organics is generally assessed by measurement of the chemical in breath samples, but some can also be found in body fluids, such as mother's milk and blood.

One of the most common volatile organic contaminants found in indoor air is formaldehyde. It is derived from various sources, as shown in Table I-4, but its use as a bonding resin in pressed wood products, such as plywood, particle board, paneling, and fiberboard commonly found in home and furniture construction, represents the single largest current use. In past years, a major source for formaldehyde was urea-formaldehyde foam insulation injected into the walls of homes. While this use has generally ended, very high indoor levels of formaldehyde are still found in homes with such insulation, where concentrations can range from 0.12 to 4 ppm compared to levels of 0.03–0.09 ppm in homes where it was not used. Homes which make extensive use of plywood, such as mobile and prefabricated houses, also have high levels, which have been measured at 1–4 ppm. It is evident that formaldehyde concentrations vary widely; they depend on the age of the structure, potential sources, and indoor temperature and humidity (e.g., high temperatures enhance offgassing).

Formaldehyde can enter the body via the respiratory system, skin, or gastrointestinal tract, but it is primarily absorbed in the respiratory tract where it is rapidly metabolized. It is an upper respiratory tract and eye irritant; may cause respiratory symptoms, reductions in lung function, and headaches; may predispose to asthma; and can also affect the nervous system. It is

TABLE I-4
Common Indoor Sources of Formaldehyde

Urea–formaldehyde foam insulation (UFFI)
Resins used as bonding agents in pressed wood products
- Particle board
- Plywood
- Paneling

Resins used as water repellants, stiffeners, or wrinkle resistors
- Paper products
  - Paper towels
  - Grocery bags
  - Waxed paper
- Permanent-press clothing
- Carpeting
- Linoleum
- Plastics
- Drapery

Consumer products
- Cosmetics
- Shampoo
- Deodorants
- Dyes

Combustion processes
- Natural gas ranges and heaters
- Kerosene heaters
- Tobacco smoke

carcinogenic in laboratory animals, but human carcinogenicity is still an open issue.

Asbestos

Asbestos is a class of fibrous silicate minerals, each type of which differs in fiber shape and chemical formulation. It was widely used for decades because of its properties as a heat and sound insulator and fireproofing material and can be found in older floor and ceiling tiles, roofing felt and shingles, dry wall patching compounds, fireproofing insulation sprayed around steel beams, and the insulation of boilers and pipes. While it can no longer be used for most applications in new buildings, it is still a major indoor contaminant in many older ones, including homes and schools. However, the mere presence of asbestos in an indoor environment does not indicate exposure. If the asbestos-containing item is intact and fibers do not escape into the air, there is no exposure, and in many cases it is better to leave the material in place if it is well contained. However, much asbestos-containing material is old and in poor condition or damaged and may be friable (i.e., sheds fibers into the air).

Exposure to certain types of asbestos fibers is associated with specific respiratory diseases. These are asbestosis, a form of lung fibrosis, and two types of malignancies, namely, mesotheliomas, which are tumors of the lung pleura or peritoneum, and bronchial carcinomas. Synthetic or man-made mineral fibers, such as fiberglass, used as asbestos substitutes for many applications seem to pose much less of a public health risk, although some have been associated with noncarcinogenic health effects in people exposed occupationally.

Radon

Radon (Rn-222) is an odorless and colorless radioactive gas. It is produced during the radioactive decay of radium-226, itself a decay product of uranium-238 found in many types of crustal materials, i.e., rocks and soils. Rn-222 has a short half-life (3.8 days) and decays into a series of solid particulate products, known as radon progeny or radon daughters, all of which have even shorter half-lives (on the order of 30 min or less). Other isotopes of radon also occur naturally, but due to differences in half-life and dosimetry their health significance is minimal compared to that from exposure to Rn-222.

The main source of indoor air radon is the soil and rock beneath a building, from which the gas penetrates indoors, primarily through cracks or openings in the foundation or basement, including drain and utility access areas. This infiltration is driven by small pressure differences between the lower parts of a building and the outdoors due, in turn, to temperature differences between indoors and outdoors and effects of wind. Thus, radon levels indoors tend to be highest in the lowest levels of a building, from which the gas can then permeate the entire structure through the ventilation system. Some well (ground) water in areas having high soil radium content may also be a source of indoor radon, as may natural gas or building materials containing radium. The highest acceptable level of residential radon has been set by the U.S. EPA at 4 pCi/liter of air, but about 5–10% of homes in the United States exceed this benchmark. Levels of 1 or 2 pCi/liter are common in average homes.

The risk from radon exposure is essentially due to inhalation of its progeny, which can attach to abundant sources of particles in indoor air that then act as carriers of these radioactive particles into the respiratory tract. Radon accounts for up to 50% of the total internal dose from all natural background radiation sources and this, in turn, is due almost completely to two of its progeny, namely, polonium-218 and polonium-214, that decay via the release of α-particles.

Radon exposure in the home likely substantially increases lung cancer risk in both nonsmokers or smokers. It has been estimated that up to 20,000 lung cancers per year in the United States can be attributed to such exposure. Furthermore, the individual risk may increase if other cancer-associated factors, especially cigarette smoke, are also present.

Biological Agents

Indoor air can contain a wide variety of biological contaminants; some examples are presented in Table I-5. While many of these are nonpathogenic, others induce disease by infection of the respiratory tract or by immunologic means, such as allergy.

Most indoor biological pollutants originally derived from outdoor sources, with indoor contamination occurring wherever the environment is conducive to

TABLE I-5
Common Indoor Biological Contaminants

Bacteria
Bacillus subtilis
Escherichia coli
Klebsiella pneumoniae
Legionella pneumophila
Mycobacterium spp.
Pseudomonas aeroginosa
Salmonella typhosa
Staphylococcus aureus
Streptococcus spp.
Viruses
Fungi
Alternarium
Aspergillus spp.
Penicilium funiculosum
Thermophilic actinomycetes
Insects and insect parts
Cockroach
Mites
Dander

growth or accumulation. For example, bacterial, mold, and fungal contamination typically occur in moist environments, such as bathrooms, kitchens, basements, and forced air ventilation systems, and in standing water found in humidifiers, evaporation pans of self-defrost refrigerators, and even toilets.

Biological agents are disseminated in indoor air by various means. Depending on the organism, this includes human actions (such as sneezing and coughing); via mechanical devices which result in the aerosolization of water spray containing these agents, such as humidification systems and whirlpool baths; via air movement induced by ventilation systems and by air currents derived from convective radiant heating systems; or by dusting or vacuuming of contaminated carpets or furniture. The risk of developing an infection or allergy from exposure to indoor air is often greater than that from outdoor air due to reduced ventilation in confined spaces resulting in the buildup of microorganisms or allergens to effective localized levels.

Infectious Agents

Infectious agents found in indoor air include viruses, bacteria, fungi, and protozoans. Viruses are internal cell parasites and can exist outside living cells for only a short period of time. On the other hand, bacteria, fungi, and protozoans can exist for extended durations on nonliving material. While bacteria are primary pathogens for humans, fungi and protozoans are generally opportunistic, i.e., they produce disease only in compromised individuals, such as those with reduced defenses due to concurrent disease or use of certain medications.

Infectious disease can be produced by any pathogen able to be aerosolized and subsequently transported into the respiratory tract at the appropriate concentration. Some common diseases which may result from airborne transmission in indoor environments are listed in Table I-6. The rate of infection within any environment is a function of the viability and virulence of the pathogen, its concentration in the inhaled air, and characteristics, such as droplet size, of the carrier aerosol within which it is contained. Some biological agents produce disease at low concentrations, while others must accumulate to a higher level. Furthermore, individual susceptibility to infection depends on a number of factors, such as age and health, as well as concomitant exposure to chemical pollutants.

While there are a number of potential sources of infectious agents in the indoor environment, humans are the principal one for pathogens responsible for most airborne viral diseases and many bacterial diseases. Nonliving sources can also harbor infectious agents. A good example is the bacterium, *Legionella pneumophila,* which becomes airborne from contaminated cooling system water and is responsible for Legion-

TABLE I-6
Some Diseases Potentially Spread by Indoor Air Exposure

Viral
Chicken pox
Colds
Influenza
Smallpox
Measles
Bacterial
Legionnaires' disease
Tuberculosis
Brucellosis
Fungal
Histoplasmosis
Cryptococcosis
Coccidiomycosis
Protozoan
Pneumocystis carinii
Acanthameoebosis

naires' disease. Water is also the main source for airborne protozoans.

Pathogenic fungi generally derive from outdoor air, but their spores are able to penetrate into buildings through air spaces or intake vents, and interior growth can then occur on damp surfaces. An example is *Aspergillus,* an opportunistic pathogen associated with infections in hospitals.

Allergens and Immunologic Agents

Indoor air may contain biological agents capable of eliciting an allergic response. Almost all microbial allergens are fungal in origin, although some bacterial components are also allergenic. Other indoor airborne allergens include dust mites (discussed later), insect parts, and dander (shed skin scales from pets or even other people). Many of these are found in common household dust, which is actually a complex mixture of a number of allergenic biological substances.

There are several different types of immune responses. For example, an allergic response is characterized by production of a specific immunoglobulin (antibody) termed IgE. Examples of respiratory allergies are rhinitis and asthma. One particular group of people who are especially susceptible to such allergies are termed atopic and show a greater tendency to produce IgE following exposure to numerous allergens present in indoor air environments.

Another type of immunologically mediated lung disease is hypersensitivity pneumonitis. This is acutely characterized by flu-like symptoms, including fevers, cough, and chills, but in a chronic state may result in a slow, progressive decline in pulmonary function. A number of antigenic materials can produce hypersensitivity pneumonitis. While they are mostly complex organic particles, a fairly common indoor antigen involved in its pathogenesis is the thermophilic actinomycetes. These organisms are found in decomposing organic matter and contaminate indoor environments through ventilation and humidification systems. Humidifier fever, which shows symptoms similar to those of hypersensitivity pneumonitis but without the chest signs, is a syndrome associated with exposure to these organisms.

Allergic asthma may be exacerbated by exposure to antigens found in indoor air, including house dust, fungal spores, and molds. The house dust mite (*Dermatophagoides farinae*), which exists in bedding and in the stuffing of upholstered furniture, contains a potent allergen which occurs at high concentrations in house dust and then becomes airborne during cleaning activities. Inhalation of dust contaminated with these mites can increase the severity of asthma or perhaps even the risk of its inception.

Sick Building Syndrome and Multiple Chemical Sensitivity

Most indoor environments are contaminated by a combination of both viable organisms and nonviable particles and gases, but little is known regarding health effects from exposure to such complex mixtures even though biological responses to the inhalation of contaminated indoor air may depend on interactions between individual substances. Examples of some potential interactions having health significance are those between radon and environmental tobacco smoke in the risk of developing lung cancer; between environmental tobacco smoke and nitrogen dioxide in the induction of respiratory infection in children; and between allergens and environmental tobacco smoke in the exacerbation of asthmatic symptoms. Exposure to mixtures of indoor air pollutants does appear to be associated with two clinical conditions, namely, sick building syndrome and multiple chemical sensitivity.

During the past 20 years, there have been numerous reports of a spectrum of nonspecific health complaints from occupants of various buildings, including schools, hospitals, and, most often, modern offices. Complaints include respiratory tract infection, irritation of the eyes, nose, and throat, headaches, neurological reactions, nausea, lethargy, and dizziness. The range and severity of the symptoms varied greatly depending on the sensitivity of exposed individuals. While a causative role of the indoor environment was strongly suggested when it became clear that the symptoms generally abated upon leaving the building, in most cases no specific cause for them has been found. The term used for this collection of clinical signs is sick building syndrome, or tight building syndrome, and it is estimated to occur in about one-third of all buildings in the United States, especially in those that have been made "tight" for energy conservation. This, in turn, allowed for the accumulation of contaminants from numerous indoor sources.

One chemical is most likely not responsible for sick building syndrome but, rather, it probably reflects exposures to various chemicals, which can differ at different sites. Because many volatile organic compounds produce similar symptoms to those noted in sick building syndrome, they are suspected to be causative agents. However, because of the large number of such chemicals in most indoor environments, it is hard to associate health problems with any one organic contaminant.

Sick building syndrome is to be distinguished from what have been termed building-related illnesses. These latter have definite etiological agents and specific clinical manifestations, e.g., hypersensitivity pneumonitis associated with bacterially mediated Legionnaires' disease. The symptoms do not abate when leaving the building, and medical treatment is generally necessary.

Multiple chemical sensitivity is a term used to describe a variety of symptoms associated, in some cases, with exposure to indoor air contaminants. Individuals with this syndrome seem to respond to very low levels of chemicals, and the condition can involve various organ systems. It appears to be induced by a wide variety of agents, but once induced it can be triggered by low-concentration exposures to numerous other chemicals.

Control of Indoor Air Contaminants

Most indoor air pollutants can be controlled by the proper measure. Once an understanding of the nature of the problem is obtained, remediation generally involves some combination of the following: changes in ventilation; source removal, substitution, or modification; air purification; or change in behavior. While details are beyond the scope of this entry, some examples of these approaches will suffice. Increased ventilation to allow dilution of indoor air with fresh outdoor air or recirculated indoor air can reduce levels of combustion by-products, biological agents, and radon gas; removal of sources or substitution of less hazardous materials for asbestos insulation and organics in consumer products and furnishings can reduce contamination by these agents; source modifications, such as reduction of contaminant emission rates through design changes or containment of emissions by some barrier, can reduce levels of combustion by-products, radon, and volatile organics; and behaviorial modifications can reduce cigarette smoke exposure to nonsmokers.

Further Reading

Gammage, R. B., and Kaye, S. V. (Eds.) (1985). *Indoor Air and Human Health*. Lewis, Chelsea, MI.

Indoor air and health effects (1991). *Environ. Health Perspect.* **95**.

Lippmann, M. (Ed.) (1992). *Environmental Toxicants. Human Exposures and Their Health Effects*. Van Nostrand Reinhold, New York.

National Research Council (1981). *Indoor Pollutants*. National Academy Press, Washington, DC.

Samet, J. M., and Spengler, J. D. (Eds.) (1991). *Indoor Air Pollution: A Health Perspective*. Johns Hopkins Univ. Press, Baltimore, MD.

Samet, J. M., Marbury, M. C., and Spengler, J. D. (1987). Health effects and sources of indoor air pollution. Part I. *Am. Rev. Respir. Dis.* **136**, 1486–1508.

Samet, J. M., Marbury, M. C., and Spengler, J. D. (1988). Health effects and sources of indoor air pollution. Part II. *Am. Rev. Respir. Dis.* **137**, 221–242.

U.S. Environmental Protection Agency (1989). *Report to Congress on Indoor Air Quality*, EPA/400/1-89/D01A. U.S. EPA, Washington, DC.

U.S. Environmental Protection Agency (1992). *Respiratory Health Effects of Passive Smoking: Lung Cancer and Other Disorders*, EPA/600/6-90/006F. U.S. EPA, Washington, DC.

Upton, A. C., and Graber, E. (Eds.) (1993). *Staying Healthy in a Risky Environment: The New York University Medical Center Family Guide*. Simon & Schuster, New York.

—Richard B. Schlesinger

Related Topics

Combustion Toxicology
Multiple Chemical Sensitivities
Pollution, Air
Psychological Indices of Toxicology
Sick Building Syndrome

Information Resources in Toxicology

Introduction

The availability of toxicological information has dramatically increased during the past 90 years, spurred by an increased awareness of how chemicals and other environmental factors influence biological systems. While during the first half of the twentieth century toxicology was considered a subset of pharmacology, it became a focused discipline largely through public awareness of toxicological issues. Recognition of the need for protection from hazardous chemical exposure, and environmental impact, resulted in legislation designed to safeguard the consumer. This legislation mandated continuing research on the effects of chemicals on man and the environment. In the past 20 years the major legislation in the United States dealing with controls on medicinals, environmental contaminants, and energy have all included provision for the collection and dissemination of data. Spurred on by these types of regulatory requirements and worldwide concern for the safety of the planet industry, research organizations, government agencies, academic centers, and international groups have all contributed to a huge body of toxicology information.

This entry provides a selection of printed and electronic information resources of use in identifying toxicological information. Technological advances and ways to communicate on a global scale have provided great opportunities for sharing knowledge. It is estimated that scientific information doubles every 4 years; in the vast toxicological arena, this figure is greatly accelerated. One of the larger U.S. catalog systems provides references to more than 1700 toxicology titles of reports, monographs, and serial titles published in the past 4 years alone. A study of the National Technical Information Service (NTIS) database titles shows that environmental health and toxicology records have increased by 600% during the past 13 years. Today there are an estimated 300 public databases and databanks that could be consulted for toxicology-related information, thousands of journal articles published each year on the effects of xenobiotics on humans and the environment, and more than a score of organizations whose primary activities are the creation of banks of available files of data and the production of research reports in specialized areas of toxicology.

This huge amount of information, scattered throughout the literature of the scientific disciplines—chemistry, biology, medicine—and present in many forms—raw data, technical reports, articles, monographs, statutes, and regulations—presents an enormous challenge to identify and retrieve relevant information. During the past decade technological developments have provided computerized systems capable of storing and providing access to information on a scale unimagined less than 20 years ago. Some systems provide access to data itself, and some are designed to provide information on sources of data. Some systems determine hazard assessment by applying sophisticated algorithms and use of mathematical modeling, and some systems are designed as interactive, multimedia instructional tools. The development of hypertext and other sophisticated software systems for navigating databases, electronic superhighways such as the Internet linking investigators to potentially valuable electronic repositories of information, the creation of local storage and retrieval systems such as those based on CD technology, and the developments in electronic communication systems provide opportunities, and frustrations, for the investigator.

Approaching the Problem

Although we have access to an enormous amount of information, the quality and reproducibility of data varies considerably. Governmental and regulatory influences have not provided any guarantees as to the accuracy of data related to xenobiotics and the researcher needs to understand the purpose and mandates behind an information resource to fully evaluate the data contained within. For example, the NIOSH Registry of Toxic Effects of Chemical Substances (RTECS) criteria for selection of data is not based on the reproducibility of that data. Other sources, like the National Library of Medicine's Hazardous Substances Databank (HSDB), present information compiled from a wide variety of source materials and are extensively reviewed by experts.

The professional is usually aware of the major texts, journals, organizations, and other standard resources in their own field. However, because of the interdisciplinary nature of toxicology, and the need to access information that may reside in the resources of other scientific areas of study, the user is frequently at a loss. Some types of sources are difficult to find. The so-called "gray literature"—for example, manufacturer's brochures, internal agency/company reports, conference proceedings, or translations, all excellent sources of potentially useful information—can be extremely difficult to identify. Other obstacles include those related to technology. Hardware limitations, varying search software and operating systems, and telecommunications problems can limit the investigator's ability to identify needed resources. There are also the common problems of interpretation of data—language barriers or varying scientific research conventions.

Valuable assistance in finding information can be obtained by consulting information intermediaries with subject expertise who can identify and access information resources unknown or unavailable locally. These individuals may be in local information centers or may be brokers who specialize in individual information services or creation of compilations of data for a fee. An example of this type of service is the Comprehensive Health and Environmental Monographs (CHEMS) division of Health and Environment International. This service creates detailed reports on the health and environmental effects of a chemical. Professional organizations, database producers, and government agencies can also be sources of experts as well as providers of direct information. An example of the former type of service is INFOTERRA, an international referral and research organization of the United Nations Environmental Program (UNEP). INFOTERRA provides access to an extensive range of information sources, as well as expert consultants, worldwide. The U.S. EPA is the National Focal Point for this organization in the United States, one of over 150 sites around the globe.

Keeping Current

Columns and review sections in journals or newsletters can help the professional keep abreast of new resources or provide comparative information on established resources in selected areas. Collections of reviews are also available on-line in such sources as *Comprehensive Core Medical Library* (CCML) by CDP, *Book Review Index* (on-line and in print) by Wilson, and the National Library of Medicine's *TOXLINE* database. Reviews of popular works dealing with consumer health or environmental concerns can also be found in newspapers, popular magazines, and consumer organization newsletters. Summaries and reviews of on-line databases and databanks can be found in the information science journals, directories of on-line resources, producer/vendor documentation, and Internet websites and listservers.

In addition to journals, texts, and newsletters, resource information can be identified by examining the program reports of government agencies, scientific organizations, or research institutions. Names of experts, identification of programs of interest, and organs for dissemination of information can all be identified in this way. An example of this type of resource is *Access EPA,* Information Access Branch, Information Management and Services, Division, U.S. Environmental Protection Agency, U.S. Government Printing Office, Washington, DC (ISBN 0-160418674). This document serves as a pathfinder to the clearinghouses, hotlines, records, databases, libraries, report series, and other resources supported by the U.S. EPA.

Guides to the Literature

There are few guides to the literature of toxicology, but many excellent guides exist in narrower areas. The following is a selection of available tools published within the past few years:

Balachandran, S. (1993). *Encyclopedia of Environmental Information Sources.* Gale Research, Detroit, MI. (ISBN 0-810385686)

This new edition to the growing Gale Research Environmental Library of publications contains 34,000 citations of print, electronic, and expert systems arranged under 1100 topics of environmental concern.

Deck, K. S., and Wright, P. (Updated periodically). *Environmental Health and Toxicology: A Selected Bibliography of Printed Information Resources.* U.S. Health and Human Services, Public Health Service, Centers for Disease Control and Prevention, National Center for Environmental Health, Information Resources Management Group.

This huge work contains citations to over 1300 books, reports, pamphlets, monographic and special series, newsletters, and includes a section giving address and telephone numbers for 200 publishers/distributors. While giving few annotations, it represents one of the most comprehensive bibliographies of sources. It is arranged alphabetically with no index; updated annually. Two more specialized bibliographies by the same author are also available: New editions: K. S. Deck and P. Wright, *Some Pub-*

licly Available Sources of Computerized Information on Environmental Health and Toxicology, and K. S. Deck and P. Wright, *Risk Assessment, Management, Communication: A Guide to Selected Sources.*

Hane, P. (Ed.) (1992). *Environment Online: The Greening of Databases.* Online, Wilton, CT. (ISBN 0-910965056)

A collection of related articles on literature sources on environmental concern, the majority of which are written by Gayle Alston and Frederick Stoss. This provides an excellent starting point for identifying on-line information resources concentrating on the environment. An update to this series, by Gayle Alston, titled "Environment Online: Update '93'," appears in the journal *Database* (December 1993, **16**(6), 42–46).

Lu, P. Y., Wassom, J. S., Farland, W. H., and DeRosa, C. (Eds.) (1990). *Access and Use of Information Resources in Assessing Health Risks from Chemical Exposure.* Oak Ridge National Laboratory, Oak Ridge, TN.

Based on a symposium of the same name held in 1990 and sponsored by the U.S. EPA and Oak Ridge, this work provides an array of 38 technical papers and abstracts of 39 poster sessions on information needs, uses, and the future of information access and retrieval in toxicology and environmental health.

Snow, B. (1989). *Drug Information: A Guide to Current Resources.* Medical Library Association, Chicago. (ISBN 0-810824302)

Designed as a self-study guide as well as a reference tool, this volume is considered the best work in the field. It is expected that Ms. Snow will produce an updated edition in 1998. Two chapters of particular interest in this context deal with side effects of therapeutic agents, adverse reactions, poisonings, and drug abuse.

Webster, J. K. (1987). *Toxic and Hazardous Materials, A Sourcebook and Guide to Information Sources.* Greenwood, Westport, CT. (ISBN 0-313245754)

This work is organized into separately authored chapters by subject (e.g., radioactive materials, laws and regulations, and transportation) listing more than 1600 sources (e.g., literature, organizations, audiovisuals, databases, agencies, research centers, and libraries). It is not as well indexed or as extensively annotated as Wexler's work but is still a useful resource.

Wexler, P. (1988). *Information Resources in Toxicology,* 2nd. ed. Elsevier, New York. (ISBN 0-444012141) (The third edition, to be published by IOS Press in the Netherlands, is expected out in 1998)

This is probably the best literature guide available today. Separate sections deal with the U.S. and foreign information resources. Printed and on-line sources, professional organizations, government agencies, regulations, education centers, and testing laboratories are covered for the United States and for selected countries. A history of toxicology and toxicology information systems developments are also included.

Texts

This section provides a very select list of classic or standard texts, dictionaries, thesauri, glossaries, directories, handbooks, encyclopedias, databooks, and some new and impressive works which can provide useful toxicology information. The focus is on works that have been published or revised within the past few years. For information on texts published prior to 1987, consult Wexler's *Information Resources in Toxicology* (listed in the previous section).

Klaassen, C. D., Amdur, M. O., Doull, J., and Casarett, L. J. (Eds.) (1996). *Casarett & Doull's Toxicology: The Basic Science of Poisons,* 5th ed. McGraw-Hill, New York. (ISBN 0-071054766)

A classic, well-documented, detailed text on general principles, toxic responses by body systems, toxic effects of major toxicant classes, and major discipline applications of toxicology.

Ballantyne, B., Marrs, T. C., and Turner, P. (Eds.) (1995). *General & Applied Toxicology,* 2 Vols. Stockton Press, New York. (ISBN 1-56159167X)

This very recent encyclopedic work provides an excellent collection of chapters dealing with toxicology theory and practice. Both U.S. and European viewpoints are presented. The chapter on information resources is written primarily from a European perspective.

Budavari, S (Ed.) (1989). *Merck Index: An Encyclopedia of Chemicals, Drugs and Biologicals,* 11th ed. Merck, Rahway, NJ. (ISBN 0-91191028X)

A compendium of quick information on over 10,000 substances—chemicals, drugs, biologicals, agricultural, and natural substances. Includes nomenclature, physical/chemical properties, patents, uses, literature references, structure, toxicity data, and related data. Available on-line on several public vendor systems and on CD-ROM.

Clayton, D. C. (Ed.) (1992). *Dictionary & Thesaurus of Environment, Health & Safety.* CRC Press, Boca Raton, FL. (ISBN 0-873718763)

This work represents the most thorough compilation to date of terminology related to the environment, health, and safety. The terminology has been extracted from numerous governmental and industry sources. Three major appendices cover acronyms, subject categorization of terms, and a mini-thesaurus of the FRASE vocabulary from the U.S. Department of Energy.

Clayton, G. D., and Clayton, F. E. (Eds.). *Patty's Industrial Hygiene and Toxicology,* 4th ed. Wiley, New York. Volume I, Parts A and B(1991) (ISBN 0-471552054 set); Volume II, Parts A–F (1993/1994) (ISBN 0-471547271 set)

Cralley, L. J., Cralley, L. V., and Bus, J. S. (Eds.) (1993). *Patty's Industrial Hygiene and Toxicology,* 3rd ed. Wiley, New York. Volume III, Part A (ISBN 0-471530662)
Volume III, Part B (1995). (ISBN 0-471530654)

This classic, giant compendium is one of the most complete in the area of occupational/industrial and general toxicological information. Volumes are updated irregularly.

Dreisbach, R. H., and Robertson, W. O. (1987). *Handbook of Poisoning: Prevention, Diagnosis, and Treatment,* 12th ed. Appleton & Lange, Norwalk, CT. (ISBN 0-8536433)

This handbook for the clinical toxicologist is a standard in emergency situations, covering all types of poison situations–agricultural, medical, industrial, and household. The work is organized to facilitate ease of use in emergency situations and as a reference source. Background chapters are on prevention, identification/diagnosis, management, and legal/medical responsibilities.

Derelanko, M. J., and Hollinger, M. A. (Eds.) (1995). *CRC Handbook of Toxicology.* CRC Press, New York. (ISBN 0-849386683)

An excellent compendium of practical reference information for the toxicologist. The focus is on providing normal values, reproductive indices, physiological parameters, regulatory requirements, procedures, values, endpoints, recommended sources, animal care, and tables/graphs of use to the practicing toxicologist. Information is presented in a loose chapter arrangement with detailed tables of contents for each. The index could be more useful.

Ellenhorn, M. J., and Barceloux, D. G. (1997). *Medical Toxicology: Diagnosis and Treatment of Human Poisoning.* Williams & Wilkins, Baltimore. (ISBN 0-683300318)

Provides an excellent reference for clinicians in emergency and occupational health settings. Medical toxicology defined here as poisoning by overdose of medication and exposure to chemicals and toxins not ordinarily used therapeutically. A good companion work to Dreisbach.

Gilman, A. G., Goodman, L. S., Rall, T. W., and Murad, F. (Eds.) (1996). *Goodman and Gilman's The Pharmacological Basis of Therapeutics,* 9th ed. McGraw-Hill, New York. (ISBN 0-070262667)

This gigantic textbook is the standard in clinical pharmacology and contains an enormous amount of information of use to the clinician and researcher. It is strong in drug interactions and mechanism of action. It is updated every 5 years. Available on CD-ROM.

Goldfrank, L. R., Flomenbaum, N. E., Lewin, N. A., Weisman, R. S., Howland, M. A., and Hoffman, R. S. (Eds.) (1994). *Goldfrank's Toxicologic Emergencies,* 5th ed. Appleton & Lange, Norwalk, CT. (ISBN 0-838531466)

This is a unique text and strong as a training manual and in clinical management settings (second in popularity to Ellenhorn and Barceloux).

Gosselin, R. E., Smith, R. P., Hodge, H. C., and Braddock, J. E. (1984). *Clinical Toxicology of Commercial Products,* 5th ed. Williams & Wilkins, Baltimore. (ISBN 0-683036327)

This tool was intended originally to assist in quick identification and handling of chemical poisonings by consumer products. It succeeds admirably–colored-coded sections, well referenced and documented, providing excellent access points to the information within. Unfortunately, a new edition is not planned by the publisher. It is available on-line on the CIS system.

Haddad, L. M., Winchester, J. F., and Shannon, M. W. (Eds.) (1998). *Clinical Management of Poisoning and Drug Overdose*, 3rd ed. Saunders, Philadelphia.

Previous editions have an emphasis on management rather than encyclopedic; the book is well documented.

Hallenbeck, W. H. (1993). *Quantitative Risk Assessment for Environmental & Occupational Health,* 2nd ed. Lewis/CRC Press, Boca Raton, FL. (ISBN 0-873718011)

This book contains a number of risk analysis models along with information on calculation of human dose rate and dose from experimental studies, confidence limits, quantitation of response, and tests of significance. It is an impressive reference text in this area.

Hamilton, A., Hardy, H. L., and Finkel, A. J. (1989). *Hamilton and Hardy's Industrial Toxicology,* 4th ed. John Wright, Boston. (ISBN 0-723670277)

This book provides historical and current reviews on the toxic effects of industrial chemicals.

Handbook of Natural Toxins. Dekker, New York.

Volume I: Keeler, R. F., and Tu, A. T. (Eds.) (1983). *Plant and Fungal Toxins.* (ISBN 0-824718933)
Volume II: Tu, A. T. (Ed.) (1984). *Insect Poisons, Allergens, and Other Invertebrate Venoms.* (ISBN 0-824772075)
Volume III: Tu, A. T. (Ed.) (1988). *Marine Toxins and Venoms.* (ISBN 0-824776674)
Volume IV: Hardegree, M. C., and Tu, A. T. (Eds.) (1988). *Bacterial Toxins.* (ISBN 0-824778405)
Volume V: Tu, A. T. (Ed.) (1991). *Reptile Venoms and Toxins.* (ISBN 0-82478376X)
Volume VI: Keeler, R. F., and Tu, A. T. (Eds.) (1991). *Toxicology of Plant and Fungal Compounds.* (ISBN 0-824783751)
Volume VII: Tu, A. T. (Ed.). (1992). *Food Poisoning.* (ISBN 0-824786521)
Volume VIII: Moss, J. (Ed.) (1995). *Bacterial Toxins and Virulence Factors in Disease.* (ISBN 0-824793811)

A series of publications describing all aspects of toxins and consequences of exposure to these agents. Includes descriptions, categorization, symptomology with exposure, treatment, and prevention of contact. All volumes in series still in print.

Hathaway, G. J., *et al.* (Eds.) (1996). *Proctor and Hughes' Chemical Hazards of the Workplace,* 4th ed. Van Nostrand Reinhold, New York. (ISBN 0-442020503)

Concise summary of 400 of the most common substances found in the industrial setting.

Hayes, A. W. (1994). *Principles and Methods of Toxicology,* 3rd ed. Raven Press, New York. (ISBN 0-781701317)

A textbook and standard reference designed to provide a thorough introduction to toxicology in the broadest sense. Strengths include coverage of methods, techniques, procedures, interpretation of data, and examination of controversial areas.

Hayes, W. J., Jr., and Laws, E. R., Jr. (Eds.) (1991). *Handbook of Pesticide Toxicology.* Academic Press, San Diego. (Vol. I, ISBN 0-123341612; Vol. II, ISBN 0-123341620; Vol. III, ISBN 0-123341639)

Comprehensive and timely compendium of scientific knowledge concerning the toxic effects or pesticides on humans and animals. In three volumes; updated and expanded version of *Toxicology of Pesticides* (1975) and *Pesticides Studied in Man* (1982) now out of print. Includes information on the diagnosis and treatment of pesticide poisonings. A true classic.

Herbicide Handbook, 7th ed. (1994). Weed Science Society of America, Champaign, IL. (ISBN 0-911733183)

This work, sponsored by the Weed Science Society of America, Herbicide Handbook Committee, contains a wealth of physical, chemical, and toxicological data on more than 150 herbicides. Extensive data are presented on each chemical. Included are producer information and references ($35.00; Weed Society of America, 1508 W. University Ave., Champaign, IL 61821-3133).

Hodgeson, E., and Levi, P. E. (Eds.) (1994). *Introduction to Biochemical Toxicology,* 2nd ed. Appleton & Lange, Norwalk, CT. (ISBN 0-838543324)

Designed as an advanced toxicology textbook and general reference source. Well-organized chapters on mechanisms of action, organ systems, interactions, and specific pathways.

LaDou, J. (Ed.) (1993). *Occupational Health and Safety,* 2nd ed. National Safety Council, Chicago. (ISBN 0-879121548)

Lewis, R. J., Sr. (Ed.) (1996). *Sax's Dangerous Properties of Industrial Materials,* 9th ed. (3 vols.). Van Nostrand Reinhold, New York. (ISBN 0-442020252)

This huge compendium provides properties, toxicity data, and regulatory status (United States) for over 20,000 chemical substances. Extensively indexed by CAS registry number and synonyms.

Koren, G. (Ed.) (1994). *Maternal–Fetal Toxicology: A Clinicians Guide,* 2nd ed. Dekker, New York. (ISBN 0-824788419)

A series of reviews of toxic effects of drugs, poisoning, radiation, and occupational hazards. A chapter on drugs of choice in pregnancy and a section on diagnosis of fetal malformations are included.

Mackay, D., Wan, Y. S., and Kuo C. M. *Illustrated Handbook of Physical–Chemical Properties and Environmental Fate for Organic Chemicals.* CRC Press, Boca Raton, FL.

Volume I: *Monoaromatics, Chlorobenzenes and PCBs* (1991). (ISBN 0-873715136)
Volume II: *Polycyclic Aromatics, Dioxins, Dibenzofurans and Phenols* (1992). (ISBN 0-837315837)
Volume III: *Volatile Organic Chemicals* (1993). (ISBN 0-873719735)
Volume IV: *Oxygen, Nitrogen and Sulfur Containing Compounds* (1995). (ISBN 0-1566700353)

This very recent collection of volumes provides physical–chemical data on compounds likely to impact the environment. The emphasis is on structure–activity and prediction of chemodynamics. Calculations are included and explained. A planned five-volume work is in progress.

Paul, M. (1993). *Occupational and Environmental Reproductive Hazards: A Guide for Clinicians*. Williams & Wilkins, Baltimore. (ISBN 0-683068016)

Focuses on assessment and action by clinician, summarizes the scientific basis for the relation between environmental hazards and reproduction, provides information for patient education, and offers recommendations for actions commensurate with evidence. It is unique in this focus.

Rom, W. N. (Ed.) (1992). *Environmental and Occupational Medicine,* 2nd ed. Little, Brown, Boston.

Covers basic and related areas of occupational medicine suitable for occupational health practitioners and readable enough for the practitioners in other medical disciplines. There are several excellent texts on environmental and occupational disciplines published within the past 2 years, any of which could serve the clinical health practitioner.

Schardein, J. L. (1993). *Chemically Induced Birth Defects,* Drug and Chemical Toxicology Series, Vol 2, 2nd rev ed. Dekker, New York. (ISBN 0-824787757)

A comprehensive literature review on mammalian (including human) exposure during organogenesis; current and readable.

Scialli, A. R., and Zinaman, M. J. (Eds.) (1993). *Reproductive Toxicology and Infertility.* McGraw-Hill, New York. (ISBN 0-071054383)

One of the most comprehensive texts in this field of study covering both male and female potential, processes, and exposure.

Shepard, T. H. (1995). *Catalog of Teratogenic Agents,* 8th ed. Johns Hopkins Univ. Press, Baltimore. (ISBN 0-801851823)

A standard text listing teratogenic potential of hundreds of substances; provides indexes, summaries of literature, and references to source materials.

Shibamoto, T., and Bjeldanes, L. F. (Eds.) (1993). *Introduction to Food Toxicology.* Academic Press, San Diego. (ISBN 0-126400253)

This work does a good job providing basic principles for the researcher.

Sittig, M. (1991/1992). *Handbook of Toxic & Hazardous Chemicals and Carcinogens,* 3rd ed. Noyes Data Corp., Park Ridge, NJ.

This easy to use 2-volume handbook presents chemical, safety, and health information on over 1000 toxic and hazardous chemicals. It provides information on potential exposure, environmental data, symptomology, medical surveillance, treatment, protection, and disposal. References are included.

Sullivan, J. B., Jr., and Krieger, G. R. (Eds.) (1992). *Hazardous Materials Toxicology: Clinical Principles of Environmental Health.* Williams & Wilkins, Baltimore. (ISBN 0-683080253)

Especially valuable in environmental health principles but uneven in terms of editorial policy (see *Casarett & Doull's Toxicology* and Ellenhorn & Barceloux).

Target Organ Toxicology Series. Raven Press/Taylor & Francis, New York/Washington, DC.
Wallace, K. B. (Ed.) (1997). *Free Radical Toxicology.*
Dixon, R. L. (Ed.) (1995). *Reproductive Toxicology,* 2nd ed.
Dean, J. H., *et al.* (Eds.) (1994). *Immunotoxicology and Immunopharmacology,* 2nd ed.
Kimmel, C. A., and Buelke-Sam, J. (Eds.) (1994). *Developmental Toxicology,* 2nd ed.
Kotsonis, F. N., Mackey, M., and Hjelle, J. J. (Eds.) (1994). *Nutritional Toxicology.*
Plaa, G. L., and Hewitt, W. R. (Eds.) (1994). *Toxicology of the Liver,* 2nd ed.

Waalkes, M. P., and Ward, J. M. (Eds.) (1994). *Carcinogenesis.*
Gardner, D. E., Crapo, J. D., and McClellan, R. O. (Eds.) (1993). *Toxicology of the Lung,* 2nd ed.
Hook, J. B., and Goldstein, R. S. (Eds.) (1993). *Toxicology of the Kidney,* 2nd ed.
Acosta, D., Jr. (Ed.) (1992). *Cardiovascular Toxicology,* 2nd ed.
Chiou, G. C. Y. (Ed.) (1992). *Ophthalmic Toxicology.*
Tilson, H. A., and Mitchell, C. L. (Eds.) (1992). *Neurotoxicology.*
Hayes, A. W. (Ed.) (1985). *Toxicology of the Eye, Ear, and Other Special Senses.*
Irons, R. D. (Ed.) (1985). *Toxicology of the Blood and Bone Marrow.*
Thomas, J. A., Korach, K. S., and McLachlan, J. A. (Eds.) (1985). *Endocrine Toxicology.*
Drill, V. A., and Lazar, P. (Eds.) (1984). *Cutaneous Toxicity.*
Schiller, C. M. (Ed.) (1984). *Intestinal Toxicology.*

This excellent, though expensive, series of works focuses on target organ toxicity and disease states. Some of the earlier volumes are currently out of print.

Threshold Limit Values for Chemical Substances and Physical Agents, and Biological Exposure Indices (1996). American Conference of Governmental Industrial Hygienists, Cincinnati, OH. (ISBN 1-882417-13-5)

This pocket-sized handbook provides Threshold Limit Values established by the ACGIH as guidelines for good practices. Main sections provide data for chemical and physical agents. Sections also include those explaining background and tests, biological exposure indices, and the role of the organization. Companion work titled *Documentation of the Threshold Limit Values and Biological Exposure Indices* provides the data and references used in developing the TLVs and BEIs.

Tomlin, C. (1995). *The Pesticide Manual,* 10th ed. British Crop Protection Council, Berkshire, UK (in the United States: Blackwell, Cambridge, MA). (ISBN 0-948404795)

Provides chemical, physical, analytical, use, and toxicity data for nearly 1200 pesticides, herbicides, and other agricultural chemicals. This edition incorporates *The Agrochemicals Handbook* from the Royal Society of Chemistry which alleviates deficiencies in the earlier editions. Environmental fate/transport, resistance information, and lists of manufacturers are now included. A companion tool from the British Crop Protection Council is the 2nd edition of *The World Directory of Pesticide Control Organizations* (ISBN 0-948404787), which gives sources of contacts in over 160 organizations worldwide involved in the control of pesticides.

Verschueren, K. (1996). *Handbook of Environmental Data on Organic Chemicals,* 3rd ed. Van Nostrand Reinhold, New York. (ISBN 0-442019165)

Provides information on properties, air pollution factors, water pollution factors, and biological effects for thousands of chemicals. All information referenced, and the introduction contains a minireview of the ecotoxicologic relevance and determination techniques for the data presented in each monograph.

Wilson, C. (1993). *Chemical Exposure and Human Health.* McFarland, Jefferson, NC. (ISBN 0-899508103)

A slim handbook designed as a symptom guide for the practitioner in identifying and diagnosing chemically induced health problems. The author's viewpoint is that of an educated consumer voicing the shortcomings of the federal and medical systems in providing adequate education and protection for the public. The bulk of the work consists of symptom–chemical and chemical–symptom–toxicity values sections, all fully referenced. Annotated listings of international, national, regional, and state organizations, research services, and related publications are included.

Periodicals

During the past 20 years there has been a steady increase in the number of journals transmitting information on toxicity, hazard, and risk. As knowledge has grown, more specialized titles have appeared reflecting the expanding literature of narrower disciplines, i.e., cellular toxicology, aquatic toxicology, food toxicology, contact dermatitis, risk analysis, drug/nutrition interactions, molecular toxicology, and target organ/system toxicity. Also, because of the cross-disciplinary nature of toxicological concerns, relevant information appears not only in the primary toxicology journals but also in those of related disciplines—medicine, epidemiology, food, biology, agriculture, and so on. This is especially true in medicine, where published data suggest that over 40% of clinical toxicology information is published in the journals of related disciplines (i.e., general medicine and pediatrics) rather than primary emergency medicine journals. New journal titles will frequently be distributed directly to professionals and announcements will appear in the review sections of professional journals. Additional titles of journals and series publications can be found in *Ulrich's International Periodicals Directory* (Bowker) or *The Serials Directory* (Ebsco). These directories are available in print and on CD-ROM, and *Ulrich's* is also available on-line through major vendors.

Generally, information published in a research journal is well-known in the scientific community long before it appears in print. The research journal is not an effective rapid communication device but one for quality control, claiming of priority, and as a mechanism of archiving research information. Because the potential sources of toxicological information are so widespread, typical hand scanning issues of journals for newly published information can be overwhelming for the investigator. Also overwhelming is the increasing cost of journal subscriptions. The average cost of a journal has increased 15–30% each year since 1980, forcing local collections to judiciously examine journal renewals.

The use of tertiary indexing and abstracting sources can provide an effective alternative to the time-consuming scanning of journal issues and limited subscription resources. These services provide regularly updated title, author, and subject access to the contents of thousands of journal titles. Enlisting the power of computerized systems can automate this process. Profiles of user interest areas are applied against large databases of journal references and results delivered to users on a recurring basis. In some services the user not only can browse the source information (and frequently an abstract) of a newly published article but also can request a full text copy of the original. An example of this type of service geared to rapid communication of journal contents is the *Current Contents* service from the Institute for Scientific Information, Inc., available in both print or electronic form.

Listed below is a sampling of the core journal titles in toxicology. They have been organized into simple subject categories. Sample copies of journals are quite easily obtained from publishers. Addresses and phone numbers for these publishers may be found in *Ulrich's* or *The Serials Directory*.

General

Advances in Modern Environmental Toxicology (Princeton Scientific)

Annual Review of Pharmacology and Toxicology (Annual Reviews)

Archives of Toxicology (Springer-Verlag)

The Banbury Report (Cold Spring Harbor Laboratory Press)

Chemical Research in Toxicology (American Chemical Society)

Concepts in Toxicology (Karger)

Critical Reviews in Toxicology (CRC Press)

Drug and Chemical Toxicology (Dekker)

Food and Chemical Toxicology (Pergamon)

Fundamental and Applied Toxicology (Academic Press)

Human and Experimental Toxicology (Macmillan)

In Vitro Toxicology (Liebert)

International Journal of Toxicology (Taylor and Francis)

Journal of Analytical Toxicology (Preston)

Journal of Applied Toxicology (Wiley)

Journal of Biochemical Toxicology (VCH)

Molecular Toxicology (Hemisphere)

Pharmacology and Toxicology (Munksgaard)

Regulatory Toxicology and Pharmacology (Academic Press)

Toxicity Review (HMSO, London)

Toxicologic Pathology (Society of Toxicologic Pathologists)

Toxicological and Environmental Chemistry (Gordon & Breach Science)

Toxicology (Elsevier Science)

Toxicology and Applied Pharmacology (Academic Press)

Toxicology and Industrial Health (Princeton Scientific)

Toxicology in Vitro (Pergamon)

Toxicology Letters (Elsevier Science)

Toxicology Methods (Liebert)

Veterinary and Human Toxicology (American Academy of Veterinary and Comparative Toxicology)

Alternative Toxicology Testing

Alternative Methods in Toxicology (Liebert)

ALTA (Alternatives to Laboratory Animals; Fund for the Replacement of Animals in Medical Experiments)

ILAR News (Institute of Laboratory Animal Resources)

Cancer and Carcinogenesis

Carcinogenesis: A Comprehensive Survey (Raven Press)

Environmental

Ambio (Royal Swedish Academy of Sciences)

Aquatic Toxicology (Raven Press)

Archives of Environmental Contamination and Toxicology (Springer-Verlag)

Archives of Environmental Health (Heldref)

Bulletin of Environmental Contamination and Toxicology (Springer-Verlag)

Chemosphere (Pergamon)

Developments in Toxicology and Environmental Science (Elsevier Science)

Ecotoxicity and Environmental Safety (Academic Press)

Environmental Mutagenesis (Wiley)

Environmental Science Research (Plenum)

Environmental Toxicology and Chemistry (Pergamon)

Hazardous Waste & Hazardous Materials (Liebert)

International Journal of Environmental Analytical Chemistry (Gordon & Breach Science)

Journal of Environmental Health (National Environmental Health Association)

Journal of Environmental Pathology, Toxicology, and Oncology (CRC Press)

Journal of Environmental Science and Health (Dekker)

Journal of Hazardous Materials (Elsevier Science)

Journal of the Air and Waste Management Association (AWMA)

Journal of Toxicology and Environmental Health (Taylor & Francis)

Pesticide and Toxic Chemical News (Food Chemical News)

Reviews of Environmental Contamination and Toxicology (Springer-Verlag)

Reviews in Environmental Toxicology (Elsevier Science)

Toxicological and Environmental Chemistry (Gordon & Breach Science)

Topics in Environmental Health (Elsevier Science)

Occupational and Industrial

American Industrial Hygiene Association Journal (American Industrial Hygiene Association)

American Journal of Industrial Medicine (Wiley)

Annals of the American Conference of Governmental Industrial Hygienists (Conference of Governmental Industrial Hygienists)

International Archives of Occupational and Environmental Health (Springer-Verlag)

Journal of Occupational Medicine (Williams & Wilkins)

Clinical

Adverse Drug Reactions and Toxicological Reviews (Oxford Univ. Press)

Association of Food and Drug Officials Quarterly Bulletin (Association of Food and Drug Officials)

Clinically Important Adverse Drug Interactions (Elsevier Science)

Drug and Chemical Toxicology (Dekker)

Emergency Medical Clinics of North America

Emergency Medicine

Human Toxicology (Macmillan)

Journal of Toxicology. Clinical Toxicology (Dekker)

Reactions (ADIS International)

Toxicon (Pergamon)

Mutagenesis

Chemical Mutagens: Principles and Methods for Their Detection (Plenum)

Mutagenesis (IRL Press)

Mutation Research (Elsevier Science)

Radiation

Advances in Radiation Biology (Academic Press)

Annals of the ICRP (Pergamon)

Radiation Research (Academic Press)

Reproduction and Teratology

Advances in the Study of Birth Defects (University Part Press)

Issues and Reviews in Teratology (Plenum)

Teratology (Wiley)

Reproductive Toxicology (Pergamon)

Series

A type of publication related to the periodical is the report series. While many of the journals listed previously provide monographic reviews (i.e., *Advances in Modern Environmental Toxicity, CRC Review Series, Methods in Toxicology,* and *Reviews of Environmental Contamination and Toxicology*) the report type of publication issues from government agencies, scientific organizations, or research institutes. They vary considerably in scope and purpose but typically provide excellent summary information compiled by panels of experts. Many of these series are irregularly produced but issue consecutively within a volume/issue framework. Identification of series entries may be found by consulting catalogs such as *CATLINE* (the catalog of the National Library of Medicine) or the *OCLC Online Union Catalog,* a list of catalog entries for materials contained in thousands of libraries in the North America and the United Kingdom. A brief, very select list of major sources of these series and their producers include:

Agency for Toxic Substances and Disease Registry, U.S. Government (ATSDR)
1600 Clinton Road, N.E., Atlanta, GA 30333
http://atsdr1.atsdr.cdc.gov:8080/atsdrhome.html
ASTDR Toxicological Profiles

Commission of the European Communities (CEC)
Rue Rasson 34, B-1040 Brussels, Belgium
http://www.cec.lu/en/comm/opoce/wel.html
EUR Report Series, Reports of the Scientific Committee on Cosmetology, Reports of the Scientific Committee for Food

Food and Agriculture Organization of the United Nations (FAO)
Via delle Terme di Caracalla, I-00100 Rome, Italy
gopher://gopher.undp.org:70/00/comm_catalogue/fao.hq
[series include those of the Joint FAO/WHO Expert Committee on Food Additives(JECFA)]
FAO Food and Nutrition Papers, FAO Plant Production and Protection Papers, JECFA Monographs on Toxicological Evaluation of Food Additives, Reports of the FAO Panel of

Experts on Pesticide Residues in Food and the Environment

International Agency for Research on Cancer (IARC)
(part of the World Health Organization)
150, cours Albert Thomas, F-69373 Lyon Cedex 08, France
http://www.iarc.fr
IARC Monographs (and supplements) *on the Evaluation of the Carcinogenic Risk of Chemicals to Humans, Scientific Publications*

British Industrial Biological Research Association (BIBRA)
Woodmansterne Road, Carshalton, Surrey SM5 4DS
Toxicity Profiles

Environmental Protection Agency, U.S. Government (EPA)
401 M Street S.W., Washington, DC 20460
http://www.epa.gov/
Too numerous to list—a resource guide to EPA services and resources: Access EPA (EPA/220-B-93-008 from GPO ISBN 0-16-041867-4)

World Health Organization
Avenue Appia, CH-1211 Geneva 27, Switzerland
http://www.who.ch/
WHO Technical Report Series, Environmental Health Criteria, Health Aspects of Chemical Safety, Food Additives Series

National Academy of Sciences/National Research Council (NRC)
2101 Constitution Ave, NW, Washington, DC
http://www.nas.edu
Medical and Biologic Effects of Environmental Pollutants, Biologic Markers, Drinking Water and Health

National Center for Toxicological Research (NCTR)
Jefferson, AK 72079
NCTR Reports

National Institute of Environmental Health Sciences (NIEHS)
Research Triangle Park, NC 27709
http://www.niehs.nih.gov
Environmental Health Perspectives

News

Newsletters can provide timely reporting of "hot" information—research findings, regulatory updating, society/organization news—all in brief reports. Most professional organizations support some kind of newsletter to communicate to its membership, but the ones of most interest here focus on current news used to inform and mobilize. Kathy Deck's *Environmental Health and Toxicology* lists over 30 newsletters of interest in environmental health, and there are dozens more which are issued from regional and state consumer groups and professional organizations in areas of interest to the toxicology professional. Some government and commercial titles in this area include:

BNA Toxics Law Reporter/Daily (Bureau of National Affairs)

Environmental Reporter (Bureau of National Affairs)

Hazardous Substances and Public Health (ATSDR)

Occupational Safety and Health Reporter/Daily (Bureau of National Affairs)

Pollution Prevention News (U.S. EPA)

Toxic Materials News (Business Publishers)

Electronic access to newsletters is provided via a number of services. These services vary in scope and how often they are updated. Examples include the *PTS Promt Newsletter* database (IAC) with a focus on business and industry and the *Newsletters in Print* database (Gale Research) available in print and on-line via several vendor systems. The *McGraw-Hill Publications Online* database carries over 45 leading publications on-line in full-text form, many of them newsletters and bulletins.

The need for extremely rapid reporting of information can be filled by specialized, and expensive, electronic "clipping services" that offer daily feeds of news items from dozens of newspapers, newsletters, newswires, and other types of information resources directly to the user's workstation or by fax. Examples of these are *P.A.S.S.PORT* from DataTimes, *//CLIP* from Dow Jones, *NewsEdge* from Desktop Data, Inc., and the *NewsFlash* service from NewsNet, Inc.

The Internet has become a very popular mechanism for disseminating timely information via newsgroups and mailing lists (listservs). At least in the United States, an increasing number of associations and interest groups are communicating directly through the use of the Internet. Government agencies, commercial producers, and research organizations are also using this network. It is estimated that more than 5000 discussion groups and 2500 electronic newsletters are available over the Internet and this figure is growing daily. One such recent effort of interest to the toxicology community is *Mid-Morning Newsbreak,* a daily summary of the news of the day concerning toxics, pollution prevention, and the chemical industry produced and distributed over the Internet by the Office of Pollution Prevention and Toxics of the U.S. EPA. The U.S. FDA also supports a publicly available server on the Internet covering staff activities, recent regulatory actions, and administrative news. The National Institute of Standards and Technology at the U.S. Department of Commerce sponsors the *Fedworld* system, which provides access to federal government bulletin boards (50 in all), government files, newsletters, and links to other government computerized systems.

Computerized Information

In the mid-1960s the first publicly available systems for accessing machine-readable databases appeared. With the explosion of information in the sciences, coupled with the vast number of resources (journals, reports, newspapers, and monographs) in which this information was appearing, the use of computers to store and retrieve information became an effective means to handle the increasing flow. It is estimated that from 1975 to 1993 records available in electronic form have grown by a factor of over 100 (52 million to 5.6 billion) and the number of electronic databases has grown from 301 to more than 8400.

Electronic files (also generically known as "databases") may be classed according to the type of information stored: bibliographic (containing references to the literature), directory (directing the user to sources of information), dictionary (providing information on nomenclature or identification of substances), bulletin boards (constantly updated news or activities), full-text, and databank information (containing actual data extracted or extrapolated from other sources). These distinctions blur as producers create composite databases, mixing full text and bibliographic and handbook and directory information. As a general observation, the availability of full-text databases has grown more than bibliographic types of file and the directory database is now as numerous as the bibliographic file. Full-text and data files are gaining as computer storage costs drop and people demand direct, rather than surrogate, information.

Files can be accessed through communication with host computers, where data are stored by producers or vendors, or by loading them locally, such as through tape or CD-ROM storage. The use of direct telephone lines or data networks is necessary to communicate with off-site files. The choice for accessing these electronic files—on-line vs local—will be influenced by the availability, cost of the products, the platforms available for use, and available expertise. No matter what medium is chosen, it is important to recognize the disadvantages of each route: On-line may mean subscriber and use charges but it is convenient and universally available via telecommunications systems like SprintNet, Internet, or DataPac; CD-ROM storage can be very cost-effective for unlimited use but production methods invariably necessitate a delay in currency over on-line. Tape requires a host search system, expert support personnel, and compatible hardware. The information science literature contains several articles providing criteria and checklists help in determining the most appropriate medium for each situation. Transparent bridges between on-line and CD, recordable CD technology, easier to use interfaces, mass market media platforms, and other developments will increase the investigator's ability to find, identify, and retrieve useful information.

Besides the development of data and text information systems, software programs are being designed to provide assistance in predicting the toxicity of substances based on structure–activity relationships, such as the TOPKAT program by Health Designs, Inc., or by an expert system, such as the CASE system by Case Western Reserve University. Computer-assisted instruction programs, incorporating text, audio, graphic, and full-motion video technologies, are an exciting use of computer-assisted instruction. Examples of this last type of CD-ROM product include the environmental health, industrial hygiene, and occupational health and safety titles of the ACTIV Series from ITC (Herndon, VA) and the hazardous materials series training program from Interactive Media Communications (Waltham, MA).

Selection and Use of Electronic Sources

To determine the value of a resource, we use a number of criterion. The scope and purpose of the database/file, the selection criteria for source materials, regular updating schedules, consistency of indexing or catagorization, standards for record creation, access points for retrieval, and quality of documentation/support are all factors to consider. With the unregulated flow of new sources on the Internet, as well as the thousands of databases available through public and subscription vendors, it becomes increasingly important to evaluate each resource as to the quality of the information content.

Directories of information on computerized sources such as the *Gale Directory of Databases* (Gale Research Inc.) and the Mekler directory *CD-ROMs in Print* give identification, coverage, content, and availability information for publicly available electronic files, as can many of the literature guides listed in the introduction to this entry. An example of a resource tool more limited in scope is the *Environmental Software Directory* (Donley Technologies). Articles and columns appearing in the information science literature (*Online, Searcher, Database, CD-ROM Professional,* and *Information Today*) can provide excellent reviews of new files and comparative studies on resources in specific subject areas. Directories of Internet resources abound these days as do on-line search engines, which allow the user to search for Internet resources on specific topics. Examples of these Internet search engines include Lycos, InfoSeek, Yahoo, Inference Find, Alta Vista, WebCrawler, and Excite.

The following is an illustrative, selected list of electronic files containing publicly available toxicology information. Represented here are databases which cover toxicology under a larger discipline—medicine, biology, and chemistry; those devoted to specific areas of toxicological concerns—occupational health, reproductive toxicology, environmental health, hazard assessment; industry-specific files such as those for specific industries—petroleum, nuclear power, agricultural, and engineering; and those that cover specific types of data—regulations, legislation, newsletter, industry or technical reports, and books. In many cases electronic databases are the counterparts to printed indexing, abstracting, or full-text source materials. Increasingly, electronic files are being developed which have no print counterparts, such as the *Hazardous Substances Databank*. In this list, the host system(s) is noted for each file, as is the availability of tape or CD-ROM formats. Many of these databases may also be available through the Internet:

Aquatic Information Retrieval (ACQUIRE):
Contains over 100,000 records of data on acute, chronic, bioaccumulative, and sublethal effects data from experimental assays performed on fresh and saltwater aquatic species. Originally produced by the U.S. EPA Office of Toxic Substances, and currently produced by CIS. (CIS, TDS Numerica)

Agricola:
Contains more than 3 million citations to all types of publications acquired, indexed, and cataloged by the U.S. National Agricultural Library. Comprehensive coverage of all areas of agriculture and related topics including agrochemicals and veterinary toxicology. Produced by the U.S. National Agricultural Library. (DIALOG, Life Science Network, EPIC)

BioBusiness:
Contains over 600,000 records covering the worldwide periodical literature on business applications of biological and biomedical research. Includes occupational health, biotechnology, bioremediation, pesticides, toxicology, and energy. Produced by BIOSIS. (OVID, Data-Star, DIALOG, Life Science Network, STN)

BIOSIS Previews:
Contains more than 8.6 million citations to the worldwide literature in the life sciences, environmental sciences, and experimental medicine. One of the largest of the science databases. Pro-

duced by BIOSIS. Selected citations contained in a subset of TOXLINE. (OVID, Data-Star, CISTI, DIALOG, DIMDI, ESA-IRS, Life Science Network, STN)

CA Search (CAS):
Contains more than 10 million references to the worldwide chemistry literature. Companion registry file allows for identification of nomenclature and structure of chemicals. In some systems the user can also search by structure or substructure. The CAS registry number is a widely used identifier for a unique chemical substance. (CAN/OLE, Data-Star, DIALOG, ESA-IRS, Life Science Network, ORBIT, STN; collective indexes available from Silver Platter)

CAB Abstracts:
Contains more than 2.9 million records to worldwide literature in the agricultural sciences and related areas of applied biology. Corresponds to the 46 abstract journals by CAB International (formerly Commonwealth Agricultural Bureaux), its producer. (CAN/OLE, DIALOG, DMIDI, ESA-IRS, Life Science Network, STN)

CERCLIS Database of Hazardous Waste:
Contains information on each hazardous waste disposal or spill site nominated or selected for the EPA National Priorities List for cleanup under Superfund (CERCLA) or SARA amendments. Over 38,000 to date. (CIS, WESTLAW)

Chemical Carcinogenesis Research Information System (CCRIS):
Contains references and data extracted from the worldwide literature on tests for carcinogenicity, cocarcinogenicity, tumor promotion, and mutagenicity of chemicals. Evaluated data on over 1450 chemicals appear in CCRIS to date. Produced by the U.S. National Library of Medicine through funding by the National Cancer Institute. (CIS, DIMDI, TOXNET)

Chemical Evaluation Search and Retrieval System (CESARS):
This on-line handbook contains toxicological data on over 370 chemicals of particular interest to the United States Great Lakes basin. Each record containing up to 120 data fields covering physical and chemical properties, toxicity, and environmental fate. Produced by the Office of Materials Control of Michigan's Department of Natural Resources. Fully evaluated and referenced data. (CCINFOline, CIS; contained in CCINFOdisc; Cores Series A2 from CCOHS)

Chemical Safety Newsbase (CSNB):
Contains 28,000 records of information on occupational hazards in the chemical industry—identification, storage, handling, transportation, emergency planning, regulations and legislation, standards and practices, and waste management. Only new information on well-known hazards is included. Produced by the Royal Society of Chemistry. (Data-Star, DIALOG, ESA-IRS, Life Sciences Network, ORBIT, STN)

Chemicals Currently Being Tested for Toxic Effects (CCTTE):
Supported by the International Programme on Chemical Safety (IPSC) and UNEP International Register of Potentially Toxic Chemicals (IRPTC). A computerized register of tests currently being performed by researchers in basic and applied toxicological research into toxic hazards. Excludes carcinogenicity tests. Annual reports available from IRPTC. (direct dial)

Chemlist:
Contains information on over 160,000 chemicals subject to legislative and regulatory control. Covers all U.S. EPA TSCA (Toxic Substances Control Act) and EINECS (European Inventory of Existing Commercial Chemical Substances). Provides citations to regulations, ITC recommendations, rule violations, safety and health studies, Superfund actions, and citizen's petitions. Produced by the Chemical Abstracts Service. (STN)

Clinical Toxicology of Commercial Products (CTCP):
On-line equivalent of the standard text by Gosselin (5th ed., 1984), this database provides information on over 20,000 consumer products (excluding food) derived from 3000 commercial products. Access by ingredient, class, trade/chemical name, and CAS registry number. Focus is on

the identification, toxicity, and care of emergency exposure. (CIS)

Compendex PLUS:
Contains over 2.1 million citations to the world's engineering and technology literature. Useful for sources of information on processes and equipment for use in analysis, remediation, and pollution control areas. Produced by Engineering Information, Inc. (CDP, CAN/OLE, Data-Star, DIALOG, ESA-IRS, ORBIT, STN; available on CD from DIALOG and Silver Platter and as part of several combined source discs)

Developmental and Reproductive Toxicology Database (DART), continues ETICBACK (Environmental Teratology Information Center Backfile):
Contains over 10,000 references to the worldwide literature of teratology and some coverage of developmental and reproductive toxicology. DART covers 1989+ and ETICBACK covers 1950–1988. Over half the references are scanned into DART from MEDLINE and it includes coverage of technical reports and conference papers. Produced by the National Library of Medicine. (both available through TOXNET)

DERWENT Drug File (RINGDOC):
Contains over 1.5 million citations with lengthy, quantitative abstracts to the worldwide journal literature of drugs and pharmaceuticals. Ability to search by structure–activity unique to Derwent files. Covers less source journals than MEDLINE or EMBASE (1500) but provides more in-depth on-line information through indexing and abstracts. Other Derwent files include Derwent Veterinary Drug File (VETDOC) and Derwent Crop Protection File (PESTDOC) providing similar in-depth analysis of the literature in these areas. The Derwent Drug Registry is the companion nomenclature file giving names, therapeutic class, and structures for chemical compounds. Formerly a subscription service, selected files are now publicly available. (Data-Star, DIALOG, ORBIT, STN)

Embase:
Contains more than 5 million records covering the world's biomedical literature related to human health and medicine. Environmental pollution and health, occupational health, and clinical toxicology are strong areas. Corresponds in part to 46 specialty abstract journals and two literature indexes produced under the Excerpta Medica specialty series titles by Elsevier Science. (CDP, Data-Star, DIALOG, DIMDI, Life Science Network, STN; entire database and sections in composite discs available from Silver Platter and DIALOG)

Energy Science and Technology (formerly DOE ENERGY):
One of the world's largest sources of literature references on energy and related topics. Produced by the U.S. Department of Energy. (DIALOG; available on CD from DIALOG)

Enviroline:
Contains over 170,000 citations to the environment and management of land and natural resources. Covers over 5,000 international sources materials. Includes journals, industry reports, conference papers, newspapers, audiovisuals, and monographs. Produced by Congressional Information Service. (Data-Star, DIALOG, DIMDI, ESA-IRS, Life Science Network, ORBIT; available on CD through Bowker)

Environmental Fate Database:
This on-line database contains four subfiles focusing on the environmental fate or behavior of chemicals released into the environment (>1 million pounds/year). Substances covered are predominantly organic compounds. The CHEMFATE subfile covers environmental fate and biodegradation data and references; DATALOG covers physical properties, reactions rates, and monitoring data; BIODEG and BIOLOG cover biodegradation and toxicity data and references, respectively. Produced by the Syracuse Research Corporation (SRC). (TDS NUMERICA)

Environmental Mutagen Information Center Data Base (EMIC):
This database is composed of two files, EMIC and EMICBACK, which provide access to the bibliographic information of chemical, biological, and physical agents which have been tested

for genotoxic activity, most of which were published since 1950. Sixty percent of the records are extracted from MEDLINE. Produced by the U.S. Oak Ridge National Laboratory. (TOXNET; available on CD as a subfile in PolTox I and Toxline, both by Silver Platter)

Food Science and Technology Abstracts:
Covers the worldwide literature of food science and technology. Includes information on occupational toxicology in the food handling and processing areas, toxicology of foods and packaging, and additives information. Produced by the International Food Service, Germany. (CAN/OLE, Data-Star, DIALOG, DIMDI, ESA-IRS, Life Science Collection, ORBIT, STN; available on CD only or with several combined files from a number of producers)

Genetox:
A relatively new database, this file provides mutagenicity data on about 3000 chemicals from 39 assays systems. This file is assembled by expert panels at the U.S. EPA Office of Toxic Substances with the cooperation of the NIEHS and the EMIC program at Oak Ridge National Laboratories. There are strict criteria for selection and review of data. Produced by the U.S. EPA (CIS, TOXNET)

Hazardous Substances Databank:
This huge chemical handbook of information covers over 5000 chemical substances. The main emphasis is to provide evaluated, current toxicology data on high-use chemicals supplemented by data on manufacturing, use, environmental fate, detection methods, U.S. regulatory information, emergency treatment, etc. It is produced by the National Library of Medicine's TOXNET program. All material is reviewed by a Scientific Review Panel drawn from major subject disciplines within the databank's scope. Data are compiled from the journal, texts, government documents, and technical report literature. (Data-Star, DIMDI, STN, TOXNET; available as part of TOMES PLUS by Micromedex)

HSELINE:
Contains over 150,000 citations to the worldwide literature on occupational health and safety. Includes physical, chemical, and medical hazards. Covers all U.K. Health and Safety Commission and Health and Safety Executive publications and a wide range of journals, conference papers, reports, and legislation (United Kingdom). Produced by the Health and Safety Executive, United Kingdom (Data-Star, ESA-IRS, ORBIT; available on CD from Silver Platter; available on CD as part of several products)

International Pharmaceutical Abstracts:
Contains more than 300,000 citations to the worldwide pharmaceutical and pharmacy literature including pharmaceutical technology, drug research and development, adverse drug reactions and toxicity, occupational health in the pharmaceutical industry, and other topics. Covers more than 800 journal sources. Produced by the American Society of Hospital Pharmacists (OVID, Data-Star, DIALOG, DIMDI, ESA-IRS, Life Science Network; available on CD from Silver Platter)

Integrated Risk Information System (IRIS):
Contains information on hazard identification and dose–response assessment of over 500 hazardous substances. Covers toxicity, carcinogenicity, chemical and physical properties, and applicable regulations. Includes the reference dose as defined by U.S. EPA, unit risk of exposure by oral and inhalation routes. Produced by the U.S. EPA. (CIS, TOXNET; available on CD as part of TOMES Plus by Micromedex and on the EPA Internet website)

Martindale Online:
This is a full-text electronic version of this standard directory of pharmaceuticals and ancillary substances. Contains reviews, physical/chemical properties, adverse reactions, toxicity, uses, actions, dosages, pharmaceutical properties, contraindications, interactions, and trade and generic nomenclature. Produced by the Royal Pharmaceutical Society of Great Britain. (Data-Star, Life Science Network; available on CD from RSGB)

Medline:
One of the largest and most popular international biomedical databases in the world. Strengths in-

clude coverage of preclinical and clinical aspects of biomedicine, drug and pharmaceuticals, human and veterinary toxicology, and the practice of medicine. Covers over 8000 sources journals and contains over 7 million references to the journal literature 1966 to present. Produced by the U.S. National Library of Medicine. (OVID, Data-Star, DIALOG, DIMDI, EPIC, Life Science Network, STN; available on CD from a number of producers)

MSDS-CCOHS:
This database contains the complete text of over 100,000 Material Safety Data Sheets compiled by the Canadian Center for Occupational Health and Safety. This information was gathered from over 500 manufacturers and suppliers in the United States and Canada. Each record covers one chemical substance and provides trade and supplier name, description, chemical/physical properties, reactivity, health hazards, storage and disposal, personal protection, cleanup and disposal, and emergency first aid. (CIS, STN; available on CD from CCOHS)

MSDS-OHS:
This collection of Material Safety Data Sheets covers over 17,000 single substances and 74,000 mixtures documented under the HCLS of OSHA. Sources include NIOSH, OSHA, and Dreisbach's *Handbook of Poisoning*. Each MSDS record contains extensive information on identification, handling, and hazard disclosure. The OHS on-line system provides a full file, a summary information file, and a file composed of records to chemicals used in the manufacture of pesticide and other agricultural chemical products. (OHS, STN gateway to OHS; available on CD from OHS)

NIOSH Technical Information Center (NIOSHTIC):
Contains more than 180,000 references to the literature of occupational health and safety from monographs, journals, and reports. Produced by the U.S. National Institute for Occupational Safety and Health (NIOSH). As of 1997, NIOSH will only add NIOSH publications and articles by NIOSH authors to the database. (DIALOG, ESA-IRS, ORBIT; available as subfile in CCINFOdisc: Core Series CI from CCOHS and several other combination products)

Oil and Hazardous Materials Technical Assistance Data System (OHM-TADS):
This handbook database contains references to published material on 1500 materials that have been designated oil or hazardous materials. Provides technical support for dealing with the handling of environmental spills (water emphasis). Each record covers information on one chemical substance—identification, physical properties, uses, toxicity, handling, and disposal. (CIS)

Phytotox:
Contains over 100,000 records of data extracted from articles published on the toxic effects of organic chemicals on terrestrial vascular plants. References included. Produced by the University of Oklahoma. (CIS)

Pollution Abstracts:
Contains references to worldwide technical and nontechnical literature on all aspects of pollution, solid waste management, and environmental quality. Covers journals, books, technical reports, conference papers, and government documents. Produced by Cambridge Scientific Abstracts. (Data-Star, DIALOG, ESA-IRA, Life Science Network; available as part of the CD PolTox I from Silver Platter)

REPROTOX:
Provides reviewed and summarized information on the reproductive risk of hundreds of chemical substances. Includes coverage of industrial and environmental chemicals, drugs, nutritional agents, and radiation. Effects noted on fertility (male and female), pregnancy, development, and lactation. Database use is included with membership in the Reproductive Toxicology Center of the Columbia Hospital for Women, Washington, DC (available by direct access to the RTC).

SEDBASE:
The on-line full text of *Meyler's Side Effects of Drugs and Side Effects of Drugs Annual* which provides references and summaries of the significant drug adverse reactions, interactions, and toxicity literature. Entries linked to the records from

EMBASE cited in the original source. Produced by Elsevier Science. (OVID, Data-Star, DIALOG, DIMDI; available on CD from Elsevier)

Registry of Toxic Effects of Chemical Substances (RTECS):
Contains toxic effects data (with citations) on over 150,000 chemicals identified by NIOSH and mandated by the Occupational Safety and Health Act of 1970. Acute and chronic effects, selected regulatory information, IARC reviews, TSCA status, GENE-TOX data, and NTP documents cited. Data selectively included, not comprehensive. Produced by the U.S. National Library of Medicine. (CIS, Data-Star, DIALOG, DIMDI, Life Science Network, TOXNET, STN; CD version contained in CCIHNFOdisc: Core Series C2 from CCOHS and CHEMBANK from Silver Platter)

Toxic Substances Control Act Test Submissions (TSCATS):
Provides over 48,000 citations to unpublished health and safety studies, chemical tests, and substantial risk data on over 5700 chemical substances submitted to the U.S. EPA under the Toxic Substances Control Act (TSCA). Copies of the original submissions available from the U.S. EPA.(CIS, subset of TOXLINE; available on CD in PolTox I and Toxline from Silver Platter)

Toxic Chemical Release Inventory (TRI):
Consists of a series of files containing information on the annual estimated releases of toxic chemicals to the environment. This information is gathered by the U.S. EPA through manufacturers/importers/users of chemicals under the provisions of the SARA amendments of CERCLA. Records contain information on storage, discharge, waste treatment, and waste transfer. TRIFACTS, a companion database, contains information from the state of New Jersey's Hazardous Substance Fact sheets collected under New Jersey Right-to-Know Act. This provides information on the safety and ecological effects of most TRI chemicals. Produced by the U.S. National Library of Medicine and the U.S. EPA. (TOXNET; CD of the 1987 TRI file available from the U.S. Government Printing Office)

TOXLINE/TOXLIT (National Library of Medicine, Toxicology Information Program):
One of the largest on-line bibliographic sources for toxicology information, these databases contain over 2.1 million citations to all areas of toxicology. The information is a collection of 17 discrete source files of journal citations, technical reports, conference papers, and research project information. Both files are available on the NLM MEDLARS system, and 14 of the 17 source records are available on other on-line vendors (Data-Star, DIALOG, Life Science Network; on CD through Silver Platter)

Nomenclature and Locator Files

Many database producers provide controlled vocabulary systems which assist the user in obtaining specific and comprehensive retrieval. Registry or nomenclature files can be useful in identifying the controlled vocabulary for a compound used in a specific file or to obtain a collection of synonyms identifying that compound (lab code, generic name, chemical name, trade names, government agency control numbers, etc.) to be used in searching other resources. The Chemical Abstracts Service **Registry** file provides structure information, provides synonyms, and a chemical identifier code (CAS registry name) used extensively worldwide. Chemical Abstracts started its identification system in the mid-1960s and has established records for over 12.7 million compounds. Derwent, producer of the *Derwent Drug File* and the *World Patents Index* provides a **Drug Registry** file and establishes its own unique registry number for chemical compounds referenced in its products. Several on-line files carry extensive nomenclature information embedded in substance records, such as the **Merck Index** and **RTECS**, for example. Some files also provide locator information for chemical substance information on files mounted on a particular vendor system along with the nomenclature of the compound. The **Chemical Identification File** (**ChemId**), for example, provides nomenclature and locator information for the MEDLARS and TOXNET systems.

Vendors

Listed below is a selected list of on-line vendors that focus on providing toxicology information files. The directories listed in the beginning of this section also give contact information for on-line vendors.

CCINFOline (Canadian Centre for Occupational Safety and Health)
250 Main Street E.
Hamilton, ON, Canada L8N 1H6
416-570-8094; in Canada, 800-668-4284

Chemical Information System (CIS)
810 Gleneagles Ct., Suite 300
Towson, MD 21286
410-321-8440; in United States, 800-247-8737

European Space Agency—Information Retrieval System (ESA-IRS)
ESRIN, Via Galileo Galilei
I-00044 Frascati, Rome, Italy
06-941801

Life Science Network
BIOSIS
2100 Arch Street
Philadelphia, PA 19103-1399
215-587-4806; in United States, 800-523-4806

Occupational Health Services (OHS)
11 W. 42nd Street, 12th Floor
New York, NY 10036
212-789-3535

STN International
FIZ Karlsruhe
P.O. Box 2465
D-76012 Karlruhe 1, Germany
07247-808555
U.S. address:
c/o Chemical Abstracts Service
2540 Olentangy River Road
P.O. Box 3012
Columbus, OH 43210-0012
614-447-3600
800-848-6533

Technical Database Services, Inc.
(TDS Numerica)
135 West 50th Street
New York, NY 10020-1201
212-245-0044

TOXNET
National Library of Medicine
Specialized Information Services Division
8600 Rockville Pike
Bethesda, MD 20894
301-496-6531

CD-ROMS

During the past 10 years computer disc technology has grown to become one of the most popular media for local electronic storage and retrieval. Studies show that the number of CD-ROM titles is growing by over 50% each year and it is estimated that 80% of all computer users will have CD-ROM desktop access by 1999. CD recordable technology is soon to be widespread and CDs may be as easy to create as floppy discs. While the most common type of CD-ROM product for bibliographic retrieval is still the single source product, producers are using this powerful storage medium to mix material into subject collection discs, combining various types of resources—handbooks, journal articles, regulations, and directories. Below are examples of these composite CD-ROM products/series of interest to the toxicology professional:

CCINFOdisc Products (CCOHS):
This collection of several CD-ROM products provides a wealth of legislative, regulatory, handbook, directory, numeric, and bibliographic information focusing on occupational health, workplace safety, environmental hazards, regulatory information, and safety topics. There are 11 titles currently available. International in scope. Vendor: Canadian Centre for Occupational Health and Safety.

Environmental Chemicals Data and Information Network (ECDIN):
This handbook-type product contains a selection of 7000 chemical records from the massive ECDIN databank (available on-line through DIMDI) created by the Joint Research Centre of the Commission of the European Communities. Each record contains data on identification, uses, health effects, treatment, prevention, environmental concentrations, and fate. Rules, regula-

tions, and recommendations covering CEC countries are included. Distributor varies.

Environmental/Safety Library:
Contains titles from the CFR (all of Title 40 and portions of 29, 42, and 49), *Federal Register* notices from 1990 to present, and industry standards from OSHA and EPA. Updated monthly. Produced by Information Handling Service, Inc.

ENVIRO/ENERGY ABSTRACTS PLUS:
Provides over 250,000 references to the world's literature on environmental and energy-related topics. Contains the contents of *Acid Rain Abstracts, Energy Information Abstracts,* and *Environment Abstracts.* Produced by Congressional Information Service; updated quarterly.

OSH-ROM:
Contains over 350,000 references to the world's literature on occupational health and safety. Consists of *CISDOC* (CIS Abstracts by the International Labour Office), *HSELine* (HSELine by the Great Britain Health and Safety Executive), *MIHIDAS* (MIHIDAS database by the United Kingdom Atomic Energy Authority), and *NIOSHTIC* (NIOSHTIC database by the U.S. National Institute for Occupational Safety and Health). Produced by Silver Platter, Inc.; updated quarterly.

PolTox:
The PolTox series from Silver Platter, Inc., provides information on pollution and toxicology. PolTox I contains *Aquatic Sciences and Fisheries Abstracts, Ecology Abstracts, Food Science and Technology Abstracts, Health and Safety Science Abstracts, Pollution Abstracts, RISKLINE, Toxicology Abstracts,* and all of *TOXLINE.* PolTox II contains information derived from EMBASE and PolTox II information from the CAB Abstracts database.

REPRORISK:
Contains a collection of reproductive risk information resources, including REROTEXT, a collection of reviews (with hazard ratings) of the health effects of industrial chemicals; REPROTOX from the Reproductive Toxicology Center at Columbia Hospital for Women; the text of Shepard's *Catalog of Teratogenic Agents;* and TERIS, the teratogen information system from the University of Washington. Produced by Micromedex, Inc.

TOMES Plus:
This title contains information on toxicology, occupational health, and environmental information with a focus on emergency situations of exposure and hazard control. It contains bibliographic, full text, and numeric information. Consists of eight files of information from various government sources—U.S. EPA, OSHA, DOT, Coast Guard, NIOSH, and others. Updated quarterly. Produced by Micromedex, Inc.

Acknowledgments

Appreciation is expressed to Kathy Deck of the Centers for Disease Control and Prevention and to Fred Stoss of Oak Ridge National Labs for their kind assistance and also to Pharmacia & Upjohn for its support of this project.

—Janet M. Everitt

Related Topics

Agency for Toxic Substances and Disease Registry
American Conference of Governmental Industrial Hygienists
Food and Agriculture Organization of the United Nations
Food and Drug Administration
International Agency for Research on Cancer
International Programme on Chemical Safety
International Register of Potentially Toxic Chemicals
National Center for Toxicological Research
National Institute for Occupational Safety and Health
National Institute of Environmental Health Sciences
National Institutes of Health
Occupational Safety and Health Administration
Toxicology, Education and Careers
Toxic Substances Control Act

International Agency for Research on Cancer

Introduction

The mission of the International Agency for Research on Cancer (IARC) is to promote, by way of international collaborative research and other means, improvement of health through reduction of the incidence and mortality from cancer throughout the world by

- Conducting research into the occurrence, impact, causes, early detection, and prevention of human cancer
- Evaluating and disseminating the results of such research
- Training personnel in relevant scientific and technical skills

Its unique role in international cancer research depends on its international status, its independence of national political interests, its experience and acceptability as a coordinator of research in developing countries, and its capacity within its own structure to combine epidemiological and laboratory approaches to cancer research.

The agency's research concentrates on the occurrence, causes, and prevention of cancer. It does not undertake research into therapy or other aspects of the care of cancer patients, nor does it develop cancer control policies or implement cancer control measures except where this is necessary to achieve its research objectives.

Selection of specific activities for the agency's scientific program is based on its mission, considerations of scientific quality, ethical issues, and the known or potential impact on public health of particular cancers or agents that may cause or prevent cancer. The agency's activities have concentrated on three main fields: (1) research into the prevention and early detection of cancer, particularly intervention studies in both developing and developed countries; (2) use of biomarkers of exposure, effects, and susceptibility in epidemiological studies; and (3) emphasis on studies with potential cancer prevention applications particularly in developing countries. For the last part of this century, there will be new research lines, focusing on genetics and cancer, cancer susceptibility genes and their interaction with environmental factors, and on cancer chemopreventive agents.

In this short review, general directions of the IARC are briefly presented.

Background

The IARC was established over 30 years ago by the World Health Assembly on May 20th, 1965. The agency was created in a spirit of altruism by several of the wealthier countries of the world to provide capacity for research on important cancer problems wherever they might occur. In the spirit of its creation, the public health-oriented mission of the IARC is to promote, by way of international collaborative research and other means, improvement of health through reduction of the incidence and mortality from cancer throughout the world by conducting research into the causes, early detection, and prevention of cancer; by evaluating and disseminating the results of such research; and by organizing training also for those parts of the world which otherwise would be somewhat deprived of the educational possibilities in cancer research and control. Research into treatment or other aspects of the care does not usually form part of the agency's mission.

Some of the agency's lines of activities are described in the following sections in general terms.

Identification, Elucidation, and Evaluation of Environmental Causes of Cancer

The IARC Monographs Programme on the Evaluation of Carcinogenic Risks to Humans is one of the cornerstones of the agency's activities. During the past few years, it has become increasingly evident that in addition to environmental chemical carcinogens, which have been the traditional target of the IARC monographs, infectious agents contribute significantly to human cancer burden. In addition, chemical carcinogens and infectious agents may interact in their adverse effects on biological systems, leading to an overproportional increase in cancer risk, as exemplified by the effects on liver cancer risk of aflatoxin B_1 exposure and Hepatitis B virus infection. Other biological agents which have been evaluated in the monographs series, and found to carry a cancer risk, include schistosomiasis (bladder cancer), liver flukes (cholangiocarcinoma of the liver), *Helicobacter pylori* (stomach cancer), and human papilloma viruses (types 16 and 18).

The use of tobacco products remains a central focus of the agency's epidemiological work since it is generally agreed that in industrialized countries, approximately 30–35% of all known cancers are related to tobacco consumption and, worldwide, one in seven cancers can be attributed to smoking. The question to which extent passive smoking constitutes a health risk has not yet been unanimously solved. The agency is involved in a multicenter case–control study in European countries to be completed in 1997. This epidemiological study has a laboratory research branch with the objective to study the interaction between genetic polymorphisms for cytochrome P450 enzymes and passive smoking-associated lung cancer. Although there is no doubt that the high incidence of all cancers in the Indian subcontinent is related to the oral use of tobacco, risk estimates are still difficult due to the lack of high-quality epidemiological data. Subject to the results of a feasibility study now in progress, the agency plans a prospective study of oral tobacco use and cancer in more than 100,000 men and women in Bombay, India.

In addition to environmental factors, carcinogens may also be formed endogenously, e.g., in the context of chronic inflammatory states. One mechanism is the production of reactive oxygen and nitrogen species which may cause tissue and DNA damage. The recently created Unit of Endogenous Cancer Risk Factors focuses on biochemical mechanisms by which oxidative stress produces DNA damage and protein oxidation/nitrosation. These studies will be conducted in a variety of conditions including inflammation and precancerous lesions.

The agency has a long and successful history of achievements in the field of DNA damage and its relationship to mutation and cancer. This has led to the development of highly sensitive methods to assess the extent of interaction between environmental agents and the human genome. Recently, scientists at the agency have succeeded in assessing specific mutations in the tumor-suppressor gene *p53* in normal human skin following UV irradiation. This methodology will be expanded during the next biennium since it opens a new and much more specific way of assessing mutations in critical cellular target molecules at a time when phenotypic changes reflecting neoplastic transformation are not yet recognizable. This methodology thus offers a new prospective on risk assessment.

It is now generally agreed that phenotypic changes occurring in cells during the process of malignant transformation reflect the sequential acquisition of genetic alterations. This applies to all tissues, but the type of oncogene and tumor-suppressor gene and the sequence in which they contribute to tumor progression show a remarkable degree of organ specificity. IARC scientists have therefore focused their attention on some organ sites (e.g. esophagus, stomach, liver, and cervix) that contribute significantly to the overall human cancer burden. Analyses of genetic alterations associated with tumor progression not only help us to understand the evolution of human cancers but, in some cases, also provide a tool to identify the environmental agent responsible for the initiation of malignant transformation. This has been shown in tumors of the skin (ultraviolet irradiation), liver (aflatoxin B_1), and hemangiosarcoma of the liver (vinyl chloride). In the case of stomach cancer, basic laboratory research will be extended into preventive measures, particularly with respect to the role of *H. pylori* in the causation of human stomach cancer. This is similarly true for cancer of the cervix, which in many parts of Central America and Asia remains the most frequent cause of cancer mortality in women. The agency has in the past conducted extensive surveys in different world regions regarding the prevalence of certain types of human papilloma viruses (HPV) and their association with cancer of the cervix. We anticipate that during the next biennium vaccines will be available for clinical trials.

Mechanisms of Carcinogenesis, Host Factors, and Their Interaction with Environmental Agents

The cytochrome P450 enzyme system has been the focus of investigation in several laboratories worldwide since these enzymes participate in the bioactivation of many environmental carcinogens. IARC scientists focus their research on the role of individual pattern of cytochrome P450 isozymes as a determinant in genetic susceptibility to environmental carcinogens, in particular tobacco smoking. Over the past few years evidence has accumulated indicating that individual susceptibility may, at least in part, be related to the individual pattern expression of genes involved in the bioactivation of xenobiotics. This question will also be pursued with respect to the genetic polymorphism of enzymes involved in the detoxification of environmental carcinogens. Individual capacity for DNA repair also appears to play a role in genetic cancer susceptibility. Methodological progress will allow us to launch, in the future, epidemiological projects to analyze the complex relationship between the bioactivation and detoxification of environmental carcinogens, DNA repair, and the production of mutations in critical target cells and transformation-associated genes.

For some human cancers, including brain tumors, our understanding of the etiology is still incomplete. The fraction of cases attributable to radiation or environmental agents is very small. The possibility exists that genetic alterations observed in the evolution of gliomas may be due to endogenous DNA damage rather than interaction with environmental factors. Also, there is strong evidence that germline mutations may play a larger role in brain tumor development than previously anticipated. The newly created Unit of Molecular Pathology will focus much of its work on the etiopathogenesis of human brain tumors, particularly in children.

In 1995, the agency started a new laboratory concentrating on genetic susceptibility to cancer, particularly in relation to smoking. Unlike familial cancer syndromes, this is probably a complex genetic trait but recent developments in the methodology of genetic epidemiology have made the analysis of such multifactorial diseases possible. Not only will these studies, if successful, help us to identify people with exceptional high risk to smoking-induced lung cancer but also the results will also increase our level of understanding of lung cancer development in general. The genetic background facilitating smoking-induced cancer may differ for different organ sites (lung, pancreas, bladder, and oral cavity) and is also likely to differ from that determining susceptibility to cardiovascular diseases associated with smoking.

A new promising line of research has evolved from the observation that in some human cancers genomic instability may be reflected in microsatellite DNA changes which commonly originate from replication errors. Effective mismatch repair may be the underlying cause, but so far only a restricted number of fragile microsatellite foci have been identified.

Research on the Prevention of Cancer and Its Consequences

The Gambia Hepatitis Intervention Study is a major effort to determine the role of chronic hepatitis B virus infection in the evolution of hepatocellular carcinomas. The vaccinated children are followed-up for serological markers of HBV infection and, later in life, the occurrence of liver tumors. This is a long-term study, but the agency is committed to lead this important work to a successful conclusion.

It is now increasingly possible to identify individuals with a high risk to cancer development, e.g., through genetic analysis, high levels of exposure to environmental carcinogens, or the occurrence of a tumor at a site where second primary tumors are frequent. It is, therefore, necessary to offer these subjects advice and treatment. More targeted screening for early neoplastic lesions is advisable but, in addition, chemoprevention may be a tool to reduce the incidence of malignant transformation and to revert early stages of cancer development. Since cancer prevention is a key element of the agency's mission, IARC scientists would like to be involved in this important research area. This is planned to be done in two ways. Similar to, but distinct from, the monographs series on the *Carcinogenic Risks to Humans,* an IARC *Handbook of Cancer Prevention* series has been launched, focusing on chemopreventive agents and other preventive strategies, such as vaccination. Again, an independent panel of experts will convene to evaluate whether there is sufficient evidence for chemoprevention and whether there is associated toxicity and carcinogenicity which would have to be taken into account in clinical trials. If the budget allows, we also plan to have a small laboratory group focusing on the mechanisms of cancer prevention.

While breast cancer incidence is higher in developed countries, changes in lifestyle make this cancer type increasingly common in developing countries as well. A significant reduction of breast cancer mortality is best achieved by early detection. However, in many developing countries diagnostic tools such as mammography may not be available for widespread tests. The agency is initiating a large project in the Philippines aiming at a reduction of breast cancer mortality by annual examination of the breasts by trained nurses. Similarly, IARC scientists are involved in projects aiming at early detection of stomach and cervical cancer.

—*Harri Vainio and Paul Kleihues*

Related Topics

Biomarkers, Human Health
Carcinogen Classification Schemes
Carcinogen–DNA Adduct Formation and DNA Repair
Carcinogenesis
Epidemiology
Food and Agriculture Organization of the United Nations
Information Resources in Toxicology
International Programme on Chemical Safety
International Register of Potentially Toxic Chemicals
International Union of Toxicology
Toxicity Testing, Carcinogenesis

International Life Sciences Institute —North America

The International Life Sciences Institute—North America (ILSI-NA) was founded in 1985. It was formerly (1991) the International Life Sciences Institute—Nutrition Foundation. It was formed by the merger of Nutrition Foundation (founded in 1941) and North American branch of International Life Sciences Institute (founded in 1978). The institute is sponsored by companies within the food, pharmaceutical, chemical, toxicology, and related industries. ILSI-NA promotes basic research and education in the areas of nutrition toxicology through support of research, scientific symposia, workshops, and monographs. It also fosters career development of outstanding young scientists.

ILSI-NA committees include antioxidant, emulsifiers, caffeine, colors, diet, and behavior; food microbiology; food nutrition and safety; oral health; and sweeteners.

Publications include *Nutrition Reviews,* which is a monthly, and *Present Knowledge in Nutrition,* which is quinquennial. ILSI-NA also publishes monographs, reprints, scientific reports, and educational materials. The institute holds a periodic symposium.

For more information contact the International Life Sciences Institute—North America, 1126 16th Street, NW, No. 300, Washington, DC 20036. Telephone: 202-569-0074.

—*David M. Krentz and Harihara M. Mehendale*

(Adapted from information supplied by ILSI-NA.)

Related Topics

Food Additives
Food and Agriculture Organization of the United Nations
Food and Drug Administration
International Register of Potentially Toxic Chemicals
Organisation for Economic Cooperation and Development

International Programme on Chemical Safety

The International Programme on Chemical Safety (IPCS) is a cooperative program of the United Nations Environment Program (UNEP), the International Labour Office, and the World Health Organization (WHO). WHO is the executing agency for the program;

the Central Unit of the IPCS, which runs the program on a day-to-day basis, is located in WHO headquarters in Geneva. A consultative mechanism, called the Inter-Secretariat Coordinating Committee, ensures close collaboration between the three cooperating organizations. Within WHO, chemical safety activities are coordinated through an Intra-WHO Coordinating Committee on Chemical Safety. The evaluation of the risks to health and the environment are the responsibility of the IPCS; activities directed toward the management of those risks are undertaken mainly by other WHO programs such as Control of Environmental Health Hazards, Food Safety, and Workers' Health, although certain risk management activities are also the responsibility of the IPCS. WHO also has regional activities on chemical safety which are run through the six WHO regional offices and their Environmental Health Centres. These offices use the outputs of the IPCS in their own chemical safety activities.

Countries or specific national agencies willing to participate in the work of the IPCS express their commitment by signing a Memorandum of Understanding. This lays down the particular areas of interest and the support which will be provided.

Many of the specific activities of the IPCS are undertaken through a network of participating institutions designated by member states. These are various types of centers of excellence, usually involved in scientific research concerned with effects of chemicals. Two international institutions also participate in the work of the IPCS: the International Agency for Research on Cancer (IARC) in the field of chemical carcinogenicity and UNEP's International Register of Potentially Toxic Chemicals (IRPTC) for chemical information. They both also participate through training activities. While many of the IPCS activities are implemented through the Central Unit, each of the three organizations cooperating in the IPCS also contributes to the program's objectives individually, for example, through the UNEP Industry and Environment Office and through the networks of the Global Environment Monitoring System. The ILO contributes through its program on chemical safety, i.e., the preparation of the codes of practice, guides and manuals, the provision of technical advisory services, and technical cooperation projects. In response to the 1989 International Labour Conference Resolution concerning the harmonization of the criteria for classification, identification, and labeling of chemicals used at places of work, the ILO contributes to the IPCS with a scientific support and use of outputs from the IPCS. All countries are encouraged to designate a focal point, through which the IPCS outputs may be disseminated in the country. Through the focal point, guidance may be given to the IPCS on the needs and views of the country.

Policy Guidance

Overall policy guidance for the IPCS is given by a Programme Advisory Committee. It consists of 20 designated advisors chosen by their personal capacity. Priorities for particular areas of work are established through a regular process of review and consultation with member states and other bodies which cooperate with the IPCS.

Collaborative Structure of the IPCS with Other Organizations

The IPCS works closely with other international governmental and nongovernmental organizations, associations, and professional bodies which have activities in the field of chemical safety. Some activities are undertaken jointly and others in consultation. In particular, the IPCS works closely with the Organisation for Economic Cooperation and Development, as well as with the Programme on Toxicology for Health Protection of the Commission of the European Communities. The evaluation of chemicals in food is a joint activity with the Food and Agricultural Organization (FAO). Some specific collaborative activities are undertaken with international scientific bodies such as the Scientific Committee on Problems of the Environment of the International Council of Scientific Unions, the International Union of Pure and Applied Chemistry, the International Union of Toxicology, and the International Life Sciences Institute.

Professional bodies and associations dealing with chemical safety are consulted in implementing many of the IPCS activities including the World Federation of Associations of Clinical Toxicology and Poison Control Centres for the work on poison control, the International Group of National Associations of Manufacturers of Chemical Products for work on agrochemicals, and the European Chemical Industry Ecology and Toxicology Centre for assessment of chemicals.

Roles and Objectives of the IPCS

IPCS roles

The IPCS has two overall roles. The first is to provide a forum for establishing an international consensus assessment of the risks of chemicals to health and the environment. The second is to promote the use nationally of these assessments and to strengthen the capabilities of member states to deal with chemical-related problems, including chemical accidents. Through the IPCS, the scientific basis is provided for member states to develop and implement their own chemical safety activities.

These roles are expressed in six objectives. The first two objectives are concerned with health and environmental risk assessment and the methodologies to undertake them. The fourth and fifth objectives deal with the prevention and medical response to the human health and environmental effects of chemicals. The third objective deals with strengthening the capabilities of member states to take effective chemical safety measures, and the final objective is directed toward the development of human resources and the training needs required to implement the other five objectives. Objectives 3 and 6 use the outputs of the other four objectives and are described after them in the following section.

IPCS Objectives

IPCS objectives are to catalyze and coordinate activities in relation to chemical safety, and in particular to:

1. Carry out and disseminate evaluations of the risk to human health and the environment from exposure to chemicals, mixtures of chemicals, or combinations of chemicals and physical and biological agents

2. Promote the development, improvement, validation, and use of methods for laboratory testing and ecological and epidemiological studies and other methods suitable for the evaluation of health and environmental risks and hazards from chemicals

3. Promote technical cooperation with member states, in particular developing countries, to (a) facilitate the use of available evaluations of health and environmental risks and hazards from chemicals, (b) improve the capabilities of national authorities in conducting their own evaluations of health and environmental risks and hazards from chemicals, and (c) strengthen infrastructures for safety aspects relating to chemicals—their production, importation, transportation, storage, use, and disposal

4. Promote effective international cooperation with respect to emergencies and accidents involving chemicals

5. Support national programs for prevention and treatment of poisonings involving chemicals

6. Promote training of the required manpower

IPCS Achievements

Risk Evaluation of Priority Chemicals

As its first objective, the IPCS prepares evaluations of the risk to human health and the environment from exposure to chemicals. In the evaluation process the scientific literature is reviewed and the first draft of a document prepared according to standard guidelines. This draft is circulated to experts, IPCS participating institutions, and national focal points for scientific peer review, comment, and further inputs. A second draft is then prepared and examined at an international meeting of independent experts where a consensus evaluation is made and is incorporated into the published document. The preparation and review of these documents represents a large coordinated effort by the IPCS staff, consultants, and scientists from all over the world. Available in several languages and distributed to all member states, these documents provide a scientific and objective basis that national health and other authorities may use for planning and for the development of regulatory actions and control measures. It must be stressed that evaluations established through international consensus, under the aegis of the three cooperating organizations of the IPCS, are much more readily acceptable, especially by countries which do not have the capacity to perform their own evaluations, than those provided by any one national authority. Chemicals for evaluation are selected through an international consultative process, guided by four main criteria: adverse effects, exposure, targets, and international concern.

Criteria for the Selection of Priority Chemicals

Adverse effects: An evaluation of scientific information leading to the conclusion that the substance presents a hazard for human health and/or the environment.

Exposure: The possible use, persistence, accumulation, or degradation of the substance shows that there may be significant exposure to man or the environment.

Targets: The size and nature of the populations at risk (both human and other species) and the risks to the environment should be taken into account.

International concern: The substance should be of major interest to several countries, where the need for an evaluation is not satisfied by current scientific documents prepared by other international bodies.

The basic scientific risk evaluation documents are published in the *Environmental Health Criteria* series. For administrators, managers, and decision makers, clear and concise summaries are published as *Health and Safety Guides*. For use in the workplace and field where several thousands of chemicals are commonly used, the IPCS publishes *International Chemical Safety Cards,* which summarize essential data, using standard phrases, on a single sheet. Specialized evaluated information for the medical profession on how to diagnose and treat victims poisoned by chemicals are published as *Poisons Information Monographs*.

Some IPCS Evaluated Outputs

Environmental Health Criteria documents are designed for scientific experts responsible for the evaluation of the risk posed by chemicals to human health and the environment, enabling relevant authorities to establish policies for the safe use of these chemicals.

Health and Safety Guides are designed for a wide range of administrators, managers, and decision makers in various ministries and governmental agencies, as well as in commerce, industry, and trade unions, who are involved in various aspects of using chemicals safety and avoiding environmental health hazards. They are short documents summarizing toxicity information in nontechnical language and provide practical advice on matters such as safe storage, handling and disposal of the chemicals, accident prevention and health protection measures, first aid and medical treatment in cases of exposure leading to acute effects, and clean-up procedures.

International Chemical Safety Cards summarizing essential product identity data and health and safety information on chemicals, are designed to provide evaluated information for use at the shop floor level, in factories, agriculture, and other workplaces. They have no legally binding status and are not intended to be used in the regulatory process in any specific country.

Poisons Information Monographs are designed for poisons information centers and others giving medical advice on prevention and treatment of poisoning. They summarize the basic chemical, physical, and toxicological properties of the chemical and provide detailed advice on diagnosis and patient management, including analytical toxicological methods.

Toxicological evaluation of chemicals associated with food are made jointly with FAO. FAO also collaborates with WHO in the preparation of data sheets on pesticides widely used in public health and those with a high or unusual toxicity. They contain not only toxicological and risk information but also guidance on first aid and laboratory analysis as well as recommendations to regulatory authorities. The two international participating institutions also contribute to the IPCS risk evaluation process: IARC produces monographs on carcinogenicity of chemicals; and the IRPTC prepares data profiles on chemicals for which risk evaluations are required. The IPCS and IRPTC also collaborate to produce a computerized listing of chemicals being tested and reviewed for toxicity.

Since its conception, the IPCS has evaluated an impressive list of commonly used and internationally traded agricultural and industrial chemicals. Furthermore, chemicals frequently found as dangerous air and water pollutants and those associated with global atmospheric changes, such as the greenhouse gases and the chlorofluorocarbons, as well as certain natural toxins have also been evaluated. Additionally, evaluations of certain physical factors, such as noise and low-frequency radiation, as well as of radioisotopes have been published in the *Environmental Health Criteria* series.

The IPCS not only disseminates its outputs in hard copy form but also is increasingly using informatics. In cooperation with the Canadian Centre for Occupational Health and Safety, the *Environmental Health Criteria* documents, *Health and Safety Guides*, the *International Chemical Safety Cards*, and the *Poisons Information Monographs* are issued on compact disk (CD-ROM).

The IRPTC also systematically incorporates IPCS risk evaluations in its data profiles and the IRPTC bulletin carries executive summaries of these evaluations. A collection of approximately 80,000 chemical safety sheets as well as information on workplace legislation and training materials are available from the LLO's International Occupational Safety and Health Information Centre.

For more information, the IPCS web site address is http://www.who.ch/programmes/pcs/pcs_home.htm.

Acknowledgment

This entry is extracted from a public information brochure published by the IPCS, CH-1211, Geneva 27, Switzerland.

Related Topics

Food and Agricultural Organization of the United Nations
Information Resources in Toxicology
International Agency for Research on Cancer
International Life Sciences Institute—North America
International Register of Potentially Toxic Chemicals
International Union of Toxicology
Organisation for Economic Cooperation and Development

International Register of Potentially Toxic Chemicals

Introduction

The International Register of Potentially Toxic Chemicals (IRPTC) was established by the United Nations Environment Programme (UNEP) in 1976, following a recommendation of the 1972 United Nations Conference on the Human Environment held in Stockholm. For the first time the world had an institution to collect information on hazardous chemicals and disseminate it to anyone who needed the data. The central unit of the register, known as the Programme Activity Centre (PAC), was set up in Geneva that same year and received its first query in March 1976 (Fig. I-4).

IRPTC is part of UNEP's Earthwatch program created to look out for environmental changes, try to establish their causes, and communicate the results. It works alongside the Global Environmental Monitoring System (GEMS) and other information exchange activities of UNEP, such as INFOTERRA.

IRPTC maintains a databank of centralized computer files linking a formal network of government-nominated institutions. Equally important, it embodies a concept for managing and exchanging information in a consistent, scientifically sound fashion, leading to information-sharing partnerships.

Ultimately, IRPTC aims to help the world community make better use of existing global resources and to give developing countries the information base to manage chemicals effectively.

IRPTC is also a scientific tool for recording and sharing data used to assess the hazards posed by chemicals to human health and the environment. It is moving toward making its resources available on personal computers, which should be of great benefit to scientists who evaluate data. This should also make contributing data to the databank much easier and more of a natural part of day-to-day activities.

National Registers of Potentially Toxic Chemicals (NRPTCs)

Assisting developing countries to establish national chemical data systems that are compatible with IRPTC is an attempt to extend the IRPTC concept to the national level. Currently involving ten countries, this activity will be a major priority for the decade.

Contributing Network Partners

These are national and international institutions engaged in the assessment of chemical hazards. Through formal or informal agreements they assist with collection and validation of data on chemicals. They often provide scientific or technical expertise on request, or links to other institutions that may be able to help. IRPTC's Contributing Network Partners include United Nations bodies, international scientific organizations, national academies of science, specialized research institutions and industrial research centres. IRPTC co-operates in programmes with the International Programme on Chemical Safety, the European Communities, the Organisation for Economic Co-operation and Development and the Council for Mutual Economic Assistance. Other partners are chemical manufacturers and industry associations.

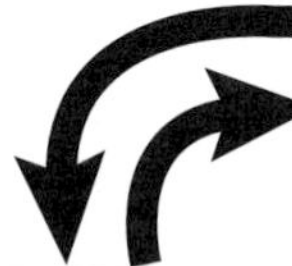

IRPTC Programme Activity Centre

The IRPTC-PAC staff consist of 19 people including consultants. Their scientific expertise covers such fields as biology, chemistry, computer science, environmental science, marine biology, microbiology, pharmacology and toxicology.

National Correspondents

By 1990 the Governments of some 110 member countries of the United Nations had each appointed at least one scientist or civil servant to assist IRPTC in information gathering and dissemination. Regular contacts and regional workshops for these National Correspondents are part of IRPTC's strategy in order to involve them and the institutions they represent in IRPTC activities.

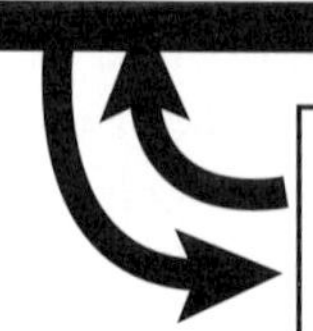

Designated National Authorities

These are specially designated government institutions which are responsible for implementing at a national level the London Guidelines for the Exchange of Information on Chemicals in International Trade. At the end of 1989, 75 countries had named their contacts, who were participating in the exchange of notifications of control actions.

FIGURE I-4. IRPTC's global network.

UNEP's Governing Council revised the objectives of IRPTC in 1989, in keeping with the center's expanding role, and set five main goals:

1. To make it easier to obtain the existing information on production, distribution, release, disposal, and adverse effects of chemicals

2. To identify the important gaps in our knowledge of the effects of chemicals and call attention to the need for research to fill those gaps

3. To help identify potential hazards from chemicals and wastes and to improve awareness of the dangers

4. To provide information about national, regional, and global policies; controls; and recommendations on potentially toxic chemicals

5. To help implement policies for the exchange of information on chemicals in international trade

As part of UNEP's targets for the 1990s, IRPTC operates its databank, oversees and helps implement the London Guidelines for the Exchange of Information on Chemicals in International Trade, assists developing countries in setting up National Registers of Potentially Toxic Chemicals, produces regular publications, and offers training. It is also involved with GEMS in producing statements on environmental problems related to chemicals.

The Databank

There are two sides to IRPTC's databank: one is data collection and validation; the other is management of these data by computer, including dissemination to users.

IRPTC aims to maintain a storehouse of information adequate for an understanding of the hazards to health and the environment associated with toxic chemicals. Pharmaceuticals and radioactive substances are not included. It offers concise overviews of selected data on chemicals for evaluation purposes, called chemical data profiles. It also contains a register index that offers a "profile of the profiles," an indication of the substances covered, their current status, and the subject areas where information exists or is absent.

Data profiles are prepared by contributing network partners, consultants, and IRPTC staff. All data are verified by IRPTC staff. The steps involved are to select the chemicals on which information is to be gathered, to search and acquire available scientific information, and to select and validate the information received.

Data Profiles

The production of data profiles remains a central activity of IRPTC. As one IRPTC staff member explains:

> Data profiles are prepared so as to present the information in concise, carefully organized and clear form. It is important that data can be easily retrieved and understood. Users must be able to see immediately what information exists on a particular aspect of a chemical. For example, if there has been a spill near a river, they need to know immediately how the substance reacts with water and its effect on aquatic organisms.

A profile is never really considered complete. IRPTC continues to monitor sources of new information with which to update and revise the files.

There are 17 categories of data entered into the register (see Table I-7). The attributes are chosen for their relevance in evaluating potential hazards. Each data record and every piece of information in the data files is referenced with a bibliography.

A data profile may also indicate when information is missing, which can act as an alert mechanism for

TABLE I-7
IRPTC Data Profile Structure

Identifiers, properties, and classification
Production/trade
Production processes
Use
Pathways into the environment
Concentrations
Loss/persistence
Concentrations
Human intake
Environmental fate tests
Biodegradation/biotransformation
Photodegradation
Hydrolysis
Sorption
Evaporation
Oxidation
Model ecosystem studies
Environmental fate
Chemobiokinetics
Absorption
Distribution
Bioconcentration factor
Metabolism
Excretion
Mammalian toxicity
Special toxicity studies
Biochemical interactions
Carcinogenicity
Mutagenicity
Neurotoxicity
Behavior
Sensitization
Interacting agents
Primary irritation
Immunotoxicity
Reproduction
Teratogenicity
Effects on organisms in the environment
Aquatic toxicity
Terrestrial toxicity
Sampling/preparation/analysis
Spills
Treatment of poisoning
Waste management
Recommendations/legal mechanisms

government officials, a stimulus to research designed to fill the gap, and a guide for scientists who want to avoid repeating the work of others.

Half of the chemicals for which full data profiles exist are used in agriculture.

Selection of Chemicals

The IRPTC Scientific Advisory Committee, a group of United Nations experts appointed by UNEP's executive director, in 1978 identified and defined the chemical attributes on which information would be needed to assess the hazards and risks of a particular substance.

IRPTC's Information Processing Unit established an open-ended working list of chemicals in 1979, drawing mainly on national and international lists of substances causing governments concern. This enabled the center to concentrate on priority substances of international significance rather than try to cover all the chemicals in common use.

The first *Working List of Selected Chemical Substances,* identifying 250 chemicals of international significance, was produced in 1979. It was distributed to IRPTC's contributing network partners and has been regularly revised and expanded.

IRPTC's current priorities are to update information on chemicals on the list, to carry out work in accordance with the priorities of the London Guidelines, to ensure that it proceeds in step with other United Nations programs such as the International Programme on Chemical Safety, and to respond to the priorities of Contributing Network Partners and the Query Response Service.

For more information, the IRPTC web site address is http://irptc.unep.ch/irptc/.

Acknowledgment

This entry is extracted from a public information brochure published by IRPTC/UNEP, Palais des Natias, 1211 Geneva 10, Switzerland.

Note: In 1996, IRPTC changed its name to UNEP Chemicals. At that time, governments thoroughly revised its program of work. Although the activities described herein remain a minor component of UNEP Chemicals' activities, its major work program involves negotiating and implementing a convention on Prior Informed Consent (PIC) jointly with the Food and Agriculture Organization of the UN, and both negotiating a global treaty for and undertaking immediate actions on Persistent Organic Pollutants (POPs).

Related Topics

European Commission
Food and Agricultural Organization of the UN
Information Resources in Toxicology
International Agency for Research on Cancer
ILSI of North America
International Programme on Chemical Safety
International Union of Toxicology
Organisation for Economic Cooperation and Development

International Union of Toxicology

The International Union of Toxicology (IUTOX) is an international body composed of 30 national/supernational toxicological societies from all parts of the world. Its creation reflects the growing awareness of the wide range of toxic threats throughout the world and the need for concerted and coordinated efforts to resolve these problems. This awareness led initially to the creation of special toxicological sections or groups within international or national associations of scientists from various fields. Although the specific toxicological concerns of these groups were different, the basic principles and approaches used to investigate them are strikingly similar, and independent bodies dedicated specifically to the discipline of toxicology were soon established in many countries. IUTOX was founded on July 6, 1980, in Brussels, Belgium, during the 2nd International Congress of Toxicology. Its purposes are to promote a full and uniform development of toxicology within and across various scientific disciplines and to provide an international platform for scientists active in toxicological research.

IUTOX is directed by a 12-member executive committee composed of the president, 1st and 2nd vice presidents, secretary general, treasurer, past president, and five directors. A new executive committee, reflecting the international membership of the Union, is elected every 3 years by a general assembly of the member societies. Each member society is allowed one vote for every 200 registered members, up to a maximum of five votes for those with more than 800 individual members. Standing commissions include those for Communications, Developing Countries, Education, and Central and Eastern European Countries. Since 1986 IUTOX has published an annual newsletter that is circulated among member societies.

IUTOX has been an associate member of the International Council of Scientific Unions since 1987 and became a full member in 1996. In 1993 it was recognized as an official nongovernmental organization of the World Health Organization (WHO) and, as such, it contributes to the activities of the WHO's International Programme on Chemical Safety (WHO-IPCS) and sends delegates to the recently established International Forum on Chemical Safety.

Every 3 years, IUTOX organizes an International Congress of Toxicology lasting 4 or 5 days with an average attendance of from 800 to 1500 persons. During these congresses, joint symposia on specific questions are organized with other international scientific bodies, such as the International Union of Pharmacology, the International Union of Pure and Applied Chemistry (IUPAC), the WHO-IPCS, the International Agency for Research on Cancer, and the International Council for Laboratory Animal Sciences. Past congresses have been held in Brussels (1980), San Diego (1983), Tokyo (1986), Brighton (1989), Rome (1992), and Seattle (1995). The VIII International Congress of Toxicology will be held in Paris in 1998 and the IX in Brisbane (2001).

IUTOX also sponsors numerous other international meetings (e.g., Joint Meeting of the Italian and French Societies of Toxicology in 1991, the Convention of the International Neurotoxicology Association in 1991, and the Second Nordic Toxicology Congress in 1992). Activities organized in developing countries include the Workshop on Prevention and Management of Poisonings in South America (Montevideo, Uruguay) in 1991, the Workshop on Development of Poison Control Programmes in South America (Montevideo, Uruguay) in 1992 (both of which were organized in conjunction with the WHO-IPCS), the Seminar and Training Course on Diagnosis, Management and Prevention of Poisoning for Francophone, Sub-Saharan Countries (Dakar, Senegal) in 1995, and the Second and Third Congresses of Toxicology in Developing Countries, held, respectively, in New Delhi, India, in 1991 and Cairo, Egypt, in 1995.

IUTOX also contributed to the *Glossary of Terms Used in Toxicology* published by the IUPAC in 1994.

As part of its continuing education program, IUTOX organizes Risk Assessment Summer Schools, which have been held every 2 years since 1984. These 1-week courses provide training for young toxicologists in strategies and skills associated with chemical risk assessment.

IUTOX Member Societies

Founding members: European Society of Toxicology, the British Toxicological Society, the Finnish Society of Toxicology, the French Society of Toxicology, the Italian Society of Toxicology, the Japanese Society of Toxicological Sciences, the Netherlands Society of Toxicology, the Norwegian Society of Pharmacology and Toxicology, the Society of Toxicology of Canada, the Indian Society of Toxicology, the Society of Toxicology—United States, the Swedish Society of Toxicology, the Swiss Society of Pharmacology and Toxicology, the Yugoslavian Society of Toxicology, and the Society of Toxicology of the Democratic Republic of Germany.

Other members: the Committee of Toxicology of the Academia Sinica (Taiwan), the American Academy of Clinical Toxicology, the Argentinean Society of Toxicology, Asiatox, the Australasian Society of Clinical and Experimental Pharmacologists and Toxicologists, the Brazilian Society of Toxicology, the Danish Society of Pharmacology and Toxicology, the Egyptian Society of Toxicology, the European Association of Poison Centres and Clinical Toxicologists, the French Society of Clinical Toxicology, the German Society for Pharmacology and Toxicology, the Hungarian Pharmacological Society, the Irish Society of Toxicology, the Korean Society of Toxicology, the Society of Toxicology—Thailand, the Society of Toxicologic Pathologists—United States, and the Spanish Society of Toxicology.

—Paolo Preziosi

Related Topics

American Academy of Clinical Toxicology
European Commission

European Society of Toxicology
Food an Agricultural Organization of the United Nations
International Agency for Research on Cancer
International Life Sciences Institute—North America
International Programme on Chemical Safety
International Register of Potentially Toxic Chemicals
Organisation for Economic Cooperation and Development
Society of Toxicology (U.S.)

Investigative New Drug Application

- TITLE: INDA
- AGENCY: U.S. FDA
- YEAR PASSED: 1962 Drug Amendment to FD&C Act
- GROUPS REGULATED: Drug and biopharmaceutical industries

Synopsis of Law

The regulations specifically applicable to human drugs are covered in Subchapter D, Parts 300–399. The definition of a new drug is covered in Part 310(g): "A new drug substance means any substance that when used in the manufacturer, processing, or packaging of a drug causes that drug to be a new drug but does not include intermediates used in the synthesis of such substances."

The regulation then goes on to discuss "newness with regard to new formulations, indications, or in combinations." For toxicologists, the meat of the regulations can be found in Section 312 (INDA) and Section 314 (applications for approval to market a new drug or antibiotic drug or NDA). The major focus for a toxicologist working in the pharmaceutical industry is on preparing the correct toxicology "packages" to be included to "support" these two types of applications. (The exact nature of these packages will be covered later).

In a nutshell, the law requires solid scientific evidence of safety and efficacy before a new drug will be permitted in clinical trails or (later) on the market. INDA (covered in 21 CFR 310) is for permission to proceed with clinical trails on human subjects. Once clinical trails have been completed, the manufacturer or "sponsor" can then proceed to file an NDA (covered in 21 CFR 314) for permission to market the new drug.

As stated in 321.21, "A sponsor shall submit an IND if the sponsor intends to conduct a clinical investigation with a new drug . . . (and) shall not begin a clinical investigation until . . . an IND . . . is in effect." Similar procedures are in place in other major countries. In the United Kingdom, for example, a clinical trails certificate (CTC) must be filed or a CTX (clinical trial exemption) obtained before clinical trails may proceed. Clinical trails are divided into three phases, as described in 312.21. Phase I trials are initial introductions into healthy volunteers primarily for the purposes of establishing tolerance (side effects), bioavailability, and metabolism. Phase II clinical trials are "controlled studies . . . to evaluate defectiveness of the drug for a particular indication or disease." The secondary objective is to determine common short-term side effects; hence the subjects are closely monitored. Phase III studies are expanded clinical trials. It is during this phase that the definitive, large-scale, double-blind studies are performed.

The toxicologist's main responsibilities in the IND process are to design, conduct, and interpret appropriate toxicology studies (or packages) to support the initial IND and then design the appropriate studies necessary to support each additional phase of investigation. The toxicologist's second responsibility is to prepare the toxicology summaries for the (clinical) investigator's brochure [described in 312.23(a)(8)(ii)]. This is an integrated summary of the toxicological effects of the drug in animals and *in vitro*.

Once an IND or CTC/X is opened, the toxicologist may have several additional responsibilities: first, to design, conduct, and report the additional tests necessary to support a new clinical protocol or an amendment to the current clinical protocol (Section 312.20); second, to bring to the sponsor's attention any finding in an ongoing toxicology study in animals, "suggesting a significant risk to human subjects, including any finding of mutagenicity, teratogenicity or carcinogenicity," as described in 21 CFR 312.32. The sponsor has a legal obligation to report such findings within 10 working days; and third, to prepare a "list of the preclinical studies . . . completed or in progress during the past year" and a summary of the major preclinical findings. The sponsor is required (under Section 312.23) to file an annual report (within 60 days of the IND anniversary date) describing the progress of the investigation. INDs are never "approved" in the strict sense of the word. Once filed, an IND can be opened 30 days after submission, unless U.S. FDA informs the sponsor otherwise. The structure of an IND is outlined in Table I-8.

If the clinical trials conducted under an IND are successful in demonstrating safety and effectiveness [often established at a pre-NDA meeting, described in (2) CFR 312.47(b)(2)], the sponsor can then submit an NDA. Unlike an IND, the NDA must be specifically approved by U.S. FDA. The toxicologist's responsibility in the NDA/Marketing Authorization Application (MAA) process is to prepare an integrated summary of all the toxicology and/or safety studies performed and be in a position to present and review the toxicology findings to U.S. FDA or its advisory bodies. The approval process can be exhausting, including many meetings, hearings, and appeals. The ground rules for all of these are described in Part A of the law. For example, all NDAs are reviewed by an "independent" (persons not connected with either the sponsor or the agency) scientific advisory board which will review the findings and make recommendations as to approval. MAAs must be reviewed by and reported on by an expert recognized by the cognizant regulatory authority. Final statutory approval in the United States lies with the commissioner of U.S. FDA.

It is hoped that few additional studies will be requested during the NDA review and approval process. When an NDA is approved, the agency will send the sponsor an approval letter and will issue a Summary Basis of Approval (SBA) (312.30), which is designed and intended to provide a public record on the agency's reasoning for approving the NDA while not revealing any proprietary information. The SBA can be obtained through Freedom of Information and can provide insights into the precedents for which types of toxicology studies are used to support specific types ofclaims.

—*Shayne C. Gad*

Related Topics

Delaney Clause
Food and Drug Administration
Food, Drug and Cosmetic Act
Good Laboratory Practices
Toxic Torts

TABLE I-8
Composition of a Standard Investigational New Drug Application

IND cover sheet (Form FDA-1571)
Table of contents
Introductory statement
General (clinical) investigation plan
(Clinical) investigators brochure
(Proposed) clinical protocol(s)
Chemistry, manufacturing, and control information
Pharmacology and toxicology information (includes metabolism and pharmacokinetic assessments done in animals)
Previous human experience with the investigational drug
Additional information
Other relevant information

In Vitro Test

In vitro test systems are those that do not employ intact higher organism as models for predicting potential human (or other target animal) toxicity. Such test systems are a (albeit) large subset of alternative models, which are addressed extensively under their own entries in this work. Varieties of these are classified in Table I-9.

The most famous *in vitro* test system is the Ames mutagenicity assay, and indeed, most mutagenicity tests employ *in vitro* systems. Though much work has gone into the development of such systems, other than

TABLE I-9
Types of *in Vitro* Models for Toxicity Testing and Research

Level/examples	*Advantages*	*Disadvantages*
Lower organisms (earthworms, fish)	Range of integrated organismic responses	Frequently lack responses typical of higher organisms Animal welfare concerns
Isolated organs	Intact yet isolated tissue and vascular system Controlled environmental and exposure conditions	Donor organism still required Time-consuming and expensive No intact organismic responses Limited duration of viability
Cultured cells	No intact animals directly involved Ability to carefully manipulate system Low cost Ability to study a wide range of variables	Instability of system Limited enzymatic capabilities and viability of system No (or limited) integrated multicell and/or organismic responses
Chemical/biochemical systems	No donor organism problems Low cost Long-term stability of preparation Ability to study a wide range of variables Specificity of response	No *de facto* correlation to *in vivo* system Limited to investigation of a single defined mechanism
Computer simulations	No animal welfare concerns Speed and low per-evaluation cost	May not have predictive value beyond a narrow range of structures Expensive to establish

mutagenicity, currently such systems are widely employed only for pyrogenicity and cytotoxicity testing in the medical device industry.

Further Reading

Gad, S. C. (1993). *In Vitro Toxicology*. Raven Press, New York.
Gad, S. C., and Kapis, M. B. (1993). *Non-Animal Techniques in Biomedical and Behavioral Research and Testing*. Lewis, Ann Arbor, MI.
Frazier, J. M. (1992). *In Vitro Toxicity Testing*. Dekker, New York.

—Shayne C. Gad

Related Topics

Ames Test
Analytical Toxicology
In Vivo Test
Microtox
Mutagenesis
Toxicity Testing, Alternatives

In Vivo Test

In vivo studies are technically those performed using any intact living organism as a model system, but in toxicology are generally considered to be only those performed in intact higher organisms (most commonly, mammals).

Eight different species are currently used with any frequency in toxicology. These are, in approximate numbers of animals utilized (from most to least), rat, mouse, rabbit, guinea pig, hamster, dog, ferret, and monkey. The cat and the frog, while common biological models, have not been used in toxicity testing for some time.

It is generally assumed that the results of animal tests on chemical toxicity are relevant to humans. In many cases, humans are considered at least as sensitive to the effects of the test agent as is the most sensitive species used in these tests. Such assumptions are necessitated by a current lack of knowledge of more appropriate methodology and reflect other assumptions made by our distant ancestors on the relevance of observations in animals to the human situation. Two series of questions arise from these assumptions. At the qualitative level, it should first be asked whether any specific animal tests are more likely than others to lead to results of questionable significance to humans. Second, it may be asked whether the risk to humans can be assessed quantitatively from animal data. The first series of assumptions are analyzed in this section.

Some test protocols are particularly liable to produce misleading results. Maternal toxicity induced by test agents, rather than the direct action of the test agent itself, may be responsible for the induction of certain patterns of teratogenic effects. Several examples of possibly confusing results obtained in carcinogenesis bioassays are presented here. Perhaps the first to be recognized concerned the induction of sarcomas following the local injection of chemicals subcutaneously in rats. Although there can be little doubt that the injection of small quantities of chemicals such as 7,12-dimethylbenz(*a*)anthracene actually induces these tumors, overloading the tissues with dyestuffs may well lead to cancer because of a mechanism dependent on factors other than the specific interactions of the test chemical. Similarly, bladder stone formation can lead to bladder cancer in rats and mice, thus making it difficult to be certain whether a chemical that leads to bladder stone formation and tumorigenesis is or is not a true carcinogen.

Perhaps the greatest cause of confusion in the interpretation of carcinogenicity bioassays occurs when a substantial background incidence of tumors is enhanced. It should be asked whether the test chemical is inducing such tumors or merely enhancing their incidence. Although this problem is clearly recognized with chemicals that enhance the already high incidence of pulmonary tumors in strain A mice, there has been little discussion of the confounding effects of naturally occurring tumors that demonstrate a lower but still appreciable incidence. The B6C3F1 male mouse used in the NCI/NTP Bioassay Program in the United States demonstrates a 15–60% incidence of hepatic cell tumors by 2 years of age. However, whether this confounds the interpretation of a bioassay or whether enhancement of the yield of such tumors, as opposed to their direct induction, is relevant to the effects of the chemical in humans is not asked; instead, these chemicals are usually uncritically accepted as carcinogens and generally regulated as such.

There are many tumors that have a naturally high incidence, such as tumors of the endocrine tissues in certain strains of rats. In each case, it is necessary to consider the overall evidence that agents increasing the yield of such tumors may or may not induce cancer in humans. Such considerations require in-depth knowledge of biological and biochemical mechanisms of carcinogenesis and development of new and testable ideas. Increased emphasis on how agents exert their effect, rather than on which agents exert an effect, will move toxicology to the forefront of integrated biological science.

One further problem needs to be addressed regarding human and animal reactions to toxic agents. Although it is possible to control the exposure of a test animal quite precisely in a well-run experiment, humans are exposed to an ever-changing multitude of chemicals as a result of the food they eat, the drugs they take, or the lifestyles they have chosen. Therefore, single-substance toxicological tests may either overemphasize or underemphasize the significance of the potential hazard to humans, except possibly in the case of massive exposures. There is very limited laboratory evidence on the effects of chemical mixtures because a single chemical assay is so expensive that the assay of mixtures becomes prohibitively costly. However, the coadministration of a carcinogen and a promoting agent may lead to far more tumors than either agent alone. By contrast, two carcinogens, such as 4-dimethylaminoazobenzene and 3-methylcholanthrene, may fail to produce tumors when given together yet they do so when given separately. More information on chemical interactions continues to be needed if we are to extrapolate animal tests to humans even with qualitative accuracy.

Further Reading

Arnold, D. L., Grice, H. C., and Krewski, D. R. (1990). *Handbook of in Vivo Toxicity Testing*. Academic Press, San Diego.

Gad, S. C., and Chengelis, C. P. (Eds.) (1992). *Animal Models in Toxicology*. Dekker, New York.

—*Shayne C. Gad*

Related Topics

Analytical Toxicology
Animal Models

Host-Mediated Assay
In Vitro Test
Mixtures
Mouse Lymphoma Assay
Toxicity Testing, Alternatives
Toxicity Testing, Aquatic
Toxicity Testing, Behavioral
Toxicity Testing, Carcinogenesis
Toxicity Testing, Dermal
Toxicity Testing, Developmental
Toxicity Testing, Inhalation
Toxicity Testing, Reproductive

Iodine

- CAS: 7553-56-2
- SYNONYMS: Iode; iodine crystals; iodine sublimed; ELEMENTAL IODINE; iodio
- CHEMICAL CLASS: Halogen
- CHEMICAL STRUCTURE: I-I

Uses

Iodine is used as an antihyperthyroid and a topical antiinfective. It is an ingredient in antiseptics and other medicinal preparations and in germicides. The latter use includes udder washes used on cattle in dairy operations; thus iodine is found in cow's milk. Other uses include disinfectants that may be added to swimming pools or drinking water. It is also used as a chemical reagent. Iodine is found naturally in seaweed and is considered a generally recognized as safe substance by the U.S. FDA. Iodine is a required element by many species, including humans. It has been recognized as preventative against goiter since 1819 and is used in iodized salt for this purpose. Iodine is also used as a dough oxidizer in commercial bread making.

Exposure Pathways

Exposure may occur via inhalation, ingestion, or dermal or ocular contact.

Toxicokinetics

Iodine is absorbed rapidly and completely as I^- from the gastrointestinal tract. It is also absorbed when applied to the skin. Surgical scrubs containing iodine compounds were found to increase the level of urinary iodine in medical personnel. Iodine compounds are efficiently trapped and concentrated in the thyroid gland. Excretion is primarily via urine, although some iodine is excreted in feces and sweat. There is some salivary recycling. The half-life of iodine in blood is 6–10 hr. Prolonged administration of large doses of iodine markedly reduces thyroidal iodine uptake.

Mechanism of Toxicity

Iodine has a direct action on cells by precipitating proteins. The affected cells may be destroyed. In addition to the primary irritant action of iodine, this compound can act as a potent sensitizer.

Human Toxicity

Ingestion of large quantities of iodine may cause burning of the mouth, throat, and stomach and abdominal pain, nausea, vomiting, and diarrhea. Sufficient exposure may result in progression of symptoms to fever, shock, delirium, and death. Ingestion of 2–4 g has been fatal. The solid element is intensely irritating to eyes, skin, and mucous membranes. Iodine vapor is more irritating than vapors of chlorine or bromine. Occupational reports indicate that concentrations of 0.1 ppm are tolerable, but concentrations of 0.15 or 0.2 ppm are less tolerable. Concentrations of 1 ppm are highly irritating. Vapor concentrations of 0.57 ppm were tolerated for 5 min without eye irritation; but 1.63 ppm caused irritation within 2 min. Symptoms of inhalation exposure include tightness in the chest, sore throat, and headache. High exposures may result in airway constriction, shortness of breath, difficulty in breathing, pulmonary edema (onset may be delayed several hours), and death. Skin contact may result in corrosive tissue destruction at the site of contact. Individual susceptibility to skin reactions varies widely. Application of tincture of iodine to one-third of the body surface was reported as fatal in one case. Iodine solutions are recognized sensitizing agents. The OSHA permissible exposure ceiling level for iodine in the air is 0.1 ppm. Excessive ingestion in humans can result in iodide goiter resulting from inhibition of the thyroid gland. The resulting lack of thyroid hormone secretion causes compensatory increase in thyrotropin secretion and thyroid enlargement. The human oral toxic dose has been estimated at 1000 times the U.S. Recommended Daily Allowance of 100–200 μg/day.

Clinical Management

Rescue workers should avoid direct contact with the chemical. The source of contamination should be removed or the victim should be moved to fresh air. Oxygen may be administered by a trained professional. A conscious victim who has ingested excess iodine should rinse his or her mouth out with water; however, vomiting should not be induced. The victim should drink 8–10 oz of water. If vomiting occurs, the victim should lean forward to reduce the risk of aspiration. If contact with the eyes occurs, the eyes should be immediately flushed with lukewarm, gently flowing water for at least 15 min, taking care not to rinse contaminated water into the eye. General supportive measures should be provided.

Animal Toxicity

Application of a 2% solution of iodine in alcohol to rabbit eyes caused reversible damage. Stronger solutions of 7% caused severe damage to rabbit and monkey eyes. Dogs exposed by injection in the trachea to vapors of iodine demonstrated inflammation of the lungs, breathing problems, and coughing which persisted for weeks. The lowest doses causing effects were 7–12 mg/kg. Doses of 14–18 mg/kg caused pulmonary edema and death within 24 hr. In guinea pigs, 0.5 ppm did not cause detectable effects, but 7 ppm caused impaired breathing capacity. Adult female rats fed 500, 1000, 1500, or 2000 ppm iodine (as potassium iodide; KI) from 0 to 35 days prior to giving birth exhibited increased neonatal mortality with increasing dose, and milk secretion was reduced as evidenced by examination of the mammary glands. Reproductive impairment was also noted in studies with rabbits and chickens. Rabbits fed 250 ppm iodine for 2–5 days in late gestation exhibited increased mortality of young, and hens fed 312–5000 ppm KI ceased egg production within 1 week. Clinical signs of excessive dietary iodide in cattle include lacrimation, nasal discharge, conjunctivitis, hair loss, dermatitis, and exopthalmia. The oral LD_{50} for mice is 2 g/kg. The oral LD_{50} for dogs is 200–500 mg/kg.

—Mary Lee Hultin

Related Topics

Generally Recognized as Safe
Sensitivity Analysis

Iron (Fe)

- CAS: 7439-89-6
- Selected Compounds: Ferrous sulfate, $FeSO_4$ (CAS: 7720-78-7); iron oxide, Fe_2O_3 (CAS: 1309-37-1)
- Chemical Class: Metals

Uses

Iron is one of the major essential elements and one of the most important commercial metals. The total number of products made from iron is greater than that of all other metals combined. Iron is the basis for various steels and is used in pigments, fuel additives, catalysts, magnetic tapes, and animal feeds. As an essential element, iron is the central atom in the heme of hemoglobin. Medicinally, it is administered to anemic patients and to many premenopausal women.

Exposure Pathways

The primary exposure pathway for iron is ingestion. Iron is present in practically all foods, in dietary supplements, and in drinking water. In some drinking water, iron concentrations may be especially high as iron pipes have been used extensively in transporting potable water. In industrial settings, inhalation is a significant exposure pathway (e.g., arc welders are exposed to a high atmosphere of metal fumes and particles). Dermal contact is not a significant exposure pathway.

Toxicokinetics

Iron is absorbed (in a complicated process) through the gastrointestinal tract as the ferrous ion, first into the mucosal cells, where it oxidizes into the ferric state, and then is carried by the plasma. It is bound to the iron protein, transferrin (a 1-globulin), which transfers the iron to the various tissues. The enzyme ferroxidase oxidizes the ferrous iron to the ferric state. Most absorbed iron is found bound to hemoglobin (66%), a small amount is found in the protein myoglobin, and a minute amount in the iron-dependent enzymes.

Iron is stored in the blood, liver, bone marrow, and spleen. The storage proteins for iron are ferritin and hemosiderin. With "iron overload" more ferritin is synthesized in the liver to bind this excess iron. Iron is a cofactor for hemoglobin and cytochromes.

The homeostasis mechanism permits up to 15% of ingested iron to be absorbed while the average person only excretes 0.01% of the intake. During periods of increased demand, such as pregnancy or childhood, absorption of iron is greatly increased. Normally excess iron is excreted and some is contained within shed intestinal cells and in bile and urine. Smaller amounts are excreted in sweat, nails, and hair. Approximately 0.5 mg/day total iron is excreted.

Mechanism of Toxicity

In some adults, iron overload can be the result of a genetic defect (idiopathic hemochromatosis) that causes malfunction of the normal homeostasis mechanism and, in turn, excessive absorption of iron. Iron overload can also be caused by too many blood transfusions, which results in too much iron in the various iron-containing organs.

Recently, it has been suggested that the presence of increased transferrin concentrations in males and excess heart attacks are associated. This must be corroborated by further research.

Excess iron can lead to diabetes mellitus, faulty liver functions, and endocrine disturbance. Iron is a catalyst for oxidative damage leading to lipid peroxidation. The latest hypotheses link peroxidation to heart disease, cancer, and accelerated aging. Iron is involved in the Fenton Reaction, which catalyzes the formation of free radicals which cause excessive damage to cells and their components.

Human Toxicity

Most iron toxicity is found in very young children who ingest iron-containing medicines with candy-like coatings. Fatalities have occurred from childhood ingestion of iron. After eating more than 0.5 g of iron, toxic symptoms can be delayed for up to 6 hr. The gastrointestinal tract can be ulcerated, which alters the limiting mechanism of iron absorption. Besides nausea, bloody vomiting (due to ulceration of the gastrointestinal tract), and black stools, acidosis and some liver damage follows; this can, in some cases, lead to cirrhosis of the liver, liver failure, or renal failure. Excess free-circulating iron damages blood vessels and hypotension can occur.

In the industrial setting, iron and its oxides can be inhaled, leaving iron deposits in the lungs. On X-rays, these deposits appear similar to silicosis. An increase in lung cancer, as well as tuberculosis and interstitial fibrosis, has been noted in hematite miners. Due to inadequate controls, it is possible that the increased incidence of lung diseases noted in the study is due to smoking or exposure to other carcinogens present in the occupational setting.

The ACGIH TLV-TWA for iron oxide dust and fume is 5 mg/m^3.

Clinical Management

Acute iron poisoning is treated by removal of ingested iron from the gastrointestinal tract using emesis (vomiting) or gastric lavage and by providing therapy for the associated systemic effects of shock and acidosis. The chelation agent, deferrioxamine, is also administered to bind iron that was not successfully removed from the gastrointestinal tract and has been absorbed.

Excess iron can be removed by either phlebotomy (letting of blood from a vein) or administration of the chelating agent, deferrioxamine, for cases of chronic excess iron. Ascorbic acid can accelerate iron excretion by about twofold.

Animal Toxicity

Iron does not seem to be mutagenic or teratogenic. In a few animal experiments, sarcomas have appeared at the site following the injection of a large dose of the dextran salt or the lactate or gluconate. However, these experimental findings of tumor formation are open to question and may be associated with "solid-state carcinogenesis" (believed to be a result of an irritation-type effect at the site of injection as opposed to a genetic mechanism).

—*Arthur Furst, Shirley B. Radding, and Kathryn A. Wurzel*

Related Topics

Blood
Metals
Poisoning Emergencies in Humans
(Deferoxomine)

Isocyanates

- Representative Compounds: Toluene-2,4-diisocyanate (TDI); methyl-isocyanate (MIC); methylene bisphenyl isocyanate (MDI); hexamethylene diisocyanate (HDI)

Uses

Isocyanates are used in polyurethane "foamed-in-place" plastics, in adhesives, and as intermediates in carbamate insecticides and herbicides.

Exposure Pathways

Inhalation, ingestion, and dermal contact are all possible routes of exposure.

Mechanism of Toxicity

Isocyanates are powerful irritants to the eyes, skin, mucous membranes, and gastrointestinal tract. They are also potent dermal and pulmonary sensitizers.

Human Toxicity

Methylene bisphenyl isocyanate was the primary lethal agent in the Bhopal accident (India; December 3, 1984), where more than 3000 people died due to pulmonary edema. More than 20,000 additional exposed individuals were seriously injured, and from 150,000 to 200,000 total were affected to some extent.

Isocyanates are severe skin and eye irritants and dermal and inhalation sensitizers. Exposure may cause pulmonary edema and corneal ulceration. With toluene-2,4-diisocyanate, mucosal irritation begins to appear at exposure concentrations between 0.05 and 0.1 ppm. Occupational asthma with reduced pulmonary function results from repeated exposures.

Clinical Management

For ocular and dermal contamination, the skin and eyes should be copiously irrigated with saline. Otherwise, treatment is symptomatic.

Animal Toxicity

IARC and the National Toxicity Program list toluene-2,4-diisocyanate as a carcinogen.

—*Shayne C. Gad*

Related Topics

Carbamate Pesticides
Sensitivity Analysis

Isoniazid

- CAS: 54-85-3
- Synonym: Isonicotinic acid hydrazide
- Pharmaceutical Class: A molecule of the pyridine class
- Chemical Structure:

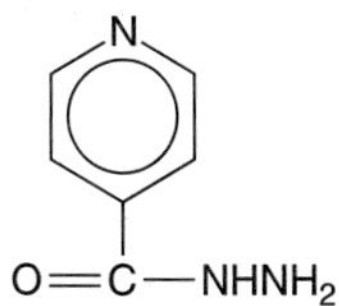

Uses

Isoniazid is used as an antituberculous antibiotic.

Exposure Pathways

Isoniazid is available only in an oral form.

Toxicokinetics

Isoniazid is rapidly absorbed from the gastrointestinal tract with peak serum concentrations attained within 1 or 2 hr of ingestion. When administered concomitantly with food or antacids, the extent of absorption and the time to peak may be reduced. Isoniazid has a volume of distribution of 0.6 liters/kg with less than 50% binding to plasma proteins. Metabolism occurs in the liver, primarily by acetylation. Metabolism follows Michaelis–Menten kinetics. Also, genetic polymorphism is responsible for phenotypic "slow" and "fast" acetylators. Fast acetylators metabolize isoniazid five or six times faster than slow acetylators; serum isoniazid concentrations are 30–50% lower in fast acetylators. The serum half-life of isoniazid is a mean 3 hr in slow acetylators and 70 min in fast acetylators. The major metabolites, acetylisoniazid, isonicotinic acid, and hydrazine, are inactive. Isoniazid and its metabolites are eliminated in the urine with 27% of unchanged drug being excreted in slow acetylators and 11% in fast acetylators.

Mechanism of Toxicity

Isoniazid has three general mechanisms of toxicity: It inhibits several enzymes, it binds pyridoxal phosphate, and it competes for nicotinic acid in the synthesis of nicotinamide adenine nucleotide (NAD).

Isoniazid is an inhibitor of several enzymes including the cytochrome P450 mixed function oxidases as well as momoamine oxidase, glutamate decarboxylase, γ-aminobutyric acid (GABA) aminotransferase, histaminase, and pyridoxine phosphokinase. The consequence of these extensive enzymatic disturbances are impaired metabolism of other drugs, mood elevation, decreased central nervous system GABA levels, and depressed catecholamine synthesis. When isoniazid binds pyridoxal phosphate, it renders it inactive. When isoniazid competes for nicotinic acid in the synthesis of NAD, the resultant NAD inhibition produces defects in glucose and fatty acid oxidation. The most important of these clinical effects is the production of pyridoxine depletion.

Human Toxicity: Acute

Acute ingestions of more than 1.5 g may produce mild symptoms of malaise, nausea, vomiting, dizziness, and tachycardia. Ingestions of more than 2–5 g produce moderate toxicity, and ingestions of >6 g are typically fatal unless there is aggressive intervention. Isoniazid intoxication is associated with a distinct clinical syndrome characterized by the appearance of recurrent seizures, coma, and metabolic acidosis. Canine studies suggest that metabolic acidosis is the direct result of seizures although other metabolic disturbances, including abnormal fatty acid metabolism, may contribute. Seizures generally occur at regular intervals. Coma may be prolonged.

Human Toxicity: Chronic

Because of its effects on enzyme activity, isoniazid is associated with many adverse effects. The most common of these are rash, fever, and abnormal liver function tests (in up to 20% of patients). Chronic use may lead to the development of autoantibody production with resulting hemolytic anemia, thrombocytopenia, arthritis, or vasculitis. Neurologic symptoms may also occur, consisting of optic neuritis or peripheral neuropathy in a stocking-glove distribution. Seizures may occur in the absence of an overdose. Important drug interactions include those with phenytoin (with resulting phenytoin toxicity), carbamazepine, and rifampin.

Clinical Management

In the patient who presents with convulsions, airway protection and seizure control are primary goals. The preferred anticonvulsant is a benzodiazepine. Disturbances in cardiac rhythm or function also require immediate attention. Gastrointestinal decontamination should consist of orogastric lavage followed by the administration of activated charcoal. Induced emesis with ipecac is contraindicated due to the risk of seizures with resulting aspiration. Administration of pyridoxine provides immediate relief from all symptoms of severe isoniazid toxicity, including seizures. Pyridoxine is given intravenously in a dose that equals the estimated isoniazid dose. If the quantity of isoniazid taken is unknown, 5 g of pyridoxine is given. Repeat doses may be necessary should severe toxicity recur or coma linger.

Animal Toxicity

When taken or administered in overdose to dogs, isoniazid produces seizures, metabolic acidosis, and, if untreated, death.

—Michael Shannon

Related Topics

Liver
Modifying Factors of Toxicity

Isoprene

- CAS: 78-79-5
- Synonyms: 2-Methyl-1,3-butadiene; 2-methylbutadiene; β-methylbivinyl; isopentadiene

- CHEMICAL CLASS: Reactive branched diene
- MOLECULAR FORMULA: C_5H_8

Uses

The isoprene unit is the most important building block for lipids, steroids, terpenoids, and a wide variety of natural products. The only chemical reaction of commercial importance (other than polymerization) is its conversion to terpenes. Isoprene is used in the manufacture of "synthetic" natural rubber, butyl rubber, and as a copolymer in the production of synthetic elastomers.

Exposure Pathways

Inhalation, ingestion, and dermal exposure are exposure pathways for isoprene.

Toxicokinetics

Hemoglobin adduct formation is linearly related to administered doses of isoprene up to approximately 55 μmols per kilogram. Mice exhaled approximately twice as much butadiene as isoprene following exposure to isoprene. The percentage of inhaled isoprene metabolized decreased with increasing exposure concentrations and vapor concentration. Approximately 75% of the total metabolites are excreted in the urine, independent of the inhaled concentration. A higher percentage of metabolites are excreted in the feces following high-concentration exposures.

Saturation kinetics are observed in rats and mice. The half-life in rats and mice is 6.8 and 4.4 min, respectively, following inhalation exposure. The presence of isoprene products in the respiratory epithelium even after short exposure durations suggests that significant metabolism occurs in this tissue.

Isoprene is metabolized to epoxides and diepoxides. Body fat appears to be reservoir for isoprene and its metabolites.

Mechanism of Toxicity

A mutagenic metabolite, isoprene dioxide, was tentatively identified in all examined tissues following exposure to isoprene. It is believed that the formation of reactive epoxides following exposure to isoprene results in tumor induction.

Human Toxicity

Acute contact with isoprene may irritate or burn the eyes and skin. Upper respiratory tract irritation is associated with exposure via inhalation. Central nervous system (CNS) depression is possible with exposure to high concentrations. A potential adverse hematological response has also been indicated.

There is inadequate evidence of carcinogenicity in humans.

Clinical Management

There is no information available specifically for isoprene. Exposed skin and eyes should be flushed with copious quantities of water following exposure. Humidified oxygen should be administered after excess inhalation exposure. Induced emesis should be avoided if ingestion has occurred. Measures to decrease gastrointestinal absorption should be instituted (gastric lavage, activated charcoal, or dilution by administration of liquids).

Animal Toxicity

A 2% isoprene air concentration did not cause CNS depression in mice exposed for a 2-hr period. Concentrations of 3.5–4.5% caused deep CNS depression and death occurred at 5% exposure concentrations.

Isoprene is nonmutagenic in bacterial test systems. However, isoprene forms adducts of blood hemoglobin in mice and rats. Increases in frequency of sister chromatid exchanges in bone marrow cells and in levels of micronucleated polychromatic erythrocytes were detected. Based on these results, isoprene is expected to induce tumors at multiple sites in exposed mice.

Mice exposed to 7000 ppm isoprene via inhalation showed decreased weight gain, testicular atrophy in males, and microscopic lesions. In addition, there is sufficient evidence of the carcinogenicity of isoprene in animals.

—Kathryn A. Wurzel

Isopropanol

- CAS: 67-63-0
- PREFERRED NAME: Isopropyl alcohol

- SYNONYMS: 2-Propanol; *sec*-propyl alcohol; dimethyl carbinol
- CHEMICAL CLASS: Alcohol
- MOLECULAR FORMULA: C_3H_8O
- CHEMICAL STRUCTURE: CH_3–CHOH–CH_3

Uses

Isopropanol is used as a solvent in numerous industrial and commercial products. It is used as a solvent for synthetic resins, coatings, and lacquers. It is also used in drug and cosmetic formulations, including rubbing compounds, perfumes, and colognes. It is also found in consumer products such as windshield cleaning fluids and glass cleaners.

Exposure Pathways

The principal routes of exposure for isopropanol are inhalation and ingestion.

Toxicokinetics

Isopropanol is rapidly absorbed and distributed throughout the body after inhalation or ingestion. Intestinal uptake of isopropanol is rapid; approximately 80% of an oral dose is absorbed in 30 min. Complete absorption and tissue distribution occurs within approximately 2 hr. Skin absorption is relatively low. Animal studies indicate that isopropanol passes the blood–brain barrier twice as effectively as ethanol.

Isopropanol is excreted either unchanged or as its oxidized metabolite, acetone. The kidney excretes 20–50% of an absorbed dose unchanged, with the lung or kidney more slowly eliminating the acetone metabolite. Biological half-lives for isopropanol and acetone in humans are 2.5–6.4 and 22 hr, respectively.

Mechanism of Toxicity

Isopropanol is a potent central nervous system (CNS) depressant. It is approximately twice as potent in this regard as ethanol and is believed to exert this effect via a similar mechanism probably involving interference with ion transport at the cell membrane. The metabolite, acetone, may potentiate and lengthen the duration of CNS symptoms observed upon isopropanol exposure.

Human Toxicity

Given its widespread use, isopropanol has resulted in relatively few reports of adverse effects in humans. In cases of poisoning or intentional ingestion, the major signs of isopropanol toxicity are those of alcoholic intoxication including nausea, vomiting, abdominal pain, hypertension, and hypothermia. In extreme cases, isopropanol depression of the CNS can produce unconsciousness, leading to coma and death due to respiratory depression. Skin absorption of isopropanol in toxic amounts has not been routinely reported, but one case involving a child intoxicated after being sponged with isopropanol suggests that dermal absorption should not be underestimated, particularly in children.

Exposure to approximately 400 ppm isopropanol vapors for 3–5 min can cause mild irritation of the eyes, nose, and throat. The lethal dose upon ingestion in an adult is roughly 240 ml.

Clinical Management

Individuals overexposed to isopropanol should be removed from exposure, affected areas of the skin should be washed with soap and water, and the eyes should be irrigated with water. Upon ingestion of large amounts of isopropanol, gastric lavage, fluids and symptomatic therapy of CNS effects should be administered. Severe isopropanol overdoses have been managed successfully with both peritoneal dialysis and hemodialysis.

Animal Toxicity

The acute toxicity of isopropanol is low for animals based on LD_{50} values for oral, dermal, and inhalation exposure. LD_{50} values obtained from rats, mice, and rabbits ranged from 4.5 g/kg (in mice) to approximately 8 g/kg (rabbits). The acute dermal LD_{50} in rabbits has been reported to be 12.9 g/kg. The 8-hr LD_{50}s for rats ranged from 16,000 to 22,000 ppm. These levels produced severe irritation of mucous membranes, CNS depression, and death caused by respiratory or cardiac arrest.

Repeated or prolonged exposure to isopropanol has generally produced negative results in animal studies with respect to systemic effects and/or developmental toxicity. Rats and mice exposed to 5000 ppm isopropanol for 13 weeks did exhibit an increase in body weight and increase in relative liver weights, as well as increased hyaline droplet formation within the kidneys of male rats. In contrast, changes were not observed in neurobehavioral functions of rats exposed to 5000 ppm isopropanol for 13 weeks, although females did exhibit an increase in motor activity.

The developmental toxicity of isopropanol has been studied in rats and rabbits at doses of up to 1200 mg per day during Gestational Days 6–15 in rats, and up to 480 mg/kg/day during Gestational Days 16–18 in rabbits. No teratogenic effects were observed in the offspring from these studies. The NOAELs for both maternal and developmental toxicity from these studies were 400 mg/kg/day in rats and 240 (maternal toxicity) and 480 mg/kg/day (developmental toxicity) in rabbits.

The reproductive toxicity of isopropanol was studied in rats in a two-generation study at exposures of 100, 500, and 1000 mg/kg. Reproductive toxicity was not observed except in the high-dose P2 males which exhibited a reduction in male mating index. In a three-generation study of rats exposed to 2.5% isopropanol in drinking water, no reproductive toxicity was observed. A similar two-generation study in rats did report reductions in parental body weight gains, fertility, litter size, and reduction in pup weights at Days 3 and 21 postpartum in animals exposed to isopropanol at 3% in drinking water. Two-percent isopropanol in drinking water did not elicit this effect.

—*Bradford Strohm*

Related Topics

Modifying Factors of Toxicity
Neurotoxicology: Central and Peripheral

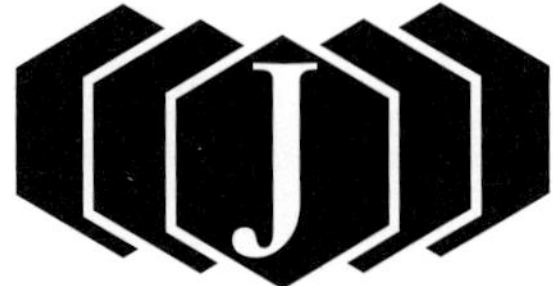

Jequirity Bean

- Synonyms: *Abrus precatorius;* deadly crab's eye; indian bean; love bean; lucky bean; mienie mienie; prayer bean; rosary bean; Seminole bead
- Chemical Class: Toxalbumins

Uses

There are no known therapeutic uses for jequirity bean.

Exposure Pathways

Ingestion of the bean is the most common route of exposure.

Toxicokinetics

The mature bean is innocuous if the hard outer coat is intact. Any interruption in the integrity of the seed coat (e.g., chewing) or ingestion of the soft-coated immature bean may cause toxicity. The inner core contains the amino acid *n*-methyltryptophan, abric acid, glycyrrhizin, and abrin. The absorption is erratic. In rats, distribution sites occur primarily in the liver (12%) and spleen. Biotransformation and elimination of toxalbumins are poorly defined.

Mechanism of Toxicity

Abrin is responsible for the toxic effects of the bean by causing inhibition of protein synthesis. The clinical effects include an initial aggregation of red blood cells within the first hour, adrenal insufficiency, hepatic and adrenal failure, endothelial damage, and in severe cases profound capillary hemorrhage. It has been determined that abrin does not inhibit mitochondrial respiration *in vitro,* but it does interfere with amino acid incorporation in the liver of rats.

Human Toxicity

Clinical effects include severe gastroenteritis accompanied by serosal hemorrhage, swelling, inflammation of Peyer's patches, and retroperitoneal lymph nodes. Hepatic and renal necrosis have been reported. Retinal hemorrhages may appear. Abrin combines with the cell stroma and agglutinates red blood cells leading to thrombus and embolus formation. Symptoms may begin after a delay of up to several days and may persist for as long as 10 or 11 days.

Clinical Management

Supportive measures, including administration of blood products, parenteral fluid, and electrolytes, are recommended. Removal of the seeds from the gastrointestinal tract with whole bowel irrigation is preferred to emesis and gastric lavage due to the necrotizing action of the abrin. Alkalinization of the urine with sodium bicarbonate has been recommended for the prevention of hemoglobin precipitates in the renal tubules.

Animal Toxicity

Acute manifestations of jequirity bean toxicity in animals are similar to those found in humans.

—Brenda Swanson Biearman

Jimsonweed

- CAS: 8063-18-1
- SYNONYMS: *Datura* species; *Datura arborea; Datura cornigera; Datura suaveolens;* angel's trumpet; downy thorn apple; horn-of-plenty; stinkweed; thornapple
- PHARMACEUTICAL CLASS: Anticholinergic

Uses

Datura species are abused for psychedelic properties. They do not have a therapeutic use.

Exposure Pathways

Exposure occurs via ingestion of the seeds or tea made from the seeds.

Toxicokinetics

Decreased gastrointestinal motility may delay absorption.

Mechanism of Toxicity

The anticholinergic effects of Jimsonweed are due to the antagonism of acetylcholine at the neuroreceptor site with cardiac muscle, exocrine glands, brain, and smooth muscle.

Human Toxicity

Common symptoms of exposure include mydriasis, sinus tachycardia, hypertension or hypotension, anxiety, hallucinations, seizures, dry mouth, flushed skin, decreased gastrointestinal motility, urinary retention, and hyperpyrexia. Anticholinergic agents may be detected in the urine, but this does not direct clinical management. Due to multiple plant variations, the alkaloid content differs greatly.

Clinical Management

Gastric decontamination with activated charcoal up to 24 hr after ingestion may be useful. Supportive care is the cornerstone of therapy. Physostigmine may be used in the presence of severe incapacitating or life-threatening anticholinergic effects that are unresponsive to conventional therapies. Propanolol may be considered for the treatment of tachyarrhythmias.

Animal Toxicity

In farm animals, muscle tremors, ataxia, drowsiness, tachypnea, and sudden death have been reported.

—*Brenda Swanson-Biearman*

Related Topic

Poisoning Emergencies in Humans

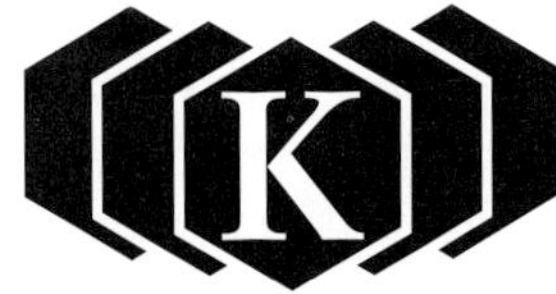

Kerosene

- CAS: 8008-20-6
- Synonyms: Straight-run kerosene (petroleum); kerosine; range oil; fuel oil No. 1; Deobase
- Chemical Class: Petroleum hydrocarbons
- Description: Kerosene, a refined petroleum product, is a complex combination of aliphatic, naphthenic, and alkyl aromatic hydrocarbons produced by the fractional distillation of crude oil between approximately 150°C (302°F) and 300°C (572°F). It consists of hydrocarbons having carbon numbers predominantly in the range of C9 through C16 and boiling in the range as listed for its fractional distillation from crude oil. The chemical composition depends on the nature of the crude oil from which the kerosene is derived.

Uses

Kerosene, originally used for lighting and heating, is also used as a diesel fuel, as a component in blending aviation fuels, as a solvent and carrier for a wide range of products (including cleaning compositions and pesticides), as a weed killer, and a as mold-release agent in the ceramic and pottery industry.

Exposure Pathways

Kerosene may enter the water or soil environment as a result of regular use (e.g., evaporation of pesticide solvent), from spills during use or transportation, or from leaking storage facilities. The relatively low vapor pressure of kerosene makes inhalation exposure unlikely under ordinary occupational conditions unless conditions of poor ventilation exist. The combustion product of burned kerosene, carbon monoxide, is of real concern when kerosene heaters are not vented. Exposure to kerosene mist can occur as kerosene is often applied in the form of a spray. Eye and skin contact with kerosene and kerosene mists and vapors can occur. The exposure pathway usually of most concern is ingestion because this is the most common means of acute poisoning, especially in children.

Toxicokinetics

None or little quantitative data were available concerning the absorption, distribution, metabolism, and excretion of kerosene. Indirect evidence suggests that kerosene may be absorbed through the respiratory tract, the gastrointestinal tract, and percutaneously.

Mechanism of Toxicity

The specific mechanism of kerosene toxicity has not been completely determined. The primary risk from ingestion of kerosene is aspiration during emesis, which may cause pneumonitis. The biochemical mechanism of the lung response to large concentrations of aerosolized kerosene (resulting in bronchoconstriction and asthma-like symptoms) may involve the parasympathetic nervous system via a direct effect on the vagus nerve or by inhibition of acetylcholinesterase. The mechanism(s) of central nervous system (CNS) depression from kerosene exposure has not been elucidated.

Human Toxicity

Kerosene is of low-order toxicity following oral, dermal, or inhalation exposure. Symptoms from exposure to high levels of kerosene may include hypoactivity, ataxia, and prostration, consistent with CNS depression, including coma and death. Pneumonia (chemical pneumonitis) is the major lethal complication after ingestion of kerosene due to aspiration into the lungs after vomiting or emesis. Tachycardia, nausea, abdominal cramps, and diarrhea have also been associated with the ingestion of kerosene. Skin irritation, which can be severe, can occur especially after prolonged or repeated exposure. Respiratory tract irritation may occur after inhalation of mists or aerosols. Slight eye irritation may occur if exposure is prolonged. Kerosene was not identified as a skin sensitizer in experimental animals. Prolonged or repeated contact of the skin with kerosene may result in drying of the skin and dermatitis, which may lead to severe skin damage with degenerative changes. Repeated inhalation of kerosene vapors may cause symptoms consistent with CNS depression such as headache and vertigo. Other symptoms reported in experimental animals and/or humans after repeated exposure to kerosene include neuralgia, loss of memory, blood changes, kidney effects, and respiratory disturbances. Kerosene has been reported to have weak cancer-promoting activity but no cancer-initiating activity. Repeated applications of kerosene to the skin of laboratory animals caused moderate to severe skin irritation with an increase in skin tumors after long latency periods. The increase in skin tumors was considered to be the result of the severe skin damage. This explanation is consistent with the general lack of activity of kerosenes in genotoxicity assays.

Clinical Management

Asymptomatic individuals should be observed for 4–6 hr after exposure for the development of symptoms. Respiratory and cardiovascular function should be supported in symptomatic individuals. If there is suspicion of aspiration, breathing should be observed and the patient treated symptomatically.

If kerosene has been ingested, nothing should be administered by mouth and vomiting should not be induced. Gastric decontamination is not usually indicated after ingestion due to the possibility of aspiration. If necessary, gastric lavage must only be performed after cuffed endotracheal intubation. Treatment should be symptomatic. Antibiotic and corticosteroid therapy may be considered for treatment of possible chemical pneumonitis resulting from aspiration. If aspiration is expected to have occurred (i.e., a coughing symptomatic individual), arterial blood should be monitored to ensure adequate ventilation. The development of pulmonary edema may be delayed in onset up to 24–72 hr after exposure.

For skin contact, affected areas should be washed thoroughly with soap and water. For eye contact, the eyes should be gently flushed with copious amounts of water for at least 10 min.

Animal Toxicity

The acute toxicities (LD_{50}/LC_{50}) for kerosene are >5 g/kg (oral; rats), >2 g/kg (dermal; rabbit), and >5 mg/liter/4 hr (inhalation; rats). Skin exposure for more than 4 hr resulted in mild to severe irritation in rabbits and other experimental animals. Prolonged eye exposure caused mild irritation in rabbits. Skin sensitization did not occur after treatment of guinea pigs with kerosene. Chronic dermal applications of kerosene caused skin carcinoma in mice.

—Gary P. Bond

Related Topics

Petroleum Hydrocarbons
Pollution, Water

Kidney

Introduction

The kidney is an organ which performs several important functions to help sustain life. Among these functions are the regulation of volume and electrolyte homeostasis, control of acid-base balance, and the excretion of waste products. The kidney also has endocrine functions including renin secretion, stimulation of erythropoietin formation, and activation of vitamin D. Numerous disease states (e.g., infections, diabetes, and gout) can affect the ability of the kidney to perform its normal functions, and if these diseases are not properly treated, serious illness or death can result.

The kidney is also a major target organ for the toxic effects induced by a wide range of chemical and physical agents. Renal toxicity or nephrotoxicity can be the result of a direct toxic effect of an agent on renal tissue (e.g., mercuric salts and cephalosporins) or a secondary event following toxicity or tissue damage at a site other than the kidney (e.g., carbon monoxide poisoning and crush injury). In addition, the nephron, the functional unit of the kidney, is composed of several distinct anatomical segments. Some compounds or their metabolites induce toxicity to only one segment of the nephron and are considered to be site-selective nephrotoxicants, while other agents may induce widespread renal damage and are considered to be non-site-selective toxicants.

An understanding of how and why chemicals induce nephrotoxicity requires some familiarity with the anatomy and physiology of the kidney. In addition, interpretation of renal toxicology studies will require a working knowledge of the various techniques used for evaluating renal function. It is also important to be aware of which nephrotoxicants require biotransformation before they induce nephrotoxicity, nephrotoxic mechanisms when known, and the site(s) of renal damage for the various nephrotoxicants.

Renal Anatomy and Physiology

In mammalian species, the two kidneys carry out the normal physiological and endocrine functions described previously. The kidney receives blood via the renal artery, and blood leaves the kidney by way of the renal vein. In adult humans, the rate of blood flow through both kidneys is about 1.2 liters/min or about 20% of the cardiac output for a 70-kg individual. Urine formed within the kidneys is transported from the kidneys through the ureters to the bladder, a reservoir for the urine until it is excreted.

Each kidney is subdivided anatomically into three zones: (1) an outer zone called the cortex, (2) an intermediate zone called the medulla, and (3) an innermost zone called the pelvis. The cortex and medulla have important characteristics which help facilitate the formation of urine and control the composition of waste products, electrolytes, and water.

Each kidney also contains over 1 million nephrons which are the functional units of the kidney. Nephrons originate in the cortex where an afferent arteriole forms a specialized capillary bed known as the glomerulus (Fig. K-1). Some nephrons originate near the surface of the kidney and are called superficial nephrons, while other nephrons originate near the cortical–medullary region and are called juxtamedullary nephrons.

The glomerulus, which forms within Bowman's capsule, is a special capillary bed with large pores, and substances which are not bound to plasma proteins and have molecular weights less than albumin (~69,000) can be filtered at the glomerulus and enter Bowman's capsule. This glomerular filtrate is essentially protein-free plasma, although a small amount of low-molecular-weight protein is also filtered by the glomerulus. The rate at which the glomerular filtrate is formed, the glomerular filtration rate (GFR), is about 125 ml/min in humans and serves as an important measure of renal function.

The glomerular filtrate flows from Bowman's capsule into the proximal tubule. The proximal tubule can be subdivided into three segments (S_1–S_3). The S_1 segment is closest to the glomerulus and is localized in the cortex, while the S_3 segment is furthest from the glomerulus and is found in both the cortex and the outer portion of the medulla. The S_1 and S_2 segments comprise the pars convoluta, while the latter portion of the S_2 segment and the S_3 segment comprise the pars recta or straight portion.

The proximal tubular cells contain numerous finger-like projections on the luminal surface which markedly increase the luminal surface area of the cells and help promote reabsorption of substances filtered at the glomerulus. Under normal conditions, approximately 65–70% of filtered sodium, chloride, calcium, and water; 80–90% of filtered bicarbonate, phosphate, and urate; and essentially all of the filtered amino acids, glucose, and low-molecular-weight proteins are reabsorbed from the glomerular filtrate as the filtrate passes the length of the proximal tubule. Reabsorption occurs without a major change in the osmolality of the filtrate such that the fluid leaving the S_3 segment of the proximal tubule has essentially the same osmolality as the fluid entering the S_1 segment. However, the quantity of the glomerular filtrate is markedly reduced during its transit through this nephron component.

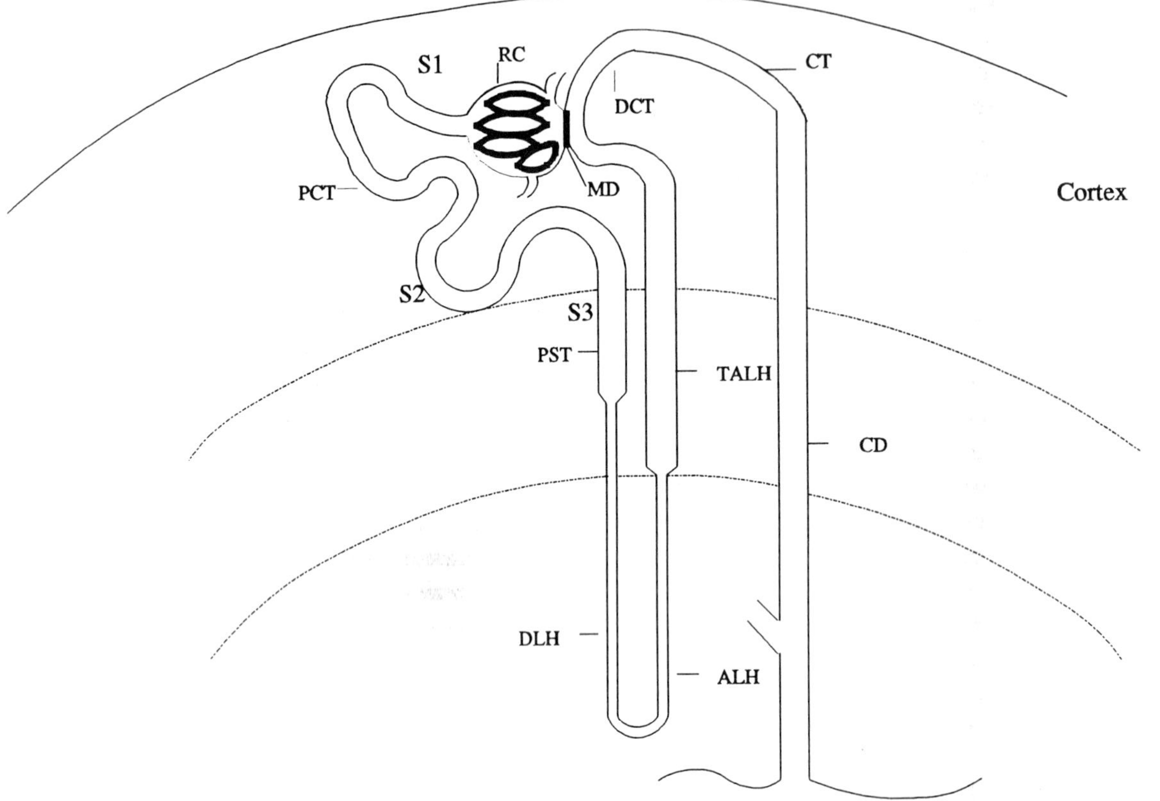

FIGURE K-1. Anatomy of the nephron. RC, renal corpuscle (includes glomerulus and Bowman's capsule); PCT, proximal convoluted tubule; PST, proximal straight tubule; DLH, descending limb of the loop of Henle; ALH, ascending limb of the loop of Henle; TALH, thick ascending limb of the loop of Henle; MD, macula densa; DCT, distal convoluted tubule; CT, connecting tubule; CD, collecting duct.

Proximal tubular cells also contain active transport systems on the basolateral or antiluminal side of the cells which are capable of transporting weakly acidic or weakly basic compounds from the interstitial space into the proximal tubular cells. These transport systems are distinct systems and transport either organic anions (weakly acidic compounds) or organic cations (weakly basic and quaternary ammonium compounds). As a result of transport into proximal tubular cells, weak acids and bases can achieve intracellular concentrations which are hundreds of times higher than the corresponding plasma concentration for the compound. The prototypic organic anion for studying the organic anion transporter is *p*-aminohippurate (PAH), and the prototypic organic cations for examining organic cation transport are *N*-methylnicotinamide and tetraethylammonium (TEA). Accumulated material can then enter luminal fluid via either passive diffusion or facilitated transport.

The location of the organic anion and cation transport systems is not homogeneous along the entire proximal tubule. In the rabbit, PAH transport is greatest in the S_2 segment and lower in the S_1 and S_3 segments. In contrast, organic cation transport is highest in the S_1 segment and lowest in the S_3 segment. In superficial nephrons, the transport of organic cations in the S_2 segment is intermediate between the S_1 and S_3 segments but is about equal to the capacity of S_1 segments in juxtamedullary nephrons. Although the organic anion and cation transporters are clearly localized in the proximal tubules for all mammalian species studied to date, the segmental localization of these transporters has not been studied in great detail in species other than the rabbit. Nevertheless, the ability of many nephrotoxicants to induce nephrotoxicity to proximal tubular segments is dependent on the compound or its metabolites being accumulated in proximal tubular cells via one of these organic transport systems. The function of these systems also serves as a sensitive measure of renal function and is routinely used to monitor renal function in animal models.

Luminal fluid leaving the proximal tubule enters the descending limb of the loop of Henle. This nephron segment passes deeper into the medulla than the proximal tubule, and the high medullary interstitial osmolality causes water to move from the luminal fluid and into the medullary interstitial space. As a result, the luminal fluid becomes more concentrated as it passes through the descending limb. Organic compounds (e.g., sulfonamides and methotrexate) which have poor water solubility can precipitate in this nephron segment, once their water-solubility limit is reached, and block luminal flow and glomerular filtration.

When the luminal fluid reaches the thick ascending limb of the loop of Henle, water no longer can freely move from the luminal fluid into the medullary interstitial space. Instead, this portion of the nephron is impermeable to water reabsorption and actively reabsorbs sodium, chloride, and potassium ions. Approximately 20–25% of filtered sodium and calcium ions are reabsorbed at this location. In addition, most, if not all, of the potassium ions reaching the thick limb of the loop of Henle are reabsorbed as well. Thus, as the luminal fluid passes through the ascending limb, the luminal fluid becomes more dilute.

Although the ascending limb of the loop of Henle begins in the medulla, it ends in the cortex where it joins the distal tubule. Sodium chloride is also reabsorbed in the early segment of the distal tubule, and the combination of this segment with the cortical portion of the thick ascending limb of the loop of Henle is referred to as the cortical diluting segment of the nephron. In the late distal tubule, sodium ions are reabsorbed in exchange for potassium or hydrogen ions. The secretion of hydrogen ions in exchange for sodium ions results in the acidification of the urine. The process of sodium exchange is partially under the control of mineralocorticoids (e.g., aldosterone) and accounts for the reabsorption of 2 or 3% of filtered sodium ions.

The kidney also has the ability to respond to changes in the glomerular filtration rate through the action of specialized distal epithelial cells called the macula densa. These cells are in close contact with the glomerular apparatus of the same nephron and can detect even small changes in the flow of luminal fluid. Increases in the flow rate activate the macula densa cells to communicate with the granular cells and vascular components of the juxtaglomerular apparatus and stimulate the release of renin. Renin release results in the formation of the vasoactive peptide angiotensin II and subsequent vasoconstriction which leads to a decrease in the GFR and the luminal flow rate. Thus, the distal tubule is not only important for urine formation but also plays a role in regulating the GFR.

Another important urinary regulatory mechanism involves the effects of vasopressin, also known as antidiuretic hormone (ADH). A decrease in blood pressure or an elevation in plasma osmolality will result in the release of ADH from the posterior pituitary. ADH is carried by the blood to the nephron, where ADH increases the reabsorption of water from the collecting tubule. Thus, in the presence of ADH, water reabsorption is increased and urine becomes more concentrated, while decreased ADH secretion will result in diuresis and a more dilute urine.

Mechanisms of Nephrotoxicity

The kidney is a target organ for many chemicals, in large part because of the physiology of the kidney described previously. The substantial amount of blood flowing through the kidneys results in the kidneys being exposed to significant amounts of chemicals and their metabolites. The ability of the proximal tubular cells to transport organic anions and cations can lead to the intracellular accumulation of weakly acidic or basic chemicals as well as amino acid conjugates and quaternary compounds (e.g., paraquat) in this renal nephron segment. Such accumulations can eventually lead to toxic levels of the chemical in proximal tubular cells. In addition, the large demand for energy to support all of the reabsorption and secretion processes makes the kidney particularly susceptible to compounds which inhibit the production of cellular energy and/or oxygen utilization.

There are several mechanisms by which renal toxicity can be induced (Table K-1). Direct tubular toxicity is one of the most common mechanisms by which chemicals or their toxic metabolites induce nephropathy. Proximal tubular cells are especially susceptible to toxicity via this mechanism because (1) they are one of

TABLE K-1
Mechanisms of Nephrotoxicity

Direct tubular toxicity
Examples: amphotericin B, aminoglycosides, cephaloridine, cisplatin, heavy metals, cysteine conjugates, 4-aminophenol, many others
Altered renal hemodynamics
Examples: angiotensin converting enzyme (ACE) inhibitors, cyclosporine, nonsteroidal antiinflammatory drugs (NSAIDs)
Tubular obstruction
Examples: sulfonamides, methotrexate, oxalic acid, acyclovir
Tubulointerstitial nephritis
Examples: analgesics, penicillins, cephalosporins, heavy metals, cisplatin, nitrosoureas, NSAIDs, cimetadine, many others
Glomerular injury
Examples: heavy metals, *d*-penicillamine, captopril, methimazole, heroin, puromycin aminonucleoside
Fluid/electrolyte imbalance
Examples: chlorpropamide, lithium, captopril, NSAIDs, fluoride, diuretics, ACE inhibitors

the first segments of the nephron to be exposed to toxicants and (2) these cells can accumulate toxicants by actively transporting the toxicants into this tubular segment and achieving high intracellular concentrations of toxic chemical species or their precursors. The exact mechanism of direct tubular toxicity or the critical cellular target is not known with certainty for most toxicants. However, nephrotoxicants can induce direct toxicity by (1) alkylation of cell macromolecules (e.g., phosgene formed from chloroform), (2) complexation with cellular sulfhydryl groups and other ligands (e.g., heavy metals), (3) generation of free radials and/or initiation of lipid peroxidation (e.g., cephaloridine and paraquat), or (4) disruption of mitochondrial function and energy production (e.g., cysteine conjugates and cyanide).

Nephrotoxicity can also occur following an alteration in renal hemodynamics. Since renal blood flow is important for maintaining a steady supply of oxygen and nutrients to renal cells, a reduction in blood flow to the kidney can result in decreased oxygen delivery (ischemia), decreased energy production, and decreased renal function. The vasodilatory prostaglandins PGE_2 and PGI_2 can be important in maintaining proper renal perfusion. Inhibition of cyclooxygenase by administration of nonsterodial antiinflammatory drugs (NSAIDs), such as indomethacin, can result in a decrease in production of the vasodilatory prostaglandins, overriding renal vasoconstriction and, ultimately, renal failure. In disease states, such as congestive heart failure and cirrhosis with ascites, where renal perfusion may be augmented by the synthesis of PGE_2, NSAIDs can cause reversible acute renal failure.

The obstruction of renal tubules can occur following the precipitation of compounds with low water solubility. The obstruction of tubules prevents the filtration of blood at the glomerulus and can lead to oliguric acute renal failure characterized by a decrease in urine volume and a rise in the blood urea nitrogen (BUN) concentration. Precipitation of the toxicant occurs as the luminal fluid passes through the descending limb of the loop of Henle and the fluid becomes more concentrated. When the solubility limit of the toxicant is exceeded, the toxicant begins to precipitate and obstruct flow. Tubular obstruction was occasionally seen following the use of some of the early sulfonamide antimicrobial agents but is less of a problem with the currently used drugs. High-dose methotrexate therapy or rapidly infused acyclovir can also result in tubular obstruction. The use of cancer chemotherapeutic agents can lead to rapid cell killing and the delivery of large amounts of uric acid to the kidney. Uric acid is particularly prone to deposit in acidic urine so that therapy to prevent uric acid deposition can include alkaline diuresis, hydration of the patient, and allopurinol, an inhibitor of xanthine oxidase, which decreases uric acid formation. Oxalic acid, which is formed from the biotransformation of ethylene glycol and other compounds, can also deposit in renal tubules and may contribute to the nephrotoxicity induced by these agents.

Tubulointerstitial nephritis can be either acute or chronic in nature. Acute interstitial nephritis is characterized by an acute renal interstitial inflammatory response with urinary eosinophils and nonoliguric acute renal failure. The more common drugs which induce acute interstitial nephritis include penicillins, rifampicin, sulfonamides, and cimetadine. Chronic tubulointerstitial nephritis is most commonly associated with the long-term use of large amounts of analgesics (e.g., aspirin and phenacetin) which are often taken in combination.

Glomerular toxicity is frequently seen as a "leaky sieve" effect. Normally, the glomerulus serves as a barrier to high-molecular-weight (>50,000–60,000) proteins; however, when the glomerulus is damaged, proteinuria can be observed. Chemically induced glomerular disease is frequently immune mediated with the observation of immunoglobulin and complement deposits in renal biopsies noted in some cases. Heavy metals such as mercuric salts may induce their glomerular effects via an immune-mediated pathway, but the exact mechanism of this effect is unclear.

Many drugs and other chemicals can adversely affect renal function by directly or indirectly affecting the reabsorption of electrolytes and water in the kidney. Chlorpropamide can enhance the secretion of ADH and promote the water conservation actions of the hormone, while lithium use can lead to a nephrogenic diabetes insipidus. NSAIDs block the formation of renal prostaglandins, which can result in hyperkalemia. Hyperkalemia may also result from the use of beta blockers, potassium-sparing diuretics, and cyclosporine.

Methods for Evaluating Nephrotoxicity

There are numerous methods to determine the nephrotoxic potential of a chemical or to study the mechanism(s) by which a chemical induces nephrotoxicity. In humans, the concern is most often related to either drug-induced or occupationally associated nephrotoxicity. Evaluation of nephrotoxicity in humans is limited primarily to the measurement of urinary changes (e.g., volume and protein), BUN, or serum creatinine concentrations, creatinine clearance, or renal biopsy. However, in laboratory animals, many techniques and models are available for monitoring renal function both *in vivo* and *in vitro*.

In Vivo Techniques

There are two general models for evaluating the nephrotoxic potential of chemicals which utilize whole animals. In one model, conscious animals are administered the test compound and renal functional parameters (Table K-2) are evaluated over a period of hours or days. Some of the urinary parameters routinely monitored in *in vivo* nephrotoxicity studies include volume, osmolality, and contents. Urine volume can increase (polyuria), decrease (oliguria), or approach a zero value (anuria). Urinary osmolality is a measure of the ability of the kidney to concentrate urine. In polyuric states, urinary osmolality usually decreases from control levels, while in oliguric states urine tends to be more concentrated and urinary osmolality values rise above the control level.

TABLE K-2
Common Parameters of Renal Function Monitored in *in Vivo* Studies

Parameter
Clearance of organic compounds; creatinine, urea, inulin, PAH, phenol red, TEA Comment: allows for the determination of GFR or RBF (PAH)
Urinary volume Comment: reflects absorption capability of nephron or altered GFR
Urinary free water/osmolality Comment: represents the ability of the kidney to concentrate urine
Enzymuria/proteinuria Comment: changes reflect cellular toxicity and/or altered glomerular function
Glucosuria/amino aciduria Comment: increasing amounts of either in urine suggest proximal tubular damage, extrarenal effects also possible (e.g., diabetes)
Electrolyte excretion; pH Comment: may be influenced by many factors
Kidney weight Comment: can increase (edema and hypertrophy) or decrease (atrophy)
Morphological changes Comment: provides information on the sight and nature of the lesion

Note. Abbreviations used: PAH, *p*-aminohippurate; TEA, tetraethylammonium; GFR, glomerular filtration rate; RBF, renal blood flow.

The urinary contents also can provide important information concerning the presence of nephrotoxicity. The presence or elevated levels of enzymes, protein, amino acids, glucose, blood, or casts in the urine can signal renal injury. Enzymuria results primarily from the loss of the brush border (microvilli) of proximal tubular cells or from the rupture of necrotic tubular cells with the release of cytosolic enzymes and organelles. The appearance of significant enzymuria has been used as an early indicator of nephrotoxicity and for predicting the injured nephron site.

Proteinuria is also an index of chemically induced nephrotoxicity. The amount of protein present in the urine can be used as a measure of the relative degree of renal damage, while the nature of the protein can provide information on the site of the lesion. Low-molecular-weight proteins such as β_2-microglobulin (12,000 Da) are freely filtered at the glomerulus and almost completely reabsorbed by the proximal tubule, while high-molecular-weight proteins (e.g., albumin, ~69,000 Da) are not normally filtered at the glomerulus. Thus, the appearance of increased amounts of albumin can indicate glomerular damage, and an increased excretion of β_2-microglobulin or a decreased ratio of albumin to β_2-microglobulin can be indicative of proximal tubular damage.

The appearance of amino acids and/or glucose in urine can also indicate proximal tubular toxicity. Both nutrients are almost entirely reabsorbed in the proximal tubule and proximal tubular damage can lead to the increased excretion of both compounds. However, reabsorption of these materials is dependent on membrane transport systems which can become saturated and lead to the increased excretion of the amino acid or glucose (e.g., uncontrolled diabetes).

Creatinine, an endogenous endproduct of muscle metabolism, is often measured in plasma and urine to determine creatinine clearance. Since creatinine is freely filtered at the glomerulus and is not reabsorbed or secreted by the proximal tubule of most species, creatinine clearance provides a good measure of the GFR. Another endogenous compound, urea, is also cleared mainly by renal filtration and excretion. Increases in the blood or serum concentration of urea are indicative of decreased GFR. However, increases in BUN concentration occur only after substantial renal toxicity has been established. Thus, BUN concentration is not a sensitive indicator of nephrotoxicity and changes usually occur later than changes in other parameters (e.g., enzymuria).

At the end of a screening protocol in animal models, the kidneys can be removed and examined for morphological changes (using light or electron microscopy) or used in an *in vitro* model as described later to further evaluate renal function following *in vivo* exposure to the test agent. Kidney weight can also be easily measured at the end of a screening period as one index of nephrotoxicity. Some nephrotoxicants induce an increase in kidney weight, while exposure to other nephrotoxicants results in decreased kidney weight.

A second *in vivo* model involves the use of anesthetized animals. The animals used in these studies are either untreated or have received the test agent or procedure before anesthesia. Changes in GFR are frequently measured by determining the urinary clearance of inulin, an exogenously administered polysaccharide which is freely filtered at the glomerulus but is not secreted or reabsorbed by the nephron. Changes in renal blood flow (RBF), a measure of renal hemodynamics, can be monitored by measuring the renal clearance of PAH or other organic compounds which are essentially 100% extracted from the peritubular fluid but poorly reabsorbed from the luminal fluid or by the use of electromagnetic flow probes placed on one or both renal arteries. In addition to determining changes in GFR and RBF, the excretion patterns of electrolytes, protein, enzymes, glucose, water, and other urinary components can be determined both before and after exposure to a nephrotoxicant to provide information on the relative renal toxicity of test compound, the temporal aspects of toxicity, and the nephron segment where toxicity occurs. Kidneys may be perfused with fixative solutions at the end of the experiment to allow for histological examination of tissue.

In Vitro Techniques

There are a large number of *in vitro* techniques available for evaluating the nephrotoxic potential of an agent or examining potential mechanisms by which an agent induces nephrotoxicity (Table K-3). These techniques employ various levels of tissue organization including whole kidneys, tubules or tubule segments, cortical slices, cells, and isolated cellular components. *In vitro* techniques offer the advantage of allowing the investigator to study the direct effects of a compound on renal function without the contribution of indirect mechanisms (e.g., extrarenal biotransformation or altered renal hemodynamics). However, many *in vitro* systems remove the integral nature of the kidney, and in other *in vitro* models the *in vivo* cellular characteristics change over time (e.g., cell culture techniques). The relative importance of these factors for the induction

TABLE K-3
Common *in Vitro* Models for Examining Nephrotoxicity

Isolated perfused kidney/tubule
Renal cortical slices
Nephron segments
Isolated renal epithelial cells
Renal cell cultures
Isolated renal organelles (e.g., mitochondria)
Membrane vesicles (basolateral or luminal)

of nephrotoxicity by a test compound will determine the toxic potential of that agent in the various *in vitro* systems. Therefore, the use of *in vitro* systems may not always provide the same results as will be obtained in whole animals. Nonetheless, valuable information can be obtained once the toxicant species has been identified and an appropriate *in vitro* model is selected for use. In the remainder of this section, a general description of the more common *in vitro* systems for examining nephrotoxicity is provided.

The isolated perfused kidney allows the investigator the ability to monitor the effects of chemicals on the intact kidney without the effects of extrarenal systems. Transport of chemicals occurs via normal mechanisms as vasculature and tubular lumen remain open in the perfused state, and renal handling and biotransformation of chemicals can be evaluated using this technique. However, to utilize an isolated perfused kidney preparation, a special apparatus must be used.

Renal cortical slices offer a convenient and sensitive model for determining the induction of nephrotoxicity following either *in vivo* or *in vitro* exposure to a nephrotoxicant. Slices can be prepared freehand or by the use of a mechanical tissue slicer. When isolated from different depths of the cortex, renal cortical slices can provide one method for examining cell- or site-specific damage. Superficial slices contain S_1 and S_2 segments of the proximal tubule, while deeper slices can be prepared which contain mainly the S_3 segment. Thus, effects of nephrotoxicants on S_1 and S_2 segments versus S_3 segments can be performed. Renal function parameters monitored in renal slices can include organic ion (PAH and TEA) accumulation, gluconeogenesis, LDH release, oxygen consumption, electrolyte levels, adenosine triphosphate (ATP) production, and morphology. In addition, the order of nephrotoxic potential of several agents (mercuric chloride > potassium dichromate > hexachloro-1,3-butadiene > cephaloridine > gentamicin) is the same *in vivo* and in renal cortical slices from Fischer 344 rats.

Renal tubules or tubular segments can be isolated from the kidneys of a variety of species and either perfused with or suspended in an appropriate medium. The rabbit is commonly used as the model for tubular perfusion studies, although renal tubules from many species, including humans, have been used. Tubular segments allow the renal cells to remain in contact, but tubular collapse may occur in nonperfused segments which could hinder absorption of toxicants from lumen. If the normal route of entry into renal tissue for a toxicant is via absorption at the luminal surface, then a reduction in the nephrotoxic potential of the toxicant might be observed using nonperfused tubular segments. However, the perfused tubule allows ready access to the luminal surface when the toxicant is added to the perfusate. Also, addition of a toxicant to the bathing media provides exposure of the basolateral membrane to the toxicant for the measurement of transport and toxicological parameters as well following exposure of this cell surface to the test compound. Thus, the perfused tubular segment can provide an *in vitro* model with many of the characteristics of the *in vivo* model.

Isolated renal cortical epithelial cells and cultured cell lines have become standard *in vitro* model systems for examining the nephrotoxic potential of toxicants, toxicant bioactivation, and direct mechanisms of toxicity. Enriched populations of freshly isolated proximal and distal tubular cells can be obtained to examine the effects of toxicants on these distinct cell populations. Cell cultures can also be obtained which are derived from proximal tubule or distal tubule/collecting duct cells. In addition, cell lines have been developed from specific segments of the proximal tubule. These cell systems allow for the rapid screening of chemicals, exposure to apical and/or basolateral surfaces, and more detailed studies of specific cell populations. However, cells in culture can exhibit reduced functional and metabolic characteristics with time. These changes might impact on the potential effects of some chemicals in cell culture systems. Therefore, toxicity in the specific cell line to be used should be validated prior to mechanistic studies.

Isolated renal cell components (cytosol, organelles, and membranes) are also commonly used *in vitro* systems. Renal microsomes and cytosol are useful in examining the renal biotransformation and bioactivation of nephrotoxicants. Since mitochondria are frequently targets for nephrotoxicants, isolated renal mitochondria are also an important model system for determining the toxic mechanism(s) of some compounds. Also, the direct effects of toxicants on renal cell membranes can be studied in vesicles prepared from either the luminal (brush border) or basolateral (antiluminal and peritubular) membrane of renal cortical cells. The use of isolated cell components is helpful in answering specific questions about mechanisms of nephrotoxicity and bioactivation of nephrotoxicants.

Nephrotoxicants

Nephrotoxicants can be classified in many different ways including chemical class (e.g., heavy metals and halogenated hydrocarbons), intended use (e.g., drugs and agricultural agents), site of toxicity (e.g., glomerular toxicants and proximal tubular toxicants), and mechanism of toxicity (e.g., acute renal failure and interstitial nephritis). Nephrotoxicants can also be considered either primary or secondary nephrotoxicants. Primary nephrotoxicants (e.g., heavy metals) are capable of inducing nephrotoxicity as the parent compound, while secondary nephrotoxicants (e.g., trichloroethylene) require bioactivation to the ultimate nephrotoxicant species. In the following sections on specific nephrotoxicants, nephrotoxic agents will be divided into therapeutic and environmental nephrotoxicants. Sites of toxicity, mechanisms of toxicity, and the ultimate nephrotoxicant species, if known, will be discussed.

Therapeutic Nephrotoxicants

Many drugs have the potential to alter renal function. In the case of the diuretic drugs, such as furosemide and hydrochlorothiazide, the increased urine flow rate and sodium excretion which these drugs induce is a desirable, therapeutic response. However, for most therapeutics, drug-induced effects on renal function are not desirable and constitute a toxic response. Examples of some drug classes whose members induce nephrotoxicity include the antimicrobials, nonsteroidal antiinflammatory agents, analgesics, cancer chemotherapeutic agents, immunosuppressives, and radiocontrast media. In addition, there are several miscellaneous drugs within other pharmacological classes which affect renal function. The nature and magnitude of the nephrotoxic response varies greatly among these drugs, and a single drug may induce more than one type of nephrotoxic response depending on dose, duration of therapy, age of the patient, and other patient variables.

Antimicrobials

Several different classes of antimicrobial agents contain members which induce nephrotoxicity. The primary groups of drugs which induce nephrotoxicity include the β-lactams (penicillins, cephalosporins, and carbapenems), aminoglycosides, the antifungal agent amphotericin B, and the tetracyclines. The spectrum of nephrotoxic effects and mechanism(s) of nephrotoxicity vary among these agents, and the potential for a nephrotoxic response can be increased by combining two antimicrobial drugs which can induce renal toxicity or by combining a nephrotoxicant antimicrobial with other nephrotoxicant drugs.

β-Lactam Antimicrobials. The β-lactam antimicrobial drugs (penicillins, cephalosporins, and carbapenems; Fig. K-2) are related chemically by the presence of a four-membered ring containing a nitrogen atom adjacent to a carbonyl group (a β-lactam ring). This β-lactam ring also confers antimicrobial activity to these drugs since hydrolysis of the ring results in inactive drugs. Because these drugs are weakly acidic drugs, they are actively secreted by the organic anion transport system of the proximal tubule and can concentrate in this nephron segment during the secretory process. The nephrotoxicity observed following administration of a β-lactam antibiotic can occur by different mechanisms depending on the antibiotic used and patient variables.

Penicillin-induced renal toxicity is most commonly seen as allergic acute interstitial nephritis (AIN). Methicillin is the most common penicillin to induce AIN, but the use of penicillin G, ampicillin, amoxacillin, oxacillin, and carbenicillin also can lead to the development of AIN. Typically, acute renal failure follows 1 or 2 weeks of treatment with fever or rashes sometimes occurring before overt renal dysfunction. Removal of the penicillin generally allows renal function to return to normal within a few days or weeks. AIN can also be induced by certain cephalosporins (e.g., cephalothin, cephalexin, cephradine, cefoxitin, and cefotaxime) and non-β-lactam antimicrobials (e.g., sulfonamides, rifampicin, tetracyclines, and erythromycin).

In addition to inducing AIN, several of the cephalosporins (e.g., cephaloridine, cephaloglycine, cefaclor, and cephalothin) are directly toxic to the proximal tubule. Accumulation in proximal tubular cells via the organic anion transporter is an important step in cephalosporin nephrotoxicity since inhibition of cephalosporin transport by probenecid also attenuates cephalosporin nephrotoxicity. In addition, the site of the cephalosporin-induced renal lesion correlates with the proximal tubular segment having the greatest capacity for organic anion transport for a particular species.

The cellular mechanism of direct cephalosporin-induced nephrotoxicity may include several possible actions of the cephalosporins. Nephrotoxic cephalospo-

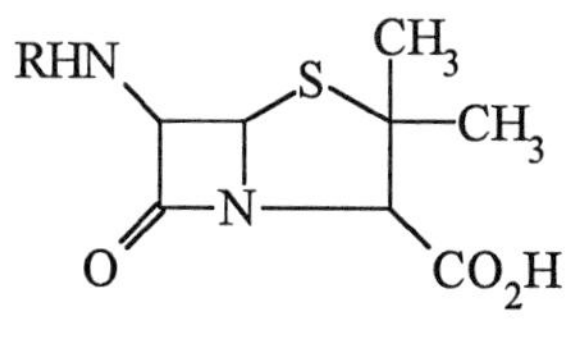

FIGURE K-2. Structures of β-lactam antimicrobials.

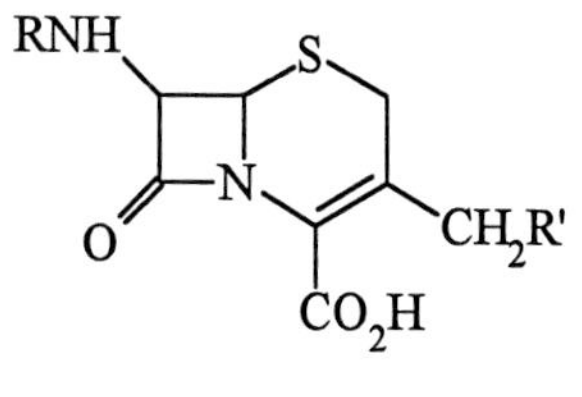

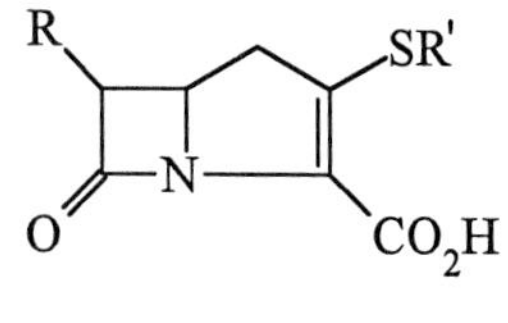

rins are known to induce lipid peroxidation and cellular membrane damage, acylate cellular proteins, and/or interfere with mitochodrial respiration. Mitochondrial respiration appears to be inhibited due to acylation of mitochondrial transporters for metabolic substrates, thereby depriving mitochondria of the necessary intermediates to utilize oxygen. Ultimately, the formation of ATP, needed to supply cellular energy, also declines to inhibit energy-dependent cellular functions.

Imipenem, a carbapenem antimicrobial, also possess nephrotoxic potential. In animal models, nephrotoxicity is dose dependent and characterized by tubular necrosis. Interestingly, imipenem nephrotoxicity is markedly attenuated by coadministration of cilastatin, an inhibitor of the cytosolic and brush border enzyme dehydropeptidase I (DHP). Although DHP is responsible for hydrolyzing imipenem to inactive metabolites, the major protective effect of cilastatin appears to be due to inhibition of renal imipenem accumulation rather than DHP inhibition.

Aminoglycosides. The aminoglycosides are important antimicrobial drugs used alone or in combination with β-lactam antibiotics for the treatment of certain serious gram-negative infections. Chemically, the aminoglycosides consist of various sugars containing amino groups and linked by glycosidic bonds. The amino groups are ionized at physiological pH and give the aminoglycosides polycationic character and a highly polar nature.

Aminoglycosides concentrate in the S_1 and S_2 segments of the proximal tubule via a high-capacity, adsorptive endocytotic mechanism following binding to cellular membrane acidic (anionic) phospholipids. This endocytotic process occurs primarily at the brush border membrane. Following adsorption, aminoglycoside-containing vesicles bind to secondary lysosomes where the drug becomes sequestered. Lysosomes become early targets for aminoglycoside-induced effects, with inhibition of phospholipid degradation and subsequent myeloid body formation being characteristic of aminoglycoside nephrotoxicity. Some lysosomes may rupture to release lysosomal enzymes into the cytosol of renal cells. Changes in brush border microvilli, alterations in rough endoplasmic reticulum, and increased numbers of cytoplasmic vacuoles also occur. Mitochondrial swelling, decreased mitochondrial respiration, and inhibition of basolateral Na^+/K^+-ATPase activity precede tubular necrosis. Ultimately, nonoliguric renal failure results which may not completely reverse following cessation of aminoglycoside administration.

Although all aminoglycosides possess the ability to induce nephrotoxicity, differences exist in the nephrotoxic potential of the various drugs. Neomycin and gentamicin are the most potent nephrotoxicant aminoglycosides, while amikacin and netilmicin are the least nephrotoxic aminoglycosides. Other aminoglycosides are intermediate in nephrotoxic potential.

The exact mechanism of aminoglycoside nephrotoxicity is unclear. As discussed previously, release of lysosomal enzymes can contribute to altered cellular function. Hydroxy radicals may also play a role in aminoglycoside mitochondrial effects since catalase inhibits *in vitro* alterations of mitochondrial function by gentamicin and the use of hydroxy radical scavengers or iron chelators reduces gentamicin nephrotoxicity *in vivo*. Additionally, aminoglycoside-induced decreases in cellular pyridoxal 5′-phosphate may contribute to nephrotoxicity by removing an important cellular cofactor.

Amphotericin B. The drug of choice for treating many serious systemic fungal infections is the broad-spectrum antifungal agent amphotericin B. Unfortunately, nephrotoxicity is a common side effect of amphotericin B administration, with up to 50–80% of amphotericin B-treated patients experiencing adverse renal effects. Amphotericin B nephrotoxicity is characterized by a distal renal tubular acidosis, potassium wasting, and a defect in urinary concentration. In some cases, nephrotoxicity may progress to renal failure with azotemia.

Amphotericin-induced renal effects are due to the ability of the drug (1) to induce renal vasoconstriction, which leads to a decrease in renal blood flow and GFR, and (2) to cause an increase in tubular permeability, particularly in the distal segments of the nephron. Tubular permeability changes are the result of the association of amphotericin B with the sterols in the cell membrane to form a pore or channel. Chemically, amphotericin B is a cyclic molecule composed of lipophilic (multiple conjugated double bonds) and hydrophilic regions (Fig. K-3) such that insertion of amphotericin B into the cell membrane facilitates passive movement of water, potassium ions, hydrogen ions, and other small molecules through the newly created pore and across the membrane. These fluxes appear to account for the decrease in urinary concentrating ability, potassium wasting, and renal tubular acidosis. Although it is not clear why the distal segments of the nephron are the major targets for amphotericin B, one explanation may be that the greater level of sterols found in distal membranes might facilitate the binding of amphotericin B to these sites.

Tetracyclines. Tetracyclines are broad-spectrum antibiotics obtained from *Streptomyces* strains or prepared semisynthetically. Use of tetracyclines has resulted in three types of renal effects. First, the use of outdated tetracyclines results in direct proximal tubular toxicity characterized by the increased excretion of amino acids, glucose and phosphate (Fanconi syndrome). The mechanism of this response is unclear but appears to be due to the formation of the degradation product anhydro-4-epi-tetracycline. Second, administration of some tetracyclines, particularly demeclocycline, can result in a dose-dependent, reversible nephrogenic diabetes insipidus which appears to result from an inhibition of ADH effects on water reabsorption. Lastly, in patients with preexisting compromised renal function, tetracyclines can induce increased sodium excretion and azotemia. The mechanism of the naturesis may be due to an effect of tetracyclines on luminal membrane sodium conductance, while the azotemia appears to result from the antianabolic effects of the tetracyclines.

Nonsteroidal Antiinflammatory Drugs

The NSAIDs as a class possess the ability to induce renal failure characterized by a rapid decrease in urine

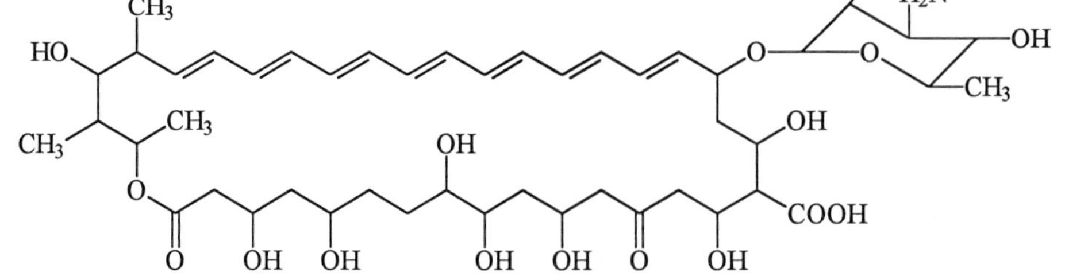

HO CH3 CH3 CH3 O O OH H2N OH CH3 OH OH COOH O OH OH OH OH O OH

FIGURE K-3. Structure of the antifungal drug amphotericin B.

volume and significant sodium and water retention which is also rapidly reversed when the drug is removed. Conditions which decrease renal perfusion (e.g., congestive heart failure, decreased blood volume, and chronic renal disease) also predispose individuals to the renal effects of NSAIDs. Under these conditions, renal blood flow and GFR are maintained by a balance of the vasoconstrictor actions of angiotensin II and the vasodilatory effects of PGE_2. NSAID-induced renal failure results as a consequence of NSAID inhibition of renal cyclooxygenase with a subsequent inhibition of PGE_2 synthesis. Renal vasoconstriction predominates under these conditions, resulting in acute oliguric renal failure. While all NSAIDs have the potential to induce acute renal failure, sulindac appears to have less of an effect on renal PGE_2 synthesis and may be the drug of choice in patients with preexisting conditions which would predispose them to NSAID-induced renal effects.

Nonnarcotic Analgesics

Nonnarcotic analgesic drugs are widely used for the relief of minor pain, to reduce fever, and/or as antiinflammatory agents. Acetaminophen (paracetamol) is perhaps the most commonly used agent in this class of drugs, which also includes aspirin and phenacetin. Analgesic use can result in acute or chronic nephrotoxicity depending on the amount of drug ingested and patient variables. Normally, acute nephrotoxicity results from acute overdose, while chronic use of single or combination products can result in renal papillary necrosis and chronic interstitial nephritis.

Acute overdose with acetaminophen (>300 mg/kg) results in hepatotoxicity and/or nephrotoxicity. Although hepatotoxicity is frequently the predominant toxicity, acetaminophen nephrotoxicity can occur in the absence of marked hepatic toxicity. In these cases, liver function returns to normal or near-normal levels before the onset of nephrotoxicity. Acute acetaminophen nephrotoxicity is generally characterized as oliguric acute renal failure with acute tubular necrosis. Acetaminophen can also induce acute nephrotoxicity in therapeutic doses, but chronic alcohol intake usually accompanies renal toxicity in these patients.

The mechanism of acute acetaminophen nephrotoxicity is related to the bioactivation of acetaminophen and/or its metabolites to highly reactive species which are capable of arylating renal macromolecules or generating reactive oxygen species. Acetaminophen hepatotoxicity is the result of conversion of acetaminophen to the reactive intermediate *N*-acetyl-*p*-benzoquinoneimine (NAPQI), which can covalently bind to hepatic macromolecules. It is less clear what role formation of NAPQI in the kidney plays in acetaminophen nephrotoxicity. In some species (e.g., the Fischer 344 rat) deacetylation appears to be an important biotransformation step in acetaminophen nephrotoxicity, while in other species (e.g., the CD-1 mouse) bioactivation does not appear to require deacetylation of acetaminophen before the ultimate nephrotoxicant species is produced. Therefore, the role of NAPQI in acute acetaminophen nephrotoxicity might be species dependent.

Biotransformation of acetaminophen by deacetylase enzymes in liver or kidney produces the metabolite 4-aminophenol (Fig. K-4). Evidence suggests that acetaminophen nephrotoxicity may result from 4-aminophenol formation. In animal studies, 4-aminophenol is a more potent nephrotoxicant than acetaminophen and

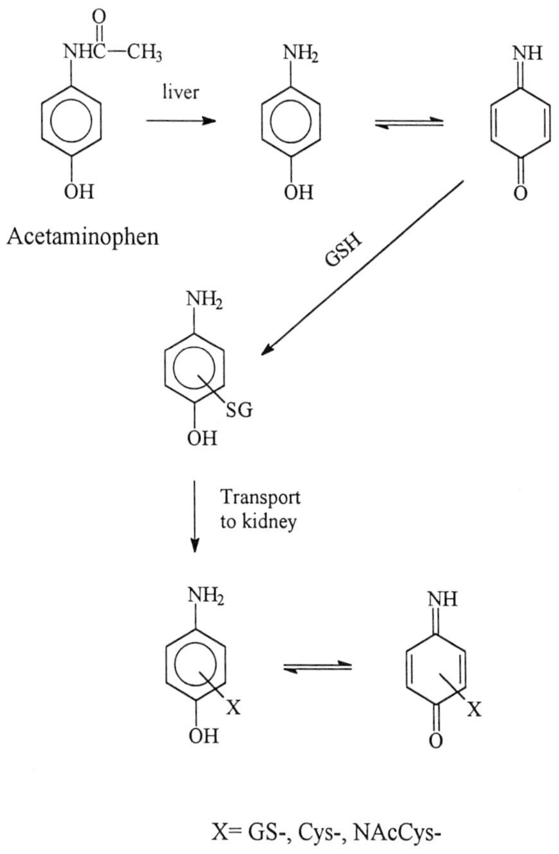

X= GS-, Cys-, NAcCys-

FIGURE K-4. Bioactivation of acetaminophen.

inhibition of deacetylase enzymes also attenuates acetaminophen nephrotoxicity. Deacetylase enzymes are also present in higher levels in renal cortex, the target for acetaminophen nephrotoxicity, than in liver or renal medulla and there is a positive correlation between renal cortex deacetylase activity and susceptibility to acetaminophen nephrotoxicity in various animal models.

The mechanism of 4-aminophenol nephrotoxicity remains to be determined with certainty. The current hypothesis suggests that 4-aminophenol is oxidized by cytochrome P450 isozymes or peroxidases to *p*-benzoquinoneimine, which can arylate renal macromolecules and/or redox cycle between 4-aminophenol and *p*-benzoquinoneimine to form reactive oxygen species. Recent studies have suggested that 4-aminophenol might be converted to a glutathione conjugate in the liver prior to transport to the kidney (Fig. K-4), and that the glutathione conjugate or one of its metabolites is the form that accumulates in kidney from extrarenal sources. Thus, acetaminophen nephrotoxicity could result from production of more than one reactive intermediate.

Chronic analgesic nephrotoxicity is characterized by renal papillary necrosis and interstitial nephritis rather than the proximal tubular necrosis observed in acute nephrotoxicity. In most cases, chronic nephropathy results from abuse of a combination of analgesic preparations (phenacetin, acetaminophen, and/or a salicylate) over a long period of time. In these situations, the primary nephrotoxicant appears to be acetaminophen, which concentrates more in the renal medulla than in renal cortex or blood. Within the medulla, acetaminophen can be converted to the reactive intermediate NAPQI by the prostaglandin hydroperoxidase component of the prostaglandin H synthase complex. NAPQI interactions within medullary tissue result in a depletion of the cytoprotective tripeptide glutathione. As glutathione becomes depleted, arylation of medullary macromolecules by NAPQI occurs. In addition, acetaminophen in therapeutic doses can increase prostaglandin hydroperoxidase activity and, therefore, stimulate formation of its own reactive metabolite NAPQI.

Aspirin also has the potential to increase acetaminophen nephropathy. Aspirin inhibits the cyclooxygenase component of prostaglandin H synthase without effect on the prostaglandin hydroperoxidase component, while salicylic acid (the deacetylated metabolite of aspirin) decreases renal glutathione concentrations. Thus, coadministration of aspirin with acetaminophen (or phenacetin) results in a synergistic nephrotoxicity.

Cancer Chemotherapeutic Drugs

Cancer chemotherapeutic drugs can be life saving in the treatment of certain cancers. Unfortunately, host systems are also a target for these agents, with several antineoplastic drugs possessing the potential to induce nephrotoxicity (Table K-4). In some cases, nephrotoxicity normally only occurs at high doses (e.g., methotrexate and 6-thioguanine) or is a low risk (e.g., 5-fluorouracil and interferon). However, nephrotoxicity can be a significant toxicity following administration of certain antineoplastic drugs (e.g., cisplatin) which can require additional efforts to minimize the development of renal failure.

Alkylating Agents. Perhaps the cancer chemotherapeutic drug which is most commonly associated with the induction of nephrotoxicity is cisplatin (Fig. K-5; also see Cisplatin). Cisplatin is a member of the platinum complex class of antineoplastic drugs which also includes carboplatin and iproplatin (CHIP). However, the nephrotoxic potential of cisplatin appears to be greater than the nephrotoxic potential of the other clinically useful platinum agents.

In rat models of cisplatin nephrotoxicity, cisplatin nephrotoxicity is observed as acute proximal tubular necrosis with the primary target being the S_3 segment.

TABLE K-4
Cancer Chemotherapeutic Drugs Capable of Inducing Nephrotoxicity

Alkylating agents
Cisplatin
Nitrosoureas
Cyclophosphamide
Antibiotics
Mitomycin C
Mithramycin
Doxorubicin
Antimetabolites
Methotrexate
5-Fluorouracil
6-Thioguanine
Cytosine arabinoside
5-Azacytidine
Miscellaneous
Interferon
Celiptinium

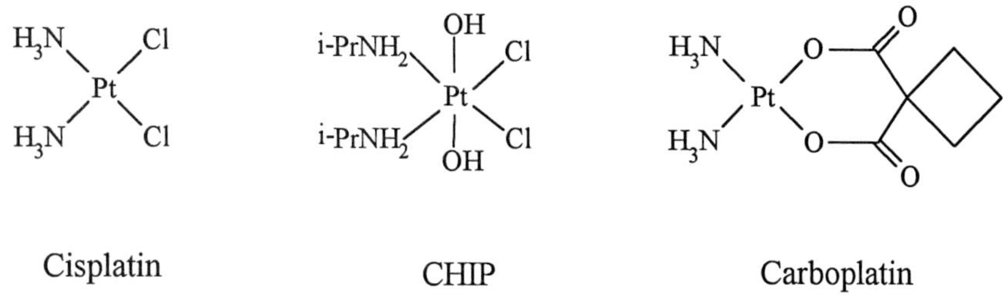

FIGURE K-5. Platinum cancer chemotherapeutic drugs.

However, in humans, cisplatin nephrotoxicity is characterized by tubular necrosis with the distal tubules and collecting ducts affected along with proximal tubules. Early changes in renal function include enzymuria (e.g., *N*-acetyl-β-glucosaminidase) and β_2-microglobinuria, which suggests that the proximal tubule is an initial target for cisplatin. Diuresis, increased BUN concentration, decreased creatinine clearance, and magnesium wasting soon develop, indicating the presence of renal failure.

The mechanism of cisplatin nephrotoxicity is unclear, although numerous hypotheses have been proposed. Cisplatin is primarily excreted via the kidneys by both filtration and secretion using the organic cation transporter, which indicates that the kidney will be exposed to a large percentage of the administered dose. It is believed that the chloride groups are replaced by water molecules *in vivo,* ultimately forming a hydrated or hydroxylated platinum species which might interact with renal macromolecules (e.g., DNA) to lead to nephrotoxicity. Other postulated targets for cisplatin are renal ATPase enzymes and renal mitochondria.

The nitrosoureas include streptozotocin, an agent useful in treating pancreatic (islet cell) tumors, and the carmustine, lomustine, and semustine group, useful in treating brain and gastrointestinal tumors. Streptozotocin induces a reversible, mild nephropathy characterized by proteinuria in 50–70% of patients and decreased creatinine clearance in 20–30% of patients. Renal phosphate wasting and proteinuria are early signs of nephrotoxicity. The primary target in the kidney for streptozotocin is the proximal tubule with glomerular abnormalities also noted. Removal of the drug results in return to normal renal function within weeks.

Semustine is the most common agent to induce nephrotoxicity among the second group of nitrosoureas. Semustine nephrotoxicity results from bioactivation of the nitrosourea to an alkylating metabolite which mainly attacks proximal tubular cells. Carbamoylating metabolites of semustine are also formed *in vivo* but do not appear to contribute to renal toxicity. Renal failure occurs most often following high-dose (>1200 mg/m^2, total dose) administration. Onset of nephrotoxicity (glomerulosclerosis, renal interstitial nephritis, and proximal tubular degeneration) can be delayed for over 1 year following therapy and may progress to irreversible renal failure.

Cyclophosphamide, a nitrogen mustard alkylating agent, is a widely used cancer chemotherapeutic drug for treating lymphomas, leukemias, multiple myeloma, and numerous solid tumors. Cyclophosphamide can induce nephrotoxicity, characterized as decreased water excretion and an inappropriate concentration of urine. These effects are due to a direct effect of one or more alkylating cyclophosphamide metabolites at distal tubules and collecting ducts. Special caution is warranted to avoid water-induced diuresis or diuretic therapy in these patients because hyponatremia can become a problem.

Antimetabolites. Nephrotoxicity is generally not a major toxicity of antimetabolite therapy, except when these drugs are administered in high doses or in susceptible patients. Acute renal failure is the most common type of nephropathy induced by the antimetabolites, with methotrexate treatment possessing the greatest risk. Acute renal failure has also been reported as a potential toxicity for 5-fluorouracil, 6-thioguanine, cytosine arabinoside, and 5-azacytidine.

Methotrexate is an antimetabolite of folic acid useful in combination therapy for a wide range of cancerous conditions. When methotrexate is administered in high doses ($\geq$50–250 mg/kg to 1–7 g/m^2), solubility limits may be exceeded with a resultant precipitation of methotrexate and its 7-hydroxy metabolite within the renal lumina. Tubular obstruction can reduce GFR by as much as 50%. Methotrexate might also have a direct effect on proximal tubular function since proximal tubular necrosis may be seen in the absence of precipitated material within the renal lumina. In addition, a direct effect of methotrexate on glomerular hemodynamics has been postulated. Renal toxicity induced by methotrexate also can enhance other methotrexate toxicities (e.g., myleosuppression) by decreasing the excretion of the drug from the body.

Antibiotics. The clinical use of three antibiotic cancer chemotherapeutic drugs (mitomycin C, mithramycin, and doxorubicin) has been associated with the development of nephrotoxicity. Each of these drugs is commonly used in combination chemotherapy which in some cases might result in additive or enhanced nephrotoxicity.

Mitomycin C is isolated from *Streptomyces caespitosis* and is used in the treatment of solid tumors. Renal failure (elevated BUN and serum creatinine concentration and proteinuria) induced by mitomycin C is dose dependent and cumulative. When administered alone, the incidence of nephrotoxicity is less than 1%, but in combination with 5-fluorouracil nephrotoxicity occurs more frequently and can be marked. The chemical species responsible for mitomycin C nephrotoxicity appears to result from the formation of alkylating metabolites.

Mithramycin is an antibiotic antineoplastic drug isolated from *S. tanashiensis*. In early studies, treatment with mithramycin (25 or 50 mg/kg/day for 1 week or three times/week each month) resulted in decreased GFR in up to 40% of patients and proteinuria in 78%. Morphological changes included proximal and distal tubular necrosis, atrophy, or swelling. Single-dose administration of mithramycin to treat the hypercalcemia sometimes associated with cancer generally does not induce renal toxicity. However, a few isolated case reports suggest that in patients with compromised renal function, nephrotoxicity may occur following single-dose therapy.

Nephrotoxicity associated with doxorubicin use is also dose dependent and occurs at the same time as doxorubicin-induced cardiotoxicity. Studies in animal models reveal glomerular effects, renal interstitial fibrosis, and vacuolization of tubules. However, clinical evidence of nephrotoxicity in the absence of cardiotoxicity is limited suggesting that dose-reduction efforts to minimize cardiotoxicity also reduce the risk of nephrotoxicity.

Miscellaneous Cancer Chemotherapeutic Agents. The lack of curative treatments for most malignancies has stimulated the search for newer, more efficacious cancer chemotherapeutic agents. Interferon-α has recently been obtained using molecular biology techniques in sufficient quantities to begin clinical testing against various cancerous conditions including hairy cell leukemia, non-Hodgkin's lymphoma, and Karposi's sarcoma. A few reports suggest that reversible acute renal insufficiency associated with proteinuria may occur following continued interferon-α administration. Morphological changes are consistent with the presence of acute interstitial nephritis.

Celiptinium is useful in the treatment of metastatic breast cancer and is useful in combination therapy because of minimal hematotoxicity. Acute and chronic renal failure have been detected in patients treated with celiptinium. Acute renal failure is dose dependent, while chronic effects appear to be cumulative in nature. The primary manifestation of celiptinium nephrotoxicity is tubular necrosis, with celiptinium-induced lipid peroxidation in proximal tubular cells proposed as the mechanism of toxicity.

Immunosuppressive Drugs

The modern development of drugs to suppress the immune system has made organ and bone marrow transplants possible and saved countless lives. Two important drugs in this class of agents are cyclosporine (cyclosporin A) and FK506, fungal products with immunosuppressive properties. Cyclosporine acts primarily by inhibiting helper T cell activation following the binding of cyclosporine to a cytoplasmic receptor protein, cyclophilin. Other effects on the immune system are also observed but appear to be less important than T cell effects. FK506 also inhibits T cell activation but via interaction with a different cytoplasmic receptor than cyclosporine. A newer drug, OKT_3, is a monoclonal antibody which can destroy effector T cells to act as an immunosuppressive drug.

Nephrotoxicity is a common toxicity and significant problem associated with the use of cyclosporine in humans. Three types of nephrotoxicity have been observed in patients receiving cyclosporine; (1) an acute, reversible renal failure; (2) acute vasculopathy or thrombotic microangiopathy; and (3) chronic renal failure with interstitial fibrosis which may not be reversible.

Cyclosporine-induced acute renal failure is characterized by decreased GFR and urine volume and elevated BUN and serum creatinine concentrations. These effects are dose dependent and rapidly reverse when cyclosporine therapy is discontinued. The mechanism of the acute renal failure appears to be related to cyclosporine-induced renal vasoconstriction to reduce glomerular filtration. The precise mechanism responsible for the resultant vasoconstriction remains to be determined with certainty. However, stimulation of the renin–angiotensin system, alteration of renal prostaglandin status (increased vasoconstrictor and/or decreased vasodilatory prostaglandin levels), and stimulation of adrenergic nerves have been proposed as possible mechanisms.

A second form of cyclosporine-induced nephrotoxicity is acute thrombotic microangiopathy. The mechanism for induction of this toxicity is unclear but may be due to a direct toxic effect of cyclosporine on renal arterioles and glomerular capillaries. Histologically, arterioles exhibit protein deposits, while glomeruli show thrombosis and endothelial cell damage. These effects are similar in nature to transplant rejection thrombotic microangiopathy, but arcuate and interlobular arteries rather than arterioles are primarily affected with transplant rejection.

Chronic cyclosporine nephrotoxicity can develop in patients receiving the drug for 1 year or longer. In these patients, there is a gradual decline in renal function. While GFR may not be markedly reduced, significant morphological changes, including vascular changes, glomerular sclerosis, interstitial fibrosis, and tubular atrophy, have been reported. Chronic effects may not be reversible upon discontinuation of cyclosporine, and the renal effects may progress to end-stage renal failure. The mechanism underlying cyclosporine-induced chronic renal failure is unclear. However, it has been proposed that the renal vasoconstriction induced by cyclosporine results in both acute and, ultimately, chronic renal failure.

FK506 nephrotoxicity can occur as proximal tubular vacuolization, proximal tubular necrosis, or glomerular capillary/arteriolar thrombi. Although there are reports that FK506 may be less potent as a nephrotoxicant than cyclosporine, FK506 potentiates cyclosporine nephrotoxicity in humans.

OKT_3, an immunosuppressive monoclonal antibody, can induce systemic vascular changes (leaky syndrome) and prerenal azotemia, presumably by stimulating the release of cytokines (e.g., tumor necrosis factor). These effects are seen more often in poorly hydrated patients. There is also evidence that OKT_3 may induce a direct tubular toxicity since significant numbers of patients developing renal insufficiency also exhibit enzymuria.

Radiocontrast Media

The use of radiocontrast media to visualize organs in the body has been a common practice for over 50 years. However, the use of these agents is now recognized as a significant cause of hospital-acquired acute renal failure, with up to 10% of all cases due to the administration of a radiocontrast agent. Numerous factors may increase the risk of acute renal failure developing following a diagnostic procedure with a radiocontrast agent, including existing renal insufficiency, diabetes mellitus, dehydration, anemia, cardiovascular disease, age, and many others.

Typically, radiocontrast-induced acute renal failure is diagnosed when oliguria or a rise of 50% or more above baseline in serum creatinine develops within 24–48 hr following the radiocontrast procedure. The most predominant morphological change seen in the kidney is extensive vacuolization of proximal tubular cells.

The agents currently used as radiocontrast media are triiodinated benzoic acid derivatives and may be ionic (e.g., sodium diatrizoate) or nonionic (e.g., iotrol, iopamidol). The mechanism of nephrotoxicity induced by radiocontrast media involves both renal hemodynamic changes and direct tubular injury, and these effects are related to the high osmolarity of the drugs (up to 1965 mOsm/liter).

Radiocontrast agents can enter the nephron by filtration and/or secretion, depending on the agent administered. The changes in renal hemodynamics induced by radiocontrast media result primarily from the large osmotic load delivered to the distal segment of the nephron. At the level of the macula densa, this osmotic load is detected and the tubuloglomerular feedback system is activated to stimulate vasoconstriction and decrease GFR. While evidence exists for direct tubular toxicity (enzymuria, naturesis, and diuresis greater than an osmotic effect), the mechanism is unclear. However, tubular injury may be exacerbated by the production of reactive oxygen species generated from mesangial cells and polymorphonuclear leukocytes and macrophages which migrate into glomerular and tubular sites following radiocontrast administration.

Environmental Nephrotoxicants

Exposure to nephrotoxicants not only occurs in the clinical setting but also occurs from environmental sources. Environmental nephrotoxicants are defined as nephrotoxicants found in the natural, home, and/or work environment which have no therapeutic utility. Unlike therapeutic nephrotoxicants, which are administered to obtain a beneficial health effect, exposure to environmental nephrotoxicants usually occurs accidentally or in suicide/intentional poisoning cases.

Although environmental nephrotoxicants differ markedly in their chemical nature, there are several distinct classes of environmental nephrotoxicants. These classes include the metals, halogenated solvents, agricultural agents, and natural products. A diverse array of miscellaneous nephrotoxicants also exists and will be discussed briefly at the end of this section.

TABLE K-5
Nephrotoxicant Metals

Aluminum
Antimony
Arsenic
Beryllium
Bismuth
Cadmium
Chromium
Cobalt
Copper
Gallium
Germanium
Gold
Indium
Iron
Lead
Lithium
Manganese
Mercury
Molybdenum
Nickel
Platinum
Silver
Thallium
Uranium
Vanadium

Metals

A wide range of metals induce nephrotoxicity in humans and/or in animal models (Table K-5). Some of these metals (e.g., iron, cobalt, and copper) are essential elements required for normal body function, while others can be useful in treating diseases. For example, gold salts are useful in treating rheumatoid arthritis, lithium salts are indicated for the treatment of manic-depressive illness, and aluminum and bismuth salts are available to treat indigestion and stomach aches. However, exposure to these and other metals can occur from environmental sources and in excessive concentrations can lead to nephropathy.

Many of the metals are potent nephrotoxicants, inducing marked renal effects at concentrations far lower than many other classes of nephrotoxicants. The proximal tubule is a major target for metal toxicity and, in some cases, renal hemodynamic changes are also important for initiating and/or maintaining the renal damage. Although metal-induced nephrotoxicity has been studied for many years, the precise cellular mechanisms which underlie the potent nature of this class of toxicants are not fully elucidated. However, there are several reasons why the kidney is susceptible to metal-induced effects.

The large reabsorptive nature of the kidney ensures that filtered proteins, electrolytes, and water will be conserved and homeostasis maintained in the body. Metals make use of these reabsorptive processes to gain entry into renal cells. For example, chromate can enter proximal tubular cells via the sulfate transporter, while cadmium binds to metallothionein, a low-molecular-weight metal-binding protein, and enters proximal tubular cells along with the protein. Once inside kidney cells, the metals may substitute for endogenous molecules. Arsenate can substitute for phosphate in oxidative phosphorylation within mitochondria to cause a decrease in ATP synthesis. Also, lead can substitute for calcium to alter a large number of calcium-mediated events within cells. Metals also have a high affinity for sulfhydryl and amino ligands and form complexes or chelates with these organic functional groups. Formation of these chelates with essential functional groups of cellular macromolecules can markedly alter cell function to eventually lead to cell death. In addition to direct interaction of metals with cellular targets, radioactive metals which accumulate in renal tissue can release radiation to initiate the formation of cellular free radicals to disrupt cell function and membrane integrity.

The chemical form of a metal that accumulates in the kidney may vary among the metals. However, the ionic form of a metal is normally much more potent as a nephrotoxicant than the elemental form. Once in the body, metal ions interact with numerous molecules (e.g., albumin, metal-binding proteins, glutathione, and amino acids) and move around the body primarily as reversible complexes. Unfortunately, little information is available on the chemical form of most metals that actually enters proximal tubular cells and additional research is needed in this area.

Mercury. The effects of various forms of mercury on renal function have been known for centuries. Therapeutically, the first class of highly efficacious diuretic drugs was the organomercurials (e.g., mersalyl), but these agents have now been replaced by the loop or high-ceiling diuretics. Toxicological interest has centered on inorganic mercury salts, primarily in the form of mercuric chloride ($HgCl_2$), and organic mercury, mainly methylmercury salts (CH_3Hg^+). In the natural environment, elemental mercury can be converted by microorganisms to both inorganic mercury salts and organic mercurials which can find their way into the food chain. Mercurials are also used agriculturally as insecticides and fungicides so that exposure to these agents can occur occupationally from industrial wastes or agricultural runoff.

Acute exposure to mercuric salts targets the S_3 segment of the proximal tubule to induce severe necrosis. Acute renal failure develops rapidly, characterized by decreased renal blood flow and GFR, oliguria, glucosuria, proteinuria, and elevated BUN concentration. Renal vasoconstriction contributes to the developing nephrotoxicity and may be due to activation of the renin–angiotensin system. At higher doses or later time points, S_1 and S_2 segments of the proximal tubule are also damaged.

The mechanism of tubular toxicity following administration of mercuric chloride has been extensively studied. However, the key sequence of events leading to cell death remains to be determined. Mercuric ions induce mitochondrial toxicity, alter cell membrane function, disrupt cell calcium homeostasis, and cause changes in membrane phospholipid composition. Binding of mercuric ions to enzymatic sulfhydryl groups and ischemia-induced mitochondrial toxicity have been proposed as the basic mechanisms leading to these cellular effects and ultimately to cell death.

In addition to tubular effects, glomerular changes are also noted. These effects are due to the formation of an autoantibody which localizes along the glomerular basement membrane. Glomerular damage then occurs from complement-mediated events or circulating lymphocytes. Chronic exposure to low levels of mercuric salts or mercury vapor can also induce immune-mediated glomerular toxicity, which is more common clinically than necrosis.

Organic mercurials are capable of inducing nephrotoxicity in S_2 and S_3 segments of the proximal tubule. Part of the S_3 damage results from the biotransformation of the organic mercurial to release mercuric ions. Methylmercury readily concentrates in renal proximal tubular cells and alters mitochondrial function and lysosomes. At least part of methymercury-induced nephrotoxicity may be due to homolytic scission of methylmercury to release methyl radicals and to lipid peroxidative toxicity.

Cadmium. Cadmium has a variety of uses including electroplating, galvanizing, as a color pigment, and in the manufacture of batteries. Industrial exposure is a major source of cadmium in humans, but cadmium is also found in food. Concentrations of cadmium in food vary widely, with shellfish (e.g., oysters, mussels, and scallops) being a major dietary source of cadmium (100–1000 μg/kg). Cigarettes also contain cadmium and it has been estimated that smoking one or more packs of cigarettes per day may double the body burden of cadmium.

Cadmium nephrotoxicity occurs when renal accumulation of cadmium exceeds 200 μg Cd^{2+}/g tissue. Nephrotoxicity is characterized by low-molecular-weight proteinuria (e.g., β_2-microglobulinuria in humans), glucosuria, calciuria, aminoaciduria, phosphaturia, and interstitial inflammatory reactions and fibrosis. These effects are due primarily to damage of the S_1 and S_2 segments of the proximal tubule. Glomerular damage may also occur since albuminuria is also occasionally observed.

Exposure to cadmium results in hepatic stimulation of the metal-binding protein metallothionein, a small protein with a molecular weight of approximately 6500–6800 Da. Metallothionein is composed of 20 cysteine residues whose sulfhydryl groups readily complex with seven metal ions such as cadmium. The metallothionein–cadmium complex is released from damaged hepatocytes and is carried via the blood to the kidney. The low molecular weight of the metallothionein–cadmium complex allows it to be readily filtered at the glomerulus and enter the tubular lumen. The complex is absorbed from luminal fluid via a pinocytotic mechanism in the S_1 and S_2 segments and degraded by lysosomal proteases to release free cadmium. The free cadmium can then bind to renal metallothionein or attack targets such as calmodulin within proximal tubular cells.

Lead. Lead is the most ubiquitous of the nephrotoxicant metals in the environment. Like mercury, the health effects of lead have been recognized for centuries, with the nervous system as well as the kidney being a target for certain forms of these metals. Sources of exposure to lead include food (100 μg or less/day for adults), lead-based paints, industrial emissions, lead dusts, and lead-glazed pottery.

Clinically, lead nephropathy is seen as either reversible tubular dysfunction or as an irreversible interstitial nephropathy. Tubular toxicity occurs most commonly in children following acute exposure and is characterized by glucosuria, phosphaturia, aminoaciduria, and occasionally proteinuria. One unique morphological feature of lead exposure is the formation of nuclear inclusion bodies within renal tubular cells. These bodies are complexes between lead and an acidic protein aggregate. Recently, it has been suggested that proteins in humans similar to rat α_{2u}-globulin bind lead in the liver (or other tissues) and transport lead to the kidney, where the lead:lead-binding protein complex is absorbed by an endocytotic mechanism. Within the renal cells, most of the lead is associated with the nuclear inclusion bodies. However, the lead–protein complex can be reversed with ethylenediamine tetraacetate and lead excretion promoted.

The cellular mechanism of lead nephrotoxicity appears to be due to an alteration of calcium homeostasis. Lead (Pb^{2+}) competes with calcium (Ca^{2+}) for transport, binding to calmodulin and at other cell calcium regulatory sites. Lead can accumulate in mitochondria using the calcium transporter and disrupt respiration. Interactions of lead with calmodulin can result in a disruption of the calcium messenger system to adversely affect normal cell function. The nuclear inclusion bodies may also alter the cellular function of DNA, although this interaction has not been fully elucidated.

Chronic exposure to low levels of lead results in lead accumulation within the body. Workers who have been chronically exposed to lead develop interstitial fibrosis, vascular and glomerular sclerosis, and tubular atrophy and/or hypertrophy. Although acute lead nephropathy is reversible with chelator therapy and/or removal from exposure, chronic effects may be irreversible. In addition, chronic exposure to lead may result in a gouty nephropathy because lead reduces uric acid excretion and elevates blood uric acid levels.

Halogenated Hydrocarbons

Halogenated hydrocarbons encompass a large group of chemicals with a wide range of applications. Many of these compounds are organic solvents (e.g., chloroform and trichloroethylene) or chemical intermediates (e.g., bromobenzene and chloroanilines) used in laboratory, industrial, or commercial applications. Halogenated hydrocarbons are also used in agriculture as pesticides (e.g., 1,2-dibromoethane). The majority of nephrotoxicant halogenated hydrocarbons contain chloro and/or bromo groups with only a few nephrotoxicants substituted with fluoro or iodo groups.

The site and severity of the nephrotoxic lesion also varies widely among the halogenated hydrocarbons depending on chemical class, number and position of halogen groups, age, sex, species, dose, and preexisting conditions. Unlike the metals, halogenated hydrocarbons are usually not direct nephrotoxicants and require bioactivation before the ultimate nephrotoxicant species is produced. Several mechanisms of bioactivation have been identified for the halogenated hydrocarbons including oxidation, free radical formation, intramolecular cyclization, and conjugation with glutathione (Table K-6). In the following sections, specific examples of halogenated hydrocarbons and their mechanisms of bioactivation will be discussed.

Chloroform. Chloroform (trichloromethane; Fig. K-6) has been used in the past as an anesthetic and as an additive in pharmaceutical preparations. Today, chloroform is used primarily as an organic solvent. Chloroform-induced nephrotoxicity is primarily seen as proximal tubular toxicity, with minimal changes in

TABLE K-6
Mechanisms of Bioactivation of Halogenated Hydrocarbons

Oxidation
  Example: Chloroform
Free radical formation
  Example: Carbon tetrachloride
Intramolecular cyclization
  Example: 2-Bromoethylamine
Glutathione conjugation
  Intramolecular cyclization
    Example: 1,2-Dibromoethane
  Cysteine conjugate β-lyase activation
    Example: Trichloroethylene
  Facilitated transport
    Example: Bromobenzene

distal tubular function and no evidence of glomerular effects. Nephrotoxicity is characterized by proteinuria, glucosuria, elevated BUN concentration and kidney weight, decreased accumulation of organic ions by renal cortical slices, and a fatty degeneration of proximal tubular cells. Species and sex differences exist in the susceptibility to the nephrotoxic effects induced by chloroform, with certain strains of male mice (e.g., DBA/2J) being particularly sensitive.

The mechanism of chloroform nephrotoxicity involves the oxidation of chloroform to trichloromethanol by renal cytochrome P450 isozymes (Fig. K-6). The trichloromethanol readily eliminates HCl to form the highly reactive toxicant phosgene ($COCl_2$). The phosgene can (1) be detoxified by conjugation with two molecules of glutathione, (2) react with water to form two molecules of HCl and one molecule of CO_2, or (3) covalently bind to renal macromolecules to disrupt cellular function and induce nephrotoxicity.

There are several lines of evidence which support the formation of phosgene as the ultimate nephrotoxicant species following exposure to chloroform in mice and rabbits. First, susceptible strains of male mice oxidize chloroform faster than resistant strains. Second, deuterium labeling of chloroform, to form $CDCl_3$, results in the formation of a chloroform derivative which is oxidized much slower than chloroform and is less potent as a nephrotoxicant. In addition, trapping experiments with cysteine have documented the formation of phosgene as a product of chloroform biotransformation. Although these results support phosgene as the toxicant species in mice and rabbits, it is not known with certainty if the same mechanism for nephrotoxicity is operating in humans. In humans, chloroform nephrotoxicity has been documented in both males and females, while only male mice exhibit nephrotoxicity following chloroform administration. Thus, additional or alternate mechanisms may be contributing to chloroform nephrotoxicity in humans.

Carbon Tetrachloride. Carbon tetrachloride (CCl_4) was widely used as a dry cleaning solvent until its potential as a hepatotoxicant, nephrotoxicant, and carcinogen was recognized. Currently, carbon tetra-

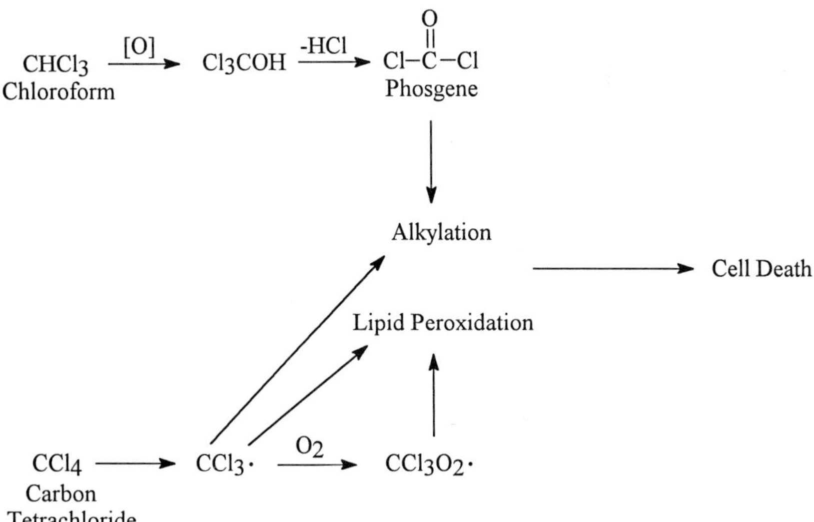

FIGURE K-6. Bioactivation of chloroform and carbon tetrachloride.

chloride is used as an organic solvent. Nephrotoxicity associated with dermal or inhalation exposure to carbon tetrachloride is seen as acute tubular necrosis, which is delayed in onset. Death occurs from acute renal failure, usually within 3 weeks of intoxication. Interestingly, humans appear to be more sensitive to acute carbon tetrachloride-induced nephrotoxicity than most animal models.

The mechanism of carbon tetrachloride nephrotoxicity involves the initial homolytic cleavage of carbon tetrachloride by cytochrome P450 to form the trichloromethyl and chlorine free radicals (Fig. K-6). The trichloromethyl free radical can then alkylate renal macromolecules or interact with membrane unsaturated fatty acids to initiate lipid peroxidation. The trichloromethyl free radical may also combine with molecular oxygen to form a peroxy free radical which is more reactive than the trichloromethyl free radical. The peroxy radical could also interact with unsaturated fatty acids in membranes to induce lipid peroxidative damage. Recently, it has been proposed that under anaerobic conditions, carbon tetrachloride is converted to a carbene metabolite (Cl_3C:) which can covalently bind to cell macromolecules in the liver. However, the role of the carbene metabolite in carbon tetrachloride nephrotoxicity is less clear.

***N*-(3,5-Dichlorophenyl)succinimide.** During the 1970s, a large number of *N*-(halophenyl)succinimides were synthesized and evaluated as agricultural fungicides. The most promising agent in this class of compounds was *N*-(3,5-dichlorophenyl)succinimide (NDPS), which had a broad spectrum of antifungal activity. NDPS, marketed as Ohric, also proved to be a nephrotoxicant and to promote the carcinogenic activity of several nephrocarcinogens. As a result of potential health hazards, NDPS has not been widely used.

Acute NDPS nephrotoxicity is characterized by diuresis, proteinuria, glucosuria, hematuria, elevated BUN concentration and kidney weight, decreased organic ion accumulation by renal cortical slices, and marked proximal tubular necrosis. Sex differences exist for NDPS nephrotoxicity with female Fischer 344 rats being twice as sensitive as males. Interestingly, the primarily sites of the renal lesion in males are the S_1 and S_2 segments of the proximal tubule, while the S_3 segment is the most affected segment in females. Chronic NDPS nephrotoxicity is seen as marked renal interstitial nephritis.

The ultimate nephrotoxicant species responsible for acute or chronic NDPS nephrotoxicity is unclear. However, oxidation of the succinimide ring in the liver via phenobarbital-inducible cytochrome P450 isozymes to form *N*-(3,5-dichlorophenyl)-2-hydroxysuccinimide (NDHS; Fig. K-7) is an essential bioactivation step in acute nephrotoxicity. Both NDHS and its hydrolysis product, *N*-(3,5-dichlorophenyl)-2-hydroxysuccinamic acid (NDHSA), are four times more potent as nephrotoxicants than NDPS, while the decarboxylation metabolite of NDHSA is a nonnephrotoxicant. However, neither NDHS nor NDHSA appear to be directly toxic to renal cortical slices, proximal tubule suspensions, or renal mitochondria. Recent studies also suggest that NDHSA can cyclize *in vivo* to form NDHS, which further clouds the identity of which NDPS metabolite ultimately gives rise to the toxicant species. Formation of sulfate and/or glucuronide conjugates of NDHS and NDHSA appears to contribute to the nephrotoxicity induced by these NDPS metabolites.

2-Haloethylamines. The 2-haloethylamines are model nephrotoxicants that target different segments of the nephron depending on the halogen atom. The bromo derivative, 2-bromoethylamine (BEA), concentrates in the renal medulla and induces renal papillary necrosis. The renal effects of BEA are dependent on the urinary concentrating ability of ADH. In the absence of ADH, urine is not concentrated in collecting ducts and BEA nephrotoxicity is diminished. The chemical species responsible for BEA nephrotoxicity is believed to be ethyleneimine formed by the intramolecular cylization of BEA, which then alkylates renal macromolecules (Fig. K-8).

The chloro derivative, 2-chloroethylamine (CEA), is less potent as a papillitoxin than BEA, presumably due to the fact that the bromo group is a better leaving group than the chloro group. Thus, the reactive intermediate, ethyleneimine, would form faster from BEA than from CEA. The fluoro derivative, 2-fluoroethylamine (FEA), is more lethal than BEA, but at nonlethal doses it is toxic to the S_3 segment of the proximal tubule rather than the renal papilla. Since the fluoro group is a poorer leaving group than chloro or bromo groups, it is not clear if FEA nephrotoxicity is due to FEA, ethyleneimine, or a FEA metabolite.

Glutathione Conjugates. Glutathione is a tripeptide (γ-Glu-Cys-Gly) which forms bonds between the

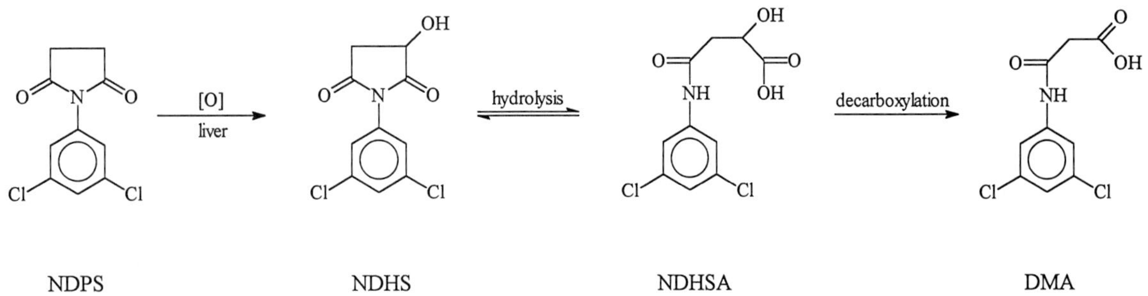

NDPS → [O] liver → NDHS ⇌ hydrolysis ⇌ NDHSA → decarboxylation → DMA

FIGURE K-7. Oxidative biotransformation of N-(3,5-dichlorophenyl)succinimide (NDPS).

sulfhydryl group of cysteine and electrophilic sites in xenobiotics or their metabolites. The formation of these glutathione conjugates is catalyzed by one or more of the glutathione *S*-transferase enzymes. The forms of glutathione *S*-transferase can also catalyze detoxification of organic peroxides to protect cells against free radical toxicity as well as electrophilic attack. Thus, interactions with glutathione serve as an important mechanism for detoxifying reactive chemical species within cells.

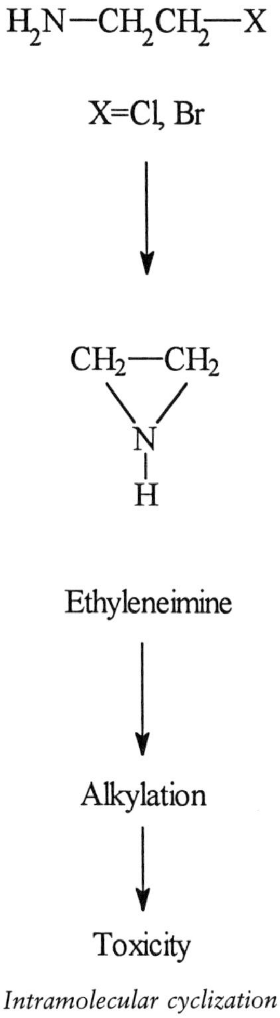

$H_2N{-}CH_2CH_2{-}X$

X=Cl, Br

↓

$CH_2{-}CH_2$ (N–H ring)

Ethyleneimine

↓

Alkylation

↓

Toxicity

FIGURE K-8. Intramolecular cyclization of haloethylamines.

Although interactions between glutathione and electrophilic molecules normally leads to detoxification, there are also several examples of bioactivation of chemicals to nephrotoxicants following glutathione conjugation. Glutathione conjugates can be formed in most segments of the kidney, with glutathione *S*-transferase activity being highest in proximal tubular cells. However, glutathione conjugates of many electrophiles are formed primarily in the liver and transported to the kidney either as the glutathione conjugate or as a glutathione conjugate metabolite.

Glutathione conjugates formed in the liver can leave hepatocytes and enter the blood or the bile. Biliary excretion of the glutathione conjugate can result in degradation of the glutathione conjugate to the cysteine conjugate within the biliary tract and small intestine. This degradation is catalyzed by γ-glutamyl transpeptidase (removes glutamate) and peptidases (remove glycine). The *N*-acetylcysteine conjugate, also known as a mercapturate, can be formed in the intestinal tract or liver following absorption of the cysteine conjugate from the small intestine by action of an *N*-acetylase enzyme. The relative amounts of the three conjugates that reach the kidney from extrarenal sites depend primarily on the chemical nature of the halogenated hydrocarbon and the animal species studied.

The kidney also can process and transport glutathione, cysteine, and *N*-acetylcysteine conjugates. Glutathione conjugates can be converted to the cysteinylglycine conjugate by γ-glutamyl transpeptidase, which is located in kidney primarily at the brush border membrane. The action of brush border dipeptidase enzymes (e.g., aminopeptidase M) then removes the glycine residue from the dipeptide conjugate to release the cysteine conjugate which is usually accumulated within proximal tubular cells. Glutathione conjugates may also be directly transported into renal cells at the basolateral membrane via a sodium-dependent uptake mechanism. Once inside the cell, the glutathione conjugate may be a substrate for γ-glutamyl cyclotransferase and peptidases to release the cysteine conjugate. Cysteine conjugates can also be substrates for amino acid uptake systems and accumulate in proximal tubular cells via the amino acid transporters, while mercapturates accumulate in proximal tubular cells via the organic anion transporter at the basolateral membrane. Accumulated mercapturates may then be secreted into the urine or deacetylated to release the corresponding cysteine conjugate. Thus, the kidney can be exposed to metabolites formed from glutathione conjugation originating at renal or extrarenal sites.

Several mechanisms have been identified for the generation of nephrotoxicants following conjugation of halogenated hydrocarbons with glutathione (Table K-6). These mechanisms include intramolecular cyclization, activation by cysteine conjugate β-lyase, and facilitated renal accumulation of the toxicant. Examples of each of these bioactivation mechanisms will be discussed in the following sections.

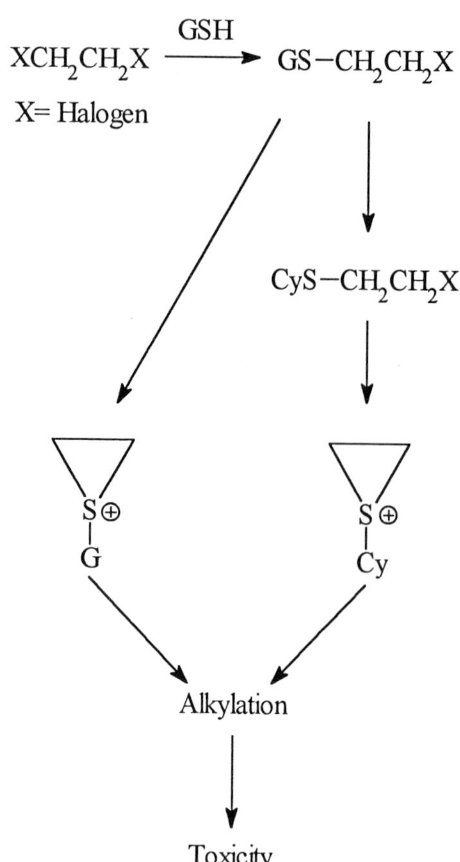

FIGURE K-9. Glutathione conjugation with 1,2-dihaloethanes.

Intramolecular Cyclization. The 1,2-dihaloethanes (XCH_2CH_2X) are used as pesticides, lead scavengers, industrial solvents, and/or grain fumigants. Both 1,2-dichloroethane and 1,2-dibromoethane are hepatotoxicants, nephrotoxicants, and potential carcinogens. Acute renal effects induced by these alkyl halides are characterized as proximal tubular necrosis, primarily in the juxtaglomerular regions. The mechanism of the nephrotoxicity induced by the 1,2-dihaloethanes is believed to initially involve conjugation of the halogenated hydrocarbon with glutathione (Fig. K-9). Both 1,2-dichloroethane and 1,2-dibromoethane form glutathione conjugates in liver, but only 1,2-dibromoethane forms a glutathione conjugate in the kidney.

The glutathione conjugate formed from 1,2-dibromoethane is relatively unstable and quickly undergoes intramolecular cyclization via displacement of the second bromo group by the glutathionyl sulfur to form an episulfonium ion (Fig. K-9). The episulfonium ion then readily forms adducts with renal cell macromolecules, including DNA, which leads to altered cell function and toxicity. Because of the highly reactive nature of the glutathione conjugate formed from 1,2-dibromoethane, it is likely that only the renally formed glutathione conjugate contributes to nephrotoxicity.

The glutathione conjugate formed in the liver from 1,2-dichloroethane is more stable than the conjugate formed from 1,2-dibromoethane and may be transported to the kidney as the glutathione or related conjugate. Within the kidney, both glutathione and cysteine conjugates appear to contribute to 1,2-dichloroethane nephrotoxicity by forming episulfonium ions which can interact with cellular macromolecules (Fig. K-9). Reactivity of the glutathione and cysteine conjugates toward DNA is greatest for the cysteine conjugate, but the relative contribution of these conjugates to the carcinogenic mechanism for 1,2-dichloroethane remains to be determined.

Two additional compounds containing 1,2-dihaloethyl groups are also nephrotoxicants. The nematocide and soil fumigant 1,2-dibromo-3-chloropropane and the flame retardant tris(2,3-dibromopropyl)phosphate both induce acute tubular necrosis. Although conjugation with glutathione may play a role in the toxicity induced by these agents, the mechanism responsible for the nephrotoxicity induced by these compounds is not known.

Cysteine Conjugate β-Lyase Activation. There are numerous glutathione and/or cysteine conjugates of unsaturated halogenated hydrocarbons that are nephrotoxicants and/or nephrocarcinogens (Table K-7). These conjugates induce nephrotoxicity following cleavage of the cysteine conjugate by the enzyme cysteine conjugate β-lyase to form pyruvate, ammonia, and a reactive thiol. Acute nephrotoxicity induced by these conjugates is characterized by diuresis, proteinuria, glucosuria, elevated BUN concentration, and proximal tubular necrosis. The site of the lesion appears to be species dependent, with most rodent models exhibiting the initial lesion in the corticomedullary region (S_3 segment of the proximal tubule). However, the initial lesion in dogs appears in the S_1 and S_2 segments of the proximal tubule. In addition, age, gender, and strain differences exist for susceptibility to the nephrotoxicity induced by these conjugates.

The nature of the ultimate nephrotoxicant species formed following the action of cysteine conjugate β-lyase is determined by the halogen substitution on the parent haloalkene. When the haloalkene is a geminal difluoroalkene (e.g., tetrafluoroethylene), then the resulting glutathione conjugate and subsequent cysteine conjugate is a saturated or alkyl conjugate (Fig. K-10). However, if the haloalkene is a geminal dichloroalkene (e.g., trichloroethylene), then unsaturated conjugates are formed (Fig. K-10). The saturated cysteine conjugates are bioactivated by β-lyase to form a thionoacyl fluoride which can rapidly acylate renal macromolecules to induce toxicity, whereas the unsaturated cysteine conjugates are bioactivated by β-lyase to the highly reactive thioketene metabolites (Fig. K-11). Primary targets for these reactive intermediates appear to be the renal mitochondria, which contain a portion of cellular cysteine conjugate β-lyase.

The reasons why the kidney is a major target for cysteine conjugate toxicity are not completely understood, particularly since cysteine conjugate β-lyase is present in organs other than the kidney. However, the ability of the kidney to (1) accumulate metabolites formed by the glutathione conjugate pathway from blood, (2) convert glutathione and *N*-acetylcysteine conjugates to cysteine conjugates, and (3) rapidly activate nephrotoxicant cysteine conjugates to their reactive intermediate may explain the susceptibility of the kidney to these agents.

The toxicity induced by nephrotoxicant glutathione, cysteine, and *N*-acetylcysteine conjugates can be modified by a variety of compounds. Probenecid, an inhibi-

TABLE K-7
Some Halogenated Hydrocarbons Whose Glutathione and/or Cysteine Conjugates Are Nephrotoxicants and/or Nephrocarcinogens

1-Chloro-1,2,2-trifluoroethylene
1,1-Dibromo-2,2-difluoroethylene
Dichloroacetylene
1,1-Dichloro-2,2-difluoroethylene
Hexachloro-1,3-butadiene
Hexafluoropropene
Tetrachloroethylene
Tetrafluoroethylene
Trichloroethylene
1,1,2-Trichloro-3,3-trifluoro-1-propene

GSH + $X_2C{=}CR_1R_2$

$R_1 = R_2 = F$ → $X_2CH{-}CF_2{-}SG$ → $X_2CH{-}CF_2{-}SCy$

$R_1 = R_2 = Cl$ → $X_2C{=}C(Cl)SG$ → $X_2C{=}C(Cl)SCy$

FIGURE K-10. Glutathione conjugation with geminal difluoro- or dichloroalkenes.

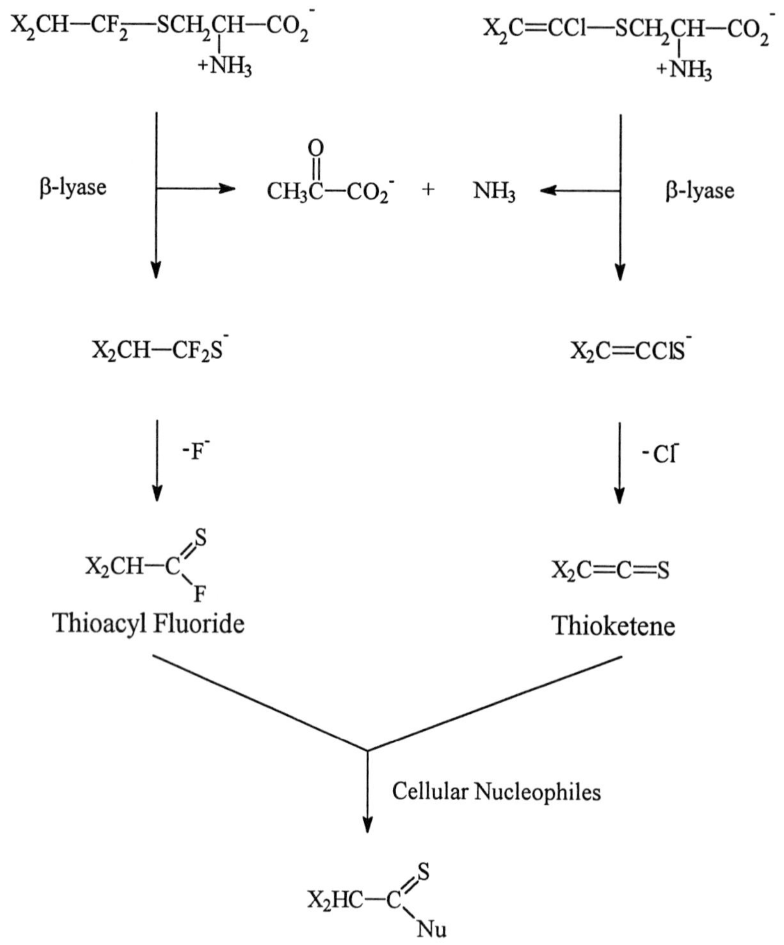

$X_2CH—CF_2—SCH_2CH(NH_3^+)—CO_2^-$ $X_2C{=}CCl—SCH_2CH(NH_3^+)—CO_2^-$

β-lyase → $CH_3C(O)—CO_2^-$ + NH_3 ← β-lyase

$X_2CH—CF_2S^-$ $X_2C{=}CClS^-$

$-F^-$ $-Cl^-$

$X_2CH—C(=S)F$ Thioacyl Fluoride $X_2C{=}C{=}S$ Thioketene

Cellular Nucleophiles

$X_2HC—C(=S)Nu$

FIGURE K-11. Cysteine conjugate β-lyase bioactivation of cysteine conjugates of haloalkenes.

tor of the organic anion transporter, can reduce the nephrotoxicity induced by glutathione conjugates, presumably by decreasing the renal accumulation of the mercapturate. Acivicin (AT-125), an anticancer agent, is an irreversible inhibitor (>97%) of γ-glutamyl transpeptidase and can attenuate the toxicity of nephrotoxicant glutathione conjugates by inhibiting conversion of the glutathione conjugate to the cysteine conjugate. In addition, aminooxyacetic acid (AOAA) inhibits the action of pyridoxal-dependent enzymes (e.g., β-lyase) and blocks the conversion of cysteine conjugates to their ultimate nephrotoxicant species. These inhibitors are useful tools in the study of glutathione and cysteine conjugate nephrotoxicity, but they may not always give clear results. Probenecid has biological effects unrelated to inhibition of organic ion transport, and acivicin pretreatment can fail to protect against haloalkene (e.g., hexachloro-1,3-butadiene) nephrotoxicity even when it is known that glutathione and/or cysteine conjugates of the parent haloalkene are nephrotoxicants. Also, AOAA not only inhibits β-lyase but can also inhibit oxidative enzymes and other pyridoxal-dependent pathways.

Facilitated Accumulation of Nephrotoxicants. Bromobenzene, a chemical intermediate, is both a hepatotoxicant and a nephrotoxicant. Bromobenzene-induced nephrotoxicity is characterized by glucosuria, enzymuria, proteinuria, elevated BUN concentration and kidney weight, and proximal tubular necrosis, with the S_3 segment exhibiting the greatest damage. Bromobenzene hepatotoxicity is due to cytochrome P450-mediated formation of a 3,4-epoxide (arene oxide) metabolite of bromobenzene which can arylate hepatic tissue. However, the formation of the ultimate nephrotoxicant species appears to require multiple biotransformation steps and possibly multiple toxicant species.

The first step in the bioactivation of bromobenzene to a nephrotoxicant is the hepatic cytochrome P450-mediated oxidation of bromobenzene to 2-bromophenol, which is further oxidized in the liver to 2-bromohydroquinone. 2-Bromohydroquinone can be activated by a renal quinol oxidase to 2-bromoquinone (Fig. K-12), which can directly arylate renal macromolecules. Although 2-bromoquinone can undergo redox cycling to potentially generate oxidative stress and reactive oxygen species, arylation appears to be more important for the cellular toxicity induced by 2-bromoquinone.

Recent studies have also demonstrated that mono- and diglutathione conjugates of 2-bromohydroquinone can be formed *in vivo* in rats (Fig. K-12). The diglutathionyl conjugate of 2-bromohydroquinone (a quinol-thioether) induces nephrotoxicity which is indistinguishable from bromobenzene, 2-bromophenol, or 2-bromohydroquinone nephrotoxicity, but occurs at a dose 10–15 times lower than with 2-bromohydroquinone. The ability of acivicin but not AOAA to attenuate nephrotoxicity induced by the diglutathionyl conjugate has suggested that γ-glutamyl transpeptidase but not β-lyase is important in activating the conjugate. Thus, entry into renal tissue via γ-glutamyl transpeptidase is a key step for diglutathionyl conjugate nephrotoxicity. Partial protection by acivicin against 2-bromohydroquinone nephrotoxicity *in vivo* suggests that the mono- and/or diglutathionyl conjugates of 2-bromohydroquinone may be formed extrarenally, and that glutathione conjugation may play a role in the transport and selective accumulation of 2-bromohydroquinone in renal tissue.

The cellular mechanism of nephrotoxicity induced by the quinol-thioethers appears to be related to the ability of the conjugates to undergo redox cycling with the concomitant formation of reactive oxygen species and oxidative stress. The cysteine conjugates of 2-bromohydroquinone are more readily oxidized than the corresponding glutathione conjugates or mercapturates and, therefore, are probably responsible for most of the conjugate-induced oxidative stress and resultant nephrotoxicity. However, the exact nature of the subcellular targets and relative contributions of the various bromobenzene metabolites to bromobenzene nephrotoxicity remain to be determined.

Mycotoxins. The mycotoxins are secondary products of fungal metabolism. Numerous mycotoxins have

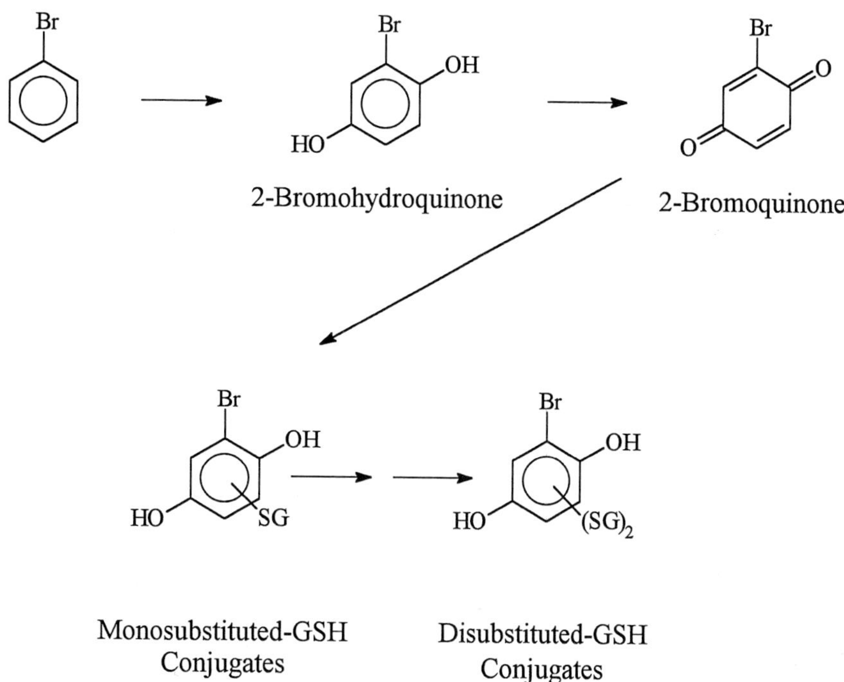

FIGURE K-12. Bioactivation of bromobenzene to nephrotoxicant metabolites.

been identified as toxicants in humans and/or animal models with several organ systems, including the kidney, being targets for these fungal products. Perhaps the two mycotoxins which have received the most attention as nephrotoxicants are citrinin and ochratoxin A. These two mycotoxins have received particular interest due to their possible role in endemic Balkan nephropathy.

Citrinin is produced by several *Penicillium* and *Aspergillus* species which may be found associated with grains (e.g., wheat and oats). Humans and animals eating the grain can experience citrinin-induced nephrotoxicity, which is characterized by diuresis, decreased urinary osmolality, glucosuria, proteinuria, and elevated BUN concentration. Morphological changes included cytoplasmic vacuolization of proximal tubular cells, mitochondrial swelling, and, ultimately, proximal tubular necrosis. The exact site of the renal lesion may vary depending on the species studied.

The mechanism of citrinin-induced nephrotoxicity has not been completely elucidated. However, it appears that citrinin accumulates in proximal tubular cells via the organic anion transporter, and that the parent compound is the nephrotoxicant species. Mitochondria are early targets for citrinin, with multiple effects on mitochondrial function observed following exposure of mitochondria to citrinin, including uncoupling of mitochondrial respiration. The subsequent loss of cellular ATP content may eventually lead to cell death.

Ochratoxin A is also produced by the *Aspergillus* species and is one of the most widely occurring mycotoxins in food and grains. Ochratoxin A nephrotoxicity is similar to citrinin nephrotoxicity but can also include renal interstitial fibrosis and glomerular changes. Like citrinin, ochratoxin A accumulates in proximal tubular cells via the organic anion transporter and appears to induce nephrotoxicity without bioactivation to a toxic metabolite. Mitochondria are also a target for ochratoxin A, with proximal tubular ATP content significantly decreased in the presence of as little as 10^{-8} M ochratoxin A. However, ochratoxin A also inhibits renal gluconeogenesis and lowers mRNA levels, and it has been suggested that these events may also contribute to ochratoxin A nephrotoxicity. While each of these cellular effects might contribute to the renal toxicity induced by ochratoxin A, the precise cellular mechanism of toxicity remains to be determined.

TABLE K-8
Miscellaneous Nephrotoxicants

Petroleum
Carbon disulfide
Oxalic acid
Venoms
Crotalus venom
Brown recluse spider venom
Decalin
Tetralin
Mushroom poisoning
d-Limonene
Carbon monoxide
1,4-Dichlorobenzene
Paraquat
Lindane
Diquat
3-Chloropropane
Glycols
Maleic acid
Ethylene glycol
Propylene glycol
Glycerol
Radiation
Physical agents
Crush injuries

Miscellaneous Environmental Nephrotoxicants

There are numerous additional agents which have been identified as nephrotoxicants, and some of these chemical and physical agents are shown in Table K-8. In addition to the compounds listed, there are hundreds of chemicals whose effects on the kidney are either unknown or are poorly characterized, and unquestionably this list will continue to grow with the ongoing development of newer drugs, agricultural agents, and industrial intermediates.

Further Reading

Anders, M. W. *et al.* (Eds.) (1993). *Renal Disposition and Nephrotoxicity of Xenobiotics.* Academic Press, New York.

Commandeur, J. N. M., and Vermeulen, N. P. E. (1990). Molecular and biochemical mechanisms of chemically induced nephrotoxicity: A review. *Chem. Res. Toxicol.* 3, 171–194.

Goldstein, R. S. (Ed.) (1997). *Comprehensive Toxicology: Renal Toxicology,* Vol. 7. Pergamon, New York.

Hewitt, W. R. *et al.* (1991). Toxic responses of the kidney. In *Casarett and Doull's Toxicology: The Basic Science of Poisons* (M. O. Amdur *et al.*, Eds.), 4th ed., pp. 354–382. Pergamon, New York.

Hook, J. B., and Goldstein, R. S. (Eds.) (1993). *Toxicology of the Kidney,* 2nd ed. Raven, New York.

—*Gary O. Rankin*

Related Topics

Cell Proliferation
Glutathione
Lipid Peroxidation
Metallothionein
Metals
Mycotoxins
Tissue Repair

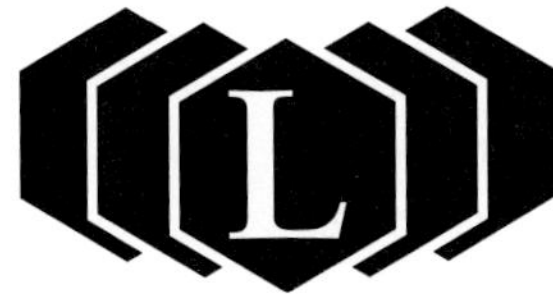

LD_{50}/LC_{50}

Introduction

The lethal dose 50% (LD_{50}) is the statistically calculated dose (or concentration) of a material (generally expressed as an amount of material per unit of body weight) which would be expected to cause the death of half the members of the target species receiving it. The lethal concentration 50% (LC_{50}) is the equivalent statistical projection for inhalation.

When did modern Western society become concerned with lethality testing? For what reasons were protocols developed for describing lethality in animals in quantitative terms for the purposes of making scientific, regulatory, or marketing decisions? Interestingly, in this age of genetic engineering, few people realize that biologically derived materials were the subject of regulations well before the passage of the Pure Food and Drug Act in 1906. In 1901, a diphtheria epidemic broke out in St. Louis because of improperly manufactured antidiphtheria toxin. In response to the resulting public outcry, the U.S. Congress passed the Virus Act of 1902. It regulated all viruses, serums, toxins, antitoxins, and other such products sold for the prevention or cure of disease in man. Among other things, the bill eventually established consistent potency criteria. In fact, by World War II the U.S. FDA was requiring batch-to-batch certification and release for biologicals, a policy that remains in effect for certain drugs. Hence, the earliest lethality testing was for the purpose of establishing consistent potencies of biologicals, such as diphtheria toxin, and not for evaluating synthetic chemicals.

One of the earliest publications discussing lethality testing was an investigation into the lethality of diphtheria toxin in guinea pigs. The Sudermerson and Glenny paper describes lethality empirically in terms of percentage of dead animals at each dosage because methods for calculating lethality curves and the median lethal dosage had not yet been developed. The authors reported that lethal response to a given dosage of toxin varied with time of the year. Hence, years before the term LD_{50} came into parlance, supposedly as an exact indicator of toxicity, data had been published attesting to the volatility and imprecision of this calculated parameter.

Because the first use of lethality testing was in describing potency of biologicals, it only makes sense that the same methods were soon applied to extracted botanicals. (Note: There is no doubt that both the Germans and English tested in animals the various poison gases employed during World War I. Little of this work, however, appears to have been published in the open scientific literature, although portions of it have recently been made public.) In 1926, de Lind van Wijngaarden published on the lethality of digitalis extracts. Interestingly, he did not plot his data as mortality vs dose. He delivered his extracts intravenously and titrated the dosage until he achieved complete heart stoppage. He was thus able to determine the precise lethal dosage for each animal and noted that these followed a bell-shaped or Gaussian distribution. His experiments took 5 years and used more than 500 cats, an effort that would have been excessive and expensive by today's standards. However, he did conclude that no more than 9 cats would normally be required to "calibrate" an extract of digitalis. Trevan, in a pivotal paper (1927), described the lethality of strophanthin, cocaine, and insulin. Modern reviews have focused a great deal of attention on the large number of frogs used by Trevan. Most of the data he discussed, however, were derived from experiments in mice using cocaine or insulin. We suspect that so little attention was given to this aspect of Trevan's paper, even though it comprised the major portions of his work (which ran 31 pages and contained 11 figures and 6 tables of data) because it has never been replicated. For some of the lethality curves reported by Trevan, well over 900 mice were dosed. Again, such efforts would be excessive and expensive by today's standards but were necessitated, in part, by the less rigorous method of deriving lethality curves and calculating the median lethal dosage (LD_{50}). Modern methods of data transformation and statistical analysis were, at that time, still in their infancy. He also recognized that it was not necessary to describe an entire dosage response curve to calculate an LD_{50}. He, in fact, recommended that lethality determinations start with small groups of two or three animals each and that larger groups be used for confirmatory purposes.

Behren confirmed the observations of both de Lind van Wijngaarden and Trevan. It is clear, from his article, that the use of animals for standardizing digitalis extracts was accepted to the point of being incorporated into the German and Dutch pharmacopoeias. The objective of his paper was to compare the cat and frog methods and develop a basis for using fewer animals. He concluded that the frog method was superior and that no more than 44 frogs needed to be used, which was considerably less than the 100–200 frogs prescribed in the German pharmacopoeia of that period. Interestingly, these early papers are often criticized with regard to the numbers of animals used, but the objectives and conclusions are often ignored.

Both Trevan and Behrens noted that when the percentage of animals that died at specific dosages were plotted against the logarithm of the dosage, the resulting curve (the lethal dosage curve) had a sigmoidal shape slope and range that was "characteristic" for the species and the test substance. Shackell (1925) first pointed out that such curves are integrated or cumulative frequency curves (or ogives) and coined the term "dose response ogive" (curve). Trevan noted that these curves owe their shape to the fact that different individual animals require different quantities of poison for death to occur. It was also Trevan who identified the midpoint on this curve as being the dosage that would kill 50% of the animals exposed. He designed that point as the median lethal dose, or LD_{50}, and, thus, is widely credited with having developed the classical LD_{50}. Trevan and Behrans essentially read the LD_{50} directly from their mortality dose–response curves.

Lethality testing of biologicals and botanicals were essentially a response to governmental regulation. It was only natural that similar methods would be applied to synthetic chemicals. Major chemical companies started establishing toxicity or industrial health laboratories during the 1930s; the lethality testing of synthetic chemicals was established by the 1930s. However, there were no regulatory requirements for such tests. In fact, there was no premarketing toxicity testing of synthetic chemicals required at all. In 1937, an elixir of sulfanilamide dissolved in ethylene glycol was introduced into the marketplace. Over 100 people died as a result of ethylene glycol toxicity. The public response to this tragedy helped prompt the U.S. Congress to pass the Federal Food, Drug, and Cosmetic Act of 1938. It was this law that mandated the premarket testing of drugs for safety in experimental animals. By the mid-1940s, most chemical and pharmaceutical companies were routinely testing new chemicals for lethality. In fact, until the 1960s, preclinical or premarketing toxicity data packages normally consisted of little more than acute lethality data. Recently, new laws, increased scientific sophistication, and greater societal concern over sublethal chronic toxicity has led to more extensive and expensive preclinical or premarketing toxicity testing packages, where acute lethality is a small, but still real, concern.

The protocols used to assess lethality have changed considerably since the 1920s. While the principles originally described by Trevan have never been questioned, the methods for calculating the LD_{50} have become more sophisticated and the need for the high degree of precision has been questioned. The practical result is that in using modern protocols, relatively few animals are required to obtain sufficient lethality data to meet most purposes.

Protocol Designs

General Considerations

Whatever type of experimental protocol one chooses to use in a lethality test, there are certain principles and criteria that should be universally applied. The principles are especially relevant in studies in which small numbers of animals will be used.

First, a wide variety of intrinsic and extrinsic factors can influence the outcome of a lethality test. These include species, strain or substrain, age, weight, and sex of the animals; husbandry practices (e.g., type of bedding and cage population); environmental conditions; feed and water quality; nutritional state; and volume and vehicles of test substance delivery. The point to be made here is that the criteria for all these factors should be specified in detail in the protocol and strict adherence to the protocol observed. Otherwise, intrastudy comparisons are invalid. Small differences in protocols can cause large differences in the LD_{50} and are probably the major cause of the considerable laboratory-to-laboratory variation in the LD_{50}s.

Second, because the animals will generally receive a single exposure, great care must be given to the preparation and delivery of the test articles. In a chronic study, occasional miscalculations or misdelivery of the dosage would not generally greatly affect the study outcome but would clearly have a greater effect on the conclusions of a lethality screen. One should always include appropriate safeguards.

Third, one must make sure that all animals are successfully dosed and that accidental deaths are identified as such. In acute rodent studies, we routinely assign spare animals to a dosing group. Permanent numbers are not assigned until we are certain that the dose has been successfully delivered (e.g., Was the supposedly intraperitoneal dose accidentally delivered intravenously? Was there reflux from the site?). Spare animals not dosed are returned to the pool of animals available for the study. Animals found dead should be examined for evidence of accidental trauma. For example, it is not uncommon for a rat to suddenly move while being gavaged. This may result in a torn esophagus that may take a day or two to become evident. Depending on the administration route, one must pay close attention to dosing techniques and the volume limitations imposed by these techniques. For example, 20 ml/kg is the maximum volume that should be given orally to a rodent. Deaths that are clearly accidental should not be considered in the final conclusions.

Fourth, lethality protocols, by the nature of the question they address, do not specify all dosages. This can sometimes result in a study in which absurdly high dosages are administered. Hence, all protocols should clearly state what the ceiling or limit dosage will be and the reasons for selection.

Classical (Traditional) Designs

The classical or traditional methods of determining the lethality of a substance have been established since the 1920s. In discussing this type of study design, it is assumed that what is desired is an LD_{50} and the slope of the lethality curve. In general, these are only necessary for meeting specific regulatory guidelines. If less precise information will suffice (which is generally the case), other protocols can be used. Briefly, this type of protocol specifies that animals (of the same species/strain, sex, and age) be divided up into groups. All the animals in a specified group receive the same dosage. Different groups are treated at different dosages. All animals are treated by the same route. The animals are then held and observed for a set and consistent period of time—usually 14 days.

Mortality in each group is calculated on the basis of the number of animals that die during the observation period and is normally presented in percentage terms: (number dead/number dosed) $\times$ 100. If mortality at each dosage is plotted against dosages, a sigmoidal dose–response curve is obtained. The LD_{50} is simply the dosage, either observed or calculated, that yields 50% mortality. Seldom are such curves reported as such because the LD_{50} is difficult to read off a curvilinear plot and the small number of dosages normally used make drawing an accurate lethal dosage curve difficult. It is most common to probit transform the data to obtain a rectilinear plot.

Traditionally, because of U.S. FDA and foreign regulatory guidelines, protocols have frequently been designed as batteries, including both sexes of two species (generally rats and mice) and two routes of administration. At least one route must be the intended or the most probable human exposure route. Hence, such protocols generally result in the generation of eight lethal dosage curves (1/route/sex/species). In the drug industry (where this approach is common), the two routes are generally oral and intraperitoneal for an oral drug and oral and intravenous for an intravenous drug.

While such extensive data packages may still be required for regulatory purposes, scientifically they are of little value. First, there is no reason to assume that either the rat or the mouse is the better predictor for humans than the other—or for each other. The only general correlation between the rat and mouse LD_{50} is that when one is high, so is the other. Obtaining lethality data from two different rodents, rather than a single species, does not generally change our conclusions nor improve our understanding of the toxicity of a drug or chemical or the potential hazard to humans. It is recommended that a simple preliminary screen be performed to pick out the most sensitive species and a rigorous protocol applied only to that species. Because the slope of the fitted line in these assays has a very large uncertainty, in relation to the uncertainty of the LD_{50} itself (the midpoint of the distribution), much caution must be used with calculated lethal doses other than LD_{50}s. It is quite possible to calculate values for other points along the lethality curve, such as the LD_{35}, a value close to the LD_{50}, but these are not precise or statistically "stable" values due to the shape of the curve in areas away from the center point.

—Shayne C. Gad

Further Reading

Gad, S. C., and Chengelis, C. P. (1997). *Acute Toxicology: Principles and Methods.* 2nd ed. Academic Press, San Diego.

Gad, S. C., and Weil, C. S. (1997), *Statistics and Experimental Design for Toxicologists,* 3rd ed. CRC Press, Boca Raton, FL.

Related Topics

Dose–Response Relationship
Federal Food, Drug and Cosmetic Act
Levels of Effect in Toxicological Assessment
Maximum Acceptable Concentration
Maximum Tolerated Dose
Structure–Activity Relationships
Toxicity Testing

Lead (Pb)

- CAS: 7439-92-1
- Selected Compounds: Lead arsenate, $Pb_3(AsO_4)_2$ (CAS: 7784-40-9); lead chromate, $PbCrO_4$ (CAS: 7758-97-6); tetraethyl lead, $Pb(C_2H_5)_4$ (CAS: 78-00-2)
- Chemical Class: Metals

Uses

Lead and its compounds are widely used throughout industry. They are found in lead-acid storage batteries, paints, sheet metal, bearings, solder, piping, and ammunition. Lead arsenate is used in insecticides and herbicides. Lead chromate is used as a yellow pigment in paints, rubber, plastics, and ceramic coatings.

Various arts and hobbies involve lead-containing materials. Lead is found in artist's paints (certain pigments), ceramic glazes (particularly reds), solder used in stained glass windows, and linings in containers used for distilling homemade whiskey. Certain Mexican, Middle Eastern, and Asian folk remedies and cosmetics contain lead.

In the past, lead solder was used to seal canned foods and lead pipes were used to carry drinking water. Tetraethyl lead was once routinely added to gasoline as an antiknock agent; certain vehicles may still use leaded gasoline (e.g., agricultural vehicles). Lead was commonly used in paint, with certain formulations containing up to 50% lead.

Exposure Pathways

Exposure to lead and its compounds may occur through ingestion, inhalation, or dermal contact. The specific characteristics of a lead compound influence how exposure is to occur through a particular route and the degree of absorption into the body through that route.

Most inorganic forms of lead are not well absorbed through the skin, whereas organic forms (e.g., tetraethyl lead) are more likely to be absorbed through skin.

For the general population, ingestion of contaminated water and food is the primary source of exposure to lead. The average adult ingests approximately 300 μg of lead each day in food. Inhalation is the most significant route of exposure to lead in the workplace.

Respirable particulate or gaseous forms of lead may be inhaled. Sources include cigarette smoke; vehicle exhaust; emissions from municipal waste incinerators, iron and steel plants, smelting and refining operations, lead-acid battery manufacturing facilities, and sandblasting and burning of surfaces coated with lead paint. Particulate air emissions may eventually deposit and contaminate soil.

Direct release of lead-containing industrial wastewater into surface water or ground-water may ultimately impact drinking water. Lead may also be present in drinking water because of leaching from old pipes, solder, water coolers, or faucets. Some historians attribute the Fall of the Roman Empire to the effects of lead leaching from drinking water pipes and wine casks.

Food may contain low levels of lead due to uptake from the environment or higher levels due to lead leaching from containers (e.g., lead crystal or lead-containing glazes on earthenware). An important cause of lead poisoning in young children is ingestion of peeling and chipping lead-based paint in older homes.

Toxicokinetics

Lead is readily absorbed through the digestive tract. Absorption becomes less efficient with age. Children absorb between 30 and 50% of ingested lead, whereas adults absorb less than one-third of that amount (between 5 and 15%). This absorption is enhanced by diets deficient in iron, zinc, and calcium. Absorption is generally greater for organic forms. Lead is well absorbed from the lung (from 50 to 70% of respirable lead particulate). Generally, inorganic forms of lead are not absorbed through the skin, while organic forms (e.g., tetraethyl lead) can be absorbed.

Once absorbed, lead distributes throughout the body tissues via the blood. Almost all (approximately 95%) of lead in the blood is found in red blood cells. There are two primary sites in the red blood cell where lead complexes: the membrane and the hemoglobin. The concentration of lead in the blood is used as an indicator of recent lead exposure.

Lead tends to accumulate in the kidneys, the brain (i.e., the gray matter and various nuclei), and the skeleton. Lead can cross the placenta and has been shown to accumulate in the developing child. Prolonged exposure to lead (>4 weeks) in young children can lead to the accumulation of lead in the growth plates at the end of the long bones.

The total body burden of lead is a function of the balance between the amount being taken in (all routes combined), the amount distributed throughout the tissues, and the amount being excreted. Most of the body burden of lead is sequestered in the bones and teeth—over 70% in children and over 90% in adults. The remainder of the body burden is distributed between soft tissue and the blood. Lead is stored in the bone for the greatest length of time. The estimated half-lives of lead range from 10 to 30 years in bone, 40 days in soft tissues, and from 28 to 36 days in blood (in adults). Children tend to retain approximately five times more absorbed lead than adults.

In young children (<3 years) the blood–brain barrier (an anatomical barrier that limits access to the brain) is not fully developed. Inorganic lead circulating in the blood is much more likely to reach the brain in an infant or very young child.

Chronic high-level exposure to lead can result in the accumulation of large stores of lead in the bone that can be slowly released over many years after the initial exposure has stopped. The release of lead from bone may be accelerated under certain conditions, including high stress, certain metabolic fluctuations, and pregnancy.

Lead is excreted from the body in bile (into feces), and in urine, sweat, sloughed off skin cells, and lost hair.

Mechanisms of Toxicity

Lead can affect most organs and systems in the body. It can interfere with certain cellular signaling processes, the generation of action potentials in certain nerve cells, and the function of a number of enzymes. Lead interferes with the sodium–potassium ATPase pump on cell membranes, the metabolism of vitamin D, heme synthesis, certain enzymes involved in oxidative phosphorylation (cytochromes), and calcium uptake and metabolism. In addition, lead can interfere with signal transmissions in nerve cells, including dopaminergic transmissions and signaling processes at the postsynaptic and presynaptic junctions. Lead can depress the function of the adrenal glands and the thyroid.

Lead binds certain active groups on protein (e.g., sulfhydral groups) and therefore may change the structure and function of certain proteins and enzymes. Lead interferes with the biosynthesis of heme in at least two steps in the multistepped process. Heme proteins are important to the structure and function of hemoglobin in red blood cells. Lead binds with δ-aminolevulinic acid dehydratase and depresses its activity. This biochemical block explains the occurrence of anemia found in chronic lead poisoning. Measurement of the blood levels of this enzyme is used as a test for lead intoxication. Lead also interferes with the incorporation of ferrous iron into the porphyrin ring. If iron is not attached to heme, then zinc will occupy the iron binding site. The concentration of zinc protoporphyrin also can be used as a diagnostic tool for lead poisoning.

Human Toxicity

Lead can disturb cellular and molecular processes in the body and affect many organs and physiological functions. The probability of adverse health effects occurring is related to the level of exposure, duration of exposure, and total body burden. The adverse effects associated with exposure to lead are a function of dose and are usually the same regardless of the route of exposure. The primary targets for toxicity are the nervous system, the blood, and the kidneys. Reproductive effects can also occur and include male infertility, abortion, and neonatal morbidity and mortality. Lead may damage sperm and parts of the reproductive tract. Chromosomal effects have been observed in lead-exposed workers. Other effects include impairment of the immune system, which has been associated with joint pains (lead arthralgia) related to gout, and myocarditis and cardiac fibrosis.

The most sensitive and vulnerable target for lead appears to be the nervous system. Exposure to high concentrations of lead can cause either encephalopathy or peripheral neuropathy. Encephalopathy is rare in adults but is more likely to occur in significantly exposed children. It has been observed in young children (1 and 3 years) following chronic lead poisoning due to ingestion of significant amounts of lead-based paint. Typically there is gastrointestinal distress (e.g., colic), disorientation, stupor, seizures, and coma.

Significant early childhood exposure has been associated with certain neuropsychiatric changes, including learning disorders, decreased IQ, behavioral abnormalities (e.g., hyperactivity), and deficits in vocabulary. In addition, decreased growth, loss of hearing acuity, deficits in reaction time, fine motor dysfunction, developmental abnormalities, deficits in hand/eye coordination, anemia, and death have been associated with exposure in children. Symptoms of acute exposure in young children include anorexia, vomiting, and irritability. In cases of very high levels of exposure, symptoms may also include slurred speech, peripheral neuropathy, paralysis, convulsions, and coma.

Exposure to lead in adults has been associated with hypertension, nephropathy, decreased hearing acuity, anemia, peripheral neuropathy, and encephalopathy. Acute exposure in adults may cause gastrointestinal effects, pain in arms and legs, and hypertension. Exposure to very high levels may cause tremor, memory loss, confusion, stupor, renal failure, convulsions, and coma. Onset of symptoms may be slow with chronic exposure.

Anemia, common in chronically exposed adults and children, tends to be more severe in children. The life span of red blood cells decreases when lead concentrations in blood increase. In the past, the morphology of various blood cells was used to diagnose lead poisoning.

Clinical Management

The decision to actively treat a patient exposed to lead is made based on a number of criteria, including patient history, symptomology, blood lead levels, and other indicators of level of exposure.

It is common to screen for exposure to lead based on blood lead levels (μg/dl). Certain exposure criteria are expressed in terms of an acceptable blood lead level. The Centers for Disease Control in Atlanta defines 9 μg/dl as a trigger for concern in young children. The concentration of erythrocyte protoporphyrin (EP; a heme-containing protein) in red blood cells is also used to indicate exposure levels. The higher the concentrations of EP, the higher the exposure. X-ray techniques may be used to estimate concentrations of lead in bone and teeth.

Chelation therapy is usually the treatment of choice. Both $CaNa_2$–EDTA (calcium disodium salt of ethylene diamine tetraacetic acid) and British Anti-Lewisite compound (BAL; 2,3-dimercaptopropanol) are commonly used to remove lead from the body. Both are administered via intramuscular injection. BAL binds lead to sulfhydral groups and chelates metal from both inside and outside the cellular space. Lead removal in the bile and urine is increased within 30 min of administration. BAL is the common choice when there is known toxicity to the kidney, but it is contraindicated if there is liver failure or glucose-6-phosphate dehydrogenase deficiency. BAL treatment has produced a number of adverse reactions, including nausea, vomiting, tachycardia, and fever.

$CaNa_2$–EDTA binds extracellular lead. After administration, excretion of lead through the kidneys may be increased 20- to 50-fold. If there is renal dysfunction, use of $CaNa_2$–EDTA may enhance toxicity. Blood lead levels may rise after the administration of $CaNa_2$–EDTA alone. BAL is usually given with $CaNa_2$–EDTA to reduce toxicity associated with the mobilization of lead stored in soft tissues. $CaNa_2$–EDTA is usually not used for patients with known low zinc stores. Sodium–EDTA is not used to treat lead poisoning because it will also chelate and reduce calcium in the body.

D-Penicillamine, a chelating agent that can be administered orally, is currently used to chelate lead on an experimental basis. Individuals who are allergic to penicillin may experience adverse reactions to this agent; toxic effects have been reported in as many as 20% of the patients treated with this compound.

2,3-Dimercapto-1-propanesulfonic acid and dimercaptosuccinic acid have mechanisms of action similar to BAL. Both are water-soluble analogs of BAL that can be administered orally, are less toxic, and have fewer unpleasant side effects than BAL. They have been found to be effective in removing lead via the kidneys. Treatment regimens may also include removal from the source of exposure and changes in the patient's diet.

Animal Toxicity

Oral exposure to certain lead compounds has been shown to induce tumors in kidneys of rats and mice in more than 20 studies. Based on this animal data, lead is classified as a probable human carcinogen by several agencies including the U.S. EPA.

The impact of environmental lead on wildlife and ecosystems has been a subject of study and concern. Water fowl may become poisoned from ingesting lead shot. Poisoning may lead to anorexia, lethargy, coma, and death. Other birds have also been shown to be impacted by environmental lead. In dogs, sheep, goats, and cattle, there have been reports of toxicity resulting from contact with environmental lead. Sources of exposure may include lead salts, lead-based paints, and waste oils.

Lead can disrupt learned behavior in certain adult animals and has been shown to disrupt learning and memory in certain young animals. Young animals tend to be more susceptible to the effects of lead than older animals. Studies on monkeys have shown fetal abnormalities and effects after lead exposure. Effects included encephalopathy and offspring that exhibited neurological and behavioral symptoms at maturity.

—Betty J. Locey, Arthur Furst, and Shirley B. Radding

Related Topics

Dimercaptopropanol, 2,3-
Behavioral Toxicology
Developmental Toxicology
EDTA
Kidney
Metals
Neurotoxicology
Occupational Toxicology
Pollution, Air
Pollution, Water
Psychological Indices of Toxicity
Reproductive System, Male
Skeletal System
Toxicology, History of
Veterinary Toxicology

Levels of Effect in Toxicological Assessment

Interpretation of data collected during a toxicological assessment study includes establishing the highest dosages levels at which toxicological effects become evident or are absent. This process is much like climbing a ladder, going from no effect to profound toxicity.

No-Observed-Effect Level (NOEL)

At this dosage level, there is (based on the data available) no identifiable difference between the control group and the treated groups.

No-Observed-Adverse-Effect Level (NOAEL)

The NOAEL is also referred to by some as the no-observed-toxic-effect level. Drugs, in particular, are expected to have biological activity of some sort. Thus, it would not be unexpected for a drug or chemical to have a biological effect that it is not necessarily adverse. For example, a drug may cause only a slight but real decrease in serum cholesterol. This would, in the absence of any other effect (based on the data available), not be considered evidence of toxicity. A new chemical may cause only a slight decrease in body weight gain, which often in rats increases survival and decreases morbidity. In rats, extensive treatment with a large variety of organic substance can cause increases in liver weight with no change in function or pathologic change in structure. This would more rightfully be considered an adaptive, not a toxic response.

Lowest-Observed-Effect Level (LOEL)

This is the dose at which some evidence of biological activity, which is not necessarily adverse, becomes apparent.

Lowest-Observed-Adverse-Effect Level (LOAEL)

This may also be considered the threshold level. This is the lowest dose at which a clear clinical sign of toxicity and/or target organ effects are noted which are part of a dose–response phenomenon.

While the aforementioned definitions are commonly used, the U.S. EPA has a slightly different official stance. This agency regulates pesticides and other chemicals that have no therapeutic benefit. The agency's primary concern is safety assessment. Thus, for the U.S. EPA, the NOEL is defined as the highest dose at which toxicological relevant or adverse effects were not detected. Thus, for the U.S. EPA, the NOEL is essentially the same as aforementioned NOAEL. The European Union uses definitions more similar to those given in the proceeding paragraphs.

—*C. P. Chengelis*

Related Topics

Dose–Response Relationship
LD_{50}/LC_{50}
Maximum Allowable Concentration
Maximum Tolerated Dose
Median Lethal Dose
Toxicity Testing

Levothyroxine

- CAS: 51-48-9
- SYNONYMS: L-Thyroxine; T4; Thyroxine; Synthroid
- PHARMACEUTICAL CLASS: Synthetic thyroid hormone
- CHEMICAL STRUCTURE:

I I NH₂ HO O CH₂C COONa · xH₂O I I H

Uses

Levothyroxine is used for thyroid replacement and in the treatment of hypothyroidism, nonendemic goiter, and chronic lymphocytic thyroiditis.

Exposure Pathways

Ingestion is the most common route of accidental and intentional exposure to levothyroxine. It is also available in an intravenous dosage form.

Toxicokinetics

Approximately 50% of levothyroxine (T4) is bioavailable. Peak serum T4 levels occur 2–6 hr after therapeutic dosing. Approximately 99% of T4 is protein bound. T4 has a volume of distribution of 8–10 liters/kg. From 75 to 85% of T4 is deiodinated in the liver, kidney, muscles, heart, and brain. Half of this is converted to active T3. Only 20% of T4 is excreted in the feces intact; 10% of conjugated T4 is excreted in the urine. The half-life of T4 is 5.3–9.4 days in euthyroid patients.

Mechanism of Toxicity

Thyroid compounds are necessary for metabolism, growth, and development. T4's primary action is related to calorigenesis and protein synthesis. Thyroid hormones potentiate the effects of catecholamines. About 40% of T4 is converted to T3. T3 is three to five times more toxic than T4. Protein binding, volume of distribution, clearance rate, half-life, and the conversion of T4 to T3 all function to maintain an euthyroid state even in acute overdose. Toxicity is an extension of the pharmacologic effects.

Human Toxicity: Acute

In general, adults and children can tolerate acute overdoses of T4. Ingestion of 3 mg of T4 is sufficient to produce symptoms in both adults and children. In acute exposures, symptomatology is generally mild. Symptoms may develop days after ingestion when T4 is converted to the more toxic T3. Symptoms may include tachycardia, nausea, vomiting, diarrhea, restlessness, and fever. Fever is usually an early symptom of toxicity, whereas restlessness and tachycardia usually develop days after exposure.

Human Toxicity: Chronic

The concern with chronic exposure is the development of thyrotoxicosis. The development of thyrotoxicosis in an acute exposure is rare. Thyrotoxicosis is characterized by tachycardia, cardiac arrhythmias, hypertension, tremors, and seizures. In patients with severe toxicity, coma and circulatory collapse can result.

Clinical Management

Basic and advanced life-support measures should be utilized as needed. Gastric emptying is recommended in ingestions of 2 mg or more of levothyroxine. Emesis, lavage, and activated charcoal can be utilized based on the time of exposure and patient's symptoms. If emesis is induced at home in the asymptomatic patient, the patient should be monitored for signs of toxicity that may develop 5–11 days after exposure. In the hospital setting, EKG and blood pressure monitoring should be performed. Propranolol should be given to treat adrenergic symptoms that occur with hyperthyroidism. Diuresis and hemoperfusion are not effective in levothyroxine overdose.

Animal Toxicity

Both dogs and cats are at risk for thyroid toxicity. Signs of toxicity in animals include vomiting, diarrhea, tachycardia, tachypnea, decreased level of consciousness, and restlessness.

—*Bridget Flaherty*

Related Topics

Endocrine System
Liothyronine
Thyroid Extract

Lidocaine

- CAS: 137-58-6
- SYNONYMS: Xylocaine; Caine-1; Delcaine; Dilocaine; Lidoject-1; Lignocaine; Nervocaine; Nulicaine; Octocaine; Solarcaine
- PHARMACEUTICAL CLASS: Amide-type local anesthetic; also used as a class IB antiarrhythmic
- CHEMICAL STRUCTURE:

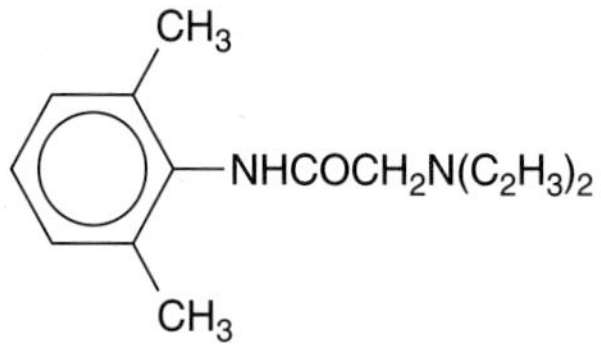

CH_3

$NHCOCH_2N(C_2H_3)_2$

CH_3

Uses

Lidocaine is used for local anesthesia and in the management of ventricular arrhythmias including premature ventricular contractions, ventricular tachycardia, and ventricular fibrillation.

Exposure Pathways

For therapeutic use, lidocaine is most often applied topically or administered locally or intravenously. Therefore, these routes are the most common routes of toxicity. Ingestion of topical lidocaine products can occur and result in toxicity.

Toxicokinetics

Lidocaine is absorbed from the gastrointestinal tract but undergoes significant first-pass metabolism (60–70%). Absorption from local sites is dependent on the dose and vascularity of the site. It is well absorbed from mucosa. Lidocaine is widely distributed to tissues. The volume of distribution is 1.1 liters/kg. Protein binding is 60–80%. Rapid hepatic metabolism to at least two active metabolites occurs. The metabolites and approximately 10% of the parent compound are excreted renally. The initial half-life is 7–30 min and the terminal half-life is 1.5–2 hr.

Mechanism of Toxicity

Lidocaine is a membrane-stabilizing antiarrhythmic which is believed to combine with fast sodium channels and inhibit recovery after repolarization. Lidocaine also increases potassium conductance resulting in decreased slope of phase 3 of the action potential. Lidocaine acts as a central nervous system (CNS) depressant that has sedative, analgesic, and anticonvulsant effects. At high doses, it depresses inhibitory effects and produces seizures.

Human Toxicity

Therapeutic lidocaine serum concentrations range from 1 to 5 μg/ml. Signs of toxicity are usually seen above 6–10 μg/ml, and death has been associated with serum concentrations above 15 μg/ml. Nausea and vomiting occur in toxicity as well as at therapeutic serum concentrations of lidocaine. The CNS toxicities of lidocaine are most common. These include lightheadedness, euphoria, dizziness, drowsiness, and confusion. Visual changes, increasing agitation, and muscle fasiculations are indicative of more serious toxicity. Severe lidocaine toxicity can result in seizures and coma. Cardiovascular effects of lidocaine include a variety of arrhythmias and hypotension. Arrhythmias include sinus arrest, sinus bradycardia, heart block, and asystole. Hypotension may be due to vasodilation or decreased cardiac output.

Clinical Management

Since lidocaine toxicity occurs most often after parenteral administration, the role of gastric decontamination is limited. If ingestion does occur, gastric lavage and activated charcoal can be used depending on the history of the ingestion and the patient's neurologic status. Serum lidocaine concentrations are helpful in assessing degree of toxicity. Seizures should be treated with benzodiazepines such as diazepam and lorazepam. If benzodiazepines are ineffective, barbiturates such as phenobarbital should be considered. Induction of anesthesia with barbiturates (i.e., pentobarbital) can be utilized for refractory seizures. Phenytoin should be avoided due to its potential to worsen lidocaine's cardiac toxicities. Atropine and a pacemaker should be considered for bradyarrhythmias and conduction disturbances. Isoproterenol will increase cardiac rate and conduction but it should be avoided due to its ability to cause vasodilation. If ventricular arrhythmias occur, the class IB antiarrhythmics should be avoided. Hypotension should be managed initially with fluids (i.e., normal saline replacement). If hypotension continues and is found to be due to vasodilation, vasopressors such as dopamine and norepinephrine should be administered. If hypotension is due to decreased cardiac output, dobutamine or amrinone should be considered.

Animal Toxicity

The clinical effects of lidocaine in animals are very similar to those observed in humans.

—Daniel J. Cobaugh

Related Topics

Cardiovascular System
Skin

Life Cycle Assessment

Introduction

During the past three decades, public recognition of environmental issues and the impact of society's activities on the environment have heightened. Society is increasingly aware of potentially adverse impacts on the environment and resource supplies from the use of manufactured products. Such effects can occur throughout the life cycle of a product or process, from its research and development stage, through raw material acquisition, manufacturing, product fabrication and use, to the ultimate management of wastes.

Pressure to improve the environmental performance of products and processes has created demands on manufacturers to consider environmental impacts early in the development of new products. It is by considering issues of environmental loading and raw material use early in the development process that companies avoid the problems and costs associated with redesign and reformulation late in the development stage. Manufacturers worldwide are beginning to address these concerns through a process called "life cycle assessment," which is often a component of product stewardship or product safety programs.

Life cycle assessment (LCA) is a tool used to evaluate the environmental burdens of a product, process, or activity throughout its entire life cycle. The assessment generally consists of three components: inventory analysis, impact analysis, and improvement analysis. The inventory analysis is a process of identifying and quantifying raw materials, energy use, and wastes. Impact analysis is a technical, quantitative or qualitative process in which the effects of resource use and environmental releases identified in the inventory analysis are characterized. The improvement analysis phase of LCA involves the application of a systematic approach to identify opportunities for improving environmental performance and reducing the impacts identified in other parts of the LCA. Before these analyses can be initiated, the purpose of the LCA, the methodologies used, and the system boundaries are defined through a process called scoping.

A key consideration in producing a meaningful life cycle inventory is the definition of the system boundaries with each product or process being represented as a system. In order to conduct an accurate inventory and interpret the data appropriately, a clear understanding of the life cycle stages is necessary. Typically, the following stages are considered part of the life cycle: raw material procurement, manufacturing (which includes materials manufacturing, product fabrication, packaging, and transportation), use, reuse and maintenance, and waste management and recycling. Processing and transportation energy requirements, environmental waste generation and management, and the contribution of coproducts to energy requirements and waste generation are characterized and quantified for each stage.

The intended applications for LCA are varied and depend on who is conducting the study. Companies may conduct analyses as part of product stewardship programs to promote improvement of products or process designs. In addition, LCA may be used in strategic planning and development to address liability or environmental issues, in developing waste minimization programs, or as part of internal environmental audit programs. Life cycle assessments or inventories may be developed for use in support of so-called "green" or "eco" labeling, for support of environmental claims, and as tools for public education. Regulators or researchers may conduct LCAs to evaluate potential environmental burdens associated with products to support public policy, assist in public education, or to identify data gaps.

Background and History of Life Cycle Assessment

Of the three components of an LCA, most of the activity in the past has been focused on the inventory analysis component. Work related to the inventory analysis component began in the 1960s as a result of increasing concerns over raw material and energy resource limitations. A number of individuals began to develop ways to calculate the current energy use and to attempt to predict resource supplies and use of energy. One such method was developed by Harold Smith, who determined the cumulative energy requirements for the production of chemical intermediates and products. This work was presented to the World Energy Conference in 1963.

Subsequently, in the late 1960s, other global modeling studies were undertaken. These studies attempted to predict the impact a changing world population would have on the demand for raw materials and energy. Two publications, *The Limits of Growth* by Meadows *et al.* and *A Blueprint for Survival* by Club of Rome concluded that such an increased demand in raw materials and energy could lead to the depletion, if not total exhaustion, of fossil fuels within the next few decades. Also predicted was the possibility of global warming and other climatological changes. In addition to these works, other studies were also conducted to examine issues such as the costs and potential environmental implications of alternative sources of energy as well as determinations of energy calculations on industrial processes.

Researchers working for the Coca Cola Company made a major contribution to many of the methods still used today for inventory analysis. They conducted a study to determine the container that had the least impact on the environment by examining releases to the environment, effects on natural resources, quantification of raw materials and fuels used in processing, and environmental loadings from the manufacturing process.

During the late 1960s and early 1970s, a number of similar studies were conducted to determine potential costs and implications of various sources of energy. During this same time period other studies were conducted by the U.S. EPA and Resource for the Future. These studies were primarily concerned with cost minimization for the pulp and paper, petroleum refining, and steel industries.

During the oil shortages of the 1970s, studies were performed to quantify resource use and releases to the environment by industrial systems and products. These analyses became known as Resource and Environmental Profile Analyses in the United States and Ecobalances in Europe. It was during this time that a more standardized methodology was developed and applied to these types of studies.

As the oil shortage crisis began to decline in the late 1970s, so too did interest in conducting these studies. Interest declined to the point that only about two energy-related studies were being conducted per year. In the 1980s, activity began to accelerate, but this time the primary focus was on hazardous waste management. The main impetus behind this activity was the establishment of a European Directorate (DGX1) by the European Commission to standardize pollution regulations in Europe. In 1985, the DGX1 also issued the Liquid Food Container Directive (85/339). The directive required European Commission member companies to monitor energy and raw materials used to produce and dispose of liquid food containers. Included in this directive was a requirement to track the generation of solid waste for this process.

With heightened interest and concern over solid waste and recycling, life cycle inventory analysis has become an important tool not only for addressing solid waste concerns but also for all areas affecting the environment. This has become very apparent, especially in the past 10 years, with a great deal of activity in both the public and private sectors.

In August 1990, SETAC organized a workshop titled "A Technical Framework for LCA." The goal of this workshop was to develop a consensus on the current state of the art and research need for conducting LCA. SETAC has since been the focal point for technical developments in LCA.

As mentioned previously, up to this time, the main emphasis in conducting LCAs had been the inventory analysis component. Current developments in LCAs indicate that a broader approach, incorporating impact analysis, is on the horizon.

Life Cycle Assessment Components

An LCA is composed of three interrelated activities: inventory analysis, impact analysis or assessment, and improvement analysis or assessment. The purpose and goals of the LCA and the process, product, or activity to be studied are defined during an initial scoping process, sometimes considered an additional component.

Scoping and Goal Definition

In the scoping process, the study goals and purpose are stated and related to the extent of the study. The system to be considered, the boundaries of the system, assumptions, and data requirements are clearly defined in this phase of the LCA. In addition, it is critical that the functional units for the analysis be defined so that systems can be compared on an equivalent basis. The functional unit must be measurable and clearly define a function of the system. Although scoping occurs early in the LCA, changes and reevaluation may become necessary during later phases of the project, especially when defining the model and collecting data.

Inventory Analysis

In inventory analysis, energy use, raw material requirements, emissions to the air and water, solid waste production, and other releases are quantified for each part of the life cycle of the product or activity. The methodology for defining systems and data collection have been under development for several years. The U.S. EPA and SETAC have published summaries of these methodologies. U.S. EPA has identified the following procedures for conducting life cycle inventories:

1. Define the purpose and scope of the inventory
2. Define the system boundaries
3. Devise an inventory checklist
4. Institute a peer review process
5. Gather data
6. Develop stand-alone data
7. Construct a computational model
8. Present the results
9. Interpret and communicate the results

To describe the system to be studied, components and subsystems are presented in a flowchart. Generally, the flowchart includes the production sequence, the ancillary materials (materials used in the system but not directly in the formation of the product), production sequence, and energy and fuel production. Data are then gathered for these components and inputs to and outputs from the system are characterized.

Data for the inventory stage may come from in-house records, such as toxicological and physical testing reports, utility and energy bills, accident and regulatory record keeping, and raw material purchasing data systems. Public information from government reports, industry associations, industry studies, toxicological data, and other available LCAs may also be used in developing the inventory analysis.

The inventory can be used to develop baseline information on the system's energy and resource consumption and environmental emissions. By identifying potential areas for improved environmental performance and allowing for comparisons to alternative processes, the inventory provides the information necessary to conduct the impact and improvement assessments.

Life Cycle Stages

The quality of a life cycle inventory is dependent on an accurate description of the product to be studied. In order to obtain that, it must be determined where each stage of the life cycle begins and ends. It is generally agreed on that the major life cycle inventory stages are

1. Raw materials acquisition
2. Manufacturing, processing, and formulation
3. Use, reuse, and maintenance
4. Recycling and waste management

Raw Materials Acquisition

Raw materials, as defined in a life cycle inventory analysis, are those materials that have been extracted from the earth without refinement or further processing. The raw material acquisition stage begins with the acquiring of raw materials at the point furthest upstream in the process and ends at the first step in the manufacturing process. This stage includes the removal of raw materials, the energy expended to obtain these materials from the earth through cultivation, harvesting, and extracting, and the transportation of these materials from their point of origin.

Deciding what materials are to be included in a life cycle inventory can be somewhat difficult because there are a number of different options. The first and most comprehensive option is to include essentially all materials, no matter how minor, in the assessment. This eliminates the need to make a decision as to what should or should not be included and also eliminates the need to document that rationale. A disadvantage to this approach is the amount of detail that is potentially involved.

The second option is to define, up front, the parameters of the study and establish a clearly defined threshold. This option establishes a more narrow scope for the assessment and, as such, reduces time and costs involved. One such method, the "1% Rule," sets a parameter that states that any material that makes up less than 1%, by weight, of the total system and contributes less than 1% to the total emissions can be considered insignificant and can be omitted from the inventory. The potential problem with such an approach is that toxic materials can be overlooked. Another method sets up the parameters based on the number of steps that the raw material is removed from the main process. This "one step back" approach eliminates secondary input into the production process. If it can be proven, mathematically, that elimination of some secondary inputs makes no significant difference in the overall analysis, then this method can be applied.

The third option is to exclude inputs that are likely to have very little effect on the overall assessment, based on a sensitivity analysis. Again, this must be defined up front, prior to performing the assessment. This proves to be a very systematic method in determining the threshold. With such an approach, much care must be used in describing how the analysis was used.

The last option excludes defined classes or types of inputs and can be used in a number of different systems. With this approach, many potentially complex subsystems can be left out. This option, like the first, may leave out potentially significant processes.

Quantification of some inputs/outputs that should be part of a raw materials system include the impact acquisition of materials and processing equipment has on the system, both point and fugitive emissions, point and nonpoint water effluent, solid waste generation, energy considerations, and other releases to the environment.

Manufacturing, Processing, and Formulation

The second stage of the life cycle is manufacturing. It is the point at which the raw materials are converted into a final product. This stage spans the time from the receipt of raw materials by the manufacturer to the transferal of the final manufactured product to distribution. This includes any on-site handling and storage of the material. Any packaging used to transfer the product before the distribution stage is also included.

The manufacturing stage is normally divided into three substages:

1. Materials manufacture
2. Product fabrication
3. Filling, packaging, and distribution

The first substage, materials manufacture, is the stage in which raw materials (or intermediates) are converted into intermediates, which will then be directly converted into the finished product. It includes any energy, materials, and water input needed for the process, as well as any releases to the environment.

Information must be gathered for each manufacturing operation and subsystem. From this, all material and energy inputs are analyzed, as are the emissions to the air and water and any solid waste generated.

The next manufacturing step is the actual fabrication of the product. This step is the conversion of intermediates into final products ready for use by consumers. As with the materials manufacture stage, this substage includes energy, materials, and water input and any environmental releases. Any transportation, up to the filling/packaging/distribution substage, is also included.

The last manufacturing step is filling, packaging, and distribution, which includes any process and transportation between the fabrication substage and delivery to the consumer. The filling step begins at the point where the finished product actually arrives at the filling/packaging location. It is interesting to note the difference between U.S. EPA and SETAC descriptions regarding this step. Whereas the U.S. EPA has included distribution and transportation as a substage in the manufacturing stage, SETAC has developed a separate distribution and transportation stage in its life cycle inventory. The difference, according the U.S. EPA, is due to the fact that its document is geared toward assembling data needed to perform an inventory study.

Use, Reuse, and Maintenance

The use/reuse/maintenance stage consists of those activities that begin after distribution of final products to the consumer until they are either recycled or discarded into a waste management system. This step also includes any packaging that reaches the consumer.

The "use" component normally includes activities such as the actual consumption of the product, any equipment operation that occurs, product storage (e.g., refrigeration), and any preparation on the product prior to use.

Reuse of a product, or package, can occur either on or off the location where use has occurred. Some products may have the capability of being reused numerous times after the product has served its original purpose. The reuse stage includes the intentional reuse of a product/package either for its original function or possibly for a whole new application. Included in this inventory is any energy used to prepare the product for reuse, such as washing out a glass container for storage of something else.

Recycle and Waste Management

Once a product has served its purpose, it is generally discarded, recycled, or composted as waste. The recycling stage begins once the product reaches the collection system. This stage includes the collection and handling of materials, any processing necessary to prepare the material to be used as a raw material again, and any transportation.

Two basic recycling systems may be considered while performing a life cycle inventory: closed-loop and open-loop recycling. With closed-loop recycling, the product can be perpetually recycled into a product similar to what it was previously; for example, aluminum cans. Open-loop recycling, on the other hand, results in an alternate product that is ultimately disposed of; for example, plastic milk bottles. Each system presents its own degree of difficulty when conducting a life cycle inventory. Closed-loop recycling can be fairly straightforward due to the limited number of inputs and outputs, once the initial data has been compiled. Open-loop recycling is generally more complicated than closed loop due to the possible variety of inputs and outputs.

The waste management component refers to the ultimate fate of solid waste generated, picked up, and discarded. This stage includes incineration, landfilling, and postconsumer wastewater treatment. With these various methods of disposal, a number of pollutants and resource use categories may be generated for a life cycle inventory.

One difficulty in trying to quantify emissions from disposal is presented by the fact that a product is not typically disposed of by itself. It is usually mixed with other solid wastes, making quantification extremely difficult. This is in contrast to recycling, in which like materials are separated prior to the actual recycling stage.

Impact Analysis

Impact analysis is the process of characterizing and assessing the environmental impacts of a process, product, or activity identified in the inventory. The purpose of this analysis is to develop an environmental profile of the system being studied. The data are assessed utilizing impact models, many of which involve hazard and risk assessment. However, methodologies and models used in impact assessment are currently evolving, making this activity among the most difficult of the phases of LCA. Many models are incomplete and many existing ones require large amounts of data and incorporate many assumptions.

The impact assessment generally involves three steps: classification, characterization, and valuation. Classification is the process of categorizing data into the following major impact categories: human health, ecological health, resource depletion, and other human welfare effects. In the characterization phase, impacts within the various categories are quantified and aggregated. This results in an impact profile, consisting of impact descriptions or measures. The various impact categories are weighted and compared in the valuation step. This allows for the comparison of different types of effects (e.g., human health effects and atmospheric effects) and for the assessment of the relative importance of each. Several expert judgment methods and participatory, or "social judgment," techniques are available to assist in making the complex evaluations and decisions necessary in the valuation step.

Within each major impact category considered in the classification step, chemical and nonchemical stressors and their impacts can be identified. Nonchemical stressors may include ionizing and ultraviolet radiation, heat, and noise. The stressors identified in the LCA may be associated with initial as well as secondary, tertiary, and additional impacts. In its conceptual framework guidance, SETAC has recognized that cause-and-effect linkage is not a necessary outcome of impact assessment and that such relationships are often difficult or impossible to prove. SETAC further points out that quantification of specific impacts is difficult within the LCA context. Therefore, the methods used for these analyses tend to link the stressors to impacts and to assess the potential quantity and potency of releases and probable environmental exposures.

Resource Depletion

The environmental and social impacts of resource use and depletion are often difficult to assess. In the impact analysis, depletion of renewable resources as well as nonrenewable, stock resources is considered. It has been noted that resource quality should also be considered during the assessment because, generally, the quality of a resource declines as it is depleted, possibly resulting in increased waste production and energy use.

Human Health and Safety

In assessing the impacts of stressors on human health and safety, acute and chronic effects are considered. These impacts are determined using hazard identification, risk assessment, exposure assessment, and risk characterization.

During hazard identification, hazardous agents and potential adverse effects are identified using physical and health effects test results. The risk assessment step involves a dose–response assessment using toxicological studies and statistical models to estimate the adverse health effects associated with different doses of the agent. Exposure assessment is utilized to determine the source, type, frequency, and duration of contact with the agent. Finally, risk characterization is the process of estimating risks associated with exposures to the agent. Methodologies and models for conducting these assessments and statistical analyses of the data are available and well described in the literature.

Ecological Health

With respect to ecological health, LCA impact analyses may address issues of population and ecosystem structure, ecological functions and processes, biodiversity, atmospheric change, and habitat degradation which may be associated with adverse impacts in interrelated species. The LCA should address whether these ecological impacts may occur on local, regional, or global scales. Although many environmental fate and media transport models are available, they are generally complex and incorporate numerous assumptions.

Human Welfare

Human welfare effects may be associated with issues that have significant impact on the quality of our lives. Impacts that may be relevant to LCA include loss of water or land resources due to environmental burdens from product or process releases and damage to buildings from air contamination. In addition, aesthetic issues, such as loss of scenic beauty, noise pollution, or poor air quality, are also considered in this impact category.

Improvement Analysis

This component of LCA involves the systematic evaluation of potential opportunities for reducing or eliminating the environmental impacts identified in other phases of the study. This process may be qualitative, quantitative, or a combination of the two, and it employs information and data gathered in the inventory analysis. Alternatives for, and improvements to, products and processes are identified, assessed, and selected during this process. Improvement analysis has not been widely discussed and standardized guidance and methodologies are not currently available.

Life Cycle Analysis Data Quality and Peer Review

Data for LCAs may be of several types and come from several sources. These data may be obtained from individual companies and may be facility specific, process specific, or aggregated. Data may be gathered from industry organizations and reflect industry averages or aggregates. In addition, the sources of data may include public documents, government reports, or other publicly available life cycle inventories or assessments. The quality of the data used will significantly impact the results and conclusions of the LCA.

U.S. EPA has described the data from life cycle inventories as being of two types: process and activity measurements that can be analyzed using standard statistical techniques and assumption and decision guidelines for combining the data sets into systems.

In its LCA guidance, SETAC discusses the importance of assessing the quality of data contained in LCAs. SETAC points out that quality indicators may be qualitative, referring to completeness, for example, or quantitative, which would include accuracy, precision, and detection limits. Generally, data obtained from individual companies should be representative, although it is doubtful that the sample will be random. The professional conducting the LCA must understand and report potential sources of bias from the data. Likewise, for data supplied for entire industries, potential sources of bias and other factors associated with grouped data must be considered. The LCA must also address other aspects of data quality, including age of the data, potential variability, and geographic specificity. These and other issues must also be addressed for secondary data, which are obtained from the literature and other published sources.

Because of the lack of standard methods for conducting LCAs, the importance of establishing an effective peer review process is especially critical; however, until LCAs are more commonly conducted, the availability of such reviewers will be limited.

LCA as Part of a Proactive Product Stewardship Program

LCAs are obviously an integral part of a proactive product stewardship program. Like risk assessment, it is a valuable initial tool to assist in designing and implementing stewardship programs, which incorporate health, safety, and environmental protection into product design, manufacture, distribution, use, recycling, and disposal. Over the years, product stewardship has been referred to as product responsibility, product integrity, environmental quality, or design for environment.

In general, interrelated components of LCA, inventory analysis, impact analysis, and improvement analysis are used to identify ways of minimizing the environmental impacts of products, materials, processes, systems, activities, and services, all of which are important sources of information for strategic planning. LCAs help focus the development and evaluation of new and existing products and their applications and allow for their incorporation into total quality management practices.

LCAs are also effective tools for incorporating changes into product and process design. Through LCA improvement assessment, a systematic evaluation can be conducted to identify ways of reducing the environmental burdens associated with energy and raw material use and waste generation. Changes throughout the life cycle of a product or process can be incorporated into the system to improve products and processes. Effective implementation of a "Design for Environment" (DfE) program (Design for Environmentally Safe Products and Processes) allows for the identification and correction of a product's potential environmental impacts at the earliest and least costly stage of its life cycle. This process also reduces costs associated with product redesign and environmental abatement measures. The DfE initiative provides a competitive advantage through superior product environmental performance. After product design changes are considered, modifications can also be incorporated into manufacturing processes to reduce the need for environmental controls.

Communication of product information is a vital component of product stewardship. LCA results must be communicated to the appropriate audience to be effective and meaningful. Effective reporting and communication begins at the onset of the LCA and continues through data processing and aggregation into a report. A complete report outlining the objectives, scope, methodology, data, results, and conclusions must be carefully and skillfully prepared. The results must be provided in a written and/or verbal format that can be clearly understood by regulators, politicians, media, consumers, and other stakeholders who may need to react to the critical information being communicated. An LCA, as part of product stewardship, can only be as effective as the message that is delivered and received by the various groups processing the information.

Therefore, a proactive product stewardship program must incorporate product LCA to continually improve the overall health, safety, and environmental performance of products. LCAs will significantly contribute to the long-term success of an effective, proactive stewardship program.

Further Reading

Curran, M. A., and Vigon, B. (1993). *EPA's Research in LCA Methodology,* EPA/600/A-93/154. U.S. Environmental Protection Agency, Cincinnati, OH.

Fava, J. A. (1993, February). Product stewardship: A proactive approach to improve environmental quality. *The Weston Way.*

Fava, J. A., Denison, R., Jones, B., Curran, M. A., Vigon, B., Selke, S., and Barnum, J. (Eds.) (1991). *Technical Framework for Life-Cycle Assessment.* SETAC Foundation for Environmental Education, Washington, DC.

Fava, J. A., Consoli, F., Denison, R., Dickson, K., Mohin, T., and Vigon, B. (Eds.) (1993). *A Conceptual Framework for Life-Cycle Impact Assessment.* SETAC Foundation for Environmental Education, Washington, DC.

Fava, J. A., Weiler, E. D., and Reinert, K. H. (1993, February). Product life-cycle assessment: A tool to implement product stewardship. *The Weston Way.*

SETAC (1993). *Guidelines for Life-Cycle Assessment: A Code of Practices.* SETAC Foundation for Environmental Education, Washington, DC.

SETAC (1994). *Life-Cycle Assessment Data Quality: A Conceptual Framework* (Fava, J. A., Jensen, A., Lindfors, L., Pomper, S., De Smet, B., Warren, J., and Vigon, B. (Eds.) (1994). SETAC Foundation for Environmental Education, Washington, DC.

U.S. EPA (1993). *Life Cycle Design Guidance Manual. Environmental Requirements and the Product System,* EPA/600/R-92/226. U.S. EPA Office of Research and Development, Washington, DC.

U.S. EPA (1993). *Life-Cycle Assessment: Inventory Guidelines and Principles,* EPA/600/R-92/245. U.S. EPA Office of Research and Development, Washington, DC.

—*Daniel C. Steinmetz, John H. Davies, and Edward J. Kerfoot*

Related Topics

Exposure Assessment
Hazard Identification
Risk Assessment, Ecological
Risk Assessment, Human Health
Risk Characterization
Risk Management
SETAC

Lily of the Valley

- Synonyms: *Convallaria majalis*; lily convalle
- Description: From the family of Liliaceae, lily of the valley is a perennial root stock with pairs of simple, broadly ovate leaves and a flowering stock. The stock bears a one-sided row of scented, waxy, bell-shaped flowers. These fragrant flowers are usually white; however, they may also be pale pink, pink, and, on rare occasions, yellow. The plant also bears a red/orange berry. Lily of the valley is commonly found in North America, the United Kingdom, and Europe.

Uses

Lily of the valley is used for bouquets, for cut flower arrangements, and as a garden perennial.

Exposure Pathways

Ingestion of the fragrant flowers or bright berries is the most common route of exposure. Drinking vase water has purportedly been described as being potentially toxic.

Mechanism of Toxicity

The whole plant contains convallarin and convallamarin, a cardiac glycoside. The glycosides are less potent than digoxin or digitalis.

Human Toxicity

Human toxic reactions are poorly reported. With significant overdosage, the sodium potassium pump mechanism is disrupted, which results in marked high-grade heart block. As intracellular potassium declines, electrical conduction falters, and progressive electrical changes occur. Potentially, this may result in a failure of the myocardial cells to act as pacemakers. Complete loss of normal myocardial electrical function and asystole can occur. The myocardium may even lose its ability to respond to electrical pacing. Potential clinical symptoms include gastrointestinal distress; hyperkalemia; bradycardia; first-, second-, or third-degree heart block; hypotension; and asystole. However, profound cardiotoxicity is unlikely.

Clinical Management

Basic and advanced life-support measures should be utilized as necessary. With significant ingestion, decontamination is advised. If the ingestion is recent (less than 30 min) and the patient is asymptomatic, syrup of ipecac may be indicated. Activated charcoal may be used to absorb plant toxins. Symptomatic and supportive therapy is indicated in cases of significant toxicity.

Animal Toxicity

Animals have the same potential for toxicity as humans. However, no reliable reports of livestock deaths exist in the literature.

—*Anne E. Bryan*

Related Topics

Aconitum Species
Cardiovascular System
Digitalis Glycosides
Foxglove
Oleander
Solanum Genus

Limonene

- CAS: 138-86-3
- SYNONYMS: Dipentene; cinene; 1-methyl-4-(1-methylethenyl) cyclohexene
- DESCRIPTION: Limonene is an essential oil that is a major constituent in oils of orange, lemon, caraway, dill, bergamot, and pine needle.
- CHEMICAL CLASS: Terpene
- MOLECULAR FORMULA: $C_{10}H_{16}$

Uses

Limonene is used in flavoring, fragrance, and perfume materials, solvents, and wetting agents. It is also used in resin manufacture.

Exposure Pathways

Dermal contact, ingestion, and inhalation are all possible routes of exposure.

Human Toxicity

Limonene is a skin irritant and dermal sensitizer. Mild local tissue (eye and skin) irritation and delayed contact dermal sensitization are common. Acute poisoning is manifested as vomiting and circulatory collapse. If ingested in sufficient quantity, albuminuria and hematuria are possible.

Clinical Management

In cases of ingestion, milk should be given to allay gastric irritation. Fluids should be given to maintain maximum urinary output to expedite elimination of limonene from the body.

Animal Toxicity

The D isomer is orally teratogenic in mice and maternally toxic in rats. The mouse oral TD_{Lo} is 67 g/kg. Limonene causes nephropathy in male rats characterized by hyaline droplet formation with degenerative intracellular changes.

—*Shayne C. Gad*

Related Topics

Sensitization
Vanillin

Lindane

- CAS: 58-89-9
- SYNONYMS: 1,2,3,4,5,6-Hexachlorocyclohexane; 666; Aparasin; Aphtiria; Ben-Hex; Borekil; γ-BHC; Gammexane; Gexane; Jacutin; Kwell; Lindatox; Lorexane; Streunex; Tri-6; Quellada
- CHEMICAL CLASS: Synthetic organochlorine insecticide
- CHEMICAL STRUCTURE:

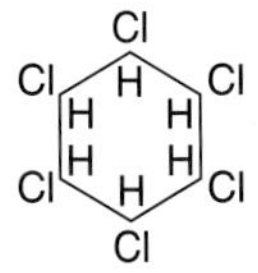

Uses

Commercially, lindane is used as an insecticide. Therapeutically, it is used against human lice and mites (scabicide).

Exposure Pathways

The most important exposure routes for lindane are oral and dermal.

Toxicokinetics

Lindane is absorbed through the gastrointestinal tract, respiratory tract, and skin.

The metabolism of lindane is extensive and cannot be fully discussed here. Lindane is metabolized in the liver by induction of microsomal enzymes. A number of pathways are involved including oxidation by cytochrome P450 as well as the formation of glucuronides by conjugation of phenol and alcohol products. Anaerobic metabolism produces benzene and chlorobenzenes through dechlorination.

Lindane is bound by serum proteins in the blood. Storage is preferentially in adipose tissue and other fat-containing tissues.

Lindane is primarily excreted in the urine. It may also be found in feces and breast milk.

Mechanism of Toxicity

Lindane has a greater inhibitory effect on Na^+,K^+-adenosine triphosphatase (ATPase) than on Mg^{2+}-ATPase in neurons. This inhibition alters ion transport and produces partial nerve depolarization and hyperexcitability.

Human Toxicity

Most instances of lindane poisoning following therapeutic use to control scabies or lice have involved gross misuse of the insecticide. Ingestion of lindane is followed by symptoms within less than 1 hr on an empty stomach to 5 hr after a full meal. Initially, faintness, dizziness, and malaise were reported followed by convulsions. Nausea and vomiting were common.

Pulmonary edema has been reported when lindane powder has been aspirated into the lungs. Deaths are not common with lindane poisoning.

Clinical Management

Management of lindane poisoning is symptomatic. Diazepam or phenobarbital are used to control convulsions. Cholestyramine or activated charcoal have been utilized to inhibit lindane uptake after ingestion. In more severe poisonings, the serum levels of lindane may be lowered by hemoperfusion over Amberlite XAD-4.

Animal Toxicity

The toxicity of lindane in animals is similar that of DDT.

—Benny L. Blaylock

Related Topics

DDT
Neurotoxicology
Organochlorine Insecticides
Pesticide
Shampoo

Liothyronine

- CAS: 6893-02-3
- SYNONYMS: L-triiodothyronine; T3; Cytomel
- PHARMACEUTICAL CLASS: Synthetic form of triiodothyronine
- CHEMICAL STRUCTURE:

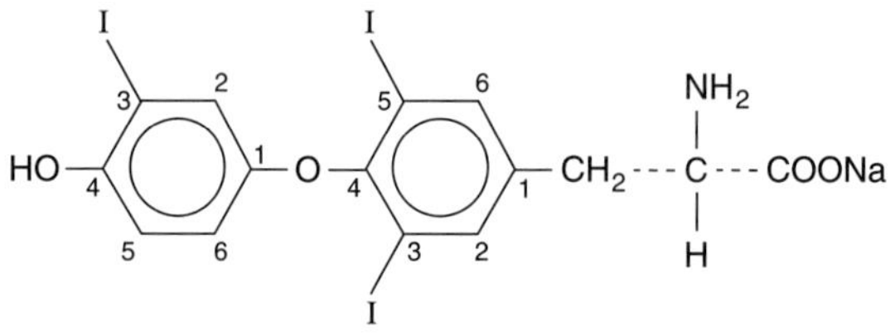

Uses

Liothyronine is used in the treatment of hypothyroidism, nontoxic goiter, cretinism, and myxedema.

Exposure Pathways

Ingestion is the only exposure route for liothyronine.

Toxicokinetics

Liothyronine (T3) is 88% absorbed. Congestive heart failure can reduce absorption by half. T3 is not firmly bound to serum protein. It has a volume of distribution in the range of 41–45 liters/kg. T3 is metabolized to deiodinated and conjugate metabolites. From 75 to 85% of T3 is deiodinated. Conjugation takes place in the kidneys. Approximately 20% of T3 is excreted in the feces and up to 10% in the urine. T3 has a half-life of 2.5 days.

Mechanism of Toxicity

The exact mechanism of action is not well understood. Thyroid hormones are needed for metabolism, growth, and development. Most organ systems are affected by thyroid hormones. Thyroid hormones cause an increase in the basal metabolic rate, in oxygen consumption, and in the metabolism of carbohydrates. T3 increases aerobic mitochondrial function causing an increased rate of utilization of high-energy phosphates. This stimulates myosin adenosine triphosphatase (ATPase) and reduces tissue acetic acid. Toxicity is an extension of the pharmacologic effects.

Human Toxicity: Acute

Ingestion of small amounts of T3-containing products produce few symptoms. Symptoms of toxicity may occur 4–12 hr following large overdoses. Symptoms of toxicity include tachycardia, nausea, vomiting, diarrhea, restlessness, and fever.

Human Toxicity: Chronic

Thyrotoxicosis is a concern with chronic exposure. Thyrotoxicosis is characterized by tachycardia, cardiac arrhythmias, hypertension, tremors, and seizures. In severe cases, coma and cardiovascular collapse can result.

Clinical Management

Basic and advanced life-support measures should be utilized as needed. Emesis, lavage, and activated charcoal can be utilized based on the patient's symptomatology and time of exposure. EKG and blood pressure monitoring should be utilized. Propranolol can be given to treat adrenergic symptoms that occur with hyperthyroidism. Diuresis and hemodialysis are ineffective.

Animal Toxicity

Dogs and cats are at risk for thyroid toxicity. Signs of toxicity include vomiting, diarrhea, tachycardia, tachypnea, decreased level of consciousness, and restlessness.

—*Bridget Flaherty*

Related Topics

Endocrine System
Levothyroxine
Thyroid Extract

Lipid Peroxidation

What Is Lipid Peroxidation?

Lipid peroxidation is an oxidative chain reaction in which one lipid molecule after another becomes oxidized to the utmost or so as to form a lipid peroxide (i.e., a lipid molecule containing one or more O–O bonds). At high temperatures, lipid peroxides decompose to produce a range of unpleasant-tasting and foul-smelling products such as epoxides, ketones, acids, and aldehydes. The development of unpleasant tastes and odors as well as changes in color, viscosity, specific gravity, and solubility of vegetable oils and animal fats are the characteristics of rancidity of lipids, a problem that has been recognized in storage of fats and oils since antiquity. It was not until 1940s that the mechanisms by which unsaturated lipids react with molecular oxygen to undergo "autoxidation," or "peroxidation," were established. Biological cell membranes are rich in polyunsaturated fatty acids (PUFAs), such as arachidonic and docoshexaenoic acid, in either the isolated form or the incorporated form in triacylglycerides and phospholipids. PUFAs are particularly susceptible to peroxidation. With increasing concerns about the potential adverse effects of lipid peroxidation in cellular membranes, the relevance of lipid peroxidation to biology and human diseases has been extensively explored since the 1950s.

Mechanisms of Lipid Peroxidation

It is now widely known that lipid peroxidation is a free radical-initiated chain oxidation of unsaturated lipids. Electrons in atoms occupy regions of space known as orbitals. Each orbital can hold a maximum of two electrons. A free radical is defined as any chemical species possessing one or more unpaired electrons and capable of independent existence. Hydroxyl (OH·) and superoxide ($O_2^{-\cdot}$) are examples of oxygen-centered radicals. There are also other types of radicals such as thiyl (RS·), trichloromethyl ($CCl_3\cdot$), and nitric oxide (NO·).

A free radical is marked by a dot, which designates the presence of one or more unpaired electrons.

Radicals can be formed in three ways: (1) by the homolytic cleavage of a covalent bond of a normal molecule, with each fragment retaining one of the paired electrons; (2) by the loss of a single electron from a normal molecule; and (3) by electron transfer or the addition of a single electron to a normal molecule. The electron transferring way is a far more common process in biological systems than is homolytic fission, which generally requires high energy input from high temperature, UV light, or ionizing radiation.

Radical formation by electron transfer: $A + e^- \longrightarrow A^-\cdot$
Radical formation by homolytic fission: $X{:}Y \longrightarrow X\cdot + Y\cdot$
Ion formation by heterolytic fission: $X{:}Y \longrightarrow X{:}^- + Y^+$

Radicals have a very short life, but are very reactive with other molecules. When two radicals meet, they can combine their unpaired electrons to form a covalent bond.

$$A\cdot + A\cdot \longrightarrow A\text{-}A$$

However, most biological molecules are nonradicals. When a radical gives one electron to, takes one electron from, or simply adds on to a nonradical, that nonradical becomes a radical. Therefore, the reaction of free radicals with nonradicals usually proceeds as chain reactions: One radical begets another. The free radicals may also attack biological macromolecules other than lipids, such as proteins, nuclear acids, and carbohydrates. Lipid peroxidation is the most studied, biologically relevant, free radical chain reaction. It takes place in two steps: initiation and propagation.

Lipid peroxidation is initiated by the attack of a radical that has sufficient reactivity to abstract a hydrogen atom from a methylene carbon in a fatty acid or in a fatty acyl side chain. The greater the number of double bond in a fatty acid side chain, the easier is the removal of a hydrogen atom; that is why PUFAs are especially susceptible to peroxidation. The hydrogen atom has one proton and a single electron and is a free radical. Removal of a hydrogen atom from a lipid molecule leaves behind an unpaired electron on the carbon to which the hydrogen was originally attached (Fig. L-1, reaction 1). The resulting carbon-centered radical can have several fates, but the most likely one in aerobic cells is to undergo molecular rearrangement, followed by reaction with O_2 to give a peroxyl radical (Fig. L-1, reaction 2). Peroxyl radicals can combine with each other or they can attack membrane proteins, but they also can attract hydrogen from adjacent fatty acid side chains to form hydroperoxides and so propagate the chain reaction of lipid peroxidation (Fig. L-1, reaction 3). Therefore, a single event of initiation can convert hundreds of fatty acids into lipid hydroperoxide.

The lipid hydroperoxide decomposition produces more radicals and noxious aldehydes.

$$\text{LOOH} \longrightarrow \text{LO}\cdot,\ \text{LOO}\cdot,\ \text{aldehydes}$$

The chain reaction can be interrupted by antioxidants (A–H), which provide an easily donatable hydrogen for abstraction by peroxyl radicals.

$$\text{A-H} + \text{LOO}\cdot \longrightarrow \text{LOOH} + \text{A}\cdot$$

The antioxidant-derived radical (A·) could be dimerized harmlessly into A_2, or it could be converted back to A–H by reaction with another molecule, it might also react with another LOO· to become a nonradical. This is the termination of lipid proxidation. The most important chain-breaking antioxidant in human lipids is α-tocopherol.

$$\text{LOO}\cdot\text{(lipid peroxyl radical)} + \alpha\text{-tocopherol-OH} \longrightarrow \text{LOOH} + \alpha\text{-tocopherol-O}\cdot$$

The resultant tocopheroxyl radical is relatively stable and, in normal circumstances, insufficiently reactive to initiate lipid peroxidation itself. It has been demonstrated *in vitro* that α-tocopherol radical can be converted back to α-tocopherol by reduction with ascorbic acid at the surface of biological membranes:

$$\text{A}\cdot + \text{ascorbic acid} \longrightarrow \text{ascorbic acid}\cdot + \text{A-H}$$

However, it is uncertain that this reaction actually happens *in vivo*. There is evidence that reduced glutathione

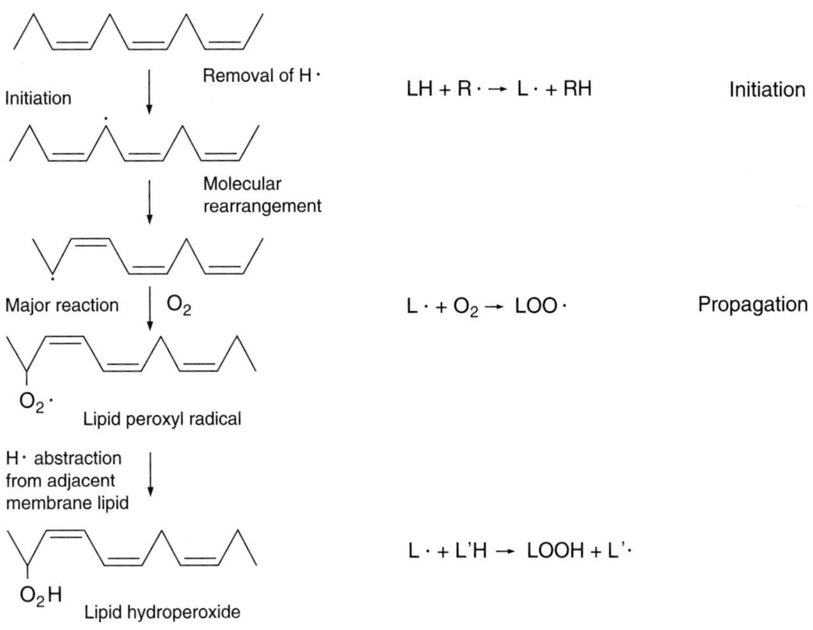

FIGURE L-1. Mechanism of lipid peroxidation.

(GSH) and ubiquinol in mitochondria may also contribute to the recycling α-tocopherol. Before its termination, the length of propagation of lipid peroxidation chain is dependent on many factors such as the lipid : protein ratio of the membrane (the higher protein content of the membrane, the higher the chance of a radical reacting with membrane protein), the fatty acid composition (more PUFAs, the longer is the propagation chain), the oxygen concentration, and the presence of chain-breaking antioxidants within the membrane.

Biological Effects of Lipid Peroxidation

Lipid peroxidation is a very destructive chain reaction and it can directly damage the structure of membrane. The occurrence of lipid peroxidation in biological membranes causes severe impairment of membrane functioning, changes in membrane fluidity, inactivation of membrane-bond receptors and enzymes, and increased nonspecific permeability to ions such as Ca^{2+}. In addition, decomposition of lipid hydroperoxides produces hydrocarbon gases (such as ethane and pentane), more radical species, and cytotoxic aldehydes. Thus, lipid peroxidation can indirectly damage other cell components by these products of its decomposition.

Lipid peroxidation has been implicated in a wide range of tissue injuries, diseases, and even in the aging process. The liver toxicity of carbon tetrachloride (CCl_4) is a classic example of the destructive effects of lipid peroxidation. A very small portion of administered carbon tetrachloride is metabolized into trichloromethyl free radical ($CCl_3\cdot$) by the action of cytochrome P450 in the liver. This radical reacts rapidly with oxygen and gives rise to the trichloromethylperoxyl radical:

$$CCl_3\cdot + O_2 \longrightarrow CCl_3O_2\cdot$$

This trichlormethylperoxyl radical can efficiently abstract hydrogen atoms from lipids and initiate lipid peroxidation.

$$L\text{-}H + CCl_3O_2\cdot \longrightarrow L\cdot + CCl_3O_2H$$

Eventually these reactions result in the oxidative destruction of cellular membrane and serious tissue damage in the liver even though $<0.5\%$ of CCl_4 is ever metabolized. An essential involvement of lipid peroxidation in the events leading to death of hepatocytes has been proved in the acute intoxication as well as with other haloalkanes such as bromotrichloromethane ($CBrCl_3$), dibromoethane, and halothane. Lipid peroxidation is also involved in the hepatotoxicity of ethanol, allyl alcohol, and some drugs like adriamycin. Liver toxicity of GSH-deplcting agents, such as bromobenzene and acetaminophen, is also associated with lipid peroxidation.

It is currently believed that lipid peroxidation is involved in the pathogenesis of atherosclerosis through oxidative modification of low-density lipoprotein (LDL). The oxidized LDL has altered receptor affinity, causing it to be scavenged by macrophages in an uncontrolled manner with the development of foam cells and the initiation of the atherosclerotic lesion. The oxidized LDL deposited in the arterial wall may continuously release highly cytotoxic lipid peroxidation products such as certain aldehydes, irritating the endothelial cell layer and causing a range of other effects that may contribute toward the development of the lesion.

Lipid peroxidation has also been suggested to be involved in the pathogenesis of several lung diseases and injuries. One of the important events for several lung diseases is arachidonic acid (AA) release induced by lipid peroxidation and metabolism of released AA to active products. Hydroperoxides have been shown to induce lipid peroxidation in the isolated perfused lung, which could lead to a perturbed plasma membrane and the activation of phospholipase A_2 (PLA_2). As a result of the activation of PLA_2, an excessive amount AA is released. The released AA and its metabolites of eicosanoids, such as prostaglandins, prostacyclin, thromboxane, and leukotriene, can lead to vasoconstriction and brochoconstriction as well as the development of edema.

Lipid peroxidation has been attributed to the pathogenesis of other human diseases such as rheumatoid arthritis, renal dysfunction, and diabetes mellitus.

However, it must be pointed out that in most cases increase in the bulk peroxidation of cell membrane lipids is not the cause of cell damage, but a consequence of cell damage. Rises in intracellular Ca^{2+}, protein damage, and DNA damage are more important events in causing cell injury than is the bulk peroxidation of membrane lipids. Lipid peroxidation is often a late event, accompanying rather than causing final cell death and often occurring after cell death, leading to putrefaction and added generation of products such as ethane.

Reactive Species That Initiate Lipid Peroxidation in Cells

High-energy irradiation of aqueous solutions produces highly reactive hydroxyl radicals (OH·) that can attack all biological molecules, including membrane lipids. This is probably a mechanism accounting for initiation of lipid peroxidation in irradiated organisms. With the exception of such an unusual circumstance, free radicals that initiate lipid peroxidation in cells are generally produced by electron transfer reactions.

It is now well established that superoxide free radical ($O_2^{-\cdot}$) and hydrogen peroxide are continuously produced *in vivo*. In normal circumstances, electron "leakage" from electron transport chains, such as those in mitochondria and the endoplasmic reticulum, to molecular oxygen can generate superoxidation radical.

$$O_2 + e^- \longrightarrow O_2^{-\cdot}$$

Superoxide can also be produced by other enzymes, such as the range of flavin oxidases located in peroxisomes, and by oxidation of certain compounds including ascorbic acid (see below), thiols, and adrenaline in the presence of transition metal ions. The autoxidation of reduced transition metal can also generate superoxide:

$$Fe^{2+} + O_2 \longrightarrow Fe^{3+} + O_2^{-\cdot}$$

$$Cu^{+} + O_2 \longrightarrow Cu^{2+} + O_2^{-\cdot}$$

Hydrogen peroxide is often produced in biological systems via the generation of superoxide: Two superoxide molecules can react together to form hydrogen peroxide and oxygen.

$$20_2^{-\cdot} + 2H^+ \longrightarrow H_2O_2 + O_2$$

This reaction can take place spontaneously and slowly or can be catalyzed by enzyme superoxide dismutase (SOD). Hydrogen peroxide can also be generated by a two-electron reduction of oxygen:

$$O_2 + 2e^- \longrightarrow H_2O_2$$

Although superoxide is a free radical, it is not a particularly damaging species and it does not appear to be capable of initiating lipid peroxidation. Its major significance is as a source of hydrogen peroxide and as a reductant of transition metal ion. Hydrogen peroxide is not a free radical but falls into the category of "reactive oxygen species." It is a source of hydroxyl radicals. In the presence of reactive transition metal ions, hydrogen peroxide can rather easily break down to produce the hydroxyl radical, the most reactive and damaging oxygen free radical that will attack most biological molecules and initiate lipid peroxidation at diffusion-controlled rates.

$$H_2O_2 + Fe^{2+} \longrightarrow OH\cdot + OH^- + Fe^{3+}$$

The generated ferric complexes (Fe^{3+}) react more slowly with H_2O_2 than do ferrous complexes (Fe^{2+}) so that reducing agents such as ascorbate can stimulate the previously mentioned reaction by recycling Fe^{3+} back to Fe^{2+}.

$$Fe^{3+} + \text{ascorbate} \longrightarrow Fe^{2+} + \text{semidehydroascorbate}$$

Therefore, mixtures of iron salts, ascorbate, and H_2O_2 are good sources of OH· radicals. Superoxide reduces certain ferric complex to ferrous complex, hence superoxide can also stimulate transition metal ion-dependent OH· generation from H_2O_2. In the absence of metal catalysts, superoxide and hydrogen peroxide are easily removed and are basically harmless.

An additional way to generate lipid peroxide is the direct combination of PUFAs or their side chains with an extremely reactive form of oxygen known as singlet oxygen. Lipid peroxidation started via this pathway does not require initiation because the singlet O_2 reacts directly with the fatty acid to give peroxide and is not attracting hydrogen atom to start a chain reaction. Singlet O_2 is produced when compounds are illuminated in the presence of oxygen: They absorb the light, enter a higher electronic excitation state, and transfer the excess energy to oxygen, converting it to the singlet state. Aromatic dyes, certain classes of drugs (e.g., tetracycline), and several substances found in human body (e.g., porphyrins, the vitamin riboflavin, and the bile pigment bilirubin) are examples of these photosensitizing agents.

In summary, the reactive species that initiate lipid peroxidation include oxygen itself, superoxide, hydrogen peroxide, transition metal ions, and the hydroxyl radical.

Defenses against Lipid Peroxidation

Because lipid peroxidation can be very damaging, organisms have evolved antioxidant defense systems to protect against it and also repair the system to prevent the accumulation of oxidatively damaged molecules. The antioxidant defenses consist of two categories: those preventing the generation of free radicals and those intercepting the generated radicals. The preventive defenses include efficiency of electron transfer (i.e., no "leakage" of electrons from the respiratory chain) and sequestration of transition metal ions. Iron, for example, is held tightly bound to special proteins such as transferrin and ferrin. Another type of preventive antioxidant defense is the removal of peroxides that react with transition metal ions to form reactive free radicals. Catalase and glutathione peroxidase are examples of this type of defense. Catalase is mainly located in peroxisomes and acts with hydrogen peroxide; glutathione peroxidase is found in the cytosol of most cells and is active toward both hydrogen peroxide and fatty acid hydroperoxides.

$$2H_2O_2 \longrightarrow \text{catalase} \longrightarrow 2H_2O + O_2$$

$$\text{ROOH} + 2\text{GSH} \longrightarrow \text{GSH peroxidase} \longrightarrow \text{ROH} + \text{GSSG}$$

The intercepting defenses "scavenge" the generated free radicals. As mentioned previously, superoxide dismutase and α-tocopherol are good examples of enzyme and nonenzyme scavengers, respectively.

The repair system removes damaged biomolecules before cell metabolism or viability has been altered due to their accumulation. Oxidatively damaged nucleic acids are repaired by specific enzymes, oxidized proteins are removed by proteolytic systems, and oxidized membrane lipids are processed by lipases, peroxidases, and acyl transferases.

Measurement of Lipid Peroxidation

The extent of lipid peroxidation can be determined by measuring (1) losses of fatty acids; (2) amounts of primary peroxidation products; (3) amounts of secondary products, such as carbonyls and hydrocarbon gases; and (4) ethane or pentane in expired air.

Some of the commonly used methods are described below. Analysis of fatty acids by gas liquid chromatography (GLC) or high-performance liquid chromatography (HPLC) is used for measuring the loss of unsaturated fatty acids, a consequence of lipid peroxidation. Iodine liberation and glutathione peroxidase methods are often used for measuring lipid peroxides. Lipid peroxides oxidize I^{-1} to I_2 for titration with thiosulfate and thus consumption of thiosulfate indirectly indicates the quantity of lipid peroxides. Hydrogen peroxides and hydroperoxides oxidize reduced GSH to oxidized glutathione (GSSG) and addition of glutathione reductase and NADPH reduces GSSG back to GSH, requiring consumption of NADPH, which can be related to peroxide content. Spin traps (phenyl *t*-butyl nitrone) are frequently used for trapping intermediate radicals. Products of lipid peroxide decomposition, such as hydrocarbon gases and cytotoxic aldehydes, can be measured by GLC or HPLC. Several techniques have been developed that use antibodies to detect protein modified by lipid peroxidation products.

The most commonly used assays for measurement of lipid peroxidation are the thiobarbituric acid (TBA) test and diene conjugation determination. In the TBA test, lipid samples are heated with TBA at low pH and malondialdehyde (MDA), a lipid peroxidation product, reacts with TBA to develop a pink color. Darkness of the color is related to the extent of lipid peroxidation. Because of its simplicity and economy, this method is very popular. During the process of lipid peroxidation, diene conjugations (a double bond–single bond–double bond structure) are formed (Fig. L-1) which absorb UV light in the wavelength range of 230–235 nm. The absorption of UV light at this wavelength range can be related to contents of diene conjugates in lipid extracts of tissues and, thus, to extent of lipid peroxidation. Endproducts of lipid peroxidation include short-chain alkanes such as ethane and pentane, which appear in expired air in trace amounts. These products can be measured by GLC in expired air.

Because all these methods measure only one stage of lipid peroxidation, and not the whole process, caution must be taken in interpreting the results from these measurements. In addition, each method has its own limitation. For example, the TBA test works well when applied to defined membrane systems but its application to body fluid and tissue extract has produced a host of problems. First, aldehydes other than MDA may react with TBA to form chromogens. Second, TBA test is supposed to measure the free MDA content in the lipid system; the actually measured MDA may partially or mostly be generated by decomposition of lipid peroxides during the acid heating stage of the test itself. Third, peroxide decomposition produces radicals that can start peroxidation of other lipid molecules during the assay, augmenting the responses. Fourth, there are many chemicals, which may vary from individual to individual, in human body fluids. Copper and iron ions have different sensitivity to the TBA reaction and will give different endproduct readings in addition to MDA contents. Colored chemicals such as bile pigments and glycoprotein may give false results. Measuring trace amounts of ethane and pentane in expired air as an *in vitro* indicator of lipid peroxidation suffers from the disadvantage of overestimating lipid peroxidation. These gases are produced normally during putrefaction. Therefore, cell death due to any cause may contribute to the production of these gases.

Further Reading

Cheeseman, K. H., and Slater, T. F. (Eds.) (1993). Free radical in medicine. *Br. Med. Bull.* **49**, 479–724.

Halliwell, B., and Chirico, S. (1993). Lipid peroxidation: Its mechanism, measurement, and significance. *Am. J. Clin. Nutr.* 57(Suppl.), 715s–725s.

—Zhengwei Cai and Harihara M. Mehendale

Related Topics

Acetaminophen
Carbon Tetrachloride
Ethanol
Liver
Kidney
Paraquat
Respiratory Tract

Lithium (Li)

- CAS: 7439-93-2
- Selected Compounds: Lithium carbonate, Li_2CO_3 (CAS: 554-13-2); lithium chloride, LiCl (CAS: 7447-41-8); lithium hydride, LiH (CAS: 7580-67-8)
- Chemical Class: Metals

Uses

The most widely known use of lithium is the use of lithium carbonate in treating manic-depressive affective disorders; the mechanism by which it alleviates depression in some people is not known. Industrially, lithium and its compounds are used in metal alloys, lubricants, nuclear reactor coolant, ceramics, alkaline storage batteries, and electronic tubes. It is also used as a catalyst and as a reducing agent.

Exposure Pathways

Ingestion is the most common exposure pathway; lithium carbonate is administered orally. Occupational exposures to lithium rarely produce toxicity.

Toxicokinetics

Lithium is readily absorbed when administered orally and is widely distributed in the body, mainly intracellularly. It is carried into the red blood cells by the sodium transport carrier and enters the central nervous system. Lithium can penetrate the placental barrier. It is excreted in the urine.

Mechanism of Toxicity

The exact mechanism of lithium toxicity is unknown. It may be related to lithium's displacement of potassium, producing an unusual equilibrium within the cells. Another hypothesis is that lithium is competitive with sodium for binding sites in various organs such as the kidney and the central nervous system.

Human Toxicity

Occupational lithium toxicity is rare. The use of lithium carbonate for depression may result in damage to the neuromuscular system resulting in ataxia and tremors. Toxicity often occurs after weeks of chronic intake. The first signs of toxicity are nausea, vomiting, and abdominal pain. The action on the central nervous system can result in tremors, epileptic-type seizures, impediment of speech, and even short blackout periods. The heart can also be affected resulting in hypertension and arrhythmias. Nephrotoxicity has been recorded in some patients.

Lithium hydride rapidly converts to lithium hydroxide in contact with water. Lithium hydroxide is corrosive to all tissues, outer skin, as well as lung cells. The ACGIH TLV-TWA for lithium hydride is 0.025 mg/m^3.

Clinical Management

There is no specific antidote for lithium toxicity. For acute overdose, administration of syrup of ipecac followed by gastric lavage is recommended. Electrolyte replacement should follow. An infusion of mannitol or urea and increasing the alkalinity of the urine will enhance lithium excretion. For abnormal motor activity, a tranquilizer such as diazepam is helpful. High salt intake protects against lithium toxicity in the kidneys.

Animal Toxicity

Lithium is neither mutagenic nor carcinogenic.

—Arthur Furst and Shirley B. Radding

Related Topics

Kidney
Metals

Liver

Introduction

The liver is the largest organ in the human body, weighing approximately 1.5 kg in human adults.

Although not an elegant organ in its structure, having (and needing) no constant form, its highly complex activities are essential for life. The liver accommodates its form to its surroundings and expands into any part of the abdominal area not occupied by other viscera. Details of arrangement and lobation vary greatly from species to species and even between individuals of the same species. Ancient priests divined the future from the liver patterns of sacrificed animals; they found plenty of scope for personalized interpretations!

The liver performs four basic functions which are essential for maintenance of homeostasis and integration of metabolism:

1. Storage and filtration of blood
2. Metabolism and storage of many xenobiotics, as well as nutrients and endogenous compounds such as bile acids, fatty acids, and steroids and other hormones
3. Secretory and excretory activities involved in bile formation and flow (exocrine functions)
4. Synthesis of a variety of important constituents of blood plasma, which are secreted directly into the blood (endocrine functions)

Liver injury by chemical substances has been recognized for more than 100 years.

Review of Liver Structure and Function

Correlation of the liver's structure with its many functions, and an appreciation of the systemic consequences of toxic injury to this vital organ, depends on an understanding of its strategic location in the circulation. The liver functions as an interface between the digestive tract and the systemic circulation. The liver's interposition between the digestive tract and the systemic circulation is responsible for both its primary role in metabolism of xenobiotics and its susceptibility to their toxic actions. It directly receives all the material (including xenobiotics) absorbed from the intestine (except the lipid chylomicrons, which are transported by lymphatic vessels). The absorbed materials are taken up and further metabolized by the liver or transformed and released to the blood for utilization or storage elsewhere.

The liver has a dual blood supply. Its principal afferent (incoming) blood vessel is the portal vein, which drains the capillary beds of the intestine and spleen at a rate of about 1100 ml per minute (about 75% of the total). A smaller volume of freshly oxygenated arterial blood (about 350 ml, or 25%) is carried by the hepatic artery. These two vessels (and the bile duct) enter the liver together at the porta (Latin for "gate") and branch together into a second capillary bed, the hepatic sinusoids. The liver is drained by the efferent (outgoing) hepatic veins into the inferior vena cava near the heart. This special arrangement of blood vessels—where blood collected from one set of capillaries passes through a larger vessel into a second set of capillaries before entering the venous circulation—is called a portal system. The hepatic blood vessels are accompanied throughout the parenchyma by bile ducts and lymphatic vessels.

The hepatic sinusoids—the second capillary bed in the hepatic portal system—differ from ordinary capillaries in several respects. They are larger and more variable in diameter, and their walls are lined with both endothelial cells and very large, actively phagocytic Kupffer cells. Unlike most other blood vessels in vertebrates, the sinusoids have actual discontinuities of as much as a micrometer in diameter between the endothelial cells, allowing the blood plasma, including plasma proteins (but not blood cells), to pass freely through into the space of Disse and directly contact the liver cells. The direct access of the plasma to the surface of the liver cell is a structural feature of great functional importance in the active exchange of materials between the liver and the bloodstream.

The Liver Serves as a Blood Filter and Reservoir

Blood entering the hepatic sinusoids carries many bacteria from the digestive tract. The phagocytic Kupffer cells interspersed among the typical endothelial cells lining this specialized capillary bed rapidly phagocytize more than 99% of bacteria and other foreign particles in the blood.

Because the liver is a soft, expansible structure, large volumes of blood can be stored in its vessels. The normal hepatic blood volume is about 450 ml, or almost 10% of the normal human total blood volume. As much as another liter can be stored when blood volume is high. Likewise, the liver can supply extra blood when the circulatory volume is diminished.

The Liver Is Composed Primarily of Hepatocytes

Although the liver consists of several cell types present which are vital for its function—endothelial cells lining the blood vessels, bile ductular cells, connective tissue cells, nerve cells, and the phagocytic Kupffer cells—the hepatocytes constitute about 80% of the cytoplasmic mass and carry out the liver's characteristic metabolic and synthetic functions. These cells are essential for life and have an extraordinary capacity to regenerate and flexibly respond to varying metabolic demands. Indeed, they are unrivaled in their functional diversity, complexity, and flexibility.

Although the hepatocyte is a highly differentiated cell that rarely divides in adult vertebrates, it possesses a tremendous capacity for compensatory hyperplasia after injury or removal of liver tissue. It appears that hepatocytes engaged in the regenerative process undergo quantitative rather than qualitative changes in gene expression. Preferentially expressed are stress proteins, the multidrug-resistance gene, and several protooncogenes.

Protooncogenes in particular are thought to play an essential role in cell proliferation and differentiation because they are highly conserved in evolution, differentially expressed during development, and known to play a role in malignant transformation. In fact, analysis of protooncogene expression during liver regeneration provided one of the first demonstrations that the expression of these genes is regulated during normal growth.

The Basic Anatomical Unit of the Liver Is the Classical Lobule

The hepatocytes are arranged in single-cell-thick plates or sheets that appear to radiate out from terminal branches of the hepatic veins. These have traditionally been termed "central veins" because of their location in the polyhedral units of liver parenchyma which constitute the classical "liver lobules," typically hexagonal structures 2 or 3 mm in length and 1 or 2 mm in diameter. Neighboring plates are separated by sinusoids, which are closely applied to the sheets of liver cells and intercommunicate through fenestrations ("windows") in them to form a labyrinthine system covering a very large area of liver parenchyma. The human liver contains 50,000–100,000 individual lobules. The corners of the polygonal lobules are each occupied by portal space containing portal triads: branches of portal venule, hepatic arteriole, and bile ductule. (See Fig. L-2 for anatomical illustration.)

It was formerly thought that blood flowed directly from the portal space vessels between plates to hepatocytes to be collected in the central veins. Although it is now clear that the actual flow of blood in these areas is not as previously envisioned, the lobule unit remains conceptually convenient because it exhibits morphologically distinguishable zones, e.g., differential deposition of glycogen and fat, referred to as centrilobular, mid-zonal, or periportal. Furthermore, toxic agents of

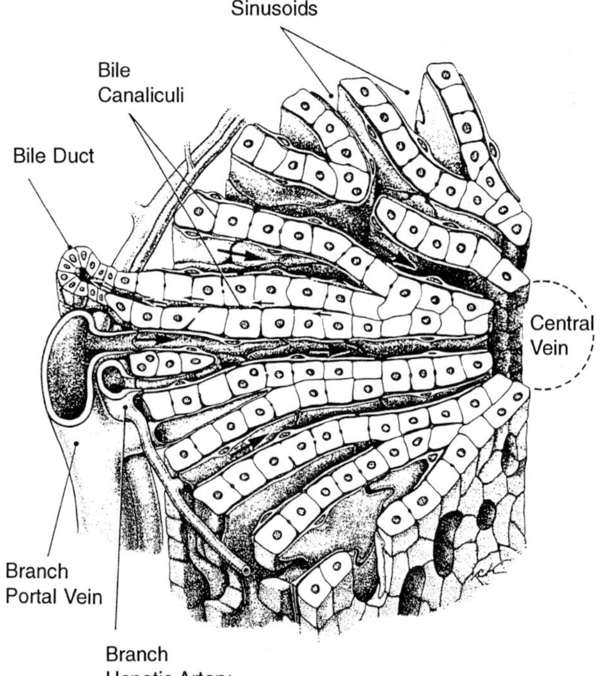

FIGURE L-2. Diagram illustrating the basic anatomical unit of the liver, the liver lobule, showing (1) the radial disposition of the liver cell plates and sinusoids around the central vein, (2) the centripetal flow of blood from branches of the hepatic artery and portal vein, and (3) the centrifugal flow of bile (small arrows) to the small bile duct in the portal space (reproduced with permission from W. Bloom and D. W. Fawcett (Eds.), A Textbook of Histology, *9th ed. Saunders, Philadelphia, 1968; redrawn and modified from Ham,* Textbook of Histology, *Lippincott, Philadelphia).*

pathological conditions may selectively show their harmful effects in these areas.

The Basic Functional Unit of the Liver Is the Acinus

We now know that blood enters the sinusoids of the parenchyma via fine terminal branches of the afferent vessels which leave the portal spaces at intervals, coursing perpendicular to the central vein and along the sides of the hexagons forming classical lobules. Each fine terminal afferent vessel supplies blood to only sectors of adjacent lobules. The associated mass of parenchymal tissue which they preferentially supply is termed an acinus (Latin for "berry") (Fig. L-3). The acinus lies between two or more terminal hepatic venules (central veins in the classical terminology), with which its vascular and biliary axis interdigitates. Acini are irregular in size and shape, and there is no physical separation between them.

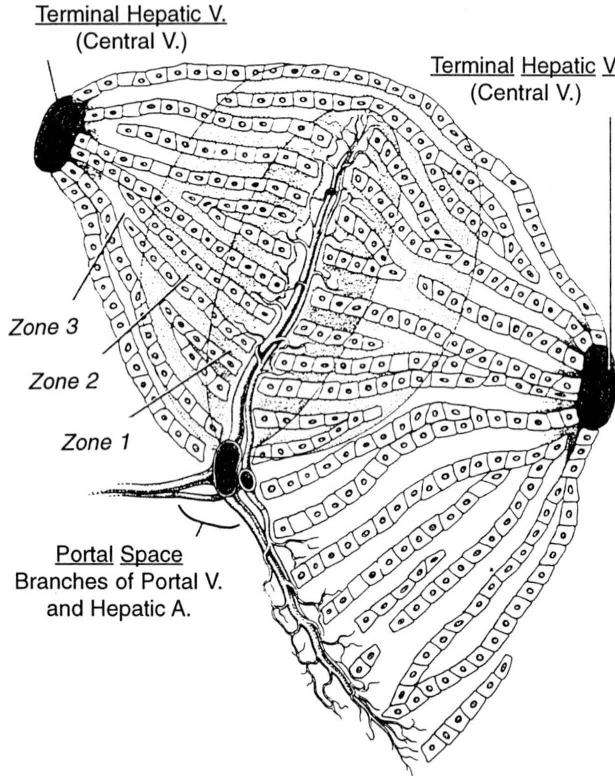

FIGURE L-3. Diagram illustrating the basic functional unit of the liver, the acinus, consisting of the tissue centered around the terminal branches of the hepatic artery and portal vein. The cells in zone 1 nearest these vessels receive the highest concentrations of oxygen and nutrients, while those in zones 2 and 3 are exposed to progressively depleted blood (reproduced with permission from W. Bloom and D. W. Fawcett (Eds.), A Textbook of Histology, *9th ed. Saunders, Philadelphia, 1968; redrawn from A. Rappaport* et al., Anat. Rec. *119, 11, 1954).*

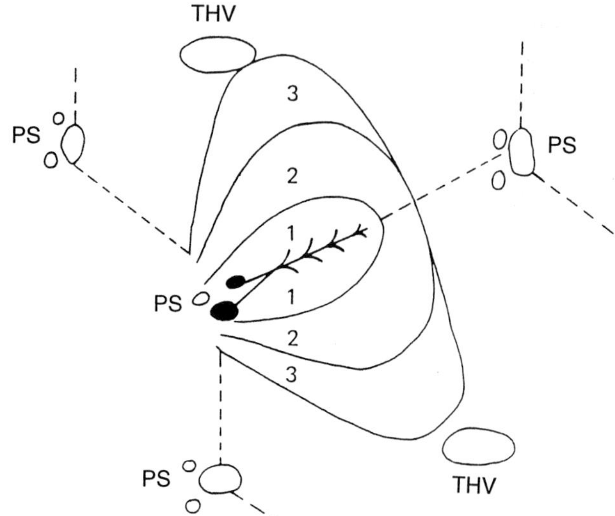

FIGURE L-4. Schematic representation of a simple hepatic acinus. PS is the portal space, consisting of a branch of the portal vein, a hepatic arteriole, and a bile duct; THV is the terminal hepatic venule (central vein); 1, 2, and 3 represent the various zones surrounding the terminal afferent vessel (reproduced with permission from Klassen, C. D., Amdur, M. O., and Doull, J. (Eds.), Casarett and Doull's Toxicology: The Basic Science of Poisons, *3rd ed., Macmillan, New York, 1986).*

As with the classical lobule, there are distinct circulatory zones within each acinus. They are typically divided into three, depending on their distance from the afferent vessels (Fig. L-4). Zone 1, being closest to the supply of fresh blood, is the first to receive oxygen and nutrients and the last to undergo necrosis. The more distal regions, zones 2 and 3, receive progressively depleted blood, and hence are possibly less resistant to hepatotoxicants and other vectors of hepatic injury. Furthermore, the fenestrations between sinusoidal endothelial cells gradually increase in number from the periportal to the pericentral end of the sinusoid, allowing the remaining nutrients greater access to the centrally located cells.

There is considerable evidence that position within the acinus also affects important aspects of hepatocyte function, including bile secretion and metabolic activity. Thus, periportal and pericentral cells differ both structurally and functionally, as summarized in Table L-1. For example, periportal (zone 1) cells take up more bile acids from sinusoidal blood, and hence secrete more biliary constituents. Pericentral (zone 3) cells are specialized to perform higher levels of metabolic and degradative activities.

The Liver Is an Exocrine Gland, Secreting Bile

The liver functions as an exocrine gland, with each hepatocyte continually secreting a small amount of bile into tiny bile canaliculi located between adjacent pairs of parenchymal cells. These tiny vessels form a continuous network from lobule to lobule throughout the organ. The canaliculi are smallest near the central vein, increasing in diameter with proximity to the portal triads. The canaliculi coalesce into biliary ductules, interlobular bile ducts, and larger hepatic ducts. The main hepatic duct joins the cystic duct from the gallbladder to form the common bile duct, which drains into the duodenum. The total secretion of bile by the human liver is approximately 700–1200 ml per day.

Important both as a digestive secretion and as a medium of excretion, bile is a complex mixture of bile salts, bile pigments, phospholipids, cholesterol, inorganic electrolytes, and endproducts of metabolism.

Bile Salts Enable the Digestion of Lipids

Cholesterol is the precursor of both steroids and bile salts and is an integral component of cell membranes. It is eliminated from the body via conversion to bile salts and direct secretion into the bile. In fact, the word cholesterol [from the Greek "chole" (bile) and "stereos" (solid)] was used originally to describe the material of which gallstones are made. In the process of degradation, it is converted to the primary bile acids cholic acid and chenodeoxycholic acid in approximately equal amounts. The salts of these acids are excreted in bile. They perform two important functions in the digestive tract:

1. They act as detergents, emulsifying large fat droplets into small ones. This action creates a much larger surface area for the action of lipase in the small intestine, thereby increasing lipid absorption.

2. They form minute complexes called micelles with the emulsified lipids. The electrical charges of the strongly ionized bile salts render these micelles highly soluble, aiding in their transport to the absorptive surfaces of the intestinal brush border. The fats readily diffuse across the membrane, leaving the charged bile salts to retrieve more fats in a "ferrying" activity.

Bile salts are extensively metabolized to secondary bile acids by intestinal microflora in the gut. Approximately 94% of the bile salts are reabsorbed at special mucosal receptor sites in the distal ileum and reused by the liver by the process of enterohepatic circulation. In enterohepatic circulation, compounds secreted in bile are reabsorbed in the gastrointestinal tract and returned to the liver. On reaching the liver in the portal blood, almost all of the bile salts are taken up across the sinusoidal membranes of hepatocytes (predominantly in periportal regions). The bile acids are then resecreted into the bile. On average, these salts make the entire circuit about 18 times before being lost in the feces. Thus, enterohepatic circulation of toxicants increases their half-life in the body and hence their opportunity to exert toxic effects.

TABLE L-1
Predominant Lobular/Acinar Localization of Major Liver Functions

Periportal zone/zone 1
Glucose release
Oxidative energy metabolism
Amino acid utilization
Protection against oxidants
Bile acid uptake and excretion
Bilirubin excretion
Centrilobular zone/zone 3
Glucose uptake
Ammonia detoxification
Biotransformation reactions

Bile Pigments Are Products of Red Blood Cell Destruction

Red blood cells circulate for about 120 days before their membranes become very fragile and they rupture in vascular "tight spots" like the spleen. The hemoglobin released when these cells rupture is rapidly taken up by tissue macrophages in many parts of the body, but especially by the Kupffer cells of the liver. The porphyrin portion of the hemoglobin molecule is oxidized in the macrophages to biliverdin, which is rapidly reduced to the yellow-green bile pigment bilirubin. The macrophages release bilirubin into the blood, where it binds tightly to albumin and is transported throughout the circulation to the liver. Inside hepatocytes, it associates with proteins which "trap" it inside the liver cells. It is subsequently removed from these holding proteins and conjugated with glucuronide (80%), sulfate (10%), and other substances (10%). These conjugated forms are then actively transported into the bile canaliculi and largely eliminated with the feces.

This pigment is highly soluble in all cell membranes and also very toxic; hence, its excretion is one of the liver's most important functions. Interestingly, however, recent studies have demonstrated that bilirubin is an effective antioxidant of possible physiological importance. Along with urate and ascorbate (vitamin C), it is one of the three principal antioxidants in plasma. In membranes, its antioxidative efficacy rivals that of vitamin E. Thus, this toxic endproduct of a degradative pathway can also perform a beneficial function.

The Liver Plays a Key Role in the Integration of Metabolism

The liver is the metabolic center of the body. In fact, most of the field of biochemistry is concerned with its metabolic reactions. The liver essentially converts ingested food into a balanced cell culture medium via metabolic interconversion of amino acids, carbohydrates, and lipids. It also synthesizes many substances that are subsequently exported for use in other areas of the body.

Carbohydrate Metabolism

The liver serves as an energy reservoir, storing glucose as glycogen for release on demand. It thus plays a very important role in maintaining a normal blood glucose concentration. In the event of severe glucose deficiency, the liver can convert amino acids into glucose.

Fat Metabolism

The liver also plays a central role in synthesis, oxidation, storage, and distribution of lipids. It not only aids in the absorption of fats through the action of the bile salts, but also (1) both synthesizes and oxidizes fatty acids, cholesterol, triacylglycerols, and phospholipids (the major components of cell membranes); (2) synthesizes most of the plasma lipoproteins; and (3) converts carbohydrates and proteins into fat.

About 80% of the cholesterol synthesized in the liver is converted into bile salts. The remainder of the cholesterol, triacylglycerols, other lipids, and hydrophobic substances (including xenobiotics) are transported to other tissues throughout the body by plasma lipoproteins. These lipoproteins, which are classified according to density, consist of apoproteins (also made by the liver) and various combinations of fat and fat-soluble compounds.

Protein Metabolism

The most important functions of the liver in protein metabolism are (1) deamination of amino acids for use as energy or conversion into fats and carbohydrates, (2) synthesis and interconversion of amino acids and other metabolically important compounds, (3) formation of urea for excretion of ammonia, and (4) formation of plasma proteins.

Approximately 90% of the plasma proteins are formed by the hepatocytes. Among these important products are albumin (involved in the maintenance of osmotic pressure), clotting and anticlotting factors, and immunoglobulins. The remaining 10% are largely γ-globulins synthesized by plasma cells.

Toxic Liver Injury

The Liver Is Often a Target of Toxic Agents

Most toxic agents enter the body via the gastrointestinal tract and after absorption are carried directly to the liver. There, the drug metabolizing enzyme systems may detoxify them or, in some cases, create reactive intermediates which injure the liver and other tissues. Even chemicals that are successfully excreted in the bile can return to the liver via the cycle of enterohepatic circulation. Furthermore, the liver has a high concentration of binding sites and therefore a tendency to accumulate certain xenobiotics. The liver's position at the interface of the digestive tract and the blood, and its central role in the metabolism and excretion of foreign chemicals, therefore renders it especially vulnerable to toxic injury.

Toxic Liver Injury Can Take Many Forms

Many chemicals are hepatotoxic, including thousands of synthetic drugs and chemicals as well as a plethora of natural compounds such as bacterial, fungal, plant, and animal toxins. Some examples of chemicals causing liver injury are shown in Table L-2.

It is clear that a variety of pathologic processes are involved in toxic liver injury, depending on causative agent and duration of exposure. The incidence of hepatotoxic injury by a given chemical differs among species and individuals; a dose–response relationship may not always be evident. The toxicity of chemicals can be significantly modified by a number of host and other variables, particularly hepatic enzyme activity. Furthermore, different biochemical alterations in the liver can lead to the same toxic effect; no single mechanism seems to govern the appearance of degenerative changes in hepatocytes or alterations in their function. Virtually all forms of drug-induced liver injury closely resemble other forms of liver disease not presently known to be produced by chemicals.

A variety of systems have been devised to impose some order on this profusion of toxic liver lesions. Our discussion resorts to the simple device of distinguishing between generally acute and generally chronic forms of toxic liver disease, followed by consideration of the mechanisms by which selected compounds exert these effects. A few other classification systems are mentioned here to provide the reader with a further conceptual framework for organization of current knowledge. In one such system, lesions are categorized by the duration of exposure to the causal agent. Some injuries typically occur after acute exposure, while others require chronic exposure. For example, an acute effect of ethanol is fatty change, metamorphosis, or accumulation (intracellular accumulation of triacylglycerols), while in the long-term cirrhosis occurs.

Some injuries may be transient, while others are irreversible. For example, fatty change is often transient and not necessarily indicative of functional compromise; under certain conditions, hepatocytes with accumulated fat function normally. Malignant transformation, on the other hand, is irreversible and seriously disrupts hepatocellular function. Necrosis (cell death) may or may not be life-threatening, depending on its extent (see previous discussion of liver regeneration).

Yet another classification system refers to the nature of the host's response to the causative agent. Some agents, referred to as intrinsic hepatotoxicants, will cause hepatotoxicity in most individuals of most species. In the case of diosyncratic hepatotoxicants, where a chemical's toxic effects are a function of unusual susceptibility of the exposed individual, it may not be clear whether the lesion is a manifestation of the hepatotoxic properties of the substance in question or a manifestation of the individual's untoward response to the agent. This response may mean hypersensitivity (allergic) reactions or exaggerated responses to minor alterations in liver function. For example, anabolic or contraceptive steroids cause diminished biliary excretion (cholestasis) in most humans, with a few showing jaundice. It is not clear whether the occasional jaundice is the result of an allergic response or an extreme reaction to diminished biliary excretion. Likewise, many drugs, for example, isoniazid and halothane, can precipitate a potentially fatal viral-like hepatitis in susceptible subjects.

TABLE L-2
Examples of Liver Toxicants Causing Specific Types of Injury

Necrosis and fatty liver
Carbon tetrachloride
Ethanol
Trichloroethylene
Acetaminophen
Cholestasis
Chlorpromazine
Diazepam
Estradiol
Sulfanilamide
Hepatitis
Isoniazid
Halothane
Indomethacin
Porphyria
Hexachlorobenzene
Cirrhosis
Ethanol
Carcinogenesis (in experimental animals)
Carbon tetrachloride
Dimethylbenzanthracene
Polychlorinated biphenyls and dioxins
Vinyl chloride

Acute Toxic Effects

Acute exposures to hepatotoxicants may result in the following:

1. Degenerative changes (lipid or water accumulation)
2. Necrosis
   Zonal, focal, or massive
   Venoocclusive disease
   Hepatitis
3. Hepatobiliary dysfunction
4. Acute porphyria

Degenerative Changes

Disturbances in cellular metabolism can cause swelling and accumulation of materials such as water or lipid. These changes are usually (but not always) reversible. Hydropic change (water accumulation) often precedes fatty metamorphosis. The fatty liver is grossly enlarged and pale yellow. Fat droplets consisting mostly of triacylglycerols and fatty acids are visible histologically using lipid stains. Fatty change may be brought about by several distinct mechanisms involving fatty acid and protein metabolism. Examples of causative agents are carbon tetrachloride, ethionine, and ethanol.

Necrosis

Cell swelling and lipid accumulation may precede cell necrosis. Necrosis can affect small groups of cells (focal), groups of cells located in discrete zones (zonal), or many cells (massive). Centrilobular necrosis refers to the death of cells surrounding the central vein of the classical lobule (zone 3 of acinar model). Typical causative agents are carbon tetrachloride, pyrrolizidine alkaloids, acetaminophen, bromobenzene, and isoniazid. An agent which causes periportal necrosis (cell death around portal spaces; zone 1 of acinus) is allyl alcohol. Mid-zonal (acinar zone 2) necrosis can be caused by beryllium and yellow phosphorus. Because of the dose-responsiveness and predictability of the lesions they cause, these agents are regarded as direct hepatotoxicants. Note, however, that many direct hepatotoxicants must undergo biotransformation to reactive forms.

Most of the unpredictable idiosyncratic forms of toxic liver injury are more diffuse, consisting of necrosis with significant inflammatory reaction. Nonspecific hepatitis, which can be caused by aspirin (acetylsalicylic acid), is characterized by a few scattered foci of necrosis. A clinical syndrome indistinguishable from viral hepatitis (hence the name viral-like hepatitis) has been associated with various drugs, e.g., isoniazid and halothane. This appears histologically as generalized parenchymal damage with disruption of the normal liver cell arrangement, often accompanied by fever, rash, arthralgias, and eosinophilia. The cells may be swollen and hydropic, especially in the centrilobular regions. There may be a progression to a massive necrosis typical of viral hepatitis. Granulomatous hepatitis, characterized by well-demarcated aggregates of inflammatory cells, occur with or without other types of hepatic injury in response to several drugs. Typical examples are sulfonamides and sulfonylurea derivatives.

Hepatobiliary Dysfunction

Interference with any step in the complex sequences of hepatic uptake and secretion could affect hepatobiliary function (see previous discussion). A number of agents cause cholestasis, generally defined as reduced bile flow. This condition can arise from extrahepatic obstruction of bile flow or intrahepatic alterations that reduce secretion and excretion of solutes and water. Because their elimination is impeded, bile substances (including bile acids and pigments, cholesterol, and various endogenous and exogenous conjugated products) accumulate within the liver and in the systemic blood. Cholestasis is generally difficult to reproduce in experimental animals using the drugs that cause it in humans. However, it is possible to produce cholestatic responses in animals following administration of certain compounds, including lithocholic acid, α-naphthylisothiocyanate, anabolic and contraceptive steroids, and chlorpromazine.

Acute Toxic Porphyria

The biochemistry of the porphyrins and the bile pigments is closely related because heme is synthesized from porphyrins and iron and the products of its degradation are bile pigments and iron. Porphyrins are cyclic compounds formed by the linkage of four pyrrole rings through methenyl bridges. Iron is complexed to the nitrogen atom of the pyrrole rings. The metalloporphyrin is in turn conjugated to proteins to form hemoglobin, cytochromes, and several other hemoproteins important in biological processes. The term "porphyrin" is derived from the Greek word porphyra (purple) because mammalian porphyrins are deep red or purple in color (due to the iron atom). They are easily detected in blood, urine, and feces due to their color and fluorescent properties.

The porphyrias are a heterogeneous group of diseases, all of which involve disorders of heme biosynthesis which result in accumulation and increased excretion of porphyrins or porphyrin precursors. The porphyrias can be divided into two kinds: the hereditary porphyrias, some of which can be exacerbated by exposure to certain chemicals, and the toxic porphyrias, which can be produced by exposure to certain chemicals alone. The pattern of excretion of porphyrins and porphyrin precursors is characteristic for each type. Clinical symptoms consist mainly of cutaneous photosensitivity and/or neurological disturbances. Hexachlorobenzene is a chemical inducer of porphyria.

Chronic Toxic Effects

Chronic exposure to certain chemicals can cause cirrhosis, a marked alteration of the entire liver structure with both degenerative and proliferative changes observed, and neoplasia.

Cirrhosis

Cirrhosis is characterized by diffuse destruction and partial regeneration of parenchymal tissue and the formation of collagen septa distributed throughout most of the liver. Separated by these fibrous sheaths, clusters of hepatocytes appear as nodules. The pathogenesis of cirrhosis is poorly understood. In most cases, the death of scattered single cells together with defective repair mechanisms appear to lead to scarring. In humans, the single most important cause of cirrhosis is chronic ingestion of alcohol. This condition is not easy to duplicate in laboratory animals with ethanol, leading to the suggestion that other factors unique to humans may play an important role in pathogenesis. A major factor might be diet since alcoholics usually suffer nutritional deficiency.

Neoplasia

Susceptibility to liver tumors differs significantly among species. A large number of chemicals, both anthropogenic and naturally occurring, are known to induce liver cancers in animals, including carbon tetrachloride, chloroform, pyrrolizidine alkaloids, dioxin, aflatoxin, and acetylaminofluorene. However, the human hepatocarcinogenicity of many chemicals has not been well established. One of the difficulties in assessing the potential risks of human exposure to chemicals is the fact that the protocols typically used in chemical risk assessment studies tend to overpredict carcinogenicity. For example, several of the commonly used rodent species have a higher natural incidence of liver tumors than do humans, and the test procedures involve long-term administration of doses very much larger than those to which humans are likely to be exposed.

Further Reading

Ellenhorn, M., and Barceloux, D. (Eds.) (1988), *Medical Toxicology: Diagnosis and Treatment of Human Poisoning*. Elsevier, New York.

Klassen, C. D., Amdur, M. O., and Doull, J. (Eds.) (1996). *Casarett and Doull's Toxicology: The Basic Science of Poisons*, 5th ed. McGraw-Hill, New York.

—Janet E. Kester

Related Topics

Acetaminophen
Acetylaminofluorine
Acetylsalicylic Acid
Aflatoxin
Biotransformation
Blood
Bromobenzene
Carbon Tetrachloride
Chloroform
Dioxins
Distribution
Ethanol
Excretion
Immune System
Isoniazid
Lipid Peroxidation
Metallothionein
Peroxisome Proliferators
Tissue Repair

Loperamide

- CAS: 53179-11-6
- Preferred Name: Loperamide hydrochloride
- Synonyms: Imodium; Imodium AD
- Pharmaceutical Class: Antidiarrheal
- Chemical Structure:

Uses
Loperamide is a nonprescription medication for the treatment of acute nonspecific diarrhea and chronic diarrhea associated with inflammatory bowel disease. It is also used to reduce the volume of discharge from ileostomies.

Exposure Pathways
Loperamide is available in capsule and liquid forms. Ingestion is the most common route of exposure.

Toxicokinetics
Loperamide is absorbed slowly from the gastrointestinal tract reaching peak levels within 4 hr. It undergoes enterohepatic circulation. Protein binding is 97%. Loperamide is primarily excreted in the urine. The half-life can range from 7 to 15 hr and is not altered as a function of dose.

Mechanism of Toxicity
Loperamide's mechanism of toxicity is related to opioid-like activity that causes depression of the central nervous system (CNS). The abuse potential for loperamide is low.

Human Toxicity
Children appear to be more susceptible than adults to the toxic effects of loperamide. These effects mimic opiate poisoning. Miosis, nausea, vomiting, and varying degrees of CNS depression exhibited by ataxia and drowsiness to prolonged coma can be seen. Loperamide is not recommended for use in children under 2 years of age. Death has occurred after misuse of loperamide in children 6.5 months and younger.

Clinical Management
Close monitoring is necessary for a minimum of 24 hr, with respiratory support as necessary. Gastric lavage and/or administration of activated charcoal is advised over the use of syrup of ipecac for gastric decontamination. Use of the narcotic antagonist naloxone may be necessary.

Animal Toxicity
In dogs 1.25–5 mg/kg/day has produced vomiting, CNS depression, severe salivation, and weight loss. Amounts >5 mg/kg/day have produced hemorrhagic enteritis and paresis.

—Linda Hart

Related Topic

Diphenoxylate

Loxapine

- Synonyms: Loxapine hydrochloride; loxapine succinate (CAS 27833-64-3); Loxitane; 2-chloro-11-(4-methyl-1-piperazinyl)-dibenz[*b,f*][1,4]oxazepine
- Pharmaceutical Class: Dibenzoxazepine, neuroleptic agent, antipsychotic, major tranquilizer

♦ CHEMICAL STRUCTURE: (Loxapine hydrochloride; loxapine succinate)

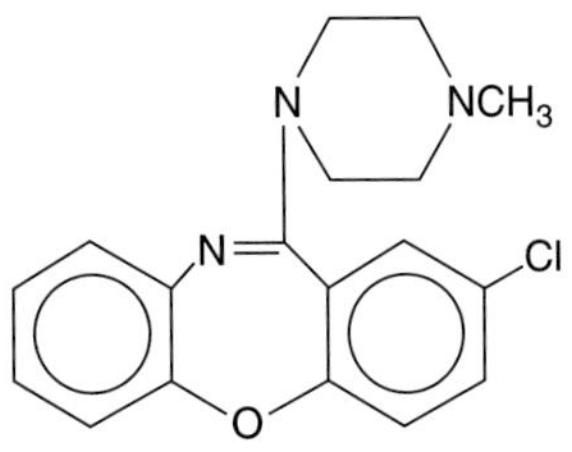

Uses

Loxapine is used to treat and control the psychotic symptoms of both acute and chronic schizophrenia. Other uses include treatment of dementia, anxiety neurosis, hostile/aggressive criminal behavior, and psychotic depression.

Exposure Pathways

Loxapine is available in oral liquid, oral capsule, and injectable dosage forms. The principal exposure pathway is intentional ingestion by adults or accidental ingestion by small children.

Toxicokinetics

Loxapine is readily but incompletely absorbed. Due to first-pass metabolism, oral bioavailability is 30% less than bioavailability after intramuscular injection. The peak blood level occurs 1 or 2 hr after oral administration and 5 hr after intramuscular injection. Loxapine is extensively metabolized in the liver through aromatic hydroxylation, N-demethylation, or N-oxidation. The metabolite amoxapine is active and marketed as an antidepressant. Loxapine is widely distributed throughout the body, including the central nervous system. The main metabolites are excreted both in the urine and feces, and 50% of a single oral dose is eliminated within 24 hr. The mean half-life of oral loxapine is 4 hr; the mean half-life of loxapine administered through intramuscular injection is 12 hr.

Mechanism of Toxicity

The exact mechanism of action of loxapine is not known. It is thought to change the level of excitability in subcortical inhibitory areas of the brain by reducing the firing threshold of some polysynaptic neurons leading to seizure activity.

Human Toxicity

The initial therapeutic dose of loxapine is 10 mg twice each day and may be increased into the normal therapeutic range of 60–100 mg per day in divided doses. The maximum dose is 250 mg per day. Clinical signs of toxicity most frequently seen include sedation, coma, seizures, extrapyramidal effects, and rarely hypotension and cardiac arrhythmias. Coma and seizures may develop rapidly following an exposure to loxapine or may be delayed for many hours. The seizures are both multiple and prolonged. Rhabdomyolysis following seizures may occur. Neuroleptic malignant syndrome has been reported after therapeutic use and acute intoxication. The most commonly reported dystonic reactions include akathisias, stiff neck, stiff or protruding tongue, and tremor. Anticholinergic effects, including dry mouth, blurred vision, and tachycardia, have been seen. Cardiac effects include prolonged Q–T interval and mild hypotension; however, the cardiac effects are less pronounced than those associated with tricyclic antidepressants. Hypokalemia has also been noted. Adverse reactions following therapeutic use include sedation, dizziness, insomnia, agitation, tardive dyskinesia, dysphoria, tachycardia, syncope, anorexia, nausea, vomiting, constipation, diarrhea, and dyspepsia.

Clinical Management

All basic and advanced life-support measures should be implemented; seizures should be anticipated. Gastric decontamination should be performed. Loxapine readily binds to activated charcoal. Aggressive supportive care should be instituted. Diazepam is the drug of choice for seizures and phenytoin to prevent recurrence. Dystonic reactions respond well to intravenous benztropine or diphenhydramine. Oral therapy with diphenhydramine or benztropine should be continued for 2 days to prevent recurrence of the dystonic reaction. For patients suffering from neuroleptic malignant syndrome, dantrolene sodium and bromocriptine have been used in conjunction with cooling and other supportive measures. Arrhythmias should be treated with lidocaine or phenytoin. Hemodialysis and hemoperfusion have not been shown to be effective.

Animal Toxicity

No specific information is available. Signs of toxicity are expected to include sedation, dullness, hypotension, respiratory depression, anorexia, colic, weakness, fever, icterus, restlessness, and seizures. Treatment consists of aggressive supportive care and gastric decontamination.

—Douglas J. Borys

Related Topics

Butyrophenones
Chlorpromazine
Neurotoxicology
Phenothiazines
Thioxanthenes

LSD

- CAS: 50-37-3
- PREFERRED NAME: Lysergic acid diethylamide
- SYNONYMS: Lysergide; *N,N*-diethyllysergamide; isolysergic acid amide; LSD-25; acid; blotter; purple microdots
- PHARMACEUTICAL CLASS: An indole alkaloid derivative that has hallucinogenic and illusionogenic activity
- CHEMICAL STRUCTURE:

$CON(C_2H_5)_2$
$N—CH_3$
N
H

Uses
LSD is a drug of abuse.

Exposure Pathways
The most common route of exposure is oral ingestion, with the dose frequently impregnated on paper. Nasal insufflation or intravenous injection are also utilized.

Toxicokinetics
The absorption of LSD is described as rapid, with peak concentrations within 60 min after ingestion. The onset of central nervous system (CNS) effects is within the first 5–10 min after ingestion. Hepatic metabolism results in the formation of numerous metabolites, and a small amount of the dose is excreted unchanged in the urine. The apparent volume of distribution is approximately 0.3 liters/kg. The drug penetrates into the CNS, concentrating in the visual brain areas and the reticular activating systems. The elimination half-life is approximately 2.5–3 hr.

Mechanism of Toxicity
LSD appears to act at postsynaptic serotonin receptors or enhance the response to serotonin. There may be dopaminergic activity and other effects in the serotonin pathways which result in starting and sustaining hallucinatory effects. LSD also has sympathomimetic, amphetamine-like activity, which accounts for much of its toxicity.

Human Toxicity: Acute
At the usual street dose of 50–300 μg, LSD produces changes in perception. These are frequently associated with distortion of what the person sees, including the appearance of Satan's face, aging of friend's faces, increasing presence of red colors, and swirling and geometric shapes. Other changes in perception include time, touch, odor, hearing, and sensation of body movement and image. These are usually identified by the intoxicated person as not real occurrences and may be considered pseudohallucinations. True hallucinations, which the individual believes are real, are less common. Other possible CNS effects include depersonalization, decreased ability to think and make judgments, and changes in mood and behavior. Patients are generally quiet and withdrawn, though aggression and bizarre behavior can less frequently occur. Acute panic attacks more commonly occur with unexpected use or less experienced users. Acute psychotic reactions can also occur. Seizures, vascular insufficiency, anisocoria, hippus, and coma are other CNS toxicities associated with LSD use. LSD toxicity is also associated with the sympathomimetic effects. Hyperthermia, rhabdomyolysis, hypertension, hyperreflexia, tremors, and muscle weakness are evidence of significant sympathetic toxicity. Death can occur, though it appears to be very infre-

quent. Plasma concentrations are very low, reported to be 5–10 ng/ml after 0.140 mg doses.

Human Toxicity: Chronic

Toxicity includes flashbacks, chronic psychosis, and possibly an increased incidence of birth defects. Flashbacks are the recurrence of the CNS changes associated with acute LSD use, which can occur up to 4 years after last use. Flashbacks occur in 15–60% of persons who use LSD and may be memory recall of the acute intoxication. Both mental and physiological stress can precipitate flashbacks. LSD may cause chromosomal aberrations and increased risk of congenital abnormalities in the fetus when used during pregnancy.

Clinical Management

The patient's airway, breathing, and circulation should be assessed and supportive care instituted as necessary. Many patients are anxious and respond to reassurance and a quiet, nonthreatening, nonstimulating environment. Benzodiazepines may be necessary for agitation or anxiety. Hyperthermia and seizures should be managed using standard therapy, a cool mist spray and fans for hyperthermia, and a benzodiazepine for seizures. Psychosis may require treatment with haloperidol. Phenothiazines, such as chlorpromazine, should probably be avoided during the acute intoxication because they have been associated with hypotension, seizures, and extrapyramidal reactions. Since the specific drug ingested is frequently unknown, non-drug therapy should be the first approach to the management of these patients.

Animal Toxicity

There is a wide range of toxicity in different species.

Further Reading

Baselt, R. C., and Cravey, R. H. (1989). *Disposition of Toxic Drugs and Chemicals in Man,* 3rd ed., pp. 470–473. Year Book Med. Pub., Chicago.

Leikin, J. B., Krantz, A. J., Zell-Kanter, M., Barkin, R. L., and Hryhorczuk, D. O. (1989). Clinical features and management of intoxication due to hallucinogenic drugs. *Med. Toxicol. Adverse Drug Exp.* **4**, 324–350.

—*William A. Watson*

Related Topics

Amphetamine
Barbiturates
Cocaine
Heroin
Jimsonweed
Marijuana
Mescaline
Morning Glory
Mushrooms, Psilocybin
Opium
Peyote
Speed
Yohimbine

Lye

- Synonyms: Caustic potash; caustic soda; actually refers to any strong alkali, usually sodium hydroxide, potassium hydroxide (CAS: 1310-58-3), or potassium carbonate (CAS: 584-08-7)
- Chemical Class: Alkali

Uses

Lye is used in household drain cleaners, ammonia, automatic dishwasher detergents, Clinitest tablets, oven cleaners, and bleaches. It is also used in the manufacture of soaps and cleaners and in chemical synthesis.

Exposure Pathways

Exposure to lye may occur via the dermal and oral routes.

Mechanism of Toxicity

The mechanisms of toxicity for lye include saponification of fats and solubilization of proteins, corrosion, reduction, and protein denaturation. The severity of corrosion is determined by pH, viscosity, concentration, volume ingested, and contact time.

Human Toxicity

Lye is a strong eye, skin, and mucous membrane irritant and corrosive. Ingestion is followed by severe pain, vomiting, diarrhea, and collapse.

Clinical Management

Alkalis penetrate the skin slowly, making the extent of damage dependent on the duration of contact. Affected skin should be washed with running water until free of alkali as indicated by the disappearance of the "soapy" feeling.

In cases of eye exposure, eyes should be washed with running water continuously for 15 min and then irrigated for 30–60 min with normal saline solution. Do not use neutralizing agents.

—*Shayne C. Gad*

Related Topics

Alkalies
Corrosives

Lyme Disease

- DESCRIPTION: Lyme disease is the most common tick-born illness in the United States. There were in excess of 9400 reported cases in 1991 and the number of cases are increasing. All age groups are affected, with children less than 10 years old at the greatest risk. The peak incidences are in the summer months.

Exposure Pathway

Lyme disease is caused by the transmission of the spirochete Borrelia burgdorferi, dammini, pacificus, or ricinus to humans by the bite of an infected *Ixodes dammini* or related ixodid tick. Deer, rabbits, rodents, and domestic animals may harbor the ticks. Humans are exposed to ticks in grass or other foliage. In the United States, the primary endemic areas are northeastern, midwestern, and western states. New York had the most reported cases between 1986 and 1989.

Mechanism of Toxicity

Lyme disease occurs due to a multisystemic spirochetal infection that attacks the skin, nervous system, heart, and joints.

Human Toxicity

Clinical stages of Lyme disease are divided into three stages. Patients may experience all three stages but may not be diagnosed until late into the disease. The average incubation period is 9 days for primary cases and 19 days for secondary cases.

Stage 1 (primary) occurs a few days to a month after the tick bite and lasts less than 2 months. This stage involves early localized infection. Clinical manifestations are erythema migrans (most characteristic feature), regional lymphadenopathy, fever, myalgias, arthralgias, fatigue, and malaise.

Stage 2 (secondary) follows within days to weeks of stage 1, although it may occur without any of the prior symptoms observed in stage 1. This stage involves disseminated infection. Clinical manifestations are intermittent and fluctuating and usually decrease or disappear in several weeks, even if untreated. The most common symptoms involve the skin. Secondary annular lesions, malar rash, diffuse erythema or urticaria, evanescent lesions, and lymphocytoma can be seen. Musculoskeletal involvement causes migratory pain in the joints, muscles, tendons, bursae, and bones; brief arthritic attacks; and myositis. Osteomyelitis and paniculitis occur but are rare. Neurologic effects can include meningitis, cranial neuritis, Bell's palsy, motor or sensory radiculoneuritis, encephalitis, or mononeuritis multiplex. Myelitis, chorea, and cerebellar ataxia occur but are rare.

Lymphatic involvement includes regional or generalized lymphadenopathy and splenomegaly. Observed cardiac effects include atrioventricular nodal block, myopericarditis, and pancarditis. Ocular symptoms usually include conjunctivitis; however, occasionally iritis, choroiditis, retinal hemorrhage or detachment, and panophthalmitis have occurred. Liver toxicity manifests as mild or recurrent hepatitis. Respiratory effects include nonexudative pharyngitis, nonproductive cough, and adult respiratory distress syndrome. Microscopic hematuria or proteinurua can occur. Orchitis has been observed but is rare. Malaise and fatigue are almost always seen in stage 2.

Late Lyme disease (stage 3) is a chronic or persistent disease that generally begins 1 year or more after the onset of the disease or may occur without any minor features. This late stage causes tertiary infection characterized by persistent inflammation of deep tissues such as the joints or nervous system for more than 2 months (arthritis, polyneuropathy, and encephalopathy).

Fetal Toxicity

Adverse outcomes of pregnancy have occurred.

Clinical Management

The tick should be removed using a blunt, curved forceps, tweezers, or fingers protected by rubber gloves. Heat should not be used because it is ineffective in dislodging the tick and may cause burns. Petroleum jelly, nail polish, alcohol, or ointments also should not be used because they may impede self-detachment. Antibiotics are the main treatment in all three stages of Lyme disease. The specific medication depends on the presenting clinical stage. Intravenous fluids are necessary for dehydration. Cardiac monitoring is advised in significant cases. Antiinflammatory drugs may be useful as adjunctive therapy. Consultation with a rheumatologist or internist, cardiologist, and orthopedist may be needed.

Animal Toxicity

Domestic animals are a potential source for ticks but have not been found to be a significant risk factor for transmission to humans.

—C. Lynn Humbertson

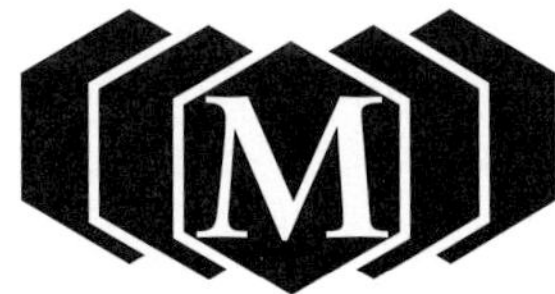

Malathion

- CAS: 121-75-5
- SYNONYMS: *O*,*O*-dimethyl-*S*-(1,2-dicarbethoxyethyl)phosphorodithioate; Chemathion; Karbophos; Cythion; Malaspray; Malathiozol
- CHEMICAL CLASS: Organophosphate insecticide
- CHEMICAL STRUCTURE:

$$(CH_3O)_2P(=S){-}S{-}CH(C(=O){-}OC_2H_5){-}CH_2{-}C(=O){-}OC_2H_5$$

Uses

Malathion is an insecticide and acaricide for control of mosquitoes, household insects, and human head and body lice.

Exposure Pathways

Poisonings have occurred mainly from accidental or intentional ingestion, although dermal exposure has resulted in systemic symptoms.

Toxicokinetics

Malathion is absorbed through the skin, lungs, and gastrointestinal tract. However, skin absorption is fairly low. Most organophosphate insecticides require activation by oxidation of the P=S bond to the more toxic P=O compound by microsomal enzymes of the liver and other organs, including the brain. However, the carboxyethyl ester groups in malathion are rapidly hydrolyzed by malathion esterases (see Carboxylesterases). This action effectively detoxifies malathion and is the reason for the relatively low mammalian toxicity compared with other organophosphates. The liver and kidney are primary sites of distribution and reflect the rapid detoxification and clearance of malathion. Malathion is rapidly excreted in the urine (>90%) after 24 hr. The half-life following intravenous administration in human volunteers was approximately 3 hr.

Mechanism of Toxicity

Malathion is converted to the toxic oxygen analog (replacement of covalent sulfur with oxygen) by microsomal enzymes. The oxygen analog then inhibits acetylcholinesterase as do other organophosphates. As a result, acetylcholine accumulates at cholinergic nerve endings with subsequent hyperstimulation of postsynaptic cells.

Human Toxicity: Acute

Malathion exhibits very low toxicity compared with other organophosphates. The lethal dose in a 70-kg man is estimated to be >60 g. However, commercial preparations of malathion may contain organophosphate impurities which can lead to increased toxicity by interference with the detoxification systems. Signs and symptoms of severe malathion poisonings are similar to those of parathion and other organophosphates.

They include an increase in secretions, gastrointestinal cramps, diarrhea, urination, slow pulse, uncontrollable muscle twitches followed by muscle weakness, paralysis, confusion, dizziness, ataxia, cyanosis, convulsions, and coma. However, life-threatening respiratory or cardiac involvement typical in parathion poisoning is usually not associated with malathion.

Human Toxicity: Chronic

Generally, the onset and course of toxicity is rapid. However, a number of poisoning cases have shown prolonged symptoms including weakness of proximal limb muscles, cranial nerve palsies, and respiratory depression.

Clinical Management

For exposure to eyes, eyelids should be held open and the eyes flushed with copious amounts of water for 15 min. For exposure to skin, affected areas should be washed immediately with soap and water. The victim should receive medical attention if irritation develops and persists.

For exposure through inhalation, the victim should be removed to fresh air and, if not breathing, given artificial ventilation. The victim should receive medical attention as soon as possible.

First aid for ingestion victims would be to induce vomiting, keeping in mind the possibility of aspiration of solvents. Gastric decontamination should be performed within 30 min of ingestion to be most effective. Initial management of acute toxicity is establishment and maintenance of adequate airway and ventilation. Atropine sulfate in conjunction with pralidoxime chloride can be administered as an antidote. Atropine by intravenous injection is the primary antidote in severe cases. Test injections of atropine (1 mg in adults and 0.15 mg/kg in children) are initially administered, followed by 2–4 mg (in adults) or 0.015–0.05 mg/kg (in children) every 10–15 min until cholinergic signs (e.g., diarrhea, salivation, and bronchial secretions) decrease. High doses of atropine over several injections may be necessary for effective control of cholinergic signs. If lavage is performed, endotracheal and/or esophageal control is suggested. At first signs of pulmonary edema, the patient should be placed in an oxygen tent and treated symptomatically.

Animal Toxicity

The acute oral and dermal LD_{50} values in rats and mice range from 1 to 12 g/kg. Domestic animals exhibit similar signs and symptoms as seen in humans. Chickens may be somewhat more sensitive to acute toxicity from malathion exposure, but delayed neurotoxicity is not caused by this agent (see Neurotoxicity, Delayed).

Further Reading

Gallo, M. A., and Lawryk, N. J. (1991). Organic phosphorus pesticides. In *Handbook of Pesticide Toxicology* (W. J. Hayes, Jr., and E. R. Laws, Jr., Eds.), Vol. 3, pp. 976–985. Academic Press, San Diego.

—Kevin N. Baer

(Clinical management section prepared by C. Pope)

Related Topics

Carboxylesterases
Cholinesterase Inhibition
Neurotoxicity, Delayed
Neurotoxicology: Central and Peripheral
Organophosphates
Pesticides
Veterinary Toxicology

Mancozeb

- CAS: 8018-01-7
- Synonyms: Ethylene bisdithiocarbamate; EBDC; Manzeb; Dithane M-45
- Chemical Class: Dithiocarbamate fungicide
- Chemical Structure:

$$\left[-\text{MnS}\overset{\overset{\text{S}}{\|}}{\text{C}}\text{NHCH}_2\text{CH}_2\text{NH}\overset{\overset{\text{S}}{\|}}{\text{C}}\text{S}- \right]_x \quad \left[\text{Zn}^{2+} \right]_y$$

x:y 10:1

Uses

Mancozeb is used as an agricultural fungicide.

Exposure Pathways

Mancozeb exposure may occur by the inhalation and dermal routes.

Toxicokinetics

Mancozeb may be absorbed via the lungs, the gastrointestinal tract, and the skin. Although detailed toxicokinetic studies are not available, there is indirect evidence (minimal tissue storage after dosing) that these chemicals are rapidly metabolized and/or excreted by humans usually within hours or days of absorption. The ethylene bisdithiocarbamate fungicides may contain ethylene thiourea (ETU) (a soil breakdown product) as a contaminant, or ETU may be formed *in vivo*. ETU is carcinogenic and teratogenic. Although little information is available, the half-life for the elimination of ETU through the kidneys was reported to be approximately 100 hr.

Mechanism of Toxicity

Unlike the carbamate insecticides, dithiocarbamates do not inhibit the cholinesterase enzyme. The ethylene bisdithiocarbamates may degrade in the environment and in mammalian tissues to ETU. This substance is a goitrogen, mutagen, and carcinogen.

Human Toxicity

There is little evidence of human toxicity associated with mancozeb. Mancozeb may be a skin sensitizer.

Clinical Management

Blood levels are not clinically useful. Emesis may be indicated in recent substantial ingestion unless the patient is or could rapidly become obtunded, comatose, or convulsing. An activated charcoal cathartic may also be administered. For inhalation exposure, the patient should be moved to fresh air and monitored for respiratory distress. If cough or difficulty in breathing develops, the patient should be evaluated for respiratory tract irritation, bronchitis, or pneumonitis. Humidified supplemental oxygen (100%) should be administered with assisted ventilation as required. For dermal exposures, the exposed area should be washed thoroughly with soap and water.

Animal Toxicity

The oral LD_{50} in rats ranges from 8 to 11 g/kg. Inhalation exposures at doses nontoxic to pregnant rats are not teratogenic. Embryotoxicity may occur at doses toxic to the dam, at concentrations of 55 mg/m^3 or above.

—*Todd A. Bartow*

Related Topics

Dithiocarbamates
Pesticides

Manganese (Mn)

- CAS: 7439-96-5
- Selected Compounds: Manganese dioxide, MnO_2 (CAS: 1313-13-9); potassium permanganate, $KMnO_4$ (CAS: 7722-64-7)
- Chemical Class: Metals

Uses

Manganese is used in ceramics, glass, dyes, dry-cell batteries, and special high-carbon steels. It is also added to fertilizers and animal food. Potassium permanganate is used as an oxidizing agent.

Exposure Pathways

Ingestion is the primary exposure pathway for the general population; sources include grains, nuts, fruits, and tea. Inhalation is a significant exposure pathway in industrial settings. Air and water pollution are minor sources in most areas.

Toxicokinetics

Less than 5% of ingested manganese is absorbed from the gastrointestinal tract. Manganese is carried in blood serum by a β-globulin, which may be specific for this metal. Manganese is a cofactor for enzymes related to synthesis of cholesterol and also fatty acids. It is necessary for phosphorylation reactions. In some cases it can substitute for magnesium. Manganese is excreted in the bile.

Human Toxicity

Available human toxicity data are limited to the industrial setting, where adverse health effects have resulted from inhalation of manganese (primarily as manganese dioxide). Acute inhalation exposure produces manganese pneumonitis; the incidence of respiratory disease among exposed workers is higher than that of the general population.

In workers with chronic inhalation exposure, iron deficiency and liver cirrhosis are commonly observed. Chronic inhalation exposure also affects the central nervous system, resulting in Parkinsonian-like symptoms. Mental aberrations are also observed. The psychiatric disturbance has been called "manganese madness." Symptoms include confusion, unusual behavior, and sometimes hallucinations. Apathy, difficulty with speech, and loss of balance are most common. Other symptoms include difficulty with fine motor movement, anxiety, and pains.

The ACGIH TLV-TWA is 0.2 mg/m^3 for elemental manganese and inorganic compounds.

Clinical Management

Many symptoms of manganese toxicity disappear after the victim is removed from the source of exposure. L-Dopa (levodopa) can reverse some symptoms, but complete recovery is not expected. Calcium–EDTA (the calcium disodium salt of ethylenediaminetetraacetic acid) will help improve an acute manganese-induced psychosis.

Animal Toxicity

Manganese per se is neither carcinogenic nor teratogenic in laboratory animals.

—*Arthur Furst and Shirley B. Radding*

Related Topic

Metals

Marijuana

- CAS: 7663-50-5
- Synonyms: Tetrahydrocannabinol (THC); δ-9-tetrahydrocannabinol; dronabinol; cannabis; marihuana; hashish; bhang; ganja; sensemilla; weed; pot; grass
- Pharmaceutical Class: Psychoactive substance
- Chemical Structure:

Uses

Dronabinol is prescribed for its antiemetic and appetite stimulant properties. Marijuana is primarily a drug of abuse, although it is currently used by patients for the same purposes as dronabinol.

Exposure Pathways

Inhalation of marijuana smoke is the most common method of use, followed by oral ingestion. Intravenous use is uncommon. Dronabinol is an oral capsule.

Toxicokinetics

Inhalation of marijuana smoke results in the systemic availability of 10–50% of the tetrahydrocannabinol (THC) dose, with peak plasma concentrations occurring in the first 10 min after initiation of inhalation. Oral absorption is high; however, large first-pass hepatic metabolism results in a systemic bioavailability of <10%, with peak concentrations occurring 3 or 4 hr after ingestion. THC is almost completely metabolized by the liver, with <1% of a dose eliminated in the urine as unmetabolized drug. The apparent volume of distribution is approximately 10 liters/kg, and tetrahydrocannabinol in plasma is primarily found bound to plasma proteins. The elimination half-life is approximately 20–40 hr. The elimination rate of the metabolites in urine is much slower and appears to be dose dependent. With chronic high-dose use of marijuana, the presence of metabolites of THC in the urine can be detected for 6–8 weeks.

Mechanism of Toxicity

The mechanisms involved in THC's central nervous system (CNS) and cardiovascular effects are not clear. They may involve altering the relationship between cholinergic, catecholaminergic, and serotonergic activity. The antiemetic effect appears to involve the CNS vomiting control center.

Human Toxicity: Acute

Toxicity primarily involves the CNS and cardiovascular system. Euphoria, increased apparent visual and auditory sensory perception, and altered perceptions of time and space are common with mild intoxication. Larger doses can impair memory, decrease attention and cognition, and result in lethargy. Impaired sensory interpretation and performance of complicated mental tasks increases the risk of trauma with activities such as operating a motor vehicle. Decreased balance, ataxia, and muscle incoordination can occur. Anxiety, panic attacks, paranoia, depression, confusion, and hallucinations can occur with high doses; these effects are more common in less experienced, younger users. Cardiovascular effects include increased heart rate and cardiac output and decreased exercise tolerance. Bronchodilation and, less frequently, bronchoconstriction may be seen. The pupils will constrict slightly and the conjunctiva will become red secondary to congestion of the blood vessels. A dry mouth is common. The intravenous administration of marijuana has been associated with severe multiple organ system failure, including renal failure, rhabdomyolysis, increased hepatic enzymes, shortness of breath, headaches, and hypotension. Plasma concentrations of THC after inhalation of marijuana smoke range from approximately 20 to 190 ng/ml over doses of 6–10 mg.

Human Toxicity: Chronic

Chronic use can result in an amotivational state, paranoid behavior, worsening muscle incoordination, chronic coughing and decreased respiratory function, slurred speech, and delusions. Fertility can be impaired in both males (decreased sperm count and activity) and females (decreased ovulation and abnormal menses). There may also be an impairment of the cell-mediated immune system. Tolerance to some CNS effects may develop with chronic use, and a withdrawal syndrome is possible after chronic high-dose use.

Clinical Management

After assessment of airway, breathing, and circulation, and any required treatment, additional treatment is generally supportive in nature. Reassurance is generally effective in treating alterations in thought process, although antipsychotics may be necessary in uncommon, severe toxicity. Correction of fluid and electrolyte abnormalities are required with intravenous marijuana toxicity.

Animal Toxicity

The beagle dog is sensitive to the effects of smoked marijuana and can be trained to smoke chronically in a manner similar to that of humans.

Further Reading

Baselt, R. C., and Cravey, R. H. (1989). *Disposition of Toxic Drugs and Chemicals in Man,* 3rd ed., pp. 780–785. Year Book Med. Pub., Chicago.

Leikin, J. B., Krantz, A. J., Zell-Kanter, M., Barkin, R. L., and Hryhorczuk, D. O. (1989). Clinical features and management of intoxication due to hallucinogenic drugs. *Med. Toxicol. Adverse Drug Exp.* **4**, 324–350.

Sullivan, M. F., and Willard, D. H: (1978). The beagle dog as an animal model for marijuana smoking studies. *Toxicol. Appl. Pharmacol.* **45**, 445–462.

—William A. Watson

Related Topics

Immune System
Neurotoxicology: Central and Peripheral

Maximum Allowable Concentration

Maximum allowable concentrations (MACs) are national consensus standards and have been established by ANSI. These values are the maximum airborne concentrations that can be justified consistent with the objective of maintaining unimpaired health or comfort of workers or both. The criteria on which the standard is established are the avoidance of (1) undesirable changes in body structures or biochemistry, (2) undesirable functional reactions that may have no discernible effects on health, and (3) irritation or other adverse sensory effects.

—*Shayne C. Gad*

Related Topics

Exposure
Exposure Assessment
Permissible Exposure Limit
Occupational Toxicology
Short-Term Exposure Limit
Threshold Limit Value

Maximum Tolerated Dose

The maximum tolerated dose (MTD) is commonly estimated to be the maximum dose that can be administered for the duration of the study that will not compromise the survival of the animals by causes other than carcinogenicity. If the MTD has been chosen appropriately, there should be no adverse effect on survival, only a modest decrement in body weight gain, and minimal overt signs of toxicity. The MTD has been exceeded if there is increased mortality, severe body weight decrement, or marked signs of toxicity.

The information used for dose selection usually comes from subchronic toxicity studies, but other information about the pharmacological effects of a drug and its metabolism and pharmacokinetics may also be considered. The maximum recommended human dose (MRHD) of the drug may be an additional criterion, if this is known when the carcinogenicity studies are being designed.

For most pharmaceutical companies, the doses selected are as follows: The highest dose is selected to be the estimated MTD, the lowest dose is usually a small multiple of the MRHD (one to five times), and the mid-dose approximates the geometric mean of the other two doses.

The procedures for dose selection described previously are generally consistent with major regulatory guidelines for carcinogenicity studies. [Note that U.S. FDA's *Redbook* applies, strictly speaking, only to food additives. It is cited here because it is a well-known toxicology guideline routinely applied to animal pharmaceuticals to which humans may be exposed. The *Redbook* has recently been updated (U.S. FDA, 1993).] There are, however, exceptions to the general approach described previously. For example, for nontoxic drugs, the difference between the high and the low doses may be many orders of magnitude if the high dose is set at the estimated MTD and the low dose is a small multiple of the clinical dose. Some guidelines request that the low dose be no less than 10% of the high dose. In this situation, it may be acceptable to set the high dose at 100 times the MRHD, even if the MTD is not achieved. Similarly, when a drug is administered in the diet, the highest concentration should not exceed 5% of the total diet, whether or not the MTD is achieved.

Metabolism and/or pharmacokinetic data, when available, should also be considered in the dose selection process. It is desirable that a drug not be administered at such a high dose that it is excreted in a different manner than at lower doses, such as the MRHD. Similarly, the high dose should not lead to the formation of metabolites other than those formed at lower (clinical) doses. If data show that a given dosage produces maximum plasma levels, administration of higher doses should be unnecessary. These considerations may be very useful when interpreting the results of the study or attempting to extrapolate the results to humans.

The dose range-finding study is necessary in most cases, but the suppression of body weight gain is a scientifically questionable benchmark when dealing with the establishment of safety factors. Physiologic, pharmacologic, or metabolic markers generally serve as better indicators of systemic response than body weight. A series of well-defined acute and subchronic studies designed to determine the "chronicity factor" and to study onset of pathology can be more predictive for dose setting than body weight suppression.

Also, the MTD may well be at a level where the metabolic mechanisms for handling a compound at real-life exposure levels have been saturated or overwhelmed, bringing into play entirely artifactual metabolic and physiologic mechanisms. The regulatory response to questioning the appropriateness of the MTD as a high level has been to acknowledge that occasionally an excessively high dose is selected, but to counter by saying that using lower doses would seriously decrease the sensitivity of detection.

Further Reading

Gad, S. C., and Chengelis, C. P. (1988). *Acute Toxicology: Principles and Methods.* Telford, Caldwell, NJ.

Gad, S. C., and Weil, C. S. (1988). *Statistics and Experimental Design for Toxicologists,* 2nd ed. Telford, Caldwell, NJ.

—Shayne C. Gad

Related Topics

Dose–Response Relationship
Food and Drug Administration
Investigative New Drug Application
Median Lethal Dose
Pharmacokinetics/Toxicokinetics
Toxicity, Acute Toxicity, Subchronic

Mechanisms of Toxicity

Toxicity is mostly caused by alterations in normal cellular physiology and biochemistry, eventually leading to cell death and tissue damage. Although many toxic responses are ultimately from cell death and loss of critical organ function, other responses may be the result of biochemical and pharmacological imbalances in normal physiological processes (genetic alterations) that do not result in cell death. Understanding of how different chemicals can affect these phenomena at biochemical and molecular level is essential to avert or prevent the toxicity. Despite a common outcome of toxicity, from all chemical-induced injury, the extent of tissue damage necessary to cause a life-threatening response varies depending on the tissue type and rate at which the injury is caused. Epithelial tissues (e.g., liver, kidney, lung, and intestine) and DNA have a great capacity to repair or regenerate in response to a loss of tissue mass or DNA architecture. Other tissues (e.g., neuronal tissues) either have a very poor capacity to regenerate or do not regenerate at all. It is also true that organs have a capacity for function that exceeds the requirements for the normal homeostasis and is referred to as functional reserve capacity. Reserve capacity allows the body to survive severe toxic insults which lead to significant loss of organ functions. Humans functioning with one kidney, a part of the lung removed, only a portion of liver, or only half of the normal amount of hemoglobin are examples of the functional reserve capacity.

There are many ways in which a chemical can interfere with the normal biochemistry and physiology of the cells and a chemical may cause toxicity to multiple tissues by multiple mechanisms. The following general categories of the mechanisms are neither comprehensive nor mutually exclusive but represent the major mechanisms of toxicity of many drugs, chemicals, and environmental agents.

Covalent Binding to Macromolecules

Many toxic substances exert their toxic effects by covalently binding to proteins, thiols, and nucleic acids. The binding can be either very tight (e.g., covalent binding by shared electrons) or loose binding through other labile bonds. Covalent binding can lead to longer lasting toxic effects. Proteins constitute many enzymes and regulate many functions and structural components of membranes that are critical to cellular function. Binding of hydrogen cyanide to the ferric atom of cytochrome oxidase and thus preventing the electron transport and, as a result, blocking the transport of oxygen by hemoglobin in the blood is a classic example of toxicity caused through protein binding. Carbon monoxide, on the other hand, principally blocks delivery of oxygen to tissues by taking the place of oxygen on hemoglobin, the oxygen carrying protein of the red blood cells. Chemically induced porphyria caused by halogenated hydrocarbons (e.g., hexachlorobenzene) and metals (e.g., lead and mercury) in part is also caused by inhibition of specific enzymes (by protein binding) of the heme biosynthetic pathway. Many toxic trace metals (e.g., arsenic, cadmium, mercury, and lead) also bind to proteins with free sulfhydryl groups (also known as thiols of proteins, amino acids, etc.), resulting in toxicity.

Many chemicals form reactive, electrophilic intermediates and free radicals during their metabolism in the body. These can be formed via enzyme-mediated reactions (many of which are oxidations) or from autoxidation of small molecules like flavins and thiols. These electrophilic intermediates covalently react with nucleophilic sites in the cell, including glutathione (GSH) and thiol-containing proteins, causing cellular dysfunction and oxidative stress to the cell. Acetaminophen is one such drug which forms a metabolite, *N*-acetyl-*p*-aminobenzoquinoneimine, which first depletes GSH and then covalently binds to protein thiols to cause toxicity. Binding to protein thiols results in the loss of activity of thiol-containing enzymes. Calcium transporting ATPase is a thiol-containing enzyme that is affected by covalent binding with many electrophilic intermediates of chemical toxicants. Binding of this enzyme results in loss of adenosine triphosphate (ATP), important for cell survival, or excessive accumulation of extracellular calcium inside the cells and this results in cell death.

Ribonucleic acid (RNA) and deoxyribonucleic acid (DNA) contain numerous nucleophilic sites that react readily with electrophilic chemicals. Binding to the nucleophilic sites of RNA leads to perturb synthesis of proteins which are very critical for the normal function of the body. Production of somatic mutations through DNA–adduct formation by certain chemicals may be responsible for chemical carcinogenesis. Adduct formation with RNA and DNA can also alter the expression of certain genes, thereby affecting the formation of certain gene products resulting in disruption of normal functions and life cycle of cells. N-7, N-2, C-2, and O-6 positions of guanine appear to be important in DNA–adduct formation and are known to cause mutagenicity and carcinogenicity.

Some chemicals may also enter normal cellular pathways of metabolism and cause perturbations in cellular metabolism. Fluoroacetate is a well-known example. Cell death occurs via interference with energy production. Fluoroacetate enters the citric acid cycle (Krebs cycle) with the formation of fluorocitrate. Isocitrate dehydrogenase, the normal enzyme in the sequential energy-producing pathway, is unable to handle the substrate, consequently blocking the energy production pathway. Another example is galactosamine, a naturally occurring amine derivative (present in high amounts in lobster shells) of sugar glucose. Galactosamine enters the normal galactose metabolism pathway of the liver cells because one of the enzymes accepts galactosamine in place of its normal substrate galactose. The impostor makes its way to form uridine diphosphogalactosamine (UDP-galactosamine), but the next enzyme (epimerase) detects the impostor and cannot act on this abnormal substrate. This results in the trapping of uridine into a useless intermediate causing cellular depletion of uridine, thereby causing depletion of UTP, inhibition of RNA and protein synthesis, and glycogen formation. This "uridyl trapping" leads to cellular death, causing liver toxicity. The toxicity can be reversed by administering orotic acid, a precursor of uridine.

Interference with Calcium (Ca^{2+}) Homeostasis

Disruption of intracellular Ca^{2+} homeostasis can result from excessive Ca^{2+} influx or release of Ca^{2+} from intracellular stores or from inhibition of extrusion of Ca^{2+} by the plasma membrane. Cellular Ca^{2+} is closely regulated by living cells. Ca^{2+} concentration is approximately 5000- to 10,000-fold higher outside the cells. If higher amounts of Ca^{2+} enter the cells (e.g., due to perturbation of plasma membrane) the Ca^{2+} ATPase pumps in the plasma membrane pump the excessive Ca^{2+} out of the cell. Additional finer regulation of Ca^{2+} inside the cell is accomplished mainly by two mechanisms—mitochondria sequester larger fraction of Ca^{2+} and endoplasmic reticulum can sequester smaller amounts of Ca^{2+}. Interference with the normal processes responsible for regulation of intracellular Ca^{2+} play a critical role in chemical-mediated cell injury and necrotic cell death. One or more of these regulatory mechanisms may be perturbed by toxic chemicals. Accumulation of Ca^{2+} in the cells has been correlated with necrotic cell injury and cell death from ischemia and a variety of toxic agents. Blebing or development membrane abnormalities with disruption of cytoskeletal structure (disruption of actin microfilaments by the activation of phospholipases and proteases) have been found *in vitro* after increased intracellular Ca^{2+}. Nitrophenols, quinones, peroxides, aldehydes, dioxins, halogenated alkenes, alkanes, and some metal ions cause toxicity by disrupting Ca^{2+} homeostasis.

Disruption of Ca^{2+} homeostasis has also been implicated in "programmed cell death" or apoptosis. An increased Ca^{2+} level in the nucleus activates some endonucleases, which result in DNA fragmentation and chromatin condensation.

Lipid Peroxidation

Carbon tetrachloride (CCl_4) toxicity is a typical example of toxicity due to lipid peroxidation. The cleavage of a carbon–chlorine bond in CCl_4 by the cytochrome P450 mixed function oxidase system generates a trichloromethyl free radical ($\cdot CCl_3$), which reacts rapidly with oxygen to form trichloromethyl peroxy radical ($\cdot CCl_3O_2$). These free radicals can initiate a process of autocatalytic lipid peroxidation by attacking the bridges of unsaturated fatty acid side chains of microsomal lipids. Also, unsaturated fatty acids in other cellular membranes are affected. Once organic free radicals are generated in this manner, a self-propagating runaway series of reactions leads to rapid destruction of cellular membranes causing cell death (see Lipid Peroxidation for a detailed discussion).

Oxyradicals and oxyradical stress may also cause lipid peroxidation. Free radical forms of oxygen include superoxide anion (O_2^-), hydroxyradical ($OH\cdot$), and hydrogen peroxide (H_2O_2). These radicals are formed by a stepwise one-electron reduction of O_2. One electron reduction of H_2O_2 leads to the formation of water (H_2O). Superoxide anion (O_2^-) is dismutated by a cellular enzyme known as superoxide dismutase, resulting in the formation of H_2O_2. Cellular iron can metabolize O_2^- to $OH\cdot$; and hydroxy anion (OH^-) radicals. Under certain circumstances a singlet O_2 (O_2) can also be formed from O_2. In the normal cellular metabolism small amounts of oxyradicals are generated. However, these are of no consequence since cellular defense mechanisms (e.g., superoxide dismutase, catalase, glutathione peroxidase, and vitamin E) mitigate these oxyradicals. Chemical toxicants may disrupt this balance to either produce excessive O_2 radicals and/or to compromise the cellular defense mechanisms.

Certain toxic chemicals may form organic radicals by being reduced by one electron, a reaction mediated by the flavin enzyme, cytochrome P450 reductase. These organic one-electron reduction products (semiradicals) can donate this electron to O_2 in the cells to form O_2^-. The organic toxic (parent) chemical is now free to be reduced again by the reductase and generate additional O_2^- radical. This reduction–oxidation cycle can continue as long as the chemical, cellular O_2, and reducing equivalents (NADPH) are available in the cell. Thus, redox cycling can generate a virtually unending supply of oxyradicals. The herbicide paraquat, anticancer agent bleomycin, and antibiotics nitrofurantoin and mitomycin are a few examples of chemicals that can undergo redox cycle.

Reperfusion injury is also thought to be associated with oxyradicals. After hypoxia during the cessation (or reduction) of blood supply to tissues (as in surgical procedures) the cells may shut down the normal defense mechanisms. When blood supply is restored after surgery, the tissue encounters a normal amount of O_2, leading to formation of oxygen free radicals. Regardless of how they are formed, free radical forms of O_2 can also initiate and propagate lipid peroxidation leading to tissue injury.

Interference with Endogenous Pathways

Many chemicals produce toxicity by interfering with different endogenous pathways (e.g., cellular energy production and excitable membrane functions). ATP is the main form of energy utilized by the living cells. ATP is thus necessary to maintain the normal functions of the cells and significant depletion will lead to loss of cell function and cell death. Cyanide, hydrogen sulfide, and azides bind to cytochrome oxidase and thus block utilization of oxygen by different tissues and thus inhibit ATP production. Rotenone and antimycin A interfere with specific enzymes in the electron transport chain necessary to generate ATP, while sodium fluoroacetate blocks Krebs cycle.

Different ion channels maintain the stability of excitable membranes which are necessary for normal function of the body. Saxitoxin, tetrodotoxin, and DDT all cause toxicity by blocking the sodium channel in excitable membranes. On the other hand, organic solvents cause toxicity by changing the membrane fluidity of the neurones in the central nervous system.

Stimulation and Blockade of Cell Cycle Progression

Regardless of the mechanisms of cell and tissue injury, toxic or physical injury elicits an endogenous cell proliferative and tissue repair response in the affected tissues and organs in the body. This is a parallel but opposing response to tissue injury. Chemicals vary in their ability to induce the compensatory tissue repair response. This response also varies depending on the strains and species. The human body is also capable of this tissue repair response. Simultaneous with the initiation of tissue injury, the surviving cells respond by receiving/sending appropriate cellular and molecular signals that lead to cell cycle progression beginning with G_0 to G_1 and G_1 to S phase synthesis. The first line of defense of tissue, however, occurs by the release of normally occurring small population of G2 cells to divide. This occurs within a few hours of exposure to toxic chemicals. When these cells divide, a host of molecular messages are expressed that facilitate surviving cells to divide. Thus, this tissue repair response usually takes the form of a biphasic cell proliferation response. At low to moderately toxic doses, tissue repair response shows a classic dose–response relationship. This allows the body to repair the injured tissue and restore the structure and function of the tissue, thereby permitting complete regression of injury, recovery, and survival. At high doses, two events occur which lead to unrestrained progression of injury initiated by the mechanisms that initiate injury. First, the tissue repair response is significantly diminished. Second, it is delayed considerably. Delay leads to unrestrained progression of injury, and diminished response is too little to cope with the progression tissue injury and destruction. There is significant interest in understanding the biological events and the molecular regulation of these events. If tissue repair response is stimulated through specific methods like partial hepatectomy, prior exposure to a low dose of a toxic chemical, nutritional supplementation with energy sources that facilitate cell division, activation of molecular signals, etc., complete protection can be demonstrated from lethal doses of toxic chemicals, even though normally lethal massive injury may be inflicted by any of the mechanisms described earlier.

Cell cycle progression is very important for the body; in newborns and young adults it helps in the normal development of the body, while in adults it is essential to replace cells that are dead or dying (either by normal aging or chemical-induced necrosis). Usually most of the cells in an adult are in resting or G0 phase of cell division. As a response to cell injury or impeding cell death, the cells go to G_1, S, G_2,and then M or mitotic phase of cell division to produce newly divided daughter cells. Cancerous growth is a result of abnormal and uncontrolled cell division. Chemical carcinogenicity (like cancers of unknown or viral etiology) leads to unregulated tumor growth due to uncontrolled cell division. Normally, each phase of cell division is finely regulated by growth factors, cytokines, and many other products of gene expression (e.g., cyclines). Cellular transduction mechanisms are also involved in the regulation of cell cycle progression. This finely regulated balance is perturbed by the cancer-causing chemicals. Many anticancer drugs cause toxicity by blocking the progression of cells through the cell cycle. They can either arrest the cells in different phases of cell division or can block specific enzymes by binding with the enzymes needed for cell cycle progression. Colchicine, a common anticancer drug, not only blocks the M phase of cell division but also inhibits the enzyme activity of thymidylate synthetase and thymidine kinase to arrest the cells in S phase of cell division. Taxol is another example of anticancer agent that works by blocking cell division. In contrast to colchicine, which blocks cell division by inhibition of S-phase synthesis and by preventing microtubular function, taxol works by interfering with microtubule aggregation.

Genetic Alterations

Chemicals that cause toxicity by genetic alterations of the somatic cells are called genotoxic carcinogens. Covalent interactions with DNA do not always lead to cell death. The vast majority of lesions in DNA are repaired; but in some cases the repair is incorrect or incomplete, leading to a mutated DNA. From this time point on, all the daughter cells produced by the mutated cell(s) are also mutated. If this mutation occurs in a somatic cell then this may eventually lead to cancer but cannot be passed to future generations. It is believed that genotoxic chemicals induce cancer by altering the protooncogenes. Protooncogenes carry a cancerous phenotype. Many of the gene products are actually responsible for determining cells' response to growth factors and cytokines.

—Sanjay Chanda and Harihara M. Mehendale

Related Topics

Carcinogenesis
Carcinogen–DNA Adduct Formation and DNA Repair
Lipid Peroxidation
Modifying Factors of Toxicity
Molecular Toxicology
Mutagenesis
Tissue Repair

Medical Surveillance

Introduction

The term medical surveillance is ambiguous and commonly used. There is no generally accepted definition of medical surveillance that differentiates it from related terms and activities of medical monitoring, biological monitoring, medical screening, and public health surveillance. The consequences of this imprecision in language are both linguistic ambiguity and, more important, substantive confusion about the purpose and content of these activities. These concepts all can contribute to the prevention of occupational disease and injury in workers or can be misused.

Surveillance in the Hierarchy of Prevention

There is a well-accepted hierarchy of prevention which includes medical surveillance and related concepts. The hierarchy includes techniques of prevention that fall into three categories: primary, secondary, and tertiary. In primary prevention, preventive actions preempt initiation of the disease process. In secondary prevention, disease is detected early and when asymptomatic—when it is more effectively treated. In tertiary prevention, clinical care including rehabilitation minimizes the adverse consequences of clinically apparent disease.

The first line of defense against occupational disease is the recognition that specific exposures are hazardous either based on prior human experience or experimental toxicologic evidence. Recognized hazards may then be eliminated from the environment through substitution, less desirably through engineering controls, or least optimally via personal protective devices that minimize exposure. These activities are examples of primary prevention because they interfere with the disease process before it is initiated.

As a fail-safe to engineering controls, exposure monitoring is useful in identifying hazards and in monitoring known exposures which in part ensures that control measures have been effective in reducing exposure; exposure monitoring is also primary prevention. Exposure monitoring based on breathing zone samples is most problematic when there is potential for percutaneous exposure or ingestion.

Biological monitoring is a fail-safe for environmental monitoring. Biological monitoring is the examination of a worker's urine, blood, or other laboratory sample for the presence of an intoxicant or its metabolite. Because the goal of biological monitoring is the detection of hazard, rather than early disease, it can also be described as primary prevention. Biological monitoring in the absence of environmental monitoring is ethically problematic; workers should not be their own canaries (referring to past practices when workers carried small birds into the mines to detect noxious environments). Laboratory advances in biological monitoring such as the detection of chemical adducts on DNA have led to expanded means of detecting exposures, which some have called molecular epidemiology.

Secondary prevention is the examination of the worker for evidence of disease before it is clinically symptomatic. Medical screening is the periodic examination of workers for preclinical disease. Examples of medical screening include use of urinary cytology in workers exposed to bladder carcinogens and mammography for asymptomatic cancer of the breast. Medical screening among workers need not be limited to the effects of occupational disease but can seek disease that may be both of an occupational and nonoccupational cause, or just the latter.

Tertiary prevention is the delivery of optimal clinical care to minimize the consequences of disease. Numerous interventions are included in tertiary prevention ranging from provision of appropriate rehabilitative services to ensuring the quality of clinical care. Once disease is symptomatic, prevention is limited to tertiary prevention.

Surveillance is the ongoing collection and timely analysis of data on exposures, disease, injury, death, and disability for the purpose of prevention. Surveillance as a term can be applied to the health of an individual or to a population. Surveillance connotes watchfulness for the purpose of prevention.

The most difficult definition is that of medical surveillance. Medical surveillance may mean medical testing of an individual or may refer to surveillance of a population. Medical surveillance for an individual may mean biological monitoring, medical screening, or the periodic assessment of an individual with clinical disease. The term medical surveillance may also be applied to a population which is biologically monitored, medically screened, or whose disease is monitored over time. As applied to a population, medical surveillance may also mean the collection, analysis, and use (e.g., public health surveillance) of health data from a population. The term medical surveillance must be used with caution to avoid inaccurate communication about the content and intent of intended activities.

Goals of Public Health Surveillance

There are four major goals of public health surveillance. The first is the estimation of the magnitude of disease occurrence and its trends over time. The second goal is the identification of new opportunities for prevention including entirely new diseases as well as old diseases in new circumstances. Cases of well established occupational disease, with known preventable etiologies, are known as Sentinel Health Events, Occupational (SHEO). Each case represents a failure of prevention. Investigation of SHEOs and intervention may lead to the identification of root causes of the failure of prevention and hence to improved prevention. The fourth goal is identifying epidemic clusters, or epidemics of diseases, so that resources can be targeted toward their prevention.

Principles for Medical Surveillance

A set of guiding principles for screening individuals in the workplace has evolved; it is similar to but somewhat different from screening of community residents. These principles are presented in the following sections.

Importance

For surveillance to play a meaningful role in prevention, the exposure or medical condition sought must be important for the individual or population that is tested. This guidance should be directed both at choosing which outcomes should become part of medical surveillance and at determination of what levels should be sought.

Accepted Intervention

Surveillance should be limited to exposures or conditions where there is an accepted intervention. For the individual's personal benefit, this means that there should be an accepted therapy if disease is detected early or that diminution of exposure can lead to a reduction in disease. For a population, diminution in exposure justifies surveillance, even if disease detected earlier is not more easily or effectively treated.

Facilities for Diagnosis and Treatment

Surveillance programs for the individual or a population should plan for the delivery of diagnostic and therapeutic medical care and industrial hygiene services for participants found to be positive.

Recognizable Latent or Early Symptomatic Stage

Some diseases, no matter how severe, do not have a substantial preclinical phase when it may be detectable through screening. These diseases are not suitable for screening and may as effectively be identified at the time of normal clinical diagnosis.

Suitable Test or Examination

When used as part of a prevention program in the community, tests must be suitable in that their cost must compete with other public health expenditures that are economical such as immunization. These constraints are relieved in occupational screening, where the costs of preventive measures do not compete with public health expenditures but rather are a cost of production.

Suitable Personnel

Successful use of medical screening requires a chain of expertise for appropriate collection and storage of samples and their transportation, analysis, and interpretation. Medical surveillance programs must have an appropriate array of suitable personnel.

Choice of Tests

Screening tests should be targeted to the specific risks of the person or population under surveillance. As knowledge about the adverse consequences of particular exposures advances, tests should be added and abandoned consistent with advancing knowledge.

Operating Characteristics of Tests

Screening tests can be described in terms of sensitivity, specificity, and predictive value. Sensitivity is the fraction of all those who in truth are positive who test positive. Specificity is the fraction of all who in truth are negative who test negative. Predictive value positive is the fraction of all positive tests that represent true positive versus false positive. Predictive value positive depends on sensitivity, specificity, and on the prevalence of the condition. True positive from a very sensitive test will be overwhelmed by false positive even from a very specific test if the condition is rare. Predictive value positive and negative are most important to the patient.

Cutoff Points

A priori decisions should be made on the level of test that constitutes a positive or negative value, and hence requires follow-up action, before the screening program is initiated.

Acceptability

The screening test and surveillance program must be acceptable to the target population for there to be participation.

Goals of Surveillance

The goals of surveillance should be delineated before initiating a screening or surveillance program. Some tests are acceptable if the goal is protection of the population which would not be worthwhile if the only goal is protection of the individual. For example, a search for untreatable disease may be of value if it leads to early reduction in exposure, but it has little value if the goal is prevention for an individual. Other tests may be acceptable, and even legal, if done for appropriate placement of employees but inappropriate if used as a condition of employment.

Challenges in Medical Surveillance

There are major challenges and opportunities that may affect the future of medical surveillance. These include fragmentation of occupational medical care, OSHA monitoring standards, the promise of molecular epidemiology, critical evaluation of medical surveillance, and growth of public health surveillance.

Fragmentation of Occupational Medical Care

It is possible that there will be major changes in the financing of medical care that may affect its organization. Interest in cost saving may lead to searches for redundancy. Regardless of its merit in preventing occupational and nonoccupational disease, work site programs for the detection of risk factors such as elevated cholesterol, hypertension, etc. may be seen as redundant and eliminated. Alternatively, there may be increased recognition of the potential of work site health promotion programs that include screening for the early detection of disease. Another noteworthy trend has been the shifting balance toward off-site contractors for the delivery of occupational medical services. It appears that the shift is due to the increase in provision of off-site services for employees rather than a diminution in on-site services. Albeit, the separation of the health care provider from the work site may lead to unfamiliarity with work site exposures and physical and intellectual separation of health care providers from specialists in industrial hygiene with a consequent decrease in appreciation for the role of medical surveillance in the continuum of prevention, especially linking medical monitoring to exposure assessment. New mechanisms for financing medical care may also lead to more critical evaluation of the role of medical surveillance in preventing disease, occupational and otherwise, leading potentially to the encouragement of some and diminution of other medical surveillance activities.

OSHA Monitoring Standard

Recent OSHA standards have included requirements and recommendations on medical screening and biological monitoring of workers. Examples include blood lead and urinary proteins for cadmium exposed workers. Future OSHA standards are likely to include medical monitoring provisions. OSHA standards require that medical surveillance data be collected for the benefit of individual employees; there is growing interest in the use of medical data, such as that required for blood lead examinations, to characterize the experience of the workforce and perhaps be used to identify those work sites with the best and worst experience in preventing exposure.

The Promise of Molecular Epidemiology

There is substantial laboratory activity in developing new methods for assessment of biomarkers of exposure, biomarkers of early biologic effect at a subcellular level, and genetic markers of variability in susceptibility that may identify workers at higher risk of disease. On the other hand, there is little evidence of the practical value of any of these approaches for routine use in protection of workers, aside from the unusual research project in which the markers are used to characterize exposure or subclinical effects at low levels of exposure. While there is substantial promise of value of molecular screening, there is also substantial possibility for damage and abuse. Examples range from inappropriate advice not to hire to anxiety associated with being told of having a marker of exposure or genetic effect of unknown consequence.

Critical Evaluation of Medical Surveillance

There has been a critical review of medical screening practices used for detection of nonoccupational disease but no concentrated effort to critically review the evidence for or against the examination of workers for occupational disease. At the same time there is substantial pressure to offer large numbers of workers at hazardous waste sites, decommissioned nuclear facilities, and other workplaces examinations that will indicate evidence of exposure or effect. A concerted effort to critically evaluate screening practices may identify useful procedures and debunk the value of others that may be misleading as currently used.

Growth of Public Health Surveillance

During the past 10 years there has been substantial progress in establishing a public health surveillance system for occupational disease and injury that is on a par with communicable disease. In this system cases of designated occupational disease and injury would be identified and reported to a regional center, usually a state health department, where the data would be analyzed and used for all the goals of surveillance enumerated previously. The best example of a national surveillance system for occupational disease is for lead poisoning. Twenty states now have regulations requiring laboratories to report to the state when a blood lead level in an adult is excessive. These data are then used to estimate the magnitude of excessive lead exposure, identify new occupations and means of exposure, assess failures of control of exposure in well-known lead hazardous industries, and identify work sites with the most excessive lead levels. Similar programs are now being developed for 12 other conditions including dermatitis, occupational burns, cadmium exposure, and silicosis.

Conclusion

The goal of medical surveillance is prevention. However, medical surveillance is an ambiguous term that includes surveillance of individuals (medical surveillance) as well as populations (public health surveillance). It includes interest in early disease (medical screening) as well as in detecting evidence of exposure (biological monitoring). Medical surveillance is most likely to lead to prevention if its role in a continuum of prevention is well understood; it is most important that medical surveillance work in conjunction with environmental monitoring. Numerous challenges face medical surveillance that make its future unpredictable.

Further Reading

Guide to Clinical Preventive Services: An Assessment of the Effectiveness of 169 Interventions (1989). Report of the U.S. Preventive Services Task Force. Williams & Wilkins, Baltimore.

Halperin, W., Ratcliffe, J., Frazier, T., Wilson, L., Becker, P., and Schulte, P. (1986). Medical screening in the workplace: proposed principles. *J. Med.* **28**, 547–552.

Halperin, W., Baker, E., and Monson, R. (Eds.) (1992). *Public Health Surveillance.* Van Nostrand Reinhold, New York.

Levy, B., and Halperin, W. (1988). Screening for occupational disease. In *Occupational Health* (B. Levy and D. Wegman, Eds.), 2nd ed. Little, Brown, Boston.

Ordin, D., and Levin, B. (1992). Medical surveillance in occupational health. In *Public Health and Preventive Medicine* (J. Last and R. Wallace, Eds.). Appleton & Lange, Norwalk, CT.

Rutstein, D., Mullan, R., Frazier, T., Halperin, W., Melius, J., and Sestito, J. (1983). The sentinel health event (occupational): A framework for occupational health surveillance and education. *Jour. Amer. Pub. Health Assoc.* **73**, 1054–1062.

Schulte, P., and Perera, F. (Eds.) (1993). *Molecular Epidemiology: Principles and Practices.* Academic Press, San Diego.

Wilson, J. M. G., and Junger, G. (1968). The principles and practice of screening for disease. WHO Public Health Papers 34, World Health Organization, Geneva.

—William Halperin

Related Topics

American Conference of Governmental Industrial Hygienists
Biomarkers, Human Health
Epidemiology
Exposure
Exposure Assessment
Occupational Safety and Health Administration
Occupational Toxicology
Poisoning Emergencies in Humans

Meperidine

- CAS: 50-13-5
- SYNONYMS: Pethidine hydrochloride; Demerol; sonipeccaine hydrochloride; pethadol; centralgion; dolantin; demex-idine; phytadon
- PHARMACEUTICAL CLASS: Synthetic opioid analgesic; a phenylpiperidine derivative
- CHEMICAL STRUCTURE:

$COOC_2H_5$
CH_3N

Uses

Meperidine is used as an analgesic for acute and severe pain, as a preoperative medication, as an obstetrical analgesic, and for support of anesthesia.

Exposure Pathways

Meperidine is commercially available in parenteral solutions for intravenous and intramuscular administration and in oral tablets and solution.

Toxicokinetics

Meperidine is well absorbed from all routes of administration. Following oral administration, meperidine undergoes extensive metabolism on first pass through the liver. Meperidine is less than one-half as effective when given orally as when given parenterally. Following oral administration peak analgesia occurs within 1 hr with a duration of 2–4 hr. Peak analgesia occurs 30–50 min after parenteral administration with a duration of 2–4 hours. Meperidine is metabolized primarily in the liver. It is demethylated to form normeperidine, which is then hydrolyzed along with meperidine to normeperidinic acid and meperidinic acid. The acid metabolites are less active than the meperidine and are further metabolized through conjugation. Normeperidine is pharmacologically active. Meperidine distributes widely into the liver, kidneys, and muscle. The volume of distribution is 3.84 liters/kg. Protein binding is 65–75%. Meperidine plasma half-life is 2.4–4.0 hr. Normeperidine half-life is 15–30 hr. Meperidine is excreted in the urine, approximately 5% as unchanged drug. The elimination half-life is biphasic: *T*½ (α) is 12 min and T½ (β) is 3.2 hr in individuals with normal renal and hepatic function.

Mechanism of Toxicity

Meperidine's chief pharmacological action is interacting with opioid receptors in the central nervous system (CNS). The highest concentration of stereospecific binding sites are in the limbic system, thalamus, striatum, hypothalamus, midbrain, and spinal cord. Meperidine's effects may result from mimicking the actions of enkephalins and endorphins and also from altering the release of neurotransmitters. Accumulation of the metabolite normeperidine can result in the toxic effects secondary to CNS stimulation such as seizures, agitation, irritability, nervousness, tremors, twitching, and myoclonus.

Human Toxicity: Acute

When greater than a therapeutic amount is administered, respiratory depression, which may progress to cessation of respirations, ensues. Pulmonary edema is a frequent complication. The patient's state of orientation goes from sedation to coma. Peripheral vasodilation can cause hypotension and possibly circulatory collapse. In addition to the usual opiate toxicity, the course is complicated by seizures. With daily doses of approximate 3 g, meperidine produces convulsions because of its conversion to normeperidine. Myoclonus will usually precede convulsions. Mydriasis often accompanies secondary to anoxia. Meperidine may also produce tachycardia through a vagolytic action which increases ventricular response.

Semiquanitative and qualitative immunoassays can measure high concentrations of meperidine in the urine. Meperidine toxicity is reported with serum levels of 10–30 μg/ml; however, drug levels do not govern treatment. Norperidine toxicity occurs with serum levels from 450 to 800 ng/ml.

Human Toxicity: Chronic

Meperidine use can produce physiologic dependence. Addicts usually demonstrate symptoms of twitching, tremors, confusion, hallucinations, and convulsions at high doses. An abstinence syndrome can begin within 3 hr after use and peak at 8–12 hr. The abstinence syndrome consists of more severe muscular twitching and restlessness and fewer autonomic symptoms than other opiates.

Clinical Management

Basic life-support measures should be instituted as necessary. Intensive support therapy may be required to correct respiratory failure and shock. Respirations must be supported and monitored until all symptoms disappear. Pulmonary edema should be managed with appropriate ventilatory support. If taken orally, gastrointestinal decontamination should be based on the patient's level of consciousness and history of ingestion. Gastric lavage is preferable to emesis if there is any evidence of loss of consciousness or decrease in gag reflex. Activated charcoal may be effective if meperidine is ingested. The specific antagonist naloxone is used to counteract respiratory depression and coma. A dose of 0.4–2.0 mg is given intravenously and can be repeated at intervals of 2 or 3 min. The therapeutic effect of naloxone may be of shorter duration than that of the opiate activity; therefore, a naloxone continuous infusion may then be of benefit. Naloxone does not antagonize the tremors or seizures caused by normeperidine. It will, however, antagonize the opiate effects. Seizures may be treated with intravenous diazepam. Arterial blood gases, vital signs, and level of consciousness should be monitored continuously until cessation of symptoms.

Animal Toxicity

Dogs act similarly to humans when exposed to opiates. Symptoms may include drowsiness, ataxia, respiratory depression, miosis, coma, seizures, and hypotension. Opiates and their derivatives have an excitatory effect on the CNS of cats and horses. Naloxone can be used at 0.02 mg/kg if needed.

—Lisa Scheuring-Mroz

Related Topic

Neurotoxicology: Central and Peripheral

Meprobamate

- CAS: 57-53-4
- SYNONYMS: Miltown; Equanil; $C_9H_{18}N_2O_4$; meprobam; meprobamatum; procalmadiol; 2,2-di(carbamoyloxymethyl)pentane; carbamic acid 2-methyl-2-propyltrimethylene ester; 2-methyl-2-propyl-1,3-propanediol dicarbamate; 2-methyl-2-propyltrimethylene carbamate
- PHARMACEUTICAL CLASS: Carbamate derivative
- CHEMICAL STRUCTURE:

$$H_2N-\overset{\overset{\displaystyle O}{\|}}{C}-OCH_2-\underset{\underset{\displaystyle CH_3}{|}}{\overset{\overset{\displaystyle C_3H_7}{|}}{C}}-CH_2O-\overset{\overset{\displaystyle O}{\|}}{C}-NH_2$$

Uses

Meprobamate is used as a minor tranquilizer and as an anxiolytic agent.

Exposure Pathways

Ingestion is the most common route of both accidental and intentional exposure to meprobamate. It is available as tablets, an oral liquid, and extended-release capsules (Meprospan-200).

Toxicokinetics

Meprobamate is readily absorbed after oral administration reaching peak serum concentrations within 1–3 hr. Meprobamate has the propensity to form a concretion (bezoar) of tablets in the gastrointestinal tract when ingested as an overdose in large amounts leading to prolonged absorption and the potential for late clinical deterioration. Meprobamate is metabolized in the liver to inactive hydroxy and glucuronide metabolites.

Meprobamate is widely distributed throughout the body. The apparent volume of distribution is 0.75 liters/kg. Protein binding is 10–20%. Only about 10% of meprobamate is eliminated unchanged in the urine. The remainder is excreted in the urine as inactive metabolites.

Mechanism of Toxicity

Meprobamate causes central nervous system depression similar to the barbiturates, but the precise mechanism of action is unknown. It reduces sensory transmission primarily in the thalamus. It also inhibits spinal reflexes. In high doses, meprobamate depresses myocardial contractility and may produce general anesthesia, respiratory depression, and relaxation of arterial smooth muscle.

Human Toxicity: Acute

The toxic dose of meprobamate is not well established. Death has resulted following the ingestion of only 12 g but patients have survived ingestion of up to 40 g. Severe intoxication and death may result with blood concentrations in excess of 100 mg/liter. Overdosage results in toxic effects similar to those produced by other sedative–hypnotic agents, which may include lethargy, ataxia, coma, hypotension, shock, respiratory depression, seizures, and death. Seizures are more likely during recovery from meprobamate overdose than during recovery from other sedative–hypnotic agents. Prolonged or possibly recurrent toxicity may result if a concretion of meprobamate forms in the gastrointestinal tract.

Human Toxicity: Chronic

Chronic use of high doses may produce psychologic and physical dependence. Abrupt discontinuation may lead to anxiety, insomnia, gastrointestinal disturbances, delirium, hallucinations, and seizures. Unlike opioid withdrawal, meprobamate withdrawal may be life-threatening.

Clinical Management

Basic and advanced life-support measures should be implemented as necessary. Gastrointestinal decontamination procedures should be used as appropriate based on the patient's level of consciousness and history of ingestion. Activated charcoal can be used to adsorb meprobamate. The patient's level of consciousness and vital signs should be monitored closely. Obtunded patients with reduced gag reflex should be intubated. Respiratory support including oxygen and ventilation should be provided as needed. There is no antidote for meprobamate. Hypotension should be treated with standard measures including cautious administration of intravenous fluids, Trendelenburg positioning, and dopamine hydrochloride by intravenous infusion. Forced diuresis is ineffective and contraindicated due to the potential to induce pulmonary edema. Hemodialysis and hemoperfusion appear to be of some benefit and may be useful in severe cases when standard supportive measures are inadequate. Withdrawal reactions should be managed with reinstitution of meprobamate followed by gradual tapering of the dose. Phenobarbital or a benzodiazepine may be substituted for meprobamate.

—Gregory P. Wedin

Mercaptoethanol, 2-

- CAS: 60-24-2
- Synonyms: 2-ME; mercaptoethanol; 1-ethanol-2-thiol; 2-hydroxy-1-ethanethiol; 2-hydroxyethyl mercaptan; monothioethyleneglycol; 2-thioethanol; thioglycol
- Chemical Class: Thiol; mercaptan
- Molecular Formula: $HSCH_2CH_2OH$
- Chemical Structure:
-

```
      H H
      | |
H—S—C—C—OH
      | |
      H H
```

Uses

2-Mercaptoethanol (2-ME) is used as an initiator for polymeric reactions; a reagent for diagnostic bioassays; a rust inhibitor for steel; a brightening agent in copper deposition; a tarnish remover for alloys and metals; an ingredient in hair permanent chemicals, and in hair and wool dyes; a stabilizer; and a mosquito control agent. It is manufactured by reacting ethylene chlorohydrin with sodium hydrogen sulfide or by reacting ethylene oxide with hydrogen sulfide. 2-ME is a white liquid with a strong unpleasant odor.

Exposure Pathways

Skin and eye contact and inhalation are the primary routes of exposure.

Toxicokinetics

2-ME is metabolized to 2-mercaptoacetate by alcohol and aldehyde dehydrogenase. Inhibition of alcohol dehydrogenase in experimental animals, blocking the formation of 2-mercaptoacetate, eliminated the adverse liver effects typically seen after exposure to 2-ME. No further metabolic data exist with respect to biological half-life.

Mechanism of Toxicity

2-ME exposure in rats induced a fatty liver condition as shown by a significant rise in liver triacylglycerol and blood-free fatty acid levels, a slight reduction of liver phospholipids, and a progressive decrease of blood triacylglycerol (25%) and blood phospholipid levels (30%), as well as a reduction of hepatic ketone body levels. 2-Mercaptoacetate induced effects similar to those produced by 2-ME on the liver and blood, consistent with the data indicating that this is the metabolite responsible for the blood and liver toxicity seen following 2-ME exposure. 2-ME has also been reported to inhibit thymus deoxycytidine formation, inhibit mitotic activity in the rat intestine, inhibit thymidine incorporation in rat DNA, and cause moderate deoxyribonuclease inhibition.

Human Toxicity

2-ME is extremely irritating to skin, eyes, and mucous membranes and may cause the development of contact dermatitis and pulmonary edema. Like other thiols, 2-ME may depress the central nervous system (CNS) and cause respiratory paralysis and death. The literature contains no information on human short-term or long-term exposure to 2-ME. One case of an accidental spill of 2-ME was reported to the CDC, with no ill effects observed in exposed individuals.

Clinical Management

If contact with 2-ME occurs, the affected areas should be flushed immediately with large amounts of water. When eye contact has occurred, the affected person should be referred to a medical facility after eye washing has been completed. Victims who are overcome with fumes should be removed to fresh air. If breathing has stopped, artificial respiration should be administered. If ingested, medical attention should be obtained immediately.

Animal Toxicity

In a number of studies, 2-ME has been reported to cause skin and eye irritation in mice and rabbits. Acute ingestion studies in mice have reported the LD_{50} at 348 mg/kg. The animals exhibited signs of CNS depression with death due to respiratory failure. Microscopic examination found lymphocyte infiltration of the liver and kidneys, destruction and hemorrhaging of the lungs, and foci inflammation of the myocardium. A 6-month inhalation study was conducted in rats in which the animals were exposed daily to 10 mg/m^3. At 3 months, neuromuscular depression, lymphopenia, neutrophilia, and decreased oxygen consumption were observed. In the fifth month, increased organic sulfate elimination, variation in weight, arterial pressure, liver function, and protein metabolism were observed. Liver damage was reported upon histological examination. Studies on the teratogenic, embryotoxic, and cytogenic effects of 2-ME have been inconclusive.

—Patricia J. Beattie

Related Topics

Respiratory Tract
Sensory Organs
Skin

Mercapturic Acid

- CAS: 616-91-1
- PREFERRED NAME: Acetylcysteine
- SYNONYMS: L-systeine; *N*-aceytyl; *N*-acetyl mercaptoalanine
- CHEMICAL CLASS: Endogenous substrate of glutathione metabolism

Uses

Mercapturic acid is used as a mucolytic agent for bronchopulmonary disorders, as an antidote to acetominophen poisoning, and as a corneal vilnerary. It is a urinary metabolite of glutathione conjugation and is produced exogenously for biomedical research.

Exposure Pathways

Ingestion is the primary exposure route; however, mercapturic acid is also endogenously produced.

Toxicokinetics

Glutathione conjugates not excreted in bile may be converted to mercapturic acids in the kidney. The two hydrolizing catalysts in the process are γ-glutamiyltranspeptidase and aminopeptidase M. The remaining cysteine conjugate interacts with *N*-acetyltransferase to break down the conjugates and release mercapturic acid.

Mechanism of Toxicity

As the body metabolizes substrates of xenobiotics, it releases cysteine conjugates which may result in metabolic activation or may bind the metabolite covalently, prolonging its time in the body.

Human Toxicity

Toxic effects from conjugation process—Cysteine *S*-conjugation of tetrafluoroethylene may release potent nephrotoxins. Symptoms from therapeutic use include stomatitis, nausea, vomiting, drowsiness, clamminess, and severe rhinorrhea. Caution should be exercised with asthamatics or patients with respiratory weakness. Pregnant or lactating women should not use mercapturic acid therapeutically.

Clinical Management

Supportive treatment should be provided. Fluid and electrolyte balance should be maintained.

Animal Toxicity

For rats, the oral LD_{50} is 5050 mg/kg and the intravenous LD_{50} is 1140 mg/kg. For mice, the oral LD_{50} is

7888 mg/kg; the intraperitoneal LD_{50} is 400 mg/kg; and the intravenous LD_{50} is 3800 mg/kg. In dogs, the oral LD_{50} is 71 g/kg; the intraperitoneal LD_{50} is 700 mg/kg; and the intravenous LD_{50} is 700 mg/kg.

—Shayne C. Gad and Jayne E. Ash

Related Topics

Cysteine
Glutathione
Kidney
Metallothionein

Mercury (Hg)

- CAS: 7439-97-6
- Selected Compounds: Mercuric chloride, $HgCl_2$ (CAS: 7487-94-7); mercuric oxide, HgO (CAS: 21908-53-2); mercurous chloride, Hg_2Cl_2 (CAS: 10112-91-1); methylmercury, CH_3Hg (CAS: 22967-92-6)
- Chemical Class: Metals

Uses

Mercury ("the liquid metal") has been known since antiquity; alchemists used it extensively. In the past century, it was used in the treatment of syphilis. Recently, mercury and its compounds have been used in electrical equipment (including disc batteries), in chloralkali plants, and in paper and pulp making, noble metal refining, photography, pyrotechnics, dentistry, and agriculture. Use of mercury has been drastically reduced in recent years.

Exposure Pathways

The primary exposure pathway for mercury is inhalation. Elemental mercury volatilizes to mercury vapor at ambient air temperatures. Atmospheric mercury pollution results from natural degassing of the earth's crust, the burning of fossil fuels, and mining, smelting, and refining processes. Most mercury pollution from industrial use has affected water.

Ingestion is another significant pathway. Extensive studies have been conducted on the consumption of mercury (as methylmercury) from fish.

Toxicokinetics

Inhaled mercury vapor crosses through the alveolar cells readily and is carried by the red blood cells. Catalase in these cells oxidizes elemental mercury almost at once to the divalent state. Alcohol inhibits the catalase activity; however, in the seconds it takes for a complete blood circulation cycle, a significant amount of free mercury can cross the blood–brain barrier.

Ingested or dermally applied elemental mercury is essentially not absorbed (an exception involved infants who absorbed mercury from disinfected diapers). It is estimated that humans absorb $<10\%$ of ingested elemental mercury; whereas absorption of ingested methylmercury can be as high as 90%.

Mercury will cross the placental barrier. In mammalian tissue, organic mercury, especially alkyl mercury, is converted to inorganic forms but not vice versa. Inorganic forms of mercury (not organic forms) induce a metallothionein. Inorganic mercury concentrates mainly in the kidney. Organic mercury compounds, being lipid soluble, concentrate in adipose tissue and the brain. All forms of mercury are excreted chiefly in the feces.

Mechanism of Toxicity

Mercury has a great affinity for sulfhydryl moieties and, hence, binds and inactivates a variety of enzymes. Methylmercury also initiates lipid peroxidation, which can produce alterations in cell membranes. Mercury damages the microtubules in the brain by reacting with the protein tubilin.

Human Toxicity

Mercury is an accumulative poison. Its toxicity depends its form.

Acute exposure to mercury vapor produces bronchitis and interstitial pneumonitis. Chronic exposure to the vapor can affect the kidneys and lead to proteinuria. The most notable effect of mercury vapor poisoning is on the central nervous system. Symptoms include loss of memory, excitability, fever, and local tremors that can progress to the entire body. Gingivitis is always associated with mercury vapor toxicity. Other symptoms are similar to toxic manifestations of inorganic mercury.

The toxicity of mercuric chloride (i.e., corrosive sublimate) has been well established. Oral ingestion causes severe abdominal cramps, possible ulceration and bleeding of the gastrointestinal tract, and a bloody diarrhea. Loose teeth are noted and hepatitis has been recorded. Nephritis is common; if the renal tubes are extensively damaged, it could lead to a possible fatal uremia. Renal failure occurs rapidly and, when patients survive, they must be maintained by dialysis. Regeneration of some kidney cells is possible but the damage is usually permanent.

Mercurous chloride is relatively insoluble and, thus, much less toxic than the soluble mercuric chloride.

Symptoms of methylmercury toxicity were noted following two Japanese disasters (Minamata Bay and Niigata) involving consumption of mercury-contaminated fish. Various ocean or river biota that had been eaten by the fish converted elemental mercury to the lipid-soluble mercury compound, methylmercury; mammalian tissue does not convert elemental mercury to methylmercury. Methylmercury resided in the muscle and liver of the fish; persons who ate the fish experienced methylmercury poisoning. Clinical symptoms included encephalitis and disease or loss of the general senses (touch, smell, taste, hearing, and vision). Children are more sensitive to methylmercury poisoning than adults.

In Iran, a local population ate bread that contained wheat seed that had been dusted with a fungicide consisting of methylmercury. The seed was intended for planting only. Symptoms of methylmercury poisoning included difficulty in walking, ataxia, paresthesia, sensory disturbance, and even deafness. A number of brain centers were damaged in the visual cortex and cerebellum.

It is obvious that methylmercury crosses the placental barrier. Pregnant women who have not displayed any signs of mercury toxicity have given birth to infants with birth defects. Some infants were mentally retarded; some had a palsy.

The ACGIH TLV-TWA for methylmercury is 0.01 mg/m^3 with a warning for skin exposure. The TLV is 0.025 mg/m^3 for mercury vapor and inorganic mercury.

Clinical Management

Normally BAL (British Anti-Lewisite; 2,3-dimercaptopropanol), administered intramuscularly, is used as an antidote for mercury poisoning. Oral D-penicillamine has been used for less severe cases. The I-acetyl derivative has been tested with good results. Experimentally, oral meso-2,3-dimercaptosuccinic acid and the less toxic 2,3-dimercaptopropane-1-sulfonate have been shown to be more effective than BAL.

Animal Toxicity

The carcinogenicity and mutagenicity of mercury have been claimed; however, further verification is needed. Although mercury is fetotoxic, the teratological aspect also needs further study.

—*Arthur Furst and Shirley B. Radding*

Related Topics

Disc Batteries
Environmental Processes
Kidney
Metals
Methylmercury
Neurotoxicology: Central and Peripheral

Mescaline

- CAS: 54-04-6
- SYNONYMS: 3,4,5-Trimethoxyphenethylamine; peyote; mescal; mescal button
- PHARMACEUTICAL CLASS: A phenylethylamine derivative alkaloid hallucinogen found in the North American cactus *Lophophora williamsii* and in several South American cacti of the trichocereus species
- CHEMICAL STRUCTURE:

CH_3O / CH_3O—(benzene ring)—$CH_2CH_2NH_2$ / CH_3O

Use

Mescaline does not have a therapeutic use. It is used as a Native American religious intoxicant. It is also a drug of abuse.

Exposure Pathways

The primary exposure pathway is oral ingestion of "buttons," the dried tops of the cactus. Ingestion usually involves three to eight buttons, for a total dose of 100–800 mg. Many substances represented as mescaline are in fact other hallucinogens such as phencyclidine.

Toxicokinetics

Mescaline appears to be well absorbed from the gastrointestinal tract, with peak concentrations at approximately 2 hr. Ninety percent of a dose is recovered in the urine during the first 24 hr, approximately 60% as unmetabolized mescaline and the remainder as hepatically produced metabolites. The apparent volume of distribution is unknown. The half-life is reported to be approximately 6 hr.

Mechanism of Toxicity

The specific mechanisms are unclear and probably include enhanced or altered central nervous system (CNS) serotonergic activity. It is structurally related to the amphetamines, which may produce similar sympathomimetic and hallucinogenic effects by increasing norepinephrine and serotonin concentrations by enhancing presynaptic release, blocking reuptake, and inhibiting monoamine oxidase.

Human Toxicity: Acute

At a hallucinogenic dose of approximately 5 mg/kg, the initial phase of nausea, vomiting, and generalized discomfort are observed followed by sympathomimetic symptoms including increased blood pressure and body temperature. Several hours after ingestion, euphoria and distortion of sensory perception begin. Visual pseudohallucinations or hallucinations are common and include bright colors and geometric patterns. Changes in taste, smell, and hearing can also be present. Depersonalization and disorientation of time can occur, and anxiety and depression may develop later during the intoxication. Larger doses can produce bradycardia, hypotension, and decreased respiration. The person will be at increased risk for trauma due to his or her altered perception of events occurring around him or her and increased emotional lability, panic attacks, and anxiety. Symptoms usually resolve over 6–12 hr. Average peak blood concentrations are approximately 4 μg/ml with a 500-mg oral dose.

Human Toxicity: Chronic

There is no evidence of genetic abnormalities with chronic use. Flashbacks have been suggested. Flashbacks appear to be much less common with mescaline than with LSD, if they occur.

Clinical Management

The patient's airway, breathing, and circulation should initially be assessed and supportive therapy provided as required. Reassurance and provision of a quiet, nonthreatening environment may be effective in decreasing anxiety. Benzodiazepines should be utilized for anxiety or panic attacks that do not respond to reassurance. If additional drug therapy is required for agitation or psychosis, which is very unlikely, haloperidol (rather than phenothiazines) should be used during the acute phase of intoxication.

Further Reading

Baselt, R. C., and Cravey, R. H. (1989). *Disposition of Toxic Drugs and Chemicals in Man,* 3rd ed., pp. 506–507. Year Book Med. Pub., Chicago.

Leikin, J. B., Krantz, A. J., Zell-Kanter, M., Barkin, R. L., and Hryhorczuk, D. O. (1989). Clinical features and management of intoxication due to hallucinogenic drugs. *Med. Toxicol. Adverse Drug Exp.* **4**, 324–350.

—*William A. Watson*

Metallothionein

Metallothionein is a metal-binding protein, rich in cysteines, that has a strong affinity to heavy metals such as cadmium and zinc. It is key in protecting organs and tissues against the toxic effects of these metals. Although found throughout the body, metallothionein is most prevalent in the kidneys and liver. Metallothionein binds with metals rendering them biologically inactive as they enter the kidneys and liver. Once within these organs, the metal–metallothionein complex breaks down, releasing the metal, which may cause toxic effects.

Outside the hepatic system, metallothionein facilitates absorption of metals such as cadmium into the kidneys and liver. Also, the induction of metallothionein via reactive metals protects hepatic enzymes against cellular damage. Without this intervention, zinc may stimulate glutathione concentration and reduce catalase activity. Cadmium reduces the amount of P450 and its activity toward testosterone oxidation. Usually, the liver can produce sufficient amounts of the protein to bind to any free metals.

However, the kidneys are at greater risk for toxicity because they must manage free metals that enter without metallothionein binding as well as those freed through biotransformation. In the kidney, the cadmium–metallothionein compound is filtered by the glomerulus and then reabsorbed by the proximal tobule. Lysomal degradation in the tubular cells may break the molecular binds and release free cadmium into the kidney, which prompts further metallothionein production. If the production within the kidney is insufficient to absorb the concentration of a free metal, it may produce kidney damage or other pathologies. Similar effects are seen with aluminum as well, which may create tubular damage in free concentrations.

Wilson disease is a specific disease associated with copper toxicity and metallothionein. Rats raised to have a large accumulation of copper had nearly 100 times greater concentration of metallothionein in their liver compared to controls (5016 μg/g versus 65 μ/g). However, bile levels for both groups did not differ significantly. This suggests that the metal may have reacted with lysomal enzymes to reduce exocytosis.

Metallothionein appears to respond to other reactive substances such as trihalomethanes. A single dose of chloroform significantly increased metallothionein levels for up to 6–12 hr following exposure. Although this indicates a response, it is not clear whether metallothionein protects against the harmful effects of this substance as well.

Toxicity due to insufficient metallothionein depends on factors such as age, gender, and health status. Young mice were found to have a fourfold greater accumulation of cadmium in their brains than adult mice and significantly less metallothionein. Because cadmium interacts with calcium, women may lose cellular calcium. Diabetics experience glomeral damage and greater sensitivity. A lung carcinogen in rats, it is a suspected human carcinogen.

In protecting the body against toxic metals, metallothionein interacts with endogenous metabolic enzymes such as glutathione and mercapturic acid. This makes sense since cysteine is a substrate of glutathione. Supplements such as cysteine may elevate levels of metallothionein and zinc in the kidneys.

—Shayne C. Gad and Jayne E. Ash

Related Topics

Glutathione
Kidney
Liver
Metals

Metals

No general principles that govern the toxicity of all metals and their compounds exist; however, a few generalizations are possible. For the purposes of this discussion, the term metals will include ions and compounds.

Oxidation state and solubility are important factors in toxic reactions. Metals can react with enzymes, cell membranes, and specific cell components. These reactions can inhibit or even stimulate the actions of these substances and components.

Metals are circulated bound to some blood protein and can concentrate; thus, metals can affect either specific target organs or multiple anatomical sites. For example, lead can deposit in the bone, affect the central nervous system (CNS), and interfere with the metabolism of the heme in hemoglobin. Cadmium appears to concentrate in the kidneys and the liver. Mercury is a CNS toxin.

The metabolic product of the metal can determine the action in the organ in which the metal is deposited. Usually metabolism of metals can lead to detoxification and often to excretion. Some metals, such as selenium metal and oxides, are converted to the volatile trimethyl derivative and are exhaled. On the other hand, mercury is converted to methyl mercury chloride, which is soluble in lipids and appears to be concentrated over time in organs with high lipid content.

Some metals (cadmium, zinc, copper, and mercury) induce special protein complexes called metallothioneines. Iron forms a number of other protein complexes (ferritin, hemosidern, and transferrin).

For the general population, inhalation is a secondary exposure route for metals. Usually, metals are ingested with food or with drinking water.

Acute toxicity from metals can follow similar patterns; these can be essentially nonspecific like nausea and vomiting. A few metals and their compounds are carcinogenic to humans; the vast majority are not.

A few metals, such as lead and mercury, can cross the placental barrier. The very young population and the older population are most susceptible to metal toxicity.

—*Arthur Furst*

Related Topics

Aluminum
Antimony
Arsenic
Barium
Beryllium
Bismuth
Boron
Cadmium
Chromium
Cobalt
Copper
Gallium
Iron
Lead
Lithium
Manganese
Mercury
Molybdenum
Nickel
Platinum
Potassium
Selenium
Silver
Sodium
Tellurium
Thallium
Tin
Titanium
Tungsten
Uranium
Vanadium
Zinc

Methadone

- CAS: 297-88-1; 76-99-3
- Synonyms: 4,4-Diphenyl-6; dimethylaminoheptan-3-one
- Pharmaceutical Class: Synthetic opioid
- Chemical Structure:

Uses

Methadone is used as a legitimate opioid alternative to prevent the advent of opioid withdrawal and as an alternative to herion. It is also used as an analgesic.

Exposure Pathways

Ingestion and parenteral administration are common routes of exposure. Ingestion is the most common route and often occurs when children accidentally ingest a parent's methadone that was prescribed as a heroin alternative.

Toxicokinetics

Methadone is rapidly absorbed after all routes of exposure. After oral doses, it is detectable in the blood within 30 min. Peak plasma levels occur in 2–4 hr. Epidural and parenteral administration result in plasma levels in 2–7 min. Methadone undergoes extensive metabolism in the liver to several inactive metabolites. Protein binding is 85%, with an approximate volume of distribution of 4 liters/kg. There is steady-state elimination by kidneys, in bile, in sweat, and at all excretion sites. Urinary excretion of methadone and its metabolic products is dose dependent and comprises the major route of excretion only in doses exceeding 55 mg/day. Methadone is excreted by glomerular filtration and undergoes renal reabsorption. Reabsorption of methadone decreases as urinary pH decreases. The half-life of methadone is 1–1.5 days.

Mechanism of Toxicity

Methadone interacts with opioid receptors in the brain, altering the rate of release of the neurotransmittors acetycholine, norepinephrine, dopamine, and substance P. It produces profound respiratory and central nervous system (CNS) depression.

Human Toxicity

Excessive CNS and/or respiratory depression are signs of methadone toxicity. Miotic, CNS, and respiratory depressant effects can persist for more than 24 hr. Seizures and pulmonary edema can occur. Rhabdomyolysis, myoglobinuria, muscle necrosis, and renal failure may all occur secondary to intoxication. In a child, 10 mg of methadone has been lethal.

Clinical Management

Gastric decontamination is recommended. Naloxone infusion may be necessary and is the preferred treatment due to the drug's long half-life, prolonged respiratory depression, and tendency toward relapse. Because of the long half-life of methadone, the patient should be monitored for at least 48 hr.

—Linda Hart

Related Topics

Poisoning Emergencies in Humans
Toxicity Testing, Reproductive

Methamidophos

- CAS: 10265-92-6
- SYNONYMS: *O,S*-dimethyl phosphoramidothioate; Tamaron-; Tamanox; Monitor-; acephate-met
- CHEMICAL CLASS: Organophosphoramidate insecticide
- CHEMICAL STRUCTURE:

$$(CH_3O)(CH_3S)P(=O)-NH_2$$

Uses

Methamidophos is used as an insecticide and acaricide.

Exposure Pathways

Poisonings can occur from inhalation, skin absorption, or ingestion.

Toxicokinetics

Methamidophos can be readily absorbed through the skin, lung, and gastrointestinal tract. The bioactivation of methamidophos (replacement of covalent sulfur with oxygen) is accomplished primarily by liver microsomal enzymes. A variety of hydrolysis reactions to alkyl phosphates and various leaving groups can occur. Methamidophos is fairly well distributed throughout the tissues, with marked accumulation in the liver, kidney, and adipose tissue. Excretion in the urine is the major elimination pathway.

Mechanism of Toxicity

See Chlorpyrifos. Methamidophos is a potent, direct acetylcholinesterase inhibitor that acts by interfering with the metabolism of acetylcholine. As a result, acetylcholine accumulates at neuroreceptor transmission sites.

Human Toxicity: Acute

Classic signs of acute toxicity include pinpoint pupils, muscular fasciculations, slow pulse, excessive salivation and lacrimation, and gastrointestinal symptoms (nausea, abdominal cramps, diarrhea, and loss of sphincter control). In severe cases, convulsions, coma, and heart block are common. Death is generally attributed to respiratory insufficiency caused by the combination of respiratory center depression, paralysis, and increased bronchial secretions. In children, the classic signs described previously may be infrequent, with the major symptoms being central nervous system depression, stupor, flaccidity, dyspnea, seizures, and coma.

Human Toxicity: Chronic

Cholinesterase inhibition may persist for 2–6 weeks. Signs of delayed neuropathy in humans have been reported following dermal and/or inhalation exposures. Progressive distal weakness, ataxia, flaccid paralysis, or quadriplegia may ensure. Additional chronic toxicities, such as memory impairment, language defects (slowed speech and slurring), and behavior disorders have been reported.

Clinical Management

For exposure to eyes, eyelids should be held open and the eyes flushed with copious amounts of water for 15 min. For exposure to skin, affected areas should be washed immediately with soap and water. Medical attention is necessary if irritation develops and persists.

For exposure through inhalation, the victim should be removed to fresh air and, if not breathing, given artificial ventilation. The victim should receive medical attention as soon as possible.

For ingestion victims, vomiting should be induced, keeping in mind the possibility of aspiration of solvents. Gastric decontamination should be performed within 30 min of ingestion to be most effective. Initial management of acute toxicity is establishment and maintenance of adequate airway and ventilation. Atropine sulfate in conjunction with 2-PAM can be administered as an antidote. Atropine by intravenous injection is the primary antidote in severe cases. Test injections of atropine (1 mg in adults and 0.15 mg/kg in children) are initially administered, followed by 2–4 mg (in adults) or 0.015–0.05 mg/kg (in children) every 10–15 minutes until cholinergic signs (e.g., diarrhea, salivation, and bronchial secretions) decrease. High doses of atropine over several injections may be necessary for effective control of cholinergic signs. If lavage is performed, endotracheal and/or esophageal control is suggested. At first signs of pulmonary edema, the patient should be placed in an oxygen tent and treated symptomatically.

Animal Toxicity

Methamidophos has high mammalian toxicity. The oral LD_{50} value in rats is about 20 mg/kg. Dermal LD_{50} values in rats and rabbits are about 100 mg/kg. Methamidophos is hazardous to bees.

Further Reading

Gallo, M. A., and Lawryk, N. J. (1991). Organic phosphorus pesticides. In *Handbook of Pesticide Toxicology* (W. J. Hayes, Jr., and E. R. Laws, Jr., Eds.), Vol. 3, pp. 917–972, 1090. Academic Press, San Diego.

—Kevin N. Baer

(Clinical management section prepared by Carey Pope)

Related Topics

Cholinesterase Inhibition
Organophosphates
Pesticides

Methane

- CAS: 74-82-8
- Synonyms: Natural gas; fire damp; marsh gas; methane (compressed, UN1971; DOT); methane (refrigerated liquid, UN1972; DOT); methyl hydride

- Chemical Class: Aliphatic hydrocarbon (C1)
- Molecular Formula: CH_4

Uses

Methane is a colorless, odorless, highly flammable gas that is lighter than air. It occurs in natural gas at a concentration of 60–80%. It evolves naturally in marshes and highly reducing sediments as a result of the microbiological decay of vegetation and organic matter. It is also found in coal deposits and is produced as a byproduct of some industrial processes, including some types of fermentation and sludge digestion. In industry, methane is used to make methanol, acetylene, hydrogen cyanide, and methyl chloride. In the form of natural gas, methane is used as a fuel, as a source of carbon black, and as a starting material for the manufacture of synthetic proteins. It is also used for gas-fired utilities and for use in the home (home heating, gas dryers, and gas cooking).

Exposure Pathways

Because methane exists as a gas at normal temperatures and pressure, exposure would occur by inhalation. It is possible to spill liquid methane from a refrigerated tank, causing frostbite upon contact with the skin due to rapid evaporation and loss of heat.

Mechanism of Toxicity

Methane acts as an asphyxiant at concentrations that are high enough to displace oxygen (87–90%).

Human Toxicity

Methane is not toxic to humans. It will, however, act as an asphyxiant at concentrations that are high enough to displace oxygen (87–90%). Methane is also highly flammable, and is therefore a fire hazard (the lower explosive limit is 5–15% by volume). ACGIH suggests that methane be treated as a simple asphyxiant. A threshold concentration of 1000 ppm is commonly assumed.

Clinical Management

Persons who are exposed to high concentrations should vacate or be removed from the source of the gas and seek fresh air. Extreme care must be taken to keep areas of high concentration free from ignition sources, such as sparks from static electricity. Explosionproof apparatus should also be used in these areas.

Animal Toxicity

The toxicity of methane in animals is similar to that in humans.

—Stephen Clough

Related Topics

Respiratory Tract
Veterinary Toxicology

Methanol

- CAS: 67-56-1
- Synonyms: Methyl alcohol; carbinol; wood spirits; wood alcohol
- Chemical Class: Alcohol
- Molecular Formula: CH_4O

Uses

Methanol is used primarily as an intermediate in the production of formaldehyde, acetic acid, and methyl-*tert*-butyl ether (MtBE). Methanol itself has been used as an oxygenated fuel additive, as well as an alternate transportation fuel in addition to its use as a solvent.

Exposure Pathways

Exposure to methanol can occur via inhalation, ingestion, and skin absorption.

Toxicokinetics

Irrespective of route of exposure, methanol distributes readily and uniformly to all organs and tissues as a function of their water content. Absorption via inhalation has been reported to be approximately 60% of the inhaled dose. Methanol is absorbed through human skin at a rate measured *in vitro* of 8.29 mg/cm^2/hr. Upon absorption, methanol is unchanged in urine, exhaled in breath, or metabolized in the liver and eventually excreted as CO_2. Greater than 90% of the administered dose is metabolized with approximately 2% excreted unchanged in expired air and 1% unchanged in urine. Depending on dose, half-lives for methanol elimination range from about 1 day or more for doses of 1 g/kg or greater to about 3 hr for doses of <0.1 g/kg.

The oxidation of methanol to CO_2 proceeds through several enzymatic steps. Methanol is first converted to formaldehyde via either a catalase/peroxidase reaction (prevalent in rats) or an alcohol dehydrogenase oxidation (predominant in humans and monkeys). Methanol-derived formaldehyde is then conjugated with glutathione to form *S*-formylglutathione via a nicotinamide adenine nucleotide-dependent formaldehyde dehydrogenase. The *S*-formylglutathione conjugate is subsequently hydrolyzed by thiolase to form formic acid and glutathione. Formic acid, in the form of formate, then enters the body's carbon pool in the liver through complexation with tetrahydrofolate, whereupon subsequent oxidation it is released as CO_2.

Mechanism of Toxicity

The toxic properties of methanol are the result of accumulation of the formate intermediate in the blood and tissues of exposed individuals. Formate accumulation produces metabolic acidosis leading to the characteristic ocular toxicity (blindness) observed in human methanol poisonings.

Humans and primates appear particularly sensitive to methanol toxicity when compared to rats. This is attributed to the slower rate of conversion in humans of the formate metabolite to CO_2 via tetrahydrofolate. This step in methanol metabolism occurs in rats at a rate approximately 2.5 times that observed in humans. Formate appears to directly affect the optic nerve. It is believed that formate acts as a metabolic poison inhibiting cytochrome oxidase. The optic nerve is composed of cells that normally have low reserves of cytochrome oxidase due to their low metabolic requirements and thus may be particularly sensitive to formate-induced metabolic inhibition.

Human Toxicity

Historically, injuries and fatalities have been reported from acute methanol overexposure via ingestion, inhalation, as well as prolonged or repeated skin contact. Clinical studies of individuals acutely poisoned by methanol ingestion have identified visual disturbances and possibly blindness as the most notable toxic effects in humans. Methanol is also a central nervous system (CNS) depressant, although less potent than ethanol, and has also been shown to produce liver damage upon overexposure.

At high doses, methanol can cause reversible or permanent blindness, and in severe cases, death. Visual problems include eye pain, blurred vision, constriction of visual field, and possibly permanent blindness which can develop in as little as 48 hr. The lethal dose of methanol in untreated individuals is estimated to be in the range of 0.8–1.5 g/kg, which translates into approximately 56–100 g, or 70–130 ml, for the average individual (70 kg). Typically, the effects noted in methanol poisoning can be divided into three stages: (1) narcosis or CNS depression similar to that observed in ethanol intoxication; (2) a latent period, generally 10–15 hr; and, (3) visual disturbances, CNS effects, nausea, vomiting, dizziness, headaches, and failing eyesight.

Clinical Management

Ingestion of methanol can be followed for up to 2 hr with syrup of ipecac or gastric lavage. Hemodialysis to remove methanol rapidly has been found to be the most effective therapy in methanol poisonings. Administration of ethanol, to competitively block the metabolism of methanol, and sodium bicarbonate, to correct acidosis, has also been successfully employed.

Animal Toxicity

The acute lethality of methanol is low based on animal testing via oral, dermal, and inhalation routes of exposure. The acute oral LD_{50}s observed in rats, rabbits, and monkeys range from approximately 7 g/kg (monkey) to 14.4 g/kg (rabbits). Acute dermal LD_{50}s in rabbits have been reported as approximately 20 ml/kg and inhalation lethal concentrations ranged from approximately 31,000 ppm (18-hr exposure, rats) to 72,000 ppm (54-hr exposure, mice).

Sublethal doses have been shown to elicit CNS effects, ocular toxicity, and liver effects. Rats receiving oral doses of 10, 100, or 500 mg/kg/day methanol for 1 month showed liver changes characterized by enlarged hepatic cells and changes in some microsomal enzymes. Rabbits exposed via inhalation to 46.6 ppm methanol for 6 months exhibited changes in the photoreceptor cells of the retina which were observed upon electron microscopic examination. Monkeys exposed to 0, 10, 100, or 1000 ppm methanol, 22 hr/day for up to 2 years exhibited slight changes in the liver and kidney at the 1000 ppm dose level. Pathologic changes in the nervous system of all animals at 1000 ppm were observed but were considered transient and probably reversible.

The developmental toxicity of methanol has been examined in rats and mice via inhalation and oral exposure. Rats exposed by inhalation to 10,000 and 20,000 ppm methanol 7 hr/day during gestation produced offspring with reduced body weights and a high incidence of malformations. Similarly, mice exposed to 4000 and 5000 ppm methanol 7 hr/day during Gestational Days 6–15 experienced a high incidence of embryotoxicity and exencephaly in surviving offspring. Single oral dosing of rats on Gestational Day 10 produced a dose-dependent increase in malformations at 1.3, 2.6, and 5.2 ml/kg methanol.

—Bradford Strohm

Related Topics

Neurotoxicology: Central and Peripheral
Sensory Organs

Methaqualone

- CAS: 340-56-7
- SYNONYMS: Methacolonum; methaqualoni; Quaalude; ludes
- PHARMACEUTICAL CLASS: Sedative–hypnotic
- CHEMICAL STRUCTURE:

Uses

Historically, methaqualone was used as a hypnotic for the treatment of insomnia. However, it is less effective than the benzodiazepines for this indication. It also has anticonvulsant, antitussive, and weak antihistaminic properties. It no longer has clinical therapeutic value and is not manufactured in the United States for legitimate pharmaceutical purposes. It is manufactured by clandestine laboratories for drug abuse purposes.

Toxicokinetics

Methaqualone is completely absorbed from the gastrointestinal tract within 2 hr. The rate of absorption of the HCl salt is faster than that of the freebase form because of faster dissolution in the stomach. Methaqualone is completely metabolized by hepatic hydroxylation. It is highly lipophilic with a volume of distribution of 2.4–6.4 liters/kg. Elimination is biphasic with a half-life of 33–40 hr for therapeutic doses and more prolonged after overdose. At least 12 metabolites are excreted in the urine and have been reported to persist as long as 7 days postingestion. These metabolites are believed to be inactive.

Mechanism of Toxicity

Methaqualone is a central nervous system depressant similar to other sedative hypnotics.

Human Toxicity

Symptoms range from gastrointestinal distress, drowsiness, ataxia, slurred speech, and paresthesias to agitation, convulsions, and coma. Unique among hypnotic drugs is methaqualone's selective depression of spinal reflexes resulting in muscular hyperactivity. The cough reflex is decreased with this drug. Methaqualone inhibits phases of platelet aggregation, prolongs prothrombin time (PT) and partial thromboplastin time (PTT), and decreases factors V and VII, all of which may lead to conjunctival, retinal, and gastrointestinal hemorrhage.

Clinical Management

Gastric decontamination with gastric lavage and/or activated charcoal should be considered. Decreased gastrointestinal motility during coma may result in lavage being effective 8–12 hr after ingestion. Conservative and supportive care with frequent monitoring of vital signs is recommended. Platelet count and PT/PTT times should be monitored as well. Muscular hyperactivity may require diazepam administration. If methaqualone has been abused chronically, the patient should be observed for withdrawal symptoms for 3–5 days after the last dose.

—Linda Hart

Methomyl

- CAS: 16752-77-5
- SYNONYMS: Nudrin; Lannate; *S*-methyl *N*-[((methylcarbamoyl)oxy)]thioacetimidate
- CHEMICAL CLASS: Carbamate insecticide
- CHEMICAL STRUCTURE:

$$CH_3-\underset{\underset{S-CH_3}{|}}{C}=N-O-\overset{\overset{O}{\|}}{C}-NH-CH_3$$

Uses

Methomyl is a broad-spectrum insecticide registered for use on several agricultural crops and commercially grown ornamental plants.

Exposure Pathways

Oral exposures are most common. Inhalation and dermal exposures are also possible, particularly in the workplace.

Toxicokinetics

Methomyl is rapidly absorbed from the oral route. Dermal exposure is less hazardous. It is biotransformed to acetonitrile and carbon dioxide. Methomyl is well distributed to the tissues. Elimination is rapid: Less than 10% remains 24 hr after an oral exposure. Approximately 75% of an absorbed oral dose of methomyl is eliminated via exhalation either as CO_2 or as acetonitrile. The remainder is excreted in urine as polar metabolites.

Mechanism of Toxicity

Methomyl exerts toxicity by inhibiting acetylcholinesterase. As with other carbamate insecticides, acetylcholinesterase inhibition is much less persistent than with organophosphate intoxication.

Human Toxicity: Acute

Methomyl is highly toxic by the oral route, moderately toxic by inhalation, and has low dermal toxicity. The primary symptom in acute methomyl poisoning is severe headaches, which may be accompanied by less severe symptoms such as nausea, vomiting, salivation, and abdominal pain. Other general symptoms are cramps, diarrhea, sweating, lassitude, weakness, runny nose, chest tightness, and blurring or dimness of vision. Sometimes the effects of acute exposure to carbamates can be long-lasting.

Human Toxicity: Chronic

Because of its rapid biotransformation, methomyl does not tend to cause cumulative toxicity.

The probable lethal oral dose in humans is 5–50 mg/kg. The actual lethal dose of methomyl depends on the route and rate of exposure and the aggressiveness of the treatment used.

Clinical Management

Basic life-support measures must be maintained. The patient should be moved to fresh air, and exposed eyes and skin should be irrigated with large amounts of water. Atropine is used to counteract muscarinic side effects. Pralidoxime is contraindicated (see Carbofuran). Charcoal may be used to absorb methomyl.

Animal Toxicity

Methomyl is also extremely toxic to animals and, as with humans, the range of toxicity depends on the route and rate of exposure. Oral LD_{50} values in laboratory rodents range from about 15 to 30 mg/kg. Methomyl is not teratogenic, mutagenic, or a reproductive toxicant.

—Janice Reeves and Carey Pope

Related Topics

Carbamate Pesticides
Carboxylesterases
Cholinesterase Inhibition
Pesticides

Methoprene

- CAS: 40596-69-8
- SYNONYMS: Altosid; Apex; Manta; Minex; Diacon; isopropyl(2e,4e)-11-methoxy-3,7,11-trimethyl-2,4-dodecadienoate
- CHEMICAL CLASS: Synthetic terpenoid
- MOLECULAR FORMULA: $C_{19}H_{34}O_3$

Uses

Methoprene is a broad-spectrum synthetic juvenile hormone which acts as an insect growth regulator. It is useful against ants, mosquitoes, flies, beetles, lice, and moths.

Exposure Pathways

Dermal contact or eye contamination are the most common routes of exposure.

Toxicokinetics

No literature is available on the toxicokinetics of methoprene in mammals. In plants, methoprene undergoes ester hydrolysis, O-demethylation, and oxidative cleavage of the double bond at the 4-position. The principal metabolite produced in plants such as rice is 7-methoxycitronellal. Methoprene is degraded in soil with an estimated half-life of 10 days.

Mechanism of Toxicity

Juvenile hormones are one of three types of internal regulators of insect growth and metamorphosis. These hormones are synthesized and released in a regulated way into the hemolymph. Immature larvae require these hormones to progress through the regular larval stages. Methoprene disrupts these hormonal processes and prevents metamorphosis.

Human Toxicity

No study has reported acute or chronic toxicity of methoprene in humans. No symptoms have been seen in humans. Because of its mechanism of action, methoprene has high selectivity for insects.

Clinical Management

Methoprene is not irritating to the skin and has very low systemic side effects if absorbed through the skin. In cases of skin exposure, the exposed area should be thoroughly washed with soap and water. Eyes should be washed with copious amounts of room-temperature water in cases of eye contamination. If small amounts are ingested, no treatment is generally needed. Low toxicity is seen in nontargeted species. Emesis is seldom necessary due to low toxicity; it is contraindicated when methoprene is in a hydrocarbon base. Activated charcoal is preferred. It can be administered as an aqueous slurry or as a mixture of charcoal with saline cathartics or sorbitol. Symptomatic treatment is recommended.

Animal Toxicity

The oral LD_{50} value in rats is $\geqq 30$ g/kg. Rats receiving 5000 ppm and mice receiving 2500 ppm methoprene in the diet for 2 years did not show any adverse effects. Methoprene has extremely low toxicity in laboratory animals.

—Sushmita M. Chanda

Related Topic

Pesticides

Methoxychlor

- CAS: 72-43-5
- SYNONYMS: 1,1,1-Trichloro-2,2-bis(*p*-methoxyphenyl)-ethane; 1,1′-(2,2,2-trichloroethylidene)bis(4-methoxy-benzene)

- Chemical Class: Organochlorine insecticide
- Chemical Structure:

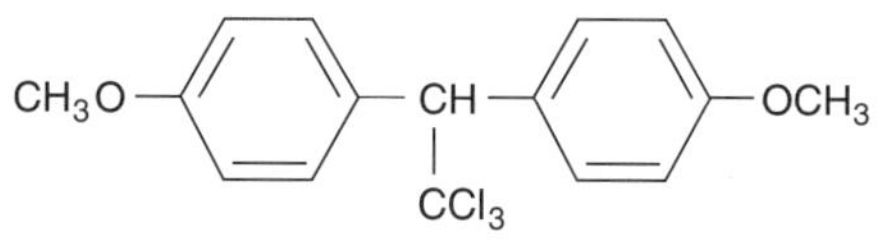

CH_3O — CH — OCH_3

CCl_3

Uses

Methoxychlor is used as an ectoparasiticide for cats and as an agricultural insecticide.

Exposure Pathways

Ingestion and dermal contact are possible routes of exposure.

Toxicokinetics

Chlorinated hydrocarbon insecticides, when dissolved in oil or other lipid, are readily absorbed by the skin and alimentary canal. Although methoxychlor is slowly metabolized to a small extent by pathways similar to those of DDT, the major pathway is by O-demethylation and subsequent conjugation. Methoxychlor has been detected in the blood of agricultural workers. All organochlorines are likely to be excreted in the milk of lactating women.

From mice fed labeled methoxychlor, 90% of recovered radioactivity was in feces and 10% in urine. Weanling rats fed a 500 mg/kg diet of methoxychlor for 4–18 weeks stored 14–36 mg/kg in fat. [^{14}C]-1-phenyl-methoxychlor in oil emulsion given intravenously to rats at a dosage of 1 mg in 0.5 ml emulsion was metabolized rapidly by the liver to unidentified hydrophilic products, which were excreted mainly in feces, by secretion from liver into bile, and to lesser extent in urine. Weanling rats fed 500 mg/kg diet methoxychlor for 4–18 weeks stored 14–36 mg/kg in fat; equilibrium was reached within 4 weeks and methoxychlor disappeared from fatty tissue within 2 weeks after the end of exposure.

Mechanism of Toxicity

Proestrogen. In addition, methoxychlor undergoes a hepatic microsomal monooxygenase(s)-mediated activation and the resultant reactive metabolites (possibly free radicals) bind covalently to microsomal components.

Human Toxicity

In extreme overdoses, central nervous system depression may occur. In general, for chlorinated hydrocarbon insecticides, aspiration of insecticide-containing petroleum distillate may result in pneumonitis. In addition, nausea, vomiting, and diarrhea may follow ingestion; blood dyscrasias, anemia, and leukemia have been associated with organochlorine exposure, and extensive contact results in dermal irritation. Organochlorine pesticides cause liver and kidney damage, microsomal enzyme induction, increased alkaline phosphotase, and aldolase activity, protein synthesis, lipid synthesis, detoxification, excretion, and liver functions are all affected. The approximate fatal dose is 6 g/kg. Chronic exposure may cause kidney damage. There is not any evidence of carcinogenicity in humans.

Clinical Management

In general, following acute exposure to chlorinated hydrocarbon insecticides, blood chlorinated hydrocarbon levels are not clinically useful; for most compounds it reflects cumulative exposure over a period of months rather than recent exposure. Emesis may be indicated in recent ingestion and is most effective if initiated within 30 min postingestion. In addition, an activated charcoal/cathartic may be given. For seizures, diazepam should be administered as an intravenous bolus. Oils should not be given by mouth. Adrenergic amines should not be administered because they may further increase myocardial irritability and produce refractory ventricular arrhythmias. If clothing is contaminated, it should be removed. The skin (including hair) should be washed three times–an initial soap washing, followed by an alcohol washing, followed by a soap washing. Leather absorbs pesticides. Hence, leather should not be worn in the presence of pesticides and all contaminated leather should be discarded.

Animal Toxicity

Ocular toxicity has been reported from systemic exposure to methoxychlor. Chronic intoxication of dogs at dosages of 2 g/kg/day in the diet led to convulsions in 6 weeks and death in 9 weeks; weight loss, high alkaline phosphatase and serum transaminase, and intestinal congestion were seen; and swine showed kidney injury and uterine and mammary enlargement. Rabbits given 200 mg/kg orally per day died after four or five doses; autopsy findings included mild liver damage and nephrosis. Atrophy of the testes was observed in rats given 1% methoxychlor in the diet. In rats given 100 or 200 mg/kg/day, arrested spermatogenesis was noted after 70 consecutive days of treatment; corpora lutea failed to develop in female rats treated with similar dosages for 14 days before and continuously after mating. Administration of 1000 mg/kg in the diet to pregnant rats caused early vaginal openings in their offspring; both male and female offspring had reduced fertility when they attained maturity. No abortions were observed in pregnant cows given methoxychlor at 10 mg/kg body weight/day. In a 27-month study in rats, 1000 ppm methoxychlor was administered in the diet; there were no differences in deaths or the incidence and distribution of benign or malignant tumors in treated animals vs controls. There is not any evidence of carcinogenicity in animals. Results were negative in the *Escherichia coli* WP2,UVRA reverse mutation assay. Injection of a 0.1% solution of methoxychlor did not induce sex-linked recessive lethals in male *Drosophila melanogaster.*

—*Robin Guy*

Related Topics

Cyclodienes
Organochlorine Insecticides
Pesticides

Methoxyethanol

- CAS: 109-86-4
- Preferred Name: Ethylene glycol monomethyl ether
- Synonyms: 2-Methoxyethanol; methyl Cellosolve; Dowanol EM glycol ether
- Chemical Class: Alkyl glycol ether
- Chemical Structure:

```
    H         H    H
    |         |    |
H — C — O — C — C — O — H
    |         |    |
    H         H    H
```

Uses

Methoxyethanol is an industrial solvent. It does not have a therapeutic application.

Exposure Pathways

Dermal contact and inhalation are likely exposure routes. Oral exposure is unlikely except by accidental or deliberate ingestion of methoxyethanol-containing liquids.

Toxicokinetics

Methoxyethanol is principally metabolized to methoxyacetic acid, presumably via methoxyacetaldehyde. Small amounts of methoxyacetylglycine are also formed. The major route of excretion of metabolites is the urine with traces in the feces. Substantial amounts are exhaled as carbon dioxide. In rats, the half-life of the compound when administered at sublethal doses is 1 to 2 hr.

Mechanism of Toxicity

High acute doses of methoxyethanol have a narcotic effect. Kidney and lung damage, accompanied by hemoglobinuria, is present. Toxicity is attributed to metabolites, including the putative intermediate methoxyacetaldehyde, and methoxyacetate. Methoxyacetate inhibits lactate production by cells in culture. Teratogenicity appears to be related to an interference by methoxyethanol, or its metabolites, with 1-carbon metabolism in the synthesis of nucleic acid precursors.

Human Toxicity

Consumption of a single dose of methoxyethanol estimated to be about 200 ml was fatal for an individual likely compromised by advanced alcoholism. Two individuals, who consumed about 100 ml of methoxyethanol, became sleepy, weak, nauseated, and acidodic but survived. Significant toxicity, involving central nervous system (CNS) depression, neurological symptoms, macrocytic anemia, and immune depression, can result from chronic inhalation of methoxyethanol. Similar symptoms occur after dermal exposure. Symptoms are reversed after cessation of exposure. The warning properties of methoxyethanol are not strong and humans tolerate inhalation levels well above the present OSHA limit.

In animal studies, reproductive effects, including depression of sperm counts, testicular atrophy, embryotoxicity, and teratogenicity, follow exposure by all routes. Although these effects have not been documented in humans, methoxyethanol exposure is considered to pose a reproductive hazard to humans.

Clinical Management

Prompt removal from the area of exposure is important. Clinical management is limited to treatment of symptoms.

Animal Toxicity

Extensive animal studies of methoxyethanol have fairly well outlined its toxic effects by oral, injection, inhalation, and dermal routes of exposure. Acute exposures to high doses can kill by severe CNS depression. Sublethal exposures cause kidney damage, thymic involution, testicular atrophy, and depression of sperm counts. High chronic exposures cause decreases in hemoglobin count, white blood cell count, platelet count, and red blood cell count. Methoxyethanol is embrytoxic in rodents, rabbits, and monkeys. The teratogenic effects of methoxyethanol are obvious in mice but effects in rabbits and rats have been attributed to maternal toxicity and fetotoxicity.

—*Michael J. Brabec*

Related Topic

Reproductive System, Male

Methoxypsoralen

- CAS: 298-81-7
- Preferred Name: Xanthotoxin
- Synonyms: 8-Methoxypsoralin; 9-methoxypsoralin; ammoidin; oxsoralen
- Chemical Class: Coumarin
- Molecular Formula: $C_{12}H_8O_4$

Uses

With long-wave ultraviolet light, methoxypsoralen is used in the treatment of psoriasis, vitiligo, and mycosis fungoides.

Exposure Pathways

Dermal contact is the most likely route of exposure.

Mechanism of Toxicity

Alkylation of DNA is the mechanism of carcinogenesis.

Human Toxicity

Methoxypsoralen is a phototoxic and photosensitizing agent. It is also a photocarcinogen. It can cause hyperpigmentation and abnormal nail pigmentation.

Animal Toxicity

Methoxypsoralen is an IARC carcinogen. It is also mutagenic in many test systems.

—*Shayne C. Gad*

Related Topics

Mutagenesis
Photoallergen

Methyl Acrylate

- CAS: 96-33-3
- Synonyms: Methyl 2-propenoate; 2-propenoic acid methyl ester; acrylic acid methyl ester
- Chemical Class: Ester
- Molecular Formula: $C_4H_6O_2$
- Chemical Structure:

$$H_2C{=}CH{-}\overset{\displaystyle O}{\overset{\|}{C}}{-}O{-}CH_3$$

Uses

Methyl acrylate is used primarily as a comonomer with acrylonitrile to produce acrylate fibers (>85% acrylonitrile by weight) and modacrylate fibers (35–85% acrylonitrile by weight). These fibers are used to manufacture carpets, clothing, blankets, and curtains. Other uses of methyl acrylate include amphoteric surfactants, textile and paper coatings, leather finish resins, and thermoplastic coatings.

Exposure Pathways

Exposures to methyl acrylate monomer are most likely to occur in an occupational environment via skin contact and inhalation. The general population is not expected to receive a significant exposure to methyl acrylate monomer due to low concentrations of residual monomer in consumer products. The public may be exposed to methyl acrylate via ingestion because it is found naturally in some foods (e.g., pineapple puree).

Toxicokinetics

Data from animal experiments indicate that methyl acrylate is readily absorbed from the gastrointestinal tract and the respiratory tract. Methyl acrylate is also absorbed through the skin but less readily because a large portion of the dermally applied dose appears to be retained in the dermis. Dermal absorption may also be impeded by the evaporation of methyl acrylate from the skin if the applied dose is unoccluded.

The primary route of methyl acrylate metabolism is its rapid hydrolysis by tissue and circulating carboxylesterases to acrylic acid and methanol which undergo further metabolism. Another route of methyl acrylate metabolism is conjugation with the sulfhydryl group of glutathione. Methyl acrylate is rapidly distributed throughout the body. Methyl acrylate and/or its metabolites can be detected in all organ systems, with the highest concentrations being present in the urine, expired air, and organ of entry (i.e., stomach, upper respiratory tract, and skin). Metabolites of methyl acrylate are excreted primarily via the lungs (as carbon dioxide) and via the kidneys.

Mechanism of Toxicity

Pretreatment of rats with a carboxylesterase inhibitor potentiates the respiratory irritation and lethality produced by the inhalation of methyl acrylate. This observation suggests that the toxicity of methyl acrylate becomes manifest when local detoxification/defense mechanisms become overwhelmed.

Human Toxicity

Methyl acrylate can be highly irritating to the skin, eyes, gastrointestinal tract, and the respiratory tract. The severity of the reaction will depend on the concentration of the applied dose as well as the duration and frequency of contact. Chronic exposures to high vapor concentrations may damage the nasal mucosa leading to decrements in the sense of smell and taste; these decrements may be reversible upon cessation of exposure. Methyl acrylate can cause an allergic contact dermatitis which may cross react with other acrylate esters.

Clinical Management

Clinical management involves removal from exposure and treatment of symptoms.

Animal Toxicity

Toxicological studies in animals indicate that methyl acrylate exposures do not generally result in systemic toxicity at sublethal doses. Although methyl acrylate concentrations approaching lethal doses may cause histopathological changes in the liver and kidneys, methyl acrylate toxicity is largely limited to irritant effects, and their sequelae, at the site of application. Methyl acrylate can produce an allergic contact dermatitis which may cross react with other acrylic esters. The acute LD_{50} varies between 200 mg/kg (rabbit, oral) and 1300 mg/kg (rabbit, dermal) depending on the species and exposure route being evaluated.

—*Ralph Parod*

Related Topics

Carboxylesterases
Glutathione Conjugation
Polymers
Respiratory Tract

Methylamine

- CAS: 74-89-5
- Synonyms: Methanamine; monomethylamine; aminomethane; carbinamine; MMA
- Chemical Class: Amine

Uses

Methylamine is used in tanning; organic synthesis of accelerators, dyes, pharmaceuticals, insecticides, surface active agents, and fungicides; and also in dyeing of acetate textiles. It is an ingredient in paint removers, solvents, photographic developers, and rocket propellants.

Exposure Pathways

Exposure may occur through oral, dermal, or inhalation routes.

Toxicokinetics

Methylamine is rapidly absorbed. Traces ($<2\%$) of the unchanged compound are excreted in the urine. Initially, the amino group is dehydrogenated to the intermediate imine, which then reacts with water forming formaldehyde and ammonia. The final metabolic products, which are excreted in the urine, are formic acid and urea. To a lesser extent, methylamine is metabolized to dimethylamine in the body. Methylamine is a normal constituent of mammalian and human urine.

Mechanism of Toxicity

The toxic effects of methylamine are due primarily to its corrosive action on tissues. Methylamine has been shown to inhibit receptor-mediated endocytosis of biologically significant molecules such as lysosomal enzymes and peptide hormones.

Human Toxicity

Methylamine is a severe skin and eye irritant. Eye exposure to methylamine can cause distortion of the ocular membranes, loss of the corneal and conjunctival lens and epithelium, and loss of the endothelium of the cornea. Respiratory tract irritation can start at concentrations as low as 25 ppm, with stridor, dyspnea, and pulmonary edema at higher concentrations. Allergic or chemical bronchitis has been reported at 2–60 ppm. An exposure of 10 ppm does not appear to cause symptoms. Ingestion of methylamine causes severe burns to the lip, tongue, oral mucosa, and esophagus, with emesis, abdominal pain, and dysphagia.

Clinical Management

Exposed skin and eyes should be irrigated with copious amounts of water. After inhalation exposures, the victim should be moved to fresh air and monitored for respiratory distress. Humidified supplemental oxygen (100%) with assisted ventilation should be administered as required. If coughing or breathing difficulties are noted, the patient should be evaluated for irritation, bronchitis, or pneumonitis, including chest X-rays and determination of blood gasses. If pulmonary edema is present, positive end expiratory pressure ventilation and steroids should be considered. For ingestion exposures, copious amounts of water should be provided for dilution. Emesis or lavage should be avoided. If symptoms are present, esophagoscopy should be performed 12–24 hr after ingestion to assess the severity; however, the esophagoscope should not be passed beyond the first circumferential burn. For visible burns, 1 mg/kg prednisone may be considered.

Animal Toxicity

Corneal damage, skin damage, and necrosis has been induced in rabbits after direct contact with methylamine. The inhalation LC_{50} in mice was 2400 mg/m^3 for 2 hr. No adverse reproductive or developmental effects were observed in mice after exposure during gestation. Liver toxicity has been reported in laboratory animals. Methylamine has been negative in *in vitro* mutagenicity assays.

—Janice M. McKee

Methyl Bromide

- CAS: 74-83-9
- SYNONYMS: Bromomethane; Embafume; MB; M-B-C Fumigant; monobromomethane
- CHEMICAL CLASS: Halogenated aliphatic hydrocarbon
- MOLECULAR FORMULA: CH_3Br

Uses

Methyl bromide is used in ionization chambers, for degreasing wool, and for extracting oils from flowers, nuts, and seeds. It is also used as an insect fumigant for freight cars, mills, ships, soil, vaults, and warehouses.

Exposure Pathways

Methyl bromide exposure may occur by inhalation, oral, or dermal routes. It has the capacity to penetrate coverings and tissues, including rubber protective gear, fabrics, neoprene, skin, and mucous membranes. Dermal penetration is so efficient that exposed workers have been poisoned even when wearing an effective, self-contained breathing apparatus.

Toxicokinetics

Methyl bromide is absorbed rapidly via the skin and mucous membranes. It is extensively metabolized and rapidly eliminated in expired air. Following oral or inhalation exposure, 75–85% of the body burden was eliminated by rats 65–72 hr postexposure. Major organs of distribution include the fat, lungs, liver, adrenals, kidneys, and brain.

Mechanism of Toxicity

Although the toxic mechanism of methyl bromide is not clear, toxic effects include pulmonary edema, increased myocardial irritability, central nervous system (CNS) depression, dermal irritation and necrosis, liver injury, and renal damage. Methyl bromide is an alkylating agent and sulfhydryl enzyme inhibitor in mammalian tissues.

Human Toxicity

Signs and symptoms of toxicity primarily involve the CNS, respiratory tract, and cardiovascular system. Coma and convulsions may occur in serious exposures. Pulmonary edema may be noted following massive exposure to the respiratory tract. Acute tubular necrosis may be noted but is delayed and generally mild. Central and peripheral neurologic sequelae such as organic brain syndrome and extrapyramidal effects may be noted. Methyl bromide is an intense vesicant and dermal exposure will result in severe burns. Symptoms generally develop 3–12 hr after inhalation of vapor. Methyl bromide exposure has been noted to exhibit species- and sex-related differences in susceptibility of specific organs. Target organ specificity of methyl bromide is similar to that of methyl chloride. The human LC_{Lo} for methyl bromide is 60,000 ppm/2 hr in the adult and 1 g/m^3/2 hr in the child.

Clinical Management

Treatment is symptomatic and supportive for respiratory and cardiovascular function. There is no specific antidote for methyl bromide poisoning.

Animal Toxicity

Rats given 200 ppm of methyl bromide for 1–6 hr developed primary olfactory mucosal lesions. The induced changes in the olfactory mucosa were associated with decreased P450-dependent alkoxy-*o*-dealkylase activities; reduced glutathione (GSH), GSH transferase, and GSH reductase activities; and lower metabolism of arachidonic acid. Methyl bromide exposure in rats resulted in a residual 15–20% olfactory epithelial damage 10 weeks following exposure. Methyl bromide tested positive for mutation in microorganisms and positive for chromosomal damage by the Micronucleus test in rats and mice. The oral LD_{50} for the rat is about 200 mg/kg. The inhalation LC_{50} for the rat is 302 ppm/8 hr.

—Todd A. Bartow

Related Topics

Mutagenesis
Respiratory Tract

*Methylcholanthrene, 3-**

- CAS: 56-49-5
- Synonyms: 3-MC; 3-MCH; 3-methyl-I,j-cyclopentabenz[*a*]anthracene; 3-methylcyclopentabenzophenanthrene
- Chemical Class: Polynuclear aromatic hydrocarbon; polycyclic aromatic hydrocarbon
- Molecular Formula: $C_{21}H_{16}$

Uses

3-Methylcholanthrene is used experimentally as a positive control in cancer research and in biochemical research to induce specific forms of cytochrome P450.

* Information Source: Hazardous Substance Data Bank, National Library of Medicine, Bethesda, MD, July 1996.

Exposure Pathways

Methylcholanthrene may be absorbed via inhalation, ingestion, or dermal contact.

Toxicokinetics

Animal studies with structurally related polynuclear aromatic hydrocarbons (PAHs), such as benzo(*a*)pyrene, benz(*a*)anthracene, and 3-methylcholanthrene, confirmed that intestinal transport readily occurs primarily by passive diffusion after oral dosing. From the partitioning parameters, the rate-limiting step involves solvation of transfer species in the interfacial water at the phospholipid surface.

Metabolic products vary with the type of enzyme induction. In fetal rat livers, several compounds, such as 1- or 2-hydroxy-, *cis*- and *trans*-dihydroxy-, 11,12-dihydroxy-11,12-dihydro-, and 1- and 2-keto-3-methylcholanthrene have been identified. Most frequently, it is the liver that produces a variety of electrophilic reactants that covalently bind to macromolecules. Metabolism or bioactivation may also be extramicrosomal or be carried out by fetoplacental tissue or gut bacteria.

PAHs are highly soluble in adipose tissue and lipids. *In vivo* binding of 3-methylcholanthrene was studied in A/J mice and demonstrated DNA binding in the liver and lung.

Mechanism of Toxicity

Metabolic activation of PAHs consists of an oxidation of the rings of unsubstituted PAHs. These oxidations are carried out by mixed function oxidases of the liver which contain cytochromes P450 and P448 and require reduced nicotine adenine dinucleotide and oxygen. In this oxidation, an epoxide intermediate is formed which has been shown to have the requisite chemical reactivity to bind covalently with DNA and histones and to serve as the ultimate carcinogenic form of PAH.

Human Toxicity

The minimum lethal human exposure and the maximum tolerated human exposure to this agent have not been delineated. PAHs are eye irritants and produce photosensitivity, respiratory irritation, cough, mild hepatotoxicity, and nephrotoxicity. Workers routinely exposed to PAHs have been reported to show increased incidences of skin, bladder, lung, and gastrointestinal cancers. Other studies also demonstrated increased incidences of lung and scrotal cancer. 3-Methylcholanthrene is a PAH and is considered to be carcinogenic in humans.

Animal Toxicity

In mice, skin application leads rather quickly to carcinoma formation. Subcutaneous injection produces sarcomas in rats or mice. Oral administration in sesame oil to female Sprague–Dawley rats results in rapid induction of breast cancer, while oral administration to mice during the last week of pregnancy produced a threefold increase in incidence of tumors in the offspring. The most common type were lymphoma and lung tumors.

3-Methylcholanthrene is a powerful irritant and is an experimental carcinogen producing neoplastic responses by various dosing routes including oral, dermal, intravenous, parenteral, subcutaneous, intrarenal, intrapleural, intratracheal, and implant. 3-Methylcholanthrene is hepatotoxic, nephrotoxic, and immunotoxic and has been reported to produce agranulocytosis, anemia, leukopenia, and pancytopenia in exposed animals. 3-Methylcholanthrene is mutagenic in a number of *in vitro* and *in vivo* assays and is used regularly as a positive control in these assays, and it has been shown to covalently bind to DNA and other macromolecules.

Treated pregnant rats produce offspring with major birth defects including open neuronal tubes, abnormal flexure rotation and proencephalic defects, among others.

—*R. A. Parent, T. R. Kline, and D. E. Sharp*

Related Topics

Carboxylesterases
Polycyclic Aromatic Hydrocarbons

Methyl Disulfide

- CAS: 624-92-0
- SYNONYMS: Dimethyl disulfide

- Chemical Class: Organic sulfur
- Chemical Structure:

$$CH_3—S—S—CH_3$$

Uses

Methyl disulfide is used as a reagent in organic synthesis especially in the α-methyl-sulfonylation of carbonyl compounds. As a natural component of brassica vegetables it is volatilized and emitted during the cooking of potatoes.

Exposure Pathways

All routes of exposure are possible. Methyl disulfide is considered an eye and skin irritant and is irritating to the gastrointestinal tract. It is considered an inhalation poison.

Toxicokinetics

The distribution and metabolic effects of methyl disulfide in humans have not been thoroughly investigated. As a sulfur-containing compound it may undergo detoxification characteristic of organic sulfur compounds. Flavin-containing monooxygenase will oxygenate several *S*-containing compounds to electrophilic-reactive metabolites. Oxidation of the alkyl methyl group (dealkylation) may also occur. The formation of Heinz bodies, indicative of oxidative stress to red cells, has been noted in chickens exposed to methyl disulfide.

Mechanism of Toxicity

The information available on the human toxicity of methyl disulfide is limited. As a sulfide it may result in toxic effects similar to cyanide exposure in which inhibition of oxidative enzymes produces tissue anoxia.

Human Toxicity

Sulfur-containing xenobiotics generally exhibit a low level of toxicity. Little is known regarding the human toxicity of methyl disulfide. It is classified as an irritant and inhalation hazard. It is not classified as a genotoxic or clastogenic hazard and is negative in the Ames *Salmonella typhimurium* mutant assay. It also produced negative results in both *in vivo* and *in vitro* mammalian DNA repair assays.

Clinical Management

Affected eyes should be flushed with copious amounts of water immediately. Exposed skin should be washed with soap and copious amounts of water. In cases of inhalation, the victim should be removed to fresh air and provided with artificial respiration if not breathing. In cases of ingestion, induction of emesis or careful gastric lavage is recommended unless tissue corrosion is noted. Administration of oxygen may be helpful to aid tissue oxygenation of the sulfide to innocuous sulfates. Providing gastric antacids, milk, or demulcents may reduce the formation potential of hydrogen sulfide gas. If symptoms suggest tissue anoxia, similar to cyanide poisoning, amyl nitrite should be administered by inhalation and sodium nitrite by intravenous route (as for cyanide therapy).

Animal Toxicity

In reports providing only lethal dose, the LC_{50} for rats was reported as 16 mg/m^3/2 hr. The acute oral LC_{50} for rats is 190 mg/kg. No mortality was noted in rabbits given a dermal dose of 2000/mg/kg, although rabbit ocular, central nervous system, and respiratory signs were observed.

—*Kathryn Kehoe*

Methyldopa

- Synonyms: Methyldopate hydrochloride; α-methyldopa; methyldopum; methyldopum hydratum [CAS: 555-30-6 (anhydrous), CAS: 41372-08-1 (sesquihydrate)]; Aldomet
- Pharmaceutical Class: Hypotensive agent, centrally acting α_2-agonist
- Chemical Structure:

$$(HO)_2C_6H_3—CH_2—C(NH_2)(CH_3)—COOH + 1\tfrac{1}{2}\,H_2O$$

Uses
Methyldopa is used in the management of moderate to severe hypertension and in the management of hypertension in pregnant women.

Exposure Pathways
Ingestion is the most common route of both accidental and intentional exposure to methyldopa. It is available in both oral dosage forms (alone or in combination with a thiazide diuretic) and parenteral dosage forms.

Toxicokinetics
About 50% of an oral dose is absorbed (from 8 to 61%) with peak plasma concentrations occurring within 3–6 hr; pharmacologic effects do not correlate with plasma concentrations. Approximately 50% of an oral dose is metabolized. Metabolism is mainly by conjugation in the gastrointestinal tract and the liver. The sulfate conjugate is therapeutically active. The rate of conjugation is decreased in patients with renal insufficiency. The volume of distribution is 0.24 liters/kg. Methyldopa and its metabolites are weakly protein bound (<15%). Methyldopa crosses the placenta; only 0.02% of a daily dose would be expected to be ingested by a nursing infant. Delayed excretion and accumulation of the metabolite occur in patients with renal insufficiency. Elimination is biphasic. The half-life of the first phase is 1.28 hr (3.6 hr in patients with renal insufficiency). The half-life of the second phase is 7–16 hr.

Mechanism of Toxicity
Methyldopa is metabolized to α-methylnorepinephrine, which stimulates central α_2-adrenoreceptor sites resulting in a decrease in sympathetic outflow and, consequently, a decrease in blood pressure. Methyldopa inhibits the decarboxylation of dihydroxyphenylalanine (dopa), the precursor of norepinephrine, in addition to 5-hydroxytryptophan, the precursor of serotonin, in the central nervous system and the peripheral tissues. These reductions in endogenous catecholamines may contribute to the drug's antihypertensive effects as may methyldopa's inhibition of plasma renin activity.

Human Toxicity: Acute
Coma, hypothermia, dry mouth, severe hypotension, bradycardia, and impairment of atrioventricular con duction may occur. The minimum lethal or toxic dose is not well defined; death has occurred in adults following ingestions of 15–25 g. Drug levels are not generally available and correlate only roughly with signs of toxicity; a toxic range has not been determined.

Human Toxicity: Chronic
Side effects occur in over 70% of patients and include drowsiness, weight gain, orthostatic hypotension, and bradycardia. Aggravation of angina pectoris and atrioventricular conduction disturbances may also occur. A positive Coomb's test is found in 10–20% of patients after 6–12 months of therapy.

Clinical Management
Gastrointestinal decontamination procedures should be used as deemed appropriate to the patient's level of consciousness and history of ingestion. Basic and advanced life-support measures should be utilized as necessary. Hemodialysis is of theoretical value but its clinical efficacy following methyldopa overdose has not been evaluated. All cases of suspected methyldopa overdose should be admitted to an intensive care unit for cardiovascular monitoring.

—Elizabeth J. Scharman

Related Topic
Cardiovascular System

---

*Methylene Chloride**

- CAS: 75-09-2
- SYNONYMS: Dichloromethane
- CHEMICAL CLASS: Chlorinated aliphatic hydrocarbon

Uses
Methylene chloride has been used as a solvent in paint stripping formulations; as a propellant in aerosols; as

* Information Source: Hazardous Substance Data Bank, National Library of Medicine, Bethesda, MD, July 1996.

a process solvent in the manufacture of drugs, pharmaceuticals, and film coatings; as a metal cleaning and finishing solvent in electronics manufacturing; and as an agent in urethane foam blowing. Aerosol products in which methylene chloride may be found include paints, automotive products, and insect sprays. Methylene chloride has also been used as an extractant solvent for spice oleoresins, hops, and for the removal of caffeine from coffee.

Methylene chloride is a clear volatile liquid having a chloroform-like odor that is detectable at concentrations from 540 to 2160 mg/m^3 in air.

Exposure Pathways

Methylene chloride is a widely used industrial chemical with reported atmospheric emissions of more than 126 million pounds annually in the United States. The principal route of exposure for the general population to methylene chloride is by inhalation. Occupational and consumer exposure to methylene chloride including exposure from spray painting and contact with other consumer products, such as paint strippers or aerosol cans, that contain methylene chloride are common sources of exposure. Exposures may occur as a result of breathing the vapors or from direct dermal contact. Occupational exposure to methylene chloride offers the most opportunity for exposure.

Toxicokinetics

Evaluation of pulmonary uptake in humans indicated that 70–75% of inhaled methylene chloride vapor was absorbed. During absorption through the lungs, the concentration of methylene chloride in alveolar air, in equilibrium with pulmonary venous blood content, approaches the concentration in inspired air until a steady state is achieved. After tissue and total body steady state is achieved through the lungs, uptake is balanced by metabolism and elimination. Steady-state blood methylene chloride concentrations appear to be reached after 2–4 hr of exposure. Once exposure ceased, methylene chloride was rapidly cleared from the blood. Uptake also increases with the percentage body fat since methylene chloride dissolves in fat to a greater extent than it dissolves in aqueous media. In animals, limited available data suggest that methylene chloride is easily absorbed from the gastrointestinal tract.

Available data suggest that there are two pathways by which methylene chloride is metabolized. One utilizes the mixed function oxidase enzymes and produces carbon monoxide, while the other pathway involves glutathione transferase and produces carbon dioxide. The mixed function oxidase pathway seems to be the preferred pathway for methylene chloride metabolism following inhalation exposures. In addition to carbon monoxide and carbon dioxide, methylene chloride is also metabolized to a lesser extent to formaldehyde and formic acid.

Human subjects exposed by inhalation to 500 ppm or greater for 1 or 2 hr experienced elevated carbon monoxide–hemoglobin concentrations indicating that methylene chloride was metabolized to carbon monoxide by the mixed function oxidase pathway. Metabolism of methylene chloride in animals is similar to that in humans. Animal data on metabolism indicate that the process is similar for both inhalation and oral exposures.

When methylene chloride is absorbed by the lungs, it is expected that it will dissolve in the lipoprotein components of the blood and be distributed from the systemic circulation to the body organs.

Distribution studies in rats demonstrate that methylene chloride and its metabolites are present in the liver, kidney, brain, lungs, muscle, and adipose tissue after inhalation exposures. One hour after exposure, the highest concentration of radioactively labeled material was found in the adipose tissue followed by the liver. The concentrations in the kidney, adrenals, and brain were less than half of that in the liver.

Methylene chloride is removed from the body primarily in expired air and urine. Methylene chloride excretion in the expired air was most evident in the first 30 min after exposure. In rats methylene chloride was excreted in the expired air, urine, and feces following a single 6-hr exposure to methylene chloride. Exhaled air accounted for 58–79% of the dose.

Human Toxicity

Case studies of methylene chloride poisoning during paint stripping operations have demonstrated that inhalation exposure can be fatal in humans. Quantitative estimates of exposure levels were not reported; however, methylene chloride was detected at autopsy in various tissues, including the liver (14.4 mg/dl), blood (50 mg/dl), serum (29 μg/ml), and brain (24.8 mg/100 g). The cause of death in these cases was uncertain; however, myocardial infarction was reported in one case.

Acute and prolonged exposures to methylene chloride have been reported to result in a number of signs and symptoms including headache, lightheadedness, nausea, vomiting, eye irritation, pulmonary irritation and cough, paresthesias, somnolence, altered sleep patterns, changing cardiac patterns, syncope, memory loss, intellectual impairment, and gastrointestinal ulceration and bleeding, the latter resulting only from oral exposure. Less common symptoms include delerium, auditory and visual hallucinations, hepatic effects, and renal effects including acute tubular necrosis. At very high levels of exposure, euphoria, central nervous system depression with associated respiratory failure, seizures, and death have been reported. Single exposures to methylene chloride at 300 ppm caused decreased visual and auditory functions. These effects were reversible once exposure ceased. Similarly, psychomotor performance was impaired, but this occurred at higher exposure levels (800 ppm for 4 hr). Alterations in visual evoked response have been observed in humans exposed to methylene chloride at 515–986 ppm for 1 or 2 hr.

Several epidemiological studies have detected no excess risk of death from malignant neoplasms in workers exposed to methylene chloride, while another study suggests an increased risk of pancreatic cancer.

Methylene chloride is considered to be a probable human carcinogen based on animal carcinogenicity studies and genotoxicity studies. Human studies are deemed inadequate in terms of establishing the human carcinogenic properties of methylene chloride.

The ACGIH TLV-TWA is 50 ppm in air.

Animal Toxicity

Studies in animals confirm that methylene chloride may be lethal after inhalation exposure at high concentrations. Acute exposure to 16,000–19,000 ppm methylene chloride for 4–8 hr caused death in rats and mice. Data suggest there is a narrow margin between concentrations causing anesthesia and those causing death. Repeated exposure in longer term studies at levels from 1000 to 16,000 ppm has been reported to cause increased deaths in rats, mice, guinea pigs, rabbits, dogs, and primates. Exposure to methylene chloride has reportedly resulted in fatty changes in the liver and elevated plasma enzymes. These effects were reversible after exposure ceased. A 28-day study in rats also showed elevated hepatic microsomal enzyme activities at 250 ppm in air. Nonspecific renal tubular degenerative and regenerative changes were observed after continuous exposure in rats at 25 and 100 ppm for 100 days, while others report splenic fibrosis and decreased cerebellar enzyme levels in rats and splenic atrophy in dogs. Methylene chloride has also been shown to cross the placental barrier.

Chronic oncogenicity studies in animal models have caused methylene chloride to be classified as an animal carcinogen. In treated mice, hepatocellular carcinomas and broncho/alveolar neoplasms have been reported to be significantly elevated over controls, while salivary gland sarcomas have been noted in male rats and increased incidences of leukemia found in female rats. Methylene chloride has been shown to be genotoxic in some short-term assays including *S. typhimurium* and *S. crevisiae,* but in other tests equivocal or negative results were reported.

—R. A. Parent, T. R. Kline, and D. E. Sharp

Methyl Ethyl Ketone

- CAS: 78-93-3
- Synonyms: MEK; 2-butanone; 2-oxobutane
- Chemical Class: Ketone
- Chemical Structure:

$$CH_3COCH_2CH_3$$

Uses

Methyl ethyl ketone (MEK) is used as a solvent in nitrocellulose coatings and vinyl films, paint removers, cements, and adhesives. It is used in printing, organic synthesis, and smokeless powder manufacturing and is found in cleaning fluids and acrylic coatings.

Exposure Pathways

Inhalation, ingestion, and dermal contact are all possible routes of exposure.

Mechanism of Toxicity

MEK is a parasympathetic central nervous system (CNS) depressant; it enhances sensitivity to epinephrine.

Human Toxicity

MEK vapor is irritating to mucous membranes and conjunctivae at 200 ppm after 15 min, but the odor is noticeable at 25 ppm. It is irritating to the skin by defatting. It is a CNS depressant and is arrhythmogenic.

Animal Toxicity

MEK causes CNS depression in animals. It potentiates the neurotoxicity of *n*-hexane and MBK in animals and in humans. It is embryotoxic and fetotoxic in rats at 1000 ppm, causing acaudia, imperforate anus, and retardation of fetal development. The oral LD_{50} in rats is 6.86 ml/kg.

—Shayne C. Gad

Related Topic

Neurotoxicology: Central and Peripheral

Methylenedioxymethamphetamine

- CAS: 69610-10-2
- Synonyms: MDMA; Ecstasy; XTC; MDM; Adam; E; Doctor; M; Ms; Essence
- Pharmaceutical Class: Synthetic phenylalkylamine derivative of amphetamine
- Chemical Structure:

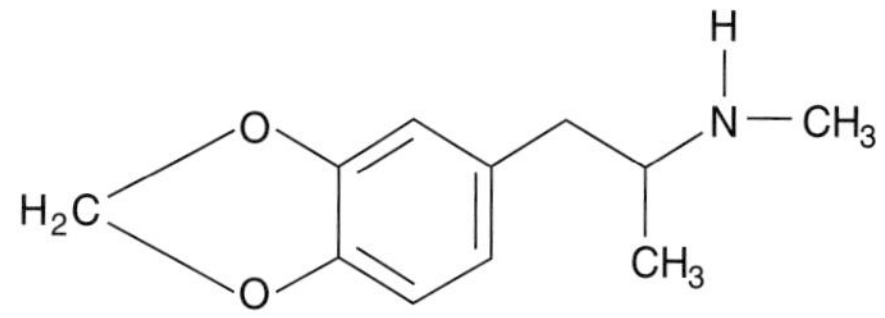

H
N — CH3
H2C
O
O
CH3

Uses

Formerly a psychotherapeutic agent, methylenedioxymethamphetamine (MDMA) is now abused as a hallucinogenic amphetamine.

Exposure Pathways

MDMA is available in tablet, capsule, and powder form in doses of 50–110 mg. It is usually ingested but occasionally sniffed or injected intravenously.

Toxicokinetics

MDMA is rapidly absorbed with the onset of effects occurring in 20–60 min. Effects peak at 1–5 hr and last 4–6 hr or as long as 48 hr with large doses. MDMA is metabolized in the liver by cytochrome P450 to form methylenedioxyamphetamine (MDA). Tissue distribution of MDMA found in a fatal overdose is as follows: heart blood, 10.9 mg/liter; femoral blood, 2.8 mg/liter; liver, 20.2 mg/liter; and brain, 13 mg/liter. MDMA is excreted via the kidneys as 65% unchanged drug and 7% MDA. Elimination is usually complete within 24 hr.

Mechanism of Toxicity

MDMA stimulates both the sympathetic nervous system and central nervous system (CNS) by catecholamine release. Methoxylation and methylenedioxylation of the catechol ring is responsible for the hallucinogenic activity. The methyl-substituted α carbon and unsubstituted β carbon make it a potent indirect sympathomimetic agent. It also depletes serotonin receptors in the brain, with a disruption in behavior.

Human Toxicity

MDMA was used in psychiatry to improve mood, introspection, and the ability to communicate. Auditory and visual hallucinations are usual. Mydriasis is always seen, and the mucous membranes are generally dry.

Acute

Most cases result in mild symptoms of anxiety, hypertension, tachycardia, increased respiratory rate, nausea, and diaphoresis. Overdoses are characterized by hyperthermia, hypotension, arrhythmias, hyperreflexia, seizures, disseminated intravascular coagulation, and rhabdomyolysis with resultant renal failure. Toxic hepatitis, metabolic acidosis, hyponatremia, hyperkalemia, coagulopathies, catatonia, pulmonary edema, and adult respiratory distress syndrome have been reported as severe toxic effects. Hallucinogenic doses are reported to be 50–150 mg. The toxic to "therapeutic" ratio is low. Severe poisonings have been seen with ingestions ranging from 60–200 mg. Sudden death is likely due to cardiac arrhythmias, seizures, and CNS depression. Deaths occurring later are from malignant hyperthermia. Blood levels do not correlate with toxicity but can confirm the ingestant.

Chronic

Chronic paranoid psychosis, depression, flashbacks, panic disorders, and some impairment of cognitive function have been related to long-term use. Psychic tolerance may occur. Withdrawal can result in somnolence and psychic disturbances.

Clinical Management

Treatment is largely supportive. Maintenance of cardiovascular and respiratory functions may be required. Gastric emptying is based on the amount ingested and the clinical condition of the patient. Diazepam can be employed to treat agitation, hallucinations, neuromuscular hyperactivity, and seizures. The use of phenothiazines is controversial. Hypothermic blankets, sponge baths, and acetaminophen may be needed to reduce body temperature. Chilled intravenous fluids and dantrolene successfully reduced hyperthermia. Cardiac arrhythmias and hypotension are managed with the usual pharmacologic agents. Alkaline diuresis may prevent myoglobin-induced renal failure.

Animal Toxicity

In animals, a toxic dose is estimated to be 10–30 mg/kg. Reported effects in small animals include hyperthermia, rapid respirations, rapid heartbeat, dilated pupils, lactic acidosis, hypertension, arrhythmias, vomiting, diarrhea, and painful urination. Renal failure, seizures, and coma are possible.

—Janet E. Bauman

Methyl Isobutyl Ketone

- CAS: 108-10-1
- Synonyms: Hexone; 4-methyl-2-pentanone; isopropyl acetone; MIBK
- Chemical Class: Solvent
- Molecular Formula: $C_6H_{12}O$; $CH_3COCH_2CH(CH_3)_2$
- Chemical Structure:

$$CH_3—\overset{\overset{\displaystyle O}{\|}}{C}—CH_2—CH_2—CH_3$$

Exposure Pathways

For the general population, inhalation and dermal contact during use of consumer products that contain methyl isobutyl ketone are the most probable routes of exposure to this compound. Such products would include coatings (i.e., paints), adhesives, rubber cements, pesticides (i.e., pyrethrins), as well as a variety of other products. Some segments of the general population may also be exposed to methyl isobutyl ketone (MIBK) by inhalation of contaminated air in source-dominated areas or areas near landfills and by ingestion of contaminated drinking water (MIBK was detected in 4 of 14 water supplies sampled between 1977 and 1979).

In the workplace, inhalation of vapors and skin and eye contact are the most likely routes of exposure.

Toxicokinetics

MIBK is absorbed by ingestion, inhalation, and dermal exposure.

A single intraperitoneal administration of 450 mg/kg MIBK to male guinea pigs yielded two serum metabolites: 4-hydroxy-4-methyl-2-pentanone and 4-methyl-2-pentanol. MIBK can be both oxidatively and reductively metabolized. Oxidation of MIBK occurs by hydroxylation of the ω-1-carbon whereby the hydroxylated ketone, 4-hydroxy-4-methyl-2-pentanone, is formed; reduction occurs at the carbonyl group forming 4-methyl-2-pentanol. The biological half-life for MIBK elimination from the serum of guinea pigs was 66 min. The elimination times for MIBK and 4-hydroxy-4-methyl-2-pentanone from these animals were 6 and 16 hr, respectively.

The toxicokinetics of MIBK was studied in human volunteers during inhalation exposure. The volunteers were exposed (2 hr per day, 50 weeks) in an exposure chamber on four different occasions to about 10, 100, and 100 mg/m^3 MIBK and to a combination of approximately 100 mg/m^3 and 150 mg/m^3 toluene. The relative pulmonary uptake of MIBK was about 60% and the total uptake increased linearly with increasing exposure concentration. The concentration of MIBK in blood rose rapidly after the onset of exposure and no plateau level was reached during exposure. No tendency for saturation kinetics could be observed within the dose interval and the apparent blood clearance was 1.61 kg/hr at all exposure levels. The concentration of unchanged MIBK in the urine after exposure was proportional with the total uptake. Only 0.04% of the total MIBK dose was eliminated unchanged via the kidneys within 3 hr postexposure. The concentrations of the metabolites 4-hydroxy-4-methyl-2-pentanone and 4-methyl-2-pentanol were below the detection limit (5 nm/liter).

Mechanism of Toxicity

No specific information regarding the mechanism of toxicity was found for MIBK. Organic solvents in general, however, have the potential on acute high-level vapor exposure to cause narcosis and death. The scenario of disorientation, euphoria, giddiness, confusion, progressing to unconsciousness, paralysis, convulsion, and death from respiratory or cardiovascular arrest is typically observed. The rapidity of the development of these symptoms almost ensures that the acute narcotic effects of solvents are due to the solvent itself and not metabolites. The similarity of the narcosis produced by solvents of diverse structure suggests that these effects result from a physical interaction of a solvent with cells of the central nervous system (CNS).

Synergism

MIBK has been observed to enhance the neurotoxicity of *n*-hexane. This may be related to its ability to induce liver microsomal cytochrome P450, resulting in increased metabolic activation of *n*-hexane to more potent neurotoxic metabolites.

MIBK has also been observed to enhance the CNS effects of ethanol by reducing alcohol dehydrogenase, thereby reducing the rate of ethanol metabolism and elimination. The pharmacological and metabolic interaction between MIBK and ethanol was studied in mice. Animals were pretreated intraperitoneally (ip) with MIBK and injected ip 30 min later with ethanol. The duration of ethanol-induced loss of righting reflex was prolonged significantly by MIBK. As the dose of solvent increased, the prolongation also increased. The activity of mouse liver alcohol dehydrogenase *in vitro* was reduced by MIBK. These data suggest that the solvents enhanced the loss of righting reflex caused by ethanol exposure by reducing the rate at which ethanol was eliminated from the body.

Human Toxicity: Acute

MIBK is an irritant to the eyes, mucous membranes, and skin. High vapor concentrations are irritating to the eyes and the respiratory tract. Vapors may cause headaches and dizziness, are anesthetic, and may have other CNS effects. Small amounts of the liquid aspirated into the respiratory system during ingestion, or from vomiting, may cause bronchiopneumonia or pulmonary edema.

An odor threshold for MIBK has been reported at 15 ppm. Workers reported no adverse effects at levels of 20 ppm. Exposure to 50–105 ppm for 15–30 min caused gastrointestinal disturbances and CNS impairment in a few workers. Workers exposed to 100 ppm developed headaches, nausea, and respiratory irritation. Exposure to 200 ppm has been reported to cause irritation of the eyes and respiratory tract. Higher concentrations cause pulmonary edema and CNS depression with dizziness, drowsiness, and unconsciousness. A concentration of 3000 ppm is immediately dangerous to life and health.

Human Toxicity: Chronic

Repeated or prolonged inhalation may cause mucous irritation. Repeated or prolonged contact may cause defatting and drying of the skin. MIBK is known to enhance the neurotoxicity of linear 6-carbon solvents.

Clinical Management

Affected eyes should be flushed immediately with large amounts of water for at least 15 min. Affected skin should be flushed immediately with large amounts of water; soap should be used if available. Contaminated clothing, including shoes, should be removed after flushing has begun.

In cases of inhalation, the victim should be removed from exposure, be kept at rest, and receive prompt medical attention. If breathing has stopped, artificial respiration should be administered.

In cases of ingestion, vomiting should not be induced. Instead, 4–8 oz of milk or water (not to exceed 15 mlkg in a child) should be given to dilute. The victim should be kept at rest and receive prompt medical attention.

Animal Toxicity: Acute

MIBK has a low acute oral toxicity. The oral LD_{50} in rats has been reported at 4500 mg/kg and the intraperitoneal LD_{50} in mice was 590 mg/kg. Oral LD_{50}s between 1600 and 3200 mg/kg for both rats and guinea pigs and intraperitonial LD_{50}s between 400 and 800 mg/kg for guinea pigs have been reported. Another study has reported a 24-hr oral LD_{50} of 1900 mg/kg for mice. In acute oral studies conducted in mice and rats, the lethal dose has been reported at 2850 and 4600 mg/kg, respectively.

Animal Toxicity: Subchronic and Chronic

Effects from chronic exposure to MIBK have included kidney damage and behavioral effects. Increased kidney weights and kidney/body weight ratios in rats occurred following exposure via inhalation to 100 ppm MIBK continuously for 2 weeks. Kidney and liver weights and the organ body weight ratios were also increased after exposure to 200 ppm for 2 weeks and to 10 ppm for 90 days. Dogs, monkeys, and mice did not demonstrate these effects after 2-week exposures. Rats exposed to 100 ppm for 2 weeks experienced kidney damage in the form of hyaline droplet tubular nephrosis. After 90 days, the rats were removed from exposure and the kidney damage was reversed.

Groups of male rats were exposed to 1500 ppm MIBK in air for 5 months. MIBK produced some minimal distal axonal changes. It has been suggested, however, that this effect may have been due to the 3% methyl *n*-butyl ketone present as a contaminant in the MIBK or was a compression neuropathy due to the type of cages used. In baboons, discriminatory behavior and memory were not affected by exposure to 20–40 ppm MIBK; however, there was an impairment on the accuracy of performance of tasks in a delayed match-to-sample discrimination test at an exposure of 50 ppm for 7 days. Rats exposed to 30 ppm for 4 hr per day for 4.5 months experienced disturbances in their conditioned reflexes. This exposure also caused an alteration in the detoxifying function of the liver.

In reproductive/developmental studies, fetotoxic effects were seen at the same exposure concentrations as those which caused maternal toxicity in both rats and mice.

—*Shayne C. Gad*

Related Topic

Neurotoxicology: Central and Peripheral

Methylmercury

- CAS: 7439-97-6 (elemental mercury)
- Synonyms: Alkyl; phenyl; alkoxyalkyl mercury compounds
- Chemical Class: Organometal
- Chemical Structure:
  The term "methylmercury" generally refers to monomethylmercury, but several organic forms can exist.
  CH_3Hg^+ (methylmercury cation is usually associated with simple anions, i.e., Cl^-)
  $(CH_3)_2Hg$ (dimethylmercury)

Uses

Organomercury compounds, such as aryl and alkoxyaryl, have been used in medicine, agriculture, and laboratory research. Their use in fungicides has been greatly reduced or eliminated.

Exposure Pathways

The general population is exposed to methylmercury through the consumption of contaminated fish and fish products. Inorganic mercury from natural or man-made sources is methylated by microorganisms in aquatic sediments. Methylmercury is then biomagnified in the food chain with relatively high concentrations accumulating in the edible tissues of fish. A minor route of exposure is through inhalation of vaporized methylmercury and organomercurials from the atmosphere or industrial workplace.

Toxicokinetics

Methylmercury from dietary and inhalation exposure is almost completely absorbed (>90%) into the bloodstream. Methylmercury may be converted to inorganic mercury in both experimental animals and humans by intestinal flora and macrophage cells. Glutathione and sulfhydryl peptide complexes have been observed in the bile. Methylmercury is rapidly distributed to all tissues, with high concentrations accumulating in the brain, the target organ of toxicity. Methylmercury moves readily across the placenta, and higher concentrations are found in cord blood compared to maternal blood. The fecal pathway is responsible for approximately 90% of the total elimination of mercury following methylmercury exposure. The majority of methylmercury resulting from biliary secretion is demethylated by intestinal flora and eliminated in the feces as inorganic mercury. The remaining methylmercury can enter the enterohepatic circulation, while a small percentage of inorganic mercury is absorbed and distributed to the tissues. The half-life in fish-eating humans is estimated to be between 39 and 70 days.

Mechanism of Toxicity

All mercury compounds exhibit high affinity for sulfhydryl groups in proteins. As a result, a variety of enzymes and structural proteins containing free sulfhydryl groups can be modified and their functions affected. Inhibition of protein synthesis is an early biochemical event following exposure. The integrity of the blood–brain barrier can be disrupted by methylmercury, which results in the alteration of amino acid uptake and subsequent brain metabolism. Methylmercury can alter cell division during critical stages of central nervous system (CNS) development, at least in part through inhibition of microtubule function. However, there is uncertainty whether methylmercury or the mercuric ion following cleavage from methylmercury is the ultimate toxicant.

Human Toxicity

Poison episodes in humans have occurred as a result of environmental contamination of fish by industrial discharge (Minamata and Niigata, Japan) and through seed grains treated with a methylmercury fungicide (Iraq). In these episodes, most of the signs and symptoms of methylmercury poisoning were attributed to damage to the CNS; effects on nonnervous tissue were absent or negligible. Recently, dimethylmercury was associated with the fatality of a research chemist. The researcher was exposed by dermal absorption after spilling a small amount of the compound on her latex gloves. Dimethylmercury was found to penetrate disposable latex and PVC gloves in 15 sec or less. Where possible, the use of inorganic mercury salts is recommended as a substitute in laboratory research. These compounds are less volatile and lipid soluble than dimethylmercury and scientists face a smaller risk of exposure to mercury.

Acute

Although methylmercury is generally recognized as a cumulative poison, acute toxicity, such as headache, gastrointestinal irritation (nausea, vomiting, abdominal pain, and diarrhea), and paresthesia of the extremities, has been reported. Severe neurologic toxicity, described below, may occur several weeks or months following exposure. Renal failure normally associated with inorganic mercury poisoning is seldom observed with methylmercury. At high concentrations, methylmercury is corrosive to the skin and eye.

Chronic

Characteristics of methylmercury poisoning in adults include a long latent period (several months) and a continuation of early nonspecific symptoms such as paresthesia, blurred vision, and malaise. Additional signs appear; they include concentric constriction of the visual field, deafness, speech difficulties, and ataxia (known as the Hunter Russell syndrome). Severely exposed patients may lapse into a coma and ultimately die, although there is no clear pattern of mercury-related deaths. Many effects in severe cases are irreversible due to destruction of neuronal cells. In less severe cases, some degree of recovery in each symptom may occur depending on the compensatory function of the

CNS. At high doses, methylmercury also causes neuromuscular weakness from effects on the peripheral nervous system. The developing CNS is more sensitive to damage than the adult CNS. Infants who have been exposed to high maternal blood levels of methylmercury were born with cerebral palsy. The main pattern is microcephaly, hyperreflexia, and gross motor and mental impairment, sometimes associated with blindness and deafness. Milder degrees of the affliction show mainly psychomotor impairment and persistence of pathological reflexes.

Clinical Management

There is no known useful treatment for methylmercury poisoning. The best approach is removal of methylmercury before absorption occurs, but due to the cumulative nature of the poison, this is usually not realistic. A variety of chelating agents, such as D-penicillamine, I-acetyl-D,L-penicillamine, thiol resins, activated charcoal, BAL (British Anti-Lewisite; 2,3-dimercaptopropanol), and meso-2,3-dimercaptosuccinic acid, have been used to treat methylmercury exposure but with limited to no success.

The best rule is prevention. The general population, especially children under 7 years and pregnant or breast-feeding women, should limit their consumption of fish that are known to have high levels of methylmercury in their edible tissues. A 5% increase in the incidence of paresthesia has been linked to a daily methylmercury intake of 3–7 μg/kg body weight. Daily intakes of 0.4 μg/kg body weight will not result in any detectable adverse effects.

Animal Toxicity

Methylmercury causes similar neurotoxicological effects in cats and dogs. Cats ingesting contaminated fish around Minamata Bay, Japan, died after paroxysmal fits (i.e., "cat-dancing disease"). Mink are particularly sensitive to the toxicity of methylmercury. Methylmercury is fetotoxic and teratogenic in laboratory mammals.

Further Reading

Clarkson, T. W. (1991). Inorganic and organometal pesticides. In *Handbook of Pesticide Toxicology* (W. J. Hayes, Jr., and E. R. Laws, Jr., Eds.), Vol. 2, pp. 515–525. Academic Press, San Diego.

Zacks, R. (1997, September). Looking for alternatives. *Sci. Am.*, p. 20.

Tsubaki, T., and Irukayama, K. (1977). *Minamata Disease*. Elsevier, New York.

World Health Organization (WHO) (1989). *Environmental Health Criteria 86: Mercury—Environmental Aspects*. WHO, Geneva.

World Health Organization (WHO) (1990). *Environmental Health Criteria 101: Methylmercury*. WHO, Geneva.

—*Kevin N. Baer*

Related Topics

Kidney
Metals
Neurotoxicology: Central and Peripheral

Methylnitrosourea

- CAS: 684-93-5
- SYNONYMS: *N*-nitroso-*N*-methylurea; *N*-methyl-*N*-nitrosourea
- CHEMICAL CLASS: Alkylating agent

Uses

Methylnitrosourea is used in experimental therapy; it has been studied for use as a cancer chemotherapy agent by a number of investigators.

Exposure Pathways

Ingestion, inhalation, and dermal contact are possible routes of exposure.

Toxicokinetics

Methylnitrosourea is rapidly absorbed from the gastrointestinal tract. To form *N*-nitroso compounds *in vivo*, there may be a reaction of nitrite with secondary amines or amides in food or water. Whole body autoradiography showed that 2 min after an intravenous dose of [^{14}C]*N*-methyl-*N*-nitrosourea to rat, ^{14}C was fairly evenly distributed in most tissues. The biological half-life of *N*-nitroso compounds appears to be less than 24 hr.

Mechanism of Toxicity

Methylnitrosourea causes dermal sensitization. It is also an inhibitor of protein and nucleic acid synthesis in tissues.

Human Toxicity

Nausea and vomiting were seen after an intravenous injection of 4 mg/kg to patients. It causes dermatitis; however, it appears to be due to sensitization rather than primary irritation. Although carcinogenicity data are not available for humans, there is sufficient evidence of carcinogenicity in animals; therefore, methylnitrosourea is probably carcinogenic to humans.

Clinical Management

Affected persons should be decontaminated with caution because methylnitrosourea is probably carcinogenic to humans. Symptoms should be treated as they appear.

Animal Toxicity

The major toxic effects result from severe damage to hematopoietic, lymphoid, and other tissues that have rapid rates of cell turnover. ICR male mice were given intraperitoneal injections at 5, 15, or 25 mg/kg/day for 5 days, then were mated on Days 1–7, 8–14, 15–21, or 64–80 after the last dose and their progeny were observed on Day 18 of pregnancy. There was an increased postimplantation loss, cleft palate, and fused ribs. There is sufficient evidence of carcinogenicity in animals. It was positive for gene mutations (HGPRT and TK genes) as well as for chromosomal aberrations, sister chromatid exchange, and DNA repair-deficient bacterial assays.

—*Robin Guy*

Related Topics

Chromosome Aberrations
Sensitivity Analysis
Sister Chromatid Exchange
Skin

Methyl Parathion

- CAS: 298-00-0
- Synonyms: Penncap-M; Bladan M; Dalf; Folidol-M; Metacide; Nitrox
- Chemical Class: Synthetic organophosphorous insecticide in the phosphorothionate class
- Chemical Structure:

S
O—P$(OCH_3)_2$
NO_2

Uses

Methyl parathion is a contact insecticide for use on a variety of crop insects.

Exposure Pathways

The dermal and inhalation routes are the most important means of occupational exposure. Accidental exposure through the oral route has also been reported. Methyl parathion is available as emulsifiable concentrates, wettable powders, and dusts of various concentrations.

Toxicokinetics

Methyl parathion is rapidly absorbed by all routes. Maximum tissue levels are achieved in 1 or 2 hr following oral exposure. Methyl parathion is activated via the P450 mixed function oxidase system to the oxygen analog, methyl paraoxon. The oxon is metabolized in the liver to *p*-nitrophenol and dimethyl phosphate and these can be conjugated as glucuronides and glycosides. Glutathione-mediated demethylation also occurs. Methyl parathion is rapidly distributed to various tissues. The water-soluble metabolites are primarily excreted through the urine. A trace amount of the unmetabolized parent compound is also eliminated through the urine. Excretion of the major metabolite, *p*-nitrophenol, is essentially complete in 24 hr following oral exposure. The excretion of dimethylphosphate is more protracted.

Mechanism of Toxicity

As with other organophosphorothionate agents, the toxicity of methyl parathion is due to inhibition of acetylcholinesterase by the active metabolite (i.e., methyl paraoxon), resulting in stimulation of the central nervous system, the parasympathetic nervous system, and the somatic motor nerves. It is generally agreed to be somewhat less toxic than its diethyl analog, parathion.

Human Toxicity: Acute

Eye contact may cause pain, moderate eye irritation, and temporary corneal injury. Prolonged exposure may cause skin irritation. Ingestion of methyl parathion has caused typical symptoms of acute organophosphorous poisoning including headache, weakness, incoordination, fasciculations, tremor, nausea, cramps, diarrhea, and sweating (see Cholinesterase Inhibition).

Human Toxicity: Chronic

With repeated exposures, acetylcholinesterase inhibition can persist without indications of toxicity. In most cases, cholinesterase inhibition is without overt effects. Methyl parathion cannot cause delayed neurotoxicity.

Clinical Management

For exposure to eyes, eyelids should be held open and the eyes flushed with copious amounts of water for 15 min. For exposure to skin, affected areas should be washed immediately with soap and water. The victim should receive medical attention if irritation develops and persists.

For exposure through inhalation, the victim should be removed to fresh air and, if not breathing, given artificial ventilation. The victim should receive medical attention as soon as possible.

First aid for ingestion victims would be to induce vomiting, keeping in mind the possibility of aspiration of solvents. Gastric decontamination should be performed within 30 min of ingestion to be most effective. Initial management of acute toxicity is establishment and maintenance of adequate airway and ventilation. Atropine sulfate in conjunction with pralidoxime chloride can be administered as an antidote. Atropine by intravenous injection is the primary antidote in severe cases. Test injections of atropine (1 mg in adults and 0.15 mg/kg in children) are initially administered, followed by 2–4 mg (in adults) or 0.015–0.05 mg/kg (in children) every 10–15 min until cholinergic signs (e.g., diarrhea, salivation, and bronchial secretions) decrease. High doses of atropine over several injections may be necessary for effective control of cholinergic signs. If lavage is performed, endotracheal and/or esophageal control is suggested. At first signs of pulmonary edema, the patient should be placed in an oxygen tent and treated symptomatically.

Animal Toxicity

The oral LD_{50} in adult rats and mice is about 20 mg/kg. Defects in reproduction at dietary levels of 10 ppm in rats were reported to be "inconsistent." In developmental studies, subacute exposures (3 mg/kg/day for 15 days) caused fetal toxicity but no teratogenic effects. As with many other organophosphate insecticides, young animals appear to be more sensitive to acute toxicity (lethality) from high doses than are adults. These age-related differences appear to be related in part to maturation of detoxification processes.

—Carey Pope

Related Topics

A-Esterase
Carboxylesterases
Cholinesterase Inhibition
Neurotoxicology: Central and Peripheral
Organophosphates
Pesticides

Methyl t-Butyl Ether

- CAS: 1634-04-4
- Preferred Name: Methyl *tert*-butyl ether

- Synonyms: MTBE; MtBE
- Chemical Class: Aliphatic ethers
- Chemical Structure:

$$CH_3—CH_2—CH_2—O—CH_3$$

Uses

Methyl *tert*-butyl ether (MTBE) is used to enhance octane in gasoline. It is used therapeutically to dissolve cholesterol calculi (gallstones).

Exposure Pathways

Ingestion and inhalation are possible exposure routes.

Toxicokinetics

Most absorption and excretion takes place through biotransformation.

Mechanism of Toxicity

Demethylation increased 4-fold by acetone treatments and 5.5-fold by phenobarbital treatment in rat livers. P450 may inhibit MTBE metabolism. Approximately 18 hr following an MTBE intraperitoneal treatment, rats displayed a 50-fold induction of dealklase activity but no change in demethylase activity.

Human Toxicity

Toxic effects for humans include kidney failure or liver damage.

Clinical Management

The affected person should be removed from exposure. Respiration should be maintained or supported as required. If ingested, emesis should be induced or gastric lavage performed.

Animal Toxicity

MTBE is an animal carcinogen and teratogen. It reduces the chance of survival in rat offspring. The oral LD_{50} in rats is 4000 mg/kg. The inhalation LC_{50} in rats is 2.35 ± 0.4 ppm. The oral LD_{50} in mice is 5960 mg/kg. The inhalation LC_{50} in mice is 141 g/m^3.

—Shayne C. Gad and Jayne E. Ash

Methyprylon

- CAS: 125-64-4
- Synonyms: Methypryl; methyprylone; 2,4-dioxo-3,3-diethyl-5-methyl piperidine; 3,3-diethyl-5-methyl-2,4-piperidinedione; Noludar; Noctan; Dimerin
- Pharmaceutical Class: Piperidinedione derivative
- Chemical Structure:

H
N
O
C_2H_5
CH_3
C_2H_5
O

Uses

Methyprylon is a sedative–hypnotic agent that was used in the treatment of anxiety, nervousness, and sleep disorders (insomnia). The drug was withdrawn from the U.S. market in 1988. It was a commonly abused sedative–hypnotic.

Exposure Pathways

Methyprylon is only available in solid oral dosage forms. Poisoning occurs following ingestion.

Toxicokinetics

Following therapeutic doses, methyprylon is rapidly absorbed, with peak plasma levels occurring within 1 or 2 hr. Greater than 95% of a dose undergoes oxidation and dehydrogenation in the liver; the remainder is excreted unchanged in the urine. There is no evidence of active metabolites. The volume of distribution with therapeutic dosing is approximately 1 liter/kg. The extent of methyprylon binding to plasma proteins is unknown. Therapeutic plasma levels occur at about 10 mg/liter, with levels above 30 mg/liter considered toxic. The metabolites and about 3% of a dose of the parent compound are eliminated in the urine. The serum elimination half-life is approximately 3–5 hr following therapeutic doses. The toxicokinetics of methyprylon are poorly understood. Both the rates of absorption and elimination are prolonged following overdose. The kinetics appear to be dose dependent, and elimination becomes nonlinear at high doses.

Mechanism of Toxicity

Methyprylon produces depression of the central nervous system (CNS) and decreases rapid eye movement sleep in a similar fashion to the barbiturates. Overdoses may also result in cardiovascular depression.

Human Toxicity: Acute

Overdose results in dose-dependent CNS depression, ranging from mild lethargy to coma. Slurred speech, ataxia, nystagmus, headache, and gastrointestinal upset may occur. Paradoxical CNS stimulation (excitement) has been reported. Severe toxicity (ingestions exceeding 3 or 4 g) may produce hypotension, shock, or pulmonary edema. Death has occurred following ingestion of 6 g, and survival has occurred following ingestion of 30 g.

Human Toxicity: Chronic

Chronic use may result in addiction, physical dependence, and withdrawal upon abrupt discontinuance of the drug.

Clinical Management

The basis of clinical management is supportive care. The airway should be secured and protected as needed. Symptomatic patients should have intravenous access and cardiac monitoring. Accidental ingestions exceeding 500–800 mg, and all intentional overdoses, should be treated with oral activated charcoal. Hemodialysis or hemoperfusion may enhance elimination of both the parent compound and metabolites, but the clinical value of extracorporeal drug removal is unknown. There is no known antidote.

—S. Rutherfoord Rose

Related Topic

Neurotoxicology: Central and Peripheral

Metronidazole

- CAS: 443-48-1
- Synonym: Flagyl
- Pharmaceutical Class: An antibiotic of the nitroimidazole class
- Chemical Structure:

CH_2CH_2OH | O_2N–(imidazole ring, N)–CH_3

Uses

Metronidazole is used as an antibiotic in antiparasitic applications.

Exposure Pathways

Metronidazole is available in oral and parenteral forms.

Toxicokinetics

At least 80% of a dose of metronidazole is absorbed after ingestion with peak concentrations found within 1–3 hr postingestion. The volume of distribution is approximately 0.74 liters/kg. Less than 20% is bound to plasma proteins. It readily crosses the placenta and is distributed into breast milk in concentrations that approximate that of serum concentrations. Thirty-sixty percent of a dose is metabolized in the liver, and the remainder is excreted unchanged in bile or urine. Biotransformation occurs through hydroxylation, oxidation of side chain, and glucuronide conjugation. The elimination half-life is unchanged by changes in renal function but may be disturbed in those with hepatic insufficiency. The half-life of metronidazole is 8 hr.

Metronidazole pigments may impart a reddish-brown color to urine.

Mechanism of Toxicity

Metronidazole is both bactericidal and amebicidal. Its mechanism of action includes interference with nucleic acid synthesis. Metronidazole is also capable of producing a disulfiram reaction through unknown means.

Human Toxicity: Acute

The acute lethal dose is unknown. Acute effects are confined to nausea, vomiting, and ataxia.

Human Toxicity: Chronic

In cases of chronic toxicity, gastrointestinal upset, headache, vomiting, and metallic taste in the mouth are not unusual. Metronidazole may produce a disulfiram reaction if ethanol is ingested. Chronic use may produce numbing or paresthesias of an extremity. Other neurotoxic effects including dizziness and vertigo may also occur. Resolution may be slow or incomplete. Reversible white blood count suppression may also occur.

Metronidazole has important drug interactions. It potentiates the effects of oral anticoagulants and produces a disulfiram-like reaction in those taking ethanol. Acute psychosis may occur in those simultaneously receiving disulfiram and metronidazole. Metronidazole may diminish the clearance of lithium. It may also produce serious adverse effects in those receiving the antihistamines astemizole or terfenadine, probably a result of cytochrome P450 inhibition.

Clinical Management

Clinical management of acute metronidazole ingestion is limited to the administration of activated charcoal (without prior gastric emptying). Laboratory tests are not beneficial. In cases of chronic metronidazole overmedication or toxicity resulting from interaction with other drugs, supportive care and symptomatic treatment with discontinuation of metronidazole are sufficient. Although disulfiram is dialyzable, the need for dialysis rarely occurs. Because the biochemical effects of metronidazole resolve slowly, clinical effects such as the disulfiram reaction with ethanol may persist for days to weeks after the last dose.

Animal Toxicity

Metronidazole is commonly used as an antiparasitic in domestic animals. Manifestations of overdose in animals include muscle fasciculations, generalized weakness, and ataxia.

—Michael Shannon

Mevinphos

- CAS: 7786-34-7
- SYNONYM: O,O-dimethyl-1-carbomethoxy-1-propen-2-yl phosphate
- CHEMICAL CLASS: Organophosphate pesticide
- CHEMICAL STRUCTURE:

$$(CH_3O)_2P(=O){-}OC(CH_3){=}CHCOOCH_3$$

Use

Mevinphos is used as an insecticide.

Exposure Pathways

Oral and dermal routes are the most common routes of accidental and intentional exposure to mevinphos.

Toxicokinetics

Mevinphos is efficiently absorbed from the gut, through the skin, and across the pulmonary membrane. The compound is hydrolyzed in the body to alkyl phosphate.

Mechanism of Toxicity

The organophosphorous insecticide, mevinphos, exerts its acute toxicity by inhibiting the hydrolytic enzyme, acetylcholinesterase. This causes an increased accumulation of acetylcholine at the synaptic nerve terminals, thereby resulting in excessive stimulation of the cholinergic nerves.

Human Toxicity

Mevinphos is a compound of high toxicity, not only orally but also dermally. It is a direct inhibitor of acetylcholinesterase. Signs and symptoms involving overstimulation of the muscarinic receptors include bronchoconstriction, increased bronchial secretion, bradycardia, salivation, lacrimation, diaphoresis, vomiting, diarrhea, and pupillary constriction (miosis). The nicotinic effects following exposure to mevinphos include tachycardia, hypertension, muscle fasciculations, weakness, muscle cramps, and respiratory paralysis. Excessive stimulation of central nervous system (CNS) receptors (both muscarinic and nicotinic) is responsible for some of the higher order symptoms such as anxiety, restlessness, CNS depression, agitation, confusion, delirium, coma, and seizures.

Clinical Management

For exposure to eyes, eyelids should be held open and the eyes flushed with copious amounts of water for 15 min. For exposure to skin, affected areas should be washed immediately with soap and water. The victim should receive medical attention if irritation develops and persists.

For exposure through inhalation, the victim should be removed to fresh air and, if not breathing, given artificial ventilation. The victim should receive medical attention as soon as possible.

First aid for ingestion victims would be to induce vomiting, keeping in mind the possibility of aspiration of solvents. Gastric decontamination should be performed within 30 min of ingestion to be most effective. Initial management of acute toxicity is establishment and maintenance of adequate airway and ventilation. Atropine sulfate in conjunction with pralidoxime chloride can be administered as an antidote. Atropine by intravenous injection is the primary antidote in severe cases. Test injections of atropine (1 mg in adults and 0.15 mg/kg in children) are initially administered, followed by 2–4 mg (in adults) or 0.015–0.05 mg/kg (in children) every 10–15 min until cholinergic signs (e.g., diarrhea, salivation, and bronchial secretions) decrease. High doses of atropine over several injections may be necessary for effective control of cholinergic signs. If lavage is performed, endotracheal and/or esophageal control is suggested. At first signs of pulmonary edema, the patient should be placed in an oxygen tent and treated symptomatically.

Animal Toxicity

The oral and dermal LD_{50} of mevinphos in male rats is 6.1 and 4.7 mg/kg, respectively. Following exposure to 50 ppm mevinphos for 60 days, rats showed reduced growth, slight tremors, and brain cholinesterase only 20% of normal. Other signs and symptoms in rats following exposure to mevinphos include nonspecific degeneration of the liver and kidneys and degeneration of the epithelial cells lining ducts and acini of salivary, lacrimal, and other exocrine glands. Dogs exposed to mevinphos at a dietary level of 0.1 mg/kg/day for 14 weeks showed a reduction in both erythrocyte and plasma cholinesterase activity; however, the brain enzyme remained normal.

—*Priya Raman*

(Clinical management section prepared by Carey Pope)

Related Topics

Cholinesterase Inhibition
Neurotoxicology: Central and Peripheral
Organophosphates
Pesticides

Microtox

Overview

Microtox is an *in vitro* test system which uses bacteria for the determination of bioreactivity and potential ocular irritancy of liquids. Microtox is used as a screening system to provide an indication of relative toxicity of a liquid sample or liquid extract from a solid material as the first phase of a test battery. It is a suitable system for the testing of industrial effluent waters and complex mixtures. (Microtox is a registered trademark of Microbics Corporation, Carlsbad, CA.)

The Microtox test system utilizes a strain of naturally luminescent bacteria, usually *Photobacterium phosphoreum*. Exposure to a test chemical causes disruption of the respiratory process of the bacteria resulting in reduced light output. The effect concentration (EC_{50}) is determined as a 50% reduction in light output. The test is fast, fairly simple to conduct, uses small sample sizes, and is relatively inexpensive. Results correlate well with those from other toxicity bioassays such as fish and crustacea. The test is used extensively in the measurement of toxicity of effluent waters and as an early screening tool for relative toxicity as part of a test battery.

Principle of Operation

Photobacterium phosphoreum is a nonpathogenic, marine, luminescent bacteria which has sensitivity to a wide range of toxicants. The organisms are supplied for use in a standard freeze-dried state, which serves to maintain the sensitivity and stability of the test cell. Disruption of the respiratory process by exposure to a toxicant affects the metabolic pathway that converts chemical energy via the electron transfer system of the bacteria to visible light. The process occurs in and close to the cell membrane so target sites are close to the cell surface. Since each test utilizes about 1 million organisms, and each is less than 1 μm in diameter, a very high surface to volume ratio is presented. Sensitivity is therefore high, the response being an integrated effect of the toxicant on the whole population.

The Microtox equipment includes a self-calibrating analyzer which incorporates a photomultiplier, a data collection and reduction system, and software. The temperature-controlled analyzer brings the test organisms and samples to a standard temperature of 15°C. It also detects the light intensity at a maximum of 490 nm, which is that wavelength emitted by the test bacteria. The EC_{50} is represented by a γ of 1, where γ is defined as the ratio of light lost to light remaining. Time, temperature, pH, salinity, and the concentration and nature of the toxicant can all affect the intensity of light output. Colored samples may also confound results by reducing light intensity. The test procedure is therefore modified using an absorbance correction cuvette which aids measurement of the color interference and the Microtox system corrects the results.

Advantages

The Microtox test has many attributes over other bioassays which make it a useful tool in monitoring programs and screening studies. These include cost-effectiveness, simplicity, rapidity, precision, and the requirement for a small sample volume. The Microtox test is one of the least volume-intensive assays, using only 3 ml of sample per test. The rapidity of the test means that real-time data can be generated as part of a monitoring program, allowing fast corrective action to be taken. Each test takes about 45 min from start to printing of the final report when conducted by a trained operator. Twenty-nine individual samples may be tested at one time for determination of relative toxicity or three complete serial dilution bioassays can be run simultaneously to provide effect concentrations.

Use as Part of a Test Battery and Correlation with Other Bioassays

No single test can ensure the detection of all toxic effects in a complex mixture. A test battery should have good sensitivity to a broad range of toxicants, while possessing unique characteristics making it a useful detector of certain types of toxicity. The Microtox test has been extensively evaluated for its correlation with other bioassays. In a comparison of the toxicity of several hundred compounds to Microtox and two freshwater species, the fathead minnow (*Pimephales promelas*) and the water flea (*Daphnia magna*), both species showed a correlation with Microtox of 0.85. The Microtox test is clearly comparable but has its own strengths that make it a valuable part of a test battery. In a test of pure compounds, the average sensitivity of Microtox (based on EC_{50} values) ranged from about 2 to 40 times less than those for the fathead minnow, rainbow trout, and water flea. The sensitivity of Microtox could be increased by selecting another EC percentage as an endpoint.

Effluent test results support the use of Microtox as part of a test battery. Uniform response of sublethal effects to 50 effluents from pulp and paper mills was obtained with the Microtox test compared to the results with fish and algae, which varied greatly with age and genetic variation within the population. The Microtox test may be a poor indicator of toxicity for effluents containing certain specific compounds highly toxic to bacteria such as ammonia and cyanide. Microtox has also been used to detect other sublethal effects (e.g., chronic toxicity). For example, the bacterial response can be used to quantify the stress on the immunological defense systems of mussels exposed to toxins in polluted rivers or wastewaters. In this case, the bacteria are exposed to hematocytes extracted from the mussels for 30 min at standard temperature. The phagocytic activity of the hematocytes on the bacteria decreases bioluminescence by a quantifiable amount.

While it alone cannot substitute for acute or sublethal hazard assessment which covers all species, Microtox could be useful in a battery of screening tests or to supplement data obtained in other well-established toxicity bioassays.

Regulatory Status

The Microtox test is recognized as an approved protocol or under consideration for acceptance by the regulatory agencies of many nations. Such countries include the United States, the Canadian Province of Quebec, and certain countries from the European Union, South America, and the Pacific Rim. The U.S. EPA has referred to Microtox as an inexpensive tool to test effluent toxicity. Test protocols involving the use of luminescent bacteria are under consideration by both the International Standards Organization and the Organization for Economic Cooperation and Development.

—Gary P. Bond and Melanie C. Thatcher

Related Topics

Effluent Biomonitoring
In Vitro Test
Toxicity Testing, Aquatic

Minoxidil

- CAS: 38304-91-5
- SYNONYMS: 2,6-Diamino-4-piperidinopyrimidine; Rogaine; Loniten
- PHARMACEUTICAL CLASS: Hypotensive agent; a direct vasodilator
- CHEMICAL STRUCTURE:

N N NH_2 N O NH_2

Uses

Minoxidil is used in the management of severe hypertension that is symptomatic or associated with end-organ damage. It is used topically to stimulate hair regrowth in patients with androgenetic alopecia or alopecia areata.

Exposure Pathways

Ingestion is the most common route of both accidental and intentional exposure to minoxidil. Toxicity may also occur via dermal exposure. It is available in an oral and a 2% topical formulation.

Toxicokinetics

Minoxidil is almost completely absorbed (95%). Peak plasma concentrations are reached within 1 hr. Plasma concentrations do not correlate with either the extent or the duration of action. The hypotensive effect begins in 30 min, is maximal in 2–8 hr, and persists for 2–5 days. About 90% of the drug is metabolized, primarily by conjugation. The metabolites are slightly active. It is widely distributed into tissues with a volume of distribution of 2.8–3.3 liters/kg. Minoxidil is not protein bound. It is distributed into breast milk.

The mean half-life of minoxidil and its metabolites is 2.77–4.4 hr. The drug and its metabolites are primarily excreted renally. In patients with renal impairment, the metabolites, but not the unchanged drug, accumulate in plasma.

Mechanism of Toxicity
Minoxidil acts as a direct vasodilator of vascular smooth muscle. The resulting hypotensive effect induces a reflex increase in heart rate, cardiac output, and stroke volume. Minoxidil's effect on arterioles is greater than that on veins. Minoxidil causes sodium and water retention and increases plasma renin activity.

Human Toxicity: Acute
Hypotension, sodium and water retention, tachycardia, and cardiac arrhythmias may be seen. Severe hypotension may result in angina pectoris secondary to myocardial ischemia. Headache and dizziness may be noted. The minimum toxic or lethal dose has not been defined because few reports of overdosage are available. It has been suggested that hypotension does not develop in patients without preexisting hypertension; however, this has not been confirmed. Serum levels are not readily available and are not correlated with clinical toxicity.

Human Toxicity: Chronic
Side effects associated with chronic toxicity include tachycardia, sodium and water retention, and hypertrichosis.

Clinical Management
Gastrointestinal decontamination procedures should be used as deemed appropriate to the patient's level of consciousness and history of ingestion. Basic and advanced life-support measures should be utilized as necessary; however, cardiac stimulating sympathomimetics such as epinephrine or norepinephrine should be avoided. Phenylephrine, vasopressin, or dopamine are the preferred agents for the management of hypotension following minoxidil overdose. There is not any clinical data to support the use of hemodialysis although minoxidil appears to be easily dialyzable.

Animal Toxicity
Long-term animal studies have demonstrated cardiac hypertrophy, cardiac dilation, and serosanguineous pericardial fluid. Short-term use of minoxidil in dogs has caused cardiac lesions (e.g., visible hemorrhagic lesions of the right atrium) and necrosis of the papillary muscles and subendocardial areas of the left ventricle. An acute toxic dose is not documented. Serum levels are not readily available and do not guide treatment.

—Elizabeth J. Scharman

Mistletoe

- SYNONYMS: *Phoradendron flavescens;* American mistletoe
- DESCRIPTION: Mistletoe is a semiparasitic shrub with ovate, opposite leaves. It is found growing on trees, especially oaks. The berries are either white or pink, round, and translucent. This plant is native to areas east of Texas and south of New Jersey to the Caribbean. The European variety, *Viscum album,* is cultivated in Sonoma County, California. This variety has pale yellowish-green leaves with white berries and grows on apple trees. It is not imported.

Uses
Native Americans chew the plant to relieve toothache pain. An extract of mistletoe is considered toxic to mosquitoes. When used as an abortifacient, its effects have been fatal.

Exposure Pathways
Exposure is by ingestion of plant parts and berries. The plant is also used in teas.

Mechanism of Toxicity
All parts of the plant contain phoratoxin and a lectin-like toxin responsible for effecting protein synthesis in the intestinal wall. The European variety, *V. album,* also has a digitalis-like effect. Sympathomimetic amnesia have both autonomic stimulant and depressant effects.

Human Toxicity
Effects begin 2 or more hours after exposure with persistent emesis, abdominal cramping, and diarrhea.

With *V. album*, it is unclear if the resulting cardiovascular collapse is due to direct cardiotoxicity or is secondary to hypovolemic shock caused by the severe gastrointestinal effects. Although severe poisonings are rare, those that occur are attributed to berry ingestions. Ingestion of less than three berries or two leaves is unlikely to produce significant effects.

Clinical Management

Initial treatment with gastric lavage or emesis, followed by activated charcoal, is indicated. Supportive care with rehydration and fluid and electrolyte replacement may be needed. Seizures can be managed with traditional anticonvulsant therapy beginning with diazepam. Pregnant patients should be monitored for premature uterine contractions.

—*Regina Wiechelt*

Mitomycin C

- CAS: 50-07-7
- Synonyms: Ametycine; MMC; mutamycin; Mit-C
- Chemical Class: Fungal metabolite
- Molecular Formula: $C_{15}H_{18}N_4O_5$

Uses

Mitomycin C is used as an antibiotic, antineoplastic, and for slowing of fibroblast formation in open-angle glaucoma.

Exposure Pathways

Mitomycin C is administered intravenously as a therapeutic agent.

Mechanism of Toxicity

Mitomycin C is an aneuploidy-inducing agent.

Human Toxicity

Intravenous administration of mitomycin C has resulted in dyspnea and lung fibrosis. It is a nephrotoxin and a male reproductive toxin. Mitomycin C causes alopecia and pulmonary damage.

Animal Toxicity

Mitomycin C is a carcinogen (IARC category 2B) in rats. It is teratogenic in mice (induces skeletal defects). The intravenous TD_{Lo} is 2.6 mg/kg in rats. It is nephrotoxic. In sister chromatid exchange assays, it is mutagenic.

—*Shayne C. Gad*

Related Topics

Kidney
Mutagenicity
Reproductive System, Male
Sister Chromatid Exchange

Mixtures

Humans are exposed to mixtures of chemicals in their environment much more frequently than they are to single chemicals and thus the consequences of interaction between the constituents of the mixture must also be considered in evaluating the potential effects of exposure to any mixture. However, toxicologic studies carried out to identify and characterize the hazards of exposure to chemicals are almost always carried out on single substances rather than on mixtures of chemicals. Epidemiologic studies are more likely to involve exposures of humans to mixtures of chemicals and such studies could provide a more reliable basis for risk assessment than the single agent toxicologic studies in animals. However, such epidemiologic data are rarely available for the specific mixtures of chemical agents and exposure situations that are of regulatory or public health interest. Thus, predictions regarding the hazards of exposure to mixtures of chemicals in our food, air, water, and elsewhere in our environment are often compromised by a lack of relevant data.

Chemicals may act jointly to elicit a toxic effect which is equivalent to (additive), less than (antagonistic), or greater than (synergistic) the sum of the individual toxicities. However, one chemical may antagonize or enhance the actions of a second chemical in a simple mixture but exhibit different effects in a complex mixture or when given by different routes, and it is also well recognized that chemicals acting via different modes of action may exhibit nonadditive interactions. Nevertheless, most standard setting bodies and regulatory agencies have adopted the assumption of additivity in the absence of known synergistic effects as the basis for estimating the adverse effects of exposure to mixtures. When these effects have dose–response thresholds or no-adverse-effect levels (NOAELs) and the allowable or tolerance dose is calculated by dividing the NOAEL by an appropriate uncertainty factor, the hazard of the mixture can be predicted by adding the ratio of exposure/threshold value for each component of the mixture. Thus, the ACGIH TLV considers that the TLV for a mixture is exceeded when the sum of all the ratios of exposure dose to TLV of the mixture constituents is >1. The assumption of additivity in the absence of synergy is also used for nonthreshold effects of mixtures, such as cancer and mutagenesis, although its utilization for these effects is more controversial both in theory and in practical application. Is it appropriate, for example, to add different tumor types within the same organ or tumors in different organs, or do these constitute different responses? The issue of concentration additivity versus response additivity also needs to be addressed. However, the assumption that doses of different agents can be treated as roughly additive in regard to producing a response appears to be reasonably consistent with the experimental evidence on the joint actions of chemicals in mixtures and the low incidence of synergism in the interactive toxicity database supports the use of assumption of additivity in mixtures. Less than 3% of the 331 studies in the U.S. EPA *Database on Toxic Interactions* (including over 600 chemicals) showed clear evidence of synergism and a similar low incidence of synergistic responses was reported in the National Research Council report, *Complex Mixtures.* However, most of these interactive studies involved only two-compound mixtures and few of them examined long-term effects. Most of the synergistic toxicologic interactions that have been identified occur as the result of the influence of one chemical on the absorption, distribution, metabolism, and excretion of another chemical and many of these effects involve induction or inhibition of various enzyme systems. It is likely that pharmacokinetic and mechanistic studies will be of greatest value in improving our ability to provide reliable predictions for the adverse effects of chemical mixtures.

Further Reading

American Conference of Governmental Industrial Hygienists (ACGIH) (1993). *Threshold Limit Values for Chemical Substances and Physical Agents and Biological Exposure Indices.* ACGIH, Cincinnati, OH.

Kodell, R. L., and Pounds, J. G. (1991). Assessing the toxicity of mixtures of chemicals. In *Statistics in Toxicology* (D. Krewski and C. Franklin, Eds.). Gordon & Breach, New York.

Krishnam, K., and Brodeur, J. (1991). Toxicologic consequences of combined exposure to environmental pollutants. *Arch. Complex Environ. Stud.* 3(3), 1–106.

National Research Council (1988). *Complex Mixtures.* National Academy Press, Washington, DC.

National Research Council (1994). Science and judgment in risk assessment. In *Aggregation.* National Academy Press, Washington, DC.

[rep]U.S. EPA (1988). *Technical Support Document on Risk Assessment of Chemical Mixtures*, EPA-600/8-90/064. U.S. EPA, Washington, DC.

—John Doull

Related Topics

American Conference on Governmental Industrial Hygienists
Levels of Effect in Toxicological Assessment
Occupational Toxicology

Modifying Factors of Toxicity

The nature and extent of the toxic manifestations in an organism that is exposed to a toxic substance depend on a variety of factors. Exposure to a substance in certain instances produces a reaction in one individual but not in another. While there may be a difference in sensitivity between these individuals, it is also possible that the responsive person was previously exposed (i.e., this individual is actually subjected to a higher concentration of chemical). Two of the factors known to modify the toxic consequences of exposure to chemicals are the dose and duration (see Exposure). This section will focus on the modification of toxicity by other factors including the species and strain of the animal, its sex and age, and its nutritional and hormonal status. Various physical factors also play a part. In addition, the toxic effect of a chemical may be influenced by simultaneous and consecutive exposure to other chemicals. The toxic effects may be modified in a number of ways: alteration of the absorption, distribution, or excretion of a chemical; an increase or decrease of its biotransformation; and changes of the sensitivity of the receptor at the target organ.

It should be remembered that the outcome of adverse effects predicted in humans is based on data generated in animals since drugs released on the market for prescription in humans must be tested in animals. Hence, a clear understanding of the existence of these factors and of their mode of action is important in designing the protocols of toxicologic investigation. It is equally important in evaluating the significance of the toxicologic data and in assessing the safety/risk to humans under specified conditions of exposure. This is not always possible, however, because in certain circumstances the testing in animals is improper (i.e., a test for toxicity is carried out in an animal, but the human responds differently). The use of thalidomide in pregnant women as a sedative resulted in fetal malformations in humans, but this drug did not produce these effects in rats. Another example of a lack of specific conditions of human exposure is related to a long latency period. Pregnant mothers were administered diethylstilbesterol to prevent miscarriage, only to discover that 20 years later female offspring developed vaginal cancer. An industrial accident involving the release of methyl isocyanate, an intermediate in carbaryl synthesis, by Union Carbide in Bhopal, India, resulted in toxicity and death. The toxicological profile of methyl isocyanate was not known, and the chemical was released under uncontrolled conditions. Industrial accidents by definition are not specified conditions of exposure but must be borne in mind as a factor to consider. With increased knowledge of chemicals and the factors that affect these chemicals, the ability to assess and react to adverse conditions is enhanced.

Modifying Factors

Species

Differences of adverse effect from one species to another have long been recognized. Knowledge in this field has been used to develop, for example, pesticides, which are more toxic to pests than to humans and other mammals. Among various species of mammals, most effects of toxicants are somewhat similar. This fact forms the basis for predicting the toxicity to humans from results obtained in toxicologic studies conducted in other mammals, such as the rat, mouse, dog, rabbit, and monkey. There are, however, notable differences in toxicity even among mammals.

Some of these differences can be attributed to variations in detoxication mechanisms. For example, the loss of consciousness induced in several species of laboratory animals by hexobarbital (a barbiturate derivative that depresses the central nervous system (CNS)) shows marked differences; these are attributable to the activity of the detoxication enzyme that inactivates this chemical. In the mouse, the activity of the detoxifying enzyme is 16-fold greater than that in the dog, which is reflected by 12 min of hexobarbital-induced sleep in the mouse versus 315 min of sleep in the dog. There are other examples of species-related differences in the ability to detoxify chemicals that consequently result in differences in toxicity. Other examples include the industrial chemicals, ethylene glycol and aniline. Ethylene glycol is metabolized to oxalic acid, which is responsible for its toxicity, or to carbon dioxide. The rank order of ethylene glycol toxicity in animals is in the following order: cat ε rat ε rabbit; this is the same for the extent of oxalic acid production. Aniline is metabolized in the cat and dog mainly to *o*-aminophenol, and these species are more prone to toxicity; however, in the rat and hamster aniline is metabolized mainly to *P*-aminophenol and thus these species are less susceptible to aniline toxicity.

A more serious example in which animal data are of little clinical relevance is the release of butadiene gas in the production of rubber products. Butadiene is converted to butadiene monoepoxide, which is believed to be responsible for carcinogenesis in rodents but not in humans. In humans, butadiene monoepoxide is further converted to butenediol and conjugation with glutathione results in no toxicity. In rodents, however, there is direct conjugation of butadiene monoepoxide with glutathione, which presumably is not adequate, and thus cancer initiation occurs. In this example it can be seen that rodent data are a poor indicator for prediction of risk in humans because the detoxification pathways differ.

Differences in bioactivation also account for many dissimilarities in toxicity. A notable example is 2-naphthylamine, which can produce bladder tumors in the dog and human but not in the rat, rabbit, or guinea pig. Dogs and humans, but not the others, excrete the carcinogenic metabolite 2-naphthyl hydroxylamine. Acetylaminofluorene (AAF) is carcinogenic in many species of animals but not in the guinea pig. The *N*-hydroxy metabolite of AAF, however, is carcinogenic to all animals including the guinea pig, demonstrating that the difference between the guinea pig and the other animals is not in their response to the toxicant but in the bioactivation, i.e., the guinea pig lacks the ability to form the toxic metabolite.

There are other factors, including absorption, distribution, and excretion of chemicals to consider, in trying to understand differences in toxicity between individuals. Paraoxon is the active metabolite of the organophosphate insecticide parathion. Hence, a difference in the rate of formation of this metabolite is attributable to a difference in toxicity. This has been reported in rats, in which females are more susceptible to parathion neurotoxicity than males and in which paraoxon formation occurs faster in the female resulting in greater toxicity in this sex. This phenomenon has been widely studied in humans with the drug isoniazid. For example, there are "slow inactivators," who are deficient in acetyltransferase. Such individuals acetylate isoniazid only slowly and are thus likely to suffer from peripheral neuropathy resulting from an accumulation of isoniazid. On the other hand, people with more efficient acetyltransferase, termed "fast metabolizers," require larger doses of isoniazid to obtain its therapeutic effect. Since large amounts of drug are needed, these individuals are more likely to suffer from hepatic damage caused by isoniazid because isoniazid also acts on the liver.

Strain

It is essential to determine the safety of new pharmaceutical agents for humans using the appropriate mammalian toxicity tests mandated by governmental regulatory agencies (e.g., U.S. FDA and Health and Welfare Canada). This necessitates the use of a species that can be compared to humans for factors such as pharmacokinetics, metabolism, excretion, absorption, and distribution of the test material. The rat is one of the species that has proven to be extremely useful in pharmacologic and toxicologic research because there are many similarities between rat and human metabolic pathways; many anatomical and physiological characteristics are similar, allowing for comparisons in absorption, excretion, and pharmacokinetics. The rat is also of a convenient size, is relatively docile, has a short life span and gestation period, and is economical to maintain. There is a large database of its characteristics which is invaluable in the interpretation of the relevance of animal data for humans.

There are three main classes of rats used in research; these are inbred strains, outbred stocks, and mutants (including transgenic stocks). It is very important that research workers understand the characteristics of these three classes of stock because they may have a profound influence on the quality of their research. For example, outbred stocks such as Wistar rats may be segregating at many genetic loci, which are important in drug metabolism, so that different individuals within a colony will react differently. In many cases it does not make much sense to do detailed pharmacological studies against such a variable genetic background. The characteristics of the three main classes of stock are briefly summarized in the following sections.

Inbred Strains

Inbred strains are produced by at least 20 generations of brother × sister mating, with all individuals being derived from a single breeding pair in the 20th or subsequent generation (this eliminates parallel sublines). For most practical purposes, an inbred strain can be regarded as an immortal clone of genetically identical individuals. Inbred strains have a number of properties that make them the animal of first choice for most types of research. Because the strain is isogenic (i.e., all individuals are genetically virtually identical), the genotype of the whole colony can be determined at a particular genetic locus by typing a single individual. Many genetic markers are fixed in each strain so that the authenticity of the strain can be determined. This can now be done using DNA markers detected by the polymerase chain reaction. This contrasts sharply with outbred rats, in which currently there are not even any genetic markers that can be used to distinguish between Wistar and Sprague–Dawley stocks.

All inbred animals are homozygous at all genetic loci, so there are no "hidden" recessive genes that could cause confusion in experiments involving breeding. As a result of this homozygosity, the strain stays genetically constant for many generations. This is valuable because it makes it possible to build up background data on genetic characteristics that should remain valid for a long period of time. Of course, the phenotype (but not the genotype) may alter if the diet, environment, or associated microorganisms change. However, over a period of several generations, an inbred strain will remain much more constant than an outbred stock.

The isogenicity and homozygosity together tend to lead to greater phenotypic uniformity of inbred animals. This is important because greater uniformity leads to more statistically powerful experiments that are able to detect a given biological effect with fewer animals. The degree of the contrast with outbred stocks depends on the character being studied. Clearly, for characters controlled by a single or small numbers of genetic loci, such as the major histocompatibility complex or the drug metabolizing enzymes, animals within an inbred strain will be uniform, whereas animals of an outbred stock will usually not. However, the greater uniformity of inbred animals may not be apparent for characters such as body and organ weights (which also depend on environmental and chance factors), unless very large numbers are studied.

Each inbred strain has its own unique pattern of behavior, growth patterns, reproductive performance, spontaneous disease (including tumors), and response to xenobiotics. Differences between strains are an indication that the observed character is under genetic control. Currently, there are over 200 inbred rat strains.

Outbred Stocks

So-called "outbred stocks" are usually maintained as closed colonies of rats of undefined genotype and sometimes known by generic names, such as Wistar, Sprague–Dawley, or Long–Evans, which indicate their historical origin. The amount of genetic variation present in any given colony depends on its history. At one extreme, if the colony has been maintained as a closed colony for many years with small numbers of breeding animals each generation, it may be genetically highly uniform to the extent that it will closely approximate an inbred strain. If the colony has become inbred, it may have gone through a period of rapid genetic drift so that it will differ from other colonies with the same historical origin. At the other extreme, a colony that has recently been crossed to an unrelated stock should be genetically highly variable.

Mutants or Transgenics

Over 300 genetic loci associated with mutants and polymorphisms of various sorts have been described in the rat. A mutant can be created by insertion of DNA from an external source, be it a virus, recombinant DNA, etc. The inserted DNA is referred to as a transgene and the recipient host a transgenic animal, and the methodology for insertion of DNA is termed transgenic technique. The sequence of DNA in the transgene can be similar to sequences already present in the host or the sequence can be different. If the inserted DNA sequence is not novel, the new mutant created is termed a "knockout" mutant or animal. Some of these, such as the polymorphisms associated with drug metabolizing enzymes and mutants such as acholuric jaundice (widely known as the "Gunn" rat) and the Rowett, a thymic nude, are important in pharmacological and toxicological research. Recently, "mutants" such as the "Big Blue" rats have been produced using transgenic techniques. Transgenic and knockout rats produced by gene targeting techniques are likely to be of increasing importance in toxicological research. Mutants and transgenes can be placed on any genetic background by suitable breeding techniques. Thus, the jaundice gene from the Gunn rat is available on the inbred ACI, LEW, R/A, and RHA genetic background, as well as on a number of outbred genetic backgrounds. For this reason, it would be incorrect to discuss drug metabolism in "the Gunn rat" (or any other mutant or transgenic) without specifying its genetic background because drug metabolism will depend on many genes in addition to the specific locus that is abnormal in the Gunn rat.

Choice of Strain in Research and Screening

There seem to be no serious disadvantages (apart from cost) and many advantages in the use of inbred strains rather than outbred stocks in academic research. These animals offer the nearest equivalent to pure reagents that is possible when using animals in research, particularly if they are also of a high health status. In disciplines other than toxicology, there has been a relentless trend toward the increased use of inbred strains. It is not entirely clear why their use is not more widespread in toxicological research. Any disadvantage in terms of initial cost should be amply compensated for by improved research quality and the need for fewer animals. In toxicological screening the relative merits of inbred strains versus outbred stocks has been debated for more than 50 years without reaching a consensus. An inbred rat strain F344 is used in the National Toxicology Program Carcinogenesis Bioassay, but most commercial screening is done using outbred stocks.

Sex

Male and female animals of the same strain and species usually react to toxicants similarly. It must be borne in mind, however, that there are marked differences in the hormonal makeup between sexes, and this can result in notable differences in responses. Chloroform produces damage to liver and kidney in humans and mice. In mice, however, chloroform produces nephrotoxicity only in males. Furthermore, administration of testosterone (male hormone) to the female mouse followed by chloroform results in kidney damage. Clearly, there are androgen (male) receptors in the kidney that sensitize males to chloroform-induced nephrotoxicity. In rats exposure to the hydrocarbon decalin results in a renal nephropathy and tumor formation in the male but not female, and this is associated with an α_2-globulin protein accumulation. Treatment of females with testosterone followed by decalin also produces renal toxicity and protein accumulation. These examples demonstrate that kidney function differs between the sexes and, consequently, toxic manifestations will vary between males and females.

There are metabolic differences between the sexes. Many barbiturates induce more prolonged sleep in female rats than in males. The shorter duration of action of hexobarbital in male rats is related to the higher activity of the liver microsomal enzymes stimulated by testosterone to hydroxylate this chemical. This higher activity can be reduced by castration or pretreatment with estrogen (female hormone).

Female rats are also more susceptible than males to such organophosphorous insecticides as azinphos-methyl and parathion. Castration or estrogen treatment of the male reverses this difference. The male rat is far more susceptible to carcinoma than the female as shown in the following examples: Males are more susceptible to the induction of pancreatic tumors by azaserine, colonic carcinoma by dimethylhydrazine, intestinal tumors by dimethylnitrosamine, renal tumors by decalin, and liver cirrhosis by acetylaminofluorene. In the case of hydroquinone, which is present in photographic material, acute exposure produced renal toxicity in the female; but in a chronic 2-year study the male and not the female was found to have tubular degeneration and adenoma.

Imbalances of non-sex hormones can also alter the susceptibility of animals to toxicants. Hyperthyroidism, hyperinsulinism, adrenalectomy, and stimulation of the pituitary–adrenal axis have all been shown to be capable of modifying the effects of certain toxicants. One of the functions of thyroid hormone involves the maintenance of normal heart activity; in hyperthyroidism, however, there is tachycardia and hypertension. In normal circumstances ingestion of caffeine, which is a cardiac stimulant, does not affect heart function but large doses of caffeine produce cardiac arrhythmias. It is thus evident that a hyperthyroid patient drinking excess coffee would be more prone to cardiac dysfunction than a normal individual. Hyperinsulinism is manifested by a hypoglycemic coma through a depletion of carbohydrate stores and lack of CNS energy supply. The insecticide DDT in toxic doses is known to produce CNS excitability, tremors, and convulsions and is associated with carbohydrate store depletion. Thus, it can be seen that in conditions of hyperinsulinemia exposure to DDT or the heavy metal cadmium, which acts in a similar fashion, results in a greater sensitivity of the CNS to toxicity.

Age

The pharmacokinetic principles applied in pediatric drug therapy are, in general, similar to those utilized for adults. Data obtained in adult studies, however, are not always applicable to rational therapy in infants or young children. The infant must be regarded as a distinct organism (not a small adult), and lack of appreciation of this fact can result in serious harm and potentially in death.

A number of important characteristics exist that distinguish drug therapy in infants from adult medication protocols. For example, after intramuscular administration, drug absorption is partially dependent on blood flow in the muscle bed. Abnormal drug absorption following intramuscular injection can occur in premature infants, in whom muscle mass is small and blood flow to the musculature is poor. Examples of adverse effects attributed to altered drug absorption are the reactions of infants to cardiac glycosides and anticonvulsants.

In the infant, absorption from the gastrointestinal tract of an orally administered drug differs from that in adults. Certain toxicants are absorbed to a greater extent by the young than by the adult. For example, young children absorb 4 or 5 times more lead than adults and 20 times more cadmium. In both adults and infants, the rate and extent of drug absorption depend on the degree of ionization, which, in turn, is influenced by pH. Within the first 24 hr of life, gastric acidity increases rapidly, and this is followed by an elevation in alkalinity over the next 4–6 weeks. These conditions result in drugs existing in the infant gastrointestinal tract in states of ionization other than might be observed in adults. The higher incidence of methemoglobinemia in young infants has been explained on the basis that their lower gastric acidity allows upward migration of intestinal microbial flora and the reduction of nitrates to a greater extent. Furthermore, infants have a higher proportion of fetal hemoglobin, which is more readily oxidized to methemoglobin. Other factors that modify gastrointestinal drug absorption in the young infant include an irregular neonatal peristalsis, a greater gastrointestinal tract surface to body ratio, and enhanced β-glucuronidase activity in the intestinal tract. The significance of the β-glucuronidase is that it converts drug-bound glucuronide to the free form and thus increases drug bioavailability.

Differences exist in the organ distribution of drugs between newborns and adults. The greater susceptibility of the young to morphine is attributable to a less efficient blood–brain barrier. In the newborn, a higher percentage of body weight is represented by water, so extracellular water space is proportionally larger. To initiate a receptor response, the distribution of drugs must occur predominantly in the extracellular space, so the amount of drug reaching the receptor sites is higher in neonates. Furthermore, the ability of newborn infants to bind drugs in plasma is significantly less than that in adults. This again suggests that neonates could be expected to be more susceptible to the effects of drugs. Differences also exist with respect to drug-metabolizing enzymes. It has been clearly demonstrated that the drug inactivation rate is generally slower in newborns. The available information indicates that the greater susceptibility of the young animals to many toxicants can be attributed to deficiencies of various detoxication enzyme systems. Both phase I and phase II reactions may be responsible. For example, hexobarbital at a dose of 10 mg/kg induced a sleeping time of longer than 360 min in 1-day-old mice compared to 27 min in the 21-day-old mice. The proportion of hexobarbital metabolized by oxidant in 3 hr in these animals was 0 and 21–33%, respectively. On the other hand, chloramphenicol (an antibiotic) is excreted mainly as a glucuronide conjugate. When a dose of 50 mg/kg was given to 1- or 2-day-old infants, the blood levels were 15 μg/ml or higher over a period of 48 hr. In contrast, children aged 1–11 years maintained such blood levels for only 12 hr.

Not all chemicals, however, are more toxic to the young. Certain substances, notably CNS stimulants, are much less toxic to neonates. The acute toxicity of DDT was reported more than 20 times smaller in newborn rats than in adults, in sharp contrast to the effect of age on malathion.

Furthermore, the ability of the neonate to eliminate drugs via the kidney, the major excretion pathway, is significantly limited by the state of development of these organs. Penicillin and tetracycline (two antiobiotics) are excreted more slowly and hence are more toxic in the young. Consideration of these factors indicates that the susceptibility and responsiveness of newborns to drug therapy are different from those of adults.

Old animals and humans are also more susceptible to certain chemicals. This problem has not been studied as extensively as in the young. The available evidence indicates that the aged patients are generally more sensitive to many drugs. A prime example is the use of antibiotics to treat infections in geriatric patients. Since the detoxification of antibiotics is dependent on renal clearance, which is generally slower in the aged, drug accumulation and toxicity are higher in the older patient. The possible mechanisms include reduced detoxication and an impaired renal excretion. In addition, the distribution of chemicals in the body may also be altered because of increased body fat and decreased body water. A number of drugs have been found to be likely to induce more severe signs of toxicity. These include most CNS depressants, certain antibiotics, cardiac glycosides, and hypotensive agents.

Pregnancy

During the course of a pregnancy a mother is likely to take a number of drugs for therapeutic reasons. In addition, with many more women in the work force, there is an increased potential of exposure to a variety of chemicals under occupational conditions. Furthermore, a large number of women indulge in a variety of recreational chemicals including cigarettes and alcohol. The consequences attributed to exposure to a pharmaceutical product can be advantageous to the mother; however, in many instances the effects are deleterious to the fetus. Exposure to occupational and/or environmental chemicals is more likely to result in adverse effects than to be beneficial. Thus, it may be stated that the fetus is at some jeopardy as a result of exposure to foreign chemicals.

Nutrients essential for fetal growth and development require an active transport system to be moved from the maternal circulation to the fetal circulation against a concentration gradient. By contrast, drugs and other chemicals cross the placenta by simple diffusion. The amount of a chemical that is transferred to the fetus is dependent on lipid solubility, the degree of ionization, and the molecular weight. Lipophilic chemicals tend to diffuse across the placenta readily, while highly ionized compounds penetrate the placental membrane slowly. The molecular weight of a chemical affects placental transfer, with the larger molecules crossing the placental barrier less readily. Protein binding of a chemical or its metabolites will affect the rate and the amount transferred to the fetus. Exposure of fetal target tissues to chemical entities may also be influenced by metabolism in the placenta or the fetal liver.

An important component to consider is the stage of fetal development at the time of chemical exposure. During the first week of development after fertilization, the embryo undergoes the process of cleavage and gastrulation. Exposure to chemicals or drugs such as antimetabolites, ergot alkaloids, or diethylstilbestrol at this stage can result in termination of pregnancy. Organogenesis is the next developmental stage covering Weeks 2–8 of gestation. Exposure to drugs or other chemicals including thalidomide, alcohol, and phenytoin during this phase can result in serious structural abnormalities. Drugs and chemicals such as cigarette smoke, heavy metals, or carbon monoxide may affect development during the remaining gestational period ranging from 9 weeks to 9 months. Predominant effects are alteration in the differentiation of the reproductive system and CNS. Consequently, altered brain function and growth retardation are some of the principal adverse effects due to exposure at this stage.

Lactation

The nursing mother can serve as a source of exposure for the neonate to drugs and environmental chemicals. Most drugs are detectable in breast milk regardless of whether they are over-the-counter medication or something prescribed by a physician. In addition, exposure of the nursing mother to environmental pollutants can result in chemical contamination of breast milk. The presence of a drug or chemical in maternal milk may be construed as a potential hazard to the infant even though only 1 or 2% of total intake is likely to be found here. Hence, the primary consideration in maternal drug therapy or exposing a lactating mother to industrial chemicals is the risk to the nursing infant rather than the mere presence of a xenobiotic in the milk.

Several factors play a role in determining the quantity of a drug or chemical that will be transferred to breast milk. The amount of drug or chemical that is actually available for transfer to milk is dependent on certain maternal factors including amount of drug or chemical absorbed, frequency and route of exposure, xenobiotic biotransformation, and protein binding and excretion.

Drug utilization can to a large extent be controlled, so the prudent use of drugs during lactation is imperative because of the potential transfer of these agents or their metabolites into the milk. Certain drugs should be totally avoided during lactation. Certain foods or nutritional supplements have also been shown to cause adverse effects in the infant as a result of lactational exposure.

It is much more difficult to control exposure to environmental chemicals. For example, a mother has no knowledge of what pesticides may have been used on the fruits or vegetables purchased for consumption. Nor is there an easy way to protect oneself from ambient industrial pollution. Some examples of environmental agents known to produce adverse effects in the nursing infant include lead and tetrachloroethylene (dry cleaning solvent).

Nutritional Status

The principal biotransformation of toxicants is catalyzed by the microsomal mixed function oxidase system (MFO). A deficiency of essential fatty acids generally depresses MFO activities. This is also true with protein deficiency. The decreased MFO has different effects on the toxicity of chemicals. For example, hexobarbital and aminopyrine are detoxified by these enzymes and are thus more toxic to rats and mice with these nutrient deficiencies. On the other hand, the toxicity of aflatoxin is lower in such animals because of their depressed bioactivation of this toxicant. MFO activities are decreased in animals fed high levels of sugar.

A number of carcinogenesis studies have demonstrated that restriction of food intake decreases tumor yield. Deficiency of protein generally lowers tumorigenicity of carcinogens, such as aflatoxin and dimethylnitrosamine. It is well-known that enzymes, derived from protein, are required to produce reactive, toxic metabolites of aflatoxin or dimethylnitrosamine. Hence, with protein deficiency less toxic metabolite will be generated. The importance of diet on carcinogenesis is further demonstrated by the fact that rats and mice fed diets rich in fats have higher tumor incidences compared to those that are given a restricted diet.

Chemical Interaction

The toxicity of a chemical in an organism may be increased or decreased by a simultaneous or consecutive exposure to another chemical. If the combined effect is equal to the sum of the effect of each substance given alone, the interaction is considered to be additive, for example, combinations of most organophosphorous pesticides on cholinesterase activity. If the combined effect is greater than the sum, the interaction is considered to be synergistic, for example, carbon tetrachloride and ethanol on the liver and asbestos exposure and cigarette smoking on the lung. In the latter example, there can be a 5-fold increase in lung cancer incidence among asbestos workers, an 11-fold increase among cigarette smokers, and a 55-fold increase among asbestos workers who are cigarette smokers. The term potentiation is used to describe the situation in which the toxicity of a substance on an organ is markedly increased by another substance that alone has no toxic effect on that organ. For example, isopropanol (a solvent) has no effect on the liver, but it can increase considerably the hepatotoxicity of carbon tetrachloride (another solvent).

The exposure of an organism to a chemical may reduce the toxicity of another. Chemical antagonism denotes the situation wherein a reaction between the two chemicals produces a less toxic product, for example, chelation of heavy metals by dimercaprol. Functional antagonism exists when two chemicals produce opposite effects on the same physiologic parameters, such as the counteraction between CNS stimulants and depressants. Competitive antagonism exists when the agonist and antagonist act on the same receptor, such as the blockade of the effects of nicotine on ganglia by ganglionic blocking agents. Noncompetitive antagonism exists when the toxic effect of a chemical is blocked by another not acting on the same receptor. For example, atropine reduces the toxicity of acetylcholinesterase (AChE) inhibitors not by blocking the receptors on the AChE, but by blocking the receptors for the ACh accumulated.

Chemical interactions are achieved through a variety of mechanisms. For instance, nitrites and certain amines can react in the stomach to form nitrosamines, the majority of which are potent carcinogens, and thus greatly increase the toxicity. On the other hand, the action of many antidotes is based on their reactivity with the toxicants; for example, thiosulfate is used in cases of cyanide poisoning. Furthermore, a chemical may displace another from its binding sites on plasma protein and thereby increase its effective concentration. A chemical may modify the renal excretion of weak acids and weak bases by altering the pH of urine. Competition for the same renal transport system by one chemical can hinder the excretion of another. A notable example is the administration of the drug probenecid along with the antibiotic penicillin to reduce the renal excretion of the antibiotic, thereby prolonging its duration of action.

One important type of interaction involves the binding of chemicals with their specific receptors. An antagonist blocks the action of an agonist, such as a neurotransmitter or a hormone, by preventing the binding of the agonist to the receptor.

Another important type of interaction results from alterations of the biotransformation of a chemical by another. Some chemicals are inducers of xenobiotic-metabolizing enzymes. They augment the activities of these enzymes, perhaps mainly by *de novo* synthesis, a fact that is consistent with the finding that repeated administrations are necessary. The common inducers include phenobarbital, 3-methylcholanthrene (3-MC), PCB, DDT, and benzo(*a*)pyrene. The inducers may lower the toxicity of other chemicals by accelerating their detoxication. For example, pretreatment with phenobarbital shortens the sleeping time induced by hexobarbital and the paralysis induced by zoxazolamine. In addition, 3-MC pretreatment greatly reduces the liver injury produced by bromobenzene, probably by increasing the activity of the epoxide hydrase. On the other hand, pretreatment with phenobarbital augments the toxicity of acetaminophen and bromobenzene, apparently by increasing the toxic metabolites formed. Repeated administration of a chemical may induce its metabolizing enzymes, as has been shown with the industrial chemical vinyl chloride.

Piperonyl butoxide, isoniazid, and SKF 525A and related chemicals are inhibitors of various xenobiotic-metabolizing enzymes. For instance, piperonyl butoxide increases the toxicity of pyrethrum (an insecticide) by inhibiting MFO activity in insects that detoxifies this agent. Isoniazid, when taken along with phenytoin, lengthens the plasma half-life of the antiepileptic drug and increases its toxicity. Iproniazid inhibits monoamine oxidase and increases the cardiovascular effects of tyramine, which is found in cheese and which is normally readily metabolized by the oxidase.

Further Reading

Lu, F. C. (1996). *Basic Toxicology: Fundamentals, Target Organs and Risk Assessment,* 3rd ed. Taylor & Francis, Washington, DC.

Kacew, S. (1990). *Drug Toxicity and Metabolism in Pediatrics.* CRC Press, Boca Raton, FL.

—Frank C. Lu and Sam Kacew

Related Topics

Absorption
Analytical Toxicology
Biotransformation
Distribution
Exposure
Mechanisms of Toxicity
Mixtures
Pharmacokinetics/Toxicokinetics
Resistance to Toxicants

Molecular Toxicology—Recombinant DNA Technology

Molecular toxicology is an emerging area of research. Currently, it consists largely of the application of recombinant DNA technology to better understand and assess mechanisms of action of substances that may adversely affect health and environmental quality.

The application of recombinant DNA technology to all areas of biology has brought about a revolution in our understanding of living organisms. This technology has enabled researchers to examine the molecular mechanisms and structures responsible for such complex processes as cell growth, metabolism, differentiation, and development. More significantly, it provides a means to manipulate molecules critical to these processes and an opportunity to examine the effects of these changes in living systems and elucidate the physiological roles of the protein under investigation. There is also general consensus among researchers that the application of recombinant DNA techniques to problems in toxicology will have a profound impact on the future direction of this field.

Molecular toxicology has enabled toxicologists to elucidate events at the molecular level and examine alterations in fundamental biological processes that lead to the manifestation of toxic responses. As a result, toxicologists are examining the mechanisms of action of toxic substances at the molecular level in order to identify molecular changes predictive of exposure to harmful substances. Consequently, this information can be used to identify susceptible groups within a population or establish safe levels of exposure using a mechanistic approach rather than through association of risk based on extrapolation of "high-dose" studies in rodent models to low-level human exposures. This molecular or "reductionist" approach is not intended to circumvent *in vivo* studies but to introduce mechanistic data into risk assessment in order to define the possible implications of exposure to potentially harmful substances. The inclusion of recombinant DNA technology in toxicological research has facilitated our understanding of the mechanisms of action of several toxic substances. This information has subsequently been used by toxicologists in risk assessment and in the development of assays to identify and assess the potential adverse effects posed by uncharacterized toxic substances.

Molecular biology has provided a dramatic expansion in our knowledge of the structure, function, multiplicity, and regulation of xenobiotic metabolizing enzyme (XME) superfamilies. Its use has resulted in the cloning of a number of complementary DNA (cDNA) sequences that encode or act as the blueprint for the synthesis of proteins that are important in toxicology. The increased availability of cDNA and deduced protein sequences has provided a rational foundation for the development of standardized nomenclatures based on amino acid sequence similarities. These systems are a welcome alternative to the multiple, laboratory-specific classifications that have led to considerable confusion particularly in the P450 superfamily, in which >200 unique cDNAs have been identified.

A major emphasis in drug metabolism research has been focused on elucidating the role of individual XMEs in the *in vivo* biotransformation of drugs and chemicals in order to understand their role in eliciting adverse drug reactions. The identification of specific XME isozymes that are responsible for adverse drug effects has been difficult since multienzyme superfamilies made up of enzymes with diverse structure and overlapping substrate specificities are involved in metabolism. A further complication has been the relatively low abundance of individual forms of XMEs. This limitation has been overcome by using heterologous expression systems to produce large quantities of specific XME isozymes. These systems use cloned XME cDNAs and take advantage of the protein production machinery in bacteria, yeast, and insect or mammalian cells in culture to overexpress large quantities of a desired protein. Depending on the system that is utilized, proteins can be generated by simply introducing the appropriate vector containing the desired cDNA into the cells of choice. The enzymatic activity of recombinant proteins can be directly measured from whole cells or isolated subcellular fractions. Heterologous expression systems have also been used to produce sufficient quantities of desired protein for subsequent purification to homogeneity and biophysical investigations. In addition, the cDNA of the desired product can be engineered so that the expressed protein contains a protein moiety that can be subsequently used with affinity chromatography to isolate the desired product or a signal instructing the cell to secrete the product into the media. The secretion signal or protein moiety is designed so that it can be removed using site-specific proteases in order to release the desired product. Many heterologous expression systems are commercially available and provide all the necessary materials to express the desired product in a variety of organisms (Table M-1).

Bacterial, yeast, and mammalian cells have been utilized in novel ways to develop or improve assays for the identification of drug metabolizing enzymes involved in the bioactivation and detoxification of xenobiotics. Historically, these systems have been supplemented with exogenous cell fractions (i.e., S9, microsomal) to confer to the system the capability of metabolizing chemicals to the ultimate carcinogen. However, the use of exogenous metabolic activation fractions such as S9 can limit the utility of mutation assays. For example, exogenous cellular fractions may generate extremely reactive intermediates that do not possess sufficient stability to enter the cell and interact with the responsive target, thus compromising the sensitivity of the assay. In addition, interspecies differences in XMEs warrant the use of human tissue fractions that may have marked interindividual variability in XME composition and

TABLE M-1
Expression Systems for Recombinant Xenobiotic Metabolizing Enzymes

	Mammalian cells	
Microorganism	*Transient*	*Stable*
Yeast	COS	V79
E. coli	Vaccinia virus	AHH-1

require appropriate handling precautions. Moreover, in order to compensate for the instability of the drug metabolizing enzymes in exogenous fractions and the short exposure times, assays are often performed at high doses of test chemicals that may create conditions of acute toxicity. Furthermore, the addition of tissue fractions containing a multiplicity of XMEs precludes the identification of the role of a specific XME isozyme in the elicited toxicological response. Nevertheless, these assay conditions have been successfully used to identify a number of carcinogenic substances.

Several of these limitations have been overcome through the development of metabolically competent cell lines that stably express a specific XME isozyme. For example, cDNAs encoding for detoxification enzymes, such as *N*-acetyltransferase and glutathione *S*-transferase, have been introduced into Ames tester strains and mammalian cells, which are naturally devoid of these enzyme activities, enabling researchers to examine the mutational specificity of a chemical following metabolism or bioactivation by specific detoxification enzymes. For instance, V79 Chinese hamster cells, which lack endogenous monooxygenase activity, have been genetically engineered to be metabolically competent by the introduction of specific P450 isozymes. In addition, a series of bioengineered lymphoblastoid cell lines expressing various human P450s and phase II enzymes have been prepared and are commercially available. Results from these *in vitro* test systems combined with data gained from experiments investigating differential regulation, tissue-specific expression, and interindividual variation in human XMEs should provide a sound mechanistic basis for assessing human risk following procarcinogen and promutagen exposure.

Molecular toxicology has also had practical applications in the development of *in vivo* assays to investigate the molecular events involved in mutagenesis. Genetic toxicity testing is performed to determine potential carcinogenicity of a substance and to assess whether it may induce inheritable genetic damage. Traditionally, these studies have used short-term *in vitro* tests such as the Ames assay or long-term *in vivo* carcinogenicity tests. Using transgenic animal technology that involves introducing new DNA sequences into the host animal's genome, researchers have combined both short-term *in vitro* tests and long-term *in vivo* carcinogenicity tests to develop a short-term *in vivo* assay. These animals possess the bacterial genes, *lacZ* or *lacl,* in all of their cells and have been used to assess the ability of a chemical to induce a mutation in any tissue. The *lacZ* and *lacl* genes have been extensively used as targets for the identification and analysis of spontaneous and induced mutations and have been designed so that they can be easily extracted from the animal's genomic DNA and subsequently introduced with high efficiency into prokaryotic cells. *LacZ* or *lacl* genes that have been mutated following treatment of the animal with a genotoxic substance can then be identified by examining the functionality of the proteins encoded by these genes in prokaryote cells using a simple colorimetric assay. By extracting DNA from specific tissues, researchers can identify potential target organs and determine the mutational spectrum introduced into the *lacZ* or *lacl* genes by automated DNA sequencing. For example, the mutational spectrums for benzo(*a*)pyrene obtained using *in vivo* and *in vitro* assays appear to correlate, thus suggesting that the mechanisms of mutagenesis are comparable in prokaryotic systems and mice. In addition to mice, transgenic rats are also commercially available and work is continuing on the development of transgenic fish.

Pharmacogenetics, the study of genetically determined variations in drug response, has been profoundly transformed by molecular biology. Genetic polymorphisms have been traditionally defined as the occurrence in a population of more than one form of a particular gene with the prevalence of the less common form being at least 1%. Prior to recombinant DNA technology, genetic polymorphisms were identified by familial and population studies following the observation of an atypical drug reaction in a population. Classification of individuals as poor or extensive metabolizers was determined by measuring drug clearance of a substance that was metabolized by a specific XME. On this basis it became evident that there were genotypic variants in a wide variety of human XMEs, including the P450s, CYP2D6 and CYP2C19, and the *N*-acetyltransferase, NAT2 (Table M-2). Using recombinant DNA technology, the major genetic defects responsible for these polymorphisms have now been identified by examining DNA sequence variations in specific XME isozymes. However, the relationship between phenotypic variants and genetic alterations for most XMEs polymorphisms remains to be clarified.

Variations in DNA sequences in the human genome randomly occur approximately every 200 base pairs.

TABLE M-2
Genetic Polymorphisms in Human Xenobiotic Metabolizing Enzymes

Polymorphic gene	*Polymorphic substrate*
CYP 2D6	Debrisoquine/sparteine
CYP 2C19	*S*-mephenytoin
NAT2	Isoniazid/sulfamethazine

These DNA sequence variations may give rise to different DNA fragmentation patterns that are known as restriction fragment length polymorphisms (RFLPs). RFLPs involve the digestion of DNA with purified bacterial enzymes, known as restriction endonucleases, that recognize and cleave specific DNA sequences (Fig. M-1). The digested DNA fragments are subsequently separated based on size using gel electrophoresis and the resultant DNA fragment lengths are determined by comparison to a known standard (Fig. M-2). RFLPs have been used in the identification of DNA sequence changes that are responsible for genetic diseases as well as in forensic science in order to establish an association between an individual and the human tissues such as blood, saliva, or semen collected at a crime scene. Genetic polymorphisms that involve changes in DNA sequence at restriction enzyme recognition sites can be directly detected following restriction enzyme digestion of both normal and variant DNA. However, polymorphisms that alter restriction endonuclease recognition sites and cause abnormalities in protein function are rare. It should also be emphasized that the majority of the DNA sequence variations located in or around a gene do not necessarily explain the observed phenotypic variants since many of the differences detected by RFLP analysis are silent polymorphisms that do not encode for changes at the protein level and, therefore, have no functional consequences. For example, in the CYP2D6 polymorphism, digestion of genomic DNA with 20 different restriction enzymes identified the presence of 14 different RFLPs. However, only 2 of these RFLPs correlated with specific DNA sequence variations that were associated with the poor metabolizer phenotype.

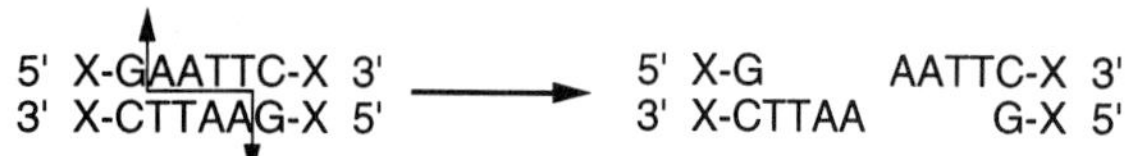

FIGURE M-1. Cleavage sequence for the restriction enzyme EcoRI (X, any nucleotide).

A

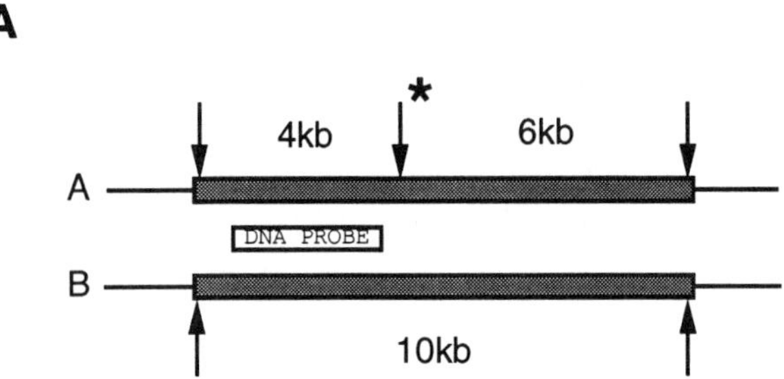

B

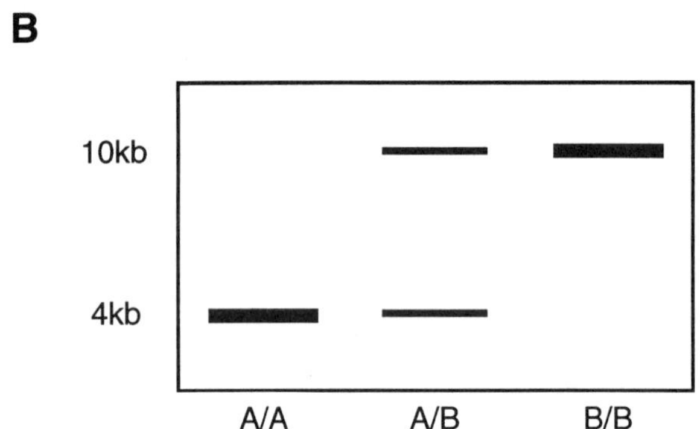

FIGURE M-2. (A) A region of chromosomal DNA that occurs as two polymorphic variants (A and B). The EcoRI *restriction enzyme sites are marked by arrows and the asterisk denotes the polymorphic restriction enzyme site found in variant A. The region of DNA detected by a radioactive probe in B is indicated. (B) Analysis of DNA digested with* EcoRI *reveals three possible banding patterns for this RFLP.*

With the incorporation of molecular technology, many DNA sequence variations responsible for these polymorphisms are now being characterized and identified at the molecular level using RFLP analysis combined with simple polymerase chain reaction (PCR)-based DNA tests. PCR exploits features of DNA replication, which provide researchers endless possibilities in the manipulation of DNA. The most powerful advantage of this technology is its ability to produce enormous numbers of copies of a specific DNA sequence from a minute sample. The technique involves two primers that are designed to be complementary to the boundaries of the desired DNA segment and DNA polymerase which produces copies of the DNA sequence between the primers (Fig. M-3). The cycling

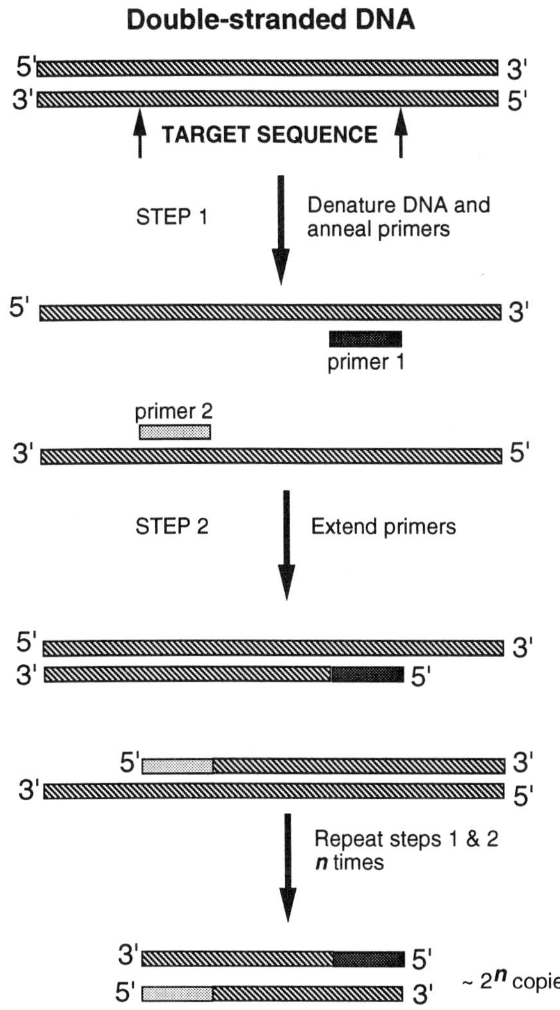

FIGURE M-3. A schematic representation of the polymerase chain reaction (PCR). Repetitive cycles of DNA denaturation followed by annealing of the primers and primer extension results in the exponential amplification of the DNA fragment whose boundaries are determined by the primers.

of this replicative reaction results in the exponential production of a DNA fragment whose boundaries are determine by the primers. PCR has applications not only in research but also in forensic toxicology, evolutionary studies, and in the diagnosis of infectious diseases, genetic abnormalities, and cancer. The technique is so sensitive that forensic scientists can obtain sufficient amounts of DNA extracted from saliva left on postage stamps or discarded cigarettes to implicate individuals in criminal activities.

By combining allele-specific DNA sequence information with PCR, noninvasive assays have been developed that can be rapidly performed to identify individuals susceptible to adverse drug reactions. The two strategies that have been successfully employed include the use of allele-specific oligonucleotide primers designed to hybridize to a sequence only if a known variation is present and the amplification of a DNA sequence that contains an RFLP which identifies a variant phenotype. For example, over 90% of poor metabolizers of the CYP2D6 polymorphism can be genotyped by RFLP analysis using an allele-specific PCR-based test. Similar tests have been developed to detect the genetic defects responsible for the polymorphisms in *S*-mephenytoin metabolism (CYP2C19) and *N*-acetyltransferase (NAT2). There are an increasing number of reports in the literature associating XME polymorphisms with susceptibility to developing certain cancers and diseases. These types of studies are important because they may provide information regarding the identification of susceptible populations and environmental agents that are involved in the pathogenesis of these diseases. Unfortunately, the results from many of these studies are equivocal, which may be due in part to small sample sizes or because of difficulties encountered in clearly identifying poor metabolizers using metabolic phenotyping. Moreover, susceptible populations may possess a series of polymorphisms that enhance their predisposition to certain environmentally induced diseases. Genotyping individuals using PCR-based assays should provide a clearer indication of the relationship between certain mutations in XMEs and the predisposition to developing these diseases.

Heterologous expression technology has been an important technique in assessing the functional consequences of XME polymorphisms. Expression of cDNAs with variant DNA sequences using heterologous systems allows one to identify protein products with altered catalytic activity without having to perform lengthy, labor-intensive purification protocols from tissue samples from multiple phenotypic populations. In addition, these studies may assist in the identification of critical residues within XMEs that are required for optimal catalytic activity. This information may lead to improved drug design and efficacy by introducing modifications that minimize metabolic transformations to reactive metabolites that are responsible for eliciting adverse reactions.

In addition to investigating the structural features of drug metabolizing enzymes, molecular biology has also enhanced our understanding of how the expression of these enzymes are regulated. The most extensively studied P450 is CYP1A1. Its expression has been linked to the bioactivation of a number of carcinogens and studies have found that it is inducible by a variety of structurally diverse compounds, including 3-methylcholanthrene, β-naphthoflavone, and halogenated aromatic hydrocarbons such as 2,3,7,8-tetrachlorodibenzo-*p*-dioxin (TCDD). The induction of CYP1A1 expression is analogous to the mechanism of action proposed for steroids such as estrogen and glucocorticoid (Fig. M-4). It is mediated by a specific cytosolic protein referred to as the aryl hydrocarbon receptor (AhR). The AhR is a ligand-inducible transcription factor that contains separable and distinct domains for ligand binding, DNA binding, and transcriptional activation for gene expression. Initially, researchers assumed that the AhR would possess structural features similar to those of steroid receptors. Its recent cloning, however, has unequivocally confirmed that the AhR possesses a basic helix–loop–helix DNA-binding domain rather than a zinc finger DNA-binding domain, which essentially precludes its membership in the nuclear receptor superfamily.

Briefly, ligand binding to the AhR causes the release of a heat shock protein, HSP90, which enables the receptor to heterodimerize with the Ah receptor nuclear translocator. The resulting complex exhibits high affinity for DNA and seeks out specific DNA sequences referred to as dioxin or xenobiotic response elements (DREs and XREs) located in the 5′ regulatory region of the CYP1A1 gene. Binding of the complex to DREs

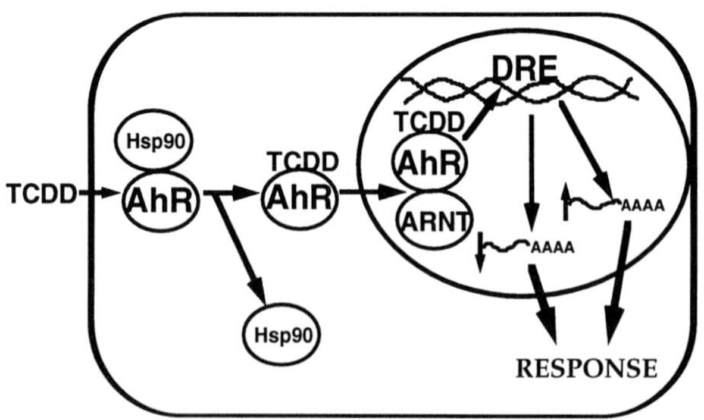

*FIGURE M-4. The proposed mechanism of action of 2,3,7,8-tetrachlorodibenzo-*p*-dioxin (TCDD, dioxin) and related compounds. AhR, aryl hydrocarbon receptor; Hsp90, heat shock protein 90; ARNT, aryl hydrocarbon receptor nuclear translocator; DRE, dioxin response element.*

results in the recruitment of factors that facilitate the increased rate of CYP1A1 gene transcription. Analysis of the CYP1A1 5′ regulatory region has identified six DREs, all of which contain the core sequence, GCGTG, and have a role in the dramatic increase in CYP1A1 activity following treatment with TCDD. In addition to CYP1A1, other TCDD-inducible genes such as the rat glutathione *S*-transferase Ya subunit, CYP1A2, and quinone oxidoreductase also possess DREs in their 5′ regulatory regions. Although the toxic effects of TCDD and related compounds have not been fully elucidated, it is generally believed that the AhR plays a role, suggesting that these effects may result from inappropriate gene expression.

The adverse effects of other compounds of toxicological significance also use a receptor-mediated mechanism of action. For example, peroxisome proliferators, such as phthalate ester plasticizers, hypolidemic drugs, and trichloroacetic acid, exert their effects through the peroxisome proliferator activated receptor (PPAR). However, no research to date has demonstrated that peroxisome proliferators directly bind to the PPAR, prompting the hypothesis that they trigger the release of fatty acids which ultimately bind and activate the PPAR. Unlike the AhR, PPAR is a member of the nuclear receptor superfamily that undergoes receptor heterodimerization with the retinoid X receptor in order to bind to peroxisome proliferator response elements found in the 5′ regulatory region of target genes including acyl CoA oxidase, CYP4A6, bifunctional enzyme, and the fatty acid-binding protein.

One of the perplexing questions in toxicology has been the normal physiological role of the AhR and PPAR as well as the identity of their endogenous ligands. Studies have demonstrated that both receptors are differentially expressed during fetal development. In the case of PPAR, three receptor subtypes exist that are conserved between species, suggesting they serve important physiological functions. In addition to the AhR and PPARs, there are a number of proteins that share amino acid sequence homologies similar to those found in members of the nuclear receptor superfamily. However, these proteins have no known physiological ligands or functions and, therefore, are collectively referred to as "orphan receptors." Conversely, there are also compounds such as phenobarbital, that might exert some of their effects through receptor-mediated mechanisms of action, although little evidence for a specific receptor exists. Consequently, it has been suggested that orphan receptors may be responsible for mediating the effects of other nongenotoxic substances.

Receptors are not the only mechanisms used by toxic substances to affect gene regulation. Reactive oxygen intermediates (ROIs), such as superoxide and hydroxyl radicals, are continuously produced in cells as side products of electron-transfer reactions. Oxidative stress occurs when abnormally high levels of ROIs are produced within a cell following exposure to physical, chemical, and biological agents including UV and gamma radiation, alkylating agents, hydrogen peroxide, metals, cytokines, and other natural ligands for cell surface receptors. In addition to causing cellular damage, ROIs also induce the expression of enzymes with radical scavenging and repair activities by the induction and activation of transcription factors such as c-*fos,* c-*jun,* and NF-κB. c-*Fos* and c-*jun* are members of the AP-1 transcription factor family, which forms *fos–jun* or *jun–jun* dimers prior to binding to specific DNA sequences located in the 5′ regulatory region of target genes. These specific DNA sequences or response elements have been found to regulate the expression of several genes including quinone oxidoreductase and glutathione *S*-transferase. Therefore, in addition to inducing repair mechanisms, oxidative stress can also induce the expression of proteins that have a protective role.

The ability of toxic substances to induce gene expression has been successfully used to develop assays that assist in the identification of substances that may cause adverse effects. In the past, toxicologists relied on physiological responses, such as decreased body weight or lethality, to assess the effects of a toxic substance. As more information regarding the mechanism of action of compounds was acquired, biochemical responses such as enzyme activities were used to determine the potential adverse health effects resulting from exposure to toxic substances. Molecular toxicology provides techniques such as the reverse transcriptase-polymerase chain reaction assay (RT-PCR), which has enabled toxicologists to directly measure subtle changes in the expression of specific target genes. For instance, RT-PCR has been reported to be 1000–10,000 times more sensitive than traditional blotting techniques for the measurement of mRNA levels. Recombinant DNA technology has also provided strategies for toxicologists to identify target genes that are directly involved in eliciting the observed toxic responses. Differential hybridization technology has been successfully used to identify structurally unrelated genes that are regulated by a common mechanism such as exposure to a specific chemical agent. The technique relies on screening duplicate filters of a cDNA library prepared from treated cells with radiolabeled cDNAs from control and treated cells and identifying those clones that hybridize more strongly to cDNA probes from treated cells. Recently, a commercially available PCR-based mRNA Differential Display assay has been developed that assists in the identification of genes whose expression is differentially regulated. The identification of these genes is important since their induction may represent the initial step leading to a toxic response.

Mechanistic studies investigating the regulation of gene expression have been exploited to develop bioassays that assist toxicologists in the detection and assessment of potentially toxic substances (Fig. M-5). These bioassays consist of reporter genes whose expression is under the control of the 5′ regulatory region of a target gene. Reporter gene expression can also be regulated by specific response elements, thus enhancing the specificity of the response, although sometimes at the expensive of overall inducibility. Reporter genes provide sensitive, rapid, and easily measured enzymatic activities that are usually absent in the host cell. Examples of reporter genes include firefly luciferase, bacterial chloramphenicol acetyltransferase, bacterial β-galactosidase, and heat-resistant mammalian alkaline phosphatase. Several different reporter gene bioassays are currently being used to assess the potential toxicity of individual chemicals as well as complex mixtures. These bioassays can detect a number of different substances including halogenated aromatic hydrocarbons, sex steroid mimetics, peroxisome proliferators, metals, and inducers of oxidative stress.

Since 1978 most of the medical research that has received international recognition has used recombinant DNA technology. Surveys of companies that are involved in biomedical research predict that this technology will be of overwhelming importance in a global economy in which economic power is derived from knowledge. Therefore, the incorporation of recombinant DNA technology into the field of toxicology will enhance both the basic and applied aspects of the discipline. This technology has already enabled toxicologists to elucidate the mechanisms of action of toxic substances at the molecular level and this information has been successfully used to engineer and improve the sensitivity and specificity of a number of assays

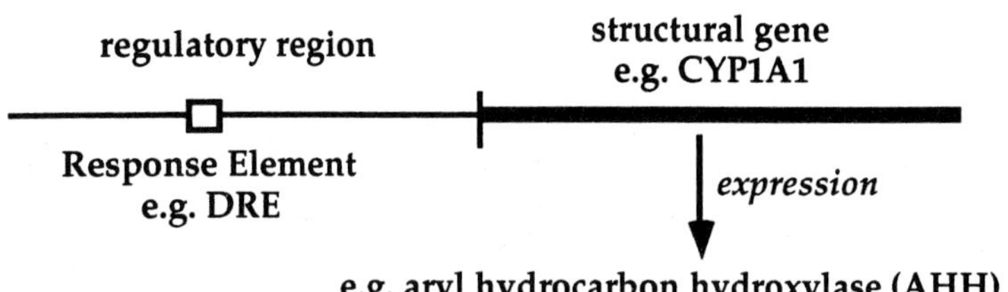

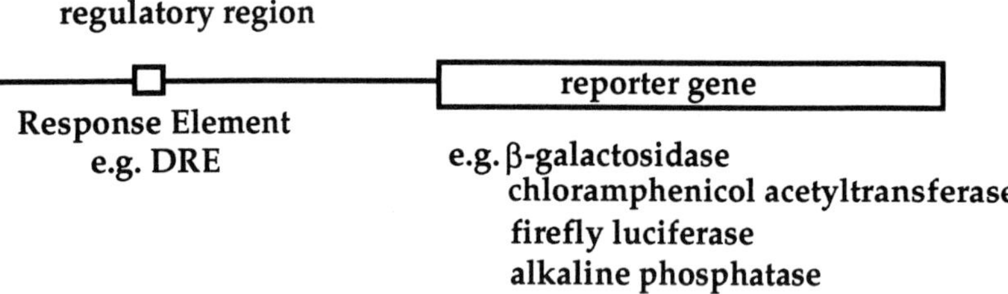

FIGURE M-5. A schematic representation of the regulatory and structural regions of a gene. The regulatory region controls the expression of the gene, while the structural region acts as a blueprint for the gene product. The structural region of the gene can be replaced by cDNAs that encode easily measurable enzyme activities that can then be used to investigate the induction of a specific protein. The open box denotes a specific DNA sequence referred to as a response element that may influence gene expression under the appropriate conditions.

commonly used to assess the potential toxicity of a substance. In addition, the use of this technology has also contributed to our understanding of the normal physiological roles of proteins and enzymes that are disrupted by toxic substances. In conclusion, the use of recombinant DNA technology will extend the comprehensive nature of toxicology and will assist toxicologists in identifying and predicting the potential risks an unknown substance may pose to human health and environmental quality.

Further Reading

de Morais, S. M., Wilkinson, G. R., Blaisdell, J., Nakamura, K., Meyer, U. A., and Goldstein, J. A. (1994). The major genetic defect responsible for the polymorphism of *S*-mephenytoin metabolism in humans. *J. Biol. Chem.* **269**, 15419–15422.

Gonzalez, F. J., and Gelboin, H. V. (1993). Role of human cytochrome P-450s in risk assessment and susceptibility to environmentally based disease. *J. Toxicol. Environ. Health* **40**, 289–308.

Gossen, J. A., de Leeuw, W. J., and Vijg, J. (1994). LacZ transgenic mouse models: Their application in genetic toxicology. *Mutat. Res.* **307**, 451–459.

Green, S., and Wahli, W. (1994). Peroxisome proliferator-activated receptors: Finding the orphan a home. *Mol. Cell. Endocrinol.* **100**, 149–153.

Hankinson, O. (1995). The aryl hydrocarbon receptor complex. *Annu. Rev. Pharmacol. Toxicol.* **35**, 307–340.

Hirvonen, A., Husgafvel Pursiainen, K., Anttila, S., Karjalainen, A., and Vainio, H. (1993). Polymorphism in CYP1A1 and CYP2D6 genes: Possible association with susceptibility to lung cancer. *Environ. Health Perspect.* **101**(Suppl. 3), 109–112.

Langenbach, R., Smith, P. B., and Crespi, C. (1992). Recombinant DNA approaches for the development of metabolic systems used in *in vitro* toxicology. *Mutat. Res.* **277**, 251–275.

MacGregor, J. T., Farr, S., Tucker, J. D., Heddle, J. A., Tice, R. R., and Turteltaub, K. W. (1995). New molecular endpoints and methods for routine toxicity testing. *Fundam. Appl. Toxicol.* **26**, 156–173.

Mirsalis, J. C., Monforte, J. A., and Winegar, R. A. (1995). Transgenic animal models for detection of *in vivo* mutations. *Annu. Rev. Pharmacol. Toxicol.* **35**, 145–164.

Watson, J. D., Gilman, M., Witkowski, J., and Zoller, M. (1992). *Recombinant DNA*, 2nd ed. Sci. Am./Freeman, New York.

—Gordon P. McCallum and Tim R. Zacharewski

Related Topics

Analytical Toxicology
Carcinogen–DNA Adduct Formation and DNA Repair
Chromosome Aberrations
Developmental Toxicology
Immune System
Mechanisms of Toxicity
Mutagenesis
Peroxisome Proliferators
Risk Assessment, Human Health
Sister Chromatid Exchanges
Structure–Activity Relationships

Molybdenum (Mo)

- CAS: 7439-98-7
- SELECTED COMPOUNDS: Molybdenum dioxide, MoO_2 (CAS: 18868-43-4); molybdenum trioxide, MoO_3 (CAS: 1313-27-5); molybdenum pentachloride, $MoCl_5$ (CAS: 10241-05-1)
- CHEMICAL CLASS: Metals

Uses

Molybdenum is an essential trace element for plants, ruminants, and humans. It must be present for plants to fix nitrogen; thus, its main commercial use is in fertilizers. Industrially, it is a component of steel alloys used in high-temperature conditions in aircraft engines and turbines.

Exposure Pathways

The primary route of exposure to molybdenum is ingestion; sources include leafy vegetables, legumes, meat, grains, and many city waters. Molybdenum does not appear to be absorbed dermally.

Toxicokinetics

Molybdenum is well absorbed from the gastrointestinal tract; it does not appear to be absorbed from the lungs. Once absorbed, it binds to the red blood cells but is cleared rapidly from the blood. It concentrates in the liver, kidneys, bones, and pancreas. Molybdenum is associated with the enzymes xanthine oxidase (which metabolizes coffee), aldehyde oxidase, and sulfite oxidase. The molybdate ion, MoO_4^{-2}, inhibits glutaminase and sulfoxidase. Molybdenum is excreted primarily in the urine although some molybdenum is excreted in perspiration.

Human Toxicity

The toxicity of molybdenum depends on the oxidation state; the molybdates are not very toxic. Hexavalent molybdenum (e.g., MoO_3) is more toxic than other compounds, such as the sulfites.

Toxic manifestations include muscular incoordination and loss of weight and hair. This is followed by fatty degeneration of the liver and kidneys. Workers exposed to molybdenum have elevated serum uric acid. The ACGIH TLV-TWA is 5 mg/m^3 for soluble compounds of molybdenum and 10 mg/m^3 for insoluble compounds.

Clinical Management

Molybdenum poisoning is treated using gastric lavage and saline catharsis.

Animal Toxicity

Cattle develop a molybdenum-related disease (teart) from grazing fields that contain from 20 to 100 ppm molybdenum. Symptoms include inadequate growth, anemia, and abnormal joint development. Removing these cattle from these pastures is necessary for their recovery; however, addition of copper (or sulfate) to the diet helps prevent teart.

Molybdenum has not been shown to be mutagenic or carcinogenic in animals.

—Arthur Furst and Shirley B. Radding

Related Topics

Metals
Veterinary Toxicology

Monoamine Oxidase Inhibitors

- Representative Compounds: Phenelzine (CAS: 51-71-8); nialamide; pheniprazine; tranylcypromine; pargyline; iproniazid; isocarboxazid; selegiline; moclobemide; clorgyline
- Synonyms: MAO inhibitors; Phenelzine—phenethylhydrazine hydrogen sulfate; Nardil; nialamide—*N*′-(2-benzylcarbamoylethyl)isonicotinohydrazide, Niamide; pheniprazine, tranylcypromine-(±)-*trans*-2-phenylcyclopropylamine, Parnate; pargyline—*N*-methyl-*N*-2-propynylbenzylamide, Eutonyl; iproniazid—2′-isopropylisonicotinohydrazide, Marsilid; isocarboxazid—2′-benzyl-5-methylisoxazole-3-carbohydrazide, Marplan; selegiline—(−)-(*R*)-*N*,α-dimethyl-*N*-(prop-2-y Eldepryl; moclobemide—4-chloro-*N*-(2-morpholinoethyl)benzamide, Avrorix; clorgyline; moclobemide
- Pharmaceutical Class: Antidepressants
- Chemical Structure: Phenelzine is the prototype monoamine oxidase inhibitor.

$CH_2CH_2NHNH_2$ $+H_2SO_4$

Uses

Monoamine oxidase inhibitors are used to treat depression, atypical depression, bulimia, posttraumatic stress reactions, obsessive–compulsive disorder, panic attacks, narcolepsy, phobias, hypochondria, anxiety, night tremors, parkinsonism, postural hypotension, headache, and aphthous stomatitis.

Exposure Pathways

Monoamine oxidase inhibitors are available orally. Accidental or intentional ingestion are the most common routes of exposure.

Toxicokinetics

Monoamine oxidase inhibitors are rapidly and completely absorbed orally reaching a peak level within 2 hr. Monoamine oxidase inhibitors are acetylated in the liver to many active and inactive metabolites. The volume of distribution is estimated to range from 1 to 4 liters/kg. The inactive metabolites are excreted by the kidneys. The elimination half-lives of monoamine oxidase inhibitor parent compounds range from 15 min to 3.5 hr. The biologic half-life often significantly exceeds the elimination half-life.

Mechanism of Toxicity

Monoamine oxidase is the enzyme principally responsible for degradation of amine neurotransmitters (norepinephrine, epinephrine, serotonin, and dopamine). In general, monoamine oxidase inhibitors irreversibly bind to monoamine oxidase leading to neurotransmitter accumulation. Moclobemide, the exception, binds reversibly. They do not have any effect on monoamine oxidase production. The enzyme then regenerates over many weeks. Monoamine oxidase inhibitors may also stimulate the release of norepinephrine from some nerve endings while having a sympatholytic effect at postganglionic terminals. In high doses, monoamine oxidase inhibitors also inhibit other enzymes which may cause many toxic effects.

Human Toxicity

Any ingestion of 2 or 3 mg/kg is potentially toxic. At therapeutic levels, the most commonly reported adverse effects are dizziness, headache, nervousness, sleep disorders, drowsiness, ataxia, constipation, dry mouth, weight gain, postural hypotension, and edema. Monoamine oxidase inhibitors combined with sympathomimetic drugs or tyramine-containing foods, in either therapeutic amounts or in overdose, may result in a hypertensive crisis characterized by severe headache, tachycardia, diaphoresis, and hyperpyrexia. In very severe cases, subarachnoid hemorrhage and death have resulted. The clinical effects of monoamine oxidase inhibitor overdose have been categorized into four phases. Phase 1 is an asymptomatic period of 12–24 hr. Sympathomimetic stimulation characterizes phase 2. Symptoms in that phase include headache, agitation, mydriasis, tachycardia, drowsiness, hyperreflexia, flushing, and nausea. Symptoms may worsen to coma, muscle rigidity, hyperpyrexia, hypotension, seizures, and cardiac arrest. Phase 3 is cardiovascular or central nervous system collapse. In the last phase, the secondary complications may include renal failure, pulmonary edema, and asystole.

Clinical Management

All basic and advanced life support measures should be implemented. Gastric decontamination should be performed. Monoamine oxidase inhibitors readily bind to activated charcoal. Aggressive supportive care should be instituted. Hypertension should be managed with intravenous sodium nitroprusside or with phentolamine. Sublingual nifedipine has also been reported to be effective in controlling hypertension. Agitation, muscle rigidity, and seizures may be controlled with intravenous diazepam. The hypotensive patient should be placed in Trendelenburg's position and given intravenous fluids. Additional hypotensive therapy may include norepinephrine or dopamine administration. Hemodialysis and hemoperfusion have not been shown to lead to any improvement in clinical status.

Animal Toxicity

Monoamine oxidase inhibitors are not used therapeutically in animals. Toxicity would be expected to resemble that observed in humans.

—Douglas J. Borys

Related Topic

Neurotoxicology: Central and Peripheral

Monosodium Glutamate

- CAS: 142-47-2
- SYNONYMS: Chinese seasoning; glutamic acid, sodium salt; α-monosodium glutamate; monosodium L-glutamate; MSG; sodium glutamate; sodium L-glutamate
- CHEMICAL CLASS: Acidic amino acid salt

Uses

Monosodium glutamate (MSG) is used as a flavor enhancer to impart a "meaty" flavor to foods.

Exposure Pathways

Exposure to MSG is usually through ingestion.

Mechanism of Toxicity

MSG is believed to exert effects on the central nervous system (CNS) and the eye through prolonged depolarization, energy depletion, and ionic imbalance in affected neurons. These conditions produce neuronal deterioration and destruction. The term "excitotoxin" is sometimes used to refer to MSG and other compounds that produce similar effects.

Human Toxicity

The toxicity of MSG in humans is generally low; however, based on animal studies, MSG is not recommended as an ingredient in baby foods. Anecdotal evidence suggests that adults who eat foods high in MSG content may experience burning sensations in the mouth, facial pressure, chest pains, and headache. This list of symptoms has been termed the "Chinese Food Syndrome" due to the reported link to Chinese foods high in MSG. The estimated dose of MSG in these reports ranged from 50 to 100 mg/kg. Symptoms similar to those which occur when individuals who are taking monoamine oxidase inhibitors are challenged with foods containing tyramine have been reported following large (4 g or less) oral exposure to MSG. CNS and reproductive effects observed in animal studies have not been confirmed in human subjects.

Clinical Management

Acute, life-threatening effects from MSG exposure are unlikely. Individuals who experience effects following oral ingestion should avoid foods containing MSG.

Animal Toxicity

MSG has been demonstrated to produce localized lesions in the CNS of neonatal mice and rats and may produce similar effects in monkeys. CNS lesions are confined to the arcuate nucleus of the hypothalamus and to areas that are not well protected by the blood–brain barrier. This effect is not believed to be specific to MSG because it may be produced by other acidic amino acids (aspartate and cysteine). Retinal lesions have also been reported in neonatal mice exposed to MSG through suckling and in mature animals injected with MSG. Male reproductive capacity effects and increased body weight have also been associated with neonatal exposure to MSG.

The oral LOAEL in rats is 1315 gm/kg for neonatal effects and 19500 mg/kg for effects on the embryo or fetus and cytological changes. The oral LD_{50} in mice is 11400 mg/kg.

—Linda Larsen

Related Topic

Neurotoxicology: Central and Peripheral

Morning Glory

- SYNONYMS: *Ipomoea violacea; Ipomoea tricolor;* pearly gates; wedding bells
- DESCRIPTION: Morning glory is a climbing vine with blue, white, or red trumpet-shaped flowers that open in the morning and close in the afternoon. The leaves are green and heart shaped. A papery thin pod holds small black seeds.

Use

Morning glory seeds are abused for their hallucinogenic effect.

Exposure Pathway

Exposure is via ingestion.

Mechanism of Toxicity

The seeds may contain up to 0.05% total alkaloids of lysergic acid amide (ergine), isolysergic acid (erginine), ergonovine, lysergic acid methyl carbinolamide, and various clavine alkaloids. The toxic effect is similar to that of lysergic acid diethylamide (LSD).

LSD acts on several sites in the central nervous system (CNS). Most notably, it is found to have an agonistic effect on presynaptic and postsynaptic seratonin receptor sites. As seratonin is displaced, sensory and higher cortical neurons experience increased electrical firing that cause perceptual and thought distortions. Hallucinations are initiated and sustained by the inhibition and potentiation of other neuron centers of the brain. Seratonin inhibition may also reduce platelet aggregation and cause bleeding disorders.

Human Toxicity

Symptoms include nausea, disorientation, delusions, hallucinations, psychosis, panic reactions, paranoia, violent behavior, prolonged changes in perception and sensation, and suicidal ideations. A few morning glory seeds are unlikely to cause significant problems. Several packages of seeds must be eaten to produce toxic effects in adults. Seeds may not release toxins unless chewed. Three hundred seeds may have a potency equivalent to 200–300 μg LSD, an amount sufficient to produce an altered state of consciousness. Twenty to fifty seeds may result in increased sociability, restlessness, and alertness followed by a period of relaxation. One hundred to one hundred and fifty seeds results in hallucinations, perceptual changes, and improved mood lasting up to 4 hr. Two hundred to five hundred seeds will cause euphoria, hallucinations, and philosophical thought. Adverse side effects are likely at this dose and include nausea, vomiting, abdominal pain, fatigue peripheral temperature, and sensation changes.

Clinical Management

Standard decontamination methods are rarely needed due to the rapid absorption of the agent and the likelihood that their use will exacerbate the patient's emotionalism. The patient's environment should be managed to prevent self-harm and to promote calmness. Acute anxiety can be managed with intravenous diazepam and haloperidol for psychotic behavior. Symptoms usually resolve in 8 hr. Close psychiatric follow-up may be needed if symptoms persist.

—Regina Wiechelt

Morphine

- CAS: 57-27-2
- SYNONYMS: 7,8-Didehydro-4, 5-epoxy-17-methylmorphinan-3,6-diol morphine acetate; morphine CHM; morphine sulfate
- PHARMACEUTICAL CLASS: Opiate analgesic; an alkaloid and phenanthrene derivative of opium
- CHEMICAL STRUCTURE:

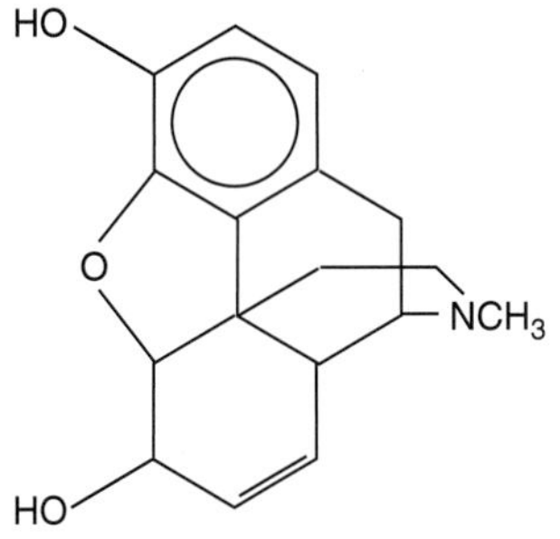

HO

O

NCH_3

HO

Uses

Morphine is used as an analgesic for acute and severe pain, as a sedative, as an antitiussive, and for treatment of dyspnea in left ventricular failure and acute pulmonary edema. It has drug abuse potential.

Exposure Pathways

Morphine is available for oral and rectal administration. Parenteral usage can be by subcutaneous, intramuscular, intravenous, or continuous infusion. It is a drug of abuse and can be nasally insufflated.

Toxicokinetics

Morphine is rapidly absorbed from the gastrointestinal tract after oral administration. The bioavailability is poor though, since it undergoes extensive first-pass metabolism in the liver and gut. Oral morphine is about one-sixth as potent as morphine administered parenterally. After parenteral injection, morphine is readily absorbed into the blood. Peak effects occur within 30 min to 1 hr. Morphine is metabolized in the liver by N-demethylation. The majority of a dose of morphine is conjugated with glucuronic acid in the liver and gut to its major metabolite morphine-3-glucuronide, which is inactive, and the active metabolite morphine-6-glucuronide. Other active metabolites include normorphine, codeine, and morphine ethereal sulfate. Enterohepatic circulation of conjugated and intestinally deconjugated morphine has been reported. Morphine is distributed throughout the body, but mainly in the kidneys, liver, lungs, and spleen. Approximately 35% is protein bound. The volume of distribution is 3 or 4 liters/kg. Mean plasma elimination half-life is 1.7 hr for morphine and 2.4–6.7 hr for morphine-3-glucuronide. Up to 10% of a dose may eventually be excreted, as conjugates, through the bile into the feces. The remainder is excreted in the urine, mainly as conjugates.

Mechanism of Toxicity

Morphine's toxicity stems mainly from its extensive effect on the central nervous system (CNS), principally that of a descending depression. Opioids interact with stereospecific and saturable binding sites mostly located in the CNS. Interaction with the opioid receptors mimics the actions of endogenous enkephlins and endorphins. Their action also appears to involve an alteration in the release of neurotransmitters, such as the inhibition of acetylcholine, norepinepherine, and dopamine. These actions result in the therapeutic effects of analgesia, sedation, euphoria, and decreased gastrointestinal motility; however, in toxic amounts they can lead to respiratory depression, coma, and cardiovascular collapse.

Human Toxicity: Acute

Symptoms of toxicity may occur in varying degrees in nontolerant adults who receive greater than a therapeutic amount of morphine. The primary insult is respiratory depression from direct depression of the CNS. This state may then progress to apnea or respiratory arrest. Pulmonary edema is a common complication. Therapeutically morphine results in analgesia; however, when toxic, neurologic depression results in coma. Miosis is frequent, but in an acidotic or asphyxiated state pupils may be dilated. From a cardiovascular perspective, morphine causes a decrease in systemic vascular resistance, which may result in a fall in systemic arterial pressure, thus leading to severe hypotension. A decrease in sympathetic tone can yield bradycardia. Hypothermia may also ensue with peripheral vasodilation. Laboratory analysis of morphine is useful only as confirmation of its presence; it does not dictate treatment. Semiquantitative and qualitative EMIT homogenous enzyme immunoassays are available for measurement of opiates in urine.

Human Toxicity: Chronic

Opiates have a high potential for abuse. Chronic users may develop tolerance, thus necessitating larger doses for the desired effect. Toxic effects in chronic abuse can yield a decrease in immunity leading to frequent infections and possible AIDS. Abrupt cessation can cause withdrawal, yielding restlessness, vomiting, and diarrhea.

Clinical Management

Basic life-support measures should be instituted as necessary. Intensive support therapy may be required to correct respiratory failure and shock. Respirations must be supported and monitored until all symptoms disappear. Pulmonary edema should be managed with appropriate ventilatory support. If taken orally, gastrointestinal decontamination should be based on the patient's level of consciousness and history of ingestion. Gastric lavage is preferable to emesis if there is any evidence of loss of consciousness or decrease in gag reflex. Activated charcoal may be used to adsorb morphine. A cathartic may be given to enhance elimination of the activated charcoal : morphine complex. The specific antagonist naloxone is used to counteract respiratory depression and coma. A dose of 0.4–2.0 mg is given intravenously and can then be repeated at intervals of 2 or 3 min. The therapeutic effect of naloxone may be of shorter duration than that of the opiate activity; therefore, a naloxone continuous infusion may then be of benefit. Arterial blood gases, vital signs, and level of consciousness should be monitored continuously until cessation of symptoms.

Animal Toxicity

Dogs act similarly to humans—symptoms may include drowsiness, ataxia, vomiting, respiratory depression, miosis, coma, and hypotension. Opiates and their derivatives have an excitatory effect on the CNS of cats and horses. Naloxone may be used at 0.02 mg/kg if needed.

—Lisa Scheuring-Mroz

Related Topic

Poisoning Emergencies in Humans

Mouse Lymphoma Assay

The L5178Y 3.7.2C $tk^{+/-}$ mouse lymphoma cell mutation assay (MLA), developed in the late 1960s and early 1970s by Donald Clive, then at the NIEHS, measures loss of heterozygosity (LOH) as a result of forward mutations ($tk^{+/-} \rightarrow tk^{-/-}$) and allele loss ($tk^{+/-} \rightarrow tk^{0/-}$) at the thymidine kinase (*tk*) locus on mouse chromosome 11b. LOH and allele loss are significant mutagenic events, particularly when tumor suppressor genes are involved, as has been found in most human tumors, and mouse chromosome 11 is homologous to human chromosome 17, with both containing the loci for the important *p53* and BRCA1 tumor suppressor genes as well as *tk*.

In the MLA, suspension cultures of 3.7.2C cells, recently "cleansed" of spontaneous mutants, are exposed for about 4 hr to a series of dilutions of the test chemical, in the absence and presence of an exogenous S9 metabolic activation system. Following chemical exposure, the cells are grown in suspension culture for an additional 2-day expression period, during which the thymidine kinase enzyme and RNA coding for thymidine kinase are depleted in cells with the mutant genotype. Following expression, the cells are immobilized by cloning them in soft agar cloning medium, or in microtiter plates, in the absence of the selective agent to assess cloning efficiency and in the presence of the selective agent to assess mutant frequency. After growth for an additional 2 weeks, the resulting colonies are counted and sized, and the results are evaluated to determine whether the test chemical induced a biologically relevant increase in thymidine kinase-deficient mutants.

The origins of the 3.7.2C cells date to the early 1950s, when L. W. Law, at NCI, induced tumors in female DBA/2 mice by painting them with 3-methylcholanthrene and isolated several leukemic cell lines, including L5178, which were then carried in mice as intraperitoneal ascites cultures (L = Law, leukemic, or lymphoma). In the late 1950s, G. Fischer at Yale University succeeded in growing the L5178 cells in a semidefined medium, which bears has name, and identified one clone of cells as L5178Y (Y = Yale). About a decade later, Clive developed the L5178Y forward mutation assay by first treating the parental $tk^{+/+}$ cell line with ethyl methanesulfonate to obtain $tk^{-/-}$ cells then selecting spontaneous revertants to $tk^{+/-}$, including clone 3.7.2C, and he suggested that the MLA would be ideally suited for use in host-mediated assays since L5178 cells had been passaged in mice.

Only a few host-mediated MLAs were conducted, however, because, in 1971, Malling defined a system to provide metabolic activation *in vitro* which was effective in the MLA. During the 1970s and early 1980s, the *in vitro* MLA was evaluated by testing a number of chemicals, including chemicals known to be rodent carcinogens, in the absence and presence of metabolic activation. Because reproducibility and a high concordance of MLA results with carcinogenicity were obtained in the validation studies, the MLA has been used extensively since that time as an initial test to assess the potential genetic hazards of chemicals. However, the MLA, and definition of mechanisms of mutagenesis operable in the MLA, has changed significantly since the early validation studies.

When the MLA was defined in 1975, bromodeoxyuridine (BUdR) was the selective agent. However, in the mid-1980s it was found that, because it is necessary for the cells to undergo one or more rounds of DNA synthesis to incorporate BudR, which results in a hazy "background lawn" of $tk^{+/-}$ cells in mutant colony plates, trifluorothymidine, which rapidly inhibits thyidylate synthetase, was a better selective agent. When the background lawns were eliminated, a bimodal distribution of mutant colony sizes was revealed, with two basic mutant phenotypes distinguished based on colony size: large (λ) colony mutants which have cytogenetically normal 11b chromosomes and small (σ, slowly growing) colony mutants which often have cytogenetic damage to chromosome 11b that can be detected in conventionally stained and banded chromosomes. Hence, λ colony mutants are generally considered to be the result of gene mutations, and chemicals that induce an elevated number of σ colony mutants are generally considered to be clastogens (chromosome-breaking chemicals).

Small colony mutants are detected in the MLA because *tk* is a homozygous locus, which permits cytogenetically damaged cells to survive, a significant feature because chromosomal mutations occupy a central role in carcinogenesis and chromosomal alterations are associated with infertility, spontaneous abortion, and congenital malformation. In contrast, cytogenetically damaged cells do not survive in mammalian cell mutagenesis assays (such as *hgprt*) that measure effects at hemizygous loci. Hence, if one of the latter assays is used for regulatory submissions, an *in vitro* cytogenetic assay is usually required to assess the potential of a test material to induce chromosomal mutations, which may increase the overall time and expense of initial testing.

Because chemicals can induce a continuous spectrum of genetic damage, from alterations at the molecular level to extensive damage (including deletions, chromosomal breakage, and rearrangements) before toxic levels are reached, it is necessary to conduct the MLA using procedures that maximize σ colony mutant recovery in order to obtain complete information on this spectrum of genetic events. Unfortunately, although the MLA has been used to test several hundred chemicals, too frequently procedures that maximize σ colony mutant recovery have not been used, resulting in an apparent failure of the assay to detect a number of clastogenic chemicals. Conversely, alarm was expressed and use of the MLA declined when common chemicals such as NaCl (i.e., table salt) were found positive in the MLA, although it was subsequently shown that, in *in vitro* assays, particularly in the presence of exogenous metabolic activation, such false-positive results are avoided if exposure conditions are monitored and adjusted to preclude acidic pH shifts and high osmolality.

In NTP testing in the mid- to late 1980s, a sizable group of chemicals were evaluated in the MLA that yielded increased mutant frequencies, but only at highly toxic levels, and the results were then evaluated by the NTP using a statistical approach that identified as significantly positive many results that were without biological relevance. Thus, when the NTP compared the concordance of results obtained in four *in vitro* tests with the outcome of rodent carcinogenicity bioassays, it was stated that, although few positive results were obtained for noncarcinogens in the Ames test in *Salmonella typhimurium* or in the test for chromosomal aberrations in CHO cells, an unacceptably high number of "false-positive" results were obtained in the *in vitro*

SCE assay and the MLA. The NTP retained the SCE assay to augment cytogenetic testing, although SCE tests have been largely discontinued by industry and are recommended by regulatory agencies only on a very limited basis. However, the NTP essentially discontinued use of the MLA which, together with the other problems noted previously, led many industrial laboratories to discontinue use of the MLA.

It has been shown, however, that the finding of apparently poor concordance of the MLA with rodent carcinogenesis was the result of the NTP's application of acceptability and evaluation criteria that are considered inappropriate by experts in this assay, who found over 40% of the NTP test results to be equivocal, inconclusive, or invalid. When the MLA results for the remaining chemicals were compared with rodent carcinogenesis, concordance was higher than for these chemicals in any of the three other short-term tests evaluated in the same comparison. Furthermore, all of the remaining chemicals that were negative in the MLA were noncarcinogens, and all of the noncarcinogens that yielded positive results in the MLA were chemicals that have been shown to induce chromosomal damage *in vitro*.

Thus, when the MLA is conducted in an appropriate manner and the results are evaluated based on generally accepted, biologically relevant criteria, the MLA has been shown to yield few positive results for noncarcinogens and to detect known carcinogens that yield negative results in bacterial mutagenesis assays, which is apparently related to the MLA's ability to detect clastogens that cannot be detected in bacteria. Hence, with strong advocacy of this system by scientists experienced in its use, the MLA has been retained (together with the Ames and micronucleus tests) as one of the three initial genotoxicity tests most frequently specified and used for national and international regulatory submissions.

—*Ann D. Mitchell*

Related Topics

Ames Test
Analytical Toxicology
Carcinogenesis
Chromosome Aberrations
Developmental Toxicology
Dominant Lethal Tests
Host-Mediated Assay
Molecular Toxicology
Mutagenesis
Sister Chromatid Exchange
Toxicity Testing

Mouthwash

- SYNONYMS: Cepacol; Listerine; Listermint; Scope; Signal
- DESCRIPTION: Commercially available mouthwashes may contain ethanol in concentrations of 14–27% (v/v), water, flavor, sweetener, preservative, color, and an astringent. Ethanol is a universal diluent that is mildly polar, able to easily cross cell membranes, and considered the toxic constituent in mouthwashes.

Use

Mouthwash is used to improve oral hygiene.

Exposure Pathways

Ingestion is the most common route of both accidental and intentional exposure to mouthwash. Ocular exposure is also a possible route of exposure.

Toxicokinetics

Ethanol absorption through the stomach wall is minimal. Since rapid absorption occurs in the small intestine, factors that delay or enhance gastric emptying will influence the rate of absorption of ethanol into the blood. The enzymatic oxidation of ethanol occurs primarily in the liver, first to acetaldehyde by the enzyme alcohol dehydrogenase and then conversion to acetic acid by the enzyme aldehyde dehydrogenase. Acetic acid is available for the formation of acetyl coenzyme A, which enters the Krebs cycle and is eventually metabolized to carbon dioxide and water. Ethanol is uniformly distributed throughout all tissues and body fluids. The volume of distribution approximates 0.47–0.6 liters/kg. Approximately 2–10% is eliminated by the kidneys and lungs. Ethanol follows Michaelis–Menton kinetics. Therefore, half-life determination is not meaningful. An average adult decreases blood ethanol levels by 15–20 mg/dl/hr.

Mechanism of Toxicity

The toxic component of commercial mouthwash products is ethanol. Ethanol is a central nervous system depressant that selectively depresses the reticular activating system, resulting in disruption of the motor and thought processes. Preferential suppression of inhibitory neurons most likely causes the excitation seen at low ethanol concentrations.

Human Toxicity: Acute

Since common commercially available mouthwashes contain only moderate concentrations of ethanol, casual ingestions will produce no toxicity. Significant ingestions, which result in blood alcohol levels of >100 mg/dl may result in ataxia, slurred speech, decreased motor skills, diplopia, and decreased attention. Unpredictable hypoglycemia may occur in children. Extreme ingestions, resulting in blood alcohol concentrations of >300 mg/dl, may result in vision impairment, stupor, or respiratory failure. Mouthwashes may be irritating to the eyes on contact.

Human Toxicity: Chronic

The complications of ethanol abuse are many. Ethanol-containing mouthwash products may be used by a chronic abuser as an alcohol substitute.

Clinical Management

Basic and advanced life-support measures should be utilized as necessary. Gastrointestinal decontamination procedures should be used as deemed appropriate to the patient's level of consciousness and the history of the ingestion. Casual ingestions of mouthwash do not necessitate treatment.

Ocular exposures require immediate flushing of the affected eye(s) with a steady stream of tepid water for a minimum of 15 min. If ocular irritation persists, an ophthalmology consult is required.

Treatment of chronic alcohol toxicity involves replacement of nutritional deficiencies such as thiamine, pyridoxine, and vitamins K and C. Correction of dehydration, electrolyte imbalance, and acid-base imbalances is of paramount importance. Chronic abuse may be associated with dependence liability.

Animal Toxicity

Animal toxicity corresponds to ethanol toxicity in humans.

—*Bonnie S. Dean*

Multiple Chemical Sensitivities

Introduction

The constellation of symptoms that has come to be known as multiple chemical sensitivities (MCS) is increasingly recognized, although the definition of the phenomenon is elusive and its pathogenesis as a distinct entity is unconfirmed. Reports of patients with MCS are increasing, but information on its natural history is lacking. Individuals diagnosed with MCS do not exhibit a specific symptom pattern; a wide range of individual symptoms have been described with the most prominent symptoms being cardiorespiratory (nasal congestions and breathing difficulties), constitutional (fatigue and weakness), and neuropsychologic (memory loss and mood or personality changes). These symptoms are similar to those seen in other syndromes such as chronic fatigue syndrome. In MCS, however, the symptoms have been attributed to chemical exposure. The diagnostic label of MCS is primarily used by a group of physicians who are called clinical ecologists. A description or diagnostic categorization of MCS, which would more readily allow animal modeling and clinical testing, has been difficult due to the involvement of multiple organ systems, lack of consistent symptomatology, and/or the absence of objective and measurable endpoints (either physical or laboratory findings). No pathophysiologic mechanism for these symptoms has been established although several speculative theories have been proposed: (1) MCS is a purely biologic or psychobiologic response to exposure to low levels of chemicals, (2) MCS is a misdiagnosis of physical or psychologic illness, or (3) MCS is a illness belief system shaped by the patient's culture and is possibly iatrogenic.

Four hypotheses with regard to the first theory have been invoked to explain the symptoms of MCS: (1) altered immune regulation, (2) neurogenic inflammation, (3) neurologic sensitization of the limbic system by odor, and (4) variations in an individual's biochemical makeup. Experimental models to test these hypotheses have not been established, thereby slowing research into mechanisms.

Definition

The first definition of MCS was created by Theron Randolph in 1962. Randolph described MCS as a condition that (1) is acquired; (2) includes physical and mental symptoms that can be triggered by chemical exposure; (3) has a specific adaptation syndrome (i.e., adaptation to chemicals is followed by chronic illness, withdrawal symptoms upon removal, and shock upon reexposure); (4) is characterized by a spreading phenomena (i.e., an intolerance to an increasing number of environmental chemicals); and (5) may be resolved by avoidance of chemicals.

Another definition was put forth by M. E. Cullen and his clinical definition is most commonly used. Although no definition is widely accepted, the Cullen definition allows physicians to distinguish MCS from other collections of similar, commonly experienced symptoms. There are four important characteristics of this definition:

> (1) MCS is acquired in relation to some documentable environmental exposure that may initially have produced a demonstrable toxic effect. This aspect excludes patients with long-standing health problems who later attribute certain symptoms to chemical exposure. (2) Symptoms involve more than one organ system, and recur and abate in response to predictable environmental stimuli. (3) Symptoms are elicited by exposures to chemicals that are demonstrable but very low. The exposures eliciting symptoms may be several standard deviations below the average exposures known to cause toxic or irritant health effects in humans and typically involve chemicals of widely varied structural classes and different mechanisms of toxicologic action. (4) The manifestations of MCS are subjective. No widely available test of organ system function can explain symptoms, and there is no objective evidence of organ system damage or dysfunction.

This definition is derived from Cullen (1987) and quoted exactly due to the need to precisely define the contribution of environmental exposure and to distinguish MCS from objectively defined illnesses such as asthma.

One problem with these definitions is that the relationship between the symptoms and the exposure is solely dependent on the patient's report. A recent definition by Ashford and Miller is an operational definition; that is, if symptoms disappear on removal from the agent and recur with specific challenges, then one can infer a causal association. In this definition, the rechallenge must be done under strictly controlled environmental conditions.

Theories of Etiology of MCS

Biologic and Psychobiologic Mechanisms

MCS, as defined by clinical ecologists, results from chemical exposure; however, the mechanisms that have been proposed include altered immune function, neurogenic inflammation, neurologic sensitization, and conditioned reflexes. To date, no mechanism has been established.

Various immunologic mechanisms have been postulated based on case reports. Alterations in various measures of antibody and cell-mediated immunity have been measured in patients with MCS, but no consistent pattern of abnormalities has been observed. Several factors, however, confound these studies: lack of standardization of protocols, wide variability (day to day and person to person) with most tests, lack of control for variables known to modulate the immune system (e.g., stress and smoking), and lack of concordance in reports of immune function response. In addition, despite some similarities in symptomatology, MCS is distinctly different from traditional allergy. Patients with allergy generally have well-defined, clinical reactions to allergens and symptoms of rhinitis, asthma, urticaria, or gastrointestinal symptoms occur shortly after exposure. In addition, if a substance acts as an allergen, a specific cell- or antibody-mediated response develops so the body will only recognize the precise antigen or one with the same structure. It is difficult to explain how structurally different chemicals could result in such diverse symptomatology and organ involvement due to an adverse effect on the immune system.

Another postulated mechanism is an altered function of the central nervous and respiratory systems through an amplification of a nonspecific inflammatory response to low-level irritants (neurogenic inflammation hypothesis). This suggests that MCS may be initiated by the interaction of chemical irritants with sensory nerves or C-fiber neurons, a nonspecific response pathway. It is proposed that inhaled chemicals stimulate irritation receptors which activate sensory nerves to release mediators producing vasodilation, edema, and other manifestations of inflammation, leading to neurogenic inflammation. There is some evidence in animals for this theory, though similar studies in humans do not generally support this theory. In animals, nasal irritation activates systemic reflexes, producing increased blood pressure and bradycardia.

Another hypothesis speculates that environmental chemicals gain access to the central nervous system via the olfactory and limbic pathways. The absence of a blood–brain barrier in the olfactory system could permit direct access of environmental chemicals through the nasal mucosa to the olfactory bulb. The olfactory and limbic systems are anatomically linked and participate directly and indirectly in the regulation of cognitive, endocrine, and immune functions. In this hypothesis, chemical exposure could induce lasting changes in limbic and neuronal activity and alter a broad spectrum of behavioral and physiological functions.

Animal studies show the olfactory and limbic pathways are particularly susceptible to kindling. Animal studies also show that acute administration of a high dose or intermittent repeated low-dose exposures to chemicals cause limbic "kindling," the ability of a stimulus previously unable to induce a seizure to later induce one, and that this response is amplified depending on the time between stimuli. Kindling without a seizure has been shown to cause affective behavior changes in animals. Kindling could amplify reactivity and lower the threshold response to low levels of chemicals.

Additionally, cacosmia, a subjective sense of altered olfactory function and feeling ill on exposure to chemical odors, which is experienced by many MCS patients, might be associated with neurocognitive dysfunction. However, MCS patients do not demonstrate a consistent or specific pattern of neurocognitive deficits and disturbances of memory and attention, which may be a result of depression and anxiety. Some have suggested that cascosmia as well as MCS may be a manifestation of a stress response. The "precipitating event" leads to stress and may lead to heightened sensitivity to chemical odors or irritants. Animal studies suggest that exposure to a stressor produces a long-lasting sensitization to some drugs. In surveys of students, individuals reporting extreme cascosmia also had higher incidences of anxiety and depression.

Biochemical mechanisms have also been suggested to explain the symptoms associated with MCS. One hypothesis states that individuals who have genetically or nutritionally defective enzyme detoxification systems might be more susceptible to exposure to low levels of chemicals. Another hypothesis states that chemicals may cause blood vessel constriction, inflammation, or leaking in multiple organ systems which would produce various combinations of symptoms.

Arguing against biologic alterations by chemicals as a cause of MCS symptoms is the observation the patients attribute their symptoms to levels of chemicals much lower than those to which others are occupationally exposed with no adverse effects. Therefore, the relationship of MCS symptoms to chemical exposure does not meet accepted toxicologic principles. In addition, the current evidence and models do not meet the criterion set forth in toxicology to establish a causal relationship between chemicals and MCS, such as strength of association, consistency, specificity, temporality, biologic gradient, and plausibility.

Misdiagnosis

As stated, some physicians believe MCS symptoms are not due to chemical exposure but may be the result of misdiagnosed physical or psychologic illness. Many investigators have concluded that MCS patients are not significantly different from psychiatric patients who do not project their disorder onto the environment. Studies show that patients with MCS met criterion for depression, anxiety, somatization, and obsessive–compulsive and personality disorders. Psychiatric evaluations have shown that MCS may be a new variant of a "somatoform disorder." In addition, studies show that psychologic mechanisms are important in the manifestation, if not the etiology, of MCS. Since it is theoretically possible that MCS produces the psychiatric symptoms, through chemical exposure, lifestyle limitations, or nonbelief of family members, studies have been conducted to attempt to evaluate the presence of psychiatric illness in patients that predated the onset of MCS symptoms. While these studies are ongoing and there is difficulty in discerning the temporal pattern of disease, most of them indicate that the prevalence of somatization symptom pattern among MCS patients prior to onset of symptoms attributed to chemical exposure was significantly greater than that in matched controls. These studies also show that there was no apparent difference in the prevalence of preexisting anxiety or depression. However, there are a small number of persons diagnosed with MCS who do not have histories of psychiatric disorders who should be more closely examined for possible mechanisms.

MCS as a Belief System

Others suggest that MCS is a belief system that is supported and reinforced by the clinical ecology subculture. Within this model, the cause of the illness is believed to be outside the control of the patients and leads to the role of a victim with adversarial interactions with those who do not share the belief system, such as conventional health care providers. MCS shares many features, such as pain, fatigue, and headache, with several syndromes, such as chronic fatigue syndrome, fibromyalgia, and neurasthenia, with few or no objective findings of pathology which encompass patients with functional disability. A factor that may contribute to this culturally shaped illness belief system is the increasing concern of the public regarding health effects of chemical exposure. It is unlikely that the majority of MCS patients are simulating their symptoms or that the symptoms result from suggestion. However, it is likely that the attribution of the symptoms to chemical exposure is due to suggestion in some cases. It is also likely that a patient's beliefs regarding illness modifies the expression of symptoms even when resulting from a direct toxic effect of a chemical.

Conclusions

To understand the phenomenon of MCS will require interaction among many disciplines to allow for the examination of the influence of the mind on the body and the influence of physical disease on the psyche. Illness should not be regarded as less "real" because psychogenic mechanisms may play a major role in causation, and this should not prevent treatment of the symptoms. It addition, patients diagnosed with MCS are heterogenous and there may be more than one causal mechanism in each person. Since none of the views described have substantial scientific support, dogmatic adherence to any one theory is unwise, particularly by the physician.

Further Reading

Cullen, M. E. (1987). The worker with multiple chemical sensitivities: An overview. In *Occupational Medicine: State of the Art Reviews* (M. R. Cullen, Ed.), pp. 655–661. Philadelphia, BC Decker.

Multiple chemical sensitivities: A symposium on the state of the science (1992). *Regul. Toxicol. Pharmacol.* 18.

National Research Council (1992). *Multiple Chemical Sensitivities.* NRC Press, Washington, DC.

—Kathleen Rodgers

Related Topics

Immune System
Neurotoxicology: Central and Peripheral
Occupational Toxicology
Psychological Indices of Toxicity

Mushrooms, Coprine

- Species Names: *Coprinus atramentarius*; *Coprinus insignis*; *Coprinus variegatus* (also known as *C. quadrifidus*); possibly other coprinus species

- Synonyms: Inky-caps; disulfiram-like; Antabuse-like
- Chemical Structure: (Coprine)

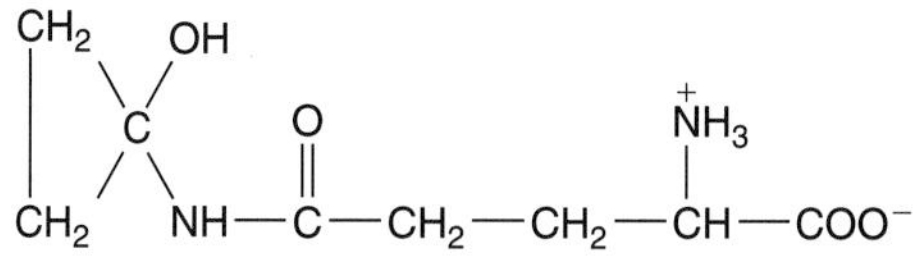

CH_2 OH
C O $\overset{+}{N}H_3$
CH_2 NH—C—CH_2—CH_2—CH—COO^-

Uses

There are not any uses for mushrooms in this group. One is usually consumed when mistaken for an edible mushroom.

Exposure Pathway

Ingestion is the route of exposure.

Toxicokinetics

Symptoms occur within 20 min to 2 hr after the ingestion of this mushroom and ethanol. The effect of coprine may persist for up to 5 days after ingestion of the mushroom.

Mechanism of Toxicity

Poisoning with mushrooms in this group occurs when ethanol is consumed shortly before or within 5 days after eating the mushrooms. Coprine [*N*(5)-(1-hydroxy cyclopropyl)-L-glutamine] is the active constituent in these mushrooms and has been shown to inhibit liver aldehyde dehydrogenase. Its active metabolite, cyclopropanone hydrate, has also been shown to possess similar activity. This inhibition of ethanol metabolism at the point of aldehyde dehydrogenase results in accumulation of acetaldehyde. In the absence of concurrent ethanol consumption, these mushrooms are edible.

Human Toxicity: Acute

When these mushrooms and ethanol are consumed within the appropriate time frame, symptoms typically develop within 20 min to 2 hr. The reaction resembles a disulfiram-ethanol reaction. Symptoms commonly include nausea, vomiting, facial flushing, throbbing headache, weakness, and paresthesias. Less frequently, chest pain, hypotension, and shortness of breath have been seen. No laboratory methods are available for determining the presence of coprine in biologic fluids.

Clinical Management

Because the syndrome is self-limiting and recovery is complete, symptomatic care is often all that is required. Emesis is not indicated because often many hours have elapsed since the ingestion of the mushroom. Also, vomiting is a prominent feature of this type of poisoning and induced emesis may worsen fluid and electrolyte losses. There is no evidence that activated charcoal and/or cathartics provide any benefit in this syndrome. Experimentally, 4-methylpyrazole inhibits the production of acetaldehyde by blocking alcohol dehydrogenase. The clinical usefulness in this type of treatment in mushroom poisoning has not been demonstrated.

Animal Toxicity

The consumption of mushrooms and ethanol concurrently is a typically human occurrence; therefore, poisoning in animals is unlikely.

—*Anthony S. Manoguerra*

Mushrooms, Cyclopeptide

- Species Names: Several genera of mushrooms contain toxic cyclopeptides; these mushrooms include but are not limited to *Amanita bisporigera; Amanita hygroscopica; Amanita ocreata; Amanita phalloides; Amanita suballiacea; Amanita tenuifolia; Amanita verna; Amanita virosa; Galerina autumnalis; Galerina fasciculata; Galerina marginata; Galerina sulcipes; Galerina venenata; Lepiota castanea; Lepiota helveola; Lepiota subincarnata; Lepiota josserandii; Conocybe filiaris.*
- Synonyms: Destroying angel (*A. virosa*); death cap (*A. phalloides*)
- Chemical Structure: (α-Amanitin)

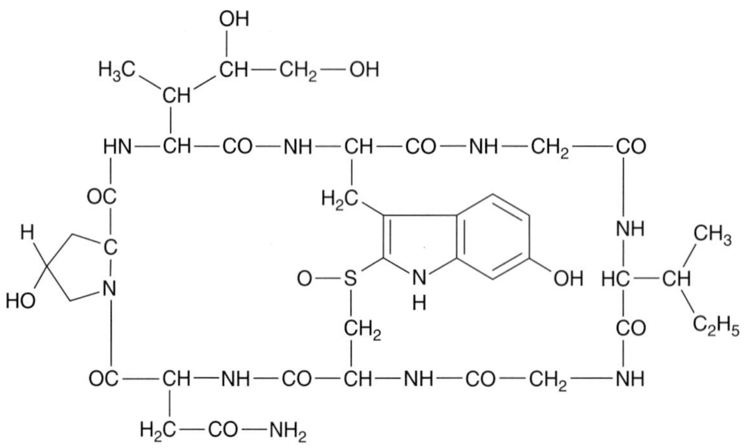

Uses

There are not any uses for mushrooms in this group. One is usually consumed when mistaken for an edible mushroom.

Exposure Pathway

Ingestion is the route of exposure.

Toxicokinetics

Amatoxins are absorbed rapidly from the gastrointestinal tract. These toxins may be detected in the urine as soon as 90–120 min after ingestion of the mushrooms. Radiolabeled amatoxins given to a dog model showed a volume of distribution equal to the volume of extracellular water (160–290 ml/kg). Amatoxins disappear rapidly from the blood because they are taken into cells rapidly. No biotransformation of amatoxins occurs. Amatoxins are found in the urine shortly after ingestion of the mushrooms and continue to be detectable for up to 96 hr after ingestion. They have also been detected in diarrhea fluid and bile.

Mechanism of Toxicity

Cyclopeptide mushrooms contain both amatoxins and phallotoxins. Studies in animals have shown that, although the phallotoxins are highly toxic when given parenterally, they are not absorbed from the gastrointestinal tract and do not produce toxicity when given orally. The toxicity of cyclopeptide mushrooms is believed to be due to the amatoxins. At least six amatoxins have been identified that differ according to amino acid substitutions on the peptide ring. The α- and β-amanitins are felt to be the predominant cyclopeptides producing systemic toxicity. The phallotoxins may contribute to gastrointestinal symptoms but this is unclear. Amatoxins interfere with RNA and DNA transcription by interfering with RNA polymerase II. Cells with the highest rate of turnover are affected most severely.

Human Toxicity

There is typically a delay of 6–24 hr between the ingestion of the mushrooms and the onset of symptoms. The first symptoms are nausea, severe vomiting, and diarrhea, which may result in severe dehydration and electrolyte imbalances. Gastrointestinal symptoms may persist for several days. Over the course of the next 24–36 hr, evidence of hepatic injury becomes evident both clinically and by laboratory measurements. Patients may progress to hepatic failure with coma, hemorrhage, and renal failure or begin to recover depending on the degree of injury. In fatal poisonings, death usually occurs after 5 or 6 days. Mortality ranges up to $\geqq 50\%$ in untreated patients and appears to be $<5\%$ in patients who receive modern intensive supportive care. The severity of poisoning also seems to correlate with the amount of toxin ingested on a body weight basis. The mortality in children appears to be greater probably because of the larger amount of toxin ingested in relation to their body size.

Clinical Management

Immediate and vigorous fluid and electrolyte replacement must be carried out. Oral activated charcoal may be given if the ingestion occurred within the previous 24 hr and severe vomiting has not yet begun. No specific antidotal therapy exists for the treatment of this ingestion, although many substances have been tried. The mainstay of therapy is meticulous supportive care.

Some authors have advocated the use of multiple dose activated charcoal or gastroduodenal drainage, but evidence for the effectiveness of these procedures is lacking. Treatment of hepatic failure follows the routine supportive procedures standard for this process. Liver transplantation has been used successfully in patients who appeared to have developed irreversible hepatic failure. Experimental studies in animals have suggested the use of high-dose penicillin G and silibinin. These substances may inhibit the uptake of amatoxins into the liver and are often given in combination in Europe. Silibinin is not available in the United States. The efficacy of these treatments in humans is unknown. Thioctic acid has also been advocated; its efficacy is unclear. It does not appear to provide any protection in experimental animal studies. It also is not available in the United States. High-dose cimetidine, high-dose vitamin C, and *n*-acetylcysteine have been studied in animals and do not provide protection against toxicity. Based on the fact that large amounts of amatoxins are found in the urine during the first 24 hr after ingestion, it has been suggested that forced diuresis may increase the excretion of the toxin. Proof of efficacy is lacking. Hemodialysis or hemoperufsion have not been shown to enhance survival and hemodialysis is only indicated as a supportive measure in patients who develop renal failure.

Animal Toxicity

Ingestions of these mushrooms in dogs have taken place both accidentally and experimentally. The toxic effects mimic those seen in humans.

—*Anthony S. Manoguerra*

Related Topic

Veterinary Toxicology

Mushrooms, Ibotenic Acid

- Species Names: *Amanita muscaria; Amanita pantherina; Amanita corthurnata*
- Synonyms: Fly-agaric; panther
- Chemical Structure:

H
O N O
CHCOOH
NH_2

Uses

There are not any uses for this mushroom. It is typically consumed for its psychopharmacologic effects.

Exposure Pathway

Ingestion is the route of exposure.

Toxicokinetics

The symptoms of intoxication seen after ingestion of this mushroom appear about 1 hr after ingestion. Ibotenic acid is converted to muscimol by decarboxylation. Ibotenic acid and muscimol can both be detected unchanged in the urine. Other metabolites found in the urine include pantherin, tricholomic acid, and solitaric acid. Intoxication with this mushroom peaks at about 5 hr after ingestion and lasts for up to 10 hr with a hangover effect the next day.

Mechanism of Toxicity

Ibotenic acid is structurally similar to glutamic acid, whereas muscimol closely resembles γ-aminobutyric acid (GABA). Muscimol has an affinity for GABA receptors in the central nervous system, functioning as a false neurotransmitter, and appears to mimic the effects of GABA.

Human Toxicity

Following the ingestion of a single mushroom, symptoms of intoxication typically appear within an hour. Nausea and vomiting are common. Users describe a typical experience where they can "view themselves from outside their own bodies along with a sense of being freed from gravity." Small objects appear large. The appearance of the user during this time may resemble someone with ethanol intoxication. On occasion, users appear to have the desire to carry out extreme physical activity followed by a deep, "death-like" sleep from which arousal is difficult. Upon wakening, users describe vivid visions during this dream period. Severe poisoning is rare, but seizures have been reported to occur in children. Deaths are said to have occurred from these mushrooms but the documentation of these occurrences is poor and the deaths may have been related to medical problems that were exacerbated by the intoxication.

Clinical Management

Most patients who ingest these mushrooms require no treatment other than observation. In recent, accidental ingestions, activated charcoal may be administered, although the efficacy of this treatment is unknown. In severe cases, when seizures occur, benzodiazepine therapy may be required. Long-term anticonvulsant therapy should not be required because the effects of the mushroom are short-lived. All other treatment is supportive and symptomatic in nature. Atropine should not be administered because these mushrooms, despite their name, contain only trace to no amounts of muscarine or other cholinergic substances.

Animal Toxicity

Animal ingestions of these mushrooms are rare and, therefore, experience is limited. Of nine puppies that supposedly had ingested *A. pantherina,* three died and the others developed seizures and the inability to walk. All survivors fully recovered by 17 hr after ingestion.

—*Anthony S. Manoguerra*

Related Topics

Neurotoxicology: Central and Peripheral
Veterinary Toxicology

Mushrooms, Monomethylhydrazine

- Species Names: *Gyromitra esculenta; Gyromitra fastigiata; Gyromitra infula; Gyromitra ambigua; Gyromitra brunnea; Gyromitra californica; Gyromitra korfii; Gyromitra sphaerospora; Gyromitra giga.* All other species of *Gyromitra* should be considered toxic unless proven edible. *Gyromitra* sp. mushrooms are nongilled mushrooms in the class Ascomycetes.
- Synonyms: False morel; beefsteak mushroom; elephant ears mushroom
- Chemical Structure:

$$CH_3—NH—NH_2$$

Uses

There are not any uses for mushrooms in this group. One is usually consumed when mistaken for an edible mushroom.

Exposure Pathways

Ingestion is the most likely route of exposure; however, it has been stated (without good documentation) that poisoning can occur from inhaling monomethylhydrazine vapors that come off in the steam during boiling of the mushrooms.

Toxicokinetics

The absorption rate is not known. Symptoms typically occur after a latent period of 6–24 hr after ingestion of the mushroom. Gyromitrin is converted to methylformylhydrazine (MFH) and then to monomethylhydrazine (MMH). Some MFH is also converted to nitrosamide, which causes liver tumors in experimental animals.

Mechanism of Toxicity

Gyromitra sp. mushrooms contain about 0.12–0.16% of the toxin Gyromitrin (*n*-methyl-*N*-formylhydrazone). This compound is very unstable and undergoes hydrolysis at low cooking temperatures to the toxic compound MMH. In some species of Gyromitra, MMH may be found in its free form and, therefore, cooking may not be required for toxicity to occur. Because MMH is highly volatile, it has been suggested that boiling of the mushroom and discarding the water may yield an edible mushroom, although cases exist in the European literature in which poisoning occurred even after the mushroom was boiled and the water discarded. MMH is thought to act similarly to other naturally occurring and synthetic hydrazines by acting as a pyridoxine antagonist. Because many enzyme systems require pyridoxine as a cofactor, hydrazines are capable of affecting numerous metabolic pathways. For example, hydrazines interfere with pyridoxine utilization by both glutamic acid decarboxylase and γ-aminobutyric acid (GABA) transaminase leading to decreased concentrations of the inhibitory neurotransmitter, GABA, in the brain and producing the resultant seizures. Hepatotoxicity is thought to result from a direct toxic action of a metabolite similar to that which occurs with isoniazid. MMH has also been shown to inhibit glycolysis; blood glucose levels fall markedly in experimental animals after exposure to MMH. MMH may also cause methemoglobinemia and hemolysis of red blood cells.

Human Toxicity: Acute

Symptoms typically appear following a 6- to-8-hr latent period; however, symptoms have been reported to occur as early as 2 hr after ingestion or as long as 24 hr after ingestion of the mushrooms. The initial symptoms are vomiting, fatigue, dizziness, and headache. In some cases, but not consistently, a watery diarrhea may also occur. In mild cases, recovery then occurs over a period of 2–5 days. In severe cases, the poisoning may progress to coma, seizures, and hepatic injury leading to hepatic coma and death. Hemolysis with a resultant anuria has also been reported.

Human Toxicity: Chronic

MMH and its precursor metabolite nitrosamide are low-grade carcinogens in experimental animals. How this relates to chronic, subacute consumption of this substance in mushrooms is unknown.

Clinical Management

Because most patients do not present for care until symptoms develop, emesis or gastric lavage are unlikely to provide much benefit. Activated charcoal administration may be considered to reduce absorption of any remaining material in the gastrointestinal tract, but proof of efficacy is lacking. Based on the resemblance to isoniazid and other hydrazine toxicity, pyridoxine has been suggested, although experience is limited. The recommended dose is 25 mg/kg given as an intravenous infusion over 15–30 min. It can be repeated to treat neurologic symptoms (seizures and coma) as needed, up to a maximum of 15–20 g a day. Seizures may also be controlled with benzodiazepines or barbiturates. Severe hemolysis may require blood transfusions and anuria may require short-term hemodialysis until renal function recovers. Hepatic injury leading to hepatic coma is treated with supportive care.

Animal Toxicity

The same pattern of toxicity that occurs in humans has been induced experimentally in small animals. The treatment is similar.

—Anthony S. Manoguerra

Related Topic

Veterinary Toxicology

Mushrooms, Muscarine

- SPECIES NAMES: Muscarine, and muscarine-like compounds, are present in varying quantities in many different species of mushrooms but reach clinically significant quantities only in certain species of *Clitocybe, Inocybe,* and *Omphalotus* mushrooms. These species include but are not limited to *Clitocybe dealbata; Clitocybe rivulosa; Clitocybe dilatata; Inocybe agglutinata; Inocybe cincinnata; Inocybe entheles; Inocybe fastigata; Inocybe geophylla; Inocybe godeyi; Inocybe griseolilacina; Inocybe lacera; Inocybe lilacina; Inocybe mixtilis; Inocybe napipes; Inocybe obscuroides; Inocybe pallidipes; Inocybe patouillardi; Inocybe pudica; Inocybe purica; Inocybe rimosus; Inocybe sororia; Inocybe subdestricta; Inocybe umbrina; Omphalotus illudens.*
- SYNONYMS: "Jack-O-Lantern" mushroom (*O. illudens*)
- CHEMICAL STRUCTURE:

H_3C ... O ... $CH_2\overset{+}{N}(CH_3)_3$, HO

Uses

There are not any uses for mushrooms in this group. One is usually consumed when mistaken for an edible mushroom.

Exposure Pathway

Ingestion is the route of exposure.

Toxicokinetics

Symptoms occur typically within 15–120 min following ingestion of the mushroom.

Mechanism of Toxicity

Mushrooms in these genera may contain varying amounts of muscarine isomers and muscarine-like compounds. L(+)Muscarine is the most potent of the muscarine isomers found. The varying amounts of these isomers in different mushrooms accounts for the diversity of reports of the severity of symptoms produced by muscarine-containing mushrooms.

Muscarine binds to the so-called "muscarinic" receptors in the parasympathetic nervous system. These are primarily postganglionic cholinergic receptors in smooth muscle and glands. Muscarine does not act on so-called "nicotinic" receptors, which are found in ganglionic synapses and at the neuromuscular junction. Muscarine is a tertiary amine structure and, therefore, does not diffuse into the central nervous system to an appreciable extent. Symptoms are, therefore, limited to the peripheral nervous system.

Human Toxicity

Stimulation of nicotinic receptors produces small pupils, blurred vision, excessive perspiration, salivation and lacrimation, bradycardia, increased intestinal peristalsis, increased pulmonary secretions, and decreased blood pressure. Acute asthma exacerbations may occur in patients with reactive airway disease. The onset is typically within 15–30 min after ingesting the mushrooms but may be delayed up to 120 min. Nausea and vomiting are often the first symptoms to occur. The rare deaths reported appear to occur from cardiovascular collapse and respiratory failure.

Clinical Management

Atropine is a competitive antagonist of muscarine at the cholinergic receptors and is therefore "antidotal" in these types of poisonings. Doses sufficient to reverse the effects of excessive pulmonary secretions and bradycardia should be administered. Activated charcoal may be useful in recent ingestions, but because most patients are having vomiting and diarrhea, its usefulness is limited and unproved.

Animal Toxicity

Toxic reactions similar to those found in humans can be induced in experimental animals and are, therefore, expected to occur following ingestion of the mushrooms. Treatment is similar to that for humans with the use of atropine.

—Anthony S. Manoguerra

Related Topics

Neurotoxicology: Central and Peripheral
Veterinary Toxicology

Mushrooms, Psilocybin

♦ Species Names: Psilocybin and psilocin have been found in the following mushroom species (as well as in others): *Psilocybe aztecorum; Psilocybe baeocystis; Psilocybe bonetti; Psilocybe caerulescens; Psilocybe caerulipes; Psilocybe candidipes; Psilocybe cambodginiensis; Psilocybe coprinifacies; Psilocybe cubensis; Psilocybe cyanescens; Psilocybe fimetaria; Psilocybe mexicana; Psilocybe pelliculosa; Psilocybe quebecensis; Psilocybe semilanceata; Psilocybe sempervira; Psilocybe serbica; Psilocybe strictipes; Psilocybe stuntzii; Psilocybe subaeruginosa; Psilocybe zapatecorum; Conocybe cyanopus; Conocybe smithii; Gymnopilus aeruginosa; Gymnopilus validipes; Panaeolus africanus;*

Panaeolus ater; Panaeolus cambodginiensis; Panaeolus fimicola; Panaeolus foenisecii; Panaeolus subalteatus; Panaeolus tropicalis.

- SYNONYMS: Hallucinogenic mushrooms; magic mushrooms; "blue legs"; "liberty caps"
- CHEMICAL STRUCTURE: (Psilocybin and Psilocin)

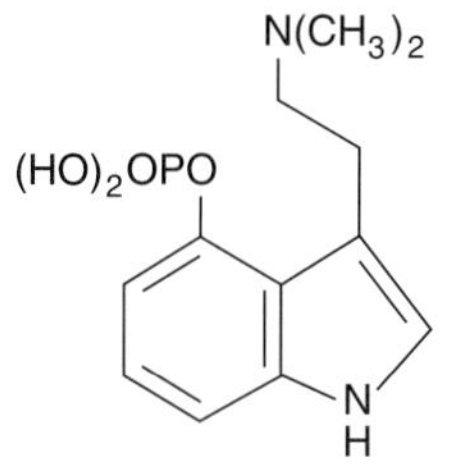

$N(CH_3)_2$

$(HO)_2OPO$

N
H

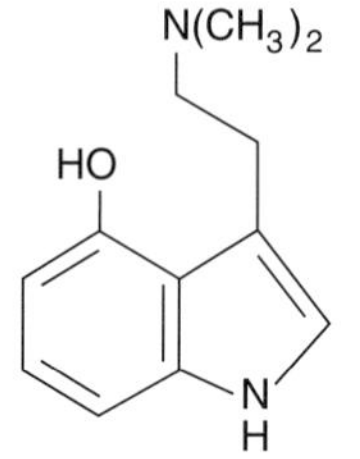

$N(CH_3)_2$

HO

N
H

Uses

There are not any uses for mushrooms in this group. These mushrooms are intentionally ingested for their hallucinogenic activity.

Exposure Pathway

Ingestion is the route of exposure.

Toxicokinetics

The onset of symptoms typically begins 20–60 min following ingestion of the mushroom, although it has been reported to be delayed up to 3 hr. The typical hallucinogenic experience lasts approximately 3 or 4 hr.

Mechanism of Toxicity

These mushrooms contain the psychoactive compound psilocybin and in some cases also the lesser active substance psilocin. Psilocybin is highly stable and is not destroyed by cooking or drying. Psilocin is rapidly destroyed by oxidation. Psilocybin can be extracted from the mushroom by boiling the mushroom in water.

The exact mechanism of action of psilocybin has not been determined, but as an indoleamine, it is thought to act similarly to LSD—as an agonist at 5-hydroxytryptamine receptors in the central nervous system.

Human Toxicity

These hallucinogenic mushrooms are small and, therefore, consumption of more than a single mushroom is required for the effects to occur. For example, two or three mushrooms of *P. cubensis* will produce the desired hallucinogenic experience, while 20–40 *P. cyanescens* are required for an equivalent experience. In addition, the concentrations of psilocybin vary significantly between species of mushrooms. Following the ingestion of an effective number of mushrooms, dizziness, giddiness, muscle twitching, restlessness, and anxiety begin within 30 min. Approximately 20% of users will also experience some nausea and vomiting. In 30–60 min, the user will begin to experience visual hallucinations and perceptual distortions. The user may experience a "good" or "bad" "trip" depending on mood, environment, and prior hallucinogenic experience. Mild tachycardia and hypertension are common during this time period. The effects of psilocybin are short-lived and recovery is typically complete in 4–6 hr. The experience usually ends with drowsiness progressing to sleep. Rare cases of flashbacks occurring 2 weeks to several months after the initial experience have been reported. Severe or life-threatening toxicity is not expected except in children or in adults who have ingested large amounts. These cases are reported to have had seizures and hyperthermia.

Clinical Management

No specific treatment is indicated for the ingestion of these mushrooms. Patients having a bad trip may require isolation in a dark, quiet environment and calm reassurance until the effects of the drug have worn off. In severe cases, sedation may be indicated. In severely symptomatic cases, seizures can be controlled with benzodiazepines and hyperthermia treated with external cooling.

Animal Toxicity

Horses and dogs have been reported to have eaten these mushrooms with predictable effects on their behavior. Treatment has included sedation or placement of the animal in a darkened, quiet environment. In severe cases seizures and hyperthermia may occur.

—Anthony S. Manoguerra

Related Topic

Neurotoxicology: Central and Peripheral

Mustard Gas

- CAS: 505-60-2
- Preferred Name: bis(2-Chloroethyl) sulfide
- Synonyms: Sulfur mustard; 1,1-thiobis(2-chloroethane); 1-chloro-2-(β-chloroethylthio)ethane; 2,2′-dichlorodiethyl sulfide; distilled mustard; S mustard; S-lost; S-yperite; Schwefel-lost; yellow cross liquid, HD, HT, H, NIOSH RETECS WQ0900000
- Chemical Class: Thioether
- Chemical Structure:

$$Cl—CH_2—CH_2—S—CH_2—CH_2—Cl$$

Uses

Mustard gas is a chemical warfare agent designed to inflict injury, principally as a skin and eye irritant, although death can result from primary and secondary effects. It does not occur naturally and has no known therapeutic application.

Exposure Pathways

Although called "mustard gas," the pure compound is a dense, yellowish oily liquid with a low vapor pressure and relatively high melting point. Hence, exposure is primarily via the skin or lungs to either the liquid or an aerosol of the agent. Exposure has resulted from the use of mustard gas as a chemical warfare agent and from accidental exposure to the agent in unexploded munitions and in manufacturing of the agent.

Toxicokinetics

Mustard gas is lipophilic and will accumulate in brain and fatty tissue. Mustard gas hydrolizes rapidly in water, although it has been detected in the blood after dermal or inhalation exposure. Products of hydrolysis and glutathione conjugation are excreted in the urine. The biological half-life of the chemical has not been published, but products are excreted in the urine for several days after acute exposure. Traces of the agent are exhaled and excreted in the feces. Several hours can pass before symptoms become manifest but this is attributed to the mechanism of action and not to direct effects of residual levels of the agent.

Mechanism of Toxicity

The mechanism of action has been attributed to the ability of the agent to directly alkylate DNA.

Human Toxicity

Mustard gas is a powerful irritant and vesicant. Dermal effects range from itching to erthema, blistering, corrosion, and necrosis. Dermal blistering is delayed in onset but slow to heal. Ocular irritation, conjunctivitis, and blindness can occur. Respiratory symptoms include a harsh and painful cough, bronchitis, sneezing, rhinorrhea, and sore throat. Mustard gas is not acutely lethal; 3 to 4% of soldiers exposed to mustard gas during World War I died of its direct effect. Death is generally due to respiratory collapse, shock, and secondary infections.

Survivors may be susceptible to bronchitis and pneumonia and may be at an increased risk to develop tumors of the respiratory tract. Mustard gas produces tumors in animal studies.

Chronic

Production workers exposed to mustard gas had increased rates of bronchitis and pneumonia. Increased incidence of tumors of the respiratory tract, lung cancer, bladder cancer, and leukemia were also found. Mustard gas is classified as a human carcinogen.

Clinical Management

It is important that the agent be washed from the skin with soap and water as soon after exposure as possible. The eyes should be thoroughly flushed. The onset of symptoms typically is delayed and an absence of immediate effect does not rule out toxicity. Although ingestion is unlikely, due to the sources of mustard gas, an emetic should not be administered because of the extreme caustic nature of the chemical. If the patient is not comatose, dilution of stomach contents with milk or water, prior to gastric lavage, may be attempted. Application of a solution of sodium thiosulfate to the skin, and inhalation of a nebulizing mist of sodium thiosulfate, may speed inactivation of mustard gas. Animal studies have shown that administration of corticosteroids (e.g., dexamethasone) and antihistamines (e.g., promethazine) may prove beneficial.

Animal Toxicity

The irritant, vesicant, and respiratory effects of mustard gas are the same in animals and humans, although the hair coat and lack of extensive sweat glands may somewhat protect the animal from the dermal effects of the agent. The grooming habits of animals may result in some exposure by the oral route.

—*Michael J. Brabec*

Related Topics

Respiratory Tract
Skin

Mutagenesis

Overview of Mutagenesis and Its Biological Significance

What is mutagenesis and why should we be concerned with this process? Mutagenesis is the process by which mutations are induced in organisms. Mutations are changes in cells that cause visible changes in hereditary traits in offspring. We know that mutations are caused by changes in the hereditary material of the cell, its deoxyribonucleic acid (DNA). These changes are transmitted to the ribonucleic acid (RNA), which is synthesized according to the instructions carried by the DNA, and then to proteins, which conduct chemical reactions in the cell or serve as structural materials, giving a cell its shape.

Mutations can have beneficial, deleterious, or no consequences. Certain mutations have a positive effect on the organism. The sickle cell mutation in hemoglobin may, for instance, give humans in Africa an ability to survive malaria better. Many mutations are neutral and have no significant effect on the organism at all. However, certain types of mutations can have deleterious consequences in organisms. An example of a deleterious mutation in humans is one that destroys the activity of an enzyme called adenosine deaminase, leading to a deficient immune system and a consequent inability to fight disease, as occurred in the famous "bubble boy." Other deleterious mutations, such as mutations in the germ cells (sperm or egg cells), can lead to a predisposition to cancer, and still others can be lethal and result in nonviable offspring. Mutation is an inevitable process, and it is occurring all the time at spontaneous rates. Mutations that lead to beneficial traits in an organism will be selected for, and mutations that lead to defects in critical cellular properties or to the death of the organism will be selected against, during the course of evolution.

During the past 90 years, we have learned a significant amount about the nature and effects of mutations on cell growth and survival and on the growth and survival of various organisms. Mutations have been most intensively studied in bacteria because bacteria grow very rapidly, and the mutations are rapidly expressed. We also know a significant amount concerning mutations in the fruitfly *Drosophila,* a significant amount concerning the effects of mutations in mice, and somewhat lesser amount concerning the effects of mutations in humans. With current methods, we can detect the presence of certain mutations believed to be deleterious in humans, and genetic counseling can occasionally help certain families.

From experimental studies, we now know that radiations and specific chemicals called mutagens can induce mutations in bacteria, in *Drosophila,* in single mouse and human cells in cell culture, in mice, and almost certainly in humans, although this has been less well studied.

A very important consideration is that radiations and specific chemical mutagens induce mutations in specific cellular genes called protooncogenes, which activate them to oncogenes. Mutagens also induce deleterious or inactivating mutations in other genes called tumor suppressor genes, inactivating them. Such mutations in somatic (nongermline) cells play a key role in carcinogenesis, or the process of cancer induction, in humans. Specific details of the types of mutations that occur in organisms and their biological significance follow.

Definition and Description of Mutations

As has been well-known since the pioneering experiments of Griffith, Avery, MacLeod, McCarty, Watson, and Crick, DNA is the genetic material of bacterial and mammalian cells. DNA encodes information in a triplet code which specifies the sequence of amino acids in proteins and the enzymatic and structural properties of cells. DNA consists of two antiparallel chains of nucleotides. Hydrogen bonds between bases on one strand and bases on the opposite strand constitute in the aggregate sufficient bond strength to keep the double helix of DNA intact. DNA is replicated in a semiconservative fashion, such that each original strand serves as a template on which a new complementary strand is replicated. In this replication, complementary DNA bases are added to bases on the original strand, such that guanine pairs opposite cytosine and thymine pairs opposite adenine.

The sequence of DNA is specified very precisely. A mutation is any change in the sequence of DNA bases from the original sequence of DNA bases. In the simplest form, during replication, the DNA polymerase enzymes can accidentally substitute an adenine for a guanine during DNA replication opposite a cytosine. This simple kind of mutation would be called a transition mutation, in which one purine, guanine, was instead replaced by another purine, an adenine base. Similarly, if during replication a pyrimidine base such as thymine was supposed to be inserted opposite an adenine base on the template strand, but instead a cytosine was inserted opposite the adenine, this would also be called a transition mutation. A transversion mutation is one in which a purine substitutes for a pyrimidine base (guanine for thymidine) or a pyrimidine base substitutes for a purine base (cytosine for adenine). These types of mutations are also called base substitution mutations.

The next more complex type of mutation is referred to as an addition or deletion mutation. In this type of mutation, either one or more bases are removed from the DNA in a deletion or one or more bases are added to the DNA in an addition mutation. Addition mutations are also called insertion mutations. Deletion mutations can be called small deletions if only a few bases are deleted from the DNA or large deletions if many bases are deleted from the DNA. The same considerations hold for small-addition and large-addition mutations.

So far, we have only considered mutations in which the genetic code is kept in register. As is commonly known, the genetic code is read in triplets, such that three nucleotides are read together to specify one specific amino acid. With base substitution mutations, one base is changed, so the amino acid specified by the new triplet nucleotide specifies a new amino acid; however, the rest of the nucleotide sequence remains the same, so the protein specified only has one amino acid changed in it. This situation is similar in the case of addition and deletion mutations, provided the addition or deletion is three bases or a multiple of three bases. Of course, in this situation, there is gain or loss of one or more amino acids, and this can have severe consequences for the resultant protein formed, depending on where in the protein the amino acids are inserted or deleted.

A special circumstance arises when one or two, or any multiple of one or two bases are deleted or inserted into a DNA sequence. In this case, as well as addition or deletion of bases, the sequence of bases encoding amino acids is now shifted. The original amino acids in the encoded protein are changed, and a new or "scrambled" protein is produced from the site of the mutation onward. Such a mutation is called a frameshift mutation since the coding frame is shifted out of its original alignment.

Another simple type of mutation that needs to be considered is gene amplification, in which a gene is copied into many more copies and these are inserted into the DNA. In mammalian cells, there is the additional complication that the DNA and its genes are arranged on discrete chromosomes. These chromosomes can be broken, and pieces from one chromosome attached to another chromosome, to form a structure known as a translocation. This can result in a deletion mutation if the sequences are not joined correctly and can also result in the translocated gene being placed next to a strong promoter element, which can cause the gene to be read more frequently, affecting the expression of this gene.

Consequences of Specific Types of Mutations

The consequences of transitions and transversions depend on where they occur in a gene coding for a protein. If they occur in a site that does not significantly change the shape of a protein used to maintain structural integrity of a cell, or in a site that does not affect the structure of an enzyme, then they do not have a significant effect on the structure of the cell or on the enzymatic activity of a protein. If, however, the transition or transversion mutation occurs in a part of the protein that significantly changes it structure or decreases its enzymatic activity, then the mutation can have severe negative consequences for the survival of the cell.

Three base additions and deletions similarly may not have severe consequences if they occur in a region of the protein that does not affect the structure of the protein or its enzymatic activity. Of course, if these deletions and additions occur in critical parts of the protein that affect its structure, or in the active site of an enzyme, they can have significant effects on cell survival and the phenotype of the cell.

In general, the frameshift type of mutation is usually deleterious to protein structure and enzymatic activity. Such mutations "scramble" the structure of the protein downstream from the mutation, and hence destroy the structural integrity of structural proteins and destroy the enzymatic activity of enzymes.

General Types of Mutagens: The Concept of Metabolic Activation

Broadly speaking, there are six general types of mutagens. First, there are mutagens that are "fraudulent" bases, or bases whose structures are similar to but somewhat different in structure than the normal bases. An example of such a base is 5-bromouracil, which is similar in structure to the normal base thymidine and can substitute for thymidine in DNA. There are a large number of base analogs that fall into this category.

Second, there is a group of mutagens called frameshift mutagens. These mutagens are, in general, large, planar aromatic molecules that can intercalate into the DNA. In the process of intercalation, the intercalators slip into the DNA and lie flat between two adjacent base pairs, with the plane of the intercalator lying flat upon the planar aromatic rings of the base pairs. Treatment of cells with this type of mutagen increases the frequency of occurrence of frameshift mutations. Examples of such mutagens include acridine orange, acriflavine, and ethidium bromide.

The third group of mutagens are the direct alkylating agents. These mutagens bind covalently to groups on the DNA bases by generating methyl and ethyl carbonium ions, which are chemically reactive and bind readily to DNA. Examples of these mutagens are *N*-methyl-*N′*-nitro-*N*-nitrosoguanidine (MNNG), methyl methanesulfonate, ethyl methanesulfonate, and epoxides such as ethylene oxide. There are also alkylating agents that have two reactive groups on the same molecule, such as nitrogen mustard. These can bind to both strands of DNA, leading to a cross-link between them, or to two places within one strand of DNA, leading to an intrastrand cross-link.

Fourth, there is a large group of mutagens referred to as premutagens or promutagens. These compounds are chemically inert and usually very hydrophobic. All organisms must metabolize these hydrophobic compounds to make them sufficiently water soluble for excretion from the cell membrane and from the organism. To do this, the organisms utilize cytochrome P450 enzymes in mammalian cells to epoxidate the hydrophobic molecules, activating them to mutagens. This step results in generation of an active mutagen. This active mutagen can cause mutation in the organism, although most of this reactive molecule will react with water via the enzyme epoxide hydrase or with glucose, sulfate, or glutathione to form water-soluble conjugates that can be excreted in the urine. Examples of such promutagens are the polycyclic aromatic hydrocarbons [e.g., benzo(*a*)pyrene], the aromatic amines(e.g., β-naphthylamine), and the fungal metabolite, aflatoxin B_1. Other examples include the large group of nitrosamines (e.g., dimethylnitrosamine).

Fifth, it must be pointed out that the polycyclic aromatic hydrocarbons can intercalate into DNA and also are metabolized to active alkylating agents such as epoxides and, hence, form a fifth set of complex mutagens that can cause base substitution and frameshift mutations. Other compounds that bind specifically to DNA in a physical sense, such as aflatoxin, and are metabolically activated to epoxides that bind covalently to DNA bases are also included in this complex mutagen group.

A sixth type of agent that is active at the DNA level are the metal salts. Metal salts cause chromosomal breakage, are carcinogenic to occupationally exposed humans, and are carcinogenic when injected into animals. Soluble hexavalent chromium compounds are mutagenic. Nickel compounds are not mutagenic in classical assays, but evidence is accumulating that nickel compounds cause deletions. Arsenic compounds are metalloids that are carcinogenic in humans.

Molecular Mechanisms of Mutagenesis

The simplest type of mutagenesis occurs when the enzyme DNA polymerase is copying one strand of DNA into its complementary strand and places the incorrect nucleotide into the newly synthesized strand of DNA. An example would be placement of the wrong base, adenine (A), opposite the DNA base cytosine (C), instead of inserting the correct base guanine (G) opposite the base C. This results in what is described as a G/C to A/T transition mutation, and it is called a spontaneous mutation.

A second type of mutation occurs when the alkylating agent MNNG reacts with the base guanine in DNA and places a methyl group on the oxygen in the 6 position of guanine. In this case, during the replication of the DNA, guanine, which is methylated on the oxygen in position 6, now incorrectly pairs with an incoming thymine instead of the cytosine with which a normal guanine would pair. This results in a G/C to A/T transition mutation.

Deletion and addition mutations are caused when the DNA "breathes" or opens its structure and occasionally a piece of this DNA loops out. When an intercalator molecule, such as acridine orange or ethidium bromide, intercalates into DNA at a looped out structure, it can stabilize this loop out. DNA repair enzymes can recognize this loop out as an aberrant structure and cut this structure out of the DNA, which would result in a deletion mutation. Addition mutations may be caused by insertion of extra DNA bases during DNA replication.

As mentioned previously , the polycyclic aromatic hydrocarbons are very complex molecules. They can intercalate into DNA and, by virtue of their being metabolized into epoxides, they can also covalently bind to DNA. Hence, they can cause base substitution mutations (transitions and transversions) and can also cause frameshift mutations when they are copied by the DNA polymerase incorrectly and incorrect nucleotides are inserted into the DNA, leading to mutations in the DNA.

Bacterial Mutagenesis Detection Systems

Two assays in bacteria are commonly used to detect and study the molecular mechanisms of mutation in bacteria. The most commonly employed assay is that of reversion of mutant *Salmonella typhimurium* bacteria back to wild-type or normal bacteria, developed by Ames and colleagues. In this assay, suspect mutagens plus a source of metabolic activation in the form of S-9 (a preparation in which rat liver has been homogenized, then centrifuged at 9000*g*, and the supernatant taken) are added to *S. typhimurium* bacteria, and the number of mutated bacteria that can now grow in medium lacking histidine are scored as mutant bacteria. This assay is very effective at detecting the mutagenicity of chemicals. It also detects 50% of all chemical carcinogens that are mutagenic carcinogens by detecting their mutagenicity. This assay is commonly used by industrial firms such as pharmaceutical companies, by governmental agencies charged with regulating the containment of carcinogenic substances, and by researchers interested in identifying new chemical mutagens and in understanding the molecular mechanisms of chemical mutagenesis. It is a rapid assay that takes only 2 or 3 days to complete and is relatively inexpensive ($500 or less per assay).

A second mutagenesis assay was derived based on the Ames assay. In this assay, the Ames *Salmonella* bacterial strains are used, but the assay is a forward mutation assay in which bacteria are treated with chemical mutagens plus or minus S-9 metabolic activation, then the number of bacterial colonies resistant to the toxicity of 8-azaguanine are scored as mutant colonies. This assay has been claimed to be more sensitive than the original Ames assay because the entire genes should be the targets for mutagenesis as opposed to small parts of histidine-synthesizing genes in the Ames assay. However, this assay is not employed as frequently as the Ames assay. A large body of work has been done to characterize and understand the molecular bases by which the Ames assay functions, and a very large number of mutagens have been detected and studied in the Ames assays.

In both assays, one plots the number of mutant colonies on the ordinate (*y*-axis) vs the concentration of test compound on the abscissa (*x*-axis). The plots are usually linear up to the point at which cytotoxicity overwhelms mutation induction, and the curves then decline. Hence, studies are usually conducted with low concentrations of compounds that induce a linear frequency of mutations but do not cause significant cytotoxicity.

Mammalian Cell Mutagenesis Assays

In mammalian cells, it is common to utilize mutagenesis assays that measure induction of mutants resistant to the cytotoxicity of toxic drugs. One of the most frequently employed mutation assays in mammalian cells is the assay detecting mutation to 6-thioguanine resistance. This assay is most frequently employed in the Chinese hamster ovary (CHO) cell line or in the V79 Chinese hamster lung fibroblast cell line. In this assay, the normal or "wild-type" cells are killed by the cytotoxic drug 6-thioguanine or its closely related analog, 8-azaguanine. This drug enters cells and reacts with the cell metabolite 5′-phosphoribosyl-pyrophosphate (PRPP) to form a toxic nucleotide which is incorporated into DNA and RNA, leading to cell death. In the mutation assays, the cells are treated with the suspect mutagen plus and minus S-9 metabolic activation, and then cells are reseeded into new cell culture medium containing 6-thioguanine or 8-azaguanine. 6-Thioguanine or 8-azaguanine kill all normal cells, but mutant cells are resistant to the cytotoxicity of 6-thioguanine and continue to grow and form discrete colonies. These mutant colonies are then stained with Giemsa stain and then scored with a microscope.

The mutant colonies are resistant to the cytotoxicity of 6-thioguanine because they have been mutated at the gene encoding the enzyme hypoxanthine guanine phosphoribosyl-pyrophosphate (HGPRT). This enzyme carries out a reaction between the DNA bases hypoxanthine or guanine and PRPP to form inosine and guanosine, which are then incorporated into DNA and RNA. In mutant cells, the gene encoding the HGPRT enzyme, hence the enzyme itself, is mutated. Therefore, the enzyme has a substantially reduced ability, or no ability, to carry out this condensation. The mutant cells cannot react toxic 6-thioguanine with PRPP to form a toxic nucleotide and are therefore resistant to the cytotoxicity of 6-thioguanine. They therefore survive and form colonies even in the presence of 6-thioguanine. Plotting the mutation frequency vs the concentration of mutagen added yields linear curves. This is a general assay and, as a forward mutation assay, it detects base substitution, addition, deletion, and frameshift mutations. It is one of the most widely used mutation assays in mammalian cells.

Induction of Morphological and Neoplastic Transformation in Mammalian Cells: Cell Culture Models for Chemically Induced Cancer Proceeding through Mutagenesis

There is a group of assays that can be used to study the ability of chemicals to convert normal cells to cancerous cells when normal cells are grown in cell culture and treated with chemical carcinogens. One property of normal cells, particularly fibroblasts, is that they divide, grow, and eventually fill a surface such as that of a tissue culture dish and then stop growing. This is because cells in contact transmit signals through their membranes, on through the cytoskeleton ("cell skeleton"), and on to the cell nucleus, which forces cells to stop growing. This property is referred to as contact inhibition of cell division. In cell culture, this property is manifested when the cells grow and fill the cell culture dish with a layer of cells one cell thick. However, when cells are treated with a chemical carcinogen that is already activated or that can be activated by the specific types of cytochrome P450 enzymes the cell possesses, then 1% or less of the cells are "transformed," or changed. They have lost contact inhibition and now grow on top of one another in arrays where the cells "criss-cross" over one another. Since the cells are changed in shape or morphology, we refer to this as "morphological transformation," or change in cell shape. This change in cell shape manifests itself as growth of the cells in small piles, referred to as foci. Foci are easily seen when cells are stained with specific dyes. The stained foci can then be counted under the microscope. Scoring foci is an assay for chemical carcinogens by which they induce one of the five steps that must be acquired for cells to become able to form tumors when injected into mice.

A second property of most normal cells is that they need to anchor to a surface such as that of a tissue culture dish in order for them to replicate their DNA and divide. This property is referred to as "anchorage dependence." Normal cells cannot grow in suspension in liquid media. An exception to this is white blood cells, which can grow in liquid suspension because this is their function in the blood. However, most cells, particularly connective tissue cells like fibroblasts, cannot grow in liquid suspension and are anchorage dependent. When fibroblasts are treated with chemical carcinogens that are already activated to alkylating agents or if the cells themselves have the cytochrome P450 enzymes to activate the carcinogens they are treated with, then a small fraction, on the order of 1 in 1 million, of the normal cells will be converted into anchorage-independent cells, which can grow and form colonies in liquid suspension. Anchorage independence is another property that must also be acquired by fibroblasts before they can become tumorigenic.

Normal cells also have a finite life span and undergo approximately 60 population doublings, then senesce or die through a process of programmed cell death. When cells are treated with chemical carcinogens, a small fraction of them (1% in mouse cells and far less in human cells) can become transformed to immortality such that they now grow forever.

A final step involves conversion of cells that have become immortal, morphologically transformed, and anchorage independent into tumor cells. This can occur spontaneously or upon treatment of cells with chemical carcinogens.

What changes in the DNA result in the induction of the changes in cell properties (phenotypes) that we refer to as morphological transformation, anchorage independence, cellular immortality , and tumorigenicity? It has been shown by many scientific workers that there are two broad classes of genes that control cell growth in a positive way: the protooncogenes and those that inhibit cell growth—tumor suppressor genes. Chemical carcinogens can react with and cause mutations in, amplification of, or translocation of protooncogenes, converting them into active cell transforming genes known as activated oncogenes. There are approximately 50 protooncogenes that can be converted into activated oncogenes.

There are four broad classes of protooncogenes. One class has protein products localized in the cell nucleus which act as factors that activate transcription of specific genes. This group is exemplified by genes such as c-*myc* and c-*jun*. A second group is located in the cell membrane or the cytoplasm and transfers biochemical signals in the cell. A prominent example of this group is the c-Ha-*ras* protooncogene. The protein product of this gene binds the high-energy molecule guanosine triphosphate, which activates this protein such that it transfers signals to other proteins and eventually toward the nucleus. The last two groups of protooncogenes' protein products are located at the membrane and are growth factors, such as the c-*sis* gene, and receptors for these growth factors. The significance of these genes is that mutational or other types of activations of two or more of these genes play a role in inducing transformed phenotypes and contribute to formation of a tumor cell.

There are approximately 10 tumor suppressor genes that have been identified to date. Chemical carcinogens cause mutations in these genes to inactivate them or can break the chromosomes on which these genes are located. Inactivation of two copies of a tumor suppressor gene renders it inactive in the cell. Inactivation by chemical carcinogens of two or more tumor suppressor genes, in concert with activation of two or more oncogenes, cumulatively leads to formation of a tumor cell. Examples of tumor suppressor genes include the retinoblastoma (Rb) gene and the *p53* tumor suppressor gene. Inactivations of tumor suppressor genes and activations of specific oncogenes have been found in all human tumors that have been studied intensively to date.

Tier Concept for Screening for and Detecting Chemical Carcinogens and Mutagens

Genetic toxicology, the science by which chemicals and agents that cause mutation and other changes to DNA are studied, has evolved substantially during the past 50 years. It is standard to detect chemical mutagens by utilizing the Ames assay and other bacterial mutagenesis assays with and without S-9 metabolic activation and to utilize assays detecting mutation to 6-thioguanine resistance in CHO or V79 mammalian cells. There are also assays that detect the ability of chemicals to cause chromosome breakage in V79 or CHO cells by examining chromosomes of these cells under a microscope after chemical carcinogen treatment.

In addition to detecting chemical mutagens, these methodologies can also be used to detect chemical carcinogens. The most certain way is to paint animals with carcinogens, feed carcinogens to animals or add carcinogens to the animals' food or water, and observe whether the animals develop tumors. Unfortunately, treating mice or rats with chemical carcinogens and assaying for tumor induction takes 2 years and costs $2 or 3 million per chemical tested. This price is simply too large and the time too long to permit scientists to use animal bioassays to screen for the carcinogenicity of the hundreds of thousands of chemicals that need to be studied. During the past 20 years, an alternate strategy to detect carcinogens has arisen. This strategy is referred to as a tier screening strategy and relies on the fact that approximately 50% of the known carcinogens are mutagens. Hence, the current strategy relied on by most government, regulatory, and academic laboratories is to use inexpensive, rapid assays to test the large number of chemicals in use today in what is referred to as a primary screen. In this screen, one would use the Ames bacterial mutagenesis assay, an assay for chromosome breakage, an assay to detect DNA repair, and perhaps a mammalian cell mutagenesis assay. Chemicals that cause mutagenesis, chromosome breakage, or DNA repair in these assays would be considered suspect carcinogens. Further product development on these chemicals would likely be halted or the chemicals would be modified in their structure. Chemicals negative in this primary screen that were proposed to be used for human applications, such as food additives or cosmetics, are then tested in cell transformation assays for the ability to induce morphological or anchorage-independent transformation. Chemicals positive in cell transformation assays are then eliminated from further development or chemically modified so they no longer cause cell transformation. Finally, chemicals to be marketed as cosmetics or food additives would then be tested in whole animal carcinogenesis assays.

Further Reading

Bishop, J. M. (1987). The molecular genetics of cancer. *Science 235*, 305–310.

Landolph, J. R. (1985). Chemical transformation in C3H/10T1/2 mouse embryo fibroblasts: Historical background, assessment of the transformation assay, and evolution and optimization of the transformation assay protocol. In *Transformation Assay of Established Cell Lines: Mechanisms and Application* (T. Kakunaga and H. Yamasaki, Eds.), Scientific Publ. No. 67, pp. 185–198. International Agency for Cancer Research, Lyon, France.

Landolph, J. R. (1990). Neoplastic transformation of mammalian cells by carcinogenic metal compounds: Cellular and molecular mechanisms. In *Biological Effects of Heavy Metals. Metal Carcinogenesis* (E. C. Foulkes, Ed.), Vol. II, pp. 1–18. CRC Press, Boca Raton, FL.

O'Neill, J. P., and Hsie, A. W. (1979). The CHO/HGPRT mutation assay experimental procedure. In *Mammalian Cell Mutagenesis: The Maturation of Test Systems* (A. W. Hsie, J. P. O'Neill, and V. K. McElhenny, Eds.), Banbury Report No. 2, pp. 55–70, 311–318, 407–420. Cold Spring Harbor Press, Cold Spring Harbor, NY.

Watson, J. D., Hopkins, N. H., Roberts, J. W., Steitz, J. A., and Weiner, A. M. (Eds.) (1987). *Molecular Biology of the Gene*, 4th ed., Vol. I, pp. 240–359, 360–464. (see Chaps. 4 and 5). Cummings, Menlo Park, CA.

—*Joseph R. Landolph*

Related Topics

Ames Test
Analytical Toxicology
Carcinogenesis
Carcinogen Classification Schemes
Carcinogen–DNA Adduct Formation and DNA Repair
Cell Proliferation
Chromosome Aberrations
Dominant Lethal Tests
Host-Mediated Assay
Molecular Toxicology
Mouse Lymphoma Assay
Radiation Toxicology
Reproductive System
Sister Chromatid Exchanges
Toxicity Testing, Developmental
Toxicity Testing, Reproductive

Mycotoxins

- Representative Compounds: Aflatoxin B; aflatoxin G; penicillinic acid; trichothecenes

- SYNONYMS: 2,3,6aα; 9aα-tetrahydro-4-methoxycyclopenta(*c*)furo[3′, 2:4,5]furo[2,3-*b*][1]benzopyran-1,11-dione
- DESCRIPTION: Mycotoxins are fungal metabolites evolving naturally during storage of a variety of plant products (e.g., cereal grains, nuts, corn, sorghum, rice, dried beans, and apples). They are also present in products derived from animals that consumed contaminated feeds.
- MOLECULAR FORMULA: $C_{17}H_{12}O_6$
- CHEMICAL STRUCTURE:

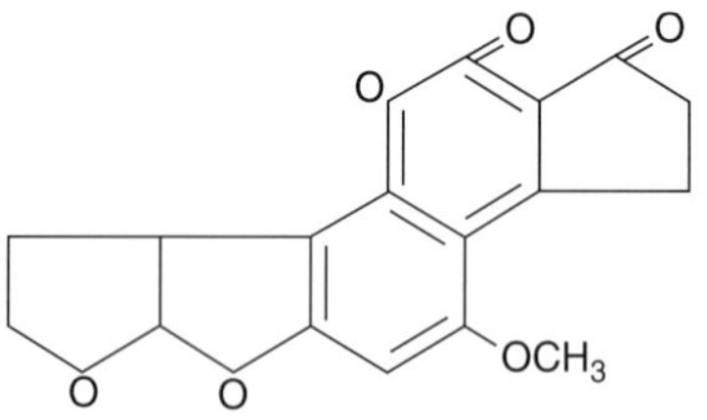

O O O O O OCH3

Exposure Pathways

Ingestion and dermal exposure are possible routes of exposure.

Toxicokinetics

Susceptibility depends on variations in moisture, temperature, the presence of metabolic substrates, and aeration. Aflatoxin B is absorbed into the blood and excreted mainly through bile. In urine, aflatoxin B is excreted as aflatoxin M_1.

Mechanism of Toxicity

Aflatoxin B is transformed in blood into a highly reactive epoxide that forms covalent bonds with DNA, RNA, and proteins. Toxicity and carcinogeneity are attributed to inhibition of nucleic acid synthesis.

Human Toxicity

Aflatoxin B is a suspected hepatocarcinogen; this association was identified in population studies. It is also associated with Reye's syndrome in children and may cause liver disease, such as hepatitis or cirrhosis, in malnourished children. The TCL in milk is 0.5 ppb.

Clinical Management

Reducing the opportunity for exposure is the first line of defense. Activated charcoal may be used to absorb the toxin. Reducing glutathione levels is suggested as a possible therapy.

Animal Toxicity

In 1960–1963, the death of turkeys in England (referred to as turkey X disease) was associated with the consumption of peanut meal feeds containing mycotoxins. Death usually occurs from hepatoxicity. Aflatoxin B is carcinogenic in rats but not in mice. The duckling LD_{50} (oral) is 0.5 mg/kg; the mouse LD_{50} is 60 mg/kg. The TCL in animal feed is 20 ppb.

—Shayne C. Gad and Jayne E. Ash

Related Topics

Kidney
Veterinary Toxicology

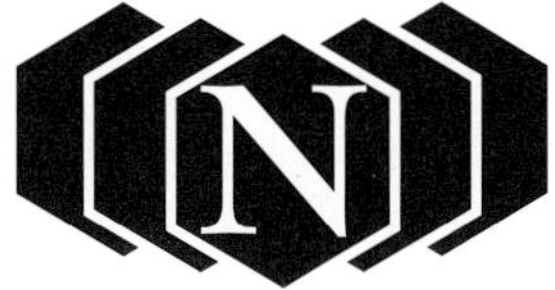

Naphthalene

- CAS: 91-20-3
- SYNONYMS: Naftalen; naphthene, NCI-C52904; albocarbon; dezodorator; mothballs; moth flakes; tar camphor; white tar; naphthalin; naphthaline; UN 2304; naftaleno
- CHEMICAL CLASS: Aromatic hydrocarbon
- MOLECULAR FORMULA: $C_{10}H_8$

Uses

Naphthalene is commonly used in the manufacture of dyes, resins, and mothballs and may also be found in association with coal tar production and in wood preservatives. It is also used as a chemical intermediate in the synthesis of pesticides.

Exposure Pathways

The primary exposure route for naphthalene is via inhalation, although it may also be absorbed orally or dermally.

Toxicokinetics

The biological distribution, metabolism, and excretion of these compounds have not been well characterized. It is a relatively volatile solid at room temperature and tends to evaporate readily. This compound has a relatively short half-life in soil and water due to its volatility and rapid degradation.

Mechanism of Toxicology

Systemic absorption of naphthalene vapor may result in cataracts. The biochemical basis for naphthalene cataract has been investigated. Naphthalene is metabolized in the liver to 1,2-dihydro-1,2-dihydoxynaphthalene. Lenticular catechol reductase biotransforms 1,2-dihydro-1,2-dihydroxylnaphthalene to 1,2-dihydroxynaphthalene, which in turn is autooxidized in air at neutral pH to 1,2-naphthaoquinone and hydrogen peroxide. Ascorbic acid reverses the latter reaction and forms dehydroascorbic acid, which diffuses out of the lens very slowly. Dehydroascorbic acid has been shown to accumulate in the lens of rabbits fed naphthalene and lens incubated *in vitro* with 1,2-dihydro-1,2-dihydroxynaphthalene. The sequence of reactions involves reduction of ascorbic acid by 1,2-naphthoquinone in the aqueous humor to dehydroascorbic acid, which rapidly penetrates the lens and is reduced by glutathione. Oxidized glutathione and 1,2-naphthoquinone may compete for enzyme glutathione reductase, which normally maintains high reticular levels of reduced glutathione. A reduction in the concentration of these coupled with the removal of oxygen from the aqueous humor due to the autooxidation of 1,2-dihydroxynaphthalene may make the lens sensitive to naphthalene toxicity.

Human Toxicity

There are no reported cases of death due to inhalation of naphthalene. Naphthalene-induced deaths are usually related to mothball ingestion during suicide attempts. Based on suicide data, the lethal dose in humans is estimated to be approximately 319–574 mg/kg. The most prominent effect of high-dose naphthalene exposure in humans is hemolytic anemia. There is a report of an infant who died of acute hemolytic anemia after being exposed to mothball-treated diapers. Another infant reportedly experienced skin rashes, systemic poisoning, and then death apparently due to naphthalene exposure from mothballs used with clothes or blankets that had been stored in or near the infant's room.

General symptoms caused by exposure to naphthalene by skin or eye surface contact, inhalation, or ingestion are described below.

Skin or eye surface contact may result in naphthalene cataracts, ocular irritation, skin irritation, and in the case of a sensitized person, severe dermatitis. Lesions will clear spontaneously, as soon as the exposure is terminated. Percutaneous absorption is inadequate to produce acute systemic reactions except in newborns.

Inhalation of vapor may result in headache, confusion, excitation, nausea, and sometimes vomiting and extensive sweating. Dysuria, hematuria, and acute hemolytic reaction are also seen.

Ingestion may cause abdominal cramps with nausea, vomiting, diarrhea, headache, profuse perspiration, listlessness, confusion, and coma with or without convulsions in a case of severe poisoning. It also may cause irritation of the urinary bladder, dysuria, the passage of a brown or black urine with or without albumin and casts, and acute intravascular hemolysis.

All reported cases of naphthalene toxicity in humans include hemolytic crisis, characterized by increased bilirubin levels, and the appearance of Heinz bodies and fragmented red blood cells. Other effects that have been associated with ingestion of lethal doses include vomiting, nausea, jaundice, proteinurea, hemoglobinuria, headache, confusion, and coma. Naphthalene ingestion or inhalation can result in massive hemolysis in glucose-6-phosphate dehydrogenase-deficient subjects; hemolysis in normal individuals occurs only with exposure to very high concentrations.

A 69-year-old female exposed to naphthalene and paradichlorobenzene developed aplastic anemia 2 months after exposure. A 36-year-old pharmacist was given 5 g of unpurified naphthalene in an emulsion of castor oil in divided doses over 13 hr. On awakening 8 or 9 hr later, he had severe pain in the bladder and found that he was nearly blind, although previously he had had good vision. After 1 year, an examination showed that his vision was reduced to the ability count fingers at 1.5 m and his visual fields were constricted 30–50°. The condition was unimproved by glasses. The development of cataracts and retinal hemorrhage in a 44-year-old man occupationally exposed to powdered naphthalene was reported. Unilateral chorioretinitis was developed in a co-worker and cataracts developed in 8 of 21 workers exposed to naphthalene fumes or dust for $\leqq 5$ years in an industrial setting.

Chronic exposure to powdered naphthalene in the workplace has been associated with an increased incidence of cataracts. However, few of these effects have been confirmed in animal studies. Human carcinogenicity data are inadequate and the U.S. EPA does not classify the potential human carcinogenicity of naphthalene at this time.

Clinical Management

There is no specific antidote for naphthalene toxicity. Treatment is symptomatic and supportive. Gastric decontamination should be considered with emesis or lavage, followed by activated charcoal. Hemolysis may require urinary alkalinization and transfusion. Methemoglobinemia may be treated with methylene blue. Emesis is more useful for mothballs because of size. Lavage may be useful for ingestion of flakes. Information on activated charcoal is scant, but adsorption is thought to occur. Mothballs dissolve slowly; gastric decontamination should be performed even in patients presenting late after ingestion. Emesis may be indicated in recent substantial ingestion unless the patient is or could rapidly become obtunded, comatose, or convulsant. It is most effective if initiated within 30 min of ingestion. The recommended dose of ipecac syrup is 30 ml for an adult and 15 ml for a child.

Gastric lavage may be indicated if performed soon after ingestion or in patients who are comatose or at risk of convulsing. The airway should be protected by placement in Trendelenburg and left lateral decubitus position or by cuffed endotracheal intubation.

Animal Toxicity

The maximum air concentration of naphthalene that can be generated (78 ppm) has not been shown to be lethal to rats. Animal studies report that the oral LD_{50} for naphthalene ranges from 354 mg/kg in mice to 2400 mg/kg in rats. In extreme circumstances, death may also occur as a result of dermal exposure.

Naphthalene does not appear to be teratogenic. Mice exposed to 300 mg/kg/day produced normal offspring, although a decrease in litter size was reported.

Oral administration of 1 g/kg/day in rabbits leads to lenticular changes, initially observed as swelling in the peripheral portion of the lens. Within 2 weeks, the whole lens is affected with mature cataract. The biochemical basis for cataract has been shown to be related to a liver metabolite of naphthalene, 1,2-dihydro-1,2-dihydoxynaphthalene.

Selective lung damage and necrosis occurred in Clara cells of mouse administered naphthalene. It produced selective depression of pulmonary monooxygenase activities without accompanying changes in hepatic monooxygenease. A dose-dependent alteration of Clara cells (bronchiolar epithelial cells) was noted.

There is no evidence that naphthalene is a carcinogen. No increased incidence of cancer was noted in a 2-year feeding study of rats exposed to naphthalene, while a 6-month study in mice produced inconclusive results. It is of interest that naphthalene was shown to inhibit skin cancer formation when it was coadministered with the carcinogen, benzo(*a*)pyrene.

—*Leyna Mulholland*

Related Topic

Sensory Organs

Naphthylisothiocyanate, 1-

- CAS: 551-06-4
- SYNONYMS: α-Naphthylisothiocyanate, ANIT
- MOLECULAR FORMULA: $C_{11}H_7NS$
- CHEMICAL STRUCTURE:

N=C=S

Uses

1-Naphthylisothiocyanate is used as an ingredient in insecticides, and as a laboratory agent for inhibiting microsomal based metabolism.

Exposure Pathways

Inhalation, ingestion, and dermal contact are all possible routes of exposure.

Mechanism of Toxicity

1-Naphthylisothiocyanate causes separation of extracellular tight junctions that seal bile canaliculi, impairing bile formation.

Human Toxicity

1-Naphthylisothiocyanate causes liver and kidney damage as well as ocular irritation and corrosion.

Animal Toxicity

A single dose can induce intrahepatic cholestasis (reduction in bile flow) in rats, producing hyperbilirubinemia. 1-Naphthylisothiocyanate inhibits microsomal drug-metabolizing activity. It is a mutagen. The oral LD_{50} in rats is 200 mg/kg.

—*Shayne C. Gad*

Related Topics

Liver
Kidney
Pesticides

National Center for Toxicological Research

The U.S. FDA's National Center for Toxicological Research (NCTR), located in Jefferson, Arkansas, conducts peer-reviewed scientific research that supports and anticipates FDA's current and future regulatory needs. This involves fundamental and applied research in the categories described below.

NCTR conducts integrated research to enhance FDA's ability to formulate science-based risk management decisions. It conducts research to study both the biological effects of potentially toxic chemicals and the complex mechanisms that govern their toxicity. Customized bioassessment of chemicals of vital interest to FDA involves the coordination of expertise in areas of: biochemical and molecular markers of carcinogenicity–solid-state toxicity (evaluation of potential toxicity of implanted materials used in medical devices); nutritional modulators of risk and toxicity (including a program focus on calorie restriction); quantitative risk assessment; transgenics (mimicking human responses in animal models by insertion of human genes into a test animal or tissue culture); neurotoxicology; and developmental toxicology.

The NCTR aim is to improve FDA's ability to find and measure contaminants and toxicants in foods and drugs through development of sensitive methods to analyze regulated products that are able to withstand legal scrutiny, quantitative biomarkers to measure effects of contaminants on human development, and methods to determine the effects of novel food additives and macronutrients on human metabolism.

One important educational focus is NCTR's contributions to enhance FDA's Life Science Education Literacy Initiative. NCTR contributes by providing continued coordination and support of an interdisciplinary toxicological program and regulatory science curriculum at two Arkansas universities and by maintaining a commitment to science education initiatives, which provide a "pipeline" from high school to postgraduate training, to help increase the limited pool of qualified scientists. In 1994, 243 people, 69 of whom represented 23 foreign countries and Puerto Rico, participated in independent or collaborative research supported by these initiatives.

The NCTR organizational structure consists of the Office of the Director, encompassing staff offices to implement EEO, training, safety, security, technology advancement, and scientific coordination functions; the Office of Planning and Resource Management, which coordinates the financial management and strategic and logistical planning for the center; the Office of Research Support, which is the management and administrative services arm; and the Office of Research, which comprises nine divisions to conduct mission research. NCTR employs approximately 240 full-time federal employees, supplemented by about 300 contractor employees providing animal diet, maintenance, and pathology; computer and information management services; facilities maintenance; on-site occupational health care; and administrative services (e.g., supplies receiving and warehousing, mail delivery, and document reproduction).

In fiscal year 1994, NCTR staff participated in more than 279 scientific protocols and published 198 manuscripts, book chapters, and books (plus abstracts) and 25 final technical reports.

For additional information, contact the National Center for Toxicological Research, 3900 NCTR Drive, Jefferson, AR 72079-9502. Telephone: 501-543-7517; fax: 501-543-7576.

—David M. Krentz and Harihara M. Mehendale

(Adapted from information supplied by NCTR.)

Related Topics

Agency for Toxic Substances and Disease Registry
American Conference of Governmental Industrial Hygienists
Environmental Protection Agency, National Health and Environmental Effects Research Laboratory
Food and Drug Administration
Information Resources in Toxicology
National Institutes of Health
National Institute for Occupational Safety and Health
National Institute of Environmental Health Sciences

National Environmental Policy Act

- Title: NEPA
- Agency: U.S. Congress

- Year Passed: 1985
- Groups Regulated: Federal regulatory agencies and, through them, all those they regulate

Synopsis of Law

The National Environmental Policy Act (NEPA; 21 CFR Part 29, April 26, 1985) requires assessment of the environmental implications of all regulatory decisions. The most significant practical impact of NEPA has been to require the development of environmental impact statements for a vast range of activities.

—*Shayne C. Gad*

Related Topic

Environmental Toxicology
RCRA
TOSCA

National Institute for Occupational Safety and Health

The National Institute for Occupational Safety and Health (NIOSH) was established by the Occupational Safety and Health Act of 1970. NIOSH is part of the Centers for Disease Control and Prevention and is the federal institute responsible for conducting research and making recommendations for the prevention of work-related illnesses and injuries. NIOSH's responsibilities include:

- Investigating potentially hazardous working conditions as requested by employers or employees;
- Evaluating hazards in the workplace, ranging from chemicals to machinery;
- Creating and disseminating methods for preventing disease, injury, and disability;
- Conducting research and providing scientifically valid recommendations for protecting workers; and
- Providing education and training to individuals preparing for or actively working in the field of occupational safety and health.

Although NIOSH and OSHA were created by the same act of Congress, they are two distinct agencies with separate responsibilities. OSHA is in the Department of Labor and is responsible for creating and enforcing workplace safety and health regulations. NIOSH is in the Department of Health and Human Services and is a research agency.

NIOSH identifies the causes of work-related diseases and injuries and the potential hazards of new work technologies and practices. With this information, NIOSH determines new and effective ways to protect workers from chemicals, machinery, and hazardous working conditions. Creating new ways to prevent workplace hazards is one of the objectives of NIOSH.

Toll-Free Technical Information Service

The NIOSH 800 number is a toll-free technical information service that provides convenient public access to NIOSH and its information resources. The 800 number combines an automated voice-mail system with direct access to NIOSH technical information staff and the NIOSH Publications Office. The automated system operates 24 hr a day. It provides recorded information on a variety of topics, including directions for ordering NIOSH publications. In addition, callers may speak directly with a technical information specialist from 9:00 AM until 4:00 PM or to a publications representative from 1:00 until 4:00 PM (EST). Callers may request information about NIOSH activities, order NIOSH publications, or request information about any aspect of occupational safety and health. However, this toll-free number is not a hotline for medical emergencies.

The service is available to anyone in the continental United States, Alaska, Hawaii, Puerto Rico, or the Virgin Islands. All information is provided free of charge within 10 working days.

The NIOSH 800 number is 1-800-35-NIOSH (1-800-356-4674). Outside the United States, the commercial toll number is (513) 533-8328.

—David M. Krentz and Harihara M. Mehendale

Related Topics

Agency for Toxic Substances and Disease Registry
Carcinogen Classification Schemes
Environmental Protection Agency, National Health and Environmental Effects Research Laboratory
Food and Drug Administration
Information Resources in Toxicology
National Center for Toxicological Research
National Institute of Environmental Health Sciences
National Institutes of Health
National Toxicology Program
Occupational Safety and Health Act
Occupational Safety and Health Administration

National Institute of Environmental Health Sciences

The National Institute of Environmental Health Sciences (NIEHS) is located in Research Triangle Park, North Carolina, and is a component institute of the federal National Institutes of Health. Since its creation in 1966, the NIEHS has been the primary source of federal efforts for studying how environmental factors affect human health. The mission of the NIEHS is to define how exposures to environmental agents affect our health, how individuals differ in their susceptibility to these effects, and how these susceptibilities change over time. Diseases and dysfunctions with an environmental component include cancer, birth defects, infertility, neurological impairments, immune disorders, and lung dysfunctions. Because environmental exposures can be controlled or avoided, they represent one of the most promising means of improving human health. Because of the broad scope of its mission, NIEHS research relies on essentially every discipline in the biological, chemical, and physical sciences. It maintains a multidisciplinary intramural research program at its Research Triangle Park facility and supports university-based research and training through a variety of grant mechanisms. Through its participation in the National Toxicology Program, NIEHS has made significant contributions in providing state-of-the-art toxicological characterization for a host of environmentally and commercially important agents. Because of the high quality of these studies, they serve to guide risk assessments both in the United States and abroad.

Basic science supported by the NIEHS attempts to identify the environmental components of human disease and to understand the basic molecular mechanisms leading to these disease states. Environmentally related diseases of special interest to the institute are those dealing with women's health, children's health, minorities' health, aging, respiratory disorders, neurological disorders, immune system disruption, and cancer. Cellular processes that hold promise for explaining environmental mechanisms for these diseases include regulatory genes that serve as targets for environmentally induced effects, cellular communication pathways, the integration of biological processes across organ systems, and the genetic basis of individual susceptibility to environmental agents and the diseases and disorders they cause. The NIEHS also is expanding its clinical research programs to enable it to more readily translate laboratory-based findings into human therapies.

Prevention and intervention efforts are a major focus of NIEHS activities. These efforts include hazard identification and characterization, both through traditional animal testing and epidemiologic studies and through incorporation of mechanistic considerations to arrive at new insights into the molecular basis of toxic effects. This improved understanding of the molecular foundation of environmentally associated effects will enable the institute to strengthen the validity of risk assessment schemes as a means of deciding regulatory policy. An improved understanding of the molecular basis of toxicant action could also lead to innovative molecular prevention and intervention therapies to circumvent clinical manifestations of environmentally caused diseases.

Finally, the NIEHS has devised a communications strategy which ensures that the findings generated by its basic and applied research reach the groups that need the information. These groups include the lay public and the institute's partners in research, governmental agencies, advocacy groups, and the international community.

—Harihara M. Mehendale

Related Topics

Agency for Toxic Substances and Disease Registry
Environmental Protection Agency, National Health and Environmental Effects Research Laboratory
Food and Drug Administration
Information Resources in Toxicology
National Center for Toxicological Research
National Institute for Occupational Safety and Health
National Institutes of Health
National Toxicology Program

National Institutes of Health

The National Institutes of Health (NIH) is the principal biomedical research agency of the U.S. federal government. Its mission is to employ science in the pursuit of knowledge to improve human health conditions. To accomplish this goal, the institute seeks to expand fundamental knowledge about the nature and behavior of living systems, to apply that knowledge to extend the health of human lives, and to reduce the burdens resulting from disease and disability. In the quest of this mission, NIH supports biomedical and behavioral research domestically and abroad, conducts research in its own laboratories and clinics, trains promising young researchers, and promotes the acquisition and distribution of medical knowledge. Focal points have been established to assist in developing NIH-wide goals for health research and training programs related to women and minorities, coordinating program direction, and ensuring that research pertaining to women's and minority health is identified and addressed through research activities conducted and supported by NIH. Research activities conducted by NIH will determine much of the quality of health care for the future and reinforce the quality of health care currently available.

Major Components

- National Cancer Institute National Heart, Lung, and Blood Institute
- National Library of Medicine
- National Institute of Diabetes and Digestive and Kidney Diseases
- National Institute of Allergy and Infectious Diseases
- National Institute of Child Health and Human Development
- National Institute on Deafness and Other Communication Disorders
- National Institute of Dental Research
- National Institute of Environmental Health Sciences
- National Institute of General Medical Sciences
- National Institute of Neurological Disorders and Stroke
- National Institute on Aging
- National Institute of Alcohol Abuse and Alcoholism
- National Institute of Arthritis and Musculoskeletal and Skin Diseases
- National Institute on Drug Abuse
- National Institute of Mental Health
- Clinical Center
- Fogarty International Center
- National Center for Human Genome Research

- National Institute of Nursing Research
- Division of Computer Research and Technology
- National Center for Research Resources
- Division of Research Grants

For additional information contact the National Institutes of Health, 6701 Rockledge Drive, Bethesda, MD 20892.

—*David M. Krentz and Harihara M. Mehendale*

Related Topics

Agency for Toxic Substances and Disease Registry
Environmental Protection Agency, National Health and Environmental Effects Research Laboratory
Food and Drug Administration
Information Resources in Toxicology
National Center for Toxicological Research
National Institute for Occupational Safety and Health
National Institute of Environmental Health Sciences
National Library of Medicine
National Toxicology Program

National Library of Medicine/TEHIP

With a collection of some 5 million items, the National Library of Medicine (NLM), part of the National Institutes of Health, in Bethesda, Maryland, is the largest medical library in the world and contains substantial holdings of books and journals on toxicology. NLM's Toxicology and Environmental Health Information Program's (TEHIP) origins date back to 1967. TEHIP offers a broad array of publicly available computer files in toxicology and environmental health, responds to queries, sponsors publications, and supports the information requirements of other federal agencies. TEHIP is one of the world's major focal points for toxicology and environmental health information resources.

TEHIP's computer files include the Chemical Carcinogenesis Research Information System, the ChemID chemical dictionary file, Developmental and Reproductive Toxicology, Environmental Mutagenesis Information Center, GENE-TOX, the Hazardous Substances Data Bank, the Integrated Risk Information System, the Registry of Toxic Effects of Chemical Substances, the TOXLINE files containing literature references, and the Toxic Chemical Release Inventory series. These files are accessible through a single nationwide toll-free number or the Internet.

For information on TEHIP's products and services, contact Toxicology and Environmental Health Information Program, Division of Specialized Information Services, National Library of Medicine, 8600 Rockville Pike, Bethesda, MD 20894. Phone: 301-496-6531; fax: 301-480-3537; e-mail:tehip@teh.nlm.nih.gov; web site: http://sis.nlm.nih.gov.

—*Philip A. Wexler*

Related Topics

Information Resources in Toxicology
National Institutes of Health

National Toxicology Program

The National Toxicology Program (NTP) was established in 1978 as a cooperative effort within the U.S. Public Health Service of the Department of Health and Human Services (DHHS) to coordinate toxicology research and testing activities within the department; to provide information about potentially toxic chemicals to health regulatory and research agencies, scientific and medical communities, and the public; and to strengthen the science base in toxicology. In its 17 years, NTP has become a world leader in designing, conducting, and interpreting various types of assays for toxicity. Through its activities, NTP provides, directly or indirectly, a large component of the basic scientific data that other federal and state scientific and regulatory agencies as well as private-sector organizations use in responding to issues relevant to the effects of chemical substances on human health and the environment.

The original contributing agencies of the NTP were the NIH's NIEHS and NCI, CDC's NIOSH, and FDA's NCTR. In 1981, the NTP component of the NCI, the carcinogenesis bioassay program, was transferred to the NIEHS. The NCI remains quite active in the program through membership on the NTP Executive Committee and in other ways. From the beginning, the director of the NIEHS has also been the director of the NTP, and the administrative staff is located at the NIEHS. Primary scientific oversight is provided by a Board of Scientific Counselors and its two subcommittees, which are composed almost entirely of nonfederal scientists comprising a broad spectra of expertise and affiliations including academia, industry, labor, public interest, and federal or state government. Primary program and policy oversight is provided by the NTP Executive Committee composed of the heads of the participating DHHS agencies (including NCI and ATSDR) as well as the heads of the major non-DHHS regulatory agencies concerned with human health.

Four overall objectives of the program remain (1) to broaden the spectrum of toxicological information obtained on selected chemicals; (2) to develop and validate improved test methods, including alternative test systems; (3) to develop improved methods for generation of scientific data useful to risk assessment; and (4) to communicate program strategies and findings to governmental agencies, the medical and scientific communities, and the public. To meet these objectives, a balanced program has been created which uses chronic bioassays, short-term tests, collection and application of mechanistic information, model development, alternative methods, and human studies. The overall aims of these initiatives are to more efficiently test chemicals for toxic effects using a broad array of test systems, to develop and validate new and better test systems, and to utilize the emerging tools of molecular biology in generating data that strengthens the scientific foundation on which risk assessments are based. Additionally, the use of predictive toxicology should play a complementary role in hazard identification. Although mechanistic approaches should and are being more frequently incorporated into toxicity testing, the chronic bioassay in rodents will continue to be used in many cases including those in which mechanistic data are not available and for the purpose of validating new methods. Thus, it must be emphasized that there is a strong and continuing commitment by the NTP to increase the number of agents entered into toxicology and carcinogenesis studies. To ensure that the agents selected for study represent the best choices from a standpoint of public or occupational health importance and/or scientific importance, the program has broadened its call for nominations from nongovernment organizations and the general public and continues to give more emphasis to noncancer endpoints.

Scientific activities are divided principally into several major program areas: carcinogenesis, genetic toxicology, risk assessment research, alternative methods, and toxicology. The general term of toxicology covers activities in immunologic, neurobehavioral, and respiratory toxicologies, as well as reproductive and developmental toxicology. There are special projects on studying toxicities of AIDS therapeutics and toxicity of superfund chemicals.

—*Harihara M. Mehendale*

Related Topics

Agency for Toxic Substances and Disease Registry
Carcinogen Classification Schemes
Environmental Protection Agency, National Health and Environmental Effects Research Laboratory
Food and Drug Administration
National Center for Toxicological Research
National Institute of Environmental Health Sciences
National Institute for Occupational Safety and Health
National Institutes of Health
Occupational Safety and Health Act
Occupational Safety and Health Administration

Nematocides

- CAS: 96-12-8 (of representative compound)
- Representative Compound: 1, 2-dibromo-3-chloropropane
- Synonyms: Nemagon; DBCP
- Other Class Members: Nem-a-tak; halogenated hydrocarbons
- Chemical Structure:

$$Cl-CH_2-\underset{}{\overset{Br}{\overset{|}{CH}}}-CH_2-Br$$

Uses
Nematocides are pesticides that kill parasitic worms such as roundworms or threadworms.

Exposure Pathways
Dermal contact, inhalation, and ingestion are possible exposure pathways.

Toxicokinetics
In rats, 98% of nemagon is absorbed into the stomach. Within 3 days, 90% of activity is excreted. Within the first 24-hr period, 49% is excreted through urine, 14% through feces, and 16.5% through expired air.

Mechanism of Toxicity
Defatting creates cell necrosis. They also reduce cell P450 content. Sulphyril, but not glutathione, mediates toxic effects. Biotransformation (hydrolysis and oxidation) via mercpturic acid route, producing α-chlorohydrin and α-bromohydrin, two antifertility agents. Further oxidation of these substances may produce oxalic acid, which causes liver and kidney damage.

Human Toxicity
Acute exposure to high concentrations produces dyspnea, gasping, and coughing. Chronic exposure affects the liver, kidneys, and heart. Other symptoms include central nervous system (CNS) depression and pulmonary congestion. It is a reproductive toxin resulting in reduced sperm count. Adverse effects are presumed to be reversible. It is a possible carcinogen. Most human exposure to nematocides is as trace residues in meat.

The OSHA PEL is 1 ppb/8 hr.

Clinical Management
The victim should be moved from exposure and given respiratory therapy. Treatment should be symptomatic.

Animal Toxicity
Chronic exposure results in eye damage, kidney degeneration, and CNS effects. It is a carcinogen to nasal passages, pharynx, and respiratory tract. A dose–response relationship exists between exposure and damage to the reproductive system. Age or stage of sexual development also mediated damage. The oral LD_{50} is 100 mg/kg in rabbits and 260 mg/kg in mice.

—Jayne E. Ash and Shayne C. Gad

Related Topic

Pesticides

Nerve Gases

- Preferred Name: Nerve agents
- Synonyms: Tabun (GA; CAS 77-81-6); sarin (GB; CAS 107-44-8); soman (GD; CAS 96-64-0); GF; G agents; organophosphates (OP); VX (CAS 20820-80-8); V agents; chemical warfare agents; irreversible cholinesterase inhibitors; anticholinesterase compounds; see Organophosphates, Sarin, Soman, Tabun, and VX
- Description: Nerve gases are clear liquids; therefore, the term "gas" is a misnomer. The preferred term is "nerve agents." Because of the chiral phosphorus in their structure, the nerve agents contain various stereoisomers. Soman,

sarin, tabun, and VX contain equal amounts of (+) and (−) enantomers. The G agents are volatile and thus present both vapor and liquid hazard. In decreasing order of volatility are sarin, soman, tabun, and VX. VX presents a negligible vapor hazard, but its volatility increases with increasing temperature. At temperatures above 40°C it also presents a vapor hazard.

- Chemical Structure:

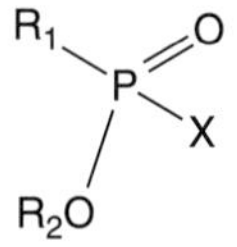

Chemical Structure: $R_1(R_2O)P(=O)X$

Chemical Structure	X	R_1	R_2
GA (Tabun)	$-CN$	$-N(CH_3)_2$	$-C_2H_5$
GB (Sarin)	$-F$	$-CH_3$	$-CH(CH_3)_2$
GD (Soman)	$-F$	$-CH_3$	$-CH(CH_3)C(CH_3)_3$
GF	$-F$		
VX		$-CH_3$	$-cyclo\ C_6H_{11}$
	$-SCH_2CH_2N(CH(CH_3)_2)_2$	$-CH_3$	$-C_2H_5$

Use

Nerve agents are used in chemical warfare.

Exposure Pathways

Casualties are caused primarily by inhalation; however, they can occur following percutaneous and ocular exposure, as well as by ingestion and injection.

Toxicokinetics

Nerve agents are absorbed both through the skin and via respiration. Because VX is an oily, nonvolatile liquid it is well absorbed through the skin (persistent nerve agent), although it can also be absorbed by inhalation. Thus, VX is more of a percutaneous threat than by inhalation, whereas the G agents (nonpersistent), which are also liquids, pose more of an inhalation hazard because of their vapor pressure.

Nerve agents are hydrolyzed by the enzyme organophosphate (OP) hydrolase. Hydrolysis of sarin, soman, tabun, and diisopropyl fluorophosphate occurs at approximately the same rate.

The isomers of the asymmetric OPs may differ in overall toxicity, rate of aging, rate of cholinesterase inhibition, and rate of detoxification. The rates of detoxification differ for different animal species and routes of administration.

The onset of effects from nerve agents depends on route, duration, and amount of exposure. They can occur within seconds to several minutes after exposure. There is no latent period following inhalation exposure of high concentrations where loss of consciousness and seizures have occurred within a minute. At low concentrations, however, miosis, rhinorrhea, and other effects may not begin for several minutes. Maximal effects usually occur within minutes after contamination ceases.

Mechanism of Toxicity

The nerve agents inhibit the enzymes butyrylcholinesterase in the plasma, the acetylcholinesterase on the red blood cell, and the acetylcholinesterase at cholinergic receptor sites in tissues. These three enzymes are not identical. Even the two acetylcholinesterases have slightly different properties, although they have a high affinity for acetylcholine. The blood enzymes reflect tissue enzyme activity. Following acute nerve agent exposure, the red blood cell enzyme activity most closely reflects tissue enzyme activity. However, during recovery, the plasma enzyme activity more closely parallels tissue enzyme activity.

Following nerve agent exposure, inhibition of the tissue enzyme blocks its ability to hydrolyze the neurotransmitter acetylcholine at the cholinergic receptor sites. Thus, acetylcholine accumulates and continues to stimulate the affected organ. The clinical effects of nerve agent exposure are caused by excess acetylcholine.

The binding of nerve agent to the enzyme is considered irreversible unless removed by therapy. The accumulation of acetylcholine in the peripheral and central nervous systems leads to depression of the respiratory center in the brain, followed by peripheral neuromuscular blockade causing respiratory depression and death.

The pharmacologic and toxicologic effects of the nerve agents are dependent on their stability, rates of absorption by the various routes of exposure, distribution, ability to cross the blood–brain barrier, rate of reaction and selectivity with the enzyme at specific foci, and behavior at the active site on the enzyme.

Red blood cell enzyme activity returns at the rate of red blood cell turnover, which is about 1% per day. Tissue and plasma activities return with synthesis of new enzymes. The rates of return of these enzymes are not identical. However, the nerve agent can be removed from the enzymes. This removal is called reactivation, which can be accomplished therapeutically by the use of oximes prior to aging. Aging is the biochemical process by which the agent–enzyme complex becomes refractory to oxime reactivation. The toxicity of nerve agents may include direct action on nicotinic acetylcholine receptors (skeletal muscle and ganglia) as well as on muscarinic acetylcholine receptors and the central nervous system (CNS).

Recently, investigations have focused on OP nerve agent poisoning secondary to acetylcholine effects. These include the effects of nerve agents on γ-aminobutyric acid neurones and cyclic nucleotides. In addition, changes in brain neurotransmitters, such as dopamine, serotonin, noradrenaline, as well as acetylcholine following inhibition of brain cholinesterase activity, have been reported. These changes may be due in part to a compensatory mechanism in response to overstimulation of the cholinergic system or could result from direct action of nerve agent on the enzymes responsible for noncholinergic neurotransmission.

Human Toxicity

The human toxicity estimates for the nerve agents are summarized in Table N-1.

Rhinorrhea may precede miosis as the first indication of exposure to even small amounts of nerve agent vapor. After exposure to high concentrations/doses by any route, rhinorrhea occurs as part of the generalized increase in secretions. Direct ocular contact to nerve agents may cause miosis, conjunctival injection, pain in or around the eyes, and dim or blurred vision.

Acute exposure of 3 mg/min/m^3 of GB vapor will produce miosis in most of the exposed population. Other routes of exposure may not cause any eye effects or cause a delayed onset of them, but will cause vomiting, sweating, and weakness.

The onset of miosis is within seconds to minutes following aerosol or vapor exposure but may not be maximal for up to an hour, especially at low concentrations. The duration of miosis varies and is dependent on the extent of exposure. The ability of the pupil to dilate maximally in darkness may not return for up to 6 weeks. There is no correlation between miosis and blood cholinesterase levels.

Respiratory distress also occurs within seconds to minutes following vapor exposure. The symptoms include tightness of the chest, shortness of breath, and gasping and irregular breathing leading to apnea. Bronchoconstriction and bronchial secretions contribute to this. With larger concentrations, cyanosis and audible pulmonary changes occur which can only be relieved by therapeutic intervention. Death due to nerve agent intoxication is attributable to respiratory failure resulting from bronchoconstriction, bronchosecretion, paralysis of skeletal muscles, including those responsible for respiration, and failure of the central drive for respiration. Nerve agent intoxication causes skeletal muscles to fasciculate, twitch, and fatigue prior to paralysis.

The cardiovascular effects of nerve agent exposure are variable. Bradycardia may occur via vagal stimulation, but other factors such as fright, hypoxia, and adrenergic stimulation secondary to ganglionic stimulation may produce tachycardia or hypertension.

Following inhalation exposure to large amounts of nerve agent, the CNS effects will cause loss of consciousness, seizure activity, and apnea within 1 min.

TABLE N-1
Human Toxicity Estimates for Nerve Agents

Agent	*Inhalation LCt_{50} (mg/min/m^3)*	*Intravenous LD_{50} (mg/kg)*	*Percutaneous LCt_{50} (mg/min/m^3)*	*Percutaneous LD_{50} (mg/kg)*
GA	135	0.08	20,000	0.014
GB	70	0.014	12,000	24.3
GD	70	—	—	5.0
GF	—	—	—	—
VX	30	0.008	—	0.143

Following skin contact to large amounts of liquid, the dermal effects may be delayed up to 30 min. Long-term exposure to an organophosphate, diisopropyl phosphorofluoridate, used in the treatment of myasthenia gravis, caused side effects including nightmares, confusion, and hallucinations.

Clinical Management

Following exposure the victim should be removed from the area to avoid further contamination and decontaminated (water/hypochlorite) by adequately protected (protective clothing and gas mask) and trained attendants. Contaminated clothing should be removed carefully so as to avoid further contamination. Respiration should be maintained and drug and supportive therapy instituted. If exposure is anticipated, pretreatment with carbamates (pyridostigmine bromide) may protect the cholinesterase enzymes before GD and possibly GA exposures, but not for GB and VX exposures. The three types of therapeutic drugs to be administered following nerve agent exposure are (1) a cholinergic blocker, anticholinergic, or cholinolytic drug such as atropine; (2) a reactivator drug to reactivate the inhibited enzyme such as the oxime, pralidoxime chloride; and (3) an anticonvulsant drug such as diazepam or other benzodiazepine. Oxygen may be indicated in respiratory failure.

Miosis, pain, dim vision, and nausea may be relieved by topical atropine in the eye. Atropine, a cholinergic blocker or anticholinergic drug, is effective in blocking the effects of excess acetylcholine at peripheral muscarinic sites. The usual dose is 2 mg for minor exposures and 6 mg for severe exposures. The dose should be repeated at 3- to 5-min until there is improvement. Pralidoxime chloride (protopam chloride) is an oxime used to break the agent–enzyme bond and restore the normal activity of the enzyme. This is most apparent in organs with nicotinic receptors. Abnormal activity decreases and normal strength returns to skeletal muscles, but no decrease in secretions is seen following oxime treatment. The usual dose is 1000 mg (intravenous or intramuscular). The injection contains 600 mg, which is not a high enough dose for a severe exposure. In a severe exposure, three of these (1800 mg) would be given. This is not an item generally used by civilians. The oxime administration may be repeated two or three times at hourly intervals either by intravenous or intramuscular injections. Diazepam, an anticonvulsant drug, is used to decrease convulsive activity and reduce brain damage that may occur from prolonged seizure activity. It is suggested that all three of these drugs be administered at the onset of severe effects from nerve agent exposure, whether or not seizures occur. The usual dose of diazepam is 10 mg.

Pyridostigmine bromide is available as a pretreatment for GD and possibly GA exposures, but not for GB and VX. It is available in 30-mg tablets, and tablets should be administered every 8 hr. When used prior to exposure, it should be followed by atropine and pralidoxime chloride after exposure. LD_{50}s in animals were increased several fold and survival rates were also increased in experiments with soman (GD) and these therapies.

Supportive therapy may include ventilation via an endotracheal airway if possible and suctioning of excess secretions from the airways.

Animal Toxicity

Small doses of nerve agents can produce tolerance.

The cause of death is attributed to anoxia resulting from a combination of central respiratory paralysis, severe bronchoconstriction, and weakness or paralysis of the accessory muscles for respiration.

Signs of nerve agent toxicity vary in rapidity of onset and severity. These are dependent on the specific agent, route of exposure, and dose or concentration. At the higher doses or concentrations, convulsions, and apnea, and neuropathies are indications of CNS toxicity. Following nerve agent exposure, animals exhibit hypothermia resulting from the cholinergic activation of the hypothalamic thermoregulatory center. In addition, plasma levels of pituitary, gonadal, thyroid, and adrenal hormones are increased during organophosphate intoxication. The nerve agents are anticholinesterases and as such inhibit the cholinesterase enzymes in the tissues resulting in the accumulation of acetylcholine at its various sites of action in both the autonomic nervous system and CNS. These include the endings of the parasympathetic nerves to the smooth muscles of the iris, ciliary body, bronchial tree, gastrointestinal tract, bladder, blood vessels, the secretory glands of the respiratory tract, the cardiac muscles, and the endings of sympathetic nerves to the sweat glands. Accumulation of acetylcholine at these sites results in characteristic muscarinic signs and symptoms, while the accumulation at the endings of the motor nerves to voluntary muscles and in the autonomic ganglia results in nicotinic signs and symptoms. The accumulation of acetylcholine in the brain and spinal cord results in the characteristic CNS signs and symptoms.

Nerve agents inhibit the activity of acetylcholinesterase by attaching to its active sites so that it cannot hydrolyze the neurotransmitter acetylcholine into choline, acetic acid, and regenerated enzyme. Thus, acetylcholine cannot attach to the enzyme, is not hydrolyzed, and continues to produce action potentials until the mechanism is fatigued. The biological effects of the nerve agents result from the excess of acetylcholine.

Animal toxicity values for nerve agents are listed in Table N-2.

Although there is a lack of information on the general toxicological effects of low-level, sublethal repeated exposures, there are studies on the behavioral effects of such exposures to nerve agents in animals free of observed signs of intoxication. These were conducted in an effort to determine whether behavioral studies can provide markers of early neurotoxicity that are more sensitive than neurochemical and neuropathological changes.

Although blood cholinesterase activity correlations with nerve agent effects are equivocal, they are indicative of exposure but do not reflect changes in the central nervous system. In rodents repeated subcutaneous injections of soman (GD) over a 5-day period at doses less than one-half the LD_{50} caused a significant decline in cholinesterase activity in all regions of the brain examined. The regional sensitivities were in agreement with the studies employing acute high-level soman exposures. In all cases, the neostriatum was the least sensitive area of the brain to nerve agent. These results are consistent with those of soman, sarin, and tabun at doses of 30, 40, 50, and 85% of the LD_{50}. No evidence

TABLE N-2
Animal Toxicity Values for Nerve Agents

		LD_{50}(μg/kg)			
Agent	LCt_{50} (mg/min/m^3) *inhalation*	SC[a]	PC[b]	IV[c]	IP[d]
Rat					
GA	3040	162	18 mg/kg	66	490
GB	1500	103	2.5	39	218
GD	30	71	7800	44.5	98
GF	—	—	—	—	—
VX	—	12	—	—	—
Rabbit					
GA	8400	375	2.5 mg/kg	63	—
GB	1200	30	925	15	—
GD	—	—	—	—	—
GF	—	—	—	—	—
VX	—	14	—	—	66
Dog					
GA	4000	—	30 mg/kg	84	—
GB	1000	—	—	—	—
GD	—	12	—	—	—
GF	—	—	—	—	—
VX	—	—	—	—	—
Monkey					
GA	2500	—	9.3 mg/kg	—	—
GB	1000	—	—	22.3	—
GD	—	13	—	—	—
GF	—	—	—	—	—
VX	—	—	—	—	—

[a] Subcutaneous.
[b] Percutaneous (depilated).
[c] Intravenous.
[d] Intraperitoneal.

of tolerance to the direct inhibitory effects of soman during 5 days of repeated injections was observed. However, a tolerance to soman-induced hypothermia was reported. Soman at 35 mg/kg injected subcutaneously up to 36 days at regular intervals reduced body temperature after the third injection, and then a steady tolerance developed to the drop in body temperature even though brain cholinesterase levels were inhibited. Brain cholinesterase levels did not parallel the recovery of serum cholinesterase following cessation of soman injection. Red blood cell cholinesterase recovery more closely reflected brain cholinesterase recovery than did serum. Daily doses of 25–54 mg/kg of soman for 5 days with survival times of 7–35 days were consistent with previous studies in that the most sensitive area of the brain to nerve agents was the piriform cortex and the least sensitive areas were the hypothalamus and neostriatum. This was demonstrated in both neurochemical and neuropathological studies. Soman-induced brain damage was similar in severity and locus whether administration was single or in repeated doses. However, the progression of brain degeneration following repeated dosing was more protracted. In rodents and nonhuman primates, the performance dose response was very steep, indicating that small changes in dose caused a large change in performance. Pretreatment plus use of antidote drugs was ineffective in preventing soman-induced performance decrements.

—Harry Salem and Frederick R. Sidell

(The views of the authors do not purport to reflect the position of the U.S. Department of Defense. The use of trade names does not constitute official endorsement or approval of the use of such commercial products.)

Related Topics

A-Esterase
Anticholinergics
Carboxylesterases
Cholinesterase Inhibition
Neurotoxicology: Central and Peripheral
Organophosphate Poisoning, Intermediate Syndrome
Organophosphates
Psychological Indices of Toxicity

Neurotoxicity, Delayed

The term "delayed neurotoxicity" may be used to describe any type of toxicity to the nervous system involving a delay between the precipitating chemical exposure and the appearance of neurological signs or symptoms. However, this designation usually refers to organophosphorus (OP) compound-induced delayed neurotoxicity (or delayed neuropathy) (OPIDN), also known as OP compound-induced delayed polyneuropathy (OPIDP). Recently, the notion has been put forward that there may be two forms of OPIDN, type I and type II, produced by absorption of a sufficiently high dose of certain pentacovalent or trivalent OP compounds, respectively. Nevertheless, pentacovalent OP compounds are more stable and more commonly used than trivalent ones, and type I OPIDN has been much more extensively studied than type II. Therefore, for the remainder of this article, OP compound will be understood to denote the pentacovalent chemical species and OPIDN will mean the type I disease.

The underlying pathology in OPIDN involves bilaterally symmetrical degeneration of sensory and motor axons in distal regions of peripheral nerves and spinal cord tracts. Generally, the longest, largest diameter fibers tend to be preferentially affected. The most prominent lesions are often found in the dorsal columns of the cervical spinal cord, especially in the fasciculus gracilis. Injury to this tract results in specific sensory deficits, including loss of recognition of limb position and vibration sensitivity. Recent pathogenesis studies indicate that the primary lesion in OPIDN is in the axon rather than the myelin sheath or the cell body of the neuron, and that demyelination occurs secondarily to axonal degeneration. The process has been likened to a "chemical transection" of the axon, with subsequent Wallerian-type degeneration, as opposed to a "dying back" of the axon following an insult to the cell body as hypothesized in earlier studies.

Signs and symptoms of axonopathy appear after a delay of about 8 days following absorption of an effective dose of an OPIDN-producing (neuropathic) OP compound and will consist of abnormal sensations (paresthesias) in the extremities, including numbness and tingling. There may also be pain, particularly in the calves of the legs. Distal reflexes may be absent or attenuated. The feet and lower legs are usually affected predominantly and prior to involvement of the hands and arms, but severe cases will involve the upper and lower limbs in a "glove and stocking" distribution. Incoordination of movement (ataxia) develops at about the same time as the sensory disturbances and may progress to partial flaccid paralysis (paresis) by Days 10–21. Recovery from severe disease is usually poor, and there is no specific treatment. Over a period of months to years, flaccidity may be replaced by spasticity, reflecting regeneration of peripheral nerve injury with residual damage to descending upper motor neuron pathways in the spinal cord.

Because of the ubiquity of OP compounds and the serious and often irreversible nature of OPIDN, much effort has been expended to develop ways to identify those OP compounds which pose a genuine risk of causing this condition. As a result, even though the pathogenic mechanism remains unknown, human OPIDN is now an extremely rare disease, with a worldwide incidence of only about two cases per year, usually from intentional ingestion of massive doses of OP compounds in attempted suicides. Sporadic episodes of OPIDN affecting domestic animals and livestock also occur, largely from misapplication of OP compounds used directly on the animals for control of insect or arachnid pests. Most of the approximately 30,000 human cases that occurred between 1930 and 1960 arose from contamination of cooking oil or beverages with tri-*o*-cresyl phosphate (TOCP; also known as tri-*o*-tolyl phosphate). Over half of the cases of OPIDN have been attributed to adulteration with TOCP of an alcoholic extract of Jamaica Ginger ("Ginger Jake") that was used as a source of alcohol during Prohibition in the United States. The resulting paralysis became known as "Jake Leg" (see Ginger Jake). Awareness of OPIDN coupled with the advent of improved methods for assessing the relative potential of OP compounds to produce the disease has led to the virtual elimination of human cases. Nevertheless, in view of the ongoing importance of OP chemistry in diverse commercial applications and the significance of understanding mechanisms of neurodegenerative diseases in neuroscience and medicine, OPIDN continues to be an active field of research.

Experimental studies have identified the adult chicken as the species of choice for testing OP compounds for their potential to cause OPIDN. Hens of greater than 8 months of age are now used in routine testing. Other species in addition to humans and chickens known to be susceptible to single doses of neuropathic OP compounds include certain nonhuman primates, water buffalo, cattle, swine, sheep, dogs, and cats. Rats and mice have been considered to be resistant to the clinical manifestations of OPIDN, but recent studies have shown that histopathological lesions, particularly in the spinal cord, can be produced in these species by compounds known to cause OPIDN in the adult hen. The apparent resistance of rodents to OPIDN may be due, at least in part, to the fact that relatively young (less than 3 months of age) animals have been used in most studies. Generally, the young of a given species are much more resistant than adults to OPIDN. For example, chicks younger than about 50 days of age will not develop OPIDN after a single dose of a neuropathic OP compound and also appear to be resistant to repeated doses if they are younger than 14 days of age. Species and age differences in susceptibility to OPIDN appear to be correlated with the greater length of axons in larger animals and more robust mechanisms for repair of neural injury in younger animals.

Although the complete mechanism of OPIDN has not been elucidated, there is good evidence that the disease is initiated by a concerted two-step reaction involving inhibition and aging of a critical amount of a protein called neurotoxic esterase (neuropathy target esterase, NTE) in target neural tissues. The net result of the aging step is the rapid formation of a negatively charged species in the active site of the enzyme (Fig. N-1). Such a reaction can take place with OP inhibitors of NTE such as phosphates, phosphonates, or phosphoramidates, which have an ester or amide group in addition to the leaving group. Compounds belonging to these structural classes that do not inhibit NTE do not cause OPIDN.

Given that inhibition and aging of NTE transpire within minutes to hours of absorption of an effective dose of a neuropathic OP compound, these events do not account for the 8- to 21-day delay between exposure and the initial signs of ataxia and paresis. However, if inhibition but no aging occurs by dosing with an NTE inhibitor that is incapable of generating a negative charge at the active site, no OPIDN ensues. Furthermore, an animal whose NTE is inhibited with a nonaging compound is protected against a subsequent dose of an OP compound that would be neuropathic in a

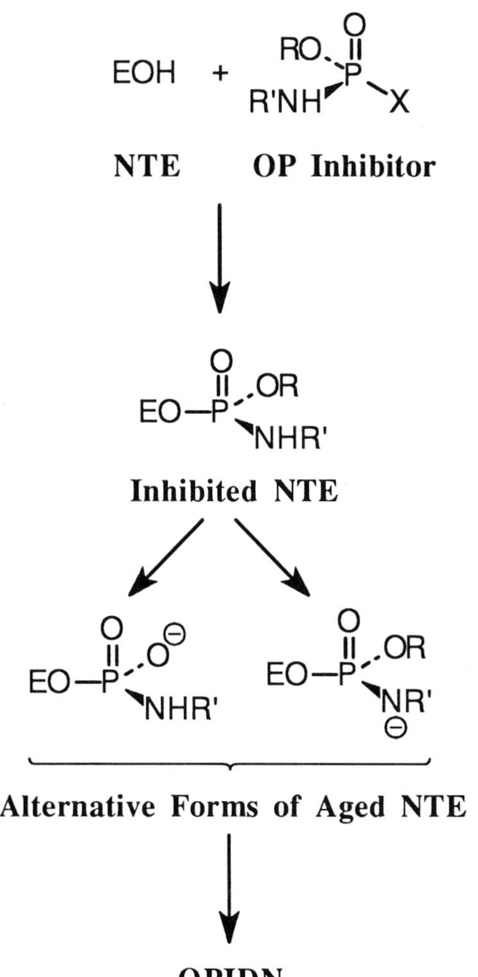

FIGURE N-1. Inhibition and aging of NTE in the initiation of OPIDN. The OP inhibitor shown illustrates two different modes of aging involving formation of a negative charge by scission of an ester (R–O-) or deprotonation of an amide (R–NH-) linkage. R may be substituted or unsubstituted alkyl or aryl; R′ may include the same groups as R or may be hydrogen. X is the leaving group displaced by reaction with the serine hydroxyl of NTE and may be, e.g., substituted or unsubstituted alkoxy or aryloxy or fluorine.

naive animal (Fig. N-2). Nonaging inhibitors of NTE include representatives from the phosphinate class of OP compounds, certain carbamates, and a sulfonyl halide, phenylmethanesulfonyl fluoride.

The threshold of NTE inhibition in target neural tissue that correlates with the development of OPIDN after a single dose of a neuropathic OP compound is approximately 70%. For many compounds, inhibition measured in brain is paralleled in spinal cord and peripheral nerve, and brain values are often used in screening tests in hens to assess relative neuropathic potency. Repeated dosing also appears to require that a high point of inhibition be reached before OPIDN will develop. The threshold appears to be the same as for acute dosing for some compounds, but for some others, the critical level of inhibition may be as low as 50%. With repeated dosing, there still appears to be a delay of about 8–21 days between the time inhibition exceeds the threshold value and the appearance of signs of OPIDN.

NTE has also been found in circulating lymphocytes and platelets, where it has found some use as a biomarker of exposure to neuropathic OP compounds. There is a reasonably good correlation between inhibition of NTE in leukocytes and brain when the measurements are carried out within 24 hr of an acute exposure. However, good correlations may not be found at later times (even by 48 hr) or under conditions of repeated exposures.

It is important to realize that OPIDN depends on a particular type of chemical modification of NTE rather

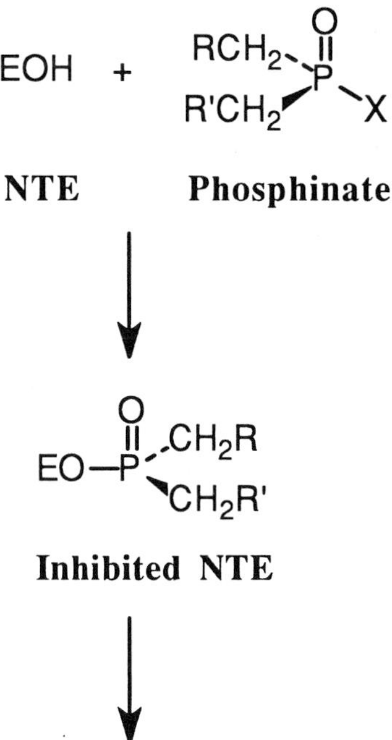

FIGURE N-2. Inhibition of NTE with a nonaging inhibitor (a phosphinate) in protection against OPIDN. The R–CH_2- linkages do not undergo scission or deprotonation and no negative charge is formed. R, R′, and X are as defined in Fig. N-1.

than mere inhibition of its enzymatic activity. Inhibition of NTE is a necessary, but not sufficient, condition for OPIDN. Aging of the inhibited enzyme results in a complete change in the toxicological outcome. Whereas inhibition without aging results in no clinically apparent injury, suprathreshold inhibition with aging triggers an inexorable neurodegenerative process leading to evident disease. The situation with NTE is completely different from that with acetylcholinesterase (AChE). Inhibition of a sufficient amount of AChE will precipitate cholinergic toxicity, regardless of whether or not aging of inhibited AChE occurs. Aging of inhibited AChE does not alter the type of toxic response, but it does change the options available for therapy against cholinergic toxicity. For example, oximes such as pralidoxime methiodide are used to reactivate inhibited AChE, but these agents are ineffective if aging of the enzyme has occurred. Moreover, oximes do not appear to affect the clinical course of OPIDN following administration of a neuropathic OP compound, except to allow survival of an otherwise lethal dose of a compound that also has cholinergic toxicity.

In a homologous series of OP compounds, increasing potency for AChE inhibition and cholinergic toxicity correlates with decreasing potency for NTE inhibition and OPIDN. The relative potency of an OP compound or its active metabolite for inhibition of NTE versus AChE *in vitro* can be used as a convenient index of probable neuropathic potential of the compound. A commonly used measure of inhibitory potency is the I_{50}, the concentration required to inhibit 50% of the enzyme activity under a standardized set of reaction conditions and time of incubation of the inhibitor with the enzyme preparation. Comparisons of NTE/AChE I_{50} ratios *in vitro* with toxicity data *in vivo* have shown that values <1 indicate that the dose required to produce OPIDN is less than the LD_{50}, whereas values >1 correspond to doses greater than the LD_{50} being required to produce OPIDN. Insecticidal OP compounds will generally be much more potent inhibitors of AChE than NTE and will not produce OPIDN except at doses that would require treatment for cholinergic toxicity. On the other hand, a compound such as TOCP is metabolized to a cyclic saligenin phosphate ester that is a more potent inhibitor of NTE than AChE and capable of producing OPIDN at doses that elicit little or no cholinergic toxicity.

Recently, it has been found that marginal or subclinical OPIDN initiated by an OP compound at a dose that is below the level required to produce obvious signs of ataxia or paresis can be potentiated to full-blown disease by subsequent treatment with nonaging inhibitors of NTE. This was initially a surprising finding, especially in view of the fact that reversing the order of dosing of the nonaging and aging NTE inhibitors affords protection against OPIDN. However, it now appears that the outcome of many types of neural injuries can be worsened by dosing with nonaging NTE inhibitors as well as with inhibitors of other serine proteases and esterases. The apparent indifference to the method of producing the initial lesion suggests a general mode of action for potentiation, such as interference with regeneration and repair. With respect to the potentiation of OPIDN and its practical significance, more data are needed to determine the following: the extent to which the NTE inhibition threshold for initiation may be lowered by potentiators, the potency of potentiators at a given dose level of initiator, the potency of initiators at a given dose level of potentiator, structure–activity relationships of potentiators, and the mechanism(s) of action of the effect.

Further Reading

Abou-Donia, M. B., and Lapadula, D. M. (1990). Mechanisms of organophosphorus-induced delayed neurotoxicity: Type I and type II. *Annu. Rev. Pharmacol. Toxicol.* **30**, 405–440.

Davis, C. S., and Richardson, R. J. (1985). Organophosphorus compounds. In *Neurotoxicity of Industrial and Commercial Chemicals* (J. L. O'Donoghue, Ed.), Vol II, pp. 1–23. CRC Press, Boca Raton, FL.

Johnson, M. K. (1990). Organophosphates and delayed neuropathy—Is NTE alive and well? *Toxicol. Appl. Pharmacol.* **102**, 385–399.

Lotti, M. (1992). The pathogenesis of organophosphate polyneuropathy. *Crit. Rev. Toxicol.* **21**, 465–487.

Pope, C. N., Tanaka, D., Jr., and Padilla, S. (1993). The role of neurotoxic esterase (NTE) in the prevention and potentiation of organophosphorus-induced delayed neurotoxicity (OPIDN). *Chem.-Biol. Interact.* **87**, 395–406.

Richardson, R. J. (1992). Interactions of organophosphorus compounds with neurotoxic esterase. In *Organophosphates: Chemistry, Fate, and Effects* (J. E. Chambers and P. E. Levi, Eds.), pp. 299–323. Academic Press, San Diego.

Zech, R., and Chemnitius, J. M. (1987). Neurotoxicant sensitive esterase. Enzymology and pathophysiology of organophosphorus ester-induced delayed neuropathy. *Prog. Neurobiol.* **29**, 193–218.

—Rudy J. Richardson

Related Topics

A-Esterase
Acetylcholine
Cholinesterase Inhibition
Neurotoxicology: Central and Peripheral
Organophosphate Poisoning, Intermediate Syndrome
Organophosphates

Neurotoxicology: Central and Peripheral

Introduction

Neurotoxicology is the study and evaluation of the effects of chemical substances on the nervous system. Humans have known that chemicals found in plants and animals can produce profound changes in the function of the nervous system and have used natural products, such as opium, cannabis, belladonna, and alcohol, for thousands of years. As people developed the capacity to extract, purify, and finally synthesize new chemical substances, the number of chemicals that could modify nervous system function grew rapidly. Occupational exposures of workers to some of these played an important role in recognizing the damage that longer term exposures could produce, even when acute effects were minimal. To date, we have learned a lot about the acute neurotoxicity of many substances and the chronic neurotoxicity of many others, yet we have barely scratched the surface. Thousands of existing chemicals have not yet been evaluated for their capacity to produce neurotoxicity. Add to that the rapid rate at which new chemicals are synthesized and it is obvious that there is much, much more to be done.

The methods by which the neurotoxicity of chemicals can be detected are numerous. The surest is to detect neurotoxicity directly in the human population. This has occurred for many chemicals which were introduced into the workplace without prior toxicity testing. Epidemiological studies of human populations have provided the initial awareness of neurotoxicity of many types. Animal testing is another, more controlled means of defining neurotoxicity. Fortunately, neurons and basic neuronal circuitry are very similar between mammalian species. Neurons from rats, cats, dogs, and humans share similar critical macromolecules with high conservation of structure and function through evolution. The enhanced intellectual capacity of humans results more from quantitative than from qualitative differences in the structure and function of neurons. It is the increase in size and complexity of the nervous system in humans that accounts for this, not the presence of a new type of neuron or other cellular element. For this reason toxic responses in humans and animals are usually similar. Thus, animals can serve as valid models for most neurotoxic responses in humans.

In the past 50 years, most of the concerns in neurotoxicology focused on the effects of acute exposures and of industrial exposures to high concentrations of chemicals. Today there is a growing recognition and concern that long-term exposures to low concentrations of chemicals in the environment may produce a cumulative type of neurotoxic response. There is suggestive evidence that polychlorinated biphenyls and lead have adversely affected intellectual development in children at levels existing in certain environments. There are hints that lifetime exposures to other chemicals may be the cause or accelerate the rate of progression of neurodegenerative diseases, including Parkinson's disease, Huntington's chorea, and Alzheimer's disease. It is incumbent on our society to determine the extent to which this is true. To not do so will either lead to unacceptable levels of neurotoxicity affecting millions of people or alternately to the indiscriminate banning of harmless chemicals with irreplaceable value to society. These concerns and directions for future research will be briefly considered at the end of this entry.

There are many reasons why the nervous system is frequently involved in toxic responses to drugs and chemical substances. The morphological and biochemical complexity of the nervous system make it a sensitive and selective target to chemical attack. One point of interest is that the brain expresses more of the total genetic information in its DNA than does any other organ, perhaps 10–20 times as much. Thus, in addition to the metabolic and maintenance machinery shared by most cell types, neurons contain many unique macromolecules, including enzymes, ion channels, neurotransmitters, and receptors, that are not found in other cells. Chemicals that target these produce selective changes in nervous system activity that are directly related in intensity and duration to the concentration of the toxicant in the brain. With exposures severe enough to kill nerve cells or parts of cells, long-term, often permanent, deficits in sensory processes, motor function, behavior, learning capacity, and memory can occur. Since neurons do not reproduce, recovery of lost function occurs only if the remaining nervous system can "take over" the functions of the cells that were killed. Less severe exposures will modify function, often profoundly, until the chemical is eliminated from the body. In most cases, normal behavior returns, and there may be no evidence of chronic consequences. With repeated exposures to some substances, however, the consequences may take on an irreversible quality. There are numerous examples in which chronic exposures to chemicals used in industry produce severe, long-lasting neuronal deficits after months or years of exposure. The same appears to be true for certain environmental exposures. Chronic effects can also be more subtle. For example, frequent use of alcohol and other drugs, particularly in children of school age, can depress nervous function for sufficiently long periods of time during critical periods of intellectual and social development so as to produce nearly irreparable changes in social and personal growth.

Bases for Selective Neurotoxicity of Chemicals

Cell Types

The nervous system is composed of three basic cellular elements: (1) neurons, (2) interstitial cells, and (3) connective tissue, blood vessels, and microglia. The neuron is the only cell type in the nervous system involved in information processing. Each neuron is, in its own right, a receiver, an integrator, and a transmitter of information. Neurons are always in contact with other neurons so that they create simple and complex channels through which many different responses can be transmitted. All behavior, no matter how complex, results from the interactive function of many, many neurons with relatively limited response potential.

Neurons vary tremendously in form and size, but they all share in common the ability to respond to stimuli and to create new stimuli to affect other cells. Regardless of their structural diversity all neurons are bounded by a plasma membrane and possess a cell body (soma), one or more axons, and, with very few exceptions, dendrites (Fig. N-3).

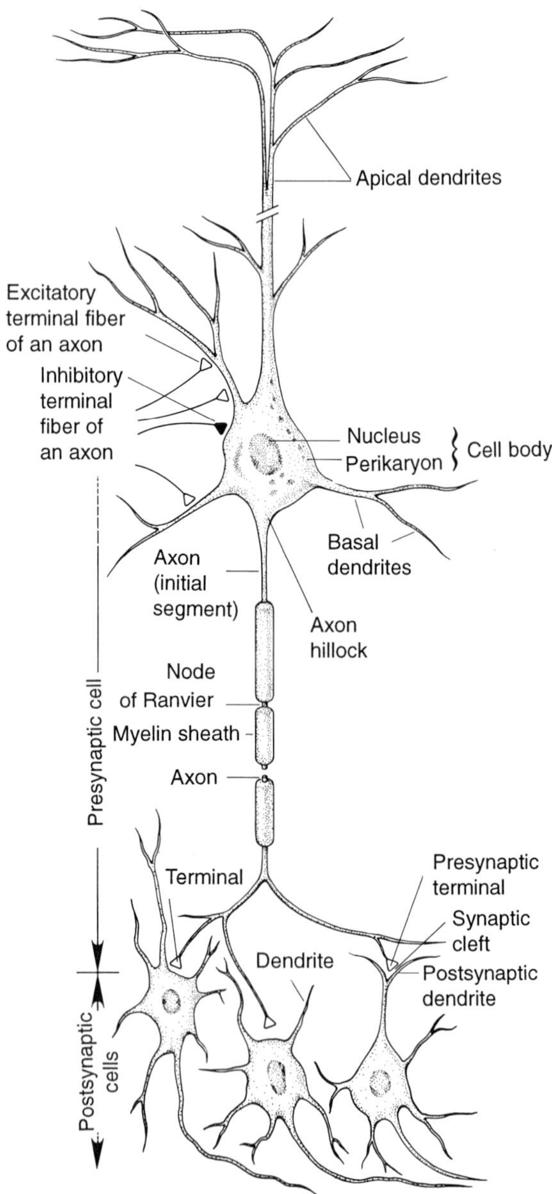

FIGURE N-3. Basic anatomy of neurons, showing the cell body (soma), axons, and dendrites, presynaptic cell, and postsynaptic cells (reproduced with permission from E. R. Kandel, J. M. Schwartz, and T. M. Jessel, Principles of Neural Science, 3rd ed., Appleton & Lange, Norwalk, CT).

The bounding membrane is typical of all cells. It is a continuous lipid bilayer sheet some 60–80 Å thick. Embedded in it or passing through it are numerous proteins and glycoproteins, many of which are found only in nerve cells. Some provide structural support to the membrane, but most form the ion channels and receptor sites that are absolutely essential to nerve function.

The membrane of the neuron is differentially specialized. The membrane of the soma and dendrites is designed to react to chemical stimuli and contains both neurotransmitter-gated ion channels and neurotransmitter-gated receptors associated with various G-proteins. The former evoke rapid changes in the cell's membrane potential, while the latter initiate slower, more persisting changes in neuronal excitability mediated via second messengers such as cyclic adenosine monophosphate (cAMP) and inositol tri-phosphate (IP_3).

The axon is specialized to react to changes in membrane potential. When the cell's membrane potential reaches a certain "threshold" the axon responds with an action potential that rapidly transmits an electrical signal from the cell body to its terminals. Finally, the axon terminal is specialized to convert the electrical signal of the action potential back into a chemical signal. It responds to depolarization by releasing a neurotransmitter which acts on the soma or dendritic membranes of the next neuron or, in the peripheral nervous system (PNS), to an effector. The membrane is absolutely essential to the electrochemical properties of neurons.

The nucleus is usually located in the center of the cell body. It contains widely dispersed, fine chromatin material. The chromatin is composed of deoxyribonucleic acid (DNA) and its associated histone proteins. The nucleolus contains the specific portion of DNA encoding the ribonucleic acid (RNA) of future ribosomes.

In the neuroplasm are located mitochondria, Nissl substance, and the Golgi apparatus. Mitochondria contain their own DNA and divide by "budding" in much the same way that bacterial cells divide. They function as the major oxidative organelles, providing energy through the production of adenosine triphosphate (ATP). The Nissl substance, which is absent from the axon, represents the nodal points of the endoplasmic reticulum which exists throughout the soma. The endoplasmic reticulum is the major protein synthesizing organelle and manufactures in 1–3 days an amount of protein equal to the total protein content of the cell. The Golgi apparatus is primarily responsible for synthesis of membrane and the incorporation of membrane-bound proteins into it. It pinches off the membrane with its associated proteins as "vesicles." Some of these vesicles contain protein needed to maintain the neurolemma, while others become secretory vesicles destined to contain neurotransmitter.

The dendrites represent all the processes of the cell body except for the specialized axonal process (axon). They are usually numerous and serve to increase the surface area of the neuron available for receiving synaptic input. Neurons will have one or more main dendrites which successively branch and branch to form many smaller processes.

The axon of the typical neuron arises from a cone-shaped region of the cell body, the axon hillock. The initial segment of the axon is both the smallest region in diameter and the region with the lowest threshold to electrical activation. Distal to the initial segment the axonal diameter enlarges and the diameter remains constant out to the terminal ending or until the axon branches. Myelinated neurons have their axons ensheathed by myelin segments, each segment provided by an oligodendrocyte or neurolemmal cell. Between segments the axonal membrane is exposed. These regions are termed the "nodes of Ranvier." Unmyelinated axons do not possess such a segmented sheath. Rather, they tend to collect in bundles which are loosely enclosed in troughs formed by neurolemmal cells or oligodendrocytes. The terminal end of an axon most often is profusely branching, with each branch ultimately terminating in a synaptic ending.

Mechanisms are available within the neuron which allow the passage of substances from the soma to axon terminal and vice versa. Most of the vesicles formed by the Golgi apparatus are transported through the axon to the nerve terminal by fast anterograde transport. Within the terminal the secretory vesicles recycle many times, binding and fusing with the terminal membrane, then being "pinched off" via endocytosis and returned to the vesicle pool. The terminal membrane is constantly being replaced by newly arriving vesicles. Old membrane and proteins are returned to the cell body for degradation by way of a fast retrograde transport system.

Fast anterograde transport can reach rates as high as 400 mm/day. It is dependent on microtubules that provide a track along which the vesicles move. The movement is energy dependent and is mediated by a specific "motor" protein, kinesin. A similar process is responsible for fast retrograde transport. A second motor protein, dynein, is needed for movement in this direction. A third type of transport process is termed slow axoplasmic transport. It ranges from 0.2 to 5 mm/day and is responsible for the transport of cytoskeletal proteins, the neurofilaments and microtubules, as well as an assortment of cytoplasmic proteins.

The interstitial cells include the astroglia (astrocytes) and oligodendroglia (oligodendrocytes) in the central nervous system (CNS) and the neurolemma cells (Schwann cells) in the PNS. These cells serve as both supportive cells and "nurse" cells from a structural and probably also a metabolic standpoint. Astroglia surround and separate neurons and often end in plate-like expansions on blood vessels, the ependyma, or on the pial surfaces. They contribute importantly to the so-called blood–brain barrier (BBB). Oligodendroglia also possess processes which appose neuronal surfaces and, most significantly, form the myelin sheaths surrounding myelinated nerve fibers in the CNS. In addition, oligodendroglia provide a looser covering through which the unmyelinated fibers course. They also appear to play a role in maintenance of extracellular ionic concentrations and actively remove and metabolize some neurotransmitters from synaptic clefts. In the periphery most neuronal elements are surrounded by processes from Schwann cells which form the multilayered myelin sheaths characteristic of peripheral myelinated nerves.

In addition to neurons and interstitial cells, the nervous system contains blood vessels, fibroblasts, and other connective tissue elements and the microglia. The latter cell type is identical with the connective tissue macrophages. They are phagocytic and remove debris throughout the CNS.

Morphological Considerations

Neurons assume a vast array of forms in accordance with the functions they serve. In most neurons the cell body and dendrites are separated from the axonal terminal by a very long tube, the axon. This creates problems unique to nerve cells. In the motoneurons that innervate the hands and feet, for example, more than 90% of the mass of the neuron is in the cell processes. An often given example is that if the cell body of that neuron were enlarged to the size of a baseball, the axon would be about 1 mile long, and the dendrites and their branches would arborize throughout a large amphitheater.

The neuron is put at a metabolic disadvantage because of this. The cell body is the only part of the neuron that can synthesize proteins, but it may make up less than 5% of the total cell mass. Because of this, very high rates of protein synthesis are required. As all proteins are synthesized in the cell body, most have to be transported long distances to their eventual target. For proteins destined for the distal portions of the axon and for the axon terminal, specialized transport systems must function continually to get them to their targets in a reasonable amount of time. These require a large, complex cytoskeleton to maintain them. Anything that compromises protein synthesis, axonal transport, or cytoskeletal integrity may reduce new functional and structural protein arrival to the point where structure and function are irreparably damaged.

Nutritional and Biochemical Aspects

The CNS is protected from certain toxic effects by the BBB. This barrier is primarily created by the tight junctions that occur in brain capillaries between neighboring endothelial cells. Nonpolar, lipid-soluble compounds can penetrate the barrier readily. However, highly polar, non-lipid-soluble compounds do not penetrate well, if at all. Thus most neurotoxic substances that target the CNS are relatively lipid soluble. The BBB is less well formed in immature brains, and children are more susceptible to certain poorly lipid-soluble substances, such as lead salts, than are adults. The patency of the BBB may also change in conditions of disease and dehydration. Although the CNS is generally well protected from certain toxicants by the BBB, the PNS does not have a comparable structure. Therefore, it is possible to have toxicity restricted to peripheral structures only, if their entry into the CNS in excluded.

The metabolic requirements of neurons often make them more susceptible than other types of cells to toxic actions. Neurons are highly active metabolically and are very susceptible to chemical actions that interfere with normal nutrient utilization. The high metabolic activity results in part from the high rates of protein synthesis needed to maintain the nerve cell and from the fact that a neuron constantly generates action potentials as part of its information processing function.

Each action potential erodes the ionic gradients existing across the nerve cell membrane which are critical to normal function. Large amounts of energy are expended by the nerve cell in restoring and maintaining these gradients. This requires the continuous formation of large amounts of ATP, which requires aerobic metabolism.

Neurons are almost entirely dependent on glucose as an energy supply. The neuron has little capacity for anaerobic metabolism and is, therefore, highly susceptible to a lack of oxygen or glucose. The oxygen consumption of neurons is nearly 10 times higher than that of glial cells, and they therefore are more often damaged by anoxic or hypoglycemic conditions. Certain large neurons, such as the pyramidal cells in the cerebral cortex, cerebellum, and hippocampus or motoneurons in the spinal cord, have a particularly high metabolic rate. Damage is often seen first at these sites when oxygen or glucose levels are not sufficiently maintained. Neuronal damage can start within minutes and become irreversible 5 or 6 min after oxygen or glucose delivery is stopped.

Role of Myelin

Myelinated nerve fibers are ensheathed by a succession of Schwann cells in the PNS or oligodendrocytes in the CNS. These form a segmental chain of myelin sheaths that completely enclose the axons except at the Nodes of Ranvier. The myelin sheath is a greatly extended and modified plasma membrane which is wrapped around the nerve axon in a spiral fashion. Each myelin-generating cell furnishes myelin for only one segment of any given axon. The axon and its myelin sheath are important to each other metabolically as well as functionally. Axons direct the formation of myelin and can provide a mitogenic stimulus for Schwann cell or oligodendrocyte cell proliferation. The myelin-forming cells can influence axonal diameter and play a role in determining the composition of the axonal membrane. Whereas in nonmyelinated fibers sodium and potassium channels are distributed uniformly across the axonal membrane, in myelinated fibers sodium channels are concentrated at the Nodes of Ranvier and potassium channels in the internodal regions. This greatly improves the efficiency of action potential propagation. As an example of the advantages imparted by myelin two different nerve fibers are compared, one myelinated and the other nonmyelinated, that both conduct action potentials at 25 m/sec. The nonmyelinated axon (squid giant axon) would be 500 μm in diameter, while the myelinated axon (human) would only be 12 μm in diameter. The nonmyelinated axon requires 5000 times as much energy to conduct an action potential and would occupy about 1500 times as much space. If the human spinal cord contained only nonmyelinated axons, it would need to be as large as a good-sized tree trunk to conduct action potentials at the same speed as it currently does.

When myelin is lost axonal function is rapidly affected. Conduction velocity slows in proportion to the degree of demyelination and, in extreme cases, conduction is blocked. Loss of myelin may also lead to the loss of the axon. Axons generally can survive some demyelination, but extensive loss of myelin can result in axonal degeneration. Because myelin-forming cells can proliferate, they generally reestablish a patent myelin sheath around an axon once the demyelinating stimulus is removed.

The Synapse

The synapse is a most important structure in the nervous system and it serves as the communication link between neurons (Fig. N-3). With few exceptions, synapses in the mammalian CNS are chemical in nature. These possess three components: a presynaptic element, a postsynaptic element, and a synaptic cleft. At a typical synapse, neurotransmission requires four steps: (1) synthesis and storage of transmitter, (2) transmitter release, (3) receptor activation, and (4) transmitter inactivation. Most neurotransmitters are synthesized within the presynaptic terminal by enzymes made in the cell body and transported to the ending by axoplasmic transport. They are subsequently stored in vesicles in the terminal. These vesicles, as well as the presynaptic terminal membrane, contain specific proteins which play essentials roles in the docking and fusing of vesicles to the membrane during the process of transmitter release.

The release of neurotransmitter is triggered by a sequence of events which begins with the propagation of an action potential into the terminal region. The depolarization that accompanies the action potential induces an increase in membrane permeability to calcium ions. A large inward electrochemical gradient exists for calcium and it moves into the terminal. The calcium which enters the terminal activates enzymes which cause the attachment of some of the vesicles to releasing sites on the terminal membrane, membrane fusion, and the release of the vesicular contents into the synaptic cleft. Transmitter release is terminated by the removal of calcium from the terminal cytoplasm, either via a calcium pump, which pumps it out of the cell, or by uptake into the endoplasmic reticulum or into mitochondria.

Once the neurotransmitter is released from the presynaptic terminal it diffuses across the synaptic cleft. On the postsynaptic side it complexes with a membrane-bound macromolecule, its receptor. This binding leads to one of two consequences. If the receptor is coupled to an ion channel, the channel is opened, ions move down electrochemical gradients, and the membrane potential is changed. If the receptor is coupled to a G-protein, the binding initiates a sequence of biochemical events that results in the production of a second messenger such as cAMP or IP_3. These evoke long-term changes that alter the excitability of the postsynaptic cell. The complexation process is usually rapidly reversible with a half-life for receptor occupancy of 1–20 msec.

The transmitter action is terminated by various means. For many neurotransmitters, the bulk is taken back up into the presynaptic terminal via an active transport process to be reused. Some of the neurotransmitter simply diffuses away and is destroyed elsewhere. In other cases enzymes may be present on the postsynaptic side of the cleft which rapidly break the transmitter down into inactive substances.

Clearly, there are many components involved in the process of neurotransmission. These can be the targets of useful drug products as well as neurotoxicants. Examples are the local anesthetics, which target sodium channels in nerve axons; neuromuscular blocking agents, which target the nicotinic receptor at the motor endplates; and some tranquilizers, such as diazepam, which target the γ-aminobutyric acid (GABA) receptor on neurons in the CNS. It is interesting that animal and plant toxins target components of the neurotransmission process more than any other aspect of neuronal function. They tend to target peripheral synapses rather than central ones because many are large, proteinaceous substances whose entry into the CNS is restricted due to a patent BBB.

Specific Neurotransmitter Systems

Certain neurotransmitter systems are more frequently involved in toxicologic responses than others. Among the neurotoxicants to be described, many target the cholinergic, glutamatergic, GABAergic, and glycinergic neurotransmitter systems, and to understand their mechanisms, a more comprehensive description of their components will be given.

Acetylcholine is the neurotransmitter released by the motoneurons which innervate skeletal muscle, all preganglionic and many postganglionic autonomic neurons which innervate smooth muscle, cardiac muscle and glands, and many neurons within the CNS. Extensive losses of cholinergic neurons in the CNS have been found in patients having Alzheimer's disease. Two distinct receptor groups have been identified for acetylcholine, the nicotinic and the muscarinic groups (Table N-3). There are at least four subtypes of nicotinic and five subtypes of muscarinic receptor. Nicotinic receptors are ubiquitous and exist at the neuromuscular junctions of skeletal muscles and on ganglion cells in the autonomic nervous system. All nicotinic receptors are parts of a cation-specific ion channel which, when opened, evokes fast, transient depolarizations of the recipient cell. Muscarinic receptors are found in smooth muscle receiving parasympathetic innervation and elsewhere. Muscarinic receptors affect second messenger systems and produce effects that vary with the specific target.

Acetylcholine is synthesized from acetyl-CoA and choline within the presynaptic terminal by the enzyme choline acetylase (Fig. N-4). The acetylcholine formed is stored in small, lightly staining synaptic vesicles which are concentrated around the synaptic contact area. The release of acetylcholine is calcium dependent. The entire content of a synaptic vesicle is released into the cleft in an all or none manner where it interacts with its receptors and then is rapidly destroyed by acetylcholinesterase.

Under normal conditions the half-life for acetylcholine in the synaptic cleft is about 1 msec. The acetylcholine is hydrolyzed to choline and acetate, and the choline is actively pumped back into the presynaptic terminal to be used to synthesize more acetylcholine.

Within the CNS there are specific neurotransmitter systems that play critical roles in controlling excitability. They, too, tend to be important target for chemicals.

Glutamate is the primary excitatory neurotransmitter in the brain. Glutamate is formed by the Kreb's cycle and is found free and stored in vesicles in synaptic terminals.

TABLE N-3
Representative Receptors and Their Actions

Receptor type	*Location, effect, and mechanism of action*
Cholinergic	
Muscarinic	Postsynaptic and presynaptic, variable effects, some increase IP_3, other inhibit adenyl cyclase
Nicotinic	Postsynaptic, excitatory, open a Na^+,K^+-selective ion channel
Adrenergic	
α_1	Postsynaptic, excitatory, linked to formation of IP_3
α_2	Presynaptic, reduce transmitter release, reduce calcium entry
β_1	Postsynaptic, depressive, ?
	Postsynaptic, excitatory, activates adenyl cyclase
β_2	Postsynaptic, depressive, activates adenyl cyclase
Dopaminergic	
D_1	Postsynaptic, variable effects, stimulates adenyl cyclase
D_2	Postsynaptic and presynaptic, variable effects, inhibits adenyl cyclase
GABAergic	
$GABA_A$	Postsynaptic, inhibitory, open a Cl^- selective ion channel
$GABA_B$	Presynaptic, inhibitory, reduce calcium entry
	Postsynaptic, inhibitory, increase K^+ conductance
Glycinergic	
	Postsynaptic, inhibitory, open a Cl^- selective ion channel
Glutamatergic	
AMPA	Postsynaptic, excitatory, open a Na^+, K^+-selective ion channel
Kainate	Postsynaptic, excitatory, open a Na^+,K^+-selective ion channel
NMDA	Postsynaptic, excitatory, open a Na^+, K^+, Ca^{2+}-selective ion channel

Its release is calcium dependent, and an uptake system exists in presynaptic terminals and in glia to terminate its action after release. It is probable that glia metabolize glutamate to glutamine and return it to the neuron for reuse.

Three subtypes of receptors are known (Table N-3). Two of these, the AMPA and kainate receptors, are part of a cation-selective ion channel that is permeable to sodium and potassium. These channels are responsible for the fast, transient excitatory postsynaptic potentials evoked by glutamate release. The third, the N-methyl-D-aspartate receptor, is part of a cation channel permeable to sodium, potassium, and calcium. Activation of this channel leads to calcium entry into the cell

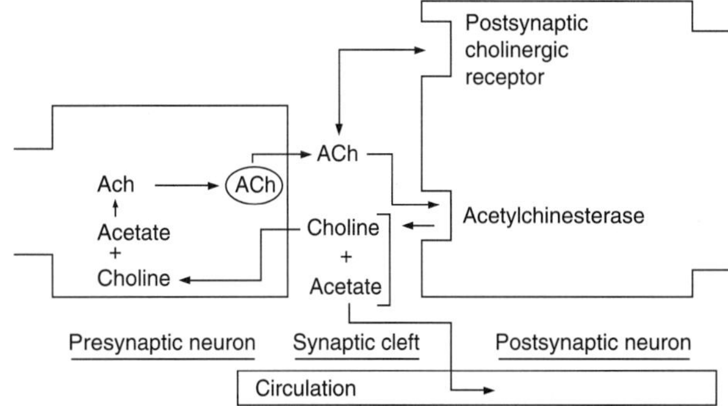

FIGURE N-4. Acetylcholine synthesized from acetyl-CoA and choline within the presynaptic terminal by the enzyme choline acetylase (reproduced with permission from D. E. Ecobichon and R. M. Joy, Pesticides and Neurological Diseases, copyright CRC Press, Boca Raton, FL.

which can act as a second messenger in its own right to modulate cellular processes. This receptor is critical to the development of neuronal plasticity in experimental model systems and is thought to be essential to higher processes of the brain, including memory and learning.

Inhibitory neurotransmission in the CNS is carried out by two substances, GABA and glycine. They are differently distributed, GABA being found primarily in the brain and glycine primarily in the spinal cord.

GABA is formed from glutamate, which is derived from the Krebs cycle, by the enzyme glutamic acid dehydrogenase. In GABAergic neurons about 10% of glutamate is converted to GABA rather than being processed further by the Krebs cycle enzymes. Synthesis occurs in the terminal cytoplasm and GABA is found free and bound in vesicles. Once released, GABA is taken up into the presynaptic terminal via a high-affinity, sodium-dependent transport system. It is also rapidly taken up into glia by a similar process where it is metabolized.

Two major subtypes of GABA receptors are known, $GABA_A$ and $GABA_B$ (Table N-3). The $GABA_A$ receptor is a part of a chloride channel. It mediates postsynaptic inhibition and gives rise to fast transient inhibitory postsynaptic potentials (IPSPs). $GABA_B$ receptors are found both pre- and postsynaptically. Presynaptically they act via a G-protein to reduce calcium entry. Postsynaptically they act via a G-protein to increase potassium conductance. In either case they mediate inhibition. The $GABA_A$ receptor–chloride channel complex is a major target for lindane- and cyclodiene-type insecticides.

Glycine is an important inhibitory transmitter in the spinal cord. The postsynaptic receptor for glycine is very similar to the $GABA_A$ receptor and forms part of a chloride channel complex. When it is activated by glycine the channel opens transiently to produce IPSPs in spinal neurons. Strychnine reversibly antagonizes the effects of glycine on spinal neurons, and this is thought to be responsible for its convulsant properties.

Actions of Selected Toxicants on the Nervous System

In this section we will consider the most common types of toxic actions known that involve the nervous system. Selective examples of toxicants will be considered and their probable mechanisms of actions will be described, where known. The intent is not to present an exhaustive list of toxic substances, but rather to focus on some of the most interesting and important agents. The substances to be discussed are listed in Table N-4. It should be remembered that most of these chemicals have nonneurological effects as well. These may be of equal or even greater importance to the larger picture of toxicity.

TABLE N-4
Representative Neurotoxicants

- Agents producing neuronal cell death (the neuropathies)
  - Secondary to anoxia or metabolic disturbances
    - Carbon monoxide
    - Cyanide
    - Fluoroacetate
  - Secondary to general cell injury
    - Mercury and mercurial compounds
    - Methanol (methyl alcohol and wood alcohol)
  - Secondary to nonspecific neuronal excitation
    - Monosodium glutamate
    - Domoic acid
    - β-*N*-methyl-L-alanine (BMAA)
  - Secondary to uptake via specific reuptake systems
    - MPTP (1-methyl-4-phenyl-1,2,3,6-tetrahydropyridine)
- Agents producing axonal degeneration (the axonopathies)
    - Ethyl alcohol
    - Acrylamide
    - Hexandione (γ ketones)
    - Organophosphorus compounds
    - Colchicine and taxol
- Agents producing demyelination
    - Diphtheria toxin
    - Triethyltin
    - Hexachlorophene
    - Lead
- Agents modifying CNS excitability in a reversible fashion
  - Generally depressing neuronal excitability
    - Alcohol
    - Organic solvents
    - Barbiturates
  - Specifically enhancing inhibition in the CNS
    - Benzodiazepines
  - Specifically blocking inhibition in the CNS
    - Lindane (γ-hexachlorocyclohexane)
    - Cyclodiene-type insecticides
    - Strychnine
    - Tetanus toxin
  - Blocking reuptake of transmitter substances
    - Cocaine
- Agents affecting axonal conduction
  - Tetrodotoxin
  - Saxitoxin
  - DDT
  - Pyrethroid insecticides
- Agents affecting peripheral neuroeffector junctions
  - Affecting transmitter release
    - Botulinum toxin
    - Black widow spider venom (latrotoxin)
  - Mimicking transmitter action
    - Nicotine
  - Enhancing transmitter action
    - Organophosphate compounds
  - Blocking transmitter action
    - Curare
    - Cobra snake venom (α-bungarotoxin)

Agents Producing Neuronal Cell Death (the Neuropathies)

As already indicated, neurons are cells having high metabolic rates which are almost totally dependent on the aerobic oxidation of glucose for energy production. They are more susceptible to anoxic damage than any other type of cell in the body. The most sensitive neurons can withstand oxygen deprivation for only a few minutes before irreversible damage takes place.

Anoxia can be produced in different ways. Anoxic anoxia occurs when there is an inadequate oxygen supply in the presence of adequate blood flow. Ischemic anoxia is the result of a decrease in arterial blood pressure to a level insufficient to provide adequate oxygen for the brain's needs. Cytotoxic anoxia occurs when oxygen and blood supplies are adequate, but the cell is unable to utilize the oxygen due to interference with cell metabolism. Regardless of cause, agents that produce anoxia produce similar changes in the nervous system.

Natural and Coal Gas and Propane

Asphyxia occurs when the concentration of oxygen in the air being breathed falls below a critical level. There are many situations in which this can occur, and the most common agents involved are propane, natural gas, and coal gas (see Propane). In mines the release of gas from coal may lead to an atmosphere too deficient in oxygen to sustain life. This may be complicated by the presence of carbon monoxide. Miners used to carry cages containing canaries when entering deep mine tunnels as a biologic indicator. Birds are even more sensitive to anoxia than humans, and symptoms will develop in them before people are seriously affected. This provided time for the miners to escape from the area before they also became asphyxiated. In the home or enclosed spaces where natural gas and propane are used for heating and cooking, leaking gases may reduce oxygen to levels no longer compatible with survival. In enclosed spaces with little air circulation prolonged use of propane heaters may burn off sufficient oxygen to lead to asphyxia. All these exposures lead to an anoxic anoxia with initial signs of giddiness and dizziness, and eventually anoxic damage and neuronal cell death. The extent of damage is related to the degree of oxygen deprivation and the duration of exposure.

Carbon Monoxide

Carbon monoxide is a colorless, odorless gas formed during the incomplete combustion of hydrocarbon fuels. It is a by-product of industrial processing and is present in exhaust fumes from internal combustion engines. Carbon monoxide decreases the oxygen transport capability of hemoglobin and produces an anoxic anoxia. This occurs because carbon monoxide competes with oxygen for binding to hemoglobin. Its affinity for hemoglobin is some 200 times greater than that of oxygen, so even small amounts displace sufficient oxygen to create an anoxic anoxia. Levels as low as 0.1% are dangerous to life. The symptoms of carbon monoxide poisoning resemble those of the gases described previously and excessive exposure can result in neuronal cell death. This leads to a chronic neuropathy (see Carbon Monoxide).

Cyanide

A disruption of aerobic metabolism can occur even when oxygen is readily available to the nerve cell. Cyanide inhibits the ability of the nerve cell to utilize the oxygen delivered to it. Cyanide (hydrocyanic acid or prussic acid) is one of the most rapid-acting poisons known. It is present in nature as an inorganic salt, as a naturally occurring glycoside in certain plants, and as free hydrocyanic acid. It is used in industry for metal cleaning, electroplating, and chemical synthesis. It has also been used as a rodenticide and a fumigant. It has been used intentionally to cause death, and it is the active agent used in "gas" chambers executions. It produces a cytotoxic anoxia by inhibiting cytochrome oxidase. Cytochrome oxidase is a critical component of the oxidative–phosphorylation process that is at the heart of ATP formation during aerobic metabolism. The inhibition depletes the cell of ATP which leads to a failure of the nerve cell to maintain ionic gradients. If prolonged, cyanide exposure can lead to cell death. When this occurs a neuropathy similar in most ways to those produced by natural gas or carbon monoxide results (see Cyanide).

Fluoroacetate

The disruption of aerobic metabolism may occur at locations other than cytochrome oxidase. Fluoroacetate (compound 1080) is a colorless, odorless, and tasteless water-soluble solid. It is used primarily for rodent and predator control where it is commonly mixed into a bait made with bran or bread. When ingested fluoroacetate can replace acetyl-CoA and combine with oxaloacetic acid to form fluorocitric acid. This product is a potent inhibitor of the enzyme aconitase, a critical enzyme participating in the Krebs's cycle. Disruption of the Krebs cycle effectively stops aerobic respiration resulting in a cytotoxic anoxia.

Neuronopathy can result from other mechanisms that interfere with energy production or protein synthesis. Regardless of cause, cell integrity is eventually lost and cell death ensues. Often these effects develop slowly over time rather than rapidly, as is the case with chemicals that interfere with aerobic metabolism.

Mercury and Organic Mercurial Compounds

The neurotoxic actions of mercury have been known for centuries. Metallic mercury is volatile, and toxicity can result from vapor inhalation. This is the primary route of entry of metallic mercury. Volatile mercury salts were used in "sizing" felt by hat makers during the last century, and many of the workers developed mercury poisoning. The effects in these workers led to the common saying, "mad as a hatter," and may have been the basis for the mad hatter characterization in the novel, *Alice in Wonderland*. Organic mercurials are particularly likely to produce neurotoxicity, in part due to their high lipid solubility which allows rapid penetration into the CNS. A classical example of mass poisoning by methylmercury was the Minamata disaster that occurred at Minimata Bay, Japan. The diet of the residents of Minamata Bay consisted primarily of fish which had become contaminated with methyl-mercury when mercury-laden industrial effluent was rerouted into the bay. The methylmercury was bioaccumulated in the fish due to its high lipid solubility so that massive amounts were ingested by the inhabitants.

The initial symptoms of mercury poisoning may be subtle and relegated to changes in behavior, mood, emotional reactivity, or aggressiveness. As exposure continues, behavior may become increasingly more abnormal. Sensory deficits may occur and paresthesias may develop, usually a tingling of the toes, fingers, or lips. Once signs and symptoms develop which include sensory or motor functional loss, there is little recovery even after removal from exposure. In children exposed to methylmercury *in utero,* profound mental retardation and paralysis can result.

The mechanism by which mercury produces a neuropathy is not well defined. A number of effects have been ascribed to it, including impaired glycolysis, impaired nucleic acid biosynthesis, and impaired protein synthesis. Mercury binds readily to sulfhydryl groups and can inactivate enzymes and alter membrane fluidity. It is likely that mercury interferes with a number of important cell functions. Before cell death, involved neurons show a loss of endoplasmic reticulum suggesting that a decrease in protein synthesis plays an important role in mercury's effects.

While the lesions produced by asphyxiants and mercury tend to be diffuse and widespread throughout the CNS, some compounds produce a much more selective cell loss restricted to small regions. Trimethyl tin is an example of a chemical that can produce a rather selective destruction of pyramidal cells in the dorsal hippocampus. Selective destruction of retinal ganglion cells can be produced by exposure to methanol (see Mercury and Methylmercury).

Methanol

Methanol or wood alcohol is a common industrial solvent. It is used as an antifreeze fluid, a solvent for paints and varnishes, and as a paint remover. Most canned fuels consist of methanol in a gel form. Methanol is the simplest of the alcohols and produces an acute CNS depression somewhat like that produced by the more common ethanol, or ethyl alcohol.

When methanol is ingested, initial symptoms include headache, vertigo, lethargy, and confusion with little or no euphoria. Even with small doses, visual disturbances are observed. Signs of visual damage include blurred vision, decreased visual acuity, and deficits in the visual field. Retinal edema develops and ganglion cells undergo a relatively selective degeneration. The result can be bilateral blindness which is usually permanent. As little as 15 ml of methanol has produced blindness, whereas the fatal dose is around 70–100 ml in untreated adults.

The cause of ganglion cell degeneration is the formation and accumulation of formate ion in the ganglion cells. Methanol is metabolized by a three-step reaction to formaldehyde then to formate and then to carbon dioxide and water. In species such as humans and other primates, the metabolism of methanol to formate is rapid, whereas the further metabolism of formate to carbon dioxide and water is slow. As a result, formate tends to accumulate with time in the body and in the eye. In most other species the conversion of formate to carbon dioxide and water occurs much more rapidly, and formate does not accumulate. These species do not develop ocular lesions after methanol exposure. Although retinal toxicity is associated with the accumulation of formate in the eye, just how formate produces retinal ganglion cell degeneration is not clear.

The treatment of methanol poisoning illustrates an interesting principle in toxicology—the use of one toxicant to "detoxify" a more dangerous one. The treatment of methanol poisoning includes the infusion of ethanol in high concentrations. The basis for this approach is that methanol and ethanol are metabolized to formaldehyde and acetaldehyde, respectively, by the same enzyme, alcohol dehydrogenase. The amount of this enzyme is small, and its capacity for metabolism is readily saturated. Ethanol has about 200 times the affinity of methanol for the enzyme and successfully competes with it for occupancy of the binding site. As a result, formate formation is greatly slowed, and its levels do not accumulate to the levels expected in the absence of ethanol (see Methanol).

Monosodium Glutamate

Excitatory neurotransmission in the brain is carried out primarily by the amino acid, glutamate. Glutamate, secreted from nerve terminals, can act on three different types of receptors in the CNS (Table N-3). The interaction of glutamate, or other substances that mimic glutamate, with these receptors leads to depolarization and increased excitability of the receptive cells. In normal function this provides the basis for excitatory neurotransmission. In excess, however, the effects of glutamate and its analogs can be damaging, leading to excessive entry of sodium, calcium, and water into the neuron. In extreme circumstances prolonged exposure to these "excitatory amino acids" can produce cell death. Cell death secondary to metabolic interruption or convulsive seizures from any cause is thought to be due primarily to a massive release of glutamate from nerve terminals.

Glutamate, in the form of monosodium glutamate (MSG), is a common ingredient in many processed foods in which it is used as a flavor enhancer. In normal circumstances, ingestion of MSG does not produce CNS effects because it is excluded from entry into the brain by the BBB. The only recognized effect of ingesting MSG in humans is the so-called "Chinese restaurant syndrome," which consists of a burning, tightness, and numbness of the neck and face, chest pain, and headache. It occurs only in susceptible individuals. Large doses of MSG, however, can produce lesions in the hypothalamus and retina, areas in which the BBB is deficient, in newborn mice and rats. On the basis of this evidence, the use of MSG as a flavor enhancer in baby foods has been discontinued.

Certain natural products can penetrate the BBB and behave as glutamate agonists in the brain. These compounds tend to be very toxic and can lead to severe cell loss after ingestion of sufficient amounts (see Monosodium Glutamate).

Domoic Acid

Domoic acid is a potent glutamate analog that has been responsible for poisoning hundreds of people. One such outbreak occurred in late 1987 in Canada among persons who had eaten cultivated mussels. It occurred following an extensive phytoplankton bloom in which the phytoplankton, *Nitzschia pungens*, was a primary component. This was the source of domoic acid which subsequently accumulated to poisonous levels in mussels ingesting the plankton. Within 24–48 hr of ingesting the poisoned mussels, people developed gastrointestinal and neurologic symptoms, including vomiting, abdominal cramps, diarrhea, headache, and loss of short-term memory. In many, the effects on memory were permanent. In the most severely poisoned individuals, seizures, coma, and death occurred. In those individuals who died, autopsy showed extensive neuronal necrosis that was most prominent in the hippocampus and the amygdaloid nuclei.

β-N-Methylamino-L-Alanine

It has been proposed that β-*N*-methylamino-L-alanine (BMAA) is responsible for the neuronal degenerative disease complex (amyotrophic lateral sclerosis–Parkinsonism–dementia) which occurred in the 1940s and 1950s in Guam. BMAA is an excitatory amino acid produced by cycad plants which were used by the Chamorro population of Guam as a foodstuff during and after World War II. The cycad was ground into a flour that was subsequently baked into a type of bread. The fruit of the cycad plant had to be washed extensively to remove the BMAA and other toxic ingredients, and this was not always accomplished successfully. In addition to the immediate toxic effects of improperly prepared cycad flour, it has been implicated in the emergence of the chronic degenerative disorder that is so prevalent in this population. Although this theory is attractive based on epidemiologic data, the only evidence in animal studies that BMAA may be the causative factor is the finding of motor deficits in monkeys exposed to tremendously large amounts of BMAA in the diet. The symptoms in monkeys bear little resemblance to the condition observed in the Chamarros.

Kainic Acid

Another potent glutamate analog is kainic acid. It was initially isolated from a seaweed in Japan which was used as an ascaricide to rid people of roundworms. This material has become an important "tool" for neuroscientists. Kainic acid interacts with receptors found only on nerve cell somas and dendrites, not on axons or glial cells. By injecting it into a specified region of the brain, it kills the nerve cells without disrupting axons traversing the area or glial cells in the same region. This chemical lesion is much more specific in its effects than is a mechanical or electrically produced lesion, which would kill nerve cells and glial cells and destroy axons with no selectivity.

In the majority of cases, we do not know why chemicals produce selective effects on certain neurons. In a few instances, however, we do. In those cases, it is usually a unique property of a neuronal subpopulation that is involved. Since a major difference between neurons relates to the neurotransmitters they synthesize and use for information transfer, the selective target is commonly some aspect of neurotransmitter synthesis or metabolism. A good example is the chemical, 1-methyl-4-phenyl-1,2,3,5-tetrahydropyridine (MPTP).

MPTP

MPTP is a chemical widely employed as an intermediate in chemical synthesis. Its neurotoxicity was sensationalized after a number of young individuals began to turn up in southern California with symptoms of advanced Parkinson's disease. These individuals exhibited the characteristic symptoms of Parkinson's disease, including an inability to walk, a mask-like facial expression, impairment of speech and skilled acts such as writing and eating, and, in the most severe cases, a rigid immobility that was life-threatening. Because Parkinson's disease is usually a progressive disease that develops in older people, its sudden, full-blown development in young adults was recognized immediately as an immanent disaster. Questioning soon revealed that the affected people had taken an illicit street "designer" drug that had properties similar to heroin. The drug unfortunately contained a small amount of MPTP as a contaminant introduced during the synthesis. Those who had ingested it or manufactured it comprised the affected population.

As soon as it was recognized that MPTP was the neurotoxicant, a number of laboratories began to investigate its mechanism of action. It was eventually shown that MPTP readily diffused into neurons and glial cells and that it was a substrate for the "B" isozyme of monoamine oxidase found predominantly in astrocytes. In the astrocyte the MPTP was successively oxidized to the primary neurotoxicant, the pyridinium ion MPP^+. Because of its structural similarity to dopamine, the MPP^+ was selectively taken up by dopaminergic neurons of the substantia nigra via the dopamine uptake system. Within these dopaminergic cells, the MPP^+ acted as a general cellular poison, ultimately blocking oxidative phosphorylation and killing the neuron.

A chilling follow-up to this acute development of Parkinson's disease was subsequently found. Some of the individuals who had taken small amounts of the illicit street drug, and therefore small amounts of MPTP, did not develop parkinsonism after its ingestion. It has been observed recently, however, that some of these individuals are beginning to show early signs of the disease years after the ingestion. The basis for this is not known for certain, but it is likely that the initial exposure killed too few dopaminergic cells to result immediately in Parkinson's disease. It takes a loss of approximately 80% of these neurons to produce symptoms of parkinsonism. Unfortunately, this cell population decreases naturally in numbers with age. The precipitous loss of a portion of cells, due to MPTP exposure, would shorten the time required for natural cell loss to reach the critical level at which symptoms of parkinsonism develop. Mechanisms such as these may be more common than currently thought, and the emergence of an increased incidence of degenerative-based conditions should be an immediate red flag to assess whether a common exposure background exists among affected individuals.

Agents Producing Axonal Degeneration (the Axonopathies)

A number of substances are known which are capable of producing rather selective effects on axons. As already indicated, the axon and its terminal are totally dependent on the cell body for the synthesis of all materials required for function and maintenance. They also require a functioning transport network to continually ferry materials in both directions, with new materials being transported into the axon and the terminal and old materials being returned to the cell body for disposal. Since the continual arrival of materials is absolutely essential, anything which compromises too much the formation of these materials or their transport can lead to the destruction of the axon and its terminal.

It was initially believed that axonopathies were of the "dying back" type. In this context, the deprivation of materials being transported into the axon would have greatest impact at points farthest away from the cell body. Thus, the first site of lesion would be expected to occur near the terminal and, with continued failure of delivery, the lesion would progress up the axon toward the cell body. Axonal loss would stop when the volume of the axon had decreased to the point where the compromised delivery of vital materials was sufficient to maintain what was left. As the toxicant was eliminated and the formation and delivery of materials returned to normal, regeneration of the axon would begin. If the lesion was not too great, it was possible for regeneration to be successful and for reinnervation of the target tissue to occur. This concept had to be modified when it was recognized that not all axonopathies started near the terminal but, depending on the particular chemical, could start anywhere along the axon. It is now thought that the toxicant produces a "chemical transection" of the axon at some point, and that the portion of the axon distal to the transection degenerates. Because long axons have more potential transection points than short axons, it is usual to find them affected more often and earlier during an axonopathic reaction.

Usually both sensory and motor axons are affected at about the same time, and neurons in the CNS and PNS of equal length and diameter tend to be equally affected. Characteristically, the longest and largest axons are affected first. These are the axons going to the distal segments of the limbs. A "glove and stocking" sensory loss is a common symptom of distal degeneration of sensory neurons. With motor axon degeneration, ataxia followed by paralysis develops, usually first in the legs and later in the arms. Microscopic examination of affected axons usually indicates a locus of transection with an accumulation of materials on the proximal side creating an enlarged, swollen region above the transection and a degenerating axon on the distal side.

Many agents can produce axonopathies. The following are some examples of the more important known toxicants.

Ethyl Alcohol

In addition to the other problems it causes, chronic intake of ethyl alcohol can produce a peripheral axonopathy. Schwann cells are spared. An alcohol-associated thiamine deficiency appears to be involved and results from the major caloric substitution of food, normally containing thiamine, by alcoholic beverages, containing no thiamine. The degenerative process rapidly responds to thiamine administration. Both sensory and motor neurons are involved.

Acrylamide

Acrylamide is the starting material for a number of polymeric products, including acrylic plastics. Various polymers of it are widely used as flocculators and purifiers of industrial wastes, strengtheners of paper and cardboard products, and as grouting and waterproofing agents. Although the various polymers are relatively nontoxic, the monomer, acrylamide, can produce an axonopathy. Exposure occurs by dermal absorption, by inhalation, or by oral ingestion. Only chronic exposure to relatively high levels produces an axonopathy.

Chronic exposure to acrylamide can produce a polyneuritis with sensory loss in the extremities and limbs and progressive ataxia and weakness. Recovery typically occurs within months of cessation of exposure, although severe exposures may result in permanent sensory and motor deficits. Affected peripheral nerves present a typical picture that includes a tremendous proliferation of smooth endoplasmic reticulum in the cell body and the presence of axonal swellings above the point of transection that are filled with clumps of neurofilaments. The mechanism by which acrylamide produces an axonopathy is still hypothetical but a failure of fast anterograde axonal transport appears to occur. Acrylamide may more selectively impair glycosylation or axonal transport of glycoproteins (see Acrylamide).

Hexanedione and Related Diketones

Two solvents widely used in industry, hexane and methyl *n*-butyl ketone, have been responsible for axonopathy in chronically exposed people. These solvents are employed in many different applications, such as the manufacture of shoes and printed fabrics, and are found in glues and cleaning fluids. Repetitive and prolonged exposure to high levels of these compounds are needed to induce neuronal damage. While most axonopathies have resulted from industrial exposures, a significant number of individuals have been poisoned by "sniffing" glues, varnishes, and lacquers containing these solvents for their inebriating properties (glue sniffer's neuropathy).

Hexane and methyl *n*-butyl ketone produce identical effects. The basis for this became apparent when it was shown that they are metabolized to the same compound, 2,5-hexanedione (2,5-H). 2,5-H was subsequently shown to be a potent neurotoxin as were all hexane derivatives capable of being metabolized to this common γ-ketone intermediate. Hexane derivatives that cannot form 2,5-H are not neurotoxic.

The primary effect of 2,5-H on axons is the production of large swellings in the axons of sensory and motor nerves both peripherally and centrally. These enlargements contain accumulations of neurofilaments. γ-Ketones are toxic because they react with amino groups of proteins to form pyrroles. A major target for this effect is the cytoskeleton of the axon, particularly the neurofilaments, which are derivativized, undergo oxidation, cross-link by forming covalent bonds with each other, then form clumps in the axoplasm. This accumulation of neurofilamentous clumps alters the anatomy of the axon and appears to disrupt axonal transport. The location at which this occurs becomes the transection point for the axonopathy which follows (see Hexane).

Organophosphate Compounds

In addition to the well-known effect of many organophosphorus compounds to inhibit cholinesterases, some of them also produce a severe axonopathy. The axonopathy develops days or weeks after exposure and is a progressive bilateral, central, and peripheral axonopathy with associated symptoms. The condition is referred to as organophosphate-induced delayed neuropathy (OPIDN). The progenitor of this type of effect is the chemical tri-*ortho*-cresylphosphate (TOCP), which was used in lacquers and varnishes; as a plasticizer in cellulose acetate, nitrocellulose, and polyvinyl chloride sheeting and tubing; as a flame retardant; and as an antiwear agent in hydraulic and lubricating fluids in aircraft and ships. Even though its toxicity was well-known many years ago, repeated incidences of massive poisonings by this compound continue to occur, with the most recent occurring in 1988 in India where some 600 people consumed TOCP-contaminated cooking oil. At least 10,000 people, worldwide, have been poisoned by TOCP.

The passage of prohibition in the United States inadvertently led to the production of OPIDN in about 50,000 people. It occurred in individuals who ingested a certain brand of an alcoholic extract of Jamaican ginger as a substitute for more traditional alcoholic beverages. The axonopathy that developed, which was called "Ginger Jake paralysis," was traced to a contaminant, TOCP, in the extract. In those affected, TOCP produced a polyneuritis with a flaccid paralysis of distal muscles of the extremities accompanied by degeneration of the axons and myelin sheaths of peripheral nerves, the spinal cord, and the medulla. The onset was delayed, with symptoms developing 1 or 2 weeks after exposure. Recovery from the axonopathy was slow at best and left many individuals permanently affected. A few other organophosphorus compounds are also capable of producing axonopathy. Human cases of paralysis have occurred after exposure to the herbicides and cotton defoliants, EPN (O-ethyl O-4-nitrophenyl phenylphosphonothioate) and leptophos [O-(4-bromo-2,5-dichlorophenyl) O-methyl phenylphosphonothioate].

These lipophilic compounds readily enter the nervous system where they can alkylate or phosphorylate many macromolecules. Earlier work indicated that organophosphates capable of producing OPIDN, but not others, selectively interacted with a particular esterase in brain tissue that was given the name neuropathy target esterase. While its structure and function have not yet been determined, it may produce OPIDN by inducing a persisting activation of an important axonal protein calcium/calmodulin kinase II. This kinase is responsible for phosphorylating a number of cytoskeletal proteins including tubulin, the substrate of microtubules. Hyperphosphorylation of cytoskeletal proteins would interfere with the normal control of cytoskeletal anatomy and affect transport of materials down the axon.

Colchicine and Taxol

Mention must be made of these two compounds because they have played important roles in the elucidation of axonal transport mechanisms. Colchicine is a plant product that binds to tubulin, the monomer subunit that associates to form the microtubules. Binding of tubulin by colchicine prevents its polymerization and leads to the dissociation of microtubules. Taxol, another plant product, has the opposite effect. Taxol binds to assembled microtubules and stabilizes them. Interestingly, both of these compounds produce an axonopathy, even though one destabilizes and the other stabilizes microtubules. The basis for this appears to be that both alter the normal dynamics by which microtubules associate and dissociate, and this leads to an impairment of axonal transport. The microscopic picture of the axon is quite different after colchicine or taxol exposure. After colchicine, the axon appears atrophied with few microtubules present. After taxol, an excessive number of microtubules are present, often aggregated in novel arrays not seen in healthy axons (see Colchicine).

Agents Producing Demyelination (the Myelinopathies)

The integrity of myelin sheaths is dependent on the normal functioning of myelin-forming oligodendrocytes in the CNS and Schwann cells in the PNS as well as on the viability of the axons that they ensheath. Agents that affect myelin-forming cells lead to either a disruption in the laminar nature of the myelin covering an axon or to frank loss of myelin in one or more internodal regions. These changes affect the electrical conductivity of the axon and lead to reductions in conduction velocity and possibly conduction block. The severity is proportional to the extent of demyelination. Extensive demyelination over many successive internodal regions can also result in the loss of the affected axon.

Diphtheria Toxin

Diphtheria toxin is a protein neurotoxin formed by certain strains of the bacterium *Corynebacterium diphtheriae*. In humans it causes a neuropathy by inducing demyelination of peripheral nerve fibers. The toxin cannot penetrate the BBB so the CNS is spared except in those locations where the barrier is inadequate. A general sensory motor neuropathy results with symptoms such as blurred vision, paresthesias, ataxia, and weakness of limb muscles. Demyelination is especially prominent in the dorsal root ganglia and adjacent dorsal and ventral roots of the spinal cord. With most exposures Schwann cells usually survive and subsequently reform the myelin sheaths. In some cases, however, a significant number of Schwann cells may be killed, and a more permanent axonopathy may result.

The Greek word, diphtheria, means skin or membrane and was given to the disease because the most characteristic lesion of diphtheria is a leathery membranous structure that forms at the back of the oral cavity after infection with the bacteria. The bacteria remain localized to the oral cavity where they multiply and form the active toxin. The toxin is released by the bacteria and is carried by the bloodstream throughout the body.

The toxin itself is fascinating and bears many similarities in structure and action to some other bacterial toxins, including botulinum toxin and tetanus toxin. It is synthesized as a single polypeptide chain with a molecular weight near 58,000. It is subsequently cleaved to produce two disulfide-linked fragments, the A fragment and the B fragment. The A fragment is actually an enzyme which catalyzes the ADP-ribosylation of a specific amino acid in elongation factor 2, an essential component in the process of protein synthesis. The B fragment binds to specific receptors on the surface of "target" cells, which include the Schwann cells. After binding, the toxin is internalized by endocytosis and is transported to endosomes where the low pH induces a conformation change in the B fragment. The change in conformation renders the B fragment much more hydrophobic and leads to its insertion into the endosome membrane. Once in the membrane the B fragment behaves as a selective monovalent cation channel promoting the movement of sodium, potassium, and hydrogen ions down their concentration gradients. These channels also appear to be the means by which the A fragment is released from the endosomes into the cytoplasm where it can act enzymatically to block protein synthesis. Because the active toxin is an enzyme, only a few A fragments need enter the cytoplasm to extensively inactivate elongation factor-2 within the cell.

It is likely that both of these activities are involved in the effects of diphtheria toxin on myelin. The formation of ion channels would tend to promote the development of intrasegmental edema and interrupt the electrical properties of the myelin. The reduction in protein synthesis would render the Schwann cell unable to maintain its large amounts of myelin in a healthy state.

Triethyltin

While the neurotoxicity of metallic tin and inorganic tin compounds is negligible, many organotin compounds are very active neurotoxicants. Organotins are used industrially as biocides, catalysts, preservatives, and polymer stabilizers. Trimethyl tin, already mentioned, is a potent neurotoxicant that selectively kills nerve cells, particularly in the cortex and hippocampus. Triethyl tin became recognized as an important hazard in the 1950s when more than 100 deaths occurred in France among 290 people who used an acne medication called Stalinon. The material contained as an active ingredient, diethyltin diiodide, which was contaminated with triethyltin. In these unfortunate individuals, nausea, vomiting, vertigo, intense headache, photophobia, altered consciousness, and visual impairment appeared after a latent period of about 4 days. Paraplegia involving the abdominal and respiratory muscles, sensory disturbances, and loss of sphincter control were also common. Postmortem studies indicated a diffuse edema of myelin formed by splitting of myelin along the intraperiod lines and degeneration of myelin sheaths around nerve axons. Triethyltin is a relatively selective agent affecting myelin-forming cells, and a selective binding of triethyltin to purified rat brain myelin has been claimed. Other cell types in the nervous system are usually spared. The mechanism of action of triethyl tin remains obscure, but it has been proposed that triethyltin acts by altering energy metabolism in glial cells.

Hexachlorophene

Hexachlorophene was widely used between 1940 and 1970 as a bacteriostatic agent. It was a common constituent of a variety of cosmetic products, including shaving creams, soaps, shampoos, deodorants, and feminine hygiene agents. It is toxic upon ingestion, and symptoms include lethargy, fever, jitteriness, convulsions, coma, and death. It was once popular as an antibacterial agent in newborn nurseries, but repeated whole body applications produced a vacuolar encephalopathy. In 1972, 204 French children developed neurotoxicity from the use of a baby talc that contained 6.5% hexachlorophene. Subsequently, the availability and use of hexachlorophene has been sharply curtailed.

A condition similar to that described for triethyl tin can be produced in animals fed large doses of hexachlorophene. Its administration results in intrameyelinic vacuoles in peripheral nerves and in the CNS. Hexachlorophene inhibits the synthesis of myelin, possibly by inhibiting oxidative phosphorylation (see Hexachlorophene).

Lead

Lead is an ubiquitous compound found throughout the environment. In adults, exposure is primarily from the workplace via inhalation. Nonoccupational sources include leaded gasoline, lead-lined containers, and improperly fired ceramic glazes. In children ingestion of lead is common. The major sources continue to be lead-based paints, lead-glazed pottery, and soils.

In adults, exposure to lead salts can produce a segmental degeneration involving the loss of myelin with a general sparing of axons. This is commonly restricted to the periphery and frequently involves motor axons only. There is usually little CNS involvement. Lead penetrates the BBB of children to a much greater extent than that of adults. In children, lead also produces a central encephalopathy which can culminate in coma and convulsions. A number of more subtle neuropsychological effects have been attributed to lead poisoning, including hyperactivity, learning disorders, and fine motor dysfunctions. There is compelling evidence demonstrating a relationship between blood lead levels and intellectual functioning in children. Whether lead is the causal factor is, however, still being debated. In one such study a 4-point reduction in mean IQ scores and significantly fewer children scoring within the "superior intelligence" range were found in asymptomatic children with elevated total body lead stores. Similar correlations have been reported in other studies (see Lead).

Agents Modifying CNS Excitability in a Reversible Fashion

For the neurotoxicants described previously, it is common that cells or parts of cells are destroyed by the intoxication, and the consequences will depend on the extent of cellular damage. If death does not occur, some recovery of function is common. While Schwann cells and axons in peripheral nerves are capable of regeneration, neurons in the CNS have essentially no capacity to regenerate and oligodendrocytes only limited capacity. Thus, peripheral deficits tend to reverse, usually slowly, with the possibility of complete recovery. Extensive damage to CNS neurons and axons produces a much more permanent and nonreversible deficit. Recovery is usually partial at best, and continuing deficits are the rule.

Many other chemical substances interact with neurons in a more specific and reversible fashion. These tend to disrupt the function of the nervous system but do not tend to result in permanent cellular damage or loss. Sublethal exposures produce effects proportional to dose and, if the poisoned individual survives the initial effects, the nervous system returns to normal when the toxicant has been removed from the body. Long-lasting deficits in function are not seen.

There are many targets available in nerve cells for this type of interaction with a neurotoxicant. Some targets are general to all nerve cells, and chemicals that affect them will produce widely dispersed effects. Others targets are found only in a subset of nerve cells, and in these cases toxicity will be restricted to them. The most common reason specific interactions occur is that neurons differ in the transmitter systems they possess.

Ethyl Alcohol (Ethanol)

Ethyl alcohol, which is the most widely consumed neurotoxicant in the United States and much of the rest of the world, is a good example of a chemical that is a global CNS depressant. Ingestion of even small amounts diminishes performance, particularly performance dependent on training and previous experience. Mood is affected and can range from euphoria to deep depression. Memory, concentration, insight, and motor function are impaired in a dose-dependent fashion. With large ingestions a state similar to general anesthesia develops. The doses that produce death are not much higher than those inducing anesthesia.

For many years it was thought that alcohol and other lipophilic solvents exerted their depressant effects by dissolving in lipid membranes, causing them to swell. This swelling was responsible for perturbing the functions of the macromolecules embedded in the membrane, including the ion channels and receptors. It is now believed that in addition to the lipid bilayer, hydrophobic domains within membrane proteins are also important targets, and lipophilic substances may have different effects on different receptor proteins. An important finding is that alcohol interacts with the $GABA_A$ receptor–chloride channel complex in the CNS and augments GABA-mediated synaptic inhibition. This occurs at levels that do not produce comparable effects on other types of neurotransmitter receptors. Normally, activation of the $GABA_A$ receptor–chloride channel complex increases the permeability of the nerve cell to chloride ion for about 10–20 msec. Inebriating amounts of ethanol prolong the time the channel remains open when GABA binds the receptor by two- or threefold. At higher concentrations neurotransmitter release is reduced from all nerve terminals, probably due to reductions in calcium entry.

The effects of alcohol on the $GABA_A$ receptor may be important to the development of tolerance and physical dependence that occurs in individuals who drink large amounts of alcohol on a daily basis. There is evidence that chronic alcohol ingestion leads to a reduction in the numbers of $GABA_A$ receptors in the brain as a compensatory response to the continual presence of an agent intensifying this type of inhibition. After that occurs, when alcohol levels in the CNS fall and its potentiating effects on $GABA_A$ receptors are lost, the brain becomes hyperexcitable and the dependent individual experiences anxiety, general malaise, and tremors. This acts as a powerful stimulus for the alcoholic to ingest more. During a prolonged withdrawal, the lack of alcohol to potentiate inhibition causes increasing hyperexcitability and frank signs of withdrawal including tremor, hyperreflexia, and convulsions (see Ethanol).

Organic Solvents

Most organic solvents possess CNS depressant actions somewhat similar to alcohol. While the basis for this has not been studied for most solvents, it is likely that the depression is due to interaction of the solvents with the lipid bilayer and the hydrophobic domains of membrane proteins. These substances are numerous (Table N-5) and are found in large quantities in the workplace and the home. They are a common cause of poisoning, especially in children, and frequently are used in suicides. Often, the odor or taste is highly unpleasant or the vapors are so irritating to mucous membranes of the eyes, nose, and throat that exposures are terminated before sufficient amount enters the body to cause CNS

TABLE N-5
Important Industrial and Household Solvents

Aliphatic hydrocarbons
Pentane
Hexane
Heptane
Gasoline
Kerosine
Halogenated aliphatic hydrocarbons
Methylene chloride
Chloroform
Carbon tetrachloride
Trichloroethylene
Aliphatic alcohols
Ethyl alcohol
Methyl alcohol
Isopropyl alcohol
Glycols
Ethylene glycol
Propylene glycol
Glycol ethers
Cellosolve
Dioxane
Aromatic hydrocarbons
Benzene
Toluene

effects. Individuals, however, who are exposed for sufficiently long periods experience headache, depression, tiredness, and show reduced work efficiency and weakness. Higher exposures can produce unconsciousness, respiratory depression, and death. Accidents in the workplace or hobby room are frequently related to the use of these solvents in poorly ventilated areas.

Many important pharmaceutical agents produce CNS depression and have been extensively studied to determine their mechanism of action. One group of drugs, exemplified by the barbiturates, effects the nervous system much like the alcohols do, whereas a second group, the benzodiazepines, are remarkably selective potentiators of $GABA_A$-mediated inhibition. Since they are commonly found in the home and are responsible for a number of suicides and alcohol-related deaths, they merit consideration.

Barbiturates

The barbiturates, like, for example, phenobarbital, were extensively used as sleeping pills and as sedative agents to reduce stress and anxiety in people. They, like alcohol, produce a spectrum of depressant effects that are dose dependent. Small doses promote tiredness and sleep and higher doses can produce a general anesthetic state and death. The barbiturates can also produce tolerance and physical dependence after chronic ingestion of high doses. The withdrawal complications are very similar to those seen for alcohol. Although not prescribed to a great extent today, barbiturates continue to be readily available on the street.

Barbiturates probably interact more specifically with hydrophobic domains of membrane proteins than do the organic solvents. Quite remarkably, they produce opposite effects on the $GABA_A$ receptor mediating inhibition in the CNS and the glutamate receptors which mediate excitation. Barbiturates enhance $GABA_A$ receptor-mediated inhibition by binding to a site within the chloride channel part of the complex. Barbiturates are more effective channel stabilizers than alcohol and can maintain the channel in its open state 2–10 times longer than normal. The same levels of barbiturates depress excitatory transmission mediated by glutamate. Why the function of one receptor complex should be enhanced while another is attenuated remains unknown (see Barbiturates, Long-Acting and Barbiturates, Short-Acting).

Benzodiazepines

The benzodiazepines are very selective neurotoxicants that target only the $GABA_A$ receptor–chloride channel complex. First discovered in the 1960s, they were soon observed to produce marked changes in animal behavior and aggressiveness and eventually were marketed for use in people. Most produce modest sedation and quite effectively alleviate anxiety resulting from any cause. Some produce a greater degree of sedation and have become the modern "sleeping pills." They are remarkably good at what they do, and the benzodiazepines are among the most widely prescribed drugs in medicine today.

The advantages benzodiazepines possess over barbiturates are due to their very selective interaction with the $GABA_A$ receptor. They bind to a location on the complex distinct from the binding site for the neurotransmitter GABA. When they bind, they alter the structure of the complex in a way that increases the affinity of the GABA binding site for GABA. This increase in affinity for GABA results in a potentiation of GABA's effects when released from GABAergic nerve terminals. The benzodiazepines do not affect the $GABA_B$ receptor or any other receptor or transmitter release.

Whereas benzodiazepines produce a selective enhancement of GABA-mediated inhibition in the CNS, there are a number of important toxicants that do exactly the opposite. They interact with the $GABA_A$ receptor–chloride channel complex in a manner that leads to a blockade of inhibition (see Benzodiazepines).

Lindane

Lindane (γ-hexachlorocyclohexane) is one of six possible isomers of hexachlorocyclohexane. The crude mixture was first synthesized by Michael Faraday in 1825, and the γ-isomer was first purified by van der Linden in 1912. Lindane is used as an insecticide and is sold in a variety of formulations. During and after World War II it was widely used in businesses and homes in "vaporizers" for local insect control. While restrictions exist today on its use in many countries, it is still widely used to control soil pests, to treat livestock and poultry, and as a fumigant. Lindane in lotion form is also used medically as a scabicide and pediculocide.

Because of its widespread use, it was soon recognized that lindane was relatively toxic to animals and people as well as to insects. In animals and humans, lindane produces hyperexcitability, muscle spasms, convulsions, and death in a dose-dependent manner. Its insecticidal and acute mammalian neurotoxic actions result when lindane binds to the $GABA_A$ receptor–chloride channel complex and blocks GABA-mediated inhibition. It binds to a site on the chloride channel and reduces the length of time the channel remains open after the complex is bound by GABA. This effect, which is the reverse of that produced by barbiturates, reduces the effectiveness of GABA and blocks inhibition in the CNS. It is of interest that the interaction of hexachlorocyclohexane with the $GABA_A$ receptor–chloride channel complex is very stereospecific, and the various isomers possess different neurotoxicological properties. The α-isomer is a weak convulsant with about one-tenth the activity of the γ-isomer. The δ-isomer is essentially inactive, whereas the β-isomer behaves as a CNS depressant (see Lindane).

Cyclodiene Insecticides

The cyclodienes are a family of chemical substances with similar chemical properties. Although they have little in common with lindane from a structural point of view, they possess insecticidal activity and produce mammalian neurotoxicity very much like that of lindane. Their mechanism of action appears the same. The evidence available suggests that they bind to the same location on the $GABA_A$ receptor–chloride channel as does lindane and affect the channel in a similar way.

Some natural products interfere specifically with glycine-mediated inhibition in the spinal cord. Strychnine and tetanus toxin are good examples (see Cyclodienes).

Strychnine

Strychnine is a natural product produced by some trees and bushes of the *Strychnos* species. Its CNS stimulant properties have been known for centuries and at one time it was widely used as an appetite stimulant, a "tonic," and an aphrodisiac. Today, poisoning results from accidental ingestion of rodenticides containing strychnine or following its use as a street drug adulterant. Unfortunately, strychnine has been used as a substitute for cocaine or amphetamine in illicit drug combinations. Its ingestion produces a dose-related sequence of hyperexcitable responses that include apprehension, muscle twitching, hyperreflexia, extensor muscle spasms (opisthotonos), convulsions, and death. Consciousness is usually retained until late in the intoxication.

After ingestion strychnine readily enters the CNS. There, it acts as a specific antagonist to the neurotransmitter glycine. Strychnine binds to glycine receptors located on the postsynaptic membranes of motoneurons. It binds at the same site that glycine does and prevents glycine from activating the complex. The result is a loss of normal inhibitory control over motoneurons which are rendered hyperexcitable and begin to discharge rapidly and repetitively to the slightest stimulation. The transmission of this activity to skeletal muscle is responsible for the bulk of the symptoms observed. The lack of effect on sensation and consciousness relate to the fact the GABA mediates most of the inhibition in the brain rather than glycine (see Strychnine).

Tetanus Toxin

Tetanus toxin is one of the most fascinating neurotoxicants. It is produced by the bacterium, *Clostridium tetani*, and is one of the most potent neurotoxins known. The bacteria and its toxin are widely distributed in soils and silts at the bottom of ponds and lakes. Tetanus toxin causes few deaths in the United States because immunization is easily accomplished. Worldwide, however, about 300,000 people are intoxicated every year and about 50,000 people die from exposure.

The disease state produced by the toxin is referred to as tetanus. In most cases it results after an individual sustains small puncture wounds or lacerations which allow the entry of bacteria into the body. The bacteria remain localized to the wound site and, if anaerobic conditions are present, form large amounts of the neurotoxin. Generally, there is an incubation period of a few days before symptoms appear. Initial symptoms consist of mild, intermittent contraction of muscles near the wound site. This is succeeded by spasms of the jaw muscles from which the common name for tetanus, lockjaw, arises. As time goes on, more and more muscles become involved, producing general rigidity, violent spasms of trunk and limb muscles, and possibly death from asphyxiation. There are no major effects on sensation or consciousness.

The toxin bears much similarity to botulinum toxin and to diphtheria toxin. It is initially formed as a single polypeptide of about 150 kDa molecular weight. It is subsequently broken by a protease to form two peptides held together by a disulfide bond. One is termed the "light chain" (about 50 kDa) and the other the "heavy chain" (about 100 kDa). This is the form in which it is released into the body.

The symptoms develop when the toxin gains access to the CNS. Its journey there is a long one. Initially the toxin is taken up, apparently in entirety, by endocytosis into spinal and brain stem motoneurons. It is transported retrogradely to the cell bodies and is somehow externalized. It then passes transynaptically and binds preferentially to synaptic terminals of inhibitory interneurons that release glycine. The heavy chain is essential to the binding of the toxin and for its subsequent internalization into the glycinergic terminal. The endocytotic vesicles containing the toxin eventually coalesce with endosomes where the internal pH of the vesicle becomes progressively more acidified. At a pH of about 4, a structural transformation of the heavy chain occurs which triggers its insertion into the vesicle membrane. The light chain is subsequently released from the vesicle into the cytoplasm of the terminal. The light chain is an enzyme, more specifically an endopeptidase, that has the potential to cleave the protein synaptobrevin. Synaptobrevin is a key protein found on the membrane of synaptic vesicles and plays an essential role in the docking and fusion of the vesicle with the plasma membrane of the terminal. Cleavage of synaptobrevin by the light chain blocks vesicle docking and fusion and thus blocks transmitter release.

We have seen that neurotoxicants affect many processes involved in neurotransmitter action in the CNS. Some (strychnine) occupy the same sight on a receptor as does the endogenous transmitter (glycine) and thus block its effects. Others (benzodiazepines) induce structural changes in receptors that increase its affinity for its transmitter (GABA). Others (barbiturates, alcohol, lindane, and cyclodienes) also bind the receptor and change the temporal kinetics of ion channel opening and closing. One (tetanus toxin) acts presynaptically to interrupt transmitter release. As a last example of yet another target, consider how cocaine produces its effects.

Cocaine

Cocaine is a natural product originally isolated from a bushy shrub, *Erythroxylon coca*, that grows in the Andes mountains of Peru. For centuries the leaves of the plant have been chewed by local natives to produce a sense of decreased hunger and fatigue and of increased well-being. Cocaine enjoyed a short popularity in human medicine as a local anesthetic, but the primary concern today is that cocaine's CNS effects appeal to many people, and cocaine is currently a major drug of abuse. Its popularity boomed in the 1980s when "freebase" cocaine or "crack" became available. The ability to achieve rapid, high brain levels of cocaine by smoking crack has greatly increased its abuse potential and also its toxicity.

Although cocaine is a local anesthetic, most of its actions relate to a second mechanism. Cocaine increases synaptic concentrations of catecholamines (dopamine, norepinephrine, and serotonin) in the brain by blocking their reuptake mechanisms. Normally, when these transmitters are released from nerve terminals, they are rapidly removed from the synaptic cleft by specific "transporter" systems that expend energy to pump them back into the terminal. By blocking these transporter systems, cocaine prolongs the time the catecholamines remain in the synapse and intensifies their actions. This increase in catecholamine concentrations at the synapse appears to be the basis for the various euphoric and related changes that occur in people who use cocaine. Cocaine also blocks the reuptake of norepinephrine in the PNS, and the combination of central and peripheral actions leads to a high probability of toxicity. The cardiovascular system is particularly sensitive to the actions of cocaine, and cardiac arrythmias, marked increases in blood pressure, cerebral hemorrhage, myocardial ischemia, and outright heart failure are not uncommon with cocaine use. Even young, otherwise healthy individuals with normal coronary and cerebral arteries have died suddenly after cocaine use from cerebral hemorrhage or ventricular fibrillation (see Cocaine).

Agents Affecting Axonal Conduction

The axon is a target for many neurotoxicants. As discussed previously, it is susceptible to actions leading to axonal death. It is also susceptible to agents which alter axonal function directly. One important group of drugs, the local anesthetics, inhibit the opening of sodium channels in axons and block action potentials. These drugs are used to create "nerve blocks." When the block is placed between the CNS and the region where pain is occurring, transmission of painful information into the CNS is disrupted and the subjective sensation of pain stops. Local anesthetics are invaluable in medicine and permit painful procedures to be done without the requirement to put the patient to sleep with a general anesthetic.

Tetrodotoxin

Tetrodotoxin is a potent neurotoxin found in various organs of the pufferfish. There are some 30 species of this fish in the world, but 28 of them are found in the waters surrounding Japan. The pufferfish is prized in Japan as a delicacy, and the meat from poisonous fish is claimed to be much more appetizing than meat from nonpoisonous varieties. Much art and skill goes into preparing "fugu" for consumption. This preparation normally extracts the tetrodotoxin. The toxin is also destroyed by sufficient cooking. Despite this, many cases of fugu poisoning and death are reported in Japan yearly.

The symptoms of poisoning with tetrodotoxin are dose dependent and progressive in nature. The first and mildest symptoms involve a loss of sensation in the lips, tongue, and fingers. Muscle weakness may follow and lead to a progressive motor paralysis. Respiratory failure and death may follow.

Tetrodotoxin blocks sodium channels in axons and interrupts action potential generation and propagation. The toxin binds to the interior of the channel much like a cork in a bottle and prohibits the passage of sodium ions. When sufficient channels are blocked in this manner, propagation of the action potential fails. In sensory nerves this leads to the loss of sensory information arriving into the CNS. In motor nerves it blocks the connection between the nervous system and muscles, leading to paralysis (see Tetrodotoxin).

Saxitoxin

Saxitoxin is a toxin produced by dinoflaggelates of the *Gonyaulax* species. These dinoflaggelates multiply rapidly in warm seawaters and, at certain times of the year, are found in high concentrations in filter-feeding shellfish such as mussels and clams. The saxitoxin that concentrates in these shellfish produces "paralytic shellfish poisoning." The symptoms of poisoning are the same as those described for tetrodotoxin. Saxitoxin acts like tetrodotoxin in blocking sodium channels (see Shellfish Poisoning, Paralytic, and Saxitoxin).

DDT

DDT is one of the most notorious neurotoxicants of the twentieth century. Although first synthesized by Zeidler in 1874, it was not until 1939 that Paul Muller discovered its insecticidal properties, a finding of such impact that Muller was awarded the Nobel Prize for it in 1948. Between 1940 and 1970, DDT and other organochlorine compounds were used in massive quantities worldwide and have been credited with saving approximately 50 million human lives and averting 1 billion cases of human disease. Unfortunately, many of the properties of DDT that made it an excellent insecticide also made it a toxicant of animals and humans. Its persistence in the environment and its tendency to accumulate along food chains led to the accumulation of high levels of DDT in some fish, bird, and mammal populations and produced injury and death. The recognition of the toxicity inherent in using DDT eventually led to the ban on DDT and most other organochlorine compounds in the United States and many other parts of the world.

DDT produces a very characteristic poisoning syndrome in animals and humans. Initial symptoms include hyperexcitability and excessive emotional and physical reactions to sensory stimuli. Persistent tremoring is almost always observed and may become so intense that purposeful movements can no longer be initiated. With sufficient exposures convulsions may develop and, rarely, death may occur.

Most of these effects of DDT appear to result from an interaction with nerve axons. DDT binds to sodium channels and keeps them in an open state longer than normal during an action potential. This allows excessive entry of sodium and leads to a persisting depolarization of the axon which promotes the development of repetitive axonal discharges. Single action potentials become converted into bursts of many action potentials. When these reach nerve terminals they greatly amplify the release of neurotransmitter and lead to hyperexcitability. When this occurs in sensory axons, paresthesias occur. When it occurs in motor axons, hyperreflexia, tremor, and muscle spasms result (see DDT).

Pyrethroid Insecticides

The pyrethroids comprise a large group of man-made chemicals that are extensively used as insecticides today. They are probably the safest agents in use because they are rapidly broken down in the environment and are rapidly metabolized by animals and humans. Toxic responses in humans are rare.

Pyrethroids produce their effects in the same way as DDT. They all interact with sodium channels in nerve axons and prolong the time the channels remain open during an action potential. Various pyrethroids hold the channels open for different lengths of time, and this may explain why some pyrethroids produce quite different symptoms during poisoning than others (see Pyrethrin/Pyrethroids).

Agents Affecting Peripheral Neuroeffector Junctions

Neuroeffector junctions are a major target of attack by neurotoxicants of biological origin. Why this area of the nervous system became such a major target is uncertain. However, these areas are not protected by a blood–brain barrier, and toxins entering the body from bites, scratches, or punctures can readily gain access to them. The junctions most often involved are those between motoneurons and skeletal muscle, the neuromuscular junctions. Neuroeffector junctions between autonomic nerve terminals and effectors such as smooth muscle, glands, and cardiac muscle may also be targets. Toxicants may act to stimulate or inhibit neurotransmitter release or they may combine directly with receptors, either mimicking or blocking the actions of the normal transmitter.

Botulinum Toxin

Botulinum toxin is a toxin produced by the bacterium, *Clostridium botulinum.* It is among the most lethal substances known, and it has been estimated that 1 or 2 oz of the pure toxin could kill the entire population of the United States. Poisoning of humans and animals occurs when food containing the toxin is ingested. The most common source is improperly prepared canned fruits and vegetables or fish products. Although only about 100 cases are reported in the United States per year, botulinum poisoning is still a world problem, particularly in Asia, where thousands of cases occur yearly. The lethality rate is 15–40%.

Clinical symptoms usually develop 18–36 hr after ingestion. Most are due to cholinergic blockade and include weakness, blurred vision, difficulty in swallowing and speaking, progressive weakness of skeletal muscles, and eventually respiratory paralysis. Sensation and consciousness are left unaffected.

There are seven distinct botulinum neurotoxins which differ somewhat in structure and potency. All are polypeptides of about 150 kDa molecular weight. Their amino acid homology is generally high. Tetanus toxin, described earlier, is also a close relative to botulinum neurotoxins and actually possesses higher structural homology with two of the botulinum toxins than with the five other botulinum toxins.

The mechanism of toxicity of botulinum neurotoxins is now well understood and is very similar to that of tetanus toxin. The toxin is synthesized as a single polypeptide chain which is proteolytically cleaved by the bacteria to form two peptides held together by a disulfide bond. One, the heavy chain, is about 100 kDa in size, and the other, the light chain, is about 50 kDa in size. When the toxin is ingested, it is absorbed from the gastrointestinal tract and distributed via the bloodstream to nerve terminals in the periphery. The toxin binds to a site on cholinergic nerve terminals and is subsequently internalized by endocytosis. The endocytotic vesicles are processed to form endosomes, which normally ferry their contents to lysosomes for destruction. In preparation for this, the endosomes contain enzymes that progressively render their contents more and more acidic. At a pH of about 4, the heavy chain of botulinum toxin undergoes a conformational change which leads to its insertion into the endosomal membrane. This insertion creates a large channel through which monovalent cations can move and through which the light chain likely leaves the endosome to gain access to the terminal cytoplasm. The light chain, when separated from the heavy chain, behaves as an enzyme which selectively cleaves a peptide associated with synaptic vesicles. This peptide, synaptobrevin, is required for docking and fusion of the vesicle with the terminal membrane during transmitter release. By enzymatically cleaving it, botulinum toxin renders vesicle docking and fusion impossible, and neurotransmission comes to a screaming halt. Because it is an enzyme, just a few molecules of toxin can catalyze the destruction of synaptobrevin on thousands of vesicles (see Botulinum Toxin).

Black Widow Spider Venom (Latrotoxin)

This venom is secreted by female spiders of the *Latrodectus* species. The venom contains a number of proteinaceous fractions, one of which is neurotoxic. The venom is highly toxic, and death can follow a single bite. When an individual is bitten, the predominant symptoms include pain, often excruciating, coupled with muscular rigidity and spasm, particularly in the abdomen and back. Abdominal tenderness and cramping are common when the bite is to the lower extremities or buttocks. These effects last from several hours to 2 or 3 days. The bite is rarely lethal, but if it is, the initial symptoms are followed by a phase of weakness and paralysis. An antiserum is available for treatment.

The mechanism of these effects is quite unique. The venom initially evokes a massive release of neurotransmitter from nerve terminals, regardless of transmitter type. This occurs after the neurotoxin binds to the terminal membrane forming an ion channel that allows the influx of calcium ion into the terminal. When a small amount of the venom is injected, the massive release of neurotransmitter is followed by the sloughing of terminals in neurons in the region of the bite. When more venom is injected, the sloughing occurs over a larger area. If degeneration occurs over large enough areas, muscle weakness and paralysis result. The return of normal function occurs only when the terminals regenerate, which takes days or weeks (see Spider, Black Widow).

Many important substances act by mimicking the action of an endogenous neurotransmitter on its receptors. An example of this is the natural alkaloid, nicotine.

Nicotine

Nicotine is an alkaloid derived from the tobacco plant *Nicotiana tabacum*. It is a liquid at room temperature and acquires a brown appearance and develops a characteristic odor when exposed to air. It is widely available in tobacco products and in certain pesticides. Tobacco products contain 1 or 2% nicotine and if ingested, especially by children, can be very toxic. Only a small amount of the nicotine found in tobacco is volatilized and absorbed during smoking.

The actions of nicotine relate to its ability to activate one of the two groups of cholinergic receptors, the nicotinic receptors. Nicotine and a second substance, muscarine (a mushroom toxin), were known long before acetylcholine was identified as a neurotransmitter, and the receptors in the PNS were initially distinguished by whether they responded to nicotine or to muscarine. Thus, the cholinergic divisions nicotinic and muscarinic were established.

Nicotinic receptors are located in autonomic ganglia, at neuromuscular junctions, and within the CNS. Activation of the latter is involved in the psychoactive and addictive properties of nicotine. Stimulation of ganglia leads to accelerations in heart rate, increases in blood pressure, and constriction of blood vessels, particularly in the skin. At high exposures a pronounced tremor develops and convulsions are possible. Even higher exposure promotes a "depolarization block" of ganglionic and neuromuscular function. Under these conditions heart rate drops precipitously, blood pressure plummets, and skeletal muscle paralysis can develop (see Nicotine).

An enhancement of acetylcholine's effects can be produced by other methods. A common neurotoxicological example is poisoning by organophosphates that inhibit cholinesterase.

Organophosphate Insecticides

There are many organophosphate compounds that have been or are still used as insecticides. Their insecticidal activity is related to their ability to irreversibly inhibit cholinesterases in insects, including the acetylcholinesterase found at cholinergic nerve terminals. This action in insects leads to uncontrolled muscular twitching and movement followed in time by prostration and death. Animals and humans are nearly as sensitive to the organophosphates as are insects. Exposure to them frequently produces toxicity associated with cholinergic blockade. The blockade of acetylcholinesterase at muscarinic and nicotinic synapses results in a sustained excess of acetylcholine which persistently activates the effector they innervate. Muscarinic stimulation results in excessive salivation, lacrimation, bronchiolar secretions, and bronchoconstriction. Nicotinic stimulation produces effects like those of nicotine. The inactivation of cholinesterase is essentially irreversible, and recovery requires the formation of new enzyme. This can take many days. Fortunately, treatment is available that can protect poisoned individuals from the most severe and potentially lethal actions.

There is an old axiom that what can be switched on can also be switched off. At peripheral synapses this is certainly the case. There are a number of chemical substances and natural products that bind to the nicotinic receptors and behave as competitive antagonists of acetylcholine.

Curare

Curare is a natural product isolated from trees and bushes of the *Strychnos* and *Chondodenron* genera. The active principle (*d*-tubocurarine) is a water-soluble and heat-stable alkaloid which can be extracted, heated, and concentrated to produce a pasty residue containing a high concentration of curare. This extract has been used for centuries in South America as an "arrow poison." Curare is not absorbed from the gastrointestinal tract nor can it penetrate the blood–brain barrier. In order for curare to produce its effects, it must be "injected" into the body.

The effects of curare develop rapidly after it enters the body. Victims develop rapid weakness of voluntary muscles followed by paralysis, respiratory failure, and death. The cause is a blockade of nicotinic cholinergic receptors at the neuromuscular junctions in skeletal muscle. Release of acetylcholine by the cholinergic terminals of the motoneurons is not affected. When curare is present, however, the acetylcholine that is released cannot bind the receptors because they are occupied by the curare. In consequence, nerve–muscle communication fails and paralysis sets in.

It is critical to the use of curare by hunters as an arrow poison that it is not absorbed from the gastrointestinal tract. Animals killed by poisoned arrows can contain many lethal doses of curare in their carcasses around the point of arrow penetration. Because curare is heat stable, it is not destroyed by cooking and is ingested by the hunters. If it were absorbed to an appreciable degree they would become paralyzed and die.

Curare has no effect on sensation, consciousness, or pain, and it does not enter the CNS. Victims injected with many lethal doses of curare will survive with no apparent damage if adequate respiration can be provided for them. Because of this, curare and derivatives of it are used in medicine to produce paralysis during delicate surgical procedures where involuntary or reflexive movement could be disastrous. The anesthetist provides artificial respiration for the patient until the curare is eliminated from the body.

Cobra Snake Venom (α-Bungarotoxin)

α-Bungarotoxin is a neurotoxin secreted by cobras and related elapid snakes. It is a potent, proteinaceous toxin. The compound is not able to penetrate the BBB, and all effects that occur do so in the peripheral nervous system. The effects of its injection (by fang) are rapid and mimic those following injection (by arrow or needle) of curare. Muscular weakness is rapidly followed by paralysis and death. The mechanism is a blockade of the nicotinic cholinergic receptors located at the neuromuscular junctions in skeletal muscle. α-Bungarotoxin binds avidly and persistently to these nicotinic receptors and occludes their occupancy by acetylcholine (see Snake, Elapidae).

Directions for the Future

It must be kept in mind that the problems that drive mankind are often determined by the level of understanding it has about a particular area at a particular time. In terms of human health, priorities during the eighteenth and nineteenth centuries were driven by attempts to avert epidemics and to develop what we would consider crude approaches to dealing with disease and sanitation. Late in the nineteenth century the discovery of bacteria, asepsis, and the general anesthetic, ether, led to rapid strides in medical and surgical approaches to disease. Until the discovery of antibiotics and insecticides suitable for vector control worldwide, the control of infectious diseases from many causes dominated health concerns, leaving little time or effort available for more subtle concerns. After infectious diseases became manageable, there was the luxury to focus on less acutely lethal problems, including chemical toxicity. Within toxicology, at least from the perspective of general human health, the priorities have changed during the past 40–50 years. Initially, the research "engine" was driven by acute toxicity and rapidly lethal exposures. This merged with concerns about longer term exposures that were not acutely lethal. The primary emphasis was with chemicals causing cancer, a disease with a latency period of many years. Recently, nonlethal, noncarcinogenic toxicity associated with specific organ systems has become a prominent concern. Much of the emphasis of the next two or three decades will focus on the consequences of long-term low-level exposures, particularly to chemicals which tend to distribute widely throughout the environment and persist there for a long time. There are many chemical substances that already fit that category. Given the relative lack of past concern in the use of many compounds, such as the chlorinated hydrocarbon insecticides and polychlorinated biphenyls, vast amounts exist in widely dispersed landfills and other dumping places.

These have or may enter into water supplies, may volatilize into the air, or may be carried into the atmosphere bound to dust particles to be returned to earth during precipitation.

With regard to neurotoxicology, it should be apparent from our coverage of specific neurotoxicants that we know much about neurotoxicity and its mechanisms for a few substances. Until 10–15 years ago, neurotoxicologists were most concerned about chemicals demonstrated to be neurotoxic in industrial or environmental exposures. Their work led to establishment of suitable exposure levels and exposure guidelines to reduce adverse effects in people and, for some chemicals, established the mechanisms by which they produced their detrimental effects. That work continues today, and there is much yet to be learned about chemicals already known to affect the nervous system. Because routine neurotoxicity testing has not been a part of required testing of chemicals reaching the workplace or environment until very recently, we have little or no data on many of the chemicals used worldwide. Current guidelines include neurotoxicity testing for new chemicals destined for environmental use. This represents a large step forward, and it can be anticipated that some minimal testing of other chemicals will also be requested in the future.

What lies ahead? The roads neurotoxicology will follow in the next 10–20 years are diverse. There will always be a continuing need to define the neurotoxic potential of chemicals which we live with daily. For the many chemicals in use that have not been adequately tested and for newly synthesized chemicals, standardized neurotoxicity testing for both high-level acute and chronic exposure needs to be done. Where potential neurotoxicity is found, more specific evaluations should be carried out in an attempt to define "safe" exposure conditions for these chemicals. There is clearly a need to establish suitable animal and *in vitro* testing procedures to avoid unnecessary human exposures.

Without a doubt, the most important problem we will face will be the assessment of the neurotoxic consequences of long-term, low-level exposure of those chemicals that have been and/or will be used widely and continually in the environment. Substances such as pesticides, herbicides, pollutants, fertilizers, and other chemicals that will find their way into our soil, air, food, and water need to be carefully evaluated for long-term effects. The lessons we are learning today about the long delay between onset of exposure and development of cancer and immunodeficiency states indicate the need for developing long-term evaluation schemes for neurotoxicity, particularly for degenerative effects brought about by facilitated aging and enhanced rates of nerve cell death.

All of this must be balanced to enable tough decisions to be made in the future. In the past, the tendency has been to ban the use of chemicals if there is the slightest possibility that they could be harmful or to set acceptable levels of exposure so low as to preclude any chance of toxicity. This was often done without regard to the financial impact of such a decision. In the future that alternative might not always be possible. It is clear that population growth and a global desire for a better standard of living will provide a continual pressure to find new and better ways, and new and better chemicals, to minimize toxic exposures. A chemical's beneficial actions will inevitably have to be balanced against its real cost to society, and part of that cost is health-related effects. A careful, appropriate assessment of toxic potential, including neurotoxic potential, will be vital to decision making.

Further Reading

Ellenhorn, M. J., and Barceloux, D. G. (1988). *Medical Toxicology—Diagnosis and Treatment of Human Poisoning*. Elsevier, New York.

Kandel, E. R., Schwartz, J. H., and Jessel, T. M. (Eds.) (1991). *Principles of Neural Science*, 3rd ed. Elsevier, New York.

Siegel, G. J., Agranoff, B. W., Albers, R. W., and Molinoff, P. B. (Eds.) (1994). *Basic Neurochemistry*, 5th ed. Raven Press, New York.

Spencer, P. S., and Schaumburg, H. H. (Eds.) (1980). *Experimental and Clinical Neurotoxicology*. Williams & Wilkins, Baltimore.

—Robert M. Joy

Related Topics

A-Esterase
Behavioral Toxicology
Carbamate Pesticides
Carboxylesterases
Cholinesterase Inhibition
Indoor Air Pollution
Metals
Multiple Chemical Sensitivities

Neurotoxicity, Delayed
Organophosphate Poisoning, Intermediate Syndrome
Organophosphates
Organotins
Pesticides
Psychological Indices of Toxicity
Pyrethrin/Pyrethroids
Sensory Organs
Sick Building Syndrome
Toxicity Testing, Behavioral

Niacin

- CAS: 59-67-6
- SYNONYMS: Vitamin B_3; nicotinic acid; nicotinamide; pellagra-preventative factor; 3-carboxypyridine
- CHEMICAL CLASS: Water-soluble vitamin
- MOLECULAR FORMULA: $C_6H_5NO_2$
- CHEMICAL STRUCTURE:

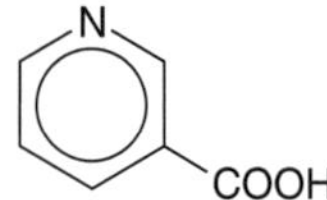

Uses

Niacin is a nutritional supplement used during periods of deficiency (pellagra). Niacin needs may increase during chronic illness such as diabetes mellitus, malignancy, metabolic diseases, hyperthyroidism, infections, chronic fever, alcoholism and during pregnancy and lactation. Niacin is also used in the treatment of hyperlipoproteinemia.

Exposure Pathways

Routes of exposure are oral and intravenous. It can also be given intramuscularly or subcutaneously but intravenous administration is recommended when possible. Dietary sources of niacin are green vegetables, eggs, milk and other dairy products, legumes, yeast, whole grains, lean meats, liver, and fish.

Toxicokinetics

Niacin is readily absorbed from the gastrointestinal tract. The peak serum concentration is usually seen within 45 min of niacin ingestion. Niacin is hepatically metabolized and widely distributed into body tissues. Niacin is renally excreted. Excess amounts of niacin, beyond daily need, are excreted largely unchanged in the urine. Plasma half-life is approximately 45 min.

Mechanism of Toxicity

In large doses peripheral vasodilation occurs.

Human Toxicity: Acute

Toxicity is unlikely even after acute ingestions of 50–100 times the recommended daily allowance. Side effects include nausea, vomiting, diarrhea, abdominal pain, headache, dizziness, and dryness of the skin. Niacin flush is a sensitivity reaction that causes warmth and flushing of the face and neck lasting approximately 2 or 3 hr. This usually occurs with doses $\geqq 1$ g.

Human Toxicity: Chronic

Chronic megadoses of niacin may be associated with hyperglycemia, hyperuricemia, cardiac arrhythmias, hepatotoxicity, cystoid maculopathy, myopathy, and hyperkeratotic pigmented skin lesions. These problems may occur with doses exceeding 3 g per day.

Clinical Management

Acute ingestions seldom require treatment. Reassurance that the niacin flush will gradually resolve over the next couple of hours should be given. In cases of chronic excessive use, the patient should be instructed to discontinue the supplement. Any toxic symptoms should be treated symptomatically.

Animal Toxicity

Acute toxicity is not expected, and it would be unlikely for animals to be given chronic niacin overdoses.

—Denise L. Kurta

Nickel (Ni)

- CAS: 7440-02-0
- Selected Compounds: Nickel subsulfide, Ni_3S_2 (CAS: 12035-72-2); nickel sulfate, $NiSO_4$ (CAS: 7786-81-4); nickel carbonyl, $Ni(CO)_4$ (CAS: 13463-39-3); nickel soluble salts
- Chemical Class: Metals

Uses

Nickel and nickel compounds are widely used in plated coatings, nickel–cadmium batteries, certain pigments, ceramic glazes, and as industrial and laboratory catalysts. Nickel subsulfide is used in refining certain ores and in smelting operations. Nickel is commonly used in alloys such as stainless steel, alloy steel, and nonferrous metal mixtures. Coins, costume jewelry, plumbing equipment, and electrodes are often made from nickel-containing alloys.

Exposure Pathways

Exposure to nickel and its compounds may occur through ingestion, inhalation, or dermal contact. The specific characteristics of the compound determine the likelihood of exposure through a particular route and the amount absorbed into the body through that route.

Nickel is ubiquitous; it is found in air, water, soil, food, certain work environments, and in certain products. Low concentrations are found in soils and in plant and animal tissues. Nickel may be released into the ambient air with emissions from certain industrial processes and with smoke from the combustion of coal and petroleum products. Cigarette smoke may contain up to 3 μg of nickel per cigarette.

Nickel is commonly ingested with food, with the average intake varying from 300 to 600 μg/day. Nickel-containing particulate (e.g., elemental nickel and nickel subsulfide) and gas (e.g., nickel carbonyl) may be inhaled. Skin exposure may occur during contact with nickel-containing products (e.g., jewelry).

Toxicokinetics

Nickel and its inorganic compounds are not well absorbed through the skin or the gastrointestinal tract. The effect of nickel particles that enter the respiratory tract depends, in part, on the size of the particles and the solubility of the compound. Once absorbed into the body, nickel is transported with the plasma, bound to serum albumin, amino acids, polypeptides, and other small organic molecules. Nickel concentrates in the kidneys, liver, and brain. Nickel has been found in adipose tissue. Nickel may act at the point of contact (e.g., in the skin or in the lung) or systemically.

The half-life of nickel in nickel platers was found to be 20–34 hr in plasma and 17–39 hr in urine. In refinery workers, the half-life in the nasal mucosa was found to be several years.

The major route of excretion for nickel is in urine. Animal studies indicate that 60% of the nickel introduced into the body via injection is excreted in the urine and to a lesser extent through the bile into the feces. Some nickel is excreted in perspiration. Ingested nickel is primarily eliminated in the feces, with only about 10% excreted in the urine.

Mechanism of Toxicity

Skin sensitization is believed to occur as a result of nickel binding to the body's natural protein (particularly on the cell surface) and changing how it appears to the immune system. The body perceives the nickel–protein complex as foreign and mounts a reaction to it. This reaction causes the allergy symptoms. For example, sweat may react with the nickel in plated jewelry that comes in direct contact with skin; dissolved metal may penetrate and react with the proteins in the skin.

Nickel may substitute for certain other metals (especially zinc) in metal-dependent enzymes. This can change their structure and activity. High nickel content in serum and tissue may interfere with both copper and zinc metabolism.

The nickel ion (Ni^{2+}) has been shown to react with DNA (genetic material). It can block certain biochemical steps in DNA repair mechanisms. Nickel has not been shown to be mutagenic.

Nickel is an essential trace nutrient in plants and certain animal species (e.g., rat and chick); however, it has not been shown to be essential in humans.

Human Toxicity

Adverse reactions to nickel exposure may occur at the site of contact (skin, respiratory tract, and gastrointestinal tract) or systemically (heart, blood, and kidneys).

Nickel compounds range from highly acutely toxic to slightly toxic.

Symptoms of exposure vary with the compound. Acute inhalation exposure to nickel may cause headache, irritation of the respiratory tract, sore throat, rapid breathing, dizziness, weakness, and toxicity to the heart, kidneys, and blood. Nickel carbonyl (gas) is highly acutely toxic. It is very irritating to the respiratory tract, and exposure may lead to pulmonary edema, pneumonia, and death. Ingestion of nickel and certain nickel compounds has been shown to cause stomach aches, increases in the number of red blood cells, and kidney damage.

Nickel is a sensitizer. Allergy-related asthma and skin reactions ("nickel itch" and contact dermatitis) have been associated with exposure. Skin sensitivity may even develop from contact with jewelry or coins made of nickel-containing alloys. Approximately 2.5–5% of the general population may be sensitized to nickel. It is likely that a higher percentage of women than men are sensitized because of direct contact with nickel-plated jewelry. Skin sensitization reactions can progress to erythema, some eruption, and in more extreme cases to pustules and ulcers. Severe skin reactions are most likely to occur in occupational settings where higher exposure is likely.

Exposure to nickel and certain nickel compounds is associated with development of cancer. Nickel particulate (e.g., elemental and subsulfide) has been associated with nasal and lung cancer after workplace exposures. ACGIH classifies nickel refinery dust and nickel subsulfide as confirmed human carcinogens (A1). U.S. EPA classifies nickel refinery dust and nickel subsulfide as known human carcinogens (A) and nickel carbonyl as a probable human carcinogen (B). IARC classifies the group, nickel and nickel compounds, as having sufficient evidence of cancer in humans (group 1); however, IARC notes that the evaluation applies to the group in general and not necessarily to all compounds in the group.

The OSHA PEL TWA for nickel metal and other nickel compounds as nickel is 1 mg/m^3; the PEL TWA for nickel carbonyl is 0.007 mg/m^3. The ACGIH TLVs for nickel metal, insoluble compounds as nickel, soluble compounds as nickel, nickel carbonyl, nickel subsulfide roasting, nickel fume, and nickel dust as nickel are 1, 1, 0.1, 0.12, 1, 1, and 1 mg/m^3, respectively. All TLVs for nickel and nickel compounds were flagged with a notice of intended change in the 1996 edition of ACGIH's booklet titled *Threshold Limit Values (TLV) for Chemical Substances and Physical Agents and Biological Exposure Indices (BEIs).*

Clinical Management

For inhalation exposure, the victim should be moved from the source of the exposure to fresh air. Contaminated clothing should be removed and contaminated skin washed. Blood, urine, and fecal nickel levels may be used as indicators of the level of recent exposure.

Chelating agents may be used to try to reduce the body burden after exposure. Diethyldithiocarbamate is the preferred chelating agent. D-Penicillamine and calcium ethylenediaminetetraacetate may also be effective in enhancing excretion of nickel.

Once sensitization has occurred, contact with nickel should be strictly avoided since reactions may occur after exposure to very low levels. This is particularly important in the workplace where high-level exposures are more likely to occur.

Animal Toxicity

Different nickel compounds have been shown to have varying toxicity in animals. Both soluble and insoluble forms of nickel have been shown to damage the lung. Chronic inhalation studies (certain forms) have shown pulmonary inflammation, damage to certain regions of the respiratory tract mucosa and epithelium, and damage to the nasal olfactory epithelium. Nickel has been shown to be carcinogenic in animals via injection and implantation. Nickel subsulfide and nickel carbonyl have been shown to be carcinogenic via inhalation.

Nickel has been shown to adversely affect the blood (e.g., severe erythrocytosis) in experimental rats. Nickel subsulfide has been shown to cause reproductive toxicity in male rats and mice.

—Betty J. Locey and Arthur Furst

Related Topics

Hypersensitivity, delayed-type
International Agency for Research on Cancer
Metals
Respiratory tract
Skin

Nicotine

- CAS: 54-11-5
- SYNONYMS: Methylpyridylpyrrolidine
- PHARMACEUTICAL CLASS: Ganglionic cholinergic-receptor agonist
- CHEMICAL STRUCTURE:

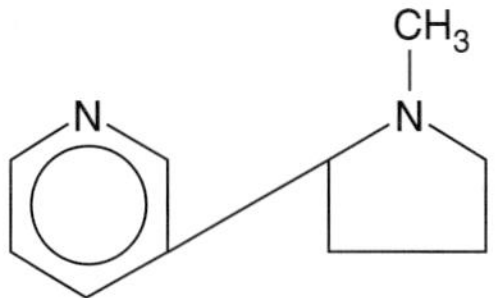

Uses

Nicotine is used in insecticides, tobacco products (cigarettes, 15–20 mg; cigars, 15–40 mg; snuff, 4.6–32 mg) and smoking cessation products such as nicotine gum (2 mg) and transdermal nicotine patches (7–52.5 mg/patch).

Exposure Pathways

Ingestion, dermal contact, and inhalation are the most common routes of accidental and intentional exposure to nicotine.

Toxicokinetics

Nicotine is readily absorbed via the oral mucosa, respiratory tract, gastrointestinal tract, and skin. It undergoes a large first-pass effect during which the liver metabolizes 80–90%. Small amounts are metabolized in the lungs and kidneys. The principal metabolites are isomethylnicotinium ion, nornicotine, cotinine, and nicotine-1′-*N*-oxide. Cotinine is present in the serum in approximately 10 times the amount of nicotine (see Cotinine). Protein binding is approximately 4.9%. Nicotine has an apparent volume of distribution in adults of about 1 liter/kg. Plasma concentrations of nicotine appear to decline in a biphasic manner. The half-life of nicotine in the initial phase is reportedly 2 or 3 min, and the half-life in the terminal phase is reportedly about 30–120 min. Nicotine and its metabolites are excreted in the urine. Approximately 10–20% of an absorbed dose of nicotine is excreted unchanged. Urinary excretion of nicotine is pH dependent, increasing in an acid urine. Nicotine-1′-*N*-oxide is reduced to nicotine by bacterial flora in the large intestine via an *N*-oxide reductase system and subsequently undergoes enterohepatic circulation and repeat metabolism in the liver.

Mechanism of Toxicity

Initially, nicotine is stimulating to the autonomic nervous system ganglia and neuromuscular junction. The prominent effects relate to stimulation of the adrenal medulla, central nervous system (CNS), cardiovascular system due to the release of catecholamines, gastrointestinal tract due to parasympathetic stimulation, salivary and bronchial glands, and the medullary vomiting center. Following these initial effects, nicotine causes blockade of the autonomic ganglia and the neuromuscular junction transmission, inhibition of catecholamine release from the adrenal medulla, and CNS depression.

Human Toxicity: Acute

Nicotine is considered to be an exceedingly lethal poison; however, few deaths have been reported from its use. The onset of symptoms is much more rapid following the ingestion of liquid nicotine-containing products than with nicotine-containing organic material. Clinical manifestations include nausea, vomiting, abdominal pain, and increased salivation. Severe toxicity might result in confusion, agitation, and restlessness, followed by lethargy, seizures, and coma. Severe toxicity with hypertension, tachycardia, and vasoconstriction has occurred from buccal absorption after biting a transdermal nicotine patch. The lethal oral dose of nicotine for adults has been established to be approximately 40–60 mg. Survival has been reported after ingestion of 1–4 g. Pediatric ingestions of 1–1.5 cigarettes resulted in episodes of weakness, limb jerking, and unresponsiveness. Children were asymptomatic if less than one cigarette was ingested.

Human Toxicity: Chronic

Chronic nicotine use can produce dependence liability. Tolerance may occur in some individuals. Withdrawal symptoms following cessation of cigarette smoking may include anxiety, impaired concentration and memory, depression, hostility, sleep disturbances, and increased appetite. Correlations between smoking and alcoholism have been observed.

Clinical Management

Basic and advanced life-support measures should be utilized as necessary. Gastrointestinal decontamination procedures should be used as deemed appropriate to the patient's level of consciousness and the history of the ingestion. Activated charcoal may be used to adsorb nicotine or concomitant ingestants. Enhanced elimination techniques of hemodialysis and hemoperfusion have not been evaluated in acute nicotine poisoning. Nicotine concentrations in the urine are not useful in management of overdosage since they fluctuate greatly with changes in pH and urine flow. The plasma nicotine level correlates well with absorbed dose and can provide a means of evaluating occupational exposure to nicotine. However, the short half-life of nicotine in plasma requires that blood be drawn shortly after exposure. Cotinine in plasma, saliva, and urine appears to have a clear dose–response relationship to passive smoke exposure.

Animal Toxicity

Nicotine causes initial hyperexcitability, hyperpnea, salivation, vomiting, and diarrhea and then depression, incoordination, and paralysis in both small and large animals.

—*Bonnie S. Dean*

Related Topics

Developmental Toxicology
Neurotoxicology: Central and Peripheral
Tobacco
Tobacco Smoke

Nitric Oxide

- CAS: 10102-43-9
- SYNONYMS: Mononitrogen monoxide; nitrogen monoxide
- CHEMICAL CLASS: Gas
- CHEMICAL STRUCTURE:

N=O

Uses

Nitric oxide is used in the manufacturing of nitric acid. It is used as a stabilizer for propylene and methyl ether. It is also used to bleach rayon. Nitric oxide is a natural product of fuel combustion and a component of smog.

Exposure Pathways

Inhalation is a possible exposure pathway. Nitric oxide is also produced endogenously.

Toxicokinetics

When exposed to air, nitric oxide may convert to nitrogen dioxide or nitrogen tetraoxide, both of which are highly toxic. Conversion is slower if below 1 ppm. Other contaminants, such as ozone in the air, expedite the conversion process.

Mechanisms of Toxicity

A cytotoxic free radical, nitric oxide impairs mitochondrial ATP synthesis by inhibiting the citrate cycle and other cellular mechanisms of electron transport.

Human Toxicity

Inhalation of nitric oxide can be toxic if converted to nitrogen dioxide or nitrogen tetraoxide. Contact with skin may be highly irritating. It is irritating to the eyes and respiratory tract. The OSHA PEL is 25 ppm.

Clinical Management

Oxygen therapy should be provided for cyanosis of dyspnea. Prednisone or predinsolone should be given at 5 mg, every 6 hr, to reduce inflammation in the lungs.

Animal Toxicity

Nitric oxide is a mutagen in somatic cells. The inhalation LC_{50} in rats is 1068 mg/m^3.

—*Jayne E. Ash and Shayne C. Gad*

Related Topics

Pollution, Air
Smog

Nitrite Inhalants

- Representative Compounds: Amyl nitrite (CAS: 110-46-3); butyl nitrite (CAS: 544-16-1); isobutyl nitrite
- Synonyms:

Amyl nitrite—*n*-amyl nitrite; nitropentane; nitrous acid; pentyl ester; pentyl nitrite; Liquid Gold

Butyl nitrite— *n*-butyl nitrite; *sec*-butyl nitrite; isobutyl nitrite; *tert*-butyl nitrite; Bang; Bolt; Bullet; Climax; discoroma; flash; Hardware; HiBall; m jack; Jungle Juice; Lightning Bolt; Locker Room; Mama Poppers; Natural Brutes; Odor of Man; OZ; Poppers; Quick Silver; Ram; Rush; Satan's Secret; snappers; Sweat; Thrust

- Chemical Class: Volatile organic nitrites
- Chemical Structures:
- Amyl Nitrite: $(CH_3)_2CHCH_2CH_2NO_2$
- Butyl Nitrite: $C_4H_9NO_3$

Uses

Amyl nitrite is used as a cyanide treatment adjunct, a diagnostic agent, and a vasodilator; it is also an abused inhalant. Butyl nitrite is an abused inhalant.

Exposure Pathways

Nitrites are usually inhaled but have been ingested, either accidentally or with suicidal intent.

Toxicokinetics

Effects following inhalation occur in 10 sec, peak at 30–60 sec, and last approximately 3–5 min. Nitrites are hydrolyzed to the nitrite ion and alcohol within seconds. Approximately 60% of the nitrite ion is biotransformed; ammonia is a metabolite. Almost 40% of the nitrite ion is excreted unchanged via the kidneys. Elimination follows first-order kinetics.

Mechanism of Toxicity

Nitrites produce relaxation of vascular smooth muscles, causing cardiovascular effects through coronary and peripheral vasodilation. They are oxidizing agents and, in excess, induce formation of methemoglobin, an abnormal hemoglobin that is unable to bind and transport oxygen or carbon dioxide. Nitrites can also precipitate an intravascular hemolysis with formation of Heinz bodies. The resulting anemia can compound the hypoxic effects of methemoglobinemia.

Human Toxicity

Users claim aphrodisiac effects from heightened stimulation, enhanced penile erection, and relaxation of the anal sphincter and rectum. Because of the rush of blood and oxygen to the brain, facial flushing and a temporary euphoria occur several seconds after inhalation. Perception of time is slowed.

Acute

Typical effects of inhalation abuse are dizziness, palpitations, blurred vision, headache, nausea, and stinging of the nasal passages, eyes, and throat. There is a fall in blood pressure with a reflexive increase in pulse rate. Pulmonary irritation, tachypnea, and shortness of breath are described. Cardiovascular collapse, coma, anion gap acidosis, and seizures can occur in severely poisoned patients. Methemoglobinemia may occur, characterized by cyanosis and respiratory depression. Ingestion of nitrites seems to produce a more rapid and malignant methemoglobinemia than inhalation. Blood methemoglobin levels should be monitored in symptomatic patients. Methemoglobin levels of 20–30% produce mild symptoms, levels of 30–45% produce moderate effects, and levels of 50–70% are associated with severe toxicity. Levels ≧70% are often lethal if untreated. Plasma nitrite levels are not clinically useful.

Chronic

Repetitive abuse can cause crusting skin lesions and telangiectasis (angioma or hyperemic spots). Tracheobronchial irritation with dyspnea and hemoptysis has been reported. Withdrawal from industrial exposure has resulted in respiratory failure, left ventricular hypertrophy, and myocardial infarctions. Nitrite inhalants are thought to be carcinogenic and immunosuppressive. Tolerance occurs.

Clinical Management

Airway management, respiratory support, and high-flow oxygen are indicated for the cyanotic patient. The cardiovascular, neurological, and metabolic effects should respond to the usual therapeutic agents. Methemoglobinemia is treated with 1–2 mg/kg of methylene blue, given intravenously over a 5-min period and repeated if needed. Methylene blue is recommended for symptomatic patients and for patients with methemoglobin levels ≧30%. Patients with preexisting anemia or cardiovascular disease may need treatment even if their methemoglobin levels are as low as 15%. Exchange transfusion has been employed in severely symptomatic patients who were unresponsive to methylene blue treatment. Hyperbaric oxygen can be supportive while preparing for exchange transfusion. Gastric decontamination is indicated for oral exposure. It will be necessary to monitor complete blood count and arterial blood gases.

Animal Toxicity

Hearing loss, lacrimation, changes in visual acuity, nausea, vomiting, decreased motor performance, tachypnea, seizures, and methemoglobinemia have been induced in animal studies.

—*Janet E. Bauman*

Nitrites

- CAS: 7632-00-0
- Synonym: Sodium nitrite
- Chemical Class: Vasodialator, hypotensive, anticholinergic
- Molecular Formula: $NaNO_2$ (sodium nitrite)

Uses

Nitrites have been used as vasodilators, as circulatory (blood pressure) depressants, as antidotes for cyanide poisoning, and to relieve smooth muscle spasm.

Exposure Pathways

Oral, dermal, ocular, and inhalation routes are all possible exposure pathways.

Toxicokinetics

Nitrites are absorbed orally and dermally. Some nitrite is transformed into nitrate. Transplacental passage of nitrite occurred in pregnant rats given doses of 2.5–50 mg/kg orally. In mice given 400, 800, or 1200 mg sodium nitrite orally in drinking water, 99.1–99.5% of the dose was eliminated. The remaining nitrite was transformed into nitrate and recovered from the liver and muscle.

Mechanism of Toxicity

Nitrites cause relaxation of smooth muscle and the conversion of hemoglobin to methemoglobin.

Human Toxicity

Fatal cases of acute sodium nitrite poisoning have been reported. Also reported are visual field defects, hypotension, tachycardia, respiratory depression, and cyanosis due to methemoglobinemia. In addition, throbbing headache, convulsions, nausea, vomiting, and diarrhea have been reported.

Acute nitrate toxicity is almost always seen in infants rather than adults when it results from ingestion of well waters and vegetables high in nitrates. Infants have an increased stomach pH (above 4) that allows nitrate-reducing organisms to enter and to reduce nitrates to nitrites. In addition, fetal hemoglobin (hemoglobin F) is oxidized by nitrite to methemoglobin at rate twice as adult hemoglobin (hemoglobin A). Furthermore, enzymatic capacity of erythrocytes of newborn infants to reduce methemoglobin to hemoglobin appears less than that of adults.

Clinical Management

In general, plasma levels of nitrites and related compounds are not clinically useful. Methemoglobinemia may be noted and is associated with a cyanosis that does not respond to oxygen therapy. Methemoglobin concentration should be determined in all cyanotic patients or patients experiencing respiratory distress. Arterial blood gases should be monitored in symptomatic or cyanotic patients; measured (not calculated) oxygen saturation will be low.

Emesis and/or activated charcoal/cathartic may be indicated. For seizures, diazepam should be administered as an intravenous bolus. For hypotension, intravenous fluids should be administered. For methemoglobinemia, methylene blue should be administered; if methemoglobinemia is not responsive, an exchange transfusion should be performed in severely symptomatic patients, especially in neonates and children. In addition, hyperbaric oxygen may be used as a supportive measure while preparations for exchange transfusion are being made.

If exposed via inhalation, the victim should be moved to fresh air and monitored for respiratory distress. Treatment should include the recommendations listed previously. Exposed eyes should be irrigated with copious amounts of tepid water for at least 15 min. Exposed areas should be washed thoroughly with soap and water.

Animal Toxicity

Rats received sodium nitrite at 100 mg/kg in drinking water daily during their entire life span over three generations and no evidence of chronic toxicity, carcinogenicity, or teratogenicity was observed. A single intravenous dose of 30 mg/kg of sodium nitrite caused methemoglobinemia in dogs. The minimum lethal dose of sodium nitrite is estimated to be 150–170 mg/kg in cattle and approximately 70–75 mg/kg in pigs. Results were positive in mammalian cytogenetics and sister chromatid exchange studies. Results were negative in DNA repair bacterial assays.

—*Robin Guy*

Related Topic

Respiratory Tract

Nitrobenzene

- CAS: 98-95-3
- SYNONYMS: Nitrobenzol
- CHEMICAL CLASS: Nitrobenzene is a chemical intermediate and is used as a solvent.
- CHEMICAL STRUCTURE:

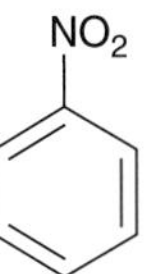

Uses

Nitrobenzene is a chemical intermediate in organic synthesis, in the manufacture of explosives, aniline, aniline dyes, and benzene. It is also used as a solvent and may be used in shoe polishes, floor polishes, and laundry marking ink.

Exposure Pathways

Dermal contact, inhalation, and ingestion are possible exposure pathways.

Toxicokinetics

Nitrobenzene is highly fat soluble and can readily be absorbed through the skin, through inhalation, or through ingestion. Nitrobenzene is metabolized via two main pathways: reduction to aniline followed by hydroxylation to aminophenols and direct hydroxylation of nitrobenzene to form nitrophenols. Further reduction of nitrophenols to aminophenols also occurs. Metabolites in urine are *p*-nitro- and *p*-aminophenol. *p*-Nitrophenol can be measured in the urine. Approximately 55% of dose was excreted as metabolites in urine, 20% in form of nitro compounds, and 35% as amino compounds. Nitro compounds found in urine were nitrobenzene, *o*-nitrophenol, and 4-nitrocatechol in very small amounts and *m*- and *p*-nitrophenol in relatively large amounts.

Mechanism of Toxicity

Gut flora present in animals may be responsible for reduction of nitrobenzene *in vivo* and subsequent methemoglobin formation.

Human Toxicity

The estimated mean lethal adult dose is about 1–5 g. Children may be much more susceptible. Nitrobenzene is toxic by all routes of exposure. Symptoms may be delayed for up to 1–4 hr. Methemoglobinemia associated with headache, nausea, lethargy, depressed respiration, and cyanosis may occur. A bitter almond odor may be present, which suggests cyanide poisoning, but cyanide produces symptoms much more rapidly than nitrobenzene. Tachycardia, hypotension, respiratory depression/failure, and cardiac arrhythmias may be observed. Repeated exposure may be followed by liver impairment up to yellow atrophy, hemolytic icterus, and anemia of varying degrees, with the presence of Heinz bodies in the red blood cells. Pregnant women may be especially at risk due to transplacental passage. Individuals with glucose-6-phosphate dehydrogenase deficiency may also be special-risk groups. Additionally, because alcohol ingestion or chronic alcoholism can lower the lethal toxic dose of nitrobenzene, individuals consuming alcoholic beverages may be at risk.

Clinical Management

Plasma nitrobenzene levels are not clinically useful. Worker exposure to nitrobenzene can be monitored by measuring *p*-nitrophenol in the urine. Methemoglobin levels should be determined in all cyanotic patients; cyanosis that does not respond to oxygen therapy will appear when the plasma methemoglobin level is $\geqq 15\%$. Treat symptomatic methemoglobinemia with methylene blue.

Nitrobenzene is toxic by all routes including skin absorption. Systemic effects may be delayed a few hours. Poisoning closely resembles aniline. Initial care should include adequate gastrointestinal (gastric lavage as indicated and activated charcoal) and dermal decontamination. The patient should be given oxygen and monitored for cyanosis. Cardiac rhythm should be monitored in symptomatic patients. The metabolites in urine, *p*-nitro- and *p*-aminophenol, can be used as evidence of exposure. For seizures, diazepam should be administered via an intravenous bolus.

Exposed eyes should be irrigated with copious amounts of tepid water for at least 15 min. Exposed areas should be washed extremely thoroughly with soap and water.

Animal Toxicity

In rabbits given subcutaneous injections of 0.75 g, hematocrit and hemoglobin levels showed marked decreases, and spherocytes, Heinz bodies, and reticulocytosis were observed. In another rabbit subcutaneous study, bone marrow showed changes ranging from hyperplasia to hypoplasia and even aplasia, with an increase in macroblasts and a decrease in reticulocytes and megakaryocytes; hyperemia of the abdominal cavity and all organs was observed. Nitrobenzene was administered at a subcutaneous dosage of 125 mg/kg/day to pregnant rats during preimplantation and placentation; delay of embryogenesis, alteration of normal placentation, and abnormalities in fetus were observed and gross morphologic defects were seen in 4 of 30 fetuses.

Pregnant rats were exposed to nitrobenzene vapor at 0, 1, 10, and 40 ppm (mean analytical values of 0.0, 1.06, 9.8, and 39.4 ppm, respectively) on Gestation Days 6–15 for 6 hr/day; at sacrifice on Gestation Day 21, fetuses were evaluated for external, visceral, and skeletal malformations and variations. Maternal toxicity was limited to decreased weight gain and absolute and relative spleen weights were increased at 10 and 40 ppm; there was no developmental toxicity (including teratogenicity) associated with exposure to nitrobenzene concentrations that produced some maternal toxicity (10 and 40 ppm) or that produced no observable maternal toxicity (1 ppm).

The embryotoxicity and teratogenicity of nitrobenzene were evaluated in mated female New Zealand White rabbits (22/group) exposed by inhalation to nitrobenzene at nominal concentrations of 0, 10, 40, or 100 ppm for 6 hr/day during Gestation Days 7–19. The animals were sacrificed on the day evidence was observed that they aborted or delivered prematurely or on Gestation Day 30, whichever occurred sooner. Significant differences between treated and control animals were observed in the following: increased absolute and relative liver weight and methemoglobin values (mid- and high-dose groups). No significant differences between treated and control animals were observed in the following areas: mortality, pregnancy, abortion or premature delivery rates, body weights, corpora lutea and uterine implantation data, fetal weight, crown–rump distance, fetal sex distribution, and external, visceral, and skeletal evaluation of fetuses.

A two-generation reproduction study was performed by exposure of rats to concentrations of 0, 1, 10, or 40 ppm of nitrobenzene vapor; at 40 ppm, a decrease in the fertility index of the F_0 and F_1 generations occurred, which was associated with decreased weights of the testes and epididymides, seminiferous tubule atrophy, spermatocyte degeneration, and the presence of giant syncytial spermatocytes. The only significant finding in the litters derived from rats exposed to 40 ppm was a decrease in the mean body weight of F_1 pups on Postnatal Day 21. Survival indices were unaltered.

The oral LD_{50} in rats was 640 mg/kg. Nitrobenzene is carcinogenic in mice and rats by the inhalation route. There was no mutagenic effect observed in tests for mutagenic activity with *Salmonella typhimurium*.

—Robin Guy

Nitroethane

- CAS: 79-24-3
- Chemical Class: Aliphatic nitro compounds
- Molecular Formula: $C_2H_5NO_2$
- Chemical Structure:

```
     H   H
     |   |
H—C—C—NO2
     |   |
     H   H
```

Uses

Nitroethane is used as a propellant; as a solvent for nitrocellulose, resins, waxes, and dyestuffs; and in chemical synthesis.

Exposure Pathways

The primary routes of occupational exposure to nitroethane are inhalation and dermal contact.

Toxicokinetics

In studies of isolated lower and upper respiratory tracts (URT) from rats, 65 and 71%, respectively, of available nitroethane was absorbed. The intact respiratory tracts of anesthetized rats absorbed 58% of the available nitroethane. Absorption was not related to water solubility or water/air partition coefficients, indicating that a complex mechanism may exist. It was concluded that the URT plays a significant role in the absorption of nitroethane vapors. In monkeys administered single dermal doses of 4.9% nitroethane in ether/ethanol, maximum blood nitroethane levels were observed at 40 min to 1 hr; however, 99.8% of the administered dose was not recovered in this study, probably due to evaporation of the test material.

Older studies indicate that nitroethane is metabolized rapidly. Recently, some mercapturic acid metabolite was detected in the urine of rabbits administered the compound. Elevated blood nitrate and nitrite levels reported in rabbits administered nitroethane by inhalation indicate that the nitrite was formed by its metabolism.

Older studies indicate that absorbed nitroethane is eliminated within 30 hr. In monkeys administered single dermal doses in ether/ethanol, 91% of total urine radioactivity was excreted within 48 hr. As stated previously, more than 99% of the administered dose was lost prior to absorption, probably as a result of volatilization.

Mechanism of Toxicity

The mechanisms of toxicity for nitroethane are unknown. It is possible that methemoglobinemia reported in some animal studies may be a result of the metabolism of nitroethane to nitrite compounds.

Human Toxicity

Nitroethane is an irritant to the eyes and respiratory tract. Overexposure to or inhalation of the vapors may cause narcosis. There are no reports of chronic overexposure.

Clinical Management

If contact with the liquid occurs, affected areas should be flushed thoroughly with water for at least 15 min and then observed for resulting irritation. In case of inhalation, the victim should be moved to fresh air, an airway should be established, and respiration should be maintained as necessary. The patient should be monitored for respiratory irritation and pulmonary edema. If ingestion occurs, emesis is not recommended; instead, the victim should be given water or milk to dilute the stomach contents. Gastric lavage may be indicated if the victim is unconscious or convulsing. Treatment for methemoglobinemia and/or monitoring for possible liver and kidney injury may be indicated.

Animal Toxicity

Nitroethane is an irritant to the eyes and mucous membranes. In animal studies, nitroethane caused narcosis in survivors and liver and kidney injury in animals that died. Acute lethality has been reported in rabbits exposed by inhalation to 1000 ppm for 2 hr. Chronic overexposure can cause inflammation of the respiratory tract, methemoglobinemia, cyanosis, and liver injury.

—*Daniel Steinmetz*

Nitrogen Mustards

- SYNONYMS: HN_1, bis(2-chloroethyl)ethylamine; HN_2, mechlorethamine hydrochloride, bis(2-chloroethyl)methylamine hydrocloride (leukeran) (CAS: 55-86-7); HN_3, tris(2-chloroethyl)amine hydrochloride (CAS: 817-09-4); 2,2′,′-trichlorotriethylamine; nitrogen mustard-3; mechlorethamine (Mustargen)
- CHEMICAL CLASS: Vesicant, alkylating agent
- MOLECULAR FORMULAS:

HN−1	HN−2	HN−3
$C_6H_{13}Cl_2N$	$C_5H_{11}Cl_2N$	$C_6H_{12}Cl_3N$

- CHEMICAL STRUCTURES:

HN-1: C_2H_5-N(CH_2CH_2Cl)(CH_2CH_2Cl)

HN-2: CH_3N(CH_2CH_2Cl)(CH_2CH_2Cl)

HN-3: CH_2CH_2Cl N(CH_2CH_2Cl)(CH_2CH_2Cl)

Uses

Nitrogen mustards are used in chemical warfare and in cancer chemotherapy.

Exposure Pathways

Ocular, percutaneous, inhalation, ingestion, and injection are all possible routes of exposure. Effects may be local, systemic, or both.

Toxicokinetics

Like sulfur mustard, the nitrogen mustards combine predominantly with the thiol group and are excreted as conjugated cysteinyl derivatives.

Both nitrogen and sulfur mustards have structural similarities and have common chemical reactions. A key reaction is the intramolecular cyclization in a polar solvent such as water to form a cyclic onium cation and a free anion. Nitrogen mustards form the immonium cation, while the sulfur mustard forms the sulfonium cation. The cyclized form is responsible for the varied effects of mustards, which are similar. In nitrogen mustard the sulfur is replaced by nitrogen.

Human Toxicity

Nitrogen mustards produce damage to the eyes, respiratory tract, and skin. Systemically they produce cytotoxicity, with the hematopoietic and lymphoid tissues being especially sensitive.

The estimated inhalation median lethal dosage (LCt_{50}) for HN-3 in humans is 1500 mg-min/m^3. The estimated percutaneous vapor LCt_{50} is 10,000 mg-min/m^3, and the estimated percutaneous liquid LD_{50} is 700 mg/70-kg. The percutaneous median incapacitating dosage (ICt_{50}) in humans has been estimated at 2500 mg-min/m^3; the dose to produce eye injury has been estimated at 200 mg-min/m^3.

Irritation of eyes following a single exposure to nitrogen mustards occurs at doses that do not affect the skin or respiratory tract and appears sooner than with sulfur mustard. Mild to moderate exposures cause slight smarting and lacrimation within 20 min, becoming persistent approximately 2.5 hr later, and reaching a maximum at 8–10 hr. The effects include erythema and edema of the palpebral and bulbar conjunctiva with superficial, steamy haziness of the cornea, irritation, lacrimation, deep eye pain, miosis, and photophobia.

Following severe exposure these symptoms progress for 24 hr or longer and are followed by spotty hemorrhagic discoloration of the iris and roughened lusterless surface of the corneal epithelium, which demonstrate punctuate fluorescein staining. The corneal epithelium may exfoliate.

Clouding and edema of the cornea and necrosis may cause rupture of the globe.

There may be no skin lesions following mild vapor exposures. However, severe vapor or liquid exposure to nitrogen mustard will produce effects similar to those of sulfur mustard (but the onset is sooner than with sulfur mustard); these effects include erythema, irritation, and itching, with blisters developing in the erythematous areas.

Exposure of the respiratory tract to nitrogen mustard produces the same effects as sulfur mustard. These include the delay in onset, irritation of the nose and throat, hoarseness progressing to aphonia, and persistent cough, fever, dyspnea, and moist rales. After 24 hr, chemical pneumonitis may appear.

Following oral administration or systemic absorption of nitrogen mustards, the intestinal tract may be damaged. In animals, severe diarrhea occurred, which may be hemorrhagic. The lesions were most marked in the small intestine and consisted of degenerative changes and necrosis in the mucosa. In humans, ingestion of 2–6 mg causes nausea and vomiting.

Following absorption of nitrogen mustard from intact skin or respiratory or gastrointestinal tract, the most specific effects are on the hematopoietic and lymphoid tissues. In bone marrow, the degenerative changes can be detected within 12 hr and may progress to severe aplasia. The thymus, spleen and lymph nodes involute rapidly with necrosis and phagocytosis of their lymphocytes. This is evident from the transient leukocytosis in the blood, which is followed by severe lymphopenia, granulocytopenia, thrombocytopenia, and lymphopenia for 5–10 days following exposure. The white blood cell count may fall to 500 cells/mm^3 or lower. The various nitrogen mustards differ in their ability to produce these changes.

The chronic physiological effects may include, for severe exposure, scarring of the cornea; the iris frequently becomes discolored and atrophied. Repeated skin burns may lead to hypersensitivity of the skin, which is an effect similar to that of sulfur mustard. That is, reexposure will cause erythema, with or without edema, and pronounced itching and burning occurring within 1 hr. Lower concentrations will produce these effects in sensitized persons. Vesication heals more rapidly. Frequent manifestations of reexposure in sensitized individuals include a morbilliform rash and eczematoid dermatitis surrounding old lesions.

Clinical Management

The victim must be removed from the source of contamination quickly by adequately protected attendants and then decontaminated using a solution of sodium hypochlorite, liquid household bleach, or Fullers' earth. Oxygen and/or artificial respiration should be administered if dyspnea is present or breathing has stopped.

Erythema should be treated with calamine or other soothing lotions or creams to reduce burning and itching. Large blisters should be unroofed and covered with a sterile dry dressing if the patient is ambulatory or left uncovered if the patient is not ambulatory. Denuded areas should be irrigated with saline or soapy water and covered with a topical antibiotic (e.g., silver sulfadiazine or mefanide acetate). Multiple or large areas of vesication require hospitalization and whirlpool irrigation.

Systemic analgesics are indicated especially prior to manipulation of the patient or irrigation of the burn areas. Systemic antipruritics (e.g., trimeprazine) may also be used.

Treatment of ocular injury includes thorough irrigation, application of homatropine (anticholinergic) ophthalmic ointment, and topical antibiotics several times daily. Vaseline or similar products should be applied regularly to the edges of the eyelids to prevent them from sticking together. Topical analgesics may be useful in severe blepharospasm for examination of the eye but should be used sparingly. Sunglasses may reduce discomfort from photophobia, and the victim must be reassured that complete healing and restoration of vision will result.

Steam inhalation and cough suppressants may relieve upper airway symptoms (sore throat, nonproductive cough, and hoarseness). Appropriate antibiotic therapy should only be instituted following confirmation of infection by positive sputum tests (gram stain and culture).

Intubation should be accomplished prior to the development of laryngeal spasm or edema so that adequate ventilation is established and suction of necrotic and inflammatory debris can be facilitated. Oxygen may be required as well. Early use of PEEP or CPAP may be useful. Bronchoscopy may be required if pseudomembrane has developed to permit suction of the necrotic debris by direct vision. Bronchodilators or steroids may also be used to relieve bronchospasm.

Death may occur between the 5th and 10th day postexposure because of pulmonary insufficiency complicated by a compromised immune response from mustard-induced bone marrow damage.

Atropine (0.4–0.6 mg intramuscular or intravenous) or other anticholinergic or antiemetic drugs may be used to control nausea and vomiting.

TABLE N-6
Animal Toxicity Values for Nitrogen Mustards

Inhalation		
Species	*Time (min)*	*LCt_{50} (mg-min/m³)*
Mouse	10	165 (vapor)
	10	345 (aerosol)
Rat	10–100	670 (vapor)
	0.25–2.0	800 (aerosol)
Cat	10	400–1000
Dog	10	400–1000

	LD_{50} (mg/kg)			
Species	*PC*[a]	*IV*[b]	*SC*[c]	*IG*[d]
Mouse	7.0	1-2	2.0	—
Rat	4.9	0.7	2.0	2.5
Rabbit	19.0	2.5	2.0	—
Dog	10.0	1.0	—	—

[a] Percutaneous.
[b] Intravenous.
[c] Subcutaneous.
[d] Intragastric.

Sterilization of the gastrointestinal tract by nonabsorbable antibiotics may reduce the possibility of infection from enteric organisms. Bone marrow transplants or blood transfusion may be indicated. The recent introduction of granulocyte colony stimulating factor may offer hope in the management of bone marrow depression.

A victim of nitrogen mustard exposure also requires the general supportive care given to a severely ill patient as well as the specific care given to a burn patient. This includes the liberal use of systemic analgesics and antipruritics and the maintenance of fluid and electrolyte balance. Parenteral food supplements and vitamins may also be beneficial.

Animal Toxicity

The animal toxicity reported for HN-3 is described in Table N-6.

—Harry Salem and Frederick R. Sidell

(The views of the authors do not purport to reflect the position of the U.S. Department of Defense. The use of trade names does not constitute official endorsement or approval of the use of such commercial products.)

Related Topics

Nerve Agents
Respiratory Tract
Sensory Organs

Nitrogen Tetraoxide

- CAS: 10544-72-6
- SYNONYMS: Liquid nitrogen dioxide under pressure.
- CHEMICAL CLASS: Nitrogen oxides
- MOLECULAR FORMULA: N_2O_4
- CHEMICAL STRUCTURE:

```
    O   O
    ‖   ‖
O═N—N═O
```

Uses

Nitrogen tetraoxide is formed by pressurizing liquid nitrogen dioxide. It is used in the manufacture of explosives and rocket fuels. It is also a component of nitric and sulfuric acid.

Exposure Pathway

Inhalation is the probable route of exposure.

Mechanisms of Toxicity

Nitrogen tetraoxide is absorbed through respiratory system and reacts with blood, reducing fluid levels and inciting massive pulmonary edema and severe reduction in hemoglobin levels.

Human Toxicity

The effects of exposure are insidious, leaving an exposed person asymptomatic for days, even at fatal dosage. The latent period may be from 5 to 72 hr.

It has an irritating odor. Exposure may inflame the lungs and cause mild chest pain. Brief exposure at a concentration of 100 ppm may cause a toxic reaction. Exposure at 200 ppm may be fatal. Nitrogen tetroxide is a class A poison. (CFR 173, Section 173.326)

Clinical Management

The victim should be treated with methylene blue and given oxygen therapy.

Animal Toxicity

The inhalation LC_{50} is 315 ppm in rabbits.

—Jayne E. Ash and Shayne C. Gad

Nitromethane

- CAS: 75-52-5
- Chemical Class: Aliphatic nitro compounds
- Molecular Formula: CH_3NO_2
- Chemical Structure:

```
     H
     |
H—C—NO2
     |
     H
```

Uses

Nitromethane is used as a solvent, chemical intermediate, fuel additive, rocket propellant, and as a chemical stabilizer for halogenated hydrocarbon solvents.

Exposure Pathways

The primary routes of occupational exposure to nitromethane are inhalation and dermal contact.

Toxicokinetics

In monkeys administered a single dermal dose of 5.5% nitromethane in ether/ethanol, blood plasma levels reached a maximum after 20 min to 6 hr; however, 99.9% of the dose was not recovered in this study, probably due to evaporation of the test material from the application site. Negligible amounts of nitrates were found in the blood of rabbits following intravenous administration of nitromethane, suggesting that it is metabolized differently than nitroethane and nitropropane. Anaerobic incubation with liver microsomes resulted in formaldehyde production. No nitrites were detected. It has been reported that nitromethane forms a complex with cytochrome P450 from rabbit liver microsomes and that it apparently competes with carbon monoxide for a common binding site. No distribution data are available for nitromethane. In monkeys administered a single dermal dose, radioactivity was detected in the urine and feces. About 90% of urine radioactivity appeared within 48 hr and 92–96% of feces radioactivity appeared within 48 hr. As discussed previously, more than 99% of the administered dose was not recovered in the study.

Mechanism of Toxicity

The mechanisms of toxicity for nitromethane are unknown.

Human Toxicity

The lethal human dose has been reported to be 0.5–5 g/kg. It is a respiratory irritant and a weak narcotic in humans.

Clinical Management

If contact with the liquid occurs, affected areas should be flushed thoroughly with water for at least 15 min. These areas should be observed for resulting irritation. In case of inhalation, the victim should be moved to fresh air, an airway should be established, and respiration should be maintained as necessary. The patient should be monitored for irritation and pulmonary edema. If ingestion occurs, emesis should be induced if the victim is conscious. Gastric lavage may be indicated if the victim is unconscious or convulsing. Treatment for methemoglobinemia and/or monitoring for possible liver and kidney injury may be required.

Animal Toxicity

Nitromethane is a mild irritant of the eyes and mucous membranes. At high concentrations (10,000–

30,000 ppm), it causes nervous system effects, including salivation, weakness, and narcosis. It does not appear to cause methemoglobinemia in animals. The acute oral LD_{50} in rats is 1210 mg/kg, indicating moderate toxicity. Acute and chronic exposures have resulted in liver and kidney injury in several animal species. In other subchronic studies, nitromethane was reported to produce adverse effects on the blood, thyroid, lung, nervous system, and sperm motility.

—*Daniel Steinmetz*

Nitrosamines

- Preferred Name: *N*-nitrosamines
- Chemical Class: Dialkylnitrosamines
- Chemical Structure: The name nitrosamines applies to a family of compounds that have an alkyl and an aryl group attached to the chemical group,

$$R_1R_2{>}N{-}N{=}O$$

=N–N=O. R_1 and R_2 are alkyl and aryl groups.

Exposure Pathways

The most common route of exposure is by oral ingestion of nitrosamines in food. Nitrosamines can be found in foods preserved with nitrates as well as in untreated foods such as mushrooms, alcoholic beverages, smoked fish, bacon, ham, and some cheeses. Nitrosamines have also been found in tobacco smoke and urban air. Nitrosamines can also be formed in the mouth or stomach if the food contains nitrosamine precursors. Under acidic pH in the mouth or stomach, nitrite or nitrates added to food or naturally occurring may combine with amines to form nitrosamines (see Nitrites).

Toxicokinetics

Physical properties of nitrosamines vary widely depending on the nature of the substituent groups R_1 and R_2. Similarly, the nature of the substituent group has an effect on the toxicological properties of the nitrosamine. For example, the LD_{50} of nitrosamine compounds is directly proportional to the carbon chain length of the substituent. Long-chain substituents have a higher LD_{50}. Also, the nature of the substituent group has an effect on the carcinogenicity properties of nitrosamines. Dimethyl and diethyl compounds cause predominantly liver tumors, while dibutyl compounds tend to cause bladder tumors.

Nitrosamines have a short half-life that has been measured in the order of minutes.

Mechanism of Toxicity

Nitrosamines are not carcinogenic at the point of application. They required bioactivation. One possible mechanism of biotransformation is by enzymatic transformation to a carbonium ion. Activation is known to proceed first by hydroxylation of an α carbon. The results of this reaction are an aldehyde, which is excreted, and an unstable primary nitrosamine.The unstable nitrosamine ultimately tautomerizes to a carbonium ion. The highly reactive carbonium ion readily alkylates with nearby cellular macromolecules. Cancer and mutagenicity may develop when reactive nitosamine metabolites alkylate to genetic macromolecules.

Human Toxicity

Dimethylnitrosamine, a member of the nitrosamine family, is highly carcinogenic to the liver and kidneys in almost all mammalian species tested. There is also a significant body of epidemiological data that links exposure to nitrosamines and human cancer.

Clinical Management

Nitrosamine exposure is not an acute hazard. Health hazards associated with nitrosamine exposure are limited to cancer and liver and kidney damage associated with chronic exposure. No specific treatment exists for nitrosamine intoxication. Supportive and symptomatic treatment should be provided.

Animal Toxicity

Nitrosamines are strong hepatotoxic agents. Large, acute doses produce liver necrosis and hemorrhages in the liver and other tissues. However, of toxicological importance is chronic, continuous exposure to low doses of nitrosamines in the diet. Nitrosamines are strong carcinogens that produce cancer of the liver and kidneys. In experiments conducted to date, 75–80% of nitrosamines tested have been found to be carcinogenic to mammals.

—*Heriberto Robles*

Related Topic

Carcinogen–DNA Adduct Formation and DNA Repair

N-Nitrosodimethylamine

- CAS: 62-75-9
- Preferred Name: Dimethylnitrosamine
- Synonyms: DMN; NDMA; *N*-methyl-*N*-nitrosomethanamine; *N*-nitrosodimethylamine; *N*-nitroso-*N,N*-dimethylamine; DMNA; *N,N*-dimethylnitrosamine
- Molecular Formula: $C_2H_6N_2O$ or $(CH_3)_2NN = O$
- Chemical Structure:

```
        O
        ‖
   H    N    H
   |    |    |
H—C—N—C—H
   |         |
   H         H
```

Uses

DMN is used commonly as an industrial solvent in the production of dimethylhydrazine. It is currently used as an antioxidant, as an additive for lubricants and gasolines, and as a softener of copolymers. Nitrosamines have been patented for use in pesticides and nematocides. They have also been found in multiple cosmetic products, hand and body lotions, and shampoos. Alarming levels have been found in soil, postulated to be from the use of triazine herbicides, which can react with nitrogenous fertilizers (which are ubiquitously used).

DMN is a research chemical, air and water pollutant, and tobacco smoke condensate. It was formerly used in the production of hypergolic rocket fuels, thiocarbonyl fluoride polymers, and as a soluble cutting oil.

Exposure Pathways

Inhalation (contaminated air), skin contact, ingestion through food and water, and *in vivo* formation from amines and nitrates are all possible exposure pathways. Maximal exposure occurs through food (e.g., nitrite-cured meat, fish, or malt beverages), household goods (e.g., rubber), tobacco and tobacco smoke, cosmetics, drugs, pesticides, and indoor air (e.g., frying of nitrite-cured meat with release of volatile nitrosamines).

Toxicokinetics

DMN is rapidly absorbed from all the routes of exposure. This chemical is dangerous because, in most instances, it is produced inside the body. DMN (and many other related compounds) is intrinsically not reactive and requires metabolic activation by the P450 system for its biological effects. Upon metabolism, very reactive electrophillic carbonium ions (e.g., methyldiazonium) are formed, which in turn attack cellular macromolecules (e.g., protein, DNA, and RNA).

No clear-cut human data are available. An intravenous bolus dose of 1.35 mmol/kg (100 mg/kg) to Fisher 344 rats revealed a predominantly hepatic clearance of 2.5 min to 3 hr. Orally administered DMN (2.02 or 4.05 mmol/kg) cleared between 5 and 120 min. Intravenously injected DMN concentrations declined in a biexponential manner with a terminal half-life of 10 min. The apparent total systemic blood clearance distribution was 39 ml/min/kg. The apparent steady-state volume of distribution was 297 ml/kg. The rate of metabolism of DMN after larger oral doses (10 mg/kg) is 5 mg/kg/hr and follows a zero-order kinetics. Terminal biological half-life is 11 min, and elimination is predominantly by the liver.

Mechanism of Toxicity

DMN is a strong alkylating agent and therefore a potent genotoxin. It is primarily metabolized (P450) in the liver and therefore a potent hepatonecrogen. Biological reactive intermediates formed after metabolism (e.g., methyldiazonium and dimethylcarbonium) may covalently bind to cellular macromolecules and jeopardize cellular functions. However, nephrotoxic and immunotoxic potential of this agent have also been well documented in the literature. DMN culminates necrosis (unprogrammed cell death) in addition to apoptosis (or programmed cell death) of the hepatocytes. Toxic concentrations of DMN elevate hepatocellular Ca^{2+} leading to endonuclease-mediated fragmentation of DNA. Low concentrations of DMN can induce DNA single- and double-strand breaks. All these events cumulatively may give rise to toxicity of a particular organ leading to organ dysfunction.

Human Toxicity: Acute

Exposure usually does not produce irritation of skin or mucous membranes. Acute poisoning may invoke headaches, malaise, fever, or general weakness. Gastrointestinal effects include abdominal cramping, nausea, and vomiting, eventually leading to diarrhea. Hepatomegaly and jaundice may follow if the exposure is severe or prolonged.

Human Toxicity: Chronic

Chronic exposure may cause liver disease with jaundice and swelling with a precipitous drop in the platelet count. The lowest lethal oral dose in humans has been reported at 10 mg/kg/80-week intermittent exposure. DMN is a suspected human carcinogen and is carcinogenic to all the other species tested upon prolonged low-level exposure.

Clinical Management

The affected person should be removed immediately from the site of exposure and respiration should be established. If exposure to mucous membranes is suspected, absorption should be prevented by repeated flushing with water. Affected parts of the body should be decontaminated with soap and water. It is necessary to evaluate hepatic and renal function tests as thoroughly as possible while paying special attention to liver size. Chest X-ray and cancer screening are necessary.

Animal Toxicity

DMN is carcinogenic to all of the 10 species tested in single bolus doses or multiple low doses. The primary target organs include the liver, kidneys, thymus, spleen, lung, skin, and trachea. Swiss mice fed a diet containing 0.005% DMN for 1 week developed tumors of the kidneys and lung. Hamsters fed a diet containing .0025% for 11 weeks developed liver tumors. ICR mice injected with 25–50 mg/kg (one dose) developed severe hepatotoxicity within 12 hr. DMN is mutagenic to several bacterial species.

—Sidhartha D. Ray

Nitrous Oxide

- CAS: 100024-97-2
- Synonyms: Dinitrogen monoxide; laughing gas; hyponitrous acid anhydride; factitious air
- Chemical Class: An oxide of nitrogen
- Chemical Structure:

$$-N{=}N^{+}{=}O$$

Uses

Nitrous oxide is used therapeutically as an anesthetic or analgesic. It is also used in the formulation of rocket fuel and as a propellant for whipped cream. It occurs endogenously.

Exposure Pathway

Inhalation is the route of exposure.

Toxicokinetics

Nitrous oxide is readily absorbed from inspired air. It is excreted in urine and expired air.

Mechanism of Toxicity

High concentrations of the gas have a narcotic and/or asphyxiatic effect.

Human Toxicity

The ACGIH TLV is 50 ppm in air. The OSHA PEL is 25 ppm.

Clinical Management

Exposure should be terminated immediately. Oxygen therapy should be provided if respiratory difficulties are present.

Animal Toxicity

Nitrous oxide is a carcinogen, mutagen, and teratogen in laboratory animals. The inhalation LC_{50} is 160/m^3 in rats.

—*Jayne E. Ash and Shayne C. Gad*

Noise: Ototraumatic Effects

Introduction

The mammalian ear is capable of responding to sound energy over a remarkably wide range of intensities, from the barely audible soft rustling of leaves to the almost painful crash of nearby thunder. In physical terms, the ear responds to pressure fluctuations ranging from approximately 0 dB sound pressure level (0.00002 Pa) under quiet listening conditions to well over a million times greater. Although the ear has a wide dynamic range, it was not designed to withstand many of the noises that are frequently encountered in modern industrialized societies. The high-level intermittent and continuous noises found in many industrial, military, and recreational settings can be potentially hazardous to hearing, particularly after years of exposure. Currently, noise-induced hearing loss (NIHL) caused by prolonged or excessive exposure to noise is considered to be one of the top 10 occupational health problems in the United States, with over 8 million workers exposed daily to noise levels of 85 dBA or greater. A 1981 OSHA report estimated that no fewer than half a million U.S. workers in the manufacturing sector had sustained moderate to severe job-related hearing impairment. The U.S. Army also recognizes NIHL as one of its most serious health problems—not simply because it costs millions in compensation costs but also because it jeopardizes the ability of trained personnel to perform their duties safely and effectively. Even individuals who are not exposed to damaging levels of noise in their workplaces may be routinely exposed to high levels of noise at home (e.g., lawn mowers, vacuum cleaners, and power tools) or recreationally (e.g., firearms, snowmobiles, rock concerts, and personal stereos).

The amount of hearing loss that an individual will develop from exposure to noise depends on a variety of factors related to both the individual and the noise environment itself. Individual factors include genetic predisposition, age, diet, general health, hormonal status, exposure history, and simultaneous exposure to other ototoxic agents, such as aminoglycoside antibiotics or industrial solvents. Environmental factors include those related to the intensity, frequency, duration, and temporal characteristics of the noise that impinges on the individual's auditory system.

Clinically, NIHL is expressed as a loss of hearing sensitivity that is typically most severe in the midfrequency range. Figure N-5 shows the audiogram typical of a patient with NIHL, showing the characteristic "4-kHz notch." The fact that the hearing loss first appears and tends to be most severe in the 4-kHz region is not a reflection of a basic weakness in that part of the ear. Rather, it is primarily the consequence of the way the external auditory meatus (EAM), or ear canal, transforms sound as it passes from the air to the middle ear. Figure N-6 is a cross section of the human temporal bone, showing the three major divisions of the auditory periphery: the external ear, consisting of the pinna and the EAM; the middle ear, an air-filled space that houses three ossicles (malleus, incus, and stapes) and two muscles (tensor tympani and stapedius); and the inner ear or cochlea, which contains contractile outer hair cells (OHC), sensory inner hair cells, and neural elements that are essential for transmitting sensory information from the cochlea to the brain. The external and middle ears transform the sound spectrum in ways that depend on their physical characteristics. Because the EAM is essentially a tube that is closed at one end by the tympanic membrane (eardrum), it acts as an acoustic resonator with a resonant frequency that is predicted by the quarter-wave formula: resonant frequency = speed

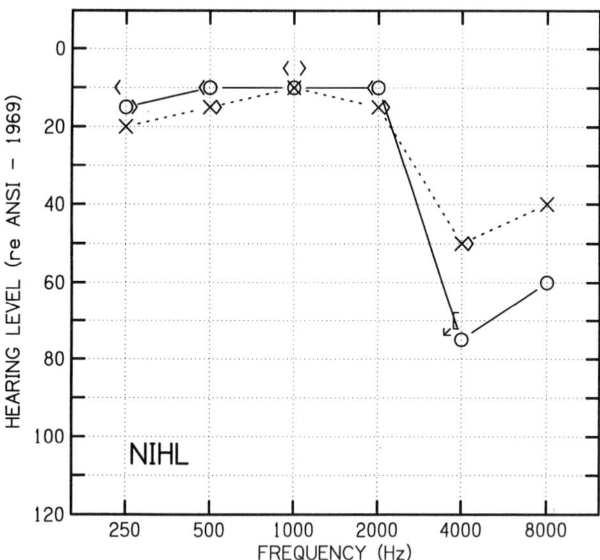

FIGURE N-5. Pure tone audiogram showing loss of sensitivity in the 4-kHz region for both the right ear (○) and the left ear (×). The "4-kHz notch" is typical of noise-induced hearing loss.

of sound/4 × length of EAM. Since the average length of the human EAM is approximately 25 mm, the resonant frequency of the ear canal is around 3200 Hz. Figure N-7 illustrates how EAM resonance serves to boost the gain of mid-frequencies at the eardrum. The resonant characteristics of the EAM amplify sounds substantially in the frequency region between approximately 2 and 4 kHz (Fig. N-7A). Since many industrial or military sound environments have broad-spectrum noises (Fig. N-7B) and the EAM selectively amplifies the mid-frequencies, the noise spectrum at the eardrum peaks in the mid-frequency range (Fig. N-7C). This results in more hearing loss in the mid-frequency region than at higher or lower frequencies.

The effects of prolonged exposure to high-level noise can accumulate over time. Although the rate of growth of hearing loss at 4 kHz slows after about 10 years of exposure, losses at the lower and higher frequencies continue to grow over a 20- to 30-year period.

Biological Effects of Noise

Hearing loss due to noise exposure is a complex function of noise parameters and individual susceptibility. When noise does cause damage to the ear, the effects are pervasive and can involve damage to all the major cell systems of the cochlea. Figure N-8 shows damaged cochlear tissue after noise exposure. Perhaps the most sensitive structures are the stereocilia, which are the transduction links between the sensory hair cells and the tectorial membrane. One of the first pathologies seen is disruption of the mechanical cross-links between individual stereocilia on a given hair cell. Stereocilia can also develop "blebs" or growths and can fuse to form "giant stereocilia."

The outer hair cells (the motile sensory cells responsible for the exquisite sensitivity and frequency selectivity of the cochlea) appear to be more vulnerable to noise damage than the inner hair cells (the sensory cells that are responsible for conveying electrochemical information to the brain via auditory nerve fibers). In most of the cochleas examined after acute exposures in experimental animals or after a lifetime of exposures in humans, the loss of OHCs is usually pervasive. When inner hair cells are missing there is usually secondary degeneration of the afferent fibers that innervated them.

The relation between cochlear blood flow and hearing loss from noise is not well understood, but there is relatively strong evidence that significant hearing losses are usually accompanied by capillary loss in stria vascularis and the spiral ligament.

Gunfire and other short-duration, high-level impulse or impact noises constitute a special hazard to the ear. The high sound pressures associated with impulse noise cause the basilar membrane to be displaced a relatively large distance in a short time, thereby developing large inertial forces that literally rip the cochlea apart. Figure N-9 is a low-power scanning electron micrograph of the cochlea following exposure to synthetic gunfire noise, showing dislocation of the organ of Corti from the basilar membrane. In addition, exposure to high-level impulse noise can lead to ripping of tight cell junctions and ejection of sensory cells from the cuticular plate.

Variability and Susceptibility

Individual variability in susceptibility to NIHL can be impressively large. In a particularly well-controlled epidemiological study of hearing loss in a foundry and forging plant, workers with ostensibly the same exposure to noise developed markedly different hearing losses. Figure N-10 shows that individuals who re-

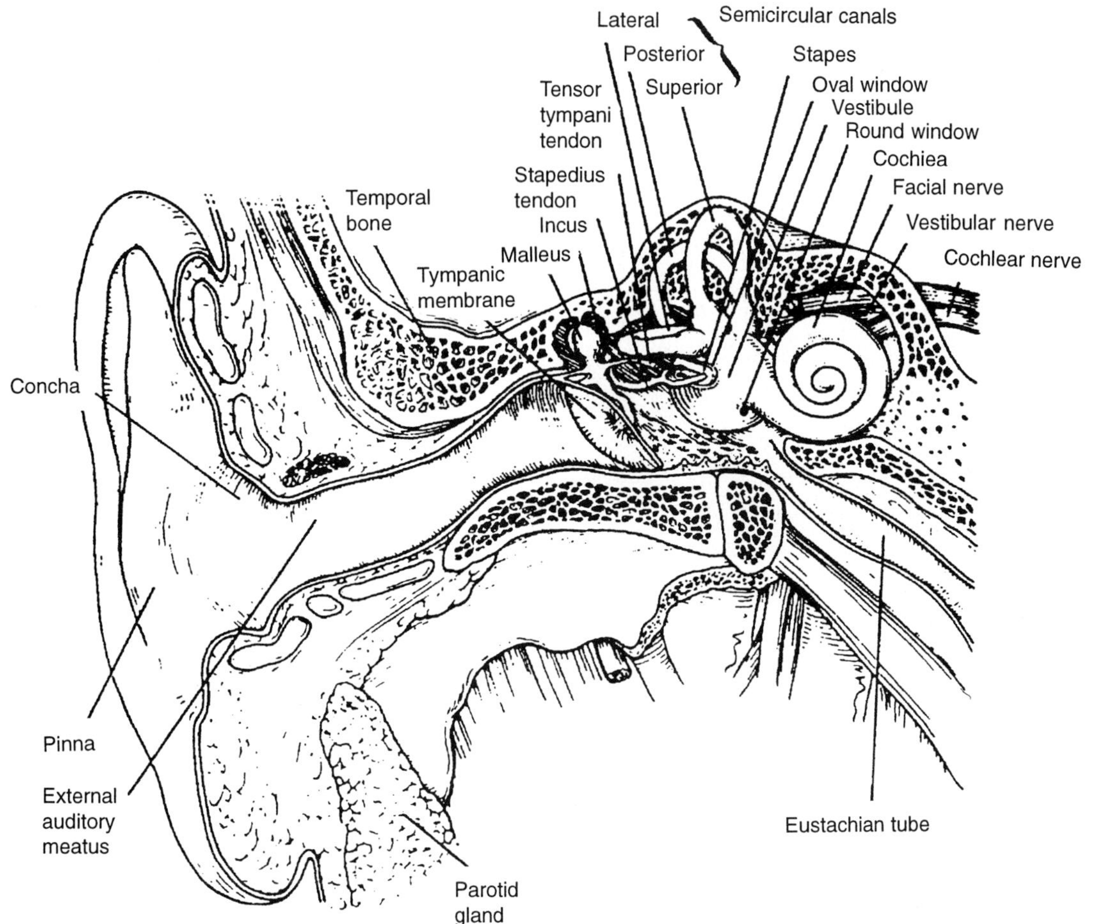

FIGURE N-6. A cross section of the human temporal bone showing the major components of the external, middle, and inner ear.

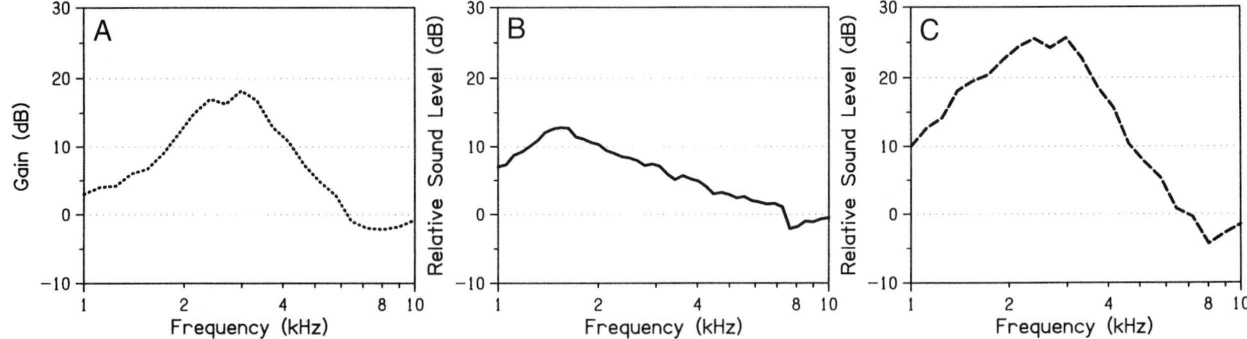

FIGURE N-7. Illustration of how the spectrum of a typical industrial noise is transformed as it passes from the air to the eardrum of a listener. (A) The resonance characteristics of a typical adult external auditory meatus, showing a peak in the gain function between 3 and 4 kHz. The precise shape of the gain function will depend on ear canal length and the angle of sound incidence. (B) The spectrum of a typical industrial noise. (C) Spectrum of the industrial noise as measured at the tympanic membrane, after passing through the external ear.

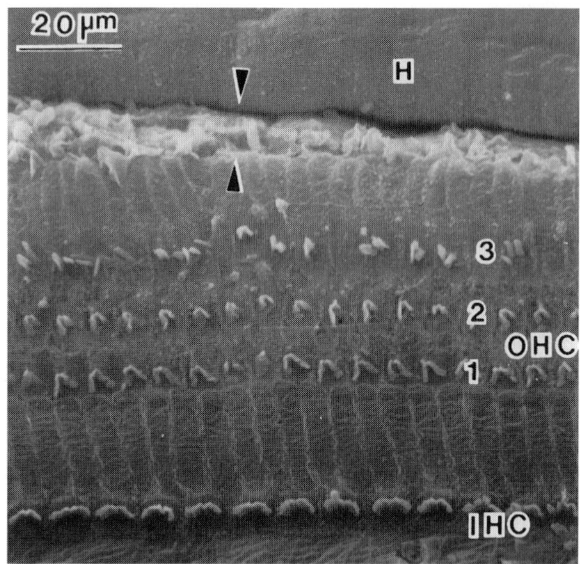

FIGURE N-8. Surface view of chinchilla cochlea showing a number of pathological changes following exposure to noise. Notice the normal orderly arrangement of stereocilia on the outer hair cells has been replaced by stereocilia that are disarrayed or fused. The inner hair cell stereocilia have growths or "blebs."

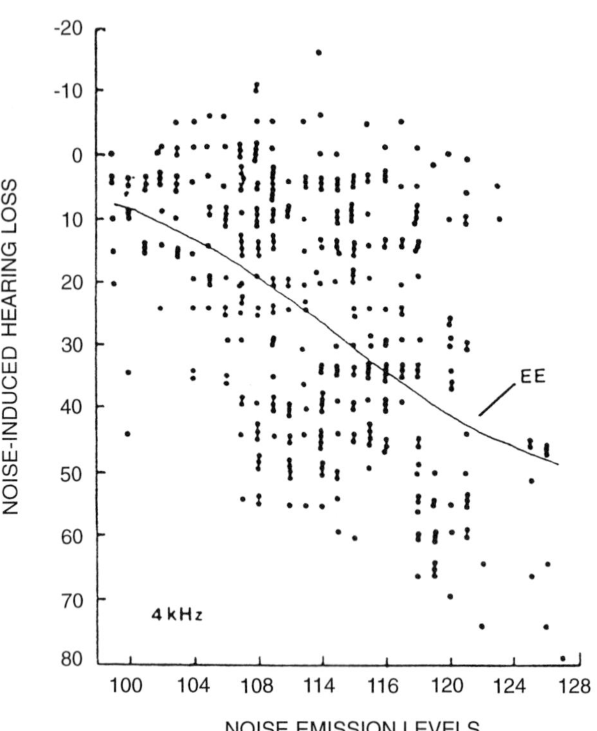

FIGURE N-10. Noise-induced hearing loss as a function of noise emission level. Individual points refer to the hearing level of a worker at 4 kHz. Note that noise emission level is an energy-related measure which reflects both the daily noise level and years of exposure. Solid line is the predicted hearing loss from an equal energy model (reproduced with permission from W. J. Taylor, A. Pearson, A. Mair, and W. Burns, Study of noise and hearing in jute weaving, J. Acoust. Soc. Am. **38**, *113–120, 1965).*

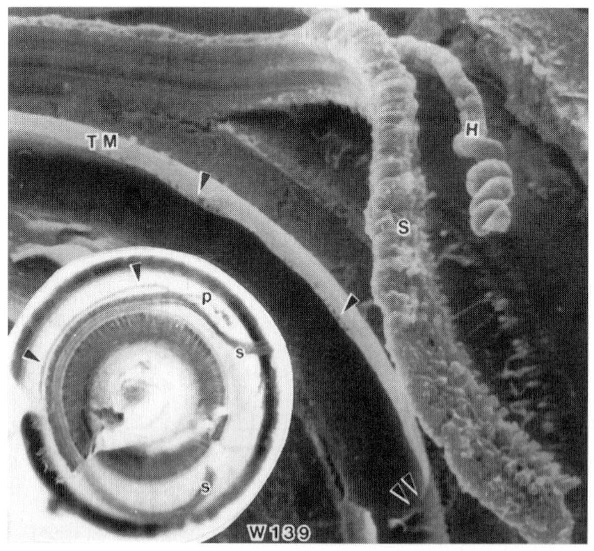

FIGURE N-9. Low-power scanning electron micrograph of the cochlea following exposure to synthetic gunfire noise. Notice that the sensory cells (S) and Hensen cells (H) are ripped from their attachment to the basilar membrane.

ceived the same overall "noise dose" (daily noise power × years of exposure) ranged from having absolutely normal hearing to having 60 dB of hearing loss. Despite careful attention to experimental details, ultimately it is difficult to control for all relevant factors that influence the amount of hearing loss a given individual will develop. Surprisingly, even when subjects are carefully screened and their noise history is known, there is still large intersubject variability in NIHL (see Fig. N-10). The large degree of intersubject variability in the amount of hearing loss caused by exposure to noise highlights the need for developing predictive measures of susceptibility to NIHL.

A number of factors that correlate with susceptibility to NIHL have been identified. For instance, an individual's concentration of melanin can be related to susceptibility, with dark-skinned individuals being more resistant to noise than fair-skinned or blue-eyed individuals.

Research has suggested that melanin plays a role in counteracting the toxic reactions produced by high-level noise exposure. Another factor related to susceptibility is acoustic reflex contraction of the middle ear muscles. Individuals with efficient acoustic reflexes (fast acting, strong contracting, and resistant to adaptation) develop substantially less NIHL than individuals with less effective reflexes. Although factors such as these have been shown to be correlated with susceptibility to NIHL in large-scale studies, there are still no practical means of assessing an individual's susceptibility to NIHL prior to noise exposure.

The high degree of variability seen in industrial survey research may be partially attributable to interactions between continuous noise and other agents, including exposure to impulse/impact noise, ototoxic drugs, and organic solvents.

Interactions between Continuous Noise and Impulse/Impact Noise

One of the more dramatic interactions is the potentiation of NIHL when continuous noise and impulse/impact noise are combined. Laboratory studies have shown that exposures to combinations of impulse and continuous noise can have large traumatic effects even though the effects of the impulse noise or continuous noise alone are minimal. Data from survey studies of industrial noise environments also indicate that continuous/impulse noise interactions in the workplace can be a potent factor influencing hearing loss. For example, two settings with the same average noise level can lead to markedly different degrees of hearing loss if one has a stationary noise and the other exposure is composed of moderate levels of noise with high peak level impulse occurring intermittently. The hypothesis is that background noise renders the ear more susceptible to the impacts.

Interactions between Noise and Ototoxic Drugs

The effects of noise can also be exacerbated when an individual is simultaneously exposed to certain ototoxic drugs. At least five general classes of ototoxic drugs have been identified: (1) aminoglycoside antibiotics (e.g., gentamycin, kanamycin, neomycin, and streptomycin), (2) antineoplastic drugs (e.g., carboplatin and cisplatin), (3) loop diuretics (e.g., furosemide and ethacrynic acid), (4) salicylates (e.g., aspirin), and (5) quinine compounds. Loop diuretics and salicylates typically produce temporary, reversible hearing loss, whereas the other types of drugs cause permanent damage to the auditory system, primarily by destroying sensory hair cells in the cochlea. Currently, there is clear evidence that noise-induced hearing loss can be exacerbated by the aminoglycosides and the antineoplastic agents. When certain doses of aminoglycoside antibiotics are given simultaneously with noise, the resultant hearing loss can be much larger than would be expected by either agent alone or even by the simple addition of effects from the drug and noise. Interactions have also been found between noise and cisplatin, a drug commonly used for treatment of solid and disseminated cancers of the head, neck, and urogenital regions despite its potential nephrotoxic and ototoxic side effects. Research has shown that animals treated with cisplatin are more vulnerable to NIHL than animals exposed to noise alone, even at low cisplatin doses that cause little or no measurable hearing loss alone. Evidence suggests that other ototoxic drugs, such as the loop diuretics and the salicylates (i.e., drugs that produce only temporary reductions of hearing sensitivity), do not interact with noise.

Interactions between Noise and Organic Solvents

Approximately 10 million workers in the United States are regularly exposed to organic solvents in the workplace. Because many of these workers are also exposed to noise, attention is beginning to be paid to ototoxic interactions between solvents and noise. Evidence suggests that in many cases, hearing loss from combined exposure is greater than hearing loss from exposure to either agent alone.

Studies have shown that combined exposures to toluene, one of the most commonly used industrial solvents, and noise results in more severe hearing losses in rats than would be produced by either agent alone. A 20-year longitudinal study of 319 workers exposed to noise or to chemicals and noise at a 10- to 20-dB lower level found a much higher incidence of hearing loss in the workers exposed to both agents than in workers exposed to higher level noise alone. A recent study of Brazilian workers from the printing and paint manufacturing industries revealed a much higher prevalence of "high-frequency" hearing loss in the group exposed to noise and toluene simultaneously than in an unexposed group, a noise-exposed group, or a group exposed to a mixture of solvents. Studies such as these suggest that the risk of developing hearing loss can be increased dramatically when various ototoxic agents are combined with noise.

Presbycusis and NIHL

Determining what percentage of a person's hearing loss is due to industrial noise exposure versus other sources is often important for workers' compensation programs. However, this is obviously a complicated task since so many factors can contribute to an individual's hearing loss. One of the greatest confounding factors in evaluating a worker's NIHL is hearing loss due to biological aging, or presbycusis. Presbycusis often becomes noticeable in middle age and becomes progressively worse with each passing decade of life. Current legal practice calls for simply subtracting some specified amount of hearing loss based on an individual's age (and sex) from the total hearing loss to determine the amount of hearing loss attributable to NIHL (Fig. N-11). This is a questionable approach for at least two reasons. First, there is tremendous variability in hearing loss exhibited by individuals as they age. Second, it is nearly impossible to determine how much age-related hearing loss can be attributed to "pure" biological aging because of the confounding contribution of a lifetime of noise exposure in a society in which noise is pervasive and its effects are insidious. Most of the animal models for presbycusis (i.e., gerbils, rats, and mice) have life spans of only 2–4 years, and studies can be difficult to interpret because the animal models rarely develop the same degree of hearing loss that people develop over 70 or more years of living. Animal studies are instructive, however, in showing that (a) presbycusis can occur even in the absence of significant noise exposure, and (b) even animals that have essentially the same noise exposure history, same diet, and a more restricted genetic pool show a wide range of hearing loss as they age. Of particular interest are studies showing that gerbils raised in a quiet environment all of their lives have hearing levels that range from normal to "flat" 60-dB losses at 3 years of age. The wide range of variability in the amount of presbycusic hearing loss displayed even in the absence of noise exposure raises the issue of whether there is a general, common susceptibility to NIHL and aging or whether the two processes are independent.

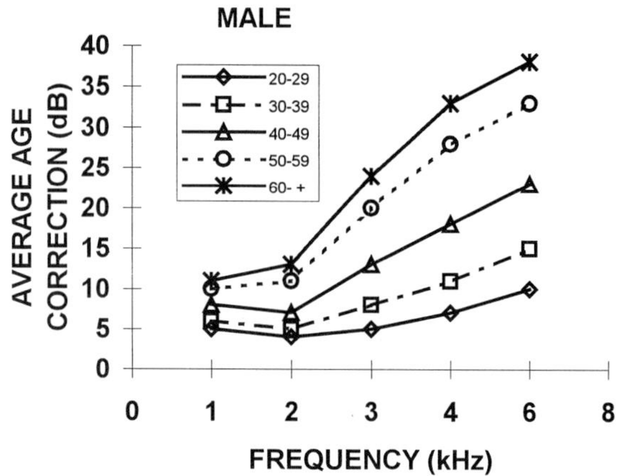

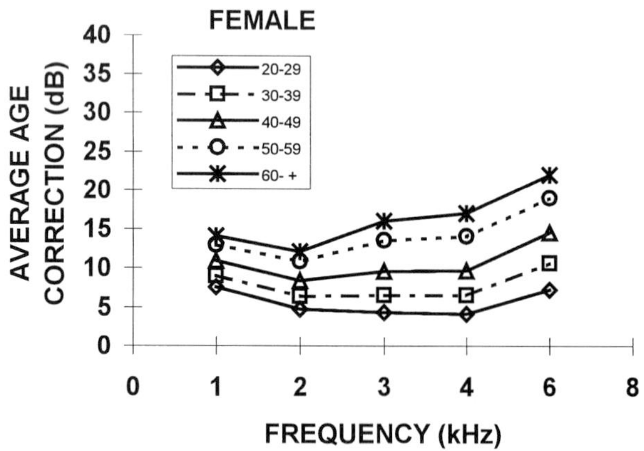

FIGURE N-11. Age correction factors suggested by OSHA for determining hearing loss attributable to noise exposure.

Much remains to be learned about the relationship between NIHL and presbycusis. For instance, does the susceptibility of the auditory system to noise increase (or decrease) as the system ages and develops presbycusis? Conversely, are noise-damaged ears more (or less) susceptible to the biological effects of aging? Is there an additive relationship between NIHL and presbycusis, as some studies have suggested?

Noise Standards

The current regulations governing exposure to noise in the United States date back to the Walsh–Healy Act of 1968. In its present form, the permissible noise exposure levels and durations are listed in Table N-7. The noise legislation requires that people working in environments with noise levels of 85 dBA or greater wear personal protection devices. At higher noise levels, the permissible amount of time a worker can remain in the exposure condition changes by a factor of 2 for each 5-dB increase in noise exposure level.

Several points should be considered when evaluating current legislation. First, the action criterion level of 85 dBA is partly a political decision, which balances protection of workers against costs to employers. Although daily 8-hr exposures to 85 dBA will be safe for most people, a small percentage (approximately 10–15%) of workers will develop hearing loss even at these levels. The noise legislation thus balances protection for the largest fraction of the population versus cumbersome regulations for industry rather than ensuring protection of all exposed workers. Second, the 5-dB trading ratio between exposure level and duration is arbitrary. The International Standards Organization recommends a more conservative 3-dB trading ratio, but putting this criterion into effect would increase costs of compliance for industry. Third, the standards are based on continuous types of noise, thereby overlooking the interaction effects between continuous and impulse noise. As noted earlier, the effects of noise are particularly related to the mix of continuous and impulse noise so that noise exposures with a combination of continuous and impulse noise may produce more hearing loss than either agent alone. Fourth, the effects of noise are also influenced by nonauditory phenomena, such as heat or exposure to industrial solvents and ototoxic drugs, while standards are based on exposure to noise alone. In summary, the current noise standards are based on 30-year-old data and could be rewritten using newer data on the biological effects of noise.

TABLE N-7
Permissible Noise Doses

Noise level (dBA)	*Permissible exposure duration*
85	Action level, hearing protection mandated
90	8 hr/day
95	4 hr/day
100	2 hr/day
105	1 hr/day
110	0.5 hr/day
115	0.25 hr/day

Future Trends

Although noise continues to be an important public health problem, there are several promising advances. First, computer-based technology has improved and it is now possible to actively cancel noise in the environment without interfering with normal communication. Second, pharmacology studies have shown that regulation of the ear's natural defense mechanisms, including heat shock proteins and free radical scavengers, may offer a means of reducing NIHL. Other studies have shown protection from NIHL with injection of drugs such as calcium blockers. Third, there is growing evidence that there may be a genetic predisposition to NIHL. Future studies are needed to clarify these issues and reduce the hazards of noise exposure in both industrial and recreational settings.

Further Reading

Boettcher, F. A., Henderson, D., Gratton, M. A., Danielson, R. W., and Byrne, C. D. (1987). Synergistic interactions of noise and other ototraumatic agents. *Ear Hearing* 8(4), 192–212.

Henderson, D., and Hamernik, R. P. (1995). Biologic bases of noise-induced hearing loss. In *Occupational Medicine: State of the Art Reviews*, Vol. 10, pp. 513–534. Hanley & Belfus, Philadelphia.

Henderson, D., Subramaniam, M., and Boettcher, F. A. (1993). Individual susceptibility to noise-induced hearing loss: An old topic revisited. *Ear Hearing* **14**(3), 152–168.

Rybak, L. P. (1992). Hearing: The effects of chemicals. *Otolaryngol. Head Neck Surg.* **106**, 677–686.

Salvi, R. J., Henderson, D., and Eddins, A. C. (1995). Effects of noise exposure on the auditory system. In *Handbook of Neurotoxicology* (L. W. Chang and R. S. Dyer, Eds.), pp. 907–961. Dekker, New York.

Taylor, W. J., Pearson, A., Mair, A., and Burns, W. (1965). Study of noise and hearing in jute weaving. *J. Acoust. Soc. Am. 38*, 113–120.

—Donald Henderson and Sandra L. McFadden

Related Topics

Occupational Safety and Health Administration
Occupational Toxicology
Sensory Organs

Norbormide

- CAS: 991-42-4
- SYNONYMS: 6-(α-hydroxy-α-2-pyridylbenzyl)-7-(α-2-pyridylbenzylidene)-5-norbor-5-ene-2,3-dicarboximide; McN-1,025; S-6,999; Shoxin; Raticate; ENT 51,76
- CHEMICAL CLASS: Heterocyclic dicarboximide
- CHEMICAL STRUCTURE:

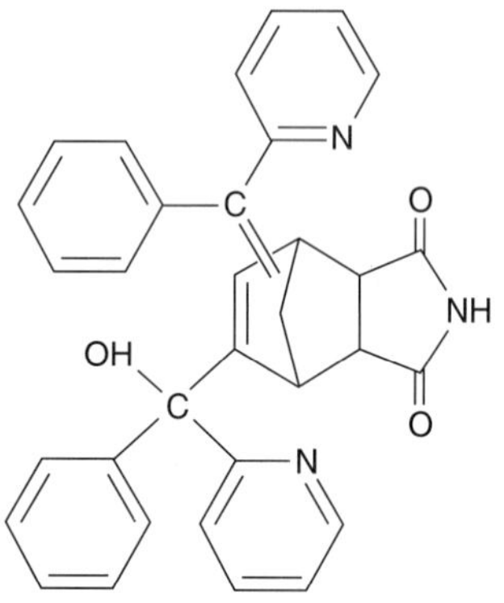

Uses

Norbormide was first introduced in the market in 1964 as a selective rodenticide. This compound is highly specific for rats.

Exposure Pathways

Norbormide can enter the body through oral, dermal, and inhalation exposures.

Mechanism of Toxicity

Norbormide causes an extreme and irreversible peripheral vasoconstriction following both systemic and local administration. This peripheral vasoconstriction subsequently reduces coronary blood flow rate, leading to cardiac arrhythmias, which can lead to death. Interestingly, this vasoconstrictive effect was not observed in other animals even at high doses. Sex- and species-related differences in sensitivity to norbormide may be attributed partially to the differences in metabolism or absorption of this compound. A lethal dose of norbormide in rats (1 g/kg) can elevate the blood glucose level twofold with a decrease in both liver and muscle glycogen. Exposed animals became comatose within 30 min to 2 hr after treatment. The hyperglycemic effect of this compound in rats is considered to be a secondary effect.

Human Toxicity

Human toxicity due to norbormide exposure is highly unlikely because of its specificity for rats. Human volunteers given 20–300 mg showed only a minimal hypotensive effect, which returned to control levels within 2 hr. A dose of 300 mg corresponds to 60 g of the 0.5% bait and 30 g of the 1% bait. Although a hypotensive effect of norbormide was cited as a potential toxic symptom, the maximum reduction in body temperature was found to be 0.7°C following 20–80 mg of norbormide in human volunteers. The hyperglycemic effect could not be demonstrated in humans.

Clinical Management

As mentioned before, human toxicity due to overdose of norbormide is not expected because of its selectivity for rats. The only symptom identified was a mild reduction of systolic blood pressure for a short period of time; therefore, only symptomatic and supportive care have been recommended in cases of norbormide ingestion. However, emesis may be induced in case of recent substantial ingestion of norbormide. Exposed eyes should be washed with tepid water for 15 min. In case of dermal exposure, the contaminated area should be washed with a sufficient amount of soap and water.

Animal Toxicity

Laboratory rats showed difficulties in locomotion and ataxia but no hindleg paralysis after treatment with norbormide. Death occurs within 15 min to 4 hr after struggling, dysnpea, hypothermia, and convulsions. Oral LD_{50} values for Norway rats ranged from 5.3 to 15 mg/kg. Rodents other than rats have considerably higher oral LD_{50} values (e.g., hamster, 140 mg/kg; guinea pigs, 620 mg/kg; mice, 2250 mg/kg). However, no effect was detected with 1000 mg/kg doses of norbormide in dogs, cats, monkey, sheep, pigs, or chickens.

—*Tamal Kumar Chakraborti*

Related Topic

Pesticides

Nutmeg

- SYNONYMS: *Myristica fragrans;* brown slime; mace; madashaunda (narcotic fruit); pala banda; spice of madness
- DESCRIPTION: Nutmeg is the seed of *M. fragrans,* an aromatic evergreen tree.
- CHEMICAL STRUCTURE:

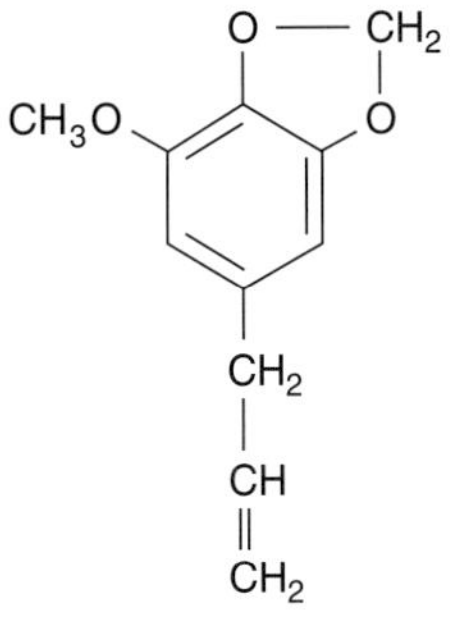

Myristicin

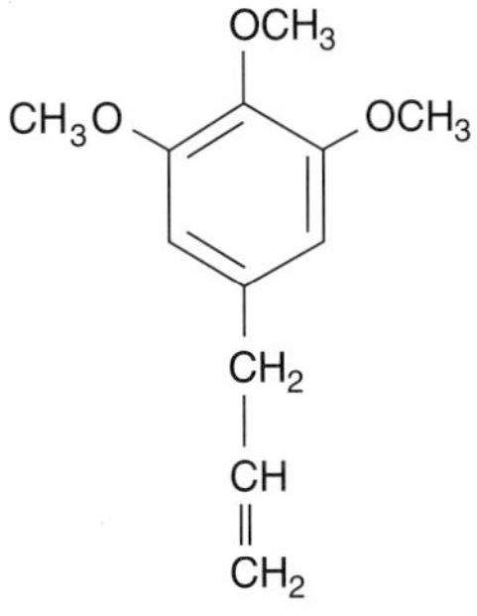

Elemicin

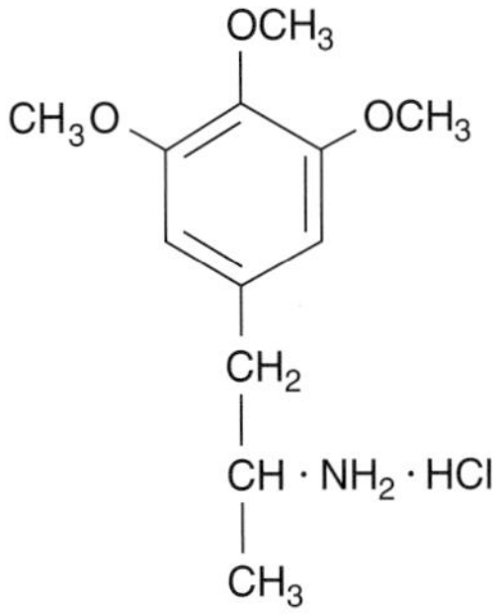

Amphetamine corresponding to elemicin

Uses

Nutmeg is used as a spice, as an herbal remedy, and as a hallucinogen.

Exposure Pathways

Nutmeg is ingested whole, in ground or grated form, or as a slurry of water and powder (brown slime). Nutmeg powder is occasionally sniffed.

Toxicokinetics

The volatile oils in nutmeg consist of allylbenzene derivatives and terpines. Myristicin, elemicin, and safrole comprise 80% of the allylbenzenes. There is some speculation that the myristicin and elemicin may be biotransformed into their amino derivatives; the percentage produced is unknown. Symptoms occur within 3–8 hr, followed by 6–24 hr of alternating periods of stupor and delirium. Recovery usually occurs within 24 hr but may take several days.

Mechanism of Toxicity

A probable metabolite of myristicin is 3-methoxy-4,5 dimethylene dioxamphetamine (MMDA). Elemicin is probably metabolized to 3,4,5-trimethoxy-amphetamine (TMA). MMDA and TMA are both psychoactive compounds related to amphetamine. Other components of the volatile oil, such as eugenol, isoeugenol, safrol, and linalool, are structurally similar to some serotonin agonists and may contribute to the psychological effects. The terpine hydrocarbons are unlikely contributors to the psychomimetic effects but may increase absorption of the allylbenzenes by irritation of the stomach. Nutmeg has weak monoamine oxidase-inhibiting abilities, which may partially account for the cardiovascular symptoms. It also inhibits the synthesis and activity of prostaglandin E_2 in the colon, giving an antidiarrheal effect. In addition, it has anti-inflammatory properties.

Human Toxicity

Nutmeg is abused for its narcotic and hallucinogenic properties. One to three seeds or 5–30 g of the ground nut are used to attain psychogenic effects. One tablespoon of ground nutmeg or one grated nutmeg yields approximately 7 g. A fatality was reported in an 8-year-old who ate two nutmegs. The initial effects are giddiness, tingling, euphoria, and hallucinations that may include distortion of time and space, detachment from reality, sensation of separation from one's limbs, and fear of impending death. This is followed by alternating delirium and extreme drowsiness or stupor. However, there are generally unpleasant side effects of headache, nausea, vomiting, and dizziness. Restlessness, chest and abdominal pain, tremor, and rapid heart rate also occur. The blood pressure may slightly increase, but a marked decrease with cyanosis and shock has been reported. Palpitations, agitation, anxiety, dry mouth, chest tightening, and blurred vision were reported in a pregnant woman in her third trimester who ingested 1 tablespoon of nutmeg. The fetal heartbeat was increased for 12 hr. Levels for myristicin and elemicin are not generally available. Myristicin has been isolated from nutmeg using high-performance liquid chromatography. Other laboratory values have been reported to be normal.

Clinical Management

Treatment should focus on keeping the patient calm while hallucinations are occurring, maintaining blood pressure, and controlling nausea and vomiting. Gastric emptying can be considered if the ingestion was recent. Activated charcoal and a cathartic may be given. Various agents, most commonly diazepam and chlorpromazine, have been used to decrease anxiety and agitation. Parenteral or rectally administered antiemetics may be indicated to treat nausea and vomiting. Nasal oxygen successfully reversed vertigo.

Animal Toxicity

The oral LD_{50} of nutmeg oil is 2600 mg/kg in rats, 4620 mg/kg in mice, and 6000 mg/kg in hamsters.

—Janet E. Bauman

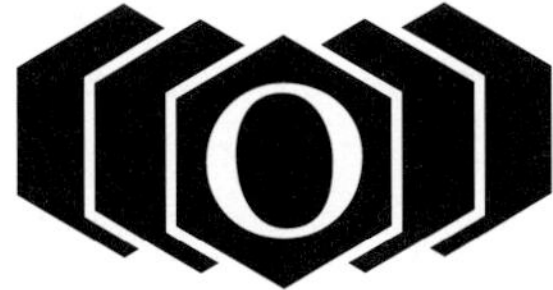

Occupational Safety and Health Act

The Occupational Safety and Health Act (OSHAct) is administered an enforced by the Occupational Safety and Health Administration (OSHA). Both OSHA and OSHAct were created in December 1970, the same month the U.S. EPA was created. Unlike the U.S. EPA, OSHA is essentially an enforcement organization and most of its employees are inspectors who perform thousands of workplace inspections per year; it is a division of the Department of Labor. The OSHAct

- Assures, as far as possible, that all working men or women have risk-free working environments; and
- Imposes on employers the obligation to provide employees with workplaces that are free from recognized health and safety hazards and to maintain compliance with specific OSHA standards.

Many states and territories also have their own plans that have been approved by OSHA and many of these are more stringent than the federal OSHA requirements.

The OSHA hazard Communication Standard, better known as the "Right-to-Know" law, requires that the hazards of all chemicals produced or imported in the United States are evaluated and that employers provide their employees with all appropriate hazard information. This involves providing employees with hazard communication/training programs and access to material safety data sheets (MSDSs) and written records. OSHA considers the MSDS the primary vehicle for transmitting detailed hazard information to downstream employers and employees.

Chemical manufacturers and importers must make a "hazard determination" of the chemicals with which they are involved. This involves an assessment of the physicochemical properties of a material (e.g., flammability, explosivity, corrosivity, and reactivity) as well as potential acute and chronic toxicity. However, manufacturers and exporters are not required to conduct additional testing. Typically, the hazard determination is made on the basis of existing company data or information from the published scientific literature.

Worker exposure to chemicals in the workplace is regulated with reference to permissible exposure limits (PELs) that are maximum allowable exposure limits or a maximum time-weighted average limit over an 8-hr working day. These are complemented by short-term exposure limits. In march 1989, OSHA reduced the PELs for many substances and set new ones for substances previously not regulated; OSHA is still in the process of developing permanent health-based workplace standards. Many of the standards are based on recommendations made in criteria documents prepared by NIOSH, although OSHA has its own standards office. Another listing of exposure limits are the TLVs recommended by ACGIH. The standards recommended by OSHA, NIOSH, and ACGIH often differ from each other and are typically quite controversial. As a result, they frequently become mired in hearings and in the courts.

—Chris F. Wilkinson

Related Topics

American Conference of Governmental Industrial Hygienists
Medical Surveillance
National Institute of Occupational Safety and Health
Occupational Safety and Health Administration
Occupational Toxicology
Permissible Exposure Limit
Short-Term Exposure Limit
Threshold Limit Values

Occupational Safety and Health Administration

With the passage of the Occupational Safety and Health Act (OSHAct) of 1970 (P.L. 91-596), the U.S. Congress created the Occupational Safety and Health Administration (OSHA) in 1971 to "assure so far as possible every working man and woman in the Nation safe and healthful working conditions."

This mandate makes OSHA responsible for saving lives, preventing injuries and illnesses, and protecting the health and safety of American workers.

In accomplishing this goal, OSHA issues and enforces regulations that cover more than 6 million workplaces and about 93 million workers in industries such as manufacturing, construction, longshoring, agriculture, law and medicine, organized labor, and private education.

The OSHAct also encourages states to develop and operate their own safety and health plans. These plans, approved under Section 18(b) of the act, must adopt standards and enforce requirements that are at least as effective as federal requirements.

In addition, OSHA has voluntary programs, such as consultation and Voluntary Protection Programs, to assist employers in developing safety and health programs to improve worker protection in their workplaces. OSHA's Training Institute in Des Plaines, Illinois, offers a broad range of safety and health training for employers and employees. The institute courses cover areas such as industries and expanded health standards. OSHA also provides funds to nonprofit organizations to conduct workplace training and education in subjects in which OSHA believes there is a current lack of workplace training.

For more information about OSHA, visit OSHA's web site at http://www.osha.gov or contact OSHA's Office of Information and Consumer Affairs at (202) 219-8615 or the OSHA Publications Office at (202) 219-4667. For information on training courses, call the OSHA Training Institute at (847) 297-4913 or write to Occupational Safety and Health Administration, Washington, DC, 20210.

—Harihara M. Mehendale

Related Topics

Information Resources in Toxicology
Medical Surveillance
Occupational Safety and Health Act
Occupational Toxicology
Permissible Exposure Limit
Short-Term Exposure Limit

Occupational Toxicology

Introduction

The aim of occupational toxicology is to prevent hazardous exposures in the workplace. Historically, occupational studies have provided some of the strongest evidence that exposure to xenobiotics (chemicals or other agents that are foreign to the body) in the environment can cause disease in humans. As early as 370 BC, Hippocrates described symptoms of lead poisoning in a metal worker. In 1775, Sir Percival Pott recognized that soot played a role in the high rate of scrotal cancer among chimney sweeps. In 1977, case studies on pesticide workers indicated that exposure to dibromochloropropane could cause infertility and sterility in men. Such observations have sparked interest in investigating how xenobiotics injure or disrupt biological systems. In turn, results from toxicological studies are used to develop methods for assessing workplace exposures and to establish occupational exposure limits.

Occupational toxicology draws from the same framework as other disciplines in toxicology (Fig. O-1). This framework outlines the major physiological steps that can influence the dose–response for a xenobiotic. A dose can be defined as the amount of a xenobiotic a worker is exposed to in an occupational setting, and a response is some overt physiological effect, such as organ damage. The growing field of molecular toxicology aims to refine the characterization of the dose–response, such that the dose reflects the amount of the xenobiotic or active metabolite that reaches a critical target in the body, and the response is an early, subtle change in cells or components of cells that precedes clinical disease.

Setting occupational exposure guidelines involves risk assessment—the evaluation of toxicological and

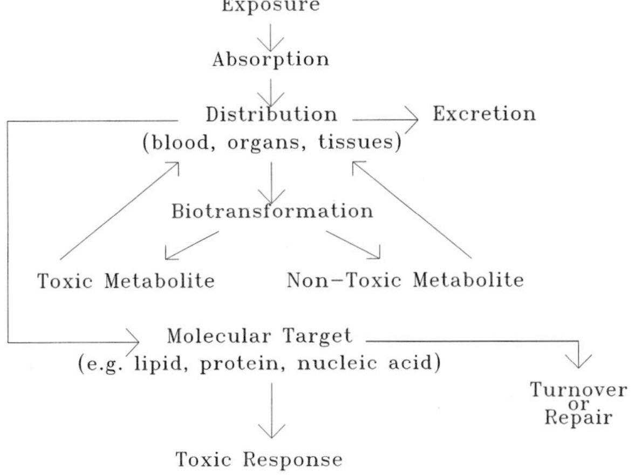

FIGURE O-1. Toxicology framework.

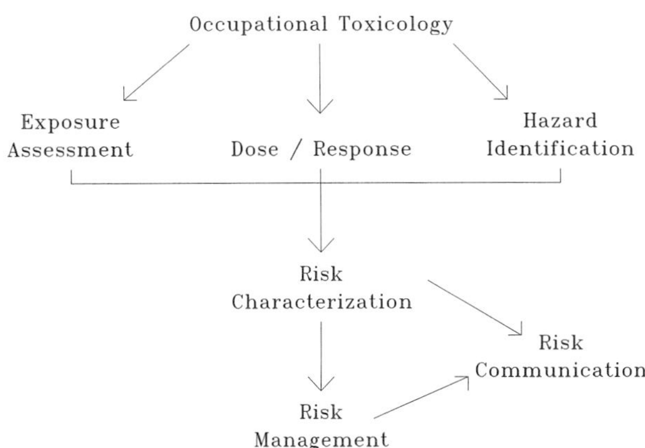

FIGURE O-2. Occupational toxicology and risk assessment.

exposure data to determine the health risks presented by using xenobiotics in the workplace. The toxicological characterization of xenobiotics contributes to the risk assessment process by providing information for the dose–response and hazard identification steps (Fig. O-2). Hazard identification describes the types of physiological effects a xenobiotic can cause—for example, reproductive toxicity, cancer, respiratory problems, or allergic reactions. Toxicology may also play an increasingly important role in exposure assessment as advances in molecular toxicology promise to improve the measurement of the dose of a xenobiotic that is absorbed by the body or that hits a critical target tissue. Risk characterization synthesizes the information gathered in the dose–response, hazard identification, and exposure assessment steps for use in risk management decisions. Risk management strategies can range from recommending the use of protective equipment to setting occupational exposure limits, or possibly to eliminating a xenobiotic from the workplace. Finally, workers, management, and other policymakers are recognizing that making informed decisions regarding worker health requires a clear understanding of health risk information.

Use of Toxicological Data

Although epidemiological data provide the strongest evidence of how chemicals affect human health, occupational exposure limits and other preventative measures cannot be based on these types of data alone. The number of chemicals to which workers are exposed far exceeds the number of solid epidemiological studies. Therefore, many occupational health standards and protective health measures must be based on data from animal studies. Consequently, one of the major challenges that faces an occupational toxicologist is how to interpret the results observed in animals for application to humans.

Occupational toxicology relies on information from both classic toxicology studies and investigations into the molecular mechanisms of xenobiotics. Classic toxicology studies involve exposing groups of animals to various doses of a xenobiotic and observing the response. These are the types of toxicology studies that are most often used to develop exposure guidelines. Very simply, toxicologists use these studies to determine what dose presents little or no risk of causing a harmful effect in humans. Classic toxicology studies also provide information on what types of effects the xenobiotic can cause, such as cancer, neurotoxicity, or organ damage.

Molecular toxicology investigates the biochemical steps that lead to the physiological response observed in the classic studies. Identifying the critical molecules and cellular processes involved in toxicity can help determine whether effects seen in animals are likely to occur in humans. For example, studies suggest that the protein α-2u-globulin plays a key role in the induction of kidney tumors by *d*-limonene. This protein is synthesized in large quantities by adult male rats, but not by humans, suggesting that although *d*-limonene causes kidney tumors in male rats, it may not cause the same effect in humans. Characterizing the molecular target of a xenobiotic can also provide clues for the prevention of toxicity or perhaps aid in developing therapies or antidotes for toxic effects. For example, neurotoxic organophosphate insecticides inactivate the enzyme acetylcholinesterase. Pralidoxime acts as an antidote for this type of pesticide poisoning by reactivating this enzyme. Finally, molecular toxicology can help identify biological markers, such as xenobiotics bound to DNA or proteins, or altered or unusual macromolecules, which can be used to indicate exposure or preclinical toxic effects.

Exposure

When choosing a study for applications in occupational toxicology, it is important that the exposure protocol be relevant to the exposure scenario in the workplace. The route, duration, and frequency of exposure can have a significant effect on the toxicity of a xenobiotic agent.

The route of exposure determines both the initial physiological barrier faced by the xenobiotic and its initial metabolic fate. Two of the primary defense mechanisms against xenobiotics are barriers, such as skin and membranes, and the biotransformation or breakdown of toxic compounds to nontoxic products. Xenobiotics must elude these defense mechanisms in order to reach the target tissue and cause damage.

Physiological barriers, such as the gastrointestinal tract, respiratory tract, or skin, determine the amount and the rate of absorption of specific xenobiotics into the body. Some xenobiotics do act directly at the site of exposure. For example, epoxy resins can cause allergic contact dermatitis, and ultraviolet light can cause skin cancer. Other xenobiotics damage tissues that are distant from the site of exposure. For example, many solvents that are inhaled, such as trichloroethylene and perchloroethylene, cause liver damage. These types of xenobiotics reach their targets by being absorbed into the circulatory system.

The toxicological effects observed due to exposure from one route cannot necessarily be used to predict the toxicological effects that would result from exposure via another route. For example, inorganic lead is almost completely absorbed through the lower respiratory tract but does not easily penetrate the skin. Ease of absorption through a particular physiological barrier depends on both the physical and chemical characteristics of xenobiotics. In contrast to inorganic lead, organic lead, such as tetraethyl lead, is readily absorbed through the skin. Therefore, the results from a dermal toxicology study on inorganic lead cannot directly predict the dose response for dermal exposure to organic lead. Likewise, reducing dermal exposure to organic lead would require stricter protective measures than that for inorganic lead.

In addition to presenting the initial physiological barrier to a xenobiotic, the route of exposure also determines the initial metabolic fate of the agent. The liver, which contains the highest concentration of enzymes involved in biotransformation, is the primary site for detoxification. In addition, some xenobiotics can be broken down by the acid pH of the stomach or enzymes present in the gastrointestinal tract. Chemicals that enter the body orally will meet both of these defense systems before they are absorbed into the general circulatory system. By contrast, xenobiotics that are absorbed through the respiratory tract or through the skin are transported to the general circulatory system without first passing through the liver. Therefore, they may reach a target tissue before meeting the detoxifying enzymes in the liver. Injection can be a particularly dangerous route of exposure since the agents bypass all of the barrier properties of the skin and directly enter the bloodstream.

The duration and frequency of exposure can also influence the physiological effect of xenobiotics. The health effects following a short-term, high-dose (acute) exposure to a xenobiotic can differ dramatically from the effects of a long-term, low-dose (chronic) exposure. For example, acute inhalation exposure to vinyl chloride causes respiratory tract irritation, lethargy, and headache. Chronic exposure to vinyl chloride can cause hepatic angiosarcoma. Whereas short-term, low-dose exposure to a specific xenobiotic may not be toxic, prolonged or frequent exposure to the same xenobiotic may deplete detoxifying or repair systems and therefore result in the accumulation of damaged tissue. Toxicologists interpret short-term animal studies with care because many xenobiotics have latent effects, such that the toxic response is not detected until long after the time of exposure. This also holds true for the interpretation of epidemiological data. For example, latency is well established for carcinogens. Tumors may not appear in animals for weeks or months, and cancer may not appear in humans until decades after exposure. Other xenobiotics, such as neurotoxins, may also have latent effects.

Exposure scenarios differ depending on the type of occupation and the physical workplace. Inhalation is a common industrial route of exposure. Some xenobiotics can be absorbed through the eyes. Many types of work involve dermal exposure to xenobiotics. Medical personnel are at risk of being exposed to a variety of agents through injection. To ensure worker safety, all of the possible pathways of exposure should be examined.

Factors That Affect Toxicity

Both environmental factors and an individual's characteristics can affect the toxicity of a given xenobiotic. For example, exposure to other xenobiotics, diet, age, sex, and genetics can alter the toxicity of a given xenobiotic, in part, by modulating its biotransformation. Biotransformation can detoxify xenobiotics, but this process can also bioactivate xenobiotics—that is, transform a relatively benign parent compound into a more toxic intermediate that can go on to interact with a target and cause damage. Ultimately, the effect of environmental agents on endogenous macromolecules, such as hormones and the enzymes and cofactors involved in biotransformation, determines the fate of a xenobiotic.

In general, biotransformation reactions convert lipophilic (fat-soluble) xenobiotics into compounds that are hydrophilic (water soluble). As a result, lipophilic xenobiotics can be excreted from the body instead of accumulating or damaging a target tissue. The biotransformation process is broadly divided into phase I and phase II reactions. Phase I reactions prime xenobiotics for phase II reactions by adding or exposing a functional group (e.g., -OH, -SH, $-NH_2$, or -COOH). Phase II reactions take advantage of the functional group produced by the phase I reactions and add a water-soluble molecule to the xenobiotic, making it even more hydrophilic and therefore more readily excreted. Xenobiotics that already have a functional group can also undergo phase II reactions. Biotransformation requires a variety of enzymes and a set of endogenous cofactors. Biotransformation takes place primarily in the liver, which contains a very high level of the enzymes involved in phase I and phase II reactions. Although biotransformation also takes place in other organs, such as the lung, stomach, intestine, skin, and kidneys, the liver generally has a wider variety of metabolic enzymes than the other tissues and therefore can modify a broader range of compounds.

Phase I reactions are primarily catalyzed by a family of enzymes called cytochrome P450s. Like the immune system, which has evolved to combat a broad range of foreign antigens, the cytochrome P450 system has evolved to modify remarkably diverse classes of xenobiotics. Specific isoenzymes of cytochrome P450 catalyze reactions involving particular classes of xenobiotics. For example, cytochrome P4501A1 catalyzes the hydroxylation of benzo[*a*]pyrene, and cytochrome P4502A6 catalyzes the oxidation of butadiene and nicotine.

Phase II reactions generally require a transferase type of enzyme and an endogenous cofactor to add a water-soluble molecule to a xenobiotic. Phase II reactions are also called conjugation reactions, and the modified products of these reactions are called conjugates. Like the cytochrome P450s, specific transferase enzymes and their associated cofactors tend to catalyze conjugation reactions with particular structural classes of compounds. For example, the enzyme UDP-glucuronosyl transferase, along with the cofactor UDP glucuronic acid, catalyzes the formation of glucuronide conjugates of aliphatic or aromatic alcohols, carboxylic acid, sulfhydryl compounds, and amines. Glutathione *S*-transferases use the cofactor glutathione to catalyze the formation of conjugates with a number of reactive intermediates, including epoxides.

Some xenobiotics can undergo competing biotransformation reactions. The extent to which a given xenobiotic will be detoxified or bioactivated depends, in part, on the physiological levels of specific enzymes and cofactors required for each biotransformation pathway. For example, nutritional status, sex, age, genetics, and the presence of previous exposure to other xenobiotics can influence the toxicological fate of xenobiotics by affecting enzyme levels or cofactor pools. If toxicologists understand how these factors modulate toxicity, they can more accurately determine if the results of animal studies can be extrapolated to humans. In addition, this information may be used to identify individuals who might be particularly sensitive to certain types of exposures.

One xenobiotic can affect the toxicity of another by either increasing enzyme activity or depleting essential cofactors. Many of the enzymes involved in biotransformation reactions are inducible, such that certain compounds can cause an increase in the levels of specific isoenzymes. An increase in the level of an isoenzyme usually results in an increase in the rate of the specific reaction catalyzed by that isoenzyme. Some xenobiotics induce the expression of enzymes that catalyze their own biotransformation. For example, polycyclic aromatic hydrocarbons induce the expression of an isoenzyme of cytochrome P450 that catalyzes the hydroxylation of benzo[*a*]pyrene, and ethanol induces the expression of an isoenzyme that catalyzes the oxidation of ethanol. Xenobiotics can also induce enzymes that catalyze the biotransformation of other compounds. For example, pretreatment of rats with 3-methylcolanthrene increases the biotransformation of aniline. Common inducers of cytochrome P450s include 2,3,7,8-tetrachlorodibenzo-*p*-dioxin (TCDD), halogenated pesticides, such as DDT, and polychlorinated biphenyls. Natural substances in the diet can also induce some of the enzymes involved in biotransformation, as can steroid hormones. Some of the enzymes involved in phase II reactions are also inducible. For example, 3-methylcholanthrene increases the expression of glutathione-*S*-transferases. Specific isoenzymes of glucuronosyltransferases are also inducible. Finally, an inadequate supply of cofactors can limit phase II reactions. Exposure to xenobiotics can deplete cofactor pools. For example, exposure to high doses of acetaminophen can deplete the supply of phase II cofactors sulfate and glutathione. Nutritional status may also affect cofactor pools.

Because many xenobiotics can modulate biotransformation pathways, it is difficult to predict the health effects or dose response that would result from exposure to multiple xenobiotics. Mixtures of xenobiotics can cause an additive response, where the mixture acts like one xenobiotic of a dose equal to the sum of the doses of the individual xenobiotics. Xenobiotics can also act synergistically; that is, cause a response that is greater than additive. The actions of different compounds may also be antagonistic such that the response is less than additive. Finally, the components of a mixture may act independently, resulting in no detectable change in response. Few xenobiotics have been tested extensively enough to determine how they might interact with other compounds. Instead, most toxicological studies investigate exposures to a single compound. Where studies on mixtures do exist, they often investigate the interaction of only two compounds. The biological response to two compounds could be altered by the presence of a third. The problem grows more complex as the number of xenobiotics increases. Finally, the type of interaction may depend on the doses of the specific components of a mixture. Clearly, there is no simple formula for accurately predicting the health risk from exposure to mixtures.

Nevertheless, workers are often exposed to more than one xenobiotic. The ACGIH has developed exposure limits for airborne substances called Threshold Limit Values (TLVs). To estimate the TLV for a mixture, the ACGIH recommends using a model based on the assumption that when xenobiotics "act upon the same organ system . . . [i]n the absence of information to the contrary, the effects of the different hazards should be considered as additive" (ACGIH, 1996). The U.S. EPA recommends using the same model in its risk assessment guidelines for mixtures. This model generates a hazard index (HI) that indicates whether a mixture has exceeded an exposure guideline:

$$HI = C_1/T_1 + C_2/T_2 + \ldots + C_x/T_x$$

C_x = atmospheric concentration of the xth (e.g., first, second) xenobiotic

T_x = Threshold Limit Value for the xth xenobiotic

A hazard index >1 indicates that the mixture exceeds the TLV. A separate hazard index is calculated for each set of xenobiotics in a mixture that cause the same type of toxicological effect. For example, a hazard index would be calculated for all liver toxicants in the mixture. A separate hazard index would be calculated for xenobiotics that cause kidney damage, etc. Further refinement of the additivity model or development of an alternative model will require more extensive research.

The ACGIH does recognize that some xenobiotics may act synergistically. For example, exposure to asbestos and cigarette smoking are synergistic for the induction of lung cancer. The ACGIH also recognizes that compounds absorbed through different routes of exposure can act synergistically. For example, drinking alcohol can affect the toxicity of a solvent like trichloroethylene that is inhaled. With regard to possible synergistic interactions, the ACGIH maintains that "[s]uch cases at present must be determined individually" (ACGIH, 1996).

The level and activity of specific enzymes involved in biotransformation can differ depending on the species, strain, age, and sex of the test animal. For example, cats cannot carry out glucuronidation reactions, newborn rats have relatively low cytochrome P450 activity, and male rats are more sensitive to carbon tetrachloride toxicity than female rats. These differences are important to consider when interpreting the results from toxicological studies. The observation that age, sex, and genetics can significantly influence biotransformation reactions in animals raises the question of whether these types of characteristics also affect the biotransformation capacity of humans.

The field of pharmacogenetics focuses on the genetic basis for differences in xenobiotic metabolism. This field has grown out of an interest in identifying individuals who may be particularly sensitive to certain types of drugs or environmental exposures. For example, sensitivity to certain compounds may differ as much as 200-fold among individuals. Individual differences in xenobiotic metabolism result from polymorphisms among the population. That is, some members of the population express different forms of enzymes involved in biotransformation. While these polymorphisms have largely been characterized in terms of drug metabolism, these differences also have implications for exposures to other types of xenobiotics.

One common polymorphism in the United States is for *N*-acetyltransferase, an enzyme involved in phase II reactions. *N*-acetyltransferase catalyzes the acetylation of aromatic amines and hydrazines, and other classes of xenobiotics. Approximately 50% of people in the United States are characterized as "slow acetylators" because they have relatively low *N*-acetytransferase activity. Consequently, slow acetylators are more sensitive to the toxic effects of certain types of drugs, including sulfa drugs. In addition, a study of workers exposed to benzidine in the dye industry suggests a link between the "slow" acetylator phenotype and the development of bladder cancer.

Polymorphisms also exist for specific isoenzymes of cytochrome P450. For example, there is a polymorphism within the human population for a cytochrome P450 isoenzyme that catalyzes the 4-hydroxylation of the drug debrisoquine. "Extensive metabolizers" hydroxylate this drug 10–200 times faster than "poor metabolizers." Poor metabolizers express much less of the isoenzyme involved in this reaction than extensive metabolizers. This polymorphism also appears to affect the metabolism of environmental agents. For example, there appears to be an association between the poor metabolizer phenotype and Parkinson's disease. By contrast, the extensive metabolizer phenotype may be correlated with an increased risk of developing cancer.

Although there is growing interest in developing simple tests for these and other types of polymorphisms in biotransformation, the use of genetic information to identify sensitive individuals raises difficult policy questions. Currently, TLVs are not developed to protect the most sensitive members of the work force. Subpopulations with certain polymorphisms might be sensitive to a xenobiotic at concentrations at or below the TLV. Some occupational medicine specialists question whether the identification of susceptible individuals could result in job discrimination. Alternatively, this information could be used to recommend additional protective measures for sensitive workers.

Male and female animals can have dramatically different responses to certain xenobiotics. For example, TCDD induces liver tumors in female rats but not in male rats. By contrast, chloroform is a more potent kidney toxin in male mice than in female mice. Female rats are more sensitive to the organophosphate insecticide parathion than male rats. Castration increases the sensitivity of the male rats to parathion. In addition to their role in xenobiotic biotransformation, cytochrome P450s are also involved in the biodegradation and synthesis of endogenous compounds, including fatty acids, prostaglandins, and steroid hormones. Therefore, it should not be surprising that hormones can regulate the activity of specific cytochrome P450 isoenzymes. The question as to what extent men and women differ in their responses to xenobiotic agents is still under investigation. The composition of the work force has changed dramatically in the past three decades, with an increasing number of women holding positions that traditionally had been held by men. Therefore, it may be important to consider possible sex-specific differences in toxic responses if results from occupational studies of male workers or other epidemiological data on men are used to set occupational standards that are applied to both men and women.

Biomonitoring: Molecular Targets

One aim of occupational toxicology is to improve exposure assessment. The field of molecular toxicology provides information on the types of molecules and macromolecules that can serve as indicators of exposure. Whereas classic toxicology studies usually examine gross effects, like changes in body weight, organ damage, or tumor development, molecular toxicology investigates the biochemical mechanism of action of xenobiotics. In other words, molecular toxicology investigates the molecular or cellular events that eventually lead to the gross effects observed in classic toxicology studies. The results from molecular toxicology studies can be used to develop biological markers, also called biomarkers. Biomarkers are generally defined as "cellular, biochemical or molecular alterations" that can be measured in "biological media such as human tissues, cells, or fluids." Biomarkers can be applied in occupational settings to measure exposure to xenobiotic agents and to detect an early response that could lead to toxic injury or disease.

The primary event in toxicology is exposure to the xenobiotic. Estimating exposure usually requires measuring the amount of the xenobiotic in the air, water, dust, or other media. These types of measurements may be technically difficult or expensive to do. In addition, concentrations of xenobiotics can vary depending on time and location. Therefore, these measurements may not give an accurate estimate of past exposures. Furthermore, monitoring the levels of xenobiotics in the workplace does not necessarily indicate how much of the xenobiotic has been absorbed into the body or how much reaches the target tissue. One potential use of biomarkers in occupational toxicology is to refine exposure assessment. Common types of biomarkers include parent compounds or metabolites that can be measured in urine or exhaled breath, and metals that can be measured in hair. Development of other types of biomarkers relies on the identification of a molecular target. For example, lead decreases ferrochelatase activity, an enzyme important in heme biosynthesis. As a result, some red blood cells contain zinc-protoporphyrin instead of hemoglobin. Therefore, zinc-protoporphyrin levels in erythrocytes are used as a biomarker of lead exposure. Likewise, since organophosphate and carbamate pesticides inhibit acetylcholinesterase, measurement of inhibition of choline esterase activity in the blood has been used as a biomarker of exposure to these pesticides. Some xenobiotic agents bind directly to DNA or to proteins. For example, benzo[*a*]pyrene forms DNA adducts and ethylene oxide forms protein adducts. Researchers continue to investigate whether measurement of DNA adducts or protein adducts in easily accessible samples, such as blood, can accurately reflect the interaction of xenobiotics with critical toxicological target tissues such as the lung.

Biomarkers can also be used to detect an early biological response to a xenobiotic agent that precedes serious damage or disease. Examples of precursory responses include mutations in critical genes, changes in hormonal status, and altered gene expression. For example, substantial evidence indicates that carcinogenesis involves the conversion of protooncogenes (normal genes, many of which code for proteins critical for regulating cellular growth control) into oncogenes—genes that can transform normal cells into cancerous cells. Some xenobiotics can cause mutations that convert protooncogenes into oncogenes. These mutations can result in the overproduction of a protein or in the expression of an altered protein, also called an oncogene product. Brandt-Rauf has proposed that oncogene products detected in the urine or serum of workers may serve as biomarkers of an early, preclinical response to carcinogen exposure and perhaps indicate if workers are at increased risk for developing cancer.

A number of parameters must be worked out in order to validate the use of biomarkers. If a biomarker is used to assess exposure, it is important to determine how long the biomarker persists following exposure. Likewise, the time interval between exposure and biomarker appearance should be determined. In addition, biomarkers often cannot be measured in the target tissue, such as lung, because the tissue is not easily accessible for sampling. Instead, the biomarker is measured in a surrogate tissue, such as red blood cells. If this is the case, it should be established that the persistence and levels of the biomarker in the surrogate tissue reflect those of the target tissue.

Regulation

The U.S. Congress passed the Occupational Safety and Health Act in 1970. This act created the Occupational Safety and Health Administration (OSHA) in the federal Department of Labor to establish and enforce safety standards for the workplace. OSHA standards are called permissible exposure limits (PELs). Many PELs have been adopted from ACGIH TLVs. TLVs are generally defined as air concentrations of chemicals that most workers can be exposed to for an 8-hr workday, 40 hr per week for a working lifetime without suffering adverse effects. TLVs are not guaranteed as safe exposure levels for the entire population. Employers may also institute voluntary exposure limits either because an OSHA standard has not been promulgated for a xenobiotic of concern or because they want to apply an exposure limit that is more protective than either the PEL or TLV.

Occupational exposure limits are not always based on toxicology alone. The way toxicological information is interpreted for the development of occupational policy can depend on economics, technology, and the sociopolitical climate. The history of occupational policies that apply specifically to women illustrates the complex meshing of toxicology and social factors in the development of occupational policy. Although some sex-specific measures were progressive and eventually led to greater occupational safety for both men and women, it has also been argued that other sex-specific measures were instituted to restrict the role of women in the workplace, and that the intent of the policies depended, in part, on whether women were considered a dispensable part of the work force.

For example, in the late nineteenth century, factory inspectors in England recognized lead poisoning as one of the most widespread industrial diseases. In 1882, the Chief Inspector of Factories, Alexander Redgrave, submitted a report that lead to the Factories (Prevention of Lead Poisoning) Act, 1883. In contrast to the Consolidating Act of 1878, which excluded children and young people from working in the white lead industry, Redgrave specifically advised against banning women from this work. He apparently recognized the economic role of women in industrial society and realized that if women lost their jobs, they would have a difficult time finding other employment. Instead of banning women from the lead industry, he recommended further protective measures that would improve working conditions. Approximately a century later in the United States, new discoveries in the toxicology of lead and a changing work force led to the implementation of just the sort of policy that Redgrave sought to avoid.

The 1970s saw an influx of women entering the United States work force. Growing numbers of women began occupying industrial positions that had been traditionally held by men, including positions in companies that manufactured lead batteries. At the same time, there was growing concern that exposure to levels of lead once considered safe could be harmful. For example, toxicological and epidemiological studies suggested that lead was not only a neurotoxin but also a reproductive toxin. As a result of both the influx of women into "nontraditional" jobs and the toxicological data on lead, some companies instituted so-called fetal protection policies. In contrast to Redgrave's recommendations a century earlier, these policies excluded fertile women from the workplace, regardless of age or intent to have children, rather than institute additional measures to lower exposure to lead. Although toxicological and epidemiological studies also indicated that lead was a reproductive toxin in men, the fetal protection policies did not apply to fertile male employees. Employees from a number of companies sued, and in 1989 the Supreme Court banned fetal protection policies on the grounds that they constitute discrimination. Although OSHA has not lowered the PEL for lead, the lead standard was amended in 1991 to include the warning that "Chronic overexposure to lead impairs the reproductive systems of both men and women."

Clearly, policymakers develop workplace standards or institute protective measures by considering health risk data along with economics, available technology, and the sociopolitical climate. The role of occupational toxicology in the development of sound and equitable safety measures is to provide the most accurate interpretation of toxicological and epidemiological data possible.

Further Reading

Craft, B. F. (1992). Occupational and environmental health standards. In *Occupational and Environmental Medicine* (W. N. Rom, Ed.), 2nd ed., pp. 1339–1345. Little, Brown, Boston.

Ecobichon, D. J. (1996). Toxic effects of pesticides. In *Casarett and Doull's Toxicology: The Basic Science of Poisons* (M. O. Amdur, J. Doull, and C. D. Klaassen, Eds.), 5th ed., pp. 643–689. McGraw-Hill, New York.

Eubanks, M. (1994). Biomarkers: The clues to genetic susceptibility. *Environ. Health Perspect.* **102,** 50–56.

Fischbein, A. (1992). Occupational and environmental lead exposure. In *Occupational and Environmental Medicine* (W. N. Rom, Ed.), 2nd ed., pp. 735–758. Little, Brown, Boston.

Flamm, W. G., and Lehman-McKeeman, L. D. (1991). The human relevance of the renal tumor-inducing potential of *d*-limonene in male rats: Implications for risk assessment. *Regul. Toxicol. Pharmacol.* **13,** 70–86.

Goyer, R. A. (1996). Toxic effects of metals. In *Casarett and Doull's Toxicology: The Basic Science of Poisons* (M. O. Amdur, J. Doull, C. D. Klaassen, Eds.), 5th ed., pp. 691–736. McGraw-Hill, New York.

—Elizabeth V. Wattenberg

Related Topics

American Conference of Governmental Industrial Hygienists
Biomarkers, Human Health
Biotransformation
Dose–Response Relationship
Exposure
Hazard Identification
Medical Surveillance
Noise: Ototraumatic Effects
Occupational Safety and Health Administration
Permissible Exposure Limits
Psychological Indices of Toxicity
Risk Assessment
Short-Term Exposure Limits
Threshold Limit Values

Octane

- CAS: 111-65-9
- SYNONYMS: Octane (ACGIH, NIOSH, OSHA, DOT); oktan (Polish); oktanen (Dutch); ottani (Italian); *n*-octane, UN1262 (DOT)
- CHEMICAL CLASS: Aliphatic hydrocarbon (C8)
- MOLECULAR FORMULA: C_8H_{18}

Uses

Octane is a colorless, highly flammable liquid that is lighter than water. It has an odor that can be detected at 400 ppm. It occurs in natural gas but is principally derived from crude oil. It is used as a solvent and raw material for organic synthesis reactions and is a very important chemical in the petroleum industry. It is also widely used in the rubber and paper processing industries. Isooctane, along with other *n*- and isoparaffins, is used in the blending of fuels to achieve desired antiknock properties. A total of 17 isomers of octane are known to exist; isooctane, or 2,2,4-trimethylpentane, is a principal ingredient of gasoline.

Exposure Pathways

Because octane can exist as a liquid and a vapor at normal temperature and pressure, exposure could occur by either dermal contact or inhalation; oral exposure would most likely be either incidental or accidental. Isooctane, an octane isomer, can comprise up to 1% of the total hydrocarbons emitted from the exhaust of diesel and gasoline engines.

Mechanism of Toxicity

The toxicity of octane is similar in potency to heptane (especially with regard to narcotic effects) but is apparently without the associated neurotoxic signs of heptane or hexane. When exposed via the oral route, octane appears to be more toxic than its lower homologs. If it is aspirated into the lungs, it may cause rapid death due to cardiac arrest, respiratory paralysis, and asphyxia. Octane is most likely converted to a hydroxy derivative (e.g., alcohol) via the cytochrome P450 oxidase system. The actual molecular mechanism of toxicity is not known, although, being a solvent, a direct physical alteration of cellular membranes and organelles would be suspect.

Human Toxicity

Most toxicological references on octane agree that it is moderately toxic if taken orally and more toxic than the lower homologs. At high acute concentrations it will have a narcotic effect (generally between 5000 and 13,700 ppm for 30 min), but no adverse effects are apparent in humans at concentrations below 500 ppm. NIOSH has the lowest recommended human exposure level of 75 ppm for octane and 350 mg/m^3 for a mixture of C5–C8 hydrocarbons. OSHA suggests a TWA PEL of 500 ppm (2350 mg/m^3), while ACGIH recommends a TWA TLV of 300 ppm (1400 mg/m^3). The lower and upper explosive limits for octane are 1 and 4.7%, respectively.

Clinical Management

Persons who are exposed to high air concentrations should vacate or be removed from the source of the gas and seek fresh air. Upon oral ingestion, persons should not be induced to vomit as pulmonary aspiration may occur, resulting in severe narcosis and/or death. Extreme care must be taken to keep areas of expected increased concentration free from ignition sources (e.g., sparks from static electricity) and to use explosion-proof apparatus in these areas.

Animal Toxicity

Octane has been shown to have narcotic effects in both mice and rats, primarily in experiments documenting acute exposure at high concentrations. One study estimated a 4-hr LC_{50} in rats of 118,000 mg/m^3 (24,780 ppm). The lowest concentration to cause an effect on righting reflexes in mice was 35 mg/liter (7350 ppm), while complete loss was seen at 50 mg/liter (10,500 ppm). For 2,5-dimethylhexane, an octane isomer, the narcotic concentration in mice was 70–80 mg/liter (14,700–16,800 ppm), and the effects were less than those seen for *n*-octane. In rats, oral administration of isooctane caused moderate toxicity, and pulmonary lesions were observed following aspiration of octane into the lungs. None of the branched octane isomers are known to have neurotoxic properties. Some types of soil-dwelling bacteria can exist using branched octanes as a sole carbon source.

—Stephen Clough

Oil, Crude

- CAS: 8002-05-9
- SYNONYMS: Crude petroleum; petroleum crude; rock oil; naphtha; petrol; seneca oil
- CHEMICAL CLASS: Petroleum hydrocarbons
- DESCRIPTION: Crude oil is a complex mixture of saturated and unsaturated aliphatic and aromatic hydrocarbons. Other carbon and hydrogen compounds are in crude oil which frequently contain significant amounts of nitrogen, sulfur, and oxygen as well as smaller amounts of nickel, vanadium, and other elements. The composition of crude oil is not fixed but varies according to the conditions associated with its generation (i.e., source of organic material, geological history, and temperature during formation). For example, at higher formation temperatures, larger molecules are broken down into smaller molecules, thereby changing the composition of the crude oil.

Uses

Crude oil is the world's main source of energy and petrochemical feedstocks. It is rarely used in the form obtained at the well but is converted or processed in refineries into a wide range of products such as lubricants and solvents, gasoline, kerosene, diesel fuel, jet fuel, domestic fuel oils, and industrial fuel oils. Petrochemical feedstocks include ethylene, propylene, the butenes, and isoprene. These feedstocks are the basis for other industrial products such as plastics, elastomers, and artificial fibers.

Exposure Pathways

Direct exposure to crude oil itself is unlikely for the general population. Exceptions are well workers and material handlers who may receive dermal exposure and inhalation exposure at elevated temperature and pressure. Unknown but possible exposure can occur by swimming in waters where spills have occurred, after leakage from storage tanks into groundwater and drinking water, and by vapors from spills which can migrate through the ground.

Toxicokinetics

None or little quantitative data were available concerning the absorption, distribution, metabolism, and excretion of crude oil. Indirect evidence suggests that crude oil may be absorbed through the respiratory tract, the gastrointestinal tract, and percutaneously.

Mechanism of Toxicity

Due to its insolubility in water and its viscosity, the ingestion of crude oil can result in aspiration during emesis, which may cause pneumonitis, pulmonary injury, and death. Any more specific mechanisms of toxicity would likely be related to individual fractions of crude oil.

Human Toxicity

Crude oil is of low-order toxicity following oral, dermal, or inhalation exposure. Eye and skin irritation may occur from repeated or prolonged contact with crude oil. Eye and respiratory tract irritation may occur after exposure to aerosols of crude oil and after exposure to vapors at elevated temperatures; these types of exposure may also cause headache and dizziness with possible anesthetic and other central nervous system (CNS) effects such as depression, including death. Small amounts of crude oil aspirated into the respiratory system during ingestion or after vomiting may cause mild to severe pulmonary injury, possibly progressing to death. These pulmonary effects may also occur from inhalation of aerosolized crude oil. Nausea, vomiting, and diarrhea may occur after ingestion. If crude oil or its components are absorbed, cardiac arrhythmias may occur. Crude oil may contain hydrogen sulfide gas in the confined spaces during transport and also low percentages of benzene. Appropriate precautionary measures for these low-level chemicals should be considered.

Crude oil has not been shown to be a sensitizer in laboratory tests but was embryotoxic to rats when dosed during gestation and was hepatotoxic to mice after repeated dosing. The relevance of these animal studies to humans is unknown. For most of the studies reported, crude oil was either equivocal or did not induce mutagenicity. In one study, an increase in the frequency of chromosomal aberrations was observed. Crude oil, and especially heavier crude oil fractions with high-boiling aromatics, caused increases in the incidence of skin cancer (carcinoma) in some laboratory tests where mice were painted during their lifetime. Repeated inhalation of crude oil vapors may cause symptoms consistent with CNS depression such as headache and vertigo.

Clinical Management

Asymptomatic individuals should be observed for 4–6 hr after exposure for the development of symptoms. Respiratory and cardiovascular function should be supported in symptomatic individuals. If there is suspicion of aspiration, breathing should be observed and the patient treated symptomatically.

If crude oil has been ingested, nothing should be given by mouth and vomiting should not be induced. Gastric decontamination is not usually indicated after ingestion due to the possibility of aspiration. If necessary, gastric lavage must only be performed after cuffed endotracheal intubation. If aspiration is expected to have occurred (i.e., a coughing symptomatic individual), arterial blood should be monitored to ensure adequate ventilation. The development of pulmonary edema may be delayed in onset up to 24–72 hr after exposure. Antibiotic and corticosteroid therapy may be considered for treatment of possible chemical pneumonitis resulting from aspiration. CNS depression should be treated as indicated.

For skin contact, affected areas should be washed thoroughly with soap and water. For eye exposure, the eyes should be gently flushed with copious amounts of water for at least 10 min.

Animal Toxicity

The acute toxicities (LD_{50}) for crude oil are $\geqq 4$ g/kg (oral, rats) and $\geqq 2$ g/kg (dermal, rabbit). Prolonged exposure caused mild eye irritation and mild to moderate skin irritation in rabbits. Skin sensitization was not observed after treatment of guinea pigs. Hepatotoxicity was observed in mice (5 ml/kg/2 weeks) and embryotoxicity was observed in rats (5 ml/kg single dose; 1 ml/kg multiple dose) dosed orally with crude oil. Chronic dermal applications of crude oil caused skin carcinoma in mice.

—Gary P. Bond

Related Topics

Pollution, Soil
Pollution, Water

Oil, Lubricating

- CHEMICAL CLASS: Petroleum hydrocarbon mixture
- DESCRIPTION: Lubricating oil consists of paraffinic oils and naphthenic oils.

Exposure Pathways

The primary exposure pathway is dermal absorption of lubricating oil through skin contact. Minor exposure pathways include ingestion of lubricating oil and inhalation of oil mist. Oil mist is defined as an airborne mist of petroleum-base cutting oils or white mineral petroleum oil.

Toxicokinetics

In general, paraffinic oils are absorbed only to a limited extent from the gastrointestinal tract. Paraffinic oil, however, was found in the liver, spleen, mesenteric and portal–hepatic lymph nodes and lungs of a man known to have ingested large amounts of liquid paraffin over many years.

Paraffinic oil injected intravenously into rabbits was noted to be taken up by the liver, bone marrow, lungs, and endothelial cells of the spleen. Liver granulomas were also observed.

Mechanism of Toxicity

Paraffin oil may enter the trachea and bronchi after oral or nasal administration to individuals (especially to those in the supine position) with redued or absent gag reflex or through its ability to inhibit the normal cough reflex. Paraffin oil inhibits the action of respiratory cilia, allowing passage to the alveoli. Paraffin oils do not produce pulmonary necrosis and are taken up by macrophages (called lipophages), which remain within the alveolar spaces.

Human Toxicity

The lungs and the skin are the major sites in humans affected by exposure to lubricant base stocks. Inhalation of greater than approximately 9 mg/m^3 of oil mist for several years or aspiration or ingestion of these materials has been reported to produce lipid pneumonia and lipid granuloma of the lung. Prolonged or repeated skin contact may produce skin irritation and dermatitis due to the defatting properties of the oils.

Ingestion of lubricating oils or subsequent vomiting that results in aspiration of light hydrocarbon liquid can cause pneumonitis. Should lubricating oil enter the lungs, the substance is very difficult to remove and can cause severe injury to the lungs and can include death.

Clinical Management

For dermal contact, it is recommended that the affected skin be thoroughly washed with soap and water and that contaminated clothing be removed and washed.

If lubricating oil is ingested, water or milk should be given and medical advice sought. The person should not be made to vomit unless so directed by medical personnel.

Animal Toxicity: Acute

Naphthenic and paraffinic lubricating base stocks were of low acute toxicity when administered to animals by the oral and dermal routes of exposure. Acute studies with these oils demonstrated an oral rat $LD_{50} \geqq 5$ g/kg and a dermal rabbit $LD_{50} \geqq 5$ g/kg. Dermal sensitization tests using 0.5 ml oil on guinea pigs showed no evidence of sensitization. Primary eye irritation and primary skin irritation tests on rabbits revealed slight to no irritation. In subacute dermal tests, rabbits were treated with 5 g/kg three times per week for 3 weeks. Skin irritation and inflammation occurred, most likely as a result of the oils' defatting properties. No mortality was reported in these studies.

Animal Toxicity: Chronic

Noncarcinogenicity

Based on the information reviewed, lubricating oil base stocks fit the definition for mineral oil mist. Oil mist is defined as an airborne mist of petroleum-base cutting oils or white mineral petroleum oil. Animals exposed to 5 mg/m^2 white mineral oil mist 6 hr per day for 1 year experienced no measured toxicity. A study conducted at 100 mg/m^3 resulted in no histological changes of significance. Slight changes occurred in some but not all species exposed. Animals exposed to 50 mg/m^3 of a sulfurized, solvent-extracted naphthenic base oil for 18 months did not show any signs of injury or indisposition.

Carcinogenicity

Two-year bioassays were conducted on a group of new and used lubricant oils submitted in 1979 and

1980 by the American Petroleum Institute. Groups of 50 C3H/HeJ mice were treated twice weekly by application of 50-mg doses to the interscapular skin after the hair was clipped. Treatment was continued for 104 weeks. Hitstopathologic examinations were conducted on the treated skin of all animals and the internal organs of half of the animals. Clinical observations were recorded for all animals. Incidence of internal lesions in all groups was not higher than expected. The naphthenic oil (64741-96-4) and two paraffinic oils (64742-65-0) did, however, cause chronic interstitial nephritis in 12, 12, and 10 animals, respectively (vs 6 animals in the control group). In addition, the naphthenic oil caused pneumonia in 11 animals vs 5 animals in the control group. The incidence of internal lesions in all groups was not higher than expected. No metastatic lesions from skin tumors were observed.

In a study by Bingham *et al.* (1965), groups of 30 C3H/HeJ male mice were give twice weekly skin applications of 50 mg of undiluted paraffinic solvent-refined oil for up to 80 weeks. The animals developed no tumors. In a similar test, a sample of undiluted naphthenic solvent-refined oils also yielded no skin tumors.

A study was performed using an unrefined dewaxed paraffinic distillate, solvent-treated distilate, and the aromatic extract from the solvent treatment. Groups of 30 Swiss female mice received skin applications of 0.05 ml of one of the samples three times per week for 1 month and two times per week for the next 11 months. Of the mice receiving the untreated sample, 13 developed skin tumors. After solvent treatment, the aromatic extract produced tumors in 25 mice. The solvent-treated sample, however, produced no tumors.

In other studies, male C3H or C3H/HeJ mice received skin application of undiluted test materials two or three times per week for approximately 80 weeks. The results showed that distillates not subjected to further treatment were generally active in the skin carcinogenesis assay. Solvent refining produces raffinates that are usually not active; however, extracts from the process were positive.

Male C3H or C3H/HeJ mice received 50 μl or 50 or 75 mg, respectively, two times per week of lubricant base oils for 98–134 weeks or 80 weeks, respectively. The results confirmed the results stated previously. The severity of solvent extraction was the major influence of carcinogenicity.

The weight of evidence suggests that severely solvent refined oils do not cause dermal carcinogenicity and that neutral oils are not likely to be mutagenic or teratogenic.

—*Shayne C. Gad*

Oleander

- Synonyms: *Nerium oleander; Nerium indicum; Nerium odorum;* common oleander; rose-bay; rose laurel
- Description: Oleander is in the Apocynaceae (dogbane) plant family. The large ornamental evergreen shrub may grow 20–25 ft in height. Leaves are long and narrow, with pointed tips. During the summer months large clusters of white, pink, or red flowers appear at the ends of the branches.

Uses

Oleander is used as an ornamental shrub along roadsides and in gardens. The plant is also used in rodenticides, insecticides, and homeopathic remedies.

Exposure Pathways

Common exposure pathways include ingestion of plant parts or oleander tea. Homeopathic extracts and insecticide and rodenticide extracts are other available sources.

Mechanism of Toxicity

Common oleander contains at least five cardiac glycosides that can exert a digitoxin-like effect by inhibiting the sodium–potassium ATPase enzyme system.

Human Toxicity

The range of toxicity from amounts of oleander is variable. Significant oleander poisoning closely resembles digitoxin poisoning. Gastrointestinal and cardiac symptoms predominate. In the first several hours, nausea and vomiting are usually present. Cardiotoxic effects, such as conduction abnormalities, ventricular arrhythmia, and asystole, can be present. Poisoned patients can present with bradycardia; first-, second-, and third-degree heart block; hypotension; and hyperkalemia.

Clinical Management

Basic and advanced life-support measures should be utilized as necessary. With significant ingestion, decontamination is advised. If the ingestion is recent (less than 30 min) and the patient is asymptomatic, syrup of ipecac-induced emesis may be appropriate in treating small amount ingestions in children. Activated charcoal may be used to adsorb plant toxins. Continuous EKG monitoring and serial potassium levels should be performed. Atropine is useful in managing bradycardia and varying degrees of heart block. Low-dose phenytoin may improve atrioventricular conduction and terminate heart block. Ventricular dysrhythmia may be managed with phenytoin and/or lidocaine. Magnesium may reverse digitalis-induced arrhythmias. Intravenous glucose and insulin should be used in life-threatening hyperkalemia. For patients who have persistent severe cardiovascular disease, an electrical pacemaker should be considered. Digoxin-immune Fab, which is used to treat severe digitalis glycoside poisoning, has been demonstrated to be effective in the management of oleander poisoning.

Animal Toxicity

Animals have the same potential for toxicity as humans. Cases involving cows, for instance, have been documented.

—*Anne E. Bryan*

Related Topics

Cardiovascular System
Digitalis Glycosides

Opium

- CAS: 8008-60-4
- Synonyms: Crude opium; gum opium; opii pulvis standardisatus; opiu pulveratum; opium titratum; powdered opium; pulvis opii; raw opium; standardized opium powder
- Description: Opium is the air-dried milky exudate obtained by incising the unripe capsules of *Papaver somniferum.*
- Pharmaceutical Class: Opiate agonist

Uses

Opium is used for analgesia, sedative–hypnotic narcosis, antiperistalsis, and in the treatment of neonatal withdrawal. It is also a drug of abuse.

Exposure Pathways

Opium can be solubilized and given parenterally. Tinctures and suspensions are available for oral administration and suppositories for rectal administration. In addition, it can be insufflated as a powder.

Toxicokinetics

Opium contains several alkaloids, including no less than 10% anhydrous morphine and small amounts of codeine and papverine. After oral administration, morphine is absorbed from the gastrointestinal tract. The drug is rapidly metabolized after oral administration and plasma concentrations of unconjugated morphine are lower than those achieved after parenteral administration. Activity following parenteral administration of concentrated opium alkaloids is similar to parentally administered morphine. Peak analgesia occurs within 60 min and can be maintained for up to 7 hr. Rectal adsorption is dependent on body hydration.

Opium preparations are metabolized in the liver. Morphine undergoes conjugation with glucuronic acid at the 3-hydroxyl group. Secondary conjugation may also occur at the 6-hydroxyl group to form the 3,6-diglucuronide. Morphine is excreted in the urine mainly as morphine-3,6-diglucuronide and smaller amounts of morphine-3,6-diglucuronide and unchanged drug. Morphine is distributed throughout the body but mainly in the kidneys, liver, lungs, and spleen. Approximately 35% is protein bound. The volume of distribution is 3 or 4 liters/kg. Opium is primarily excreted in the kidneys as metabolites. Approximately 75% of a dose of morphine is excreted in the urine within 48 hr. A secondary mode of elimination is biliary secretion.

Mechanism of Toxicity

Morphine, the major active principle of powdered opium, is responsible for the action of opium, although other alkaloids contribute to it. Morphine's toxicity is a result of its extensive effect on the central nervous system (CNS), mainly that of a descending depression. Opiates interact with stereospecific and saturable binding sites primarily located in the CNS. Interaction with these receptors mimics the actions of endogenous enkephalins and endorphins. Their action also appears to involve an alteration in the release of neurotransmitters, such as the inhibition of acetylcholine, norepinephrine, and dopamine. In therapeutic amounts, this yields analgesia, euphoria, sedation, and decreased gastrointestinal motility. In toxic amounts, it can lead to respiratory depression, coma, and cardiovascular collapse.

Human Toxicity: Acute

Symptoms of toxicity may occur in varying degrees in nontolerant individuals who receive greater than a therapeutic dosage. The primary insult is respiratory depression from direct depression of the CNS. This state may then progress to apnea or respiratory arrest. Pulmonary edema is a common complication. Therapeutically, opium results in analgesia; however, when toxic, neurological depression ensues and can progress to coma. Miosis is frequent, but in an acidotic or asphyxiated state pupils may be dilated. From a cardiovascular perspective, opium can cause hypotension and bradycardia. Hypothermia may also develop if there is peripheral vasodilation. Laboratory analysis does not dictate treatment but can confirm its presence.

Human Toxicity: Chronic

Opiates have a high potential for abuse. Chronic users may develop tolerance, thus necessitating larger doses for the desired effect. Toxic effects in chronic abuse can yield a decrease in immunity leading to frequent infections and possible AIDS. Abrupt cessation can cause withdrawal, yielding restlessness, vomiting, and diarrhea.

Clinical Management

Basic life-support measures should be instituted as necessary. Intensive support therapy may be required to correct respiratory failure and shock. Respirations must be supported and monitored until all symptoms disappear. Pulmonary edema should be managed with appropriate ventilatory support. If taken orally, gastrointestinal decontamination should be based on the patient's level of consciousness or decrease in gag reflex. Activated charcoal may be used to adsorb the opium. A cathartic may be given to enhance elimination of the activated charcoal–opium complex. The specific antagonist naloxone is used to counteract respiratory depression and coma. A dose of 0.4–2.0 mg is given intravenously and can be repeated at intervals of 2 or 3 min. The therapeutic effect of naloxone may be of shorter duration than that of the opiate activity; therefore, a naloxone continuous infusion may then be of benefit. Arterial blood gases, vital signs, and level of consciousness should be monitored continuously until cessation of symptoms.

Animal Toxicity

Dogs act similarly to humans—symptoms may include drowsiness, ataxia, vomiting, respiratory depression, miosis, coma, and hypotension. Opiates and their derivatives have an excitatory effect on the CNS of cats and horses. Naloxone may be used at 0.02 mg/kg if needed.

—*Lisa Scheuring-Mroz*

Organisation for Economic Co-operation and Development

The Organisation for Economic Co-operation and Development (OECD), based in Paris, France, is an intergovernmental organization. Its aims and responsibilities are: achieving the highest sustainable economic growth and employment, promoting economic and social welfare throughout the OECD region by coordinating policies of its member countries, and stimulating and harmonizing the efforts of member countries in favor of developing countries. At the time of writing, there were 29 member countries: Australia,

Austria, Belgium, Canada, the Czech Republic, Denmark, Finland, France, Germany, Greece, Hungary, Iceland, Ireland, Italy, Japan, Luxembourg, Mexico, the Netherlands, New Zealand, Norway, Poland, Portugal, Republic of Korea, Spain, Sweden, Switzerland, Turkey, the United Kingdom, and the United States. The European Commission also participates in the organization's work.

Within the OECD the governments of these industrialized countries compare and, if they so decide, coordinate their domestic policies. Monitoring international economic trends is one of the organization's best known activities. However, since the OECD was established in 1960 the number of policy areas in which it functions as a center for cooperation and exchange of views has steadily increased. Since 1971, work in the OECD related to chemical safety has been organized under the Chemicals Programme. The policy direction and priorities of the Chemicals Programme are determined by member country representatives, chosen by each country's government, who take part in the Joint Meeting of the Chemicals Group and Management Committee of the Special Programme on the Control of Chemicals. The Chemicals Programme is supported by the Environmental Health and Safety Division of the OECD Secretariat's Environment Directorate. Technical work on chemicals is carried out for the most part by experts from government, industry, and academic institutions in member countries who attend workshops and other meetings.

The main objectives of the Chemicals Programme are to assist member countries in identifying, preventing, and reducing the risks of chemicals; promote sustainable development concerning activities related to chemicals within OECD and non-OECD countries; prevent unnecessary distortions in trade; facilitate optimal use of national resources available for chemicals management; and assist member countries in working toward an integrated chemicals management approach which incorporates economic and environmental policy considerations.

Since the 1970s, the OECD has been in the forefront in developing policies and instruments to control chemicals and chemical products. Work in the Chemicals Programme on the development, updating, and expansion of scientifically valid harmonized methods for testing and assessment helps OECD countries (and, increasingly, non-OECD countries that use these methods) to prevent new chemicals that might present unacceptable risks from entering the market and to assess the safety of chemicals already in use.

Chemicals Programme activities are carried out in cooperation with other relevant bodies of the OECD and, as appropriate, with other international organizations including the International Programme on Chemical Safety (IPCS), International Register of Potentially Toxic Chemicals (IRPTC), United Nations Environment Programme, and World Health Organization (WHO).

Mutual Acceptance of Data

One of the most significant achievements of cooperative work in the OECD aimed at the harmonization of national chemicals control procedures and policies is the 1981 Council Act on the Mutual Acceptance of Data in the Assessment of Chemicals. This act contains a decision that

> Data generated in the testing of chemicals in an OECD Member country in accordance with OECD Test Guidelines and OECD Principles of Good Laboratory Practice shall be accepted in other Member countries for purposes of assessment and other uses relating to the protection of man and the environment.

The Council is the OECD's highest authority, in which the governments of all member countries participate. Once member countries have adopted a Council decision, they are under a legal obligation to implement it. Consequently, when data developed in an OECD country under the conditions set out in this decision are submitted in other OECD countries to fulfill regulatory requirements, the data cannot be refused and so do not have to be developed over again for notifications in each country. (The OECD Test Guidelines and OECD Principles of Good Laboratory Practice are described later.)

The intention of this act is to ensure that data generated in the safety testing of chemicals are of high quality and are based on internationally harmonized methods. Such data can then be used to assess chemical hazards and to make decisions on appropriate activities to prevent or reduce risks to human health or the environment. Where the need for duplicative testing is minimized through Mutual Acceptance of Data, testing costs can be reduced for both governments and industry. Test facilities and specialist personnel can be utilized more efficiently, and fewer animals will be used in testing (an important consideration in OECD countries, where animal welfare is an issue of concern). Harmonized safety testing can also help prevent non-tariff barriers arising in the trade of chemicals and chemical products as a result of differences in national chemicals control regulations.

The OECD Test Guidelines

The *OECD Guidelines for the Testing of Chemicals* is a collection of standard methods used by professionals in governments, industry, academic institutions, and independent laboratories for safety testing of chemical substances. They cover tests for physical–chemical properties, effects on biotic systems (ecotoxicity), environmental fate (degradation/accumulation), and health effects (toxicity) (Table O-1). The test guidelines are systematically updated to respond to scientific progress or to address new needs identified by member countries. They are published in two loose-leaf binders and are also available in a CD-ROM version.

The OECD test guidelines began to be developed in the late 1970s by several expert groups, with the goal of enhancing the validity and international acceptability of test data. Since their adoption in 1981, they have become recognized in both OECD and non-OECD countries as the authoritative reference tool for testing chemicals in a regulatory context.

The Test Guidelines Programme is overseen by national coordinators, who work to achieve consensus on draft versions of new and revised test guidelines. Proposals for new or updated guidelines can be made by a national coordinator, by the international scientific community, or by the OECD secretariat. To become effective, any new or updated guideline must be adopted by member countries in the council. Procedures for test guideline development and updating are described in detail in *Guidance Document for the Development of OECD Guidelines for Testing of Chemicals* (OECD Environment Monograph No. 76).

A special activity within the Test Guideline Programme addresses animal welfare issues, in particular the reduction, refinement, and replacement of animal use in the OECD test guidelines. The overall objective of this activity is to promote test methods that do not require the use of animals (or that require fewer test animals than existing methods) as well as to

TABLE O-1

OECD Guidelines for the Testing for Chemicals

Section 1:	Physical–chemical Properties
101	UV–VIS Absorption Spectra
102	Melting Point/Melting Range
103	Boiling Point/Boiling Range
104	Vapor Pressure Curve
105	Water Solubility
106	Adsorption/Desorption
107	Partition Coefficient (*n*-octanol/water)
108	Complex Formation Ability in Water
109	Density of Liquids and Solids
110	Particle Size Distribution/Fiber Length and Diameter Distributions
111	Hydrolysis as a Function of pH
112	Dissociation Constants in Water
113	Screening Test for Thermal Stability and Stability in Air
114	Viscosity of Liquids
115	Surface Tension of Aqueous Solutions
116	Fat Solubility of Solid and Liquid Substances
117	Partition Coefficient (-*n*-octanol/water), HPLC Method
Section 2:	Effects on Biotic Systems
201	Alga, Growth Inhibition Test
202	*Daphnia* sp. Acute Immobilisation Test and Reproduction Test
203	Fish, Acute Toxicity Test
204	Fish, Prolonged Toxicity Test: 14-Day Study
205	Avian Dietary Toxicity Test
206	Avian Reproduction Test
207	Earthworm, Acute Toxicity Tests
208	Terrestrial Plants, Growth Test
209	Activated Sludge, Respiration Inhibition Test
210	Fish, Early Life Stage Toxicity Test
Section 3:	Degradation and Accumulation
301	Ready Biodegradability
301 A	DOC Die-Away Test
301 B	CO_2 Evolution Test
301 C	Modified MITI Test (I)
301 D	Closed Bottle Test
301 E	Modified OECD Screening Test
301 F	Manometric Respirometry Test
302 A	Inherent Biodegradability: Modified SCAS test
302 B	Inherent Biodegradability: Zahn–Wellens/EMPA Test
302 C	Inherent Biodegradability: Modified MITI Test (II)
303 A	Simulation Test–Aerobic Sewage Treatment: Coupled Units Test
304 A	Inherent Biodegradability in Soil
305 A	Bioaccumulation: Sequential Static Fish Test
305 B	Bioaccumulation: Semi-Static Fish Test
305 C	Bioaccumulation: Degree of Bioconcentration in Fish
305 D	Static Fish Test
305 E	Flow-Through Fish Test
306	Biodegradability in Seawater
Section 4:	Health Effects
401	Acute Oral Toxicity
402	Acute Dermal Toxicity
403	Acute Inhalation Toxicity
404	Acute Dermal Irritation/Corrosion
405	Acute Eye Irritation/Corrosion

(*continues*)

TABLE O-1 (*Continued*)

406	Skin Sensitization
407	Repeated Dose 28-Day Oral Toxicity Study in Rodents
408	Subchronic Oral Toxicity—Rodent: 90-Day
409	Subchronic Oral Toxicity—Non-Rodent: 90-Day
410	Repeated Dose Dermal Toxicity: 21/28-Day
411	Subchronic Dermal Toxicity: 90-Day
412	Repeated Dose Inhalation Toxicity: 28/14-Day
413	Subchronic Inhalation Toxicity: 90-Day
414	Teratogenicity
415	One-Generation Reproduction Toxicity
416	Two-Generation Reproduction Toxicity
417	Toxicokinetics
418	Delayed Neurotoxicity of Organophosphorus Substances Following Acute Exposure
419	Delayed Neurotoxicity of Organophosphorus Substances: 28-Day Repeated Dose Study
420	Acute Oral Toxicity—Fixed Dose Method
421	Reproduction/Developmental Toxicity Screening Test
451	Carcinogenicity Studies
452	Chronic Toxicity Studies
453	Combined Chronic Toxicity/Carcinogenicity Studies
471/472	Genetic Toxicology: Reverse Mutation Assay Using Bacteria
473	Genetic Toxicology: *In vitro* Mammalian Chromosomal Aberration Test
474	Genetic Toxicology: Mammalian Erythrocyte Micronucleus Test
475	Genetic Toxicology: Mammalian Bone Marrow Chromosomal Aberration Test
476	Genetic Toxicology: *In vitro* Mammalian Cell Gene Mutation Test
477	Genetic Toxicology: Sex-Linked Recessive Lethal Test in *Drosophila melanogaster*
478	Genetic Toxicology: Rodent Dominant Lethal Test
479	Genetic Toxicology: *In vitro* Sister Chromatid Exchange Assay in Mammalian Cells
480	Genetic Toxicology: *Saccharomyces cerevisiae,* Gene Mutation Assay
481	Genetic Toxicology: *Saccharomyces cerevisiae,* Mitotic Recombination assay
482	Genetic Toxicology: DNA Damage and Repair, Unscheduled DNA Synthesis in Mammalian Cells *in vitro*
483	Genetic Toxicology: Mammalian Germ-Cell Chromosomal Aberration Test
484	Genetic Toxicology: Mouse Spot Test
485	Genetic Toxicology: Mouse Heritable Translocation Assay

further the development and international acceptance of such methods. A number of test guidelines have been developed or revised with a view to reducing the number of animals used and/or introducing a framework of testing that allows alternative methods to be applied first.

The OECD Principles of Good Laboratory Practice

The OECD Principles of Good Laboratory Practice (GLP) set out managerial concepts concerning the organization of test laboratories and the conditions under which laboratory studies are planned, performed, monitored, and reported. Like the test guidelines, the Principles of Good Laboratory Practice began to be developed at the end of the 1970s and were established in the 1981 Council Decision on Mutual Acceptance of Data.

The purpose of the GLP principles is to make certain that test data are reliable. In 1989, the OECD council adopted an act on Compliance with Principles of Good Laboratory Practice. This act contains a decision that member countries shall establish national procedures for monitoring compliance with GLP principles, based on laboratory inspections and study audits; designate national compliance monitoring authorities; and require the management of test facilities to issue a declaration, where applicable, that a study was carried out according to GLP principles. It also contains a decision that member countries shall, under specific conditions, recognize other member countries' assurance that test data have been generated in accordance with GLP principles, and that they shall designate authorities for international liaison, exchange relevant information on compliance monitoring procedures, and implement procedures whereby, if good reason exists, information on GLP compliance by a test facility in one member country can be sought by another member country. Annexed to this act are "Guides for Compliance Monitoring Procedures for Good Laboratory Practice," "Guidance for the Conduct of Laboratory Inspections and Study Audits," and "Guidance for the Exchange of Information Concerning National Procedures for Monitoring Compliance."

Information exchange takes place within the OECD on technical and administrative matters related to the application of the GLP principles and the implementation of the compliance monitoring procedures. The Panel on Good Laboratory Practice, made up of representatives of national GLP compliance monitoring authorities, oversees the Programme on Good Laboratory Practice and develops common positions on the administration of compliance monitoring. One of the panel's responsibilities is to find solutions to problems involving the acceptance of compliance monitoring results.

OECD training courses are held for GLP inspectors, who perform laboratory inspections on behalf of national GLP monitoring authorities. Several OECD expert working groups have met to produce consensus documents on the harmonized application and interpretation of the GLP principles in specific areas or in relation to specific points.

The "OECD Series on Principles of Good Laboratory Practice and Compliance Monitoring," published in the form of short free-on-demand booklets, includes the GLP principles, the 1981 and 1989 Council Acts, and the consensus documents. At the time of writing, there were eight booklets in the series (see Further Reading).

Cooperative Investigation of High Production Volume Chemicals

Much of the work in the Chemicals Programme in the 1970s and early 1980s involved the development of anticipatory policies to prevent chemicals that would present unacceptable risks to human health or the environment reaching the market. In 1987, however, the OECD council adopted an act on the Systematic Investigation of Existing Chemicals. Existing chemicals are the many thousands of industrial chemicals already in use. Adequate safety data or hazard assessments for these chemicals (some of which have been in use for a long time) are often unavailable. This council act contains a decision that member countries "shall establish or strengthen national programs to systematically investigate existing chemicals, in order to identify those which need to be managed and/or controlled." For the purposes of the act, systematic investigation could include the following steps: identification of relevant chemicals; priority-setting, including collection or estimation of information needed for setting priorities; generation of necessary further information, including testing; and performance of hazard assessments.

The 1987 Council Act was intended to strengthen and harmonize member countries' policies in regard to existing chemicals. To avoid duplication of efforts, and to facilitate sharing the financial and administrative burden (for governments and chemical companies) of investigating these chemicals, the Council decided in a 1990 follow-up act that member countries shall: cooperatively investigate high production volume (HPV) chemicals in order to identify those which are potentially hazardous; cooperatively select the HPV chemicals to be investigated; agree on a set of data needed to make an informed judgment concerning the potential hazards of each chemical, through collection of available data or by ensuring that testing is undertaken; and cooperatively make an initial assessment of the potential hazards of each chemical using that basic data set. These decisions are contained in the act on Cooperative Investigation and Risk Reduction of Existing Chemicals (also see Risk Reduction).

Following the adoption of this 1990 Council Act, high production volume chemicals were defined as those produced in volumes of at least 1000 tons/year in two or more OECD countries, or 10,000 tons/year in one country. Governments, in consultation with the chemical industry, provided the OECD with information on the chemicals produced in these volumes in their countries. A consolidated OECD representative list of 1500 HPV chemicals was subsequently prepared, representing an estimated 90–95% of the total volume of chemicals produced in member countries. While there was already adequate information concerning the health and environmental effects of many of the chemicals on this HPV list, little or no information of this type was available for some chemicals despite their high production volume. It is these chemicals which have been chosen for cooperative investigation by member countries, thereby efficiently sharing the burden of the enormous task of systematically investigating existing chemicals.

Information on each chemical being investigated is first gathered by a "sponsor" country through searching the scientific literature. The chemical industry, both within and outside the sponsor country, provides information that may include data not freely available before. The sponsor country evaluates the collected information. At a minimum, the OECD's Screening Information Data Set (SIDS) should be available. The SIDS is a list of data elements similar to those which governments in most OECD countries require from industry before a new chemical can be marketed. It includes information on the chemical's identity, its physical and chemical properties, the sources and likely extent of exposure and use, environmental fate and how the chemical might be disseminated in the environment, as well as toxicological data. All of these data elements are essential if an initial assessment is to be made of a chemical's risks.

In order to fill identified data gaps, or replace data whose quality is considered insufficient, a SIDS Testing Plan is prepared. The chemical industry then undertakes the necessary testing on a voluntary basis, in consultation with the sponsor country. Any single test is performed only once, by a single company. In accordance with the 1981 council decision on mutual acceptance of data, all member countries will accept the results as long as testing has been done according to the OECD test guidelines and GLP principles.

When (through a combination of data collection and testing) a complete SIDS has been compiled, the sponsor country prepares a SIDS Initial Assessment Report. The Initial Assessment Report is discussed, in the presence of observers from companies producing the chemical, at a SIDS Initial Assessment Meeting. At this meeting a cooperative assessment of the chemical is made. Based on an initial assessment of the effects and exposure data provided in its SIDS dossier, the chemical is assigned to one of three categories:

1. The chemical can be considered to present a low potential for risk to humans and the environment. Thus, there is no current priority for undertaking post-SIDS testing and/or exposure analysis or an in-depth assessment.

2. The chemical may present a potential for risk to humans and/or the environment. Thus, there is a priority for undertaking post-SIDS testing and/or exposure analysis and/or an in-depth assessment. [The hazard(s) identified and specific further activities to be undertaken should be provided when this category is used.]

3. The chemical presents a potential for risk to humans and/or the environment. Depending on the exposure situation and current risk reduction measures, further risk management actions might be necessary. These could range, as appropriate, from responsible care activities by the chemical industry to national or international risk reduction activities. [The hazard(s) identified and proposals for any further action should be provided when this category is used.]

It is conceivable that a chemical could be placed in category 3 due to its risk potential based on a specific hazard, and that it could also be placed in category 2 because further activities, for example more detailed exposure analysis or testing of other endpoints, need to be undertaken.

At the time of writing, about 350 HPV chemicals were undergoing systematic investigation of their potential health and/or environmental effects and 109 SIDS Initial Assessment Reports had been completed for these chemicals. Many more HPV chemicals will be assessed in the near future.

The Steering Group on Existing Chemicals, composed of member country representatives, provides guidance on the OECD Existing Chemicals Programme and makes operational decisions concerning the investigation of priority HPV chemicals. There is close cooperation with the European Union's (EU) Existing Chemicals Programme, which was initiated in 1993. The work undertaken in the EU is fully integrated in that of the OECD.

All nonconfidential data that become available through the OECD Existing Chemicals Programme are made publicly available. It has been agreed that SIDS Initial Assessment Reports will be forwarded to the IRPTC for database input and joint publication with the OECD, under the auspices of IPCS.

The Hazard Assessment Programme

Work in the Chemicals Programme on hazard assessment is closely related to the work on test guidelines and on existing chemicals. The objectives of OECD hazard assessment activities are to promote awareness, improvement and, to the extent possible, harmonization of hazard assessment procedures for chemicals (including pesticides), and to encourage member countries' mutual use and acceptance of hazard assessments. These activities include the development and compilation of practical methods and procedures; promotion of their application in conjunction with cooperative investigations of chemicals; and promotion of the harmonization of assessment reports. In recent years, workshops have been held (and documents produced) on aquatic exposure assessment, initial assessment of occupational and consumer exposure, and data estimation methods.

Risk Reduction

The reason for testing and assessing chemicals is ultimately to prevent or reduce their risks. In addition to decisions on the cooperative investigation of HPV chemicals, the 1990 Council Act on Cooperative Investigation and Risk Reduction of Existing Chemicals sets out three objectives in regard to risk reduction activities. It contains a decision that "Member countries shall establish or strengthen national programs aimed at the reduction of risks from existing chemicals to the environment and/or the health of the general public or workers." Moreover, it recommends that member countries collaborate to develop common criteria for determining which chemicals are suitable for concerted risk reduction activities, and that they undertake concerted activities, as appropriate, to reduce the risks of selected chemicals taking into account their entire life cycle.

Reducing the overall or collective risks of chemicals is the principal objective of cooperative work on risk reduction in the OECD. Support is given to member countries in the development of their national risk reduction policies and actions, through compiling up-to-date information on national and international appraisals of the risks of specific chemicals or groups of chemicals, as well as on national risk reduction strategies in place or planned. Such information can be the basis for considering concerted responses to unacceptable health and environmental risks, when this is considered appropriate.

Other Activities Related to Environmental Health and Safety

Other OECD activities in the environmental health and safety area are concerned with pesticides; harmonization of regulatory oversight in biotechnology; and chemical accident prevention, preparedness, and response. These activities are closely connected with the work in the Chemicals Programme and are carried out in cooperation with other parts of the OECD and other international organizations. Current OECD environmental health and safety activities are described in greater detail in the brochure, *The OECD Chemicals Programme,* available from: OECD Environment Directorate, Environmental Health and Safety Division, 2 rue André-Pascal, 75775 Paris Cedex 16, France. E-mail: ehscont@oecd.org.

Nearly all the Programme's publications are available on the Internet, as are its three major data bases (on existing chemicals, pesticides, and products of biotechnology) and the text of relevant OECD Council Acts. Information about all the Programme's activities is regularly updated. Consult http://www.oecd.org/ehs/.

Further Reading

OECD Council Acts

OECD Council Decision concerning the Mutual Acceptance of Data in the Assessment of Chemicals (1981)

OECD Council Decision on the Minimum Premarketing set of Data in the Assessment of Chemicals (1982)

OECD Council Recommendation on the Protection of Proprietary Rights to Data Submitted in Notifications of New Chemicals (1983)

OECD Council Recommendation on the Exchange of Confidential Data on Chemicals (1983)

OECD Council Recommendation on Information Exchange Related to Export of Banned or Severely Restricted Chemicals (1984)

OECD Council Decision–Recommendation on the Systematic Investigation of Existing Chemicals (1987)

OECD Council Decision–Recommendation on Compliance with Principles of Good Laboratory Practice (1989)

OECD Council Decision–Recommendation on the Co-operative Investigation and Risk Reduction of Existing Chemicals (1990)

Articles

Brydon, J. E., Morgenroth, V. H., III, Smith, A. M., and Visser, R. (1990, June). OECD's work on investigation of high production volume chemicals. *Int. Environ. Rep.* 263–270.

Koeter, H. B. W .M. (1993). Test Guideline development and animal welfare: Regulatory acceptance of in vitro studies. *Reprod. Toxicol.* 7, 117–123.

Koeter, H. B. W. M. (1995). International harmonisation of immunotoxicity testing. *Hum. Exp. Toxicol.*

Smith, A. M., Arai, S., Tanaka, K., and Visser, R. (1993, November 3). Review of the SIDS Project of the OECD Existing Chemicals Program. *Int. Environ. Rep.*

Turnheim, D. (1994, August/September). Evaluating chemical risks. *OECD Observer (Paris)* **189.**

OECD Publications

OECD Guidelines for the Testing of Chemicals, 2nd ed. (2 vols.), Paris, 1993 (updated 1996). Also available in CD-ROM version.

Documents Related to the Test Guidelines Programme

Guidance Document for the Development of OECD Guidelines for Testing of Chemicals, Environment Monograph No. 76, Paris, 1993.

OECD Series on the Test Guidelines Programme No. 1: Detailed Review Paper on Biodegradability Testing, Environment Monograph No. 98, Paris, 1995.

Scientific Criteria for Validation of in Vitro Toxicity Tests, Environment Monograph No. 36, Paris, 1990.

Documents Published in the OECD Series on Principles of Good Laboratory Practice and Compliance Monitoring (also Available in French, Spanish, and German Translations; Russian Translations Are Underway)

1. *The OECD Principles of Good Laboratory Practice,* Environment Monograph No. 45, Paris, 1992.
2. *Guides for Compliance Monitoring Procedures for Good Laboratory Practice,* Environment Monograph No. 110, Paris, 1995.
3. *Guidance for the Conduct of Laboratory Inspections and Study Audits,* Environment Monograph No. 111, Paris, 1995.
4. *Quality Assurance and GLP,* Environment Monograph No. 48, Paris, 1992.
5. *Compliance of Laboratory Suppliers with GLP Principles,* Environment Monograph No. 49, Paris, 1992.
6. *The Application of the GLP Principles to Field Studies,* Environment Monograph No. 50, Paris, 1992.
7. *The Application of the GLP Principles to Short-Term Studies,* Environment Monograph No. 73, Paris, 1993.
8. *The Role and Responsibilities of the Study Director in GLP Studies,* Environment Monograph No. 74, Paris, 1993.

Documents Related to the Hazard Assessment Programme

Application of Structure–Activity Relationships to the Estimation of Properties Important in Exposure Assessment, Environment Monograph No. 67, Paris, 1993.

Guidance Document for Aquatic Effects Assessment, Environment Monograph No. 92, Paris, 1995.

Report of the OECD Workshop on the Application of Simple Models for Exposure Assessment, Environment Monograph No. 69, Paris, 1993.

Report of the OECD Workshop on Ecological Effects Assessment, Environment Monograph No. 26, Paris, 1989.

Report of the OECD Workshop on Effects Assessment of Chemicals in Sediment, Environment Monograph No. 60, Paris, 1992.

Report of the OECD Workshop on the Extrapolation of Laboratory Aquatic Toxicity Data to the Real Environment. Environment Monograph No. 59, Paris, 1992.

Report of the OECD Workshop on Quantitative Structure Activity Relationships (QSARS) in Aquatic Effects Assessment, Environment Monograph No. 58, Paris, 1992.

Report of the OECD Workshop on Environmental Hazard/Risk Assessment, Environment Monograph No. 105, Paris, 1995.

Structure–Activity Relationships for Biodegradation, Environment Monograph No. 68, Paris, 1993.

US EPA/EC Joint Project on the Evaluation of (Quantitative) Structure Activity Relationships, Environment Monograph No. 88, Paris, 1994.

Documents Related to Risk Reduction

Risk Reduction Monograph No. 1: Lead. Background and National Experience with Reducing Risk, Paris, 1993.

Risk Reduction Monograph No. 2: Methylene Chloride. Background and National Experience with Reducing Risk, Paris, 1994.

Risk Reduction Monograph No. 3: Selected Brominated Flame Retardants. Background and National Experience with Reducing Risk, Paris, 1994.

Risk Reduction Monograph No. 4: Mercury. Background and National Experience with Reducing Risk, Paris, 1994.

Risk Reduction Monograph No. 5: Mercury. Background and National Experience with Reducing Risk, Paris, 1994.

Documents Related to Work on Pesticides

Data Requirements for Biological Pesticides, Environment Monograph No. 106, Paris, 1995.

Data Requirements for Pesticide Registration in OECD Member Countries: Survey Results, Environment Monograph No. 77, Paris, 1994.

—Robert Visser

(The opinions expressed in this article do not necessarily represent the opinions of the OECD or its member countries and should therefore be viewed as solely those of the author.)

Related Topics

Analytical Toxicity
Emergency Response
Good Laboratory Practice
Hazard Identification
International Programme on Chemical Safety
International Register of Potentially Toxic Chemicals
Pesticides
Toxicity Testing, Alternatives

Organochlorine Insecticides

The organochlorine insecticides are chlorinated hydrocarbon compounds that fall into three basic structure classifications: aryl (aromatic), carbocyclic, and heterocyclic.

They may be differentiated from other chlorinated hydrocarbon compounds (e.g., solvents) by molecular weight. Organochlorine insecticides, by virtue of their cyclic structure, have molecular weights ranging from 291 to 545, whereas chlorinated hydrocarbon solvents and fumigants have molecular weights that generally are less than 236.

Organochlorine insecticides may be divided into three broad groups: dichlorodiphenylethanes, such as DDT and methoxychlor; cyclodienes, such as chlordane and dieldrin; and hexachlorocyclohexanes, such as lindane. Mirex and chlordecone, however, are organochlorine insecticides whose caged structures do not fit well into the previous groups.

The first organochlorine synthesized was DDT. Although it was first synthesized by Zeidler in 1874, it was not produced or used for many years. Mueller rediscovered DDT in 1939 and won the Nobel Prize for his efforts in 1948. The first major uses for DDT were vector control of typhus and malaria and control of lice and other pests during World War II (see DDT).

Other organochlorine compounds were synthesized and came into general use during the late 1940s, thus introducing the synthetic insecticide era. From the 1940s through the 1960s, organochlorine insecticides were used extensively to control insect pests in both agricultural and domestic settings and for vector control for malaria, typhus, and other diseases affecting human health. Head and body lice are still treated effectively today with lindane.

Low volatility, lipid solubility, and environmental persistence are characteristic of organochlorine insecticides. Initially, these properties helped make organochlorines very useful and effective. However, starting in the 1960s and 1970s, environmental problems began to emerge as a result of the environmental persistence of these insecticides. Bioaccumulation in the food chain and the resulting toxicity led to decreased use of these insecticides and eventually to their general ban in the United States and Europe. By 1973, DDT use had ceased in the United States. By 1988, chlordane and heptachlor were no longer produced for use in the United States.

Biologically, the organochlorine insecticides are generally nervous system stimulants, although there are distinct differences in the activities of the individual chemicals. The mode of action for organochlorine insecticides in general is alteration of enzymatic and electrophysiological properties of nerve cell membranes. Ion flow is altered by inhibiting Na^+-, K^+-, and Ca^{2+}-adenosine triphosphatases that pump ions across neuronal membranes. The Na^+ channel activation is normal but its closing is prolonged. Additionally, the cyclodiene group inhibits the uptake of Cl^- ions by γ-aminobutyric acid. These activities inhibit the repolarization of neurons after excitation. The nerve remains partially depolarized and extremely sensitive to complete depolarization by very small stimuli.

All organochlorine insecticides may be absorbed through the gastrointestinal tract, respiratory tract, and skin, although there is variation among classes. Organochlorine insecticides are, in general, very lipophilic and tend to accumulate in the mammalian system in adipose tissue and/or organs with high fat content. Biotransformation of organochlorine insecticides is slow. Metabolism is by liver microsomal P450 enzymes to hydroxyl derivatives by dechlorination, conversion to stable epoxides, and/or O-dealkylation and hydroxylation, depending on the class. Excretion of the parent compound is usually in bile or through the intestinal wall. In either case, final elimination is usually in the feces. Urinary excretion after glutathione conjugation is also an important route of excretion. Organochlorine insecticides have been found in both cows' milk and human milk. In the liver, most organochlorine insecticides induce cellular hypertrophy, granule margination, and the production of lipospheres containing fat droplets. Focal necrosis is observed with high doses. Nodules of hypertrophied hepatocytes appear in the centrilobular area with a loss of lobular architecture.

Although generally negative in mutagenicity tests, organochlorine insecticides are associated with liver tumors in rodents. Whether this is a direct carcinogenic effect or due to promotion of spontaneous tumorigenic events is not currently known. Conclusive proof of carcinogenicity in humans is lacking but tumor potential, based on animal data, cannot be totally discounted in humans.

Symptomatology includes paresthesia, ataxia, nausea, vomiting, fatigue, and, in more acute cases, tremor, convulsions, coma, respiratory arrest, and death.

Clinical management is generally symptomatic. Convulsions are usually controlled using diazepam, pentobarbital, or phenobarbital. In some instances, treatment with activated charcoal is effective in increasing the excretion of the pesticide. Cholestyramine has been proven effective in chlordecone poisoning. In severe cases, mechanical maintenance of cardiac function and respiration is necessary.

—*Benny L. Blaylock*

Related Topics

Carbamate Pesticides
Federal Insecticide, Fungicide, and Rodenticide Act
Neurotoxicology: Central and Peripheral
Organochlorine Insecticides
Organotins
Psychological Indices of Toxicity

Organophosphate Poisoning, Intermediate Syndrome

The organophosphate (OP) insecticide-induced Intermediate Syndrome (IMS) was reported for the first time in human patients in Sri Lanka in 1987. Thereafter, this syndrome has been diagnosed in OP-poisoned patients in South Africa (1989), Turkey (1990), and Belgium (1992).

IMS is clearly a separate clinical entity from acute cholinergic crisis and delayed neuropathy. The acute cholinergic crisis usually emerges within a few minutes to a few hours and is due to acetylcholinesterase (AChE) inhibition resulting in acetylcholine accumulation. Patients acutely poisoned with OPs exhibit muscle fasciculations, convulsions, seizures, salivation, lacrimation, tracheobronchial secretion, and diarrhea due to overstimulation of muscarinic and nicotinic receptors within the peripheral and central nervous systems. Delayed neuropathy, commonly referred to as organophosphate-induced delayed neurotoxicity (OPIDN), a neurologic manifestation of some OPs, usually occurs about 2 or 3 weeks after exposure to OPs. OPIDN occurs due to inactivation of neurotoxic or neuropathy target esterase and is characterized by predominantly sensory, motor, distal, and symmetrical polyneuropathy.

IMS in OP-poisoned patients appears 24–96 hr after an apparently well-treated acute cholinergic crisis phase. By definition, OP-poisoned patients should completely recover from the cholinergic crisis and then develop a syndrome. Clinically, the IMS is characterized by acute respiratory paralysis and weakness in the territories of several cranial motor nerves, neck flexors, facial, extraocular, palatal, nuchal, and proximal limb muscles. Generalized weakness, depressed deep tendon reflexes, ptosis (drooping of the upper eye lids due to the paralysis of the third cranial nerve), and diplopia (double vision of an object) are also evident. These symptoms may last for several days or weeks depending on the OP involved. Despite severe AChE inhibition, muscle fasciculations and muscarinic receptor-associated hypersecretory activities are absent.

To date, OPs including fenthion, dimethoate, monocrotophos, methamidophos, trichlorfon, and a combination of parathion and methyl parathion have been reported to produce the IMS. Parathion alone is incapable of producing IMS. There have been many reports in the past that some OPs, such as diazinon, dicrotophos (bidrin), and malathion, also elicit symptoms quite similar to those associated with IMS.

Based on electromyographic (EMG) findings from OP-poisoned patients and experimental studies on laboratory animals, scientists have found that the defect in IMS is at the neuromuscular endplate and postsynaptic level, but the effects of neural and central components in producing muscular weakness have not been ruled out. EMG in the early stages reveals marked decrements at low rates of repetitive nerve stimulation and increments at a high rate, suggesting diverse types of impaired neuromuscular transmission. IMS seems to be due to persistent AChE inhibition at the endplate presumably leading to combined pre- and postsynaptic impairment of neuromuscular transmission.

Perhaps there are gradations of IMS and genetic or environmental factors which influence its onset. Some OPs may have higher affinity for nicotinic acetylcholine receptors or distribute selectively to muscle, producing a neuromuscular dysfunction that is longer lasting than at muscarinic sites. It would follow that there may be differences in the onset of IMS, which would depend on OP distribution or metabolism to active metabolite. Perhaps the lesions produced at the neuromuscular junction are more permanent than the muscarinic lesions. Currently, very little is known about the type of damage at the motor endplate or about risk factors associated with IMS. Thus, more detailed laboratory and clinical tests are necessary to determine the exogenous and endogenous factors contributing to its development. Hematologic, renal, and electrocardiographic values are reported to be normal in IMS patients.

Some studies have suggested that atropine and oxime treatment apparently do not influence its clinical course, as paralysis of the respiratory muscles occurs. In fact, the syndrome is refractory to treatment with atropine and oxime. Other studies have suggested that IMS may be an artifact of insufficient oxime therapy. The existence of IMS makes the management of OP poisoning even more complicated since the clinician must observe patients who have recovered from the initial cholinergic insult for an additional 3 or 4 days for possible respiratory arrest. In such cases, urgent respiratory support is absolutely necessary.

In most instances, recovery from IMS is complete, though a few deaths have been reported due to severe respiratory insufficiency. Only a few patients have developed delayed neuropathy. The risk of death in IMS is as dangerous as it is in the cholinergic crisis phase. Due to development of severe respiratory distress, tracheostomy is recommended for ventilatory support. Patients may remain on a respirator for 7 days or even more.

Further Reading

Bleecker, J. D., Neucker, K. V. D., and Willems, J. (1992). The intermediate syndrome in organophosphate poisoning: Presentation of a case and review of the literature. *Clin. Toxicol.* **30**, 321–329.

Bleecker, J. D., Willems, K. V. D., Reuck, J. D., and Vogelaers, D. (1992). Prolonged toxicity with intermediate syndrome after combined parathion and methyl parathion poisoning. *Clin. Toxicol.* **30**, 333–345.

Karademir, M., Erturk, F., and Kocak, R. (1990). Two cases of organophosphate poisoning with development of intermediate syndrome. *Hum. Exp. Toxicol.* **9**, 187–189.

Routier, R. J., Lipman, J., and Brown, K. (1989). Difficulty in weaning from respiratory support in a patient with the intermediate syndrome of organophosphate poisoning. *Crit. Care Med.* **17**, 1075–1076.

Senanayake, N., and Karalliedde, L. (1987). Neurotoxic effects of organophosphorus insecticides. An intermediate syndrome. *N. Engl. J. Med.* **316,** 761–763.

—*Ramesh C. Gupta*

Related Topics

A-esterase
Cholinesterase Inhibition
Neurotoxicity, Delayed
Neurotoxicology: Central and Peripheral
Organophosphates

Organophosphates

The term "organophosphates" (organophosphorus compounds and organophosphorus esters) generally refers to chemicals that are organic derivatives of phosphoric acid. These compounds contain both phosphorus and carbon atoms, which may be linked directly or through another atom such as oxygen. Each phosphorus has three such linkages, and the terms "phosphate," "phosphonate," and "phosphinate" refer to the number of linkages made through oxygen atoms (three, two, and one, respectively). Phosphorus linkages to carbon can also be made through nitrogen atoms ("phosphoroamidates" if one such linkage; "phosphorodiamidates" if two) or through sulfur atoms ("phosphorothiolates" if one such linkage; "phosphorodithiolate" if two). Some organophosphates have a phosphorus-fluoride linkage ("phosphorofluoridates"). As derivatives of phosphoric acid, four atoms are directly attached to the phosphorus atoms—three by single bonds, as described previously, and one represented as a double bond. The doubly bonded linkage to the phosphorus atom of organophosphates is with an oxygen atom or with a sulfur atom. The nature of the atom linked with a double bond to the phosphorus atom also affects the chemical nomenclature of the compound, with "thio" used in the chemical name to identify the S-containing phosphorothionate compounds. It is generally recognized that these phosphorothionate compounds are not active toxicants but rather protoxicants. Oxidation, which results in exchange of the doubly bonded sulfur for a doubly bonded oxygen, is necessary for conversion of the protoxicant phosphorothionate compounds to active neurotoxicants.

Organophosphates first gained notoriety during World War II, when they were synthesized by German chemists for use as highly toxic nerve gases. The potential for their use as chemical warfare agents continues today. However, other less volatile, less toxic organophosphates have since been synthesized, and these are used as insecticides, defoliants, herbicides, therapeutic agents in human and veterinary medicine (e.g., as ophthalmic agents and antiparasitics, respectively), flame retardants, fuel additives, lubricants, and plasticizers. They are in especially widespread use as insecticides, with formulations prepared for use in homes and gardens, on pets and livestock, and on crops and fields. Their popularity as insecticides is based on their effectiveness and on their biodegradability.

Examples of organophosphates include the insecticides malathion, parathion, diazinon, fenthion, azinphos methyl, terbufos, dichlorvos, and chlorpyrifos; the nerve gases soman, sarin, tabun, and VX; the ophthalmic agents echothiophate and isoflurophate; the anthelmintic trichlorfon; tricresyl phosphate-containing industrial chemicals; and the herbicides/defoliants DEF and merphos.

Most organophosphates are lipid soluble and all can be hydrolyzed, a reaction that results in detoxification. Some of them are gases or volatile liquids. These chemical properties contribute to their usefulness and to their toxicity by affecting their absorption and metabolism. Lipid-soluble substances more readily pass membrane barriers than compounds which are less lipid soluble, resulting in more complete absorption regardless of the route by which humans or animals are exposed. This lipid solubility aids the passage of organophosphate insecticides through the chitin exoskeleton of insects. Due to their lipid solubility, however, most organophosphates can pass through the skin of humans and animals as well, although the extent of absorption and the time in which it occurs varies from compound to compound. Volatility means that exposure to some organophosphates can be by inhalation, with absorption via the lungs. Organophosphates are esters, which means that they can be split into their component acid and an alcohol by the addition of water across the ester bond. This degradatory reaction (hydrolysis) occurs when organophosphates are in the presence of water and, in particular, in the presence of enzymes (esterases) that catalyze this reaction. That organophosphates are subject to hydrolysis increases the probability that they will biodegrade in the environment and that they will not accumulate in the environment or in the bodies of exposed subjects.

Organophosphate insecticides inhibit neural acetylcholinesterase, an enzyme responsible for the degradation of the neurotransmitter acetylcholine. This is the means by which they are effective as insecticides and the means by which they are toxic to humans and animals. Acetylcholine is a neurotransmitter found in the brain, spinal cord, and peripheral nervous system. In the peripheral nervous system, it is the neurotransmitter at effector organs of the parasympathetic nervous system, at ganglia of the autonomic nervous system (both sympathetic and parasympathetic ganglia), and at junctions between nerves and skeletal muscles. The presence of excess acetylcholine, due to inhibition of acetylcholinesterase, at muscarinic receptors (which are at the effector organs of the parasympathetic nervous system) results in clinical signs that include blurred vision due to pupil constriction, tearing, breathing difficulty due to excessive respiratory secretions, vomiting and diarrhea due to increased activity of the gastrointestinal tract, increased frequency of urination, and slowing of the heart rate. The presence of excess acetylcholine, due to inhibition of acetylcholinesterase, at nicotinic receptors found in autonomic ganglia can result in exaggeration of the effects seen by stimulation of parasympathetic muscarinic receptors and, in addition, can cause hypertension and tachycardia due to concurrent stimulation of the sympathetic nervous system. The presence of excess actylcholine at nicotinic receptors of neuromuscular junctions of skeletal muscles can result in muscle twitching, tremors, and cramps. This may be followed by muscle weakness and flaccid paralysis. Excess acetylcholine in the brain and spinal cord (central nervous system) may cause anxiety, restlessness, emotional instability, confusion, ataxia, weakness, convulsions, and/or coma. Death is usually due to respiratory failure, which may be the result of a combination of effects in the peripheral and central nervous systems. Some organophosphates are very toxic; others are not. Toxicity resulting from organophosphate exposure is dependent on the chemical structure, lipid solubility, formulation and formulation vehicle, dosage, and the absorption, distribution, metabolism, and excretion of the substance to which subjects are exposed.

The acetylcholinesterase enzyme contains two sites for binding of acetylcholine, its natural substrate. Organophosphates combine with one of these sites, called the esteratic site, preventing the attachment of acetylcholine. Treatment of acetylcholinesterase inhibition is directed toward protecting the acetylcholine receptor from excess neurotransmitter and toward removal of the organophosphate from the inhibited enzyme. Atropine competes with acetylcholine for the muscarinic receptors at which it acts in the parasympathetic nervous system; this drug is used to reduce symptoms associated with overstimulation of those receptors with the acetylcholine that accumulates as acetylcholinesterase is inhibited. Symptomatic treatment of organophosphate toxicity may also include diazepam, a tranquilizer and anticonvulsant. Oxime drugs (e.g., pralidoxime or 2-PAM) attach to the organophosphate itself, removing it from acetylcholinesterase. Oximes must be given in a relatively short time frame after exposures occur, however. Although initially reversible, with time the attachment between the organophosphate and the enzyme can become irreversible, a condition generally referred to as "aging." Once aging has occurred, treatment of toxicity with oximes is ineffective. Time is needed for synthesis of new acetylcholinesterase molecules before enzyme activities return to preexposure levels.

Prevention of organophosphate toxicity is aimed at protecting the acetylcholine receptor and/or acetylcholinesterase itself. Atropine can be used to prevent as well as to treat organophosphate poisonings. In addition, use of "reversible" inhibitors of acetylcholinesterase have been used to prevent organophosphate toxicity. The rationale behind use of such compounds (carbamates such as physostigmine) is that they occupy the site at which organophosphates could bind to acetylcholinesterase and, consequently, provide time for the organophosphate to be metabolized and excreted before sites become free for occupancy on acetylcholinesterase. Carbamates may actually be given after exposure to organophosphates, with the assumption made that absorption will take some time, so the carbamates can be used to occupy sites on acetylcholinesterase until the danger of further absorption of organophosphates is past. After sufficient time, the carbamate is withdrawn and the carbamylated enzyme is given time to spontaneously reactivate.

Esterases other than neural acetylcholinesterase may also be inhibited by organophosphates, although this is dependent on the compound and the species of animals exposed. These esterases include acetylcholinesterase of mammalian erythrocytes; pseudocholinesterases found primarily in nonneural sites, such as the liver and plasma; neurotoxic esterase (also known as neuropathy target esterase) found primarily in the nervous system; and carboxylesterases (also known as aliesterases), which are relatively nonspecific enzymes found in many cells, including those of the nervous system and liver. That organophosphates can inhibit esterases other than neural acetylcholinesterase provides opportunity to monitor exposure using red blood cell acetylcholinesterase and/or serum pseudocholinesterase as markers. Organophosphate-induced signs of toxicity generally only occur after significant inhibition of neural acetylcholinesterase or significant inhibition and aging of neurotoxic esterase; inhibition of pseudocholinesterases or carboxylesterases causes no apparent clinical signs. The organophosphates that inhibit neurotoxic esterase do not include commonly used insecticides; toxicity that follows inhibition of this enzyme differs considerably from that caused by inhibition of acetylcholinesterase. Weeks after exposure, humans and certain species of animals develop progressive degenerative changes that can be seen on microscopic examination of peripheral nerves and/or the spinal cord. This organophosphate-induced delayed neuropathy can result in incoordination, ataxia, and paralysis. Specific treatments for this disorder have not been developed (see Neurotoxicity, Delayed).

The capability of organophosphates to inhibit pseudocholinesterases and carboxylesterases without causing clinical signs provides a mechanism by which serial exposures to nontoxic dosages can result in toxicity. These enzymes provide sites additional to those on acetylcholinesterase at which organophosphates can attach, but once inhibited, they may not be available when humans or animals are exposed to organophosphates for a second time. Thus, more organophosphate is available to attach to acetylcholinesterase, resulting in toxicity at dosages that would not be toxic without prior exposure. Instead of the potentiation of toxicity seen with subsequent dosing as described previously, however, multiple administration of low dosages of organophosphates over a sufficient period of time may result in tolerance as receptors for acetylcholine become desensitized or downregulated. Metabolism of a compound may also increase with repeated exposure.

Due to their widespread use, especially as insecticides, exposure to organophosphates may be intentional, accidental, or environmental. Once exposure occurs, regardless whether the route is dermal, oral, or by inhalation, absorption is likely because organophosphates have considerable lipid solubility. This property also increases the potential that they will be generally distributed throughout the body, and that they will easily pass into the nervous system, where they exert their toxic effects. Many organophosphates, especially the insecticides, enter the body as S-containing phosphorothionate protoxicants. These protoxicants are readily activated to esterase inhibitors by mixed function oxidase enzymes of the liver. Organophosphates are metabolized by a variety of esterases, including those that they may inhibit (pseudocholinesterases, carboxylesterases, or other B-esterases) and those that they do not inhibit [arylesterases or A-esterases (also known as organophosphorus acid anhydrases, phosphohydrolases, phosphorotriester hydrolases)]; metabolites may be excreted in urine, feces, and milk. Organophosphates are readily hydrolyzed in aqueous solutions with high pH; therefore, soapy water is useful for decontamination of skin and clothing.

Although the primary mechanism of toxicity associated with exposure to organophosphates has to do with inhibition of acetylcholinesterase, signs can still occur after the cholinergic crisis has resolved. Such signs include the delayed neuropathy that can occur weeks after inhibition of neurotoxic esterase, an intermediate paralytic syndrome that may occur several days after severe acetylcholinesterase inhibition (see Organophosphate Poisoning, Intermediate Syndrome), muscle damage that may begin during the cholinergic crisis and which may develop into a myopathy that can reverse within weeks of exposure, and cardiotoxicities that may be part of or occur after the acute syndrome. Residual effects that may follow recovery from acetylcholinesterase inhibition, or effects that may occur as a result of repeated low-dose exposures that are insufficient to inhibit acetylcholinesterase in humans, have been reported to include anxiety, confusion, impairment of judgment, visual disturbances, behavioral changes, memory deficits, and incoordination. Certain organophosphates have also been reported to have immunotoxic or teratogenic effects.

Species differences in susceptibility to organophosphate toxicities are notable. For example, significant neurotoxic effects that remain after recovery of acetylcholinesterase activity have not been reported for studies performed in animals, but a number of reports suggest that a variety of long-lasting behavioral and functional changes could occur in some humans. Species differences in clinical manifestations of organophosphate-induced delayed neuropathy are also notable. Although locomotor difficulties occur in humans, hens, cats, sheep, cattle, and a variety of other species, they are not obvious in the rodent species commonly used for toxicity testing (rats and mice). Other species differences may be related to the pharmacokinetics (absorption, distribution, and clearance) of organophosphates. For example, insects, due to their small size and to their chitin exoskeleton (which does not provide an impediment to organophosphate insecticide absorption), are much more likely to succumb to organophosphate toxicity than are other animal species. Absorption also contributes to species differences among mammals. Cats are more likely to absorb organophosphates after exposure by the dermal route, and the propensity of this species to groom also increases the likelihood of oral exposure even when the original exposure was by the dermal route. Metabolic differences among species are a significant factor associated with species differences. Avians, for example, are more susceptible to organophosphate toxicity because they have less capability to hydrolyze these chemicals by enzymes that are not inhibited by the organophosphates (see A-esterase).

Pesticide assessment guidelines under the Federal Insecticide, Fungicide, and Rodenticide Act stipulate that organophosphates proposed for use as insecticides be tested both for their capability to cause acute toxicities due to inhibition of acetylcholinesterase and for their potential to cause inhibition of neurotoxic esterase and subsequent delayed neuropathy. Testing may be performed in laboratory rodents because they, like all species, are susceptible to acetylcholinesterase inhibition, but rodents do not develop notable ataxia, and neuropathological manifestations are very restricted if these species are exposed to organophosphates that cause delayed neuropathy. Testing for the toxicity of organophosphates includes, therefore, adult hens as the animal model for organophosphate-induced delayed neuropathy. Inhibition of neurotoxic esterase, ataxia, and neuropathy are detectable in hens, and the relationship between dosages causing acetylcholinesterase inhibition and delayed neuropathy can be determined.

Further Reading

Ballantyne, B., and Marrs, T. C. (1992). *Clinical and Experimental Toxicology of Organophosphates and Carbamates*. Butterworth-Heinemann, Oxford, UK.

Chambers, J. E., and Levi, P. E. (Eds.) (1992). *Organophosphates. Chemistry, Fate, and Effects.* Academic Press, San Diego.

Ecobichon, D. J., Davies, J. E., Doull, J., Ehrich, M., Joy, R., McMillan, D., MacPhail, R., Reiter, L. W., Slikker, W., Jr., and Tilson, H. (1990). Neurotoxic effects of pesticides. In *The Effects of Pesticides on Human Health* (S. R. Baker and C. F. Wilkinson, Eds.), pp. 131–199. Princeton Scientific, Princeton, NJ.

Extension Toxicology Network (EXTOXNET) (1994). *A Pesticide Information Project of Cooperative Extension Offices of Cornell University, The University of California, Michigan State University, and Oregon State University*. Cornell Distribution Center, Cornell University, Ithaca NY.

Gallo, M. A., and Lawryk, N. J. (1991). Organic phosphorus pesticides. In *Handbook of Pesticide Toxicology Vol. 2: Classes of Pesticides* (W. J. Hayes, Jr., and E. R. Laws, Jr., Eds.), pp. 917–1123. Academic Press, San Diego.

Manahan, S. E. (1992). *Toxicological Chemistry*, 2nd ed., pp. 401–414. Lewis, Boca Raton, FL.

Marrs, T. C. (1993). Organophosphate poisoning. *Pharmacol. Ther.* **58**, 51–66.

U.S. EPA (1989). *Recognition and Management of Pesticide Poisonings*, 4th ed. EPA Health Effects Division, Office of Pesticide Programs, Washington, DC.

U.S. EPA (1991). *Pesticide Assessment Guidelines*, Subdivision E. Hazard evaluation: Human and domestic animals. Addendum 10: Neurotoxicity, Series 81, 82, and 83. EPA Office of Prevention, Pesticides and Toxic Substances, Washington DC. EPA 540/09–91–123. Available from NTIS, Springfield, VA, PB91-154617.

—Marion Ehrich

Related Topics

Anticholinergics
Carbamate Pesticides
Carboxylesterases
Behavioral Toxicology
Cholinesterase Inhibition
Federal Insecticide, Fungicide, and Rodenticide Act
Nerve Gases
Neurotoxicity, Delayed
Neurotoxicology: Central and Peripheral
Organochlorine Insecticides

Organophosphate Poisoning, Intermediate Syndrome
Organotins
Psychological Indices of Toxicity

Organotins

The organotins comprise a large class of organometallic compounds containing one or more Sn atoms bound covalently to one or more carbon-containing moieties (R groups), which can be either alkyl or aryl groups. Because Sn may take on either a +2 or +4 valence state, up to four R groups may replace inorganic anions, yielding mono-, di-, tri-, and tetra-substituted organotin compounds. As of 1982, 259 organotin compounds were described in the *CRC Handbook of Chemistry and Physics;* this variety far exceeds that of any other metal, including mercury, lead, arsenic, and germanium. The large number of organotin compounds attests to their broad utility as industrial catalysts and stabilizers, as preservatives in construction material, and as agricultural and marine pesticides. More than 1000 patents have been granted for organotin stabilizer formulations alone, and approximately 25,000 metric tons of organotin compounds have been used annually in the United States since the middle of the twentieth century. A major use of organotins involves stabilization of polyvinyl chloride plastics during heated polymerization and catalysis of the polymerization of urethane foams; a variety of dibutyl and dioctyl tin derivatives are used for these purposes. Pesticidal usage relies primarily on trialkyl and triaryl tins, which provide effective rodent repellents, fungicides, insecticides, and molluscicides; bis(tri-*n*-butyltin) oxide (TBTO) is used as a preservative for wood, paper, leather, and textiles.

Exposure to organotins may occur occupationally during manufacturing processes or during application of biocidal agents containing the compounds. The general public may also receive exposure from this latter route (e.g., during spray application of paints and wood preservatives). In addition, significant leaching of tin stabilizers from plastic packaging into foodstuffs has been demonstrated; thus, the U.S. FDA closely regulates the use of organotins in the manufacture of these materials. Again, plastic tubing used for medical procedures may also contain organotin stabilizers, leachates of which may gain entry directly into the body. Finally, inorganic tin may be biomethylated by microflora in marine and estuarine sediments.

In contrast to the low toxicity of inorganic tin salts, the toxic properties of organotins have been recognized since their discovery in the latter part of the nineteenth century. Investigation of the mammalian toxicology of organotins was spurred by several case reports of severe reactions to inhalation of trimethyltin vapors and by the "Stalinon" disaster in France in 1954. In this latter episode, preparations of inorganic tin, designed for the treatment of skin disorders, were contaminated with diethyltin and triethyltin. More than 100 people died and a similar number were disabled after taking this medication.

Subsequent studies of the toxicity of organotins have provided several generalizations based on the chemical characteristics of the compounds. First, organotins primarily affect the nervous system, the immune system, and the skin, with less dramatic effects on the liver and kidneys. Second, the toxicity of organotins tends to increase with the number of organic ligands. For example, trialkyl forms appear to be the most toxic of the alkyl tins, and tetraalkyl tins are metabolically dealkylated to trialkyl forms. Further dealkylation to the dialkyl and monoalkyl forms probably does not occur in mammals. Third, toxicity tends to decrease with increasing size and complexity of the R group because of reduced penetration into target organs with increasing chain length and because tetraalkyl compounds with large alkyl groups are less readily dealkylated than those with small alkyl groups. Thus for example, dioctyltin or triphenyltin are not readily absorbed from the gut, whereas trimethyltin and triethyltin are absorbed with high efficiency. Furthermore, tetraethyl tin is rapidly converted to triethyltin, whereas tetrabutyltin is slowly converted to tributyltin. Fourth, the anionic component contributes to the toxicity of the compound by affecting its volatility and solubility in water; those compounds more soluble and volatile will naturally gain access to target organs in preference to those less so. Fifth, among the highly toxic trialkyltins, the primary target of toxicity appears to be the nervous system for trimethyltin and triethyltin, whereas the immune, renal, and hepatic systems are more sensitive to tripropyltin and tributyltin. The only aryltin with documented toxicity is triphenyltin, whose actions resemble those of tributyltin.

The neurotoxicity of trialkyltins has been well studied, using primarily trimethyltin and triethyltin. These highly toxic compounds are not used commercially but have proven to be useful tools for the study of the nervous system and its response to organotins. Trimethyltin (TMT) is readily absorbed by any route and readily penetrates the central nervous system (CNS), where it destroys neurons. Like other alkyltins, it appears to interfere with cellular and mitochondrial respiration; for unknown reasons its target cells tend to be large pyramidal neurons. Damage is most prominent in the hippocampus but can be detected in many regions of the CNS and spinal cord as well. Because the affected cells die and are not replaced, many functional changes caused by TMT (including emotional disorders, cognitive dysfunction, and hearing loss) are permanent. Like TMT, triethyltin (TET) is also neurotoxic; however, its primary target cells are the neuroglia, which generate the myelin sheath surrounding the axons of large neurons in the CNS. Thus, TET toxicity involves cerebral edema and demyelination as opposed to neuronal cell loss. Because these effects are reversible, recovery after TET intoxication is more likely than after TMT intoxication. Damage to the peripheral nervous system has not been reported following alkyltin intoxication.

The primary toxic effect of higher chain-length alkyltins in mammals involves immune suppression. For example, TBTO in the diet of rats has been shown to cause atrophy of the thymus and lymphoid organs, to deplete stores of iron in the spleen, to reduce hormonal activity of the pituitary–thyroid axis, and to decrease resistance to bacterial and parasitic infections. In rats, thymic atrophy also follows from dietary exposure to diphenyltin and triphenyltin and to dialkyltins with alkyl chains of length 2, 3, and 8, but not to alkyltins with chain lengths of 12 or 18.

All of the common low-weight organotins are potent irritants to the skin and mucous membranes, and even brief contact will cause severe chemical burns and dermatosis. Despite high acute toxicity, no organotins appear to be carcinogenic. Indeed, some evidence exists for a potential therapeutic role for organotin compounds in the diagnosis and treatment of tumors.

Further Reading

Aschner, M., and Aschner, J. L. (1992). Cellular and molecular effects of trimethyltin and triethyltin: Relevance to organotin neurotoxicity. *Neurosc. Biobehav. Rev.* **16,** 427–535.

McMillan, D. E., and Wenger, G. E. (1985). Neurobehavioral toxicology of trialkyltins. *Pharmacol. Rev.* **37,** 365–378.

Piver, W. T. (1973). Organotin compounds: Industrial applications and biological investigation. *Environ. Health Perspect.* **1,** 61–79.

Thayer, J. S. (1984). *Organometallic Compounds and Living Organisms.* Academic Press, Orlando, FL.

Tilson, H. A., and Sparber, S. B. (1987). *Neurotoxicants and Neurobiological Function: Effects of Organoheavy Metals.* Wiley-Interscience, New York.

Winship, K. A. (1988). Toxicity of tin and its compounds. *Adverse Drug Reactions Poisoning Rev.* **7,** 19–38.

—Philip J. Bushnell

(The research described in this entry has been reviewed by the Health Effects Research Laboratory, U.S. EPA and approved for publication. Approval does not signify that the contents necessarily reflect the views and policies of the agency nor does mention of trade names or commercial products constitute endorsement or recommendation for use.)

Related Topics

Metals
Neurotoxicology: Central and Peripheral
Pesticides

Oxygen

- CAS: 7782-44-7
- Chemical Class: Elemental gas (symbol O)
- Molecular Formula: O_2

Uses

Oxygen produces flame for welding and lighting. It is also used in the production of fuels. Therapeutically, it is used to relieve hypoxia and as a component of the gas mixture for respiratory support.

Exposure Pathway
Inhalation is the route of exposure.

Toxicokinetics
Toxicity occurs at elevated pressures (e.g., deep sea diving). The latent period is 2 hr at 3 atm and 30 min at 4 atm. It rapidly equilibrates with external atmosphere.

Mechanism of Toxicity
Oxidation is a mechanism of toxicity. Oxygen is essential for life in appropriate ranges of pressure and concentration.

Human Toxicity
The human TC_{Lo} is 100 pph/14-hr exposure. Concentrations of over 60% cause respiratory/pulmonary irritation, reduce vital capacity, and cause substernal distress. Oxygen poisoning causes nervousness, muscular twitch, hilarity, convulsions, or unconsciousness.

Clinical Management
In cases of pulmonary irritation, the O_2 concentration should be reduced to 60% or less. With O_2 poisoning, the O_2 concentration should be reduced to 200 mm/kg.

Animal Toxicity
Mutation was observed in the lungs of hamsters at oxygen concentrations of 95 pph.

—Shayne C. Gad and Jayne E. Ash

Related Topic

Respiratory tract

Ozone

- CAS: 10028-15-6
- SYNONYM: Triatomic oxygen
- CHEMICAL CLASS: Elemental gas
- MOLECULAR FORMULA: O_3

Uses
Ozone is used as a disinfectant for air and water. It is also used as a bleaching agent.

Exposure Pathways
Inhalation and exposure to mucous membranes are possible exposure routes.

Toxicokinetics
Ozone rapidly reacts, resulting in full oxygen.

Mechanism of Toxicity
Ozone is an oxidizing agent.

Human Toxicity
Exposure to high concentrations of ozone may cause severe irritation of the eyes or the respiratory tract. Insufficient atmospheric ozone reduces protection against ultraviolet radiation from the sun. The TC_{Lo} is 50 ppm. The ACGIH TLV is 0.1 ppm.

Clinical Management
The victim should be removed from exposure.

Animal Toxicity
Ozone is a mutagen, carcinogen, irritant, and reproductive toxicant in experimental animals. The LC_{50} in rats is 4.8 ppm.

Shayne C. Gad and Jayne E. Ash

Related Topics

Pollution, Air
Pollution, Water

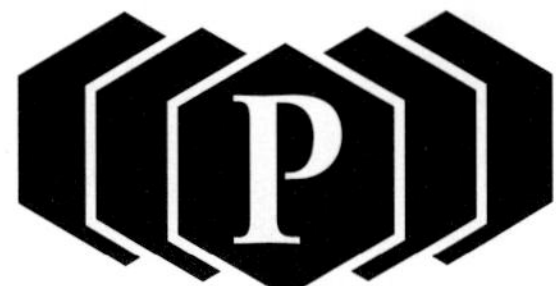

Paraquat

- CAS: 1910-42-5 (dichloride)
- SYNONYMS: Paraquat dichloride; methyl viologen; 1,1′-dimethyl-4,4′-bipyridinium ion; Gramoxone
- CHEMICAL CLASS: Quaternary nitrogen (bis pyridinium) compound
- CHEMICAL STRUCTURE:

$CH_3-{}^{+}N$ … $N^{+}-CH_3$

Use

Paraquat is used as a broad-spectrum herbicide.

Exposure Pathways

Accidental or intentional ingestion is the most common route of exposure. Poisonings from inhalation and dermal exposure have also occurred.

Toxicokinetics

Paraquat has low but rapid gastrointestinal absorption (5–10%) and low skin absorption. Peak plasma concentrations occur in less than 2 hr following ingestion. Generally, paraquat is not metabolized to any large extent. In animal studies, metabolites have been detected in urine, possibly resulting from the action of intestinal microflora. Paraquat is actively transported to alveolar cells, where it is reduced to form highly reactive free radicals. The volume of distribution is large and has been estimated at 2.75 liters/kg. Paraquat tends to attain higher and more prolonged levels in the lung. Clearance is rapid by the kidneys with 80–90% of the dose excreted in the urine after 6 hr. The terminal half-life increases from 12 to 120 hr or longer as renal failure begins.

Mechanism of Toxicity

Paraquat produces lung damage by all routes of exposure. Progressive and generalized proliferation of fibrous connective tissue is observed in the pulmonary alveoli where paraquat is selectively concentrated. While the exact mechanism remains to be elucidated, lipid peroxidation is believed to result from free radical formation by a cyclic single reduction–oxidation of paraquat. Superoxide radicals are formed and attack unsaturated lipids of cell membranes. This in turn produces lipid free radicals, resulting in membrane damage and loss of the functional integrity of the cell.

Human Toxicity: Acute

Paraquat may result in severe toxicity to all organ systems and death within 24 hr after ingestion, inhalation, and dermal exposure. The initial symptoms after ingestion are burning in the mouth and throat with vomiting and diarrhea and subsequent fluid and electrolyte loss. Depending on the dose (≧60 ml), esophageal perforation, renal failure, cardiac arrhythmias, convulsions, and coma can occur. Early death is usually due to hepatic and renal toxicity.

Human Toxicity: Chronic

Survivors of the initial poisoning or from poisonings from as little as 10–15 ml of the concentrate often develop a progressive pulmonary fibrosis associated with dyspnea and pulmonary edema several days or weeks after exposure. As a result, death is due to asphyxia. The lethal dose in humans is estimated to be about 40 mg/kg.

Clinical Management

No specific treatment is known. All cases of paraquat exposure should be managed as a potentially fatal exposure. Basic life-support measures should be instituted; however, the administration of supplemental oxygen is not advised. Treatment must be instituted early, within 10 hr after ingestion. Treatment involves removal of paraquat from the alimentary tract by gastric lavage and cathartics, prevention of further absorption by Fuller's earth (30% w/v), and removal of absorbed paraquat by hemodialysis or hemoperfusion. Use of various drugs, such as *d*-propranolol, prednisone, and vitamins E and C, has provided little benefit.

Animal Toxicity

Signs of toxicity in animals are similar to those in humans. The oral and dermal LD_{50} values reported in rats and mice range from about 20 to 150 mg/kg. Paraquat has been shown to be mutagenic, carcinogenic, and teratogenic in experimental animals.

Further Reading

Ecobichon, D. J. (1991). Toxic effects of pesticides. In *Casarett and Doull's Toxicology* (M. O. Amdur, J. Doull, and C. D. Klaassen, Eds.), 4th ed., pp. 602–603. Pergamon, New York.

Stevens, J. T., and Sumner, D. D. (1991). Herbicides. In *Handbook of Pesticide Toxicology* (W. J. Hayes, Jr., and E. R. Laws, Jr., Eds.), Vol. 3, 1356–1376.. Academic Press, San Diego.

—Kevin N. Baer

Related Topics

Lipid Peroxidation
Pesticides
Pollution, Water
Respiratory Tract

Parathion

- CAS: 56-38-2
- SYNONYMS: Bayer E-605; Corthion; *O,O*-diethyl-O-(*p*-nitrophenyl) phosphorothioate; diethyl 4-nitrophenyl phosphorothionate; DNTP; DDPP; ethyl parathion; nitrostigine; paraphos; pethion; sulphos; thiophos
- CHEMICAL CLASS: Organophosphate insecticide
- CHEMICAL STRUCTURE:

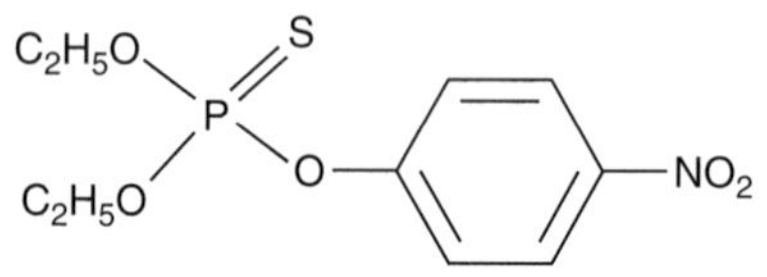

Use

Parathion is an effective insecticide for a range of insect pests.

Exposure Pathways

Fatal poisonings have occurred after oral, dermal, and inhalation exposure to parathion. The vapor pressure of the pure compound is generally not sufficient to cause respiratory exposure alone. Fine dusts or aerosol preparations may allow severe poisoning through the respiratory route, however.

Toxicokinetics

Parathion is efficiently absorbed through any route of exposure. Signs of toxicity due to parathion generally appear within several hours following dermal exposure. The rate of dermal absorption in rabbits was found to be 0.059 $\mu g/min/cm^2$. There is considerable individual variation in dermal absorption rates in animals and humans. About 0.1–2.8% of the applied compound was absorbed through skin in human volunteers. The kinetics of absorption were studied in isolated perfused porcine skin flaps and the results suggested a linear, three-compartment model of absorption.

Parathion is preferentially distributed in the liver, the kidneys, and ordinary adipose tissue. It is also concentrated to a fairly high degree in gastric and intestinal walls, thyroid, spleen, and lungs. It can cross the blood–

brain barrier because of its nonpolar nature and it accumulates to a lesser extent in the central nervous system. Parathion is metabolized in the liver and other extrahepatic sites by the mixed function oxidase enzyme system to paraoxon, which is considerably more toxic than the parent compound. The conversion of parathion to paraoxon requires the presence of NADPH and oxygen. The sulfur atom released in the metabolism of parathion to paraoxon may bind to and inactivate the cytochrome P450 enzyme, resulting in progressive impairment of parathion metabolism. Parathion is also metabolized to O-ethyl phosphoric acid, phosphoric acid, and inorganic sulfate.

Metabolites of parathion are exclusively eliminated through urine. However, some of the unmetabolized parent compound may also be excreted through sebum. The elimination half-life of parathion was found to be 2.1 days. It was reported that, following oral administration of parathion (1 or 2 mg/day) in humans, 60% of *p*-nitrophenol was excreted within 4 hr and 86% within 8 hr. The rate of excretion of diethyl phosphate was found to be slower than that of *p*-nitrophenol. Following dermal exposure of 5 g of a 2% dust for 2 hr, the *p*-nitrophenol concentration reached a peak level by 5 or 6 hr after initial exposure. In case of dermal exposure, the rate of excretion of the metabolites of parathion increases with temperature.

Mechanism of Toxicity

The mechanism of toxicity for parathion is similar to that of chlorpyrifos (see Chorpyrifos).

Human Toxicity

The toxic effects of parathion in humans are similar to those of chlorpyrifos (see Chorpyrifos).

Clinical Management

Oral Exposure

Induction of emesis is contraindicated in case of parathion poisoning due to the early onset of respiratory depression and seizures. Gastric lavage may be indicated if performed immediately after parathion ingestion. Activated charcoal/cathartic therapy may be adopted to retard the absorption from gastrointestinal tract. Atropine should be administered intravenously until atropinization is achieved. In adults, administer 2–5 mg/kg every 10–15 min and in children give 0.05 mg/kg at the same frequency. Atropinization may require several hours to days depending on the severity of poisoning. 2-PAM (Pralidoxime) may be combined with atropine in case of severe poisoning (adult, 1 or 2 g intravenously at 0.5 g/min; children, 25–50 mg/kg over 5–30 min). Seizures may be treated with conventional anticonvulsants (e.g., diazepam, phenobarbital, and phenytoin).

Inhalation Exposure

The affected person should be moved immediately to fresh air and should be administered with 100% humidified supplemental oxygen with assisted ventilation.

Eye Exposure

Exposed eyes should be irrigated with copious amount of tepid water for 15 min. If irritation, photophobia, pain, or swelling persists, the patient should be admitted to a health care facility.

Dermal Exposure

The contaminated clothing should be removed and the contaminated area of the skin should be washed repeatedly with soapy water.

Animal Toxicity

The acute oral toxicity of parathion varies from about 2 to 30 mg/kg, depending on the species and route of exposure. Sex-related differences in sensitivity to parathion were observed in rats (i.e., female rats are more sensitive than male rats). It is reported that estrogen treatment increases the susceptibility of male rats, whereas administration of androgens decreases the sensitivity of female rats to parathion.

—*Tamal Kumar Chakraborti*

Related Topics

A-Esterase
Carboxylesterases
Neurotoxicity, Delayed
Organophosphate Poisoning, Intermediate Syndrome
Organophosphates
Pollution, Water
Psychological Indices of Toxicity

Paregoric

- Synonyms: Opium; opium tincture; hydrochloride of opium alkaloids
- Pharmaceutical Class: Paregoric is an opium preparation. It is composed of several alkaloids, including anhydrous morphine (9.5% or more) and smaller amounts of codeine and papaverine.

Uses

Paregoric affects the gastrointestinal tract by inhibiting motility and propulsion and increasing smooth muscle tone. Therefore, it has been used as an antidiarrheal agent. It also decreases digestive secretions.

Exposure Pathway

Paregoric is usually taken orally.

Toxicokinetics

Paregoric is well absorbed from the gastrointestinal tract. Peak serum levels are detectable approximately 1 hr after ingestion. Opium preparations are metabolized in the liver by demethylation. Morphine undergoes conjugation with glucoronic acid at the 3-hydroxyl group. Secondary conjugation may also occur at the 6-hydroxyl group to form 3,6-diglucuronide. Paregoric is 34–37.5% protein bound. The volume of distribution is 3 or 4 liters/kg. From 8.5 to 12% is excreted unchanged in the urine, 7 to 10% excreted in feces as glucuronide conjugate, and 7 to 10% in the bile. The half-life is 1.9–2.6 hr.

Mechanism of Toxicity

Opium and its derivatives cause depression of the central nervous system (CNS) and respiratory depression.

Human Toxicity: Acute

Paregoric produces CNS depression ranging from drowsiness to coma. These symptoms may be cyclic due to decreased gastric emptying. Respiratory depression occurs and may progress to Cheyne–Stokes respirations, cyanosis, and respiratory arrest. Pulmonary edema may also be noted. Cardiac status may be compromised by bradycardia, hypotension, circulatory collapse, and cardiac arrest. Other symptoms include hypothermia, cold and clammy skin, flaccid skeletal muscles.

Human Toxicity: Chronic

Chronic use may produce psychological and physical dependence. Discontinuation of paregoric causes withdrawal symptoms.

Clinical Management

Life-support measures should be provided. Gastric decontamination with activated charcoal may be effective in recent ingestions. Respiratory and CNS depression may be counteracted with naloxone. Naloxone administration may precipitate the opioid withdrawal syndrome.

Animal Toxicity

Cats and horses experience excitability and increased CNS effects. Dogs exhibit drowsiness, ataxia, seizures, coma, respiratory depression, hypotension, and vomiting. Treatment consists of decontaminating the gastrointestinal tract, maintaining the airway, administering naloxone, and controlling seizures with diazepam and/or phenobarbital. Hypotension may be counteracted with use of intravenous fluids. If ineffective, norepinephrine is the drug of choice. Dopamine and dobutamine can also be used. Monitoring needs to be provided for at least 8 hr after cessation of symptoms since relapse can occur.

—Regina M. Rogowski

Related Topic

Veterinary Toxicology

Penicillin

- Synonyms: Amoxicillin; ampicillin; azlocillin; bacampacillin; carbenicillin; cloxacillin;

dicloxacillin; methicillin; mezlocillin; nafcillin; oxacillin; penicillin G; penicillin V; piperacillin; ticarcillin

- ♦ Pharmaceutical Class: Antibiotic

Use

Penicillin is used to treat infections caused by gram-positive cocci, gram-negative aerobic cocci, and anaerobic bacteria.

Exposure Pathways

Penicillin is available in tablet and suspension form for oral use and in injectable form for intravenous and intramuscular use. Ingestion of tablets and the suspension forms are the most common poisoning exposures.

Toxicokinetics

Following oral administration, absorption of penicillins occurs mainly in the duodenum and upper jejunum, with a small percentage absorbed in the stomach. The extent of absorption is variable and depends on several factors including the penicillin derivative, the dosage form administered, gastric and intestinal pH, and the presence of food in the gastrointestinal tract. Peak concentrations are generally seen within 1 or 2 hr. Protein binding and the volume of distribution vary with each derivative. Following absorption from either the gastrointestinal tract or from injection sites, penicillins are widely distributed into most body tissues. Most penicillins and their microbiologically active metabolites are excreted primarily unchanged in the urine by renal tubular secretion. Nonrenal elimination includes hepatic inactivation and biliary excretion. Renal clearance of penicillins is delayed in the neonate due to an immature tubular secretion mechanism. Children older than 3 months generally excrete drugs similarly to adults. Excretion is also delayed in geriatric patients because of diminished tubular secretion ability. Patients with renal impairment may also have altered tubular secretion ability and, therefore, have higher and more prolonged serum concentrations of penicillins.

The rate of absorption from parenteral administration depends on the dose, concentration, and solubility of the particular salt being administered. The elimination half-life depends on the derivative, but ranges from 0.5 to 2.5 hr in the parent compound.

Mechanism of Toxicity

The primary toxic manifestations of penicillin overdose are due to inability of renal excretion due to age, kidney disease, or anaphylaxis.

Human Toxicity

Hypersensitivity reactions may follow exposure to any amount of penicillins and could result in anaphylaxis. Acute ingestion of large amounts of penicillins ($\geqq$250 mg/kg) in children less than 6 years of age may result in nausea, vomiting, diarrhea, and abdominal pain. Acute oliguric renal failure, hematuria, and crystalluria have been reported. Intravenous use of penicillin in doses exceeding 10 million units may cause seizures and coma. Cardiac conduction defects have occurred after rapid infusion of potassium penicillin G and procaine penicillin G. Electrolyte abnormalities have been associated with large doses of potassium and sodium salts. Toxicity associated with chronic ingestions is expected to be similar.

Clinical Management

Acute ingestion mandates gastric decontamination and administration of activated charcoal. Urinalysis, renal function tests, and evaluation of electrolytes may be indicated in large exposures. In chronic ingestion, activated charcoal may be beneficial if there has been recent ingestion. In all cases, regardless of the route of exposure, the mainstay of therapy is supportive care and discontinuation of the drug. Dialysis has rarely been needed. Ocular exposures necessitate thorough irrigation with water for 15 min. Anaphylaxis is treated with supportive care and the administration of epinephrine and diphenhydramine.

Animal Toxicity

Toxic amounts of penicillin in animals are not established.

—Brenda Swanson Biearman

Pentachloronitrobenzene

- ♦ CAS: 82-68-8
- ♦ Preferred Name: Quintozene (BSI, ISO)

- SYNONYMS: Avicol; Brassicol; Folosan; Terraclor; Tilcarex; Tritisan
- CHEMICAL CLASS: Chlorinated nitrobenzenoid fungicide
- CHEMICAL STRUCTURE:

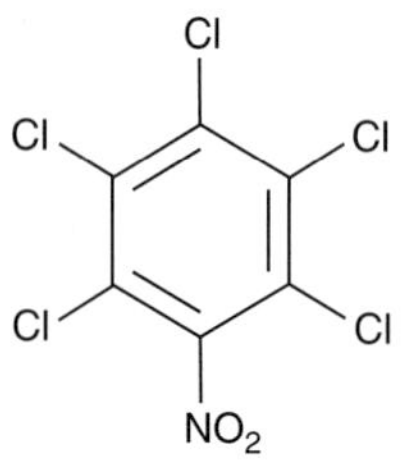

Cl Cl Cl Cl Cl NO_2

Use

Quintozene is used as a fungicide on seed and soil.

Exposure Pathways

Dermal, oral, and inhalation exposures are possible.

Toxicokinetics

Quintozene is poorly absorbed from the gastrointestinal tract in rats. In contrast, it is well absorbed from the gastrointestinal tract in monkeys. Quintozene is rapidly metabolized both in rats and in monkeys. The main metabolite of quintozene is pentachloroaniline. In rats, unabsorbed quintozene following oral exposure is excreted in the feces and the metabolites of quintozene are primarily excreted in the urine. In monkeys, metabolites of quintozene are mainly excreted in the bile.

Mechanism of Toxicity

Quintozene is an irritant. Nitrobenzenoid and anilino fungicides are also methemoglobinemic agents.

Human Toxicity

Responses to dermally applied quintozene included erythema, itching, edema, and the formation of small vesicles. Conjunctivitis occurs with ocular exposure.

Clinical Management

Treatment is symptomatic.

Animal Toxicity

The oral LD_{50} value of quintozene in rats is about 1.5 g/kg. Dogs are somewhat resistant. Quintozene can cause hepatotoxicity and liver tumors in mice. Oral administration of quintozene causes methemoglobinemia and Heinz body formation in erythrocytes. No effects on reproduction were observed in rats that received quintozene orally.

—Jing Liu

Pentachlorophenol

- CAS: 87-86-5
- SYNONYMS: PCP; penchlorol; penta; pentacon; penwar; Dowicide EC-7
- CHEMICAL CLASS: Halogenated phenol
- CHEMICAL STRUCTURE:

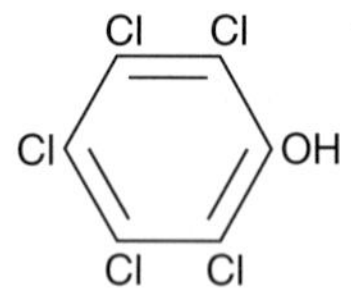

Cl Cl Cl OH Cl Cl

Uses

Pentachlorophenol is used as an insecticide, herbicide, and fungicide. It also has a major application as a wood preservative.

Exposure Pathway

Dermal contact is the most frequent route of exposure and the majority of poisonings are occupational in origin.

Toxicokinetics

Pentachlorophenol is readily and almost completely absorbed through the skin and gastrointestinal tract. The majority of the compound is excreted primarily unchanged in the urine, although glucuronide conjugates have been detected. In humans, there is conflicting evidence as to whether pentachlorophenol is metabolized in the liver to any significant extent. One metabolite, tetrachlorohydroquinone, was produced in human liver homogenates and was detected in the urine of exposed workers, while in other studies no metabolites were found. Pentachlorophenol is well distributed throughout the tissues, with high concentrations found in the urine, liver, and kidneys. Greater than 90% in blood is bound to serum proteins. The kidney is the primary route of elimination with about 80% excreted in the urine and a smaller amount in the feces. In humans, discrepancies exist concerning the elimination half-life with values ranging from 10 hr to 20 days. Although the exact reasons are not known for the long half-lives, high protein binding with tubular reabsorption and possible enterohepatic circulation may be contributing factors.

Mechanism of Toxicity

Pentachlorophenol increases metabolic rate and elevates body temperature by uncoupling oxidative phosphorylation in tissues. The circulatory system and heart are particularly affected.

Human Toxicity: Acute

Characteristic symptoms of poisoning are extremely high body temperature and profuse sweating. In fatal cases, rapid pulse, coma, heart failure, and death can occur within 3–30 hr after initial symptoms appear. Symptoms in nonfatal poisonings include weakness, gastrointestinal upset, headache, dizziness, and seizures. Pentachlorophenol is a potent skin, eye, and upper respiratory tract irritant.

Human Toxicity: Chronic

Chloracne has been reported in chronic occupational exposure to pentachlorophenol. However, commercial preparations are commonly contaminated with dioxins and furans, and chloracne may be linked to these compounds. In addition, hemolytic and aplastic anemia and weight loss have been reported in humans.

Clinical Management

Rapid decontamination is important, especially with skin exposure. The primary treatment is supportive and symptomatic and consists of promoting heat loss, reducing anxiety, and replacing fluids and electrolytes lost during sweating. Following oral exposure, emesis, activated charcoal, and cathartics are recommended. Administration of salicylates to reduce the high body temperature is contraindicated. Single-exchange transfusions have been successfully performed in infants poisoned by pentachlorophenol.

Animal Toxicity

The acute oral LD_{50} value for pentachlorophenol in rats, mice, and rabbits is about 30–200 mg/kg. Dermal LD_{50} values in rats are somewhat higher (about 100–300 mg/kg). Pentachlorophenol has been demonstrated to be fetotoxic, mutagenic, and carcinogenic in experimental animals.

—Kevin N. Baer

Pentane

- Synonyms: Pentane (ACGIH, NIOSH, OSHA, DOT); pentan (Polish); pentanen (Dutch); pentani (Italian); UN1265 (DOT)
- Chemical Class: Aliphatic hydrocarbon (C_5)
- Molecular Formula: C_5H_{12}
- Description: Pentane is a colorless, flammable liquid (the first liquid member of the alkanes) that is lighter than water. It has a pleasant odor that can be detected at 900 ppm. It occurs as two other isomers, including isopentane [$(CH_3)_2CHCH_2CH_3$] and neopentane [$C(CH_3)_4$].

Uses

Pentane is present in volatile petroleum fractions and is used as a fuel; in the production of ammonia, olefin, and hydrogen; in the manufacture of ice; in low-temperature thermometers; as a blowing agent for plastics and foams; and in solvent extraction processes. Neopentane is important in the manufacture of rubber.

Exposure Pathways

As pentane may exist as a vapor or liquid at normal temperature and pressure, exposure would be expected to occur either by inhalation or dermal contact. Oral ingestion would be expected to be incidental or accidental. Typical background concentrations that have been detected in major cities within the United States range from 0.05 to 0.35 ppm.

Mechanism of Toxicity

As seen with other short-chain alkanes, upon inhalation, pentane is moderately toxic and may cause irritation of the respiratory tract and narcosis. The narcotic action of pentane (observed in 1 hr at 90,000–120,000 ppm) is, however, much less pronounced than effects seen following exposure to the C1–C4 alkanes. Although the actual biochemical mechanism of toxicity has not been discerned, the narcotic effects seen are most likely related to its physical solvent properties. The effect is similar to the "high" experienced upon exposure to other aliphatic hydrocarbon solvents.

Human Toxicity

Human exposure for 10 min at 5000 ppm does not cause any adverse effects or irritation of mucous membranes. In humans, lethal effects have been observed in estimated air concentrations of 130,000 ppm; the lowest concentration known to cause a toxic effect is 90,000 ppm. Some studies have implicated pentane as a neurotoxicant, but these study results are confounded by the presence of other compounds in the mixture. NIOSH recommends a workplace standard of 350 mg/m^3 (120 ppm) for the C5–C8 alkanes, and a STEL of 1800 mg/m^3 (610 ppm). ACGIH suggests a workplace environmental standard of 1770 mg/m^3 (600 ppm) and an STEL of 750 mg/m^3 (2210 ppm). Pentane is also highly flammable and is therefore an explosion and/or fire hazard. The upper and lower explosive limits are 1.5 and 7.8% by volume, respectively.

Clinical Management

Persons exposed to high concentrations should vacate or be removed from the source of the liquid or vapor and seek fresh air. Extreme care must be taken to keep areas of high concentration free from ignition sources, such as sparks from static electricity and use of explosionproof apparatus.

Animal Toxicity

Pentane exposure in dogs will sensitize the heart to epinephrine. Narcosis (some authors use the term anesthesia) has been observed in mice at air concentrations ranging from 66,000 to 120,000 ppm, with death occurring at a concentration of 128,000 ppm after 37 min. In rats, air concentrations of 10.4, 50.9, and 94.7 mg/m^3 resulted in brain damage in the offspring. As with other aliphatic hydrocarbons, studies have shown that pentane can be utilized by certain microorganisms as a nutrient.

—Stephen Clough

Pentazocine

- CAS: 359-83-1
- Synonyms: Algopent; Fortal; Fortalgesic; Fortral; Fortralin; Fortwin; Pentalgina; Sosegon; Talwin NX; Talwin
- Pharmaceutical Class: Synthetic opiate partial antagonist analgesic, pharmacologically similar to butorphanol and nalbuphine.

Uses

Pentazocine is used as an analgesic and weak opiate antagonist.

Exposure Pathways

Pentazocine is available in oral and parenteral dosage forms. Exposures occur with ingestion or injection of solubilized tablets.

Toxicokinetics

Oral absorption is slow and at times incomplete. The onset of action can be seen in 15–30 min, but peak blood levels occur at 1–3 hr. Following parenteral administration, the onset of effects can be observed in 2 or 3 min with peak serum levels at 30 min. Pentazocine is largely metabolized in the liver to pentazocine glucuronide. Metabolites detected include *cis*-hydroxypentazocine (11.6%) and *trans*-carboxypentazocine (38.9%). Protein binding is 61%. The volume of distribution is 4.4–7.8 liters/kg. From 60 to 70% is excreted unchanged in the urine. The half-life ranges from 2 to 6 hr.

Mechanism of Toxicity

Pentazocine is a narcotic agonist and a partial antagonist. It produces an analgesic effect by stimulating the κ and σ opioid receptors. It blocks dopamine receptors and increases norepinephrine turnover. Pentazocine is also a γ-aminobutyric acid antagonist that potentially increases the potential for seizures.

Human Toxicity: Acute

Acute toxicity is often an extension of adverse pharmacologic effects. Central nervous system (CNS) effects include dizziness, anxiety, hallucinations, mood alterations, and seizures. Respiratory effects, depression, decreased respiratory rate, increased $PaCO_2$ levels, and apnea may occur. Tachycardia, increased systolic and diastolic blood pressure, pinpoint pupils, nausea, vomiting, and abdominal pain are common.

Human Toxicity: Chronic

Psychological and physical dependence may occur. Tolerance may develop, resulting in the need for higher and more frequent dosing. Oral preparations contain a small amount of naloxone (an opiate antagonist) to reduce parenteral abuse. However, the naloxone does not affect the efficacy of pentazocine administered via the oral route. Since pentazocine can produce dependence, abrupt withdrawal may precipitate the withdrawal syndrome. Pentazocine may be abused as a heroin alternative in a combination known as "Ts and Blues" (Talwin and blue-colored pyribenzamine tablets) in a ratio of two pentazocine tablets and one pyribenzamine tablet. They are dissolved and injected intravenously. With the advent of Talwin NX (naloxone), this type of abuse is unlikely in the United States.

Clinical Management

Cardiac and respiratory stabilization are the first priorities, followed by gastric decontamination with gastric lavage and/or activated charcoal if the tablets are ingested. Naloxone can be used to reverse respiratory and CNS depression. Naloxone administration may precipitate the opioid withdrawal syndrome in acute or chronic cases. However, opioid withdrawal is not life-threatening.

Animal Toxicity

In cases of acute exposure, dogs have experienced mild to moderate salivation, slight transient ataxia, fine tremors, and (infrequently) tonic convulsions. Horses, following intravenous administration, have experienced slight to moderate ataxia, localized muscular twitching, slight perspiration, unsteady gait, excitability, and nervousness.

—*Regina M. Rogowski*

Perchloric Acid

- CAS: 7601-90-3.
- Chemical Class: Halogenated acid
- Chemical Structure:

$$O{=}\overset{\overset{\displaystyle O}{\|}}{\underset{\underset{\displaystyle O}{\|}}{Cl}}{-}OH$$

Uses

Perchloric acid is used to separate potassium from sodium. The salts are used for explosives and plating metals.

Exposure Pathway

Contact with skin and mucous membranes is the exposure pathway.

Mechanism of Toxicity

Perchloric acid's corrosive properties and ability to cause tissue oxidation are mechanisms of toxicity.

Human Toxicity

Perchloric acid is corrosive to skin and mucous membranes. The estimated human lethal dose is 1 ml.

Clinical Management

Exposed body surfaces should be washed thoroughly. Treatment is the same as for exposure to any strong inorganic acid.

Animal Toxicity

Perchloric acid is a severe irritant and is corrosive to eyes and skin. The oral LD_{50} is 1100 mg/kg in rats and 400 mg/kg in dogs.

—Shayne C. Gad and Jayne E. Ash

Related Topics

Acids
Corrosives

Periodic Acid

- CAS: 10450-60-9
- SYNONYM: Paraperiodic acid
- Chemical class: Inorganic acid; a periodate
- MOLECULAR FORMULA: H_5IO_6
- CHEMICAL STRUCTURE:

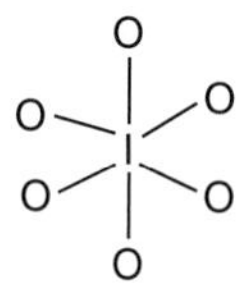

Uses

Periodic acid is used in organic synthesis. It is also used to fortify the wet strength of papers such as photographic paper.

Exposure Pathways

Dermal contact and inhalation are possible routes of exposure.

Mechanism of Toxicity

Periodic acid is corrosive. It is also an oxidizing agent.

Human Toxicity

The estimated lethal dose in humans is 1 ml/kg. Periodic acid is a strong corrosive to the skin and mucous membranes.

Clinical Management

Wash affected areas with copious amounts of water.

—Shayne C. Gad and Jayne E. Ash

Related Topics

Alkalies
Corrosives

Permethrin

- CAS: 52645-53-1
- SYNONYMS: 3-Phenoxybenzyl-(1R,1S)-*cis,trans*-3-(2,2-dichlorovinyl)-2,2-dimethyl-cyclopropanecarboxylate; Ambush; Eksmin; Kafil; Pounce; FMC 33297; OMS 1821; NRDC 143. The *cis* isomer is cispermethrin (NRDC 148) and the *trans* isomer is biopermethrin (NRDC 147).
- CHEMICAL CLASS: Type I pyrethroid insecticide
- CHEMICAL STRUCTURE:

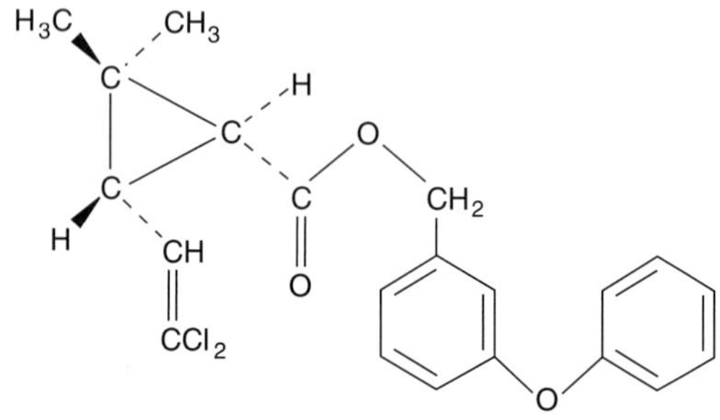

Uses

Permethrin is used as a broad-spectrum insecticide. It is also combined with sulfur in the treatment of human scabies and is the recommended treatment for scabies in patients with AIDS.

Exposure Pathways

Human exposure to permethrin most commonly occurs through dermal contact.

Toxicokinetics

Pyrethroids are poorly absorbed through the skin and are only moderately absorbed in the gastrointestinal tract. One study estimated dermal absorption of permethrin to be <2 mg/12 hr. Metabolism of permethrin occurs rapidly through ester cleavage and hydroxylation. Permethrin is slowly released from lipid tissues with a half-life of 4 or 5 days. Urinary excretion is the primary route of elimination.

Mechanism of Toxicity

Pyrethroids have a selective high affinity for membrane sodium channels. Closing of the channel, which ends the action potential, is slowed, resulting in a prolonged "tail" current and repetitive firing of presynaptic and accompanying postsynaptic cells following a single action potential. High enough doses can cause complete depolarization and blockade of nerve conduction. Permethrin has also been shown to inhibit Ca^{2+}, Mg^{2+}-ATPase and calmodulin.

Human Toxicity: Acute

In mammals, permethrin produces type I motor symptoms generally characterized by hyperexcitation, enhanced startle response, tremors, and prostration. Reports of human exposure have indicated only skin irritation.

Human Toxicity: Chronic

Chronic effects following permethrin exposure have not been reported.

Clinical Management

Oral exposures may be treated with syrup of ipecac-induced emesis, activated charcoal, or gastric lavage. Emesis is contraindicated in cases of unconsciousness or convulsions. In cases of dermal exposure, contaminated clothing should be removed and disposed of. Any exposed areas of skin should be repeatedly washed with soap and water. Paresthesia may be treated with topical application of vitamin E. For contact with the eyes, the eyes should be flushed with generous amounts of lukewarm water for a minimum of 15 min. Seizures can be treated with intravenous diazepam; phenytoin or phenobarbital may be helpful for recurrent seizures. Atropine can be used to control excessive salivation. No specific antidotes for pyrethroid-induced neurotoxic effects have been approved for use in humans. Spontaneous recovery usually occurs with mild or moderate intoxication.

Animal Toxicity

Fish and crustaceans are extremely sensitive to pyrethroid compounds in laboratory settings. However, various factors (e.g., sediment binding) may reduce pyrethroid toxicity to these nontarget organisms in a natural environment.

—Paul R. Harp

Related Topics

Neurotoxicology: Central and Peripheral
Pyrethrins/Pyrethroids

Permissible Exposure Limit

A permissible exposure limit (PEL), under U.S. Occupational Safety and Health Administration (OSHA) standards, is a worker exposure level for an airborne chemical substance which may not be exceeded. The OSHA PELs are applied to exposures levels averaged over an 8-hr period unless otherwise specified in a particular regulation. The term "Permissible Exposure Level" is used by government agencies to designate limits on exposure of their own employees, such as the

PELs developed by the National Academy of Sciences Committee on Toxicology for the U.S. Army and Navy.

Further Reading

Occupational Safety and Health Standards for General Industry (1993). *Code of Federal Regulations,* Title 29, Part 1910.1000–1050.

Occupational Safety and Health Standards for Shipyard Employment (1993).. *Code of Federal Regulations,* Title 29, Part 1915.1000–1050.

Subcommittee on Permissible Exposure Levels (1991). *Permissible Exposure Levels and Emergency Exposure Guidance Levels for Selected Airborne Contaminants.* Committee on Toxicology, National Research Council, Washington, DC.

—Charles Feigley

Related Topics

Levels of Effect in Toxicological Assessment
Occupational Safety and Health Administration
Occupational Toxicology
Short-Term Exposure Limit
Threshold Limit Value

Peroxisome Proliferators

Introduction

The process of xenobiotic-induced proliferation of the cytoplasmic organelle, the peroxisome, in mammalian liver cells has received considerable attention because of the proposed relationship between the induction of hydrogen peroxide (H_2O_2)-producing peroxisomal enzymes and the development of hepatocellular carcinomas in mice and rats. Peroxisome proliferators encompass a diverse group of compounds with dissimilar structures capable of producing pleiotropic responses in experimental animals. The pleiotropic responses are predominantly observed in hepatocytes and are characterized by enlargement of the liver, increases in a relative number of peroxisomes in a cell, marked induction of fatty acid β-oxidation, carnitine acetyltransferase, lauric acid ω-hydroxylation activities, and hypolipidemia. Long-term exposure to peroxisome proliferators is associated with the induction of hepatocellular carcinoma. Currently, there are over 100 known peroxisome proliferators in use including herbicides, industrial solvents, plasticizers, and hypolipidemic agents. Peroxisome proliferation can occur in many organs and tissues. The effects of peroxisome proliferators have been also reported in the kidneys, the heart, the prostate, the pancreas, and the thyroid. Immune reaction may also be observed. Although a significant advance has been made in this area over the past few years, there is much yet to be investigated to elucidate the molecular and cellular mechanisms underlying peroxisome proliferators associated with hepatocellular carcinoma.

Peroxisomes

The term "peroxisome" was first introduced by deDuve in 1965 to emphasize the biochemical property of H_2O_2 production by the peroxisomes as a result of respiration mediated by peroxisomal oxidases such as D-amino acid oxidase and fatty Acyl-CoA. Peroxisomes are ubiquitous subcellular organelles both in animal and plant cells which exhibit numerous oxidases involved in several catalytic and anabolic pathways such as β-oxidation of very long fatty acids. Peroxisomes are also involved in bile acid biosynthesis, a part of plasmalogen synthesis and glyoxylate transamination. Furthermore, literature indicates that peroxisomes participate in cholesterol biosynthesis, hydrogen peroxide-based cellular respiration, purine, fatty acid, long-chain dicarboxylic acid, prostaglandin, and xenobiotic metabolism. Currently, there are about 50 known enzymes associated with mammalian peroxisomes including catalase, oxidases (H_2O_2 generators), acetyl transferases (carnitine acetyl-CoA and carnitine octanoyl-CoA), dehydrogenases (NAD and NADP), and others (enoyl-CoA hydratase, thiolase, fatty acetyl-CoA synthetase). Thus, any chemical capable of disrupting these enzymes perturbs the normal functioning of peroxisomes, leading to long-term adverse health effects. Several techniques are available to identify these organelles in hepatocytes and other cells. One such technique is the recently developed immunohistochemical protocol using antibodies raised against peroxisomal enzymes, or the "protein A-gold" method.

Peroxisome Proliferators

The term "peroxisome proliferator" was introduced by Reddy and co-workers in 1975 to designate a drug or xenobiotic which induces the proliferation of peroxisomes in the liver cells. Peroxisome proliferators are structurally diverse compounds which induce peroxisome proliferation. Earlier studies with the hypolipidemic agent clofibrate revealed that it induced a marked hepatomegaly in male rats. Fine structural changes seen primarily as a massive increase in the number of dense particles or "microbodies" were first described by Paget. Catalase and three H_2O_2-producing oxidases (urate oxidase, *d*-amino acid oxidase, and 1-α-hydroxy acid oxidase) had been found to cosediment with liver cell fractions containing particles identical to microbodies, and the term "peroxisome" was coined to describe this organelle as a site of compartmentalized peroxide metabolism.

Currently, over 100 compounds have been identified as peroxisome proliferators. Literature indicates that induction of peroxisome proliferation is not limited to exogenous chemicals. A number of endogenous substances, such as the steroid hormones, thyroid hormones, morphogenes, and fatty acids, are also involved in peroxisome proliferation. Peroxisome proliferation in hepatic parenchymal cells of rats and mice following the administration of clofibrate has been reported by numerous investigators. Compounds that are structurally unrelated to clofibrate, such as acetaminophen and Wy-14,643, can also cause peroxisome proliferation (Table P-1). The industrial solvent trichloroethylene, the industrial plasticizer di(2-ethyl hexyl) phthalate (DEHP), and di(2-ethyl hexyl) adipate (DEHA) have also been found to be hepatic peroxisome proliferators.

Newer compounds of interest include the perfluoroalkanoic acids, the steroid hormones, and anticarcinogen dehydroepiandrosterone; some structurally related leukotriene D_4 antagonists; certain chlorinated hydrocarbons, primarily those metabolized to tri- or dichloro acetic acid; as well as structurally unrelated herbicides such as tridiphane, lactofen, and several of the chlorophenoxy acids (2,4-dichlorophenoxy acetic acid and 4-chloro-2-methylphenoxy acetic acid) (Table P-1). Peroxisome proliferators comprise chemicals of wide structural dissimilarity (Fig. P-1) and share a common property of inducing characteristic effects in the liver of treated rats and mice. Within a few days of exposure they produce a striking dose-dependent hepatomegaly accompanied by characteristic proliferation of the peroxisomal and microsomal compartments as assessed morphologically and biochemically.

Peroxisomes are also responsive to dietary and hormonal changes such as high-fat diets, particularly those with long-chain fatty acids; high-cholesterol diets; and

TABLE P-1
Selected Representative Peroxisome Proliferators

Fibric acid hypolipidemic agents
Beclobric acid
Ciprofibrate
Clofibrate
Gemfibrozil
Simfibrate
Other xenobiotics
Bleached kraft mill effluents
Citral
Dimethrin
Garlic, ether extracts
Trichloroethylene
Non-fibric acid hypolipidemic agents
Gemcadiol
Niadenate
Tiadenol
Tibric acid
Wy-14, 643
Herbicides
2,4-D (2,4-dichlorophenoxyacetic acid)
MCPA (2-methy-4-chlorophenoxyacetic acid)
2,4,5-T (2,4,5-trichlorophenoxyacetic acid)
Lactofen
Tridiphane
Other drugs
Acetylsalicyclic acid
Benzobromarone
Bifonazole
Flurbiprofen
Valprioic acid
Other chlorophenoxy acids
2-Phenyopropionic acid
4-Chlorophenoxypropionic acid
4-Chlorophenoxybutyric acid
Fatty acid analogs
2,2,4,4,6,8,8-Heptamethylnonane
Perfluorobutyric acid
Perfluorodecanoic acid
Sorbic acid
Tetradecylthioacetic acid

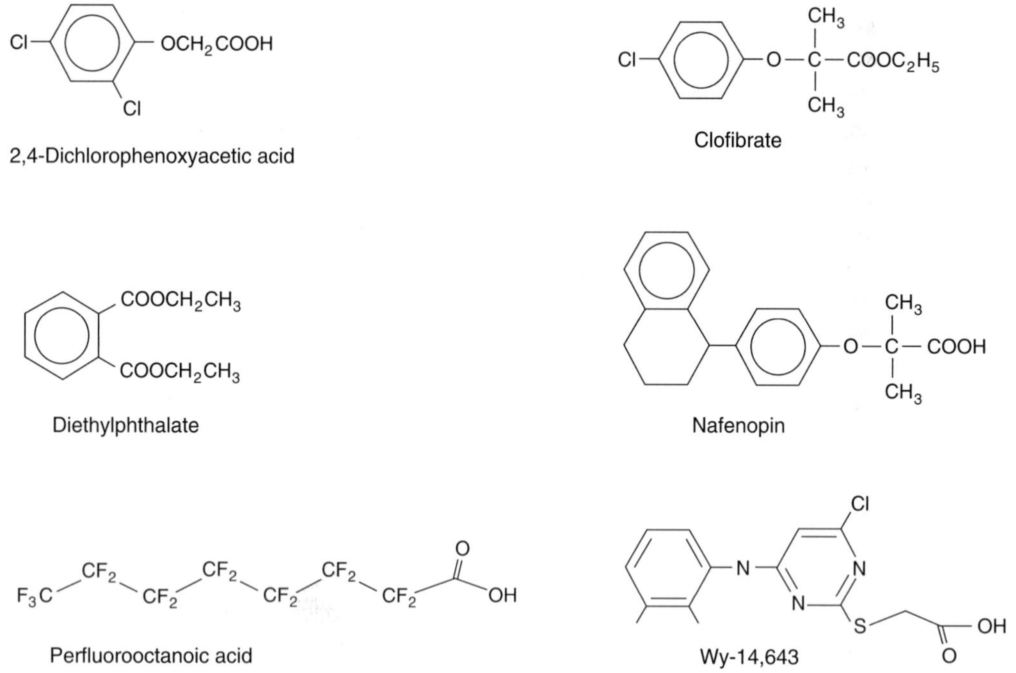

2,4-Dichlorophenoxyacetic acid

Clofibrate

Diethylphthalate

Nafenopin

Perfluorooctanoic acid

Wy-14,643

FIGURE P-1. Structures of representative peroxisome proliferators.

vitamin E deficiency.Thyroid hormones produce moderate increases in the content of hepatic peroxisomes and peroxisomal enzymes. While these diets and physiological influences rarely induce changes in peroxisomes to the same extent as many xenobiotics, they are useful in exploring the mechanisms of regulation of peroxisomal proliferation.

Biomedical Responses to Acute Toxicity of Peroxisome Proliferators

Peroxisome proliferation is consistently associated with hepatomegaly, which arises from a combination of cellular hypertrophy and hyperplasia. Studies on fine structure of hepatocytes revealed that the increase in hepatocyte size was associated with the predominant increase in peroxisomes and modest increase in smooth endoplasmic reticulum (SER). Rats exposed to peroxisome proliferators exhibit 7- to 10-fold increases in peroxisomal relative volume and surface area as evidenced by morphometric analysis of liver sections. The increase in peroxisomal relative volume is due to increases in both volume and number of peroxisomes. In contrast, the increase in SER surface area and volume rarely exceeds 2-fold. The magnitude of increase in cellular DNA and peroxisomes is dose and compound dependent and correlates with the extent of hepatomegaly. Hyperplasia, however, does not correlate with the extent of peroxisomal proliferation. For example, clofibrate and DEHP produce little hyperplasia, while nefenopin and Wy-14,643 produce relatively extensive hyperplasia. Hypolipidemia is one of the characteristic responses to peroxisome proliferators. This can be evidenced by remarkable decrease in triglyceride and cholesterol levels following exposure to nonhypolipidemic agents. Because of these properties, hypolipidemic drugs are primarily used to lower serum cholesterol and triglyceride. Earlier studies showed that clofibrate treatment increases liver carnitine acetyltransferase activity, but no correlation was established with peroxisome proliferation. It has also been reported by Moody and Reddy that an increase in carnitine acetyltransferase is a conforming response to a wide variety of peroxisome proliferators, with increase in specific activity ranging from 10- to 25-fold, the most predominant increase being in the peroxisomes. Increases in the medium- (5- to 10-fold) and long-chained (2- to 5-fold) carnitine acetyltransferases also occur. Another obvious peroxisome response to peroxisome proliferators is increased β-oxidation of fatty acids in glyoxysome, a specific form of peroxisome, in germinated seeds which later was also reported to be present in rat liver peroxisome. Studies have shown that clofibrate treatment increases β-oxidation of fatty acids by about 10-fold. Based on such studies, it has been concluded that β-oxidation of fatty acids is a generalized response to peroxisome proliferators.

Peroxisome proliferators are also involved in two other metabolic pathways of importance to lipid metabolism. Peroxisomes contain the most of dihydroxyacetone phosphate acetyltransferase and alkyldihydroxyacetone phosphate synthetase activities. Therefore, they are responsible for initiating most ether glycerolipid biosynthesis. These enzymes are also moderately induced by peroxisome proliferators. Induction of cytochrome P450s by peroxisome proliferators will be addressed separately.

Mechanism of Induction of Peroxisome Proliferation

Two widely accepted possible mechanisms for the induction of peroxisome proliferation are (1) activation of specific genes by the chemical or its metabolites, either directly or mediated by a specific receptor, and (2) substrate overload, either as a result of lipolysis occurring outside the liver and causing an influx of fatty acids into the liver or as a consequence of the peroxisome proliferators or their metabolites perturbing lipid metabolism.

The most likely mechanism of induction of peroxisome enzymes is interaction of peroxisome proliferators with a cytoplasmic receptor of the hepatocytes. The peroxisome proliferator–receptor complex interacts with the chromatin to elicit selective increases in protein, translation of mRNA, and peroxisome-specific mRNAs. The second mechanism of peroxisome proliferation may be related to substrate overload in the hepatocytes of animals treated with various peroxisome proliferators. In rats, feeding of high-fat diet results in a very slight increase in peroxisome number. The administration of clofibrate or other peroxisome proliferators may lead to an influx of fatty acids into the liver as a result of lipolysis occurring outside the liver, or these compounds and their metabolites enhance the breakdown of triglycerides in the liver cell thereby causing an intrahepatic excess of fatty acids. The fatty acid overload may then trigger an increase in peroxisomal β-oxidation pathway.

In addition to the two previously mentioned mechanisms, some investigators have proposed another mechanism for induction of peroxisome proliferation. Peroxisomes contain a fatty acid β-oxidation system which preferentially oxidizes long-chain fatty acids (C_8–C_{20}). For example, the physicochemical properties of clofibric acid, the hydrolytic product of clofibrate, are very closely similar to those of naturally occurring C_{16}–C_{18} fatty acids. It is important, therefore, to examine whether the hypolipidemic drugs and/or their metabolites serve as substrates for the peroxisomal β-oxidation, thereby causing peroxisomal enzyme induction and possibly leading to increased production of H_2O_2 and other active oxygen species which ultimately lead to peroxisome proliferation.

Induction of Cytochrome P450s by Peroxisome Proliferators

Induction of the enzymes involved in xenobiotic biotransformation (phases I and II) is one of characteristic responses to peroxisome proliferators. Attention has focused on these compounds initially because they were identified as epigenetic hepatocarcinogens in rodents. In addition, peroxisome proliferators received further attention as inducers of members of cytochrome P450 gene superfamily known to readily metabolize fatty acids. These metabolites have marked physiological activity, particularly those of arachidonic acid, which are vasoactive, regulate hormone release, and control renal ion flux. Therefore, regulation of cytochrome P450-dependent fatty acid hydroxylases by peroxisome proliferators is of particular interest in the field of physiology and pathophysiology. The cytochrome P450 gene superfamily consists of nearly 250 known different genes which have substrate specificity in metabolizing a range of xenobiotics, including drugs, pesticides, food flavors and additives, and environmental chemicals. Furthermore, peroxisome proliferator-induced cytochrome P450s can also metabolize endogenous compounds other than fatty acids such as steroids, vitamins, and eicosanoids. It should be noted that only few of the cytochrome P450s induced by peroxisome proliferators have been isolated and studied. Cytochrome P450 4A1 in rat liver and P450 4A7 in rabbit lung are two such isozymes isolated and extensively characterized. Because a vast majority of endogenous and exogenous chemical substances are metabolized by cytochrome

P450, their metabolism and effects can be modulated by exposure to peroxisome proliferators.

Mechanisms of Peroxisome Proliferator-Induced Cytochrome P450s and Other Enzymes

In general, the cytochrome P450 gene superfamily exhibits a range of induction mechanisms, including transcriptional gene activation, mRNA processing and mRNA stabilization, translational regulation, and protein stabilization. Current understanding indicates that xenobiotic-dependent transcriptional gene activation is the most common induction mechanism, and direct experimental evidence using nuclear run-on experiments has demonstrated that cytochrome P450 4A1 undergoes transcriptional gene activation by clofibrate. However, it is not clear whether or not the same induction mechanism is involved in the other cytochrome P450 4A gene superfamily. The question is then, do peroxisome proliferators directly activate the cytochrome P450 4A1 gene or do they require the intermediary of a protein factor/receptor to interact with the 5′ flanking regulatory element of the gene? Recent experimental findings suggest that peroxisome proliferator-induced cytochrome P450 and other enzymes are mediated through a receptor, better known as peroxisome proliferator activated receptor (PPAR). The existence of multiple PPARs (PPAR-α, -β, and -γ) has been recently reported. These receptors are members of a superfamily that comprises at least 30 mammalian genes encoding receptors for the classical steroid hormones, thyroid hormones, vitamin D_3, and retinoic acid. These receptors have been implicated in the activation of some enzymes and have also been implicated in the activation of CYP4A6. Investigators have shown that the peroxisome proliferator complex interacts with chromatin to result in selective increases in the transcription of peroxisomal fatty acid β-oxidation gene enzymes. There is also evidence to indicate that the PPAR is inducible by the peroxisome proliferator fenofibrate in rat liver as assessed by immunochemical methods and PPAR mRNA analysis by Northern blotting.

Species Differences in Response to Peroxisome Proliferation

Studies with a number of peroxisome proliferators have shown considerable variation in the responsiveness of species to peroxisome proliferators. Peroxisome proliferation, cytochrome P450 induction, and induction of peroxisomal enzymes by hypolipidemic agents and other chemicals such as DEHP is well established in rats and mice. Hamster liver is also responsive to these compounds, although to a lesser extent. Examination of human liver biopsy material, obtained from patients receiving clofibrate, gemfibrozil, or fenofibrate, has demonstrated marginal or no increase in peroxisomal volume densities or numbers. These studies suggest that there is a marked species difference in sensitivity to chemicals that cause hepatomegaly and peroxisome proliferation. In general, rats and mice are most responsive; hamsters, chickens, and pigeons exhibit an intermediate responsiveness; and dogs, rabbits, marmosets, and rhesus monkeys are least responsive to peroxisome proliferators. Human peroxisomes are also insensitive to these compounds. In contrast, hypolipidemic effect is quite evident in all of the primates and most other species studied. One of the reasons for interspecies differences in response to peroxisome proliferators may be attributed to the existence of multiple PPARs, each having different ligand-binding specificity and being differentially regulated and expressed in a tissue- and species-specific manner. In addition, species differences in response to peroxisome proliferators are reproducible in cell cultures since hepatocytes from rats and mice respond *in vitro* to peroxisome proliferators, whereas monkey and human hepatocytes are far less sensitive. In sharp contrast, guinea pigs do not respond to peroxisome proliferators in both *in vivo* and *in vitro* systems. Therefore, this cell culture system may provide a good method to study the effects of peroxisome proliferators in humans.

Gender Differences in Peroxisome Proliferation

There appears to be a general misconception that female rats are not responsive to the peroxisome proliferators such as clofibrate. This misconception was based on an earlier studies in which male F-344 rats but not females maintained on 0.25% clofibrate diet for up to 4 weeks exhibited hepatic peroxisome proliferation. However, subsequent studies adequately demonstrated that clofibrate, when given at 0.5, 1, and 2% in a diet, resulted in a marked peroxisome proliferation in liver parenchymal cells of both male and female rats. Therefore, gender differences can be obviated by increasing the dose of the inducing agent. On the other hand, it would be interesting to investigate the nonresponsiveness of female rats to the low dose of clofibrate in terms of risk assessment. No gender differences in the induction of peroxisome were seen in adult, fetal, and neonatal rats treated with nafenopin or other potent peroxisome proliferators. In terms of gender-related differences in cytochrome P450 induction, recent studies have shown that P450 4A1 and 4A3 mRNAs are induced to a much greater extent in male compared in female rats following clofibrate treatment. Cytochrome P450 4A2 mRNA is altogether absent from female rat liver. Male-specific expression of P450 4A2 mRNA was also observed in kidneys. These observations suggest that the lower responsiveness of female rats to clofibrate-induced peroxisome proliferation may reflect the lower inducibility of the P450 4A fatty acid hydroxylase enzyme in female rats. There is no gender difference in the induction of P450 4A12 mRNA in mice treated with the potent peroxisome proliferator methylclofenapate. Thus, gender-related differences in chemical-induced peroxisome proliferation are dependent by and large on species, strains, and doses of a given agent.

Recent studies indicate that there are gender-related differences in the induction of hepatic catalase activity by clofibrate. Catalase, which is located in peroxisomes, catalyzes the reduction of hydrogen peroxide to water either directly or using small molecules, such as ethanol, formate, or methanol, as electron donors. Basal and clofibrate-induced hepatic catalase activity in male Sprague–Dawley rats was reported to be higher as opposed to the corresponding levels in females. Induction of hepatic catalase activity by clofibrate was decreased by 50% in castrated males compared to intact male rats. Clofibrate-fed castrated male rats challenged with estradiol benzoate showed greatly diminished induction of catalase activity. It has also been reported that uninduced ovariectomized female rats had hepatic catalase activity levels comparable to those of induced intact females. Marginal increase in hepatic catalase activity was observed in induced ovariectomized females compared to ovariectomized control females. Furthermore, substantial increase in hepatic catalase activity was seen in induced ovariectomized females challenged with testosterone propionate. These observations clearly demonstrate gender-related differences in the induction of hepatic catalase activity by clofibrate in rats depending on the exposure level. A basis for these different responses could be attributed to factors such as gender-dependent metabolic pathways. Induction of acetyl-CoA oxidase activity by peroxisome proliferators has recently been shown to be receptor mediated. If induction of hepatic catalase activity by peroxisome proliferators is shown to also be receptor mediated, then hormonal status could potentially interact with signal transduction pathways, resulting in differences in induction of catalase and other biochemical endpoints between the genders. On the other hand, findings on the gender differences in the induction of catalase activity in other species and with other peroxisome proliferators are less compelling. Unlike clofibrate, other peroxisome proliferators show no consistent pattern of gender differences in induction of hepatic catalase activity in either mice or rats. Therefore, the observed differences may relate to effective dose of the inducer rather than responsiveness to peroxisome induction.

Peroxisome Proliferators and Hepatocarcinogenesis

In recent years a growing concern has developed about long-term exposure to hypolipidemic drugs and industrial plasticizers (DEHP and DEHA) and the possible effect on human health. These concerns have basically centered on the tumorigenic property of peroxisome proliferators. There is a large body of evidence to indicate an association between peroxisome proliferation and hepatocarcinogenesis in rats and mice. Hepatocellular carcinogenesis is a property of all peroxisome proliferators, with few exceptions after discounting any direct genotoxic action of these compounds. The increased production of H_2O_2, which may overwhelm protective enzymes within the hepatocyte and produce indirect genotoxic injury, and the propensity of peroxisome proliferators to induce hepatocyte replication have both been argued to contribute to the carcinogenic action of these compounds. Furthermore, there is no evidence for the covalent binding of peroxisome proliferators to DNA in experimental animals. The lack of covalent DNA binding and mutagenic activity suggests that peroxisome proliferators do not react directly with DNA to produce injury and that electrophilic species generated by peroxisome proliferators interact with non-DNA target. Therefore, since peroxisome proliferators do not directly interact with and impair DNA, their mechanism of action is considered to be epigenetic (nongenotoxic). The understanding of the carcinogenic process induced by peroxisome proliferators is a continuing challenge. Epigenetic carcinogens operate by mechanisms such as chronic tissue injury, immunosuppression, solid-state effects, hormonal imbalance, cocarcinogenesis, or promotional activity. In the presence of tumor-initiating agents, peroxisome proliferators accelerate tumor formation. The distinctive phenotypic markers (GGT-positive foci) of the early stages of hepatocarcinogenesis are not observed, suggesting that pathways specific to peroxisome proliferators underlie the transformation of rodent hepatocytes. Peroxisome proliferators such as Wy-14,643 and clofibrate have been demonstrated to promote tumors after cell initiation. Recent developments also indicate that commonly used phthalate ester plasticizers DEHA and DEHP are capable of inducing hepatocellular carcinoma in rats and mice. These observations are of a serious concern since about 400 million pounds of DEHP plasticizers are used every year in the United States and many more million pounds elsewhere in the world.

The molecular and cellular mechanism of peroxisome prolifertor-mediated hepatocarcinogenecity is not understood well. However, several hypotheses have been proposed for the hapatocarcinogenecity of these compounds. Accumulated experimental evidence does not favor any single triggering event to explain the hepatocarcinogenic process by peroxisome prolifertors. Some of the hypotheses are calcium mobilization, a cascade of oncogene activation, sustained cell growth, increased turnover of specific hepatocyte population, the effect of the activated PPAR on the differentiation state, and the long-term consequences of the metabolic imbalance resulting from increased peroxisomal enzyme activities; oxidative stress may also be involved in the carcinogenic process. Ames and associates have proposed that chemical carcinogens or promoters that are not mutagenic in *Salmonella* mutagenicity tests interact with cellular membranes and may cause DNA damage through stimulation of arachidonic acid cascade or the induction of an oxidative burst and lipid peroxidation. It is likely that the carcinogenicity of halogenated compounds is owing to their ability to form radicals which cause lipid peroxidation. Because lipid peroxidation is a chain reaction, it causes the production of a considerable number of reactive oxygen species, such as the hydroxyl radicals (OH·), H_2O_2, and the superoxide radical (O_2^-), which can damage DNA.

Chronic exposure to peroxisome proliferators results in accumulation of autofluorescent lipofuscin pigments. The accumulation of lipofuscin pigments is indicative of increased lipid peroxidation and is generally related to increased production of biologically damaging free radicals such as OH˙. Furthermore, peroxisome proliferators can alter the peroxisomal enzyme profile such that the output of the oxygen species produced can be enhanced in that the increase in the H_2O_2 destructive enzyme catalase is proportionally small compared to the peroxisomal volume and H_2O_2 generating fatty acid β-oxidation is increased by peroxisomal proliferators. Peroxisome proliferators also increase the activity of uricase, which results in decreased levels of uric acid, a powerful antioxidant which is a scavenger for oxygen radicals. While it is known that excessive H_2O_2 is formed in the liver as a result of sustained proliferation, it is not well-known whether H_2O_2 or other reactive oxygen species are directly involved in hepatocarcinogenesis.

Relevance to Public Health

A fundamental toxicological issue from a public health perspective is the ultimate outcome from chronic occupational exposure to industrial plasticizers, or long-term therapeutic effects of hypolipidemic drugs. The available evidence indicates that potent peroxisome proliferators are carcinogenic in rats and mice. However, neither the mechanism of proliferation nor the events leading to the development of hepatocellular carcinomas are sufficiently well understood. Since peroxisomal proliferation was not observed in subhuman primates and certain other species in a preliminary screening study conducted several years ago with clofibrate, the peroxisome proliferator-induced carcinogenic effects have been readily dismissed by some as being of no importance to humans. Rat liver peroxisomal proliferation was characterized as a unique atypical phenomenon restricted to the biology of peroxisomes in these species. However, in light of recent evidence that peroxisomal proliferation can be induced in a wide range of species, including subhuman primates, it seems appropriate to consider the biological implications of peroxisomal proliferators and assess their risk to humans.

Hypolipidemic drugs are being developed with the assumption that reduction of elevated serum lipid is necessary in order to control mortality and morbidity associated with cardiovascular disease. Although the causal relationship between the level of certain serum lipids and the development of the atherosclerotic lesion and its ischemic complications is supported by the experimental and human studies, there is little proof that either prevention or amelioration of coronary heart and peripheral atherosclerotic disease is achieved by lipid-lowering therapy. Studies have shown that newer lipid-lowering agents reduce the short-term risk of nonfatal and fatal myocardial infarcts and other debilitating complications of hypolipidemias. However, this has to be balanced with any long-term delayed carcinogenic risk which usually develops in 10–20 years. Thus, patients should be informed of the risks/benefits related to hypolipidemic long-term therapy. In contrast to the hypolipidemic agents, there is limited evidence for carcinogenicity of industrial plasticizers such as DEHP and DEHA in experimental animals. However, because the two compounds are widely used in the formulation of plastics, they may present a wider danger to the general public. Additional studies are needed to establish the carcinogenicity of these industrial plasticizers.

Accumulated experimental evidence suggests that carcinogenic and proliferative effects of peroxisome proliferators may not be related. Thus, the assumption that lack of or a minimal peroxisome proliferative response observed in the liver of some animals or humans to therapeutic dose levels of hypolipidemic drugs poses no danger to humans could be misleading if carcinogenesis by these drugs is not mediated by proliferated peroxisomes. On the other hand, if carcinogenesis is directly related to their ability to induce both hepatomegaly and peroxisome proliferation, carcinogenic risk to humans could be predicted with some assurance by quantitative morphometric analysis of the alterations in peroxisome volume, numerical densities, and by changes in the levels of H_2O_2-generating peroxisomal oxidases including the β-oxidation system.

In summary, substantial progress has been made over the past few years in understanding the cytoplasmic organelle peroxisome and factors that alter its normal functions. Peroxisome proliferator-induced increase in the liver peroxisomes is associated with an approximately twofold increase in catalase activity and several-fold increases in the activity of the peroxisomal fatty acid β-oxidation system. It is also evident from the available literature that hepatic peroxisomal proliferation appears to be a carcinogenic event in rodents, and this may depend on the potency of the inducer. However, there is no single mechanism that is attributed to the peroxisome proliferation or carcinogenesis induced by these agents. The hypothesis that peroxisome proliferator-induced carcinogenesis is mediated by disturbances in subcellular organelle homeostasis requires continued investigational attention because of the importance of these hypolipidemic drugs and industrial plasticizers to our society. In conclusion, because of our limited knowledge of the complex molecular changes occurring during liver cancer, it would be inappropriate and far too premature to amend scientific risk assessment procedures for nongenotoxic chemical carcinogens based on oversimplified or incompletely tested speculations.

Further Reading

Bieri, F., and Lhuguenot, J. C. (1993). Toxicity of peroxisome proliferators. *Biochimie* **75**, 263–268.

Chen, H., Huang, C., Wilson, M. W., Lay, L. T., Robertson, L. W., Chow, C. K., and Glauert, H. P. (1994). Effect of the peroxisome proliferators and perfluorodecanoic acid on hepatic cell proliferation and toxicity in Sprague–Dawley rats. *Carcinogenesis* **15**(12), 2847–2850.

Green, S., and Wahli, W. (1994). Peroxisome proliferator-activated receptors: Finding the orphan a home. *Mol. Cell. Endocronol.* **100**, 149–153.

Lock, E. A., Mitchell, A. M., and Elcombe, C. R. (1989). Biochemical mechanisms of induction of hepatic peroxisome proliferation. *Annu. Rev. Pharmacol. Toxicol.* **29**, 145–163.

Moody, D. E. (Ed.) (1994). *Peroxisome Proliferators: Unique Inducers of Drug-Metabolizing Enzymes.* CRC Press, Ann Arbor, MI.

Reddy, J. K., and Lalwai, N. D. (1983). Carcinogenesis by hepatic peroxisome proliferators: Evaluation of the risk of hypolipidemic drugs and industrial plasticizers to humans. *Crit. Rev. Toxicol.* **12**(1):1–58.

—Abraham Dalu and Harihara M. Mehendale

Related Topics

Chlorophenoxy Herbicides
Liver

Pesticides

The word pesticide literally means an agent used to kill an undesirable organism. In the amended U.S. Federal Insecticide, Fungicide and Rodenticide Act, the definition of an "economic poison" or pesticide was expanded to include

> (1) Any substance or mixture of substances intended for preventing, destroying, repelling, or mitigating any pest [insect, rodent, nematode, fungus, weed, other forms of terrestrial or aquatic plant or animal life or viruses, bacteria, or other microorganisms, except viruses, bacteria, or other microorganisms on or in living man or other animals, which the Administrator declares to be a pest] and (2) any substance or mixture of substances intended for use a plant regulator, defoliant or desiccant.

The major classes of pesticides in use today include herbicides, fungicides, rodenticides, insecticides, nematocides, acaricides, and molluscides. Prior to about 1940, pesticides were primarily inorganic chemicals (e.g., arsenic) and a few natural agents from plant origin (e.g., nicotine and pyrethrum). With the discovery of the insecticidal activity of DDT, however, a burgeoning increase in the development and utilization of synthetic organic chemicals occurred. From about 1940 to 1980, an exponential increase in the production and use of these synthetic pesticides was evident worldwide. The major chemical classes of pesticides in use today include inorganic and organic metals, chlorinated hydrocarbons, organophosphorus compounds, carbamates, pyrethroids, substituted phenols, substituted ureas, coumarins, organic acids, organic amides, and triazines. Currently, over 1 billion pounds of about 600 different pesticides (active ingredients) are produced each year in the United States alone, with total worldwide production estimated at around 5 billion pounds.

Insects were the first major focus of pest control, whether to prevent the destruction of food or fiber crops or to limit the spread of insect vectors of disease. There is little doubt that the use of insecticides had a profound impact on the further development of civilization. The control of anopheline mosquitoes and malarial infection, as well as vectors for typhus, plague, and yellow fever, by DDT undoubtedly saved millions of lives. Over the past several decades, however, the use of herbicides has dramatically increased and such efforts have markedly altered the methods of modern agriculture. As a result, herbicides now represent the most extensively used class of pesticides in the United States. Some food and fiber crops reportedly increased yields by 300–600% after the introduction and widespread use of synthetic herbicides.

While the public health and economic benefits of synthetic pesticide use over the past 50 years are indisputable, these benefits have not been without costs. Widespread environmental contamination by DDT and other organochlorine pesticides, reaching global proportions, with concomitant deleterious effects on some members of the food web heralded the end of an era for their extensive use. DDT was banned from use in the United States in 1972 and most other organochlorines were subsequently banned, being replaced by the less environmentally persistent organophosphates and carbamates. While these agents had considerably lower abilities to accumulate in environmental and biological media, they tended to be much more acutely toxic and thus more hazardous to utilize. The pyrethroids are generally regarded as safer than the anticholinesterase organophosphates and carbamates, but still constitute a smaller proportion of total insecticidal use. In general, herbicides exhibit markedly lower acute mammalian toxicity than other classes of pesticides. The relative toxicities of these agents is generally scaled, however, on the basis of acute reactions. Knowledge of the long-term health consequences of prolonged, low-level exposure to various pesticide classes is still limited. A major challenge for toxicologists in the future is the continued acquisition of data pertaining to the long-term effects of low-level pesticide exposures.

—Carey Pope

Related Topics

Bioaccumulation
Bioconcentration
Carbamate Pesticides
Chlorophenoxy Herbicides
Federal insecticide, Fungicide, and Rodenticide Act
Nematocides
Occupational Toxicology
Organochlorine Insecticides
Organophosphates
Pollution, Soil
Pollution, Water
Psychological Indices of Toxicity

Pyrethrin/Pyrethroids
Veterinary Toxicology

Petroleum Distillates

- PREFERRED NAMES: Petroleum distillates; petroleum naphtha; naphtha
- SYNONYMS: The term "petroleum distillates" generally refers to petroleum naphtha or petroleum ether, which contain the lower boiling fractions (boiling point range, 86–140°F) of petroleum, principally pentanes and hexanes, with minor amounts of paraffins ranging up to 13 carbons. Petroleum naphtha is also known by the following synonyms: Amsco H-J; Amsco H-SB; Benzin B-70; HI-Flash naphtha; hydrotreated naphtha; naphtha coal tar; naphtha; petroleum naphtha; solvent naphtha; petroleum benzin; petroleum-derived naphtha; petroleum oil; Super VMP; UN1255; UN1256; UN1270; UN2553.

  A solvent obtained from higher boiling distillates (boiling point range, 203–320°F), generically known as ligroin or "varnish-makers' and painters' naphtha" (VM&P naphtha), may also occasionally be referred to as "petroleum distillates." Other synonyms for this solvent include benzin; benzine (light petroleum distillate); benzoline; canadol; ligroin; painters naphtha; petroleum ether; petroleum spirit; refined solvent naphtha; Skellysolve F; Skellysolve G; UN1271; varnish makers' naphtha; VM and P naphtha; VM&P naphtha.

  Mineral spirits, also known as petroleum spirits, is another commonly used solvent that distills at an even higher temperature than naphtha (boiling point range, 302–392°F). It is also known as Stoddard solvent; refined petroleum spirits; white spirits; Amsco 140; Soltrol; Soltrol 50; Soltrol 100; Soltrol 180.

  Thus, the term petroleum distillates may be used generically and interchangeably for two different types of petroleum distillation fractions. It can be confusing in that many commercial products will list the term as an ingredient even though it does not contain petroleum naphtha (e.g., the label of a solvent may say "contains petroleum distillates" simply because some of the components were derived from crude oil).
- CHEMICAL CLASS: Aromatic hydrocarbons

Uses

Petroleum distillates are used as general extractants and universal solvents for paints, varnishes, fats, furniture polishes, and waxes. They are also used as vehicles for medication and pesticide applications, as counterirritants, and as degreasers, detergents, and fuel.

Exposure Pathways

The primary exposure pathway for these solvents would be inhalation of volatile components or absorption through skin. Inhalation of fumes can be hazardous, especially in environments with poor ventilation.

Toxicokinetics

Because distilled fractions are mixtures, the toxicokinetics would be different for the different types of naphthas or spirits. It can be assumed, based on the adverse effects following exposure to these mixtures, that the central nervous system (CNS) is a primary target organ; i.e., effects are similar to those seen with the methane series. For more information on these individual components, see Pentane, Hexane, Heptane, or Octane.

Human Toxicity

The naphtha mixtures that are distilled at a lower boiling temperatures have a higher volatility and, generally speaking, a higher degree of toxicity than the higher boiling fractions. In some occupational settings, chronic exposure to petroleum distillate resulted in damage to the CNS, sometimes irreversible. Adverse effects on blood-forming components have also been observed, although the frequency of this effect has decreased considerably since the removal of benzene from these mixtures.

Petroleum ether (ligroin) consists primarily of *n*-pentane and *n*-hexane. Therefore, the primary effects seen are on the CNS, including peripheral nerve damage and depression (see Petroleum Ether, Pentane, and Hexane). Irritation of the skin and respiratory tract is also a common symptom of exposure to petroleum ether. Ingestion may cause aspiration pneumonia and pneumatoceles in children. Reactions of human skin include edema (swelling), erythema (reddening), and disruption of the horny layer. Acute inhalation of high concentrations of petroleum ether may cause cerebral edema. Effects related to *n*-hexane intoxication, including paresthesia, loss of appetite, muscle weakness, and impaired motor function have been seen in workers chronically exposed to petroleum ether in inadequately ventilated buildings. The occupational threshold limit for petroleum distillates is 350 mg/m^3 (NIOSH), with a maximum ceiling concentration of 1800 mg/m^3. The lower explosive limit is 1.1%.

VM&P naphtha, also known as "light naphtha" and "spotting naphtha," is used extensively in the thinning of lacquers, varnishes, and rapidly evaporating paint thinner. It is a mildly irritating to the nose and eyes. Workers exposed to this mixture have been known to experience symptoms typical of intoxication with aliphatic compounds, including lightheadedness, labored breathing, tremors, hyperactivity, and nausea. The occupationally safe air concentration recommended by NIOSH for VM&P naphtha is 350 mg/m^3, with a ceiling limit of 1800 mg/m^3. The ACGIH TLV is 1370 mg/m^3 (300 ppm) for VM&P naphtha. The lower explosive limit is 1.2%.

None of the petroleum-derived distillates have ever been shown to be carcinogenic in humans.

Clinical Management

Persons who are exposed to high concentrations should vacate or be removed from the source of the vapor and seek fresh air. Care should be taken to keep areas of high concentration free from ignition sources, such as sparks from static electricity and use of explosion-proof apparatus.

Animal Toxicity

Toxicity tests on laboratory animals using different types of petroleum distillate forumulations have shown oral LD_{50} values ranging from 4.5 to ≧25 ml/kg. Inhalation LC_{50} values have ranged from 1600 to ≧73,000 ppm. The majority of laboratory rats subjected to chemical aspiration experiments (up to 0.2 ml) do not survive. In experiments with VM&P naphtha, temporary hematological effects are observed. As in humans, CNS depression is commonly seen following exposure; at high concentrations, convulsions are sometimes seen.

—Stephen Clough

Related Topic

Neurotoxicology: Central and Peripheral

Petroleum Ether

- CAS: 8032-32-4
- SYNONYMS: Ligroin; refined solvent naphtha; varnish makers' and painters' naphtha (VM&P naphtha); Skellysolve
- CHEMICAL CLASS: Petroleum ether is a petroleum distillate made up primarily of aliphatic and alicyclic hydrocarbons in the C_5–C_{10} range.
- DESCRIPTION: Petroleum ether is a complex mixture. The following is a typical composition; however, this will vary depending on petroleum feedstock and refining process:

  50–80% paraffins (C_5–C_{10}) (% by volume)

  20–40% monocycloparaffins

  2–10% aromatics

  The boiling point range is 38–150°C; the flash point range is −18–13°C

  The most common production process used today results in petroleum ether with <0.002% benzene and <5.0% *n*-hexane.

Uses

Petroleum solvents are typically grouped into three classes based on volatility and aromatic content. They are (1) special boiling range solvents, (2) white spirits, and, (3) high boiling aromatics. Petroleum ether is in the special boiling range solvent class. It is used in the rubber industry and as a degreasing agent. Petroleum ether is a common constituent in adhesives, inks, paints, varnishes and lacquers.

Exposure Pathways

Exposure occurs most commonly by either inhalation or through skin contact.

Toxicokinetics

Petroleum ether is absorbed by the lungs following inhalation exposure. It is metabolized by the liver with a biological half-life of 46–48 hr.

Mechanism of Toxicity

The acute toxicity from overexposure to petroleum ether is manifested primarily in central nervous system (CNS) effects. The mechanism of toxicity is unknown; however, the general anoxia observed is most likely due to oxygen deprivation. The mechanism of toxicity from long-term overexposure to petroleum ether is dependent on the chemical makeup of the distillate. For example, if peripheral neuropathy is observed, it is most likely due to a high concentration of *n*-hexane in the petroleum ether. *n*-Hexane is known to cause axonal damage in peripheral nerves.

Human Toxicity

Skin contact with petroleum solvents can cause allergic contact dermatitis. Overexposure via inhalation of petroleum ether affects primarily the CNS. Short-term, high overexposure is associated with an excitatory phase followed by a depressive phase. Exposures of 100–400 ppm for 7 hr have resulted in headaches, fatigue, and incoordination with dose-associated effects on equilibrium, reaction time, visuomotor coordination, and memory. Inhalation exposures of 445–1250 ppm resulted in blurred vision, a cold sensation in extremities, fatiguability, headache, fatty demylination of muscle fibers, and demylination and mild axonal degeneration. Several cross-sectional epidemiology studies have investigated the CNS effects observed in industrial painters, house painters, car painters, shipyard painters, and floor layers. Subjective symptoms such as headache, fatigue, poor coordination, emotional instability, impaired memory, and other intellectual functions and impaired psychomotor performance have been reported. Because most of these workers were exposed to a multitude of chemicals, in addition to petroleum ether, it is difficult to evaluate the cause of the reported effects. Exposure to 880 ppm produced eye and throat irritation with temporary olfactory fatigue.

Clinical Management

Overexposure to vapors of petroleum ether is treated by removing the patient to fresh air. If skin or eye contact occurs, the affected areas should be flushed with water for at least 15 min to remove residual solvent. Good personal hygiene and regular washing of skin and clothes minimizes the potential for developing allergic contact dermatitis. If ingestion of petroleum ether occurs, vomiting should not be induced. This could result in aspiration of solvent into the lungs, leading to chemical pneumonitis and pulmonary edema, which can be fatal. If ingestion is suspected and the patient is coughing, there is a good possibility that aspiration has occurred. The patient should be monitored closely; hospitalization may be indicated.

Animal Toxicity

In general, the toxicity reported from exposure to petroleum ether is more pronounced with samples containing higher concentrations of aromatic compounds. The irritation potential of petroleum ether to skin and eyes as tested in rabbits in the Draize protocol ranged from minimally to moderately irritating. Inhalation toxicity of VM&P naphtha was studied in mice, rats, cats, and dogs at concentrations ranging from 280 to 15,000 ppm. Acute exposure to high concentrations resulted in loss of motor coordination and CNS depression. Eye irritation was reported in rats at 3400 ppm after 4 hr and dogs at 3400 ppm after 2 hr. Respiration rate was decreased in mice after exposure for 1 min to >2600 ppm. The 4-hr LC_{50} in rats was reported to be 3400 ppm. Beagle dogs were exposed to 1200 ppm of petroleum ether for 6 hr/day, 5 days/week for 13 weeks. No significant toxicity was reported. The majority of data would suggest that petroleum ether is not mutagenic, based on *in vitro* tests using cultured mammalian cells, yeast, or bacterial test systems.

—*Patricia J. Beattie*

Related Topic

Neurotoxicology: Central and Peripheral

Petroleum Hydrocarbons

Petroleum is a naturally occurring, oily, flammable liquid composed principally of hydrocarbons; it is occasionally found in springs or pools but is usually obtained from beneath the earth's surface by drilling wells. Formerly called rock oil, unrefined petroleum is now usually termed crude oil. Crude oil is a highly complex mixture of paraffinic, cycloparaffinic (naphthenic), and aromatic hydrocarbons, containing a low percentage of sulfur and trace amounts of nitrogen and oxygen compounds (see Oil, Crude).

The most important petroleum fractions, obtained by cracking or distillation, are various hydrocarbon gases (butane, ethane, and propane), naphtha of several grades, gasoline, kerosene, fuel oils, gas oil, lubricating oils, paraffin wax, and asphalt. From the hydrocarbon gases, ethylene, butylene, and propylene are obtained; these are important industrial intermediates, being the source of alcohols, ethylene glycols and monomers for a wide range of plastics, elastomers, and pharmaceuticals. Benzene, phenol, toluene, and xylene can be made from petroleum. Hundreds of other products, including biosynthetically produced proteins, are petroleum-derived.

Petroleum is separated by distillation into fractions designed as (1) straight-run gasoline, boiling at up to about 390°F (200°C); (2) middle distillate, boiling at about 365–653°F (185–345°C), from which are obtained kerosene, heating oils, and diesel, jet, rocket, and gas turbine fuels; (3) wide-cut gas oil, which boils at about 653–1000°F (345–540°C), and from which are obtained waxes, lubrication oils, and feedstock for catalytic cracking to gasoline; and (4) residual oil, which may be asphaltic.

The physical properties and chemical composition of petroleum vary markedly, depending on its source. As it comes from the earth, it ranges from an occasional nearly colorless liquid consisting chiefly of gasoline to a heavy black tarry material high in asphalt content. Most crudes are black; many are amber, red, or brown by transmitted light and show a greenish fluorescence by reflected light and have a specific gravity in the range about 0.82–0.95.

Hydrocarbons constitute 50–98% of petroleum, and the remainder is composed chiefly of organic compounds containing oxygen, nitrogen, or sulfur and trace amounts of organometallic compounds. The hydrocarbon types found in petroleum are paraffins (alkanes), cycloparaffins (naphthenes or cycloaldanes), and aromatics. Olefins (alkenes) and other unsaturated hydrocarbons are usually absent.

The number of carbon atoms in hydrocarbons of a given boiling range depends on the hydrocarbon type. In general, gasoline will include hydrocarbons having 4–12 carbon atoms; kerosene, 10–14; middle distillate, 12–20; and wide-cut gas oil, 20–36. Five main classes of compounds are present in the gasoline fraction: straight-chain paraffins, branched-chain paraffins, alkylcyclopentanes, alkylcyclohexanes, and alkylbenzenes.

Asphalt is a dark-brown to black solid or semisolid consisting of carbon, hydrogen, oxygen, sulfur, and sometimes nitrogen. It is made up of three components: (1) asphaltene, a hard, friable, infusible powder, (2) resin, a semisolid to solid ductile and adhesive material, and (3) oil, which is structurally similar to the lubricating oil fraction from which it is derived.

Acute exposure to unleaded gasoline and a variety of light hydrocarbons present in gasoline produces a nephropathy in male rats characterized by (1) an excessive accumulation of protein (hyaline droplets) in epithelial cells of proximal tubule, (2) accumulation of casts at the corticomedullary junction, and (3) evidence of mild tubular regeneration. This nephropathy only occurs in male rats; female rats and mice do not show any renal pathology. A number of chemicals present in unleaded petrol when tested alone have been shown to produce nephropathy and, in particular, 2,2,4-trimethylpentane and decalin have been used as model compounds. Certain other industrial chemicals (1,4-dichlorobenzene and isophorone), natural products (D-limonene), and pharmaceuticals (levamisole) also produce this male-rat-specific nephropathy. Chronic exposure of male rats to unleaded petrol, 1,4-dichlorobenzene, isophorone, or D-limonene ultimately leads to the induction of a low incidence of renal adenomas and carcinomas.

Studies on the mechanism of pathogenesis have shown that the protein which accumulates in the proximal tubular cells is α_{2u}-globulin, a low-molecular-weight protein of 18,700 Da) that is synthesized in the liver of adult rats and is freely filtered at the glomerulus. Female rats excrete less than 1% of the α_{2u}-globulin that male rats excrete. The chemical itself or a metabolite has been shown to bind reversibly to α_{2u}-globulin and this chemical–protein complex is then thought to be taken up by the proximal tubular cells (primarily in the S_2 segment) by endecytosis. These complexes appear to be quite resistant to, or impair, lysosomal degradation, which leads to their accumulation a polyangular droplets. Lysosomal overload is thought to lead to individual cellular necrosis which is followed by repair and regeneration. It has been suggested that a sustained increase in renal cell proliferation can promote initiated cells to form preneoplastic foci and lead to renal neoplasia. The development of the renal toxicity and increased cell proliferation is dependent on the presence of α_{2u}-globulin The NCI Black–Reiter strain of male rat cannot synthesize α_{2u}-globulin and, by inference, would not be expected to be at risk. However, it is not known whether these hydrocarbons or their metabollites can bind to other low-molecular-weight proteins and, if so, whether the same bichemical events as those observed with α_{2u}-globulin could occur.

Products with viscosity in the range of 30–35 or lower present an extreme aspiration risk and include agents such as mineral seal oil, which is found in furniture polishes. It is important to realize that even small amounts of a low-viscosity material, once aspirated, can involve a significant portion of the lung and produce a chemical pneumonitis. Oral ingestion of hydrocarbons often is associated with symptoms of mucous membrane irritation, vomiting, and CNS depression. Cyanosis, tachycardia, and tachypnea may appear as a result of aspiration, with subsequent development of chemical pneumonitis. Other clinical findings include albuminuria, hematuria, hepatic enzyme derangement, and cardiac arrhythmias. Doses as low as 10 ml orally have been reported to be potentially fatal, whereas other patients have survived the ingestion of 60 ml of petroleum distillates. A history of coughing or choking in association with vomiting strongly suggests aspiration and hydrocarbon pneumonia. Hydrocarbon pneumonia is an acute hemorrhagic necrotizing disease that can develop within 24 hr after the ingestion. Pneumonia may require several weeks for complete resolution.

Activated charcoal and/or emesis may be indicated in some hydrocarbon ingestions in which absorption may produce systemic effects. Agents such as asphalt, tar, heavy lubricants, Vaseline, and mineral oil are considered relatively nontoxic and do not require removal. Chlorinated hydrocarbon solvents or any hydrocarbon or petroleum distillate with a potentially dangerous additive (camphor, pesticide, and heavy metals) in some cases may be treated with activated charcoal or emesis. Petroleum naphtha derivatives, gasoline, kerosene, and mineral seal oil (or signal oil) as found in furniture polish and oil polishes produce severe and often prolonged chemical pneumonitis. These compounds are poorly absorbed from the stomach but are very damaging to the lung if inhaled. They should not be removed by emesis unless very large amounts are ingested ($\geqq$12–18 ml/kg). Gastric lavage is not indicated for hydrocarbon ingestion because of the risk of aspiration if the patient vomits around the lavage tube. X-rays taken early in the course of ingestion may not demonstrate chemical pneumonia; even if it is demonstrated, the clinical severity does not correlate well with the degree of X-ray findings. However, X-rays should be repeated on follow-up to detect the development of pneumonitis or demonstrate pneumatoceles. Patients who arrive coughing probably already have aspirated and should be monitored closely for the development of pneumonitis. The decision for hospitalization should be based on clinical criteria (e.g., cyanosis and respiratory distress) rather than on X-ray findings alone. Steroid therapy may be harmful. Antibiotics, oxygen, and positive end expiratory pressure should be instituted as indicated.

The usual cutaneous response to oil-based materials is an oil folliculitis that arises as a result of chemical irritation and mechanical plugging of the follicular canals. Onset of the problem usually occurs soon after the first exposure and is marked by acute reactions starting on the dorsal surfaces of the hands and fingers, the extensor surfaces of the forearms and thighs, and the abdomen (i.e., those surfaces that are in contact with oil or oil-soaked clothing). Comedones and perifollicular papules and pustules ("oil boils") develop. Secondary infections may occur, but the bacteria in the oil are rarely primary skin pathogens and are rarely the single cause of the folliculitis. Melanosis may appear later. Clinical manifestations clear rapidly with the termination of exposure and do not resolve if the exposure is continued. Exposure is controlled through proper machine design to prevent spattering, clean clothing, protective garments, and careful attention to handwashing and other aspects of personal hygiene.

Since emulsion and synthetic fluids are potent defatting agents, the skin reaction to them may include maceration, dryness and "chapping," reddening, and vesiculation. Bacterial growths in the fluid do not appear to be directly injurious to workers, but rancid fluids and products of bacterial action can lead to skin disorders. As in the case of insoluble oils, both treatment and prevention are based on the control of exposure. Corticosteroid creams may be used as an adjunct in the treatment. The value of "barrier" creams and other protective gels is not universally accepted, but they do offer modest usefulness in certain situations and have been shown to reduce ultrastructural and cytoarchitectural changes in human epidermis after applications of acetone and kerosene.

Individual additives in cutting fluids can be a cause of either primary irritative or hypersensitive dermatitis. Detergents, soaps, and wetting agents defat the skin, and alkaline materials damage the keratin of the upper, protective skin layers. Ulcerative and erythematous lesions on the genitals and buttocks have been reported for workers wearing coveralls that had been drycleaned with Stoddard solvent, a mixture of petroleum distillates. Formalin in germicides is a sensitizer. Additives containing sulfur and chlorine are direct irritants, although so-called chloracne is not associated with cutting fluids. Nickel or chromates derived from metals being cut can be a source of allergic dermatitis. Harsh abrasive soaps and solvents, such as gasoline and kerosene, may contribute to chemical and traumatic dermatitis since these cleaning materials are common in machine shops. While grime and grease can certainly be removed from the skin with these substances, it is safer to utilize less injurious cleansers available commercially.

Certain petroleum oils have carcinogenic constituents; this is especially the case with shale oils, which are currently extracted and used outside of the United States. Since American potential supplies of oil shale tars constitute 94% of the known world resources, these substances may present toxic problems in the United States in the future. There are no good data that would establish the prevalence of skin cancers among machinists in this country, but scrotal and other skin cancers have been reported among British cotton mule spinners prior to 1953 and more recently among toolsetters and machine operators in the British Midlands. Knowledge of occupational malignancies of the skin has a long and important history that dates back to 1775 when Pott identified scrotal cancer in English chimney sweeps. A particular set of carcinogenicity bioassays, the mouse skin painting studies, were developed specifically to assess the carcinogenic potential of petroleum products.

Exposure to mist sprays or insoluble oils used as coolants, cutting fluids, and lubricants in machine operations are usually not harmful to the respiratory tract, although worker discomfort occurs at oil mist levels above 5 mg/m^3. Mineral oil droplets $<5\ \mu m$ in diameter may be inhaled and result in fibrotic nodules, paraffinomas, or in lipoid pneumonitis. There was no evidence that machinists exposed to cutting-oil mists had any unusual mortality from respiratory tract cancer.

—*Shayne C. Gad*

Related Topic

Polycyclic Aromatic Hydrocarbons

Peyote

- CAS: 11006-96-5
- Synonyms: *Lophophora williamsii;* mescaline; peyotl; 3,4,5-trimethoxyphenethylamine; mescal button; mescal; anhalonium; mesc; big chief
- Description: Peyote is the common name given to *L. williamsii,* the North American dumpling cactus.
- Chemical Class: Mescaline, peyote's major active alkaloid, is a narcotic hallucinogen (see Mescaline).
- Chemical Structure: (Mescaline)

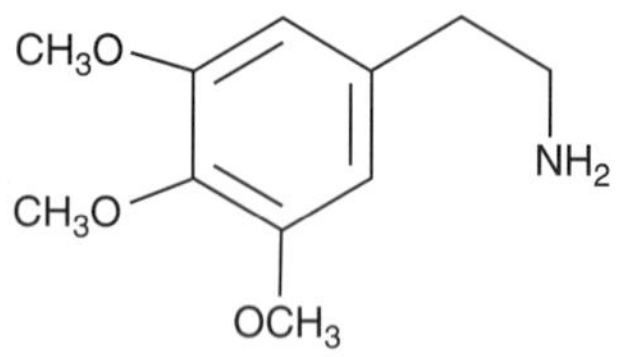

Uses

Peyote is used as a Native American religious intoxicant, a hallucinogenic agent, and a folk remedy.

Exposure Pathways

Peyote is ingested in various forms, including dried buttons, tincture of peyote (70% alcohol extract), and panpeyote (chloroform extract of ground peyote). Synthetic mescaline has been administered intravenously, orally, subcutaneously, and intramuscularly.

Toxicokinetics

Mescaline is rapidly absorbed, with peak blood levels noted in 2 hr. Gastrointestinal effects occur in 30–60 min and sensory effects peak between 4 and 6 hr postingestion. Symptoms usually resolve in 12–14 hr. Mescaline is metabolized in the liver to a number of inactive metabolites. Mescaline is widely distributed to peripheral tissues. Brain and blood levels are nearly equal; concentrations in the kidneys, liver, and spleen are three to five times greater. Approximately 60% of a dose is excreted unchanged in a 24-hr urine, and the remainder is eliminated as metabolites.

Mechanism of Toxicity

The precise mechanism of action is unknown. Mescaline is thought to stimulate both serotonin and dopamine receptors in the central nervous system, resulting in behavioral effects and hallucinations. The peripheral effects may be due to changes in catecholamine metabolism and adrenal medullary function. Peripheral effects are probably also centrally mediated. Mescaline can produce cerebral vasospasm.

Human Toxicity

A dose of 5–8 mg/kg by any route causes the desired psychedelic effects. Dried peyote buttons provide approximately 45 mg of mescaline. Nausea, chills, and vomiting, which are often accompanied with anxiety and terror, occur first in most users. Diaphoresis, mild tachycardia, and hypertension are common. Photophobia related to mydriasis, nystagmus, tremors, ataxia, and hyperreflexia are also seen. The sympathomimetic effects are followed by vivid visual hallucinations (consisting of brilliant colors) and exaggerated sensitivity to sound and other sense impressions. There is a clarity and intensity of thought. Doses of 20 mg/kg or more can result in vasodilation, bradycardia, hypotension, and respiratory depression. Death from mescaline has not been reported. It is likely that the unpleasant taste of peyote and the spontaneous vomiting limits the amount ingested and absorbed. Hallucinations may lead to death from trauma. The qualitative presence of mescaline in urine can confirm the diagnosis; blood levels do not correlate with toxicity.

Chronic

Flashbacks have occurred. Persistent psychosis, anxiety, and depression have been described following mescaline use. Tolerance, but not physical dependence, are reported. Chromosomal abnormalities have not been found in life long users.

Clinical Management

Treatment is supportive. A nonthreatening environment should be maintained and calm reassurance provided. Because mescaline is rapidly absorbed and vomiting is common, gastric decontamination is usually not necessary. However, activated charcoal can be used prior to the occurrence of symptoms. Diazepam is the sedative of choice. Haloperidol can be used for acute psychosis or hallucinations unresponsive to diazepam. Patients with massive mescaline ingestion may require ventilatory support.

Animal Toxicity

The lethal dose of mescaline in animals ranges from 150 to more than 500 mg/kg, depending on the route of administration and the species.

—Janet E. Bauman

Pharmacokinetic Models

Pharmacokinetics/toxicokinetics is the area of toxicology that is concerned with the role of absorption, distribution, metabolism, and excretion of toxicants in the body. These events, some of which may be interdependent, often have a very significant impact on the toxicity of a chemical in a specific species. Quantitative characterization of the time profile of absorption, distribution, metabolism, and excretion of xenobiotic compounds is included in the area of pharmacokinetics. In this sense, pharmacokinetics is used synonymously with toxicokinetics.

One of the methods of examining the kinetics of absorption, distribution, metabolism, and excretion of a xenobiotic involves a description of the body as a series of relevant physiological compartments in contact with the venous and arterial supplies of blood. Pharmacokinetic models are mathematical models that permit predictions about body burdens, clearance profiles for chemicals following cessation of the exposure, and other information that may aid in assessing the hazards of chemicals to humans. In these models, physiological information, such as blood flow rates to each compartment, the partition coefficients between the blood and organ tissues, and the different volumes of the various compartments, can be used to build differential mass-balance equations that describe the rate of change of concentrations of the chemical of interest in the compartments. Pharmacokinetic models are especially useful for characterizing tissue-level doses when external exposures [i.e., exposures contacting the biological barriers or membranes of the organism (e.g., skin)] are repeated or intermittent in nature. Such models utilize physiological parameters and biochemical transformation data to determine the temporal relationships of the distribution and disposition of an administered dose.

Pharmacokinetic models require three different types of information: (1) partition coefficients that describe the relative solubility or affinity of the compound for blood versus other tissues; (2) physiological constants, such as tissue and organ volumes and the relevant blood flows; and (3) rate constants for the key biochemical/biotransformation pathways. Partition coefficients are generally obtained by measurement in the laboratory, tissue volume/blood flow data are mostly available from the scientific literature (with allometric scaling from species to species), and biotransformation data are usually obtained from *in vivo* and *in vitro* kinetic studies. Biochemical constants for metabolic pathways are captured using the maximum rate of reaction, or V_{max}, and the binding affinity of the particular substrate for the metabolizing enzyme.

Two limiting cases relating to permeability of the cell membrane should be considered in developing a pharmacokinetic model for a given chemical. In the flow-limited model, transport of the chemical across the cell membrane is assumed to be so rapid that the rate of blood flow is taken to be the limiting process that determines the rate of uptake. In the membrane-limited model, cell permeability is assumed to be low, and thus the rate-limiting step, compared with the blood perfusion rate. The pharmacokinetics of volatile hydrocarbons and halogenated hydrocarbons, such as methylene chloride, are adequately described by a flow-limited model. Larger molecular weight compounds and many drugs, such as digoxin and methotrexate, are most appropriately described by a membrane-limited model.

In constructing a pharmacokinetic model, it is not necessarily critical to place each tissue or organ into a separate compartment; rather, organs with similar blood flows, diffusion characteristics, and permeability properties can often be combined into single compartments. For example, the adrenals, kidneys, thyroid, brain, heart, and heptoportal system are sometimes pooled into one compartment because their perfusion-to-volume ratios are relatively high, facilitating their classification as a vessel-rich group). The liver, lungs, and gastrointestinal tract are usually represented separately. In using a pharmacokinetic model of uptake, distribution, and elimination, an exponential power (e.g., 0.75) of the body weight is used to scale the cardiac output and ventilation rate between the laboratory species (typically rat) and humans.

Pharmacokinetic models can vary in complexity from a simple two-compartment model to a multicompartment physiologically based pharmacokinetic (PBPK) model. PBPK models describe the body in terms of tissue compartments, blood supply flow rates, partition coefficients, and tissue binding characteristics. PBPK models are particularly useful for interspecies extrapolations of dose–response data. A PBPK model will contain adequate logic to account for routes of administration, storage tissues and residence time therein, elimination rates, and sufficient mathematical detail to mimic the integration of these processes. It is important that the model parameters (e.g., elimination rates) be validated as much as possible by separate kinetic studies in the relevant species. The ultimate test of the model is how close the model predictions are for parameters such as blood levels, rate of metabolism, and tissue concentrations relative to real-life animal data for the chemical.

The simplest model is a two-compartment model in which there is a blood compartment and tissue compartment which have reversible flows of compound or metabolites or both between them. The general forms of the equations for a two-compartment model are as follows for describing the rate of change in the concentration of chemical of interest in compartment 1 (C_1) and in compartment 2 (C_2):

$$\frac{dC_1}{dt} = (k_{21}C_2) - (k_{12} + k_e)C_1$$

$$\frac{dC_2}{dt} = (k_{12}C_1) - (k_{21}C_2)$$

where k_{21} and k_{12} are the unidirectional rate constants for movement of chemical between the two compartments, and k_e is the elimination rate constant. Simultaneous integration of these two equations gives the explicit solution as a multiexponential equation, the exponents being expressed as a function of the rate constants and time, and factoring in the volumes of the compartments. A number of computer programs have been developed to integrate the differential equations and solve them by iterative processes. Although the number of compartments and corresponding differential equations that can be used in a PBPK model are virtually unlimited, there is a practical limitation in the number of rate constants and other parameters that can be adequately quantified for the model; some of these parameters are unknown and virtually unquantifiable experimentally.

Pharmacokinetic models have been developed and parameters defined for a number of chemicals, including methylene chloride, perchloroethylene, and pharmaceuticals (including anticancer drugs). U.S. EPA commonly uses the Integrated Exposure Uptake Biokinetic Model for Lead to estimate the blood lead levels in children (up to 6 years) associated with multipathway environmental exposures. Acceptability of the concentration of lead in various environmental media is linked to a blood lead level in children believed to be protective of health. For methylene chloride, the mass-balance equations that form the model adequately account for the removal of the compound by the liver as well as the significant excretion through the lungs and incomplete retention ($<15\%$) of an inhaled dose, and they are useful for comparing organ-specific doses between different routes of exposure (e.g., oral and inhalation). Because of these features, the PBPK model prevents overestimation of dose which would be obtained, for example, if total absorption of an inhaled dose were assumed and if removal by the liver were ignored. Thus, such a model provides an effective tool for exposure assessment by quantifying the internal doses that are ultimately the most appropriate dose metrics to use in route-to-route comparisons.

—*Gary Whitmyre*

Related Topics

Absorption
Distribution
Excretion
Pharmacokinetics/Toxicokinetics

Pharmacokinetics/ Toxicokinetics

It is generally accepted that the intensity of toxic effects exerted by foreign chemicals (xenobiotics) is related to the concentration of the toxic moiety at the site of action in a target tissue or organ, whereas in many cases, the duration of the toxic effects depends on the time during which the toxic moiety remains at the site of action. However, there are numerous examples showing that the administration of two xenobiotics, at the same dose and with similar toxic potential, does not yield the same concentration of the toxic moiety for the same duration of time at a given site of action. The most plausible reason for such behavior is that the respective disposition of the two chemicals in the body can differ one from one another. Disposition may be regarded as the result of the absorption, distribution, and elimination processes acting on xenobiotics. In other words, disposition is what governs the fate of chemicals in the various compartments of the body and as such plays a key role in determining the concentration and toxicity of these chemicals at the site of action.

Pharmacokinetics/toxicokinetics may be defined as the study of the dynamic movements of xenobiotics during their passage through the body and as such encompass the concept of disposition described previously (Fig. P-2). In simpler words, it tells us what the body does to foreign chemicals. To that end, pharmacokinetic/toxicokinetic analysis uses mathematical terms, or equations, to describe the time course of the absorption and disposition of xenobiotics in the body and proposes simplified representations (models) of the re-

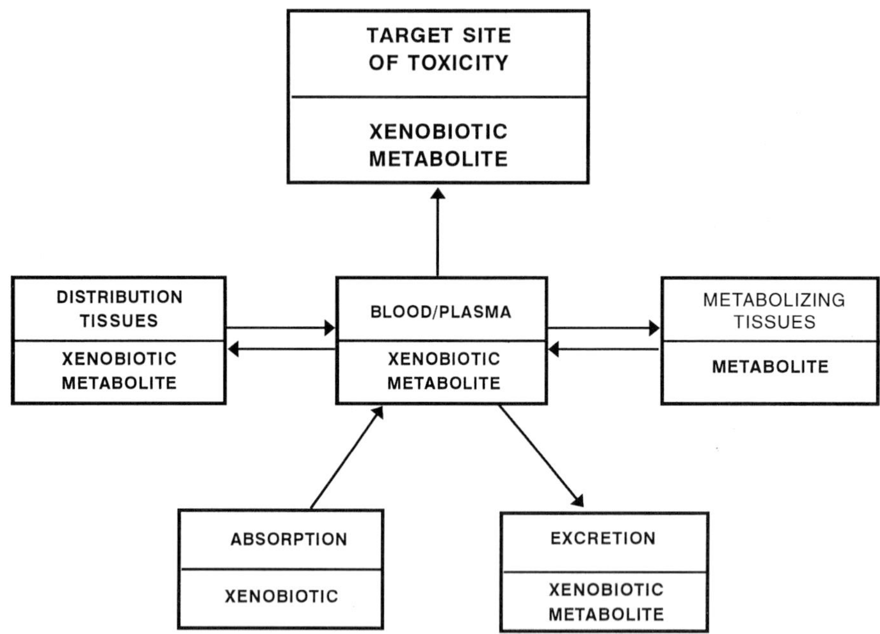

FIGURE P-2. Schematic representation of the main biological processes involved in the disposition of xenobiotics in the body.

lationship between time and movements of xenobiotics. Once the information on the concentration of a chemical in biologically relevant parts of the body is provided by pharmacokinetic/toxicokinetic studies, it then usually becomes possible to better understand, interpret, and even predict the nature and the extent of the biological effects of xenobiotics.

Etymologically, the term pharmacokinetics relates to the study of the movements of medicines or therapeutic agents within the body. From an historical point of view, principles and methods dealing with the study of the movements of chemicals within the body have evolved from data pertaining precisely to medication. For example, pharmacokinetic data are used for optimal adjustment of dosage regimen to obtain the best therapeutic effect without eliciting adverse side effects. The term toxicokinetics has a wider meaning in that it consists of applying pharmacokinetic principles and methods for the prediction of occurrence and time course of toxic events related to foreign chemicals (medication, food additives, workplace products, environmental contaminants, etc.) encountered at levels of exposure likely to induce toxicity.

In order to facilitate the description of the biological fate of xenobiotics, toxicologists represent the body as compartments that correspond to the various tissues, organs, or fluids of the body. Such functional representation is known as pharmacokinetic modeling. Two types of models are currently available to toxicologists for that purpose: compartmental models and physiologically based pharmacokinetic (PBPK) models. Compartmental models have been extensively studied and used in pharmacokinetic modeling, but recently PBPK modeling has received increasing attention.

The purpose of this entry is to introduce the reader to simple basic concepts and principles of pharmacokinetic/toxicokinetic analysis using both types of models—compartmental and physiologically based.

Pharmacokinetic Models

Compartmental Models

Compartmental models, also known as data-based models, are essentially used to fit curves to experimental data on blood, plasma, or urine concentrations of a chemical or its metabolite(s). In this approach, the body is represented as a single or a series of compartments which do not necessarily correspond to any physiological or anatomical reality. As mentioned previously, toxicologists are mainly concerned with avoiding toxicity in target organs/tissues that are presented with time-dependent concentrations of a chemical. It is not feasible, at least in humans, to determine the time course concentration of a xenobiotic at a target site (e.g., brain, liver, and kidneys). To overcome this problem, it is assumed, when using the compartmental modeling approach, that the biological effects which depend on the concentration at target site are also related to the concentration of a chemical in blood or plasma. This is the reason why almost all pharmacokinetic analyses are based on blood concentration.

Compartmental modeling consists of finding the proper mathematical equation of the curve that allows a best fit to the kinetic behavior of a xenobiotic. In the simplest case, the body is represented as a single compartment (e.g., one-compartment model). When necessary, however, additional and usually limited numbers of compartments can be added to achieve a better description of the kinetic behavior of a particular xenobiotic (e.g., two- and three-compartment models).

When using such models, it is assumed that the disposition of a chemical is governed by first-order processes. This means that the rate of disappearance of a xenobiotic from the body, as a result of excretion and/or biotransformation, is proportional to the amount of the xenobiotic in the body at that time. In other words, the quantity of a xenobiotic that leaves the body is large when the amount of xenobiotic in the body is large (e.g., immediately after exposure), whereas this quantity is small when the amount in the body is small (e.g., several hours after exposure). Most xenobiotics exhibit this type of behavior, provided that the several biological mechanisms responsible for disposition are not saturated, i.e., not overwhelmed by large concentrations of xenobiotics (see Dose-Dependent Kinetics).

One-Compartment Open Model

In this simple model, the body is treated as an homogenous unit with an entry and an exit (i.e., open model) (Fig. P-3A). It is assumed that changes occurring in blood concentrations reflect similar changes in tissue levels as the xenobiotic rapidly equilibrates between blood and all the various tissues of the body.

Figure P-3B illustrates the time dependency of the concentration of a xenobiotic in blood, following rapid intravenous administration. It is seen that the blood concentration decreases rapidly at the beginning and then falls more slowly thereafter. This is typical of first-order elimination as described previously. This curve can be described by using the following exponential term:

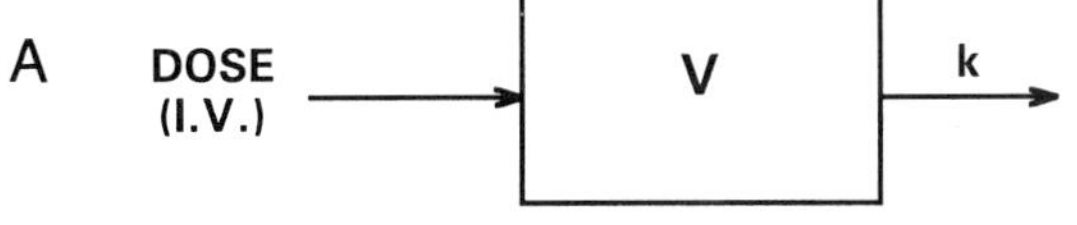

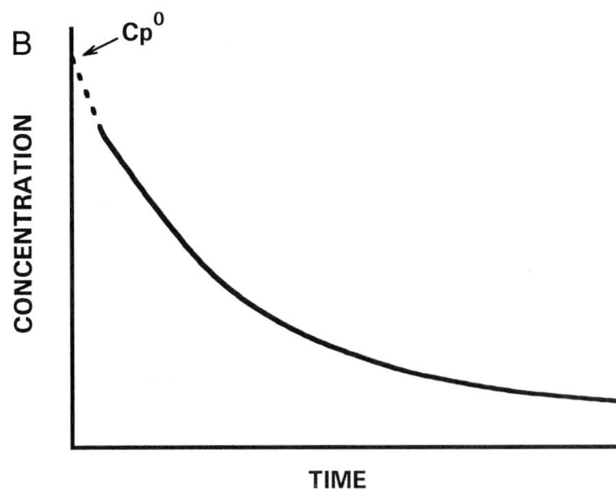

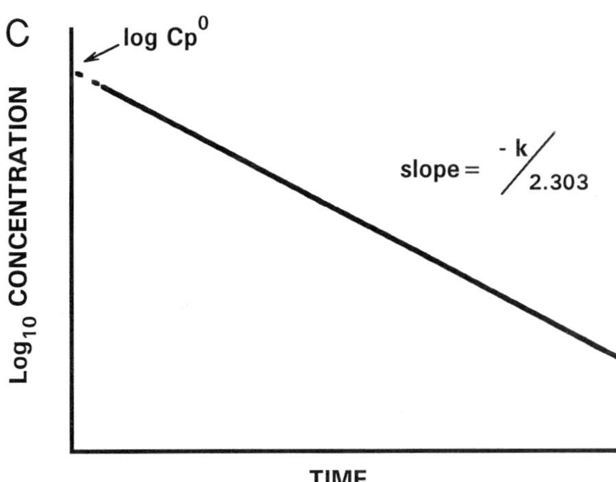

FIGURE P-3. (A) Schematic representation of a one-compartment open model: iv, intravenous administration; V, *volume of the compartment;* k, *elimination rate constant (see text). B and C represent the time course of blood concentration of a xenobiotic following intravenous administration (B, linear scale; C, logarithmic scale); Cp^0, blood concentration at time zero.*

$$Cp = Cp^{o} \cdot e^{-k.t}$$

where Cp represents the blood (plasma) concentration of a xenobiotic at time t, Cp^{o} is the blood initial concentration (i.e., extrapolated at time 0), and k is the first-order elimination rate constant. A more practical form of this equation is obtained by substituting the base 10 logarithm (Fig. P-3C):

$$\log_{10} Cp = \log_{10} Cp^{o} - \frac{k \cdot t}{2.303}$$

This simple mathematical description is very useful for determining a series of various kinetic parameters that characterize the kinetic behavior of a given xenobiotic. These kinetics parameters are the volume of distribution, the elimination rate constant, the half-life of elimination, the clearance, the area-under-the-blood-concentration curve, and the bioavailability.

Volume of Distribution **(V_D).** The volume of distribution is defined as the apparent volume (e.g., liter and milliliter) into which a chemical appears to have been dissolved, once it has penetrated in the body, to give an initial blood concentration equal to Cp^{o}:

$$V_D = DOSE / Cp^{o}$$

Usually, V_D does not correspond to any real biological volume and as such has no direct physiological meaning. In some cases, V_D may show values even larger than the volume of a standard human body. Indeed, since the value of V_D is inversely proportional to the blood concentration, chemicals showing an especially high affinity for fatty tissues (e.g., insecticides of the DDT family and several industrial solvents) and therefore having a strong tendency to leave the blood pool may exhibit large V_D values. On the other hand, a chemical that is firmly bound to blood components, such as the red cells and the proteins (e.g., warfarin, a blood anticoagulant), will remain in the blood pool and exhibit V_D values close to blood volume only.

Elimination Rate Constant (k). The elimination rate constant (i.e., usually a first-order rate constant) is a very useful value that represents the fraction of an agent that is eliminated from the body during a given period of time. For instance, when the value of the elimination rate constant of a xenobiotic is 0.25 per hour, this means that 25% of the amount remaining in the body is excreted each hour. The rate constant is calculated from the slope ($^{-k}/2.303$) of the curve relating blood concentration with time as shown in Fig. P-3C. Its value is affected by all processes (e.g., distribution, biotransformation, and excretion) that contribute to clear the substance from the blood.

Half-Life of Elimination ($t_{1/2}$). This is the time period (e.g., minutes, hours, and days) during which the blood concentration of a xenobiotic falls to one-half of its original value as a result of all processes of distribution, biotransformation, and excretion. The determination of $t_{1/2}$ is based on the calculation of the elimination rate constant described above (k):

$$t_{1/2} = 0{,}693 / k$$

Xenobiotics that show small $t_{1/2}$ values (i.e., short half-lives) are those that are cleared rapidly from the body, whereas those with high values (i.e., long half-lives) are cleared more slowly and in some cases may accumulate in the body. Insecticides of the DDT family and heavy metals like lead, cadmium, and mercury all display long half-lives, whereas aspirin is a drug that exhibits a short half-life.

Clearance (CL). Clearance represents the volume of blood (e.g., milliliter and liter) that is completely cleared of a xenobiotic during a given period of time, usually 1 min or 1 hr (e.g., ml/min, liter/hr). As such, the clearance is a quantitative measure of the rate of removal of a compound from the body. All routes of elimination (e.g., hepatic biotransformation, urinary, biliary, and pulmonary excretion) contribute to the clearance of a chemical from the body, and each one exhibits a specific clearance value. Specific clearance values provide an indication of the ability of a particular organ to dispose of a substance. When the value for clearance is high, it suggests that the compound is removed rapidly from the body, whereas a low clearance value indicates slower removal. The value of the clearance is the product of the elimination rate constant

(k) with the apparent volume of distribution (V_D) as described by the following equation:

$$CL = K \cdot V_D$$

Therefore, CL may be regarded as the volume of blood from which the compound is apparently removed during a given period of time.

Bioavailability (F). Bioavailability is a term used to describe the percentage (or the fraction F) of an administered dose of a xenobiotic that reaches the systemic circulation. Bioavailability is practically 100% ($F = 1$) following an intravenous administration. Bioavailability could be lower ($F < 1$) and in some cases almost negligible for other routes (e.g., oral, dermal, and pulmonary), depending on how efficiently a xenobiotic crosses various biological membranes (e.g., lungs, skin, and stomach) or whether or not tissues or organs (e.g., lungs, skin, and liver) through which xenobiotics pass before reaching the systemic circulation are capable of metabolizing the substance; the latter phenomenon is known as a first-past effect. Bioavailability may vary considerably between compounds or even between batches of a given compound. For example, drugs commonly used as therapeutic agents must undergo bioavailability testing in order to ensure reliable dosing throughout treatment. The blood concentration of the administered drug is used as an index of bioavailability.

Area under the Curve (AUC). The area-under-the-blood-concentration-time curve reflects the amount of a xenobiotic that has effectively reached the systemic circulation and as such is influenced both by the degree of bioavailability and by the rate at which a chemical is removed from the body. AUC is a good indicator of the internal exposure dose in the body since it takes into consideration not only the blood concentration of a xenobiotic but also the time a xenobiotic is present in the blood compartment and thus in the body.

In summary, the kinetic parameters referred to previously are used to describe the behavior of xenobiotics in the body following exposure via several routes: the extent of distribution within the body, the amount available for action and elimination, the contribution of specific organs in elimination, and the rate of elimination. Such information can be used to establish therapeutic drug regimens or to predict the extent and duration of contamination of exposed organisms.

Two-Compartment Open Model

In certain circumstances, following the completion of the absorption phase, the curve that describes the time course of the blood concentration of a xenobiotic does not exhibit a single straight line but rather two segments (Fig. P-4B). Such biexponential decline can best be described by a two-compartment model (Fig. P-4A): a central compartment that usually refers to the blood pool and a peripheral compartment that represents various fluids and tissues of the body for which a xenobiotic may have a particular affinity. This system can be described mathematically by a differential equation

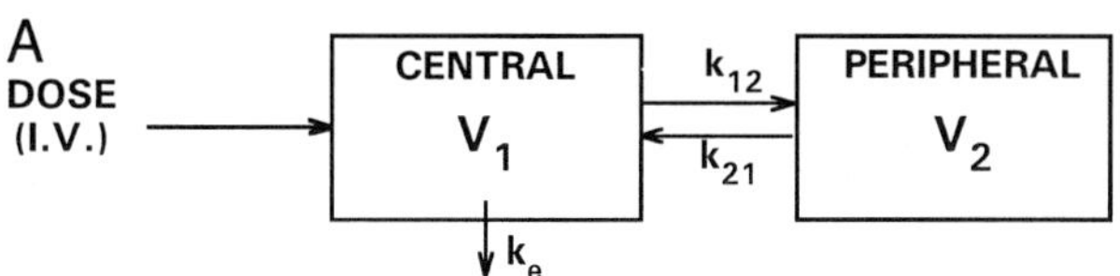

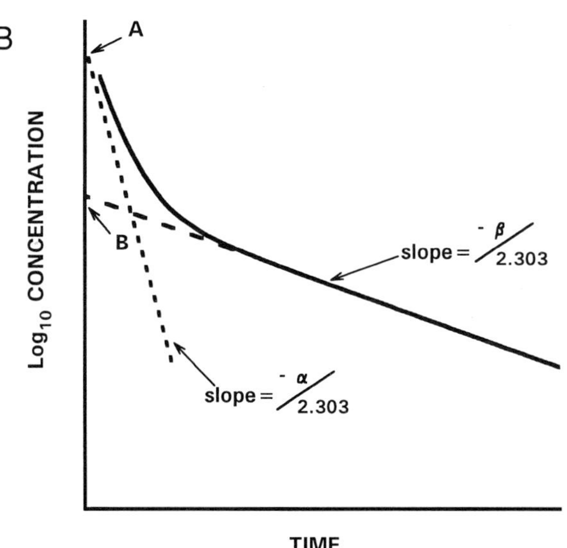

FIGURE P-4. (A) Schematic representation of a two-compartment open model: iv, intravenous administration, V_1 and V_2, respective volume of compartments 1 and 2; k_{21} and k_{12}, transfer rate constants between compartments 1 and 2; k_e, elimination rate constant. (B) Time course of blood concentration following intravenous administration: A and B, proportionality constants; α and β, elimination rate constants corresponding to each segment of the curve.

comprising two exponential terms, one for each segment of the curve. Taken individually, each one of these terms is essentially similar to the one used to describe the curve corresponding to the one-compartment model:

$$\log_{10} Cp = \log_{10} A - \frac{\alpha \cdot t}{2.303} + \log_{10} B - \frac{\beta \cdot t}{2.303}$$

where A and B are proportionality constants for each compartment ($A + B = Cp^{o}$), and α and β are composite rate constants that can be regarded as the elimination rate constant of each segment of the curve (i.e., each compartment). The first segment is known as the α-phase, during which a chemical leaves the blood circulation to be distributed among the various organs and tissues, whereas the second segment corresponds to the β-phase, which mainly characterizes the processes leading to the elimination of a chemical. Accordingly, the $t_{1/2}$ of a xenobiotic displaying such kinetic behavior is calculated from the β-phase using an equation similar to the one previously described for a one-compartment model:

$$t_{1/2} = 0.693 / \beta$$

How values A, B, α, and β are calculated falls beyond the scope of this text. Suffice it to say that these parameters represent values that contribute additively to the equation describing the two-compartment open model.

In order to facilitate the understanding of the pharmacokinetic concepts, the examples given previously are for the simplest and the most effective route of administration, i.e., intravenous administration. Regarding exposure to toxic compounds (e.g., occupational or environmental exposure), however, other routes are frequently involved. These routes imply respiratory, cutaneous, mucous, or oral uptake. In such cases, pharmacokinetic analyses are more complex since they should take into account the various processes responsible for the uptake of a xenobiotic. Usually, it consists of introducing into equations an additional term that contains a rate constant describing the uptake, operating in a direction opposite to, yet not conceptually different from, the elimination rate constant.

Physiologically Based Models

Whereas compartmental models are abstract mathematical representations of an animal or a human body, in the form of a certain number of boxes, PBPK models describe the behavior of xenobiotics on the basis of the actual anatomy, physiology, and biochemistry of human beings and animals. Being realistically modeled on how the body functions, PBPK models take into consideration the complex relationships that exist between critical biological and physicochemical determinants such as blood flow, ventilation rates, metabolic rate constants, tissue solubilities, and binding to proteins (e.g., albumin and glycoproteins) or other macromolecules (e.g., DNA and hemoglobin).

Contrary to compartmental models, PBPK models allow one to describe the time course of xenobiotic concentration in any organ or tissue represented in the model. Since these models include anatomical, physiological, and biochemical determinants, they can account for any quantitative alterations of such determinants—for example, ventilation rates, organ pathology, or metabolic enzyme activity. Not only can they describe and model what is actually occurring under a given set of exposure conditions but also they can build on such a description and expand to any other condition likely to happen within the range of variation of the anatomical, physiological, and biochemical parameters.

A PBPK model comprises a series of anatomically well-defined compartments that represent organs or tissues in which a xenobiotic distributes or exerts its toxic effects (Fig. P-5). These anatomical compartments are interconnected by the blood circulation (i.e., arterial blood to and venous blood from the tissues). The physiological and anatomical determinants for different species, including humans (e.g., alveolar ventilation rate, blood flow rates, and tissue volumes), are usually abundantly documented in the literature. Physicochemical parameters—namely partition coefficients that describe the relative solubility of a xenobiotic between air present in the lungs and blood, on the one hand, and between blood and tissues, on the other hand—may be obtained in some cases from the literature or otherwise determined experimentally in the laboratory. Usually, biochemical parameters, namely metabolic rate constants that describe the metabolic capacity of a tissue toward a given xenobiotic, are determined experimentally in the laboratory.

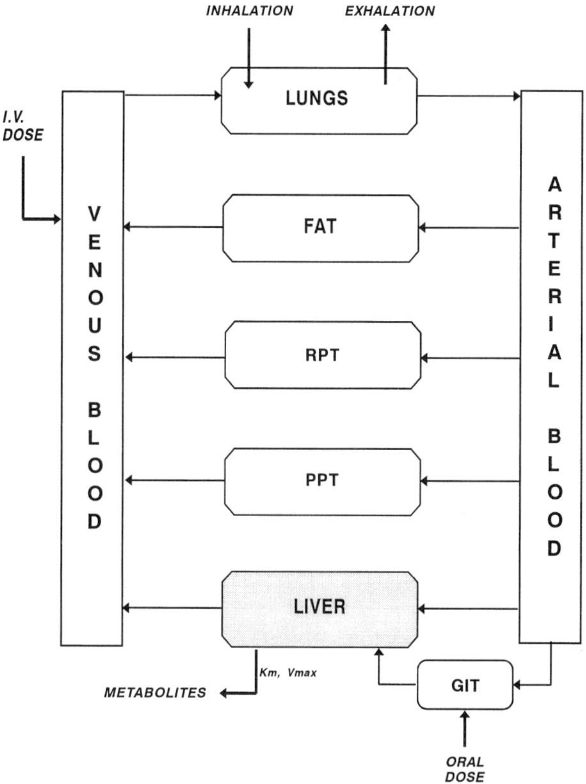

FIGURE P-5. Schematic representation of a PBPK model with different routes of entry. RPT, richly perfused tissues (e.g., brain, kidneys, and spleen); PPT, poorly perfused tissues (e.g., muscles, skin, and bone; GIT, gastrointestinal tract. K_m and V_{max} are constants that characterize metabolizing tissues like the liver.

To each compartment corresponds a mass-balance differential rate equation that describes the rate of change in the amount (Amt) of a xenobiotic in each tissue compartment, as the xenobiotic enters in, distributes within, and exits a tissue:

$$\frac{d\,Amt_i}{dt} = Q_i\,(Ca - Cvi)$$

where Q_i represents the volume of blood circulating throughout the tissue i per unit of time, C_a is the concentration of the xenobiotic in arterial blood entering the tissue, and C_{vi} is the concentration of the xenobiotic in venous blood leaving the tissue. For metabolizing tissues (e.g., liver), an additional term that takes into account the capacity of such tissues to operate the metabolic transformation of the xenobiotic is added to the basic differential equation described previously. Since the capacity of the liver and other metabolizing tissues is limited when large amounts of a xenobiotic are presented to the tissues, the basic equation contains terms (K_m and V_{max}) that account for such limitations:

$$\frac{d\,Amt_i}{dt} = Q_i\,(Ca - Cv_i) - \frac{Vmax \bullet Cvi}{Km + Cv_i}$$

where the new terms K_m and V_{max} describe respectively the affinity of a xenobiotic for metabolizing enzymes and the maximum velocity of the enzymatic reactions.

The previously described equations are characteristic of blood flow rate-limited models; it is assumed that xenobiotics cross the cell membrane by simple diffusion and that equilibrium takes place instantaneously between blood and tissue compartments. This assumption is valid for a great number of chemicals. For certain xenobiotics, however, the kinetics of tissue uptake is not consistent with blood flow rate-limited processes since their distribution in a given tissue is limited by the resistance of the cell membrane to the passage of a xenobiotic. In these cases, the basic equation should account for such phenomena in order to describe adequately the time course of the xenobiotic disposition in the tissue.

Of course, various exposure routes (e.g., inhalation, intravenous, oral, and dermal) can be accounted for in PBPK models by incorporating the proper equation describing these uptake processes.

Once formulated, a PBPK model can be used to simulate the kinetic behavior of a xenobiotic (e.g., amount metabolized, blood or tissue concentrations, percentage of dose excreted, etc.) in animals or humans. An important step in the development of PBPK model is its validation. Validation is usually based on the visual or statistical comparison of model predictions with experimental observations in humans or animals.

Once validated, PBPK models can be used by toxicologists for many purposes. For example, PBPK models can (1) provide an estimate of the time course distribution of xenobiotics and their metabolites in various parts of the body, including target organs/tissues; (2) allow various types of metabolic extrapolations between various species, from high doses of exposure to low doses, or from one route of exposure to another; (3) allow the examination of pharmacokinetic differences between species; (4) facilitate the setting and adjustment of exposure standards since it becomes possible to better estimate the concentration of a xenobiotic and its metabolite(s) in various body fluids or tissues, according to various exposure scenarios; and (5) predict changes in the disposition kinetics of xenobiotics resulting from physiological and pathological alterations in body function.

For all these reasons, PBPK models are and will continue to be increasingly used in toxicology. This is especially true in risk assessment studies since, by better defining the internal tissue dose, they may contribute to reduce the uncertainty associated with extrapolation to human beings of responses observed in animal toxicity studies in which animals usually receive high doses of xenobiotics by routes often different from the one(s) anticipated in human exposures.

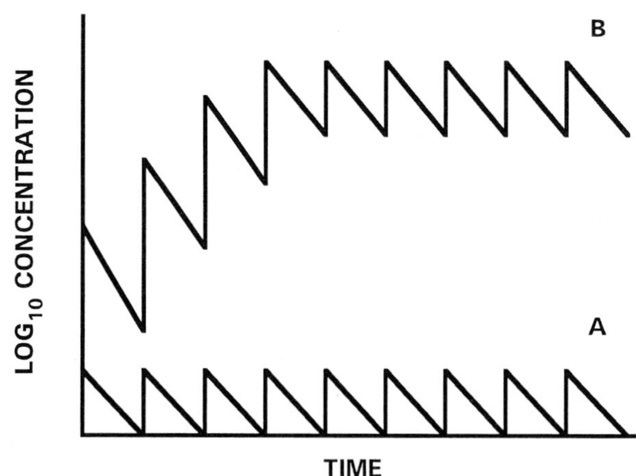

FIGURE P-6. Time-course blood concentration of a xenobiotic following repeated intravenous administration. A, xenobiotic half-life shorter than the period of time between exposures; B, xenobiotic half-life longer than the period of time between exposures.

Repetitive Exposures

Frequently, individuals are exposed repetitively to xenobiotics, be they medication, food additives, or environmental contaminants.

In general, chemicals exhibiting a short half-life (i.e., smaller than the period of time between each new exposure) are almost completely eliminated between exposures. Inversely, chemicals with a long half-life (i.e., longer than the period of time between exposures) tend to accumulate in the body leading eventually to toxicity. In the latter case, if exposure continues at a relatively constant level, the accumulated chemical will reach a plateau, also called a steady-state level, when the amount of a xenobiotic that enters the body equals the amount eliminated during a given period of time.

Figures P-6A and P-6B illustrate the accumulation of a xenobiotic in blood resulting from repeated intravenous exposures. The time that is necessary to reach the steady state depends on the half-life of the xenobiotic and corresponds to about five times the half-life value, whereas the amount present in blood is a function of the absorbed dose.

Contrasting with the sawtooth pattern of blood concentrations during repeated, noncontinuous exposure to xenobiotic (Figs. P-6A and P-6B), the pattern resulting from continuous exposure is characterized by a single stable line (Fig. P-7). However, for both situations, the time to reach a plateau concentration and the amount present in blood obey the same rules of kinetics.

Thus, for a compound administered intravenously and described by a one-compartment model, the average steady-state blood concentration (C_{ss}) is determined by the following equation:

$$Css = \frac{\text{Dosing rate}_{i.v.}}{V_D \cdot k \cdot \tau}$$

where V_D is the apparent volume of distribution, k is the elimination rate constant, and τ is the time interval between administered doses. As can be seen, the blood concentration is related proportionally to the administered dose but bears an inverse relationship to all other parameters.

Dose-Dependent Kinetics

As seen earlier, exposure conditions amenable to pharmacokinetic/toxicokinetic analysis are such that the

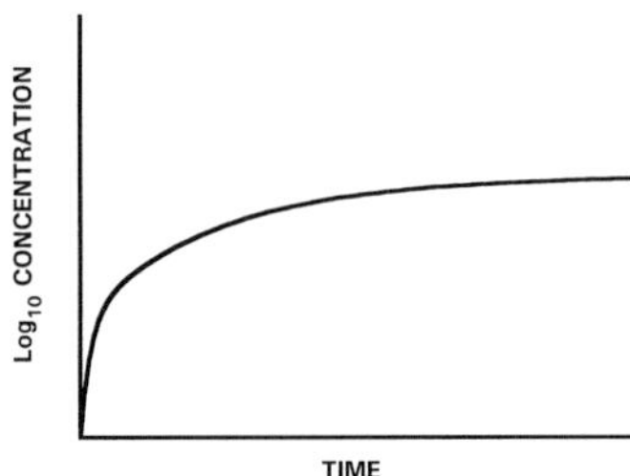

FIGURE P-7. Time-course blood concentration of xenobiotic following continuous intravenous infusion or pulmonary inhalation until steady state.

rate of the biological processes (e.g., diffusion across membranes, biotransformation, excretion by glomerular filtration, etc.) is proportional to the concentration or amount of a xenobiotic in a given compartment such as blood: The rate is then said to be governed by first-order kinetics (see Figs. P-3 and P-4).

There are biological processes, however, that involve saturable carrier or enzymatic systems, with a finite capacity for transport or catalysis. For instance, processes like active uptake at absorption sites, renal tubular secretion, or hepatic biotransformation of xenobiotics may become saturated at high exposure levels, yielding rates of disposition that are constant and independent of the concentration in blood. This is characteristic of zero-order kinetics. Biotransformation of ethanol in the liver and active tubular renal secretion of penicillin in urine are examples of biological processes that obey zero-order kinetics. Figure P-8 illustrates the blood concentration of a chemical eliminated by zero-order kinetics. Since at high concentrations, the amount of a chemical that is biotransformated or excreted is limited by saturable processes, blood concentration falls less rapidly than when first-order kinetics prevail. This may result in a more or less important accumulation of that chemical in several tissues, including those that are especially sensitive to its toxic action.

Conclusion

Pharmacokinetic/toxicokinetic analysis is a very important tool that can help toxicologists understand how the body handles foreign chemicals. With a good knowledge of the time course relationship between exposure to chemicals and their concentration in various tissues and organs, toxicologists are in a position to better interpret and predict the nature and extent of toxicity.

More specifically, data pertaining to toxicokinetics are, and will increasingly continue to be, essential to properly:

- Predict the body burden of toxic chemicals in a critical organ or tissue
- Understand the dose–response relationship of toxic chemicals
- Assist in the selection of animal species that can act as a surrogate of human toxicity
- Make rationale extrapolations from high doses, as used in animal toxicity studies, to low doses, as encountered in the human environment
- Set exposure limits to toxic chemicals for all kinds of living organisms, including humans
- Identify potentially at-risk subgroups of exposed living organisms

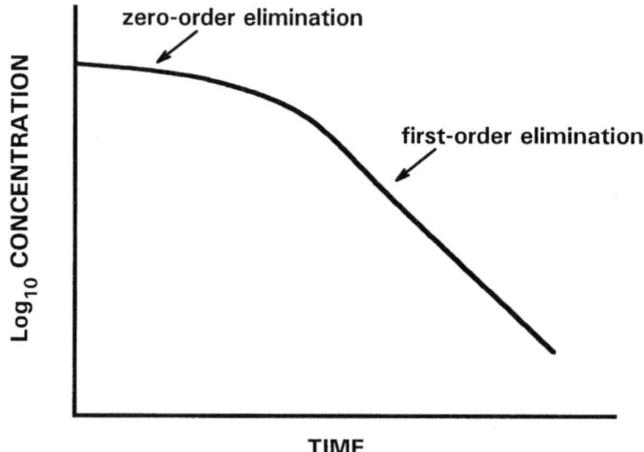

FIGURE P-8. Time-course blood concentration of a xenobiotic exhibiting nonlinear (zero-order) kinetics following intravenous administration; when the biological processes responsible for the disposition of the xenobiotic are no longer saturated, first-order kinetics resume.

Further Reading

Rozman, K., and Klaassen, C. D. (1996). Absorption, distribution, and excretion of toxicants. In *Casarett and Doull's Toxicology. The Basic Science of Poisons* (C. D. Klaassen, Ed.), 5th ed., pp. 50–87. McGraw-Hill, New York.

Krishnan, K., and Andersen, M. E. (1994). Physiologically based pharmacokinetic modeling in toxicology. In *Principles and Methods in Toxicology* (W. Hayes, Ed.), 3rd ed., pp. 149–188. Raven Press, New York.

Renwick, A. G. (1994). Toxicokinetics-pharmacokinetics in toxicology. In *Principles and Methods of Toxicology* (W. Hayes, Ed.), 3rd ed., pp. 101–147. Raven Press, New York.

—Robert Tardif and Jules Brodeur

Related Topics

Absorption
Distribution

Excretion
Pharmacokinetic Models

Related Topics

Polycyclic Aromatic Hydrocarbons
Skin

Phenanthrene

- CAS: 85-01-8
- Chemical Class: Polynuclear aromatic hydrocarbon
- Chemical Structure:

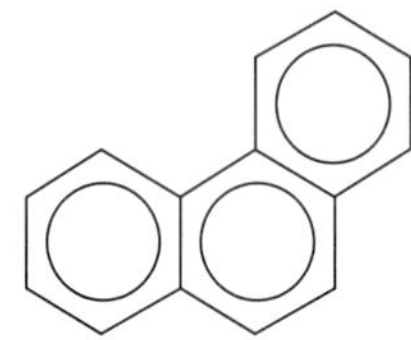

Uses

Phenanthrene is used in the production of dyes and explosives. It is used in drug manufacturing and biochemical research. Phenanthrene is a volatile component of coal tar.

Exposure Pathways

Dermal contact and inhalation are possible routes of exposure.

Mechanism of Toxicity

Phenanthrene absorbs ultraviolet light and causes production of singlet oxygen, which in turn leads to free radical production.

Human Toxicity

Phenanthrene increases the photosensitivity of skin. It is phototoxic. The PEL is 0.2 mg/m^3.

Animal Toxicity

Phenanthrene is a tumorigen (skin) and mutagen. In mice, the oral LD_{50} is 700 mg/kg and the intravenous LD_{50} is 56 mg/kg.

—*Shayne C. Gad and Jayne E. Ash*

Phencyclidine

- CAS: 77-10-1
- Synonyms: PCP; 1-phenylcyclohexylpiperidine; phencyclidine hydrochloride (CAS: 956-90-1); Sernyl; Sernylan; angel dust; peace pill; animal tranquilizer; embalming fluid; rocket or jet fuel; hog; superkool; whacky weed; kristal joint; love boat; DOA; zombie dust; star dust; murder-1; selma; mint dew; surfer; busy bee; lovely
- Phencyclidine analogs with similar pharmacologic effects include phencyclohexamine (PCE), phenylcyclohexylpyrrolidine (PHP), phenycyclopentylpiperidine (PCPP), and thienycyclohexylpiperidine (TCP).
- Pharmaceutical Class: Synthetic arylcyclohexylamine closely related to ketamine, a medically approved dissociative anesthetic
- Chemical Structure: (Phencyclidine hydrochloride)

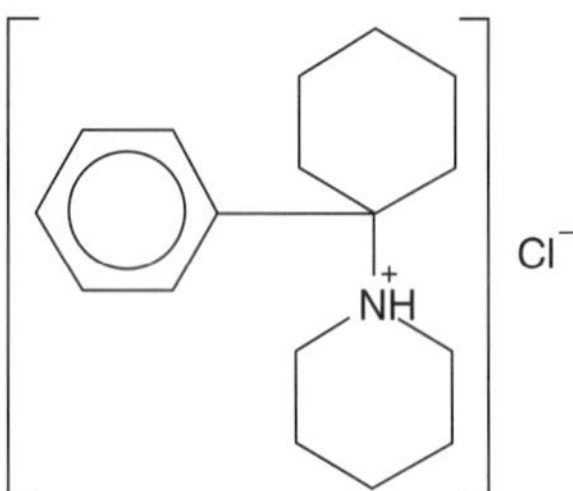

Uses

Phencyclidine is used as a veterinary analgesic and anesthetic. It is also a psychedelic drug of abuse.

Exposure Pathways

Phencyclidine is sold illicitly as powder, tablets, liquid, rock crystal, or mixed with leaves (marijuana, oregano, mint, and parsley). Phencyclidine is ingested, smoked, snorted, and injected intravenously.

Toxicokinetics

When smoked or snorted, phencyclidine has an onset of action of from 2 to 5 min; when ingested, effects are apparent within 30–60 min. Peak effects are achieved 15–30 min after onset; some effects persist for 24–48 hr. There is also evidence that phencyclidine is absorbed percutaneously. Phencyclidine undergoes hepatic degradation by oxidative hydroxylation to two metabolites that have little psychotropic activity. The volume of distribution of phencyclidine is large, averaging 6.2 liters/kg. Plasma protein binding is approximately 65%. Because of high lipid solubility, levels found in tissue far exceed those found in plasma. Phencyclidine follows first-order elimination kinetics. It undergoes enterohepatic recycling with subsequent excretion by the kidneys. The half-life of small doses is 1 hr, increasing to 17.6 hr (range, 7–50 hr) in overdose.

Mechanism of Toxicity

Phencyclidine modifies neuronal transmission, with the greatest effects on the parasympathetic and sympathetic nervous systems. It is thought that α-adrenergic receptors are stimulated, potentiating the effects of serotonin, epinephrine, and norepinephrine. The resultant sympathomimetic and hallucinogenic effects are dose related.

Human Toxicity

Phencyclidine use results in excitation with marked paranoid or aggressive behavior, which is often self-destructive. Effects include distortion of body image, no pain perception, illusions, and delusions, including a perception of superhuman strength and invulnerability.

Acute

Miosis and nystagmus (horizontal, vertical, and rotary) may be seen in association with ataxia, bizarre behavior, and hallucinations. Tachycardia, hypertension progressing to hypotension, increased reflexes, seizures, respiratory depression, and coma are reported with high doses. Dystonias and dyskinesias have occurred. Hypoglycemia is frequent. Rhabdomyolysis and resultant renal failure, embolism, disseminated intravascular coagulation, liver necrosis, and traumatic injury are reported complications. The anesthetic dose of phencyclidine is 0.25 mg/kg intravenously. Doses of 1–5 mg cause euphoria and numbness, 5–10 mg cause excitation and hallucinations, and 20 mg or more cause coma and serious toxicity or death. Plasma concentrations of phencyclidine vary widely after overdose and are not clinically useful. Phencyclidine crosses the placenta resulting in hyperirritability, tremors and hypertonia, depressed reflexes, and nystagmus in neonates; anatomic abnormalities are also possible.

Chronic

Cognitive and memory difficulties, speech problems, depression, anxiety, violent behavior, and weight loss are reported. Prolonged psychosis has been seen; it can mimic acute schizophrenia and persist for 4–6 weeks. Tolerance to the psychoactive effects necessitates increased doses. Psychological dependence has been noted, but no withdrawal symptoms have been reported.

Clinical Management

Isolation of the patient from all sensory stimuli is advised. The patient should be protected from self-inflicted injury, but the use of restraints should be avoided if possible since they can contribute to rhabdomyolysis. Hydration with intravenous fluids will minimize the precipitation of myoglobin in the urine. Although urine acidification theoretically enhances phencyclidine elimination, it is not recommended because of the frequency of rhabdomyolysis (myoglobinuric renal failure and closed head injury seen with phencyclidine intoxication). Diazepam can be employed to treat agitation or convulsions. Severe agitation may be reversed by haloperidol. Hypertensive crisis can be managed with nitroprusside. Basic and advanced life-support measures may be needed. Gastric decontamination is of little or no value since phencyclidine is customarily snorted or smoked. Multiple-dose activated charcoal administration can be employed to enhance elimination of phencyclidine since it is enterohepatically recycled regardless of the route of administration; however, there is not any data to support its use. Renal function, blood pressure, blood sugar, blood gases, electrolytes, serum creatine phosphokinase, and urine myoglobin should be monitored.

Animal Toxicity: Doses in excess of 1 mg/kg produce convulsions in dogs. Dose-dependent effects include depressed reflexes, tachycardia, twitching, dilated pupils, and hyperthermia. There are marked species differences in behavior.

—*Janet E. Bauman*

Phenol

- CAS: 108-95-2
- Synonyms: Carbolic acid; hydroxybezene; phenic acid; benzenol; phenol alcohol
- Chemical Class: Phenol
- Molecular Formula: C_6H_5OH
- Chemical Structure:

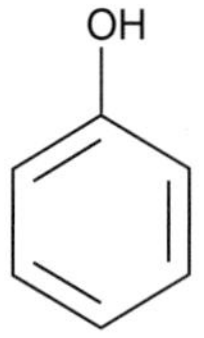

Uses

Industrially, phenol is used in the manufacture of pharmaceuticals, plastics, rubber, and plywood. Due to its antiseptic, germicidal, and anesthetic properties, it is a component of some disinfectants and preservatives. It is also a common reagent in nucleic acid/molecular biology research and is used to denature and remove protein from preparations of DNA and RNA. Phenol is a waste product of the oil refinery and coal conversion industries.

Exposure Pathways

Phenol is readily absorbed from all surfaces of the body. Acute exposures by all routes (inhalation, skin contact, and ingestion) can be fatal. Exposure may not be initially painful due to phenolic anesthetic properties; however, in skin exposure, deep dermal damage is common with subsequent gangrene.

Toxicokinetics

Phenol will undergo biotransformation to oxidation and conjugated products. Phenol and phenolic compounds can be oxidized by the peroxidase-dependent prostaglandin H synthase to phenoxyl radicals. It is a reactive intermediate in the P450 oxidation of benzene to hydroquinone. Phenol that is not oxidized will undergo conjugation to etheral, sulfate, or glycuronate species and subsequently excreted through the kidneys. A smaller amount may be eliminated through the lungs, as detected by an aromatic odor to the breath.

Mechanism of Toxicity

Phenol is a general protoplasmic poison. It can be oxidized to a reactive electrophile that combines with protein and DNA. The binding to hepatic or renal proteins leads to centrilobular and medullar damage, respectively.

Human Toxicity

Significant exposure to phenol by absorption through skin, by inhalation, or by ingestion can lead to death within minutes. It is extremely destructive to tissues of the mucus membranes and to the upper respiratory tract, skin, and eyes. Rapid death of nerve endings and tissue necrosis produces anesthesia and paralysis. Gastrointestinal, cardiovascular, and pulmonary symptoms will appear. Phenol effects on the gastrointestinal tract will result in pain, nausea, vomiting, and diarrhea. There may be cardiovascular collapse and subsequent shock. Pulmonary exposure can produce spasm, inflammation, and general edema. The central nervous system may have a transitory stimulation, followed by depression. Exposure to small amounts of phenol may result in a respiratory alkalosis similar to salicylate poisoning. This will be followed by an acidosis. Phenol has been shown to be mutagenic in several mutation test systems. Literature reports of the human LD_{Lo} by the oral route range from 0.14 to 14 g/kg. Phenol is a known mutagen; however, conclusive carcinogenic data are not available. In experiments, it does show teratogenic and reproductive effects.

Clinical Management

Individuals exposed to phenol by inhalation should be removed to fresh air and given artificial respiration/cardiopulmonary resuscitation if necessary. Prompt transport to a medical facility is recommended with observation for up to 48 hr. Treatment should be symptomatic, keeping in mind that effects such as pulmonary edema may be delayed. After ingestion, absorption should be delayed by giving milk, olive oil, castor oil, or polyethylene glycol 300, followed by repeated gastric lavage. Mineral oil or alcohol should not be administered because these can increase gastric absorption. Other therapy should be utilized as necessary noting edema and shock acidosis as predicted outcomes. After skin exposure, the affected area should be washed with soap and copious amounts of water for at least 10 min. Water alone may be harmful. Caster oil or polyethylene glycol should be applied with cotton swabs or dressings.

Animal Toxicity

Phenol shows high toxicity by all routes of exposure. The LD_{50}s in rats are as follows: 384 mg/kg (oral), 669 mg/kg (skin), 250 mg/kg (interperitoneal), and 316 mg/kg (inhalation).

—*Kathryn Kehoe*

Related Topic

Skin

Phenothiazines

- Representative Compounds: Chlorpromazine (CAS: 50-53-31); triflupromazine; thioridazine; mesoridazine; piperacetazine; ethopropazine; fluphenazine; perphenazine; prochlorperazine; promazine; promethazine; acetophenazine; trifluoperazine; clozapine; risperidone
- Synonyms: Chlorpromazine—3-(2-chlorophenothiazin-10-yl) propyldimethylamine, Thorazine; triflupromazine—*N,N*-dimethyl-3-(2-trifluoromethylphenothiazin-10-yl) propylamine, Vesprin; thioridazine—10-(2-(1-methyl-2-piperidyl)ethyl)-2-methylthiophenothiazine, Mellaril; mesoridazine—10-(2-(1-methyl-2-piperidyl)ethyl)-2-(methylsulphinyl) phenothiazine, Serentil; piperacetazine—10-{3-(4-(2-hydroxyethyl)piperidino) propyl}phenothiazin-2-yl methyl ketone, Quide; ethopropazine—10-(2-diethylaminopropyl)phenothiazine, Parsidol; fluphenazine—2-{4-(3-(2-trifluoromethylphenothiazin-10-yl)propyl)piperazin-1-yl}ethanol, {Prolixin; perphenazine—2-4-(3-(2-chlorophenothiazin-10-yl)propyl)piperazin-1-yl}ethanol, Trilafon; prochlorperazine—2-chloro-10-(3-(4-methylpiperazin-1-yl)propyl)phenothiazine, Compazine; promazine—*N,N*-dimethyl-3-phenothiazin-10-yl propylammonium chloride, Sparine; promethazine—1-*N,N*-trimethyl-2-(phenothiazin-10-yl)ethylamine, Phenergan; acetophenazine—10-{3-(4-(2-hydroxyethyl)pipeazin-1-yl) propyl}phenothiazin-2-yl methyl ketone dimaleate, Tindal; trifluoperazine—10-(3-(4-methylpiperazin-1-yl)propyl)-2-trifluoromethylphenothiazine, Stelazine; clozapine—8-chloro-11-(4-methylpiperazin-1-yl)-5H-dibenzo(*b,e*)(1,4) diazepine, Clozaril; risperidone—3-{2-(4-(6-fluoro-1,2-benzisoxazol-3-yl)piperidino)ethyl}-6,7,8,9-tetrahydro-2-methylpyrido)ethyl}-6,7,8,9-tetrahydro-2-methylpyrido(1,2-a)pyrimidin-4-one, Risperidal
- Pharmaceutical Class: Neuroleptic agent, antipsychotic, major tranquilizer
- Chemical Structure: Chlorpromazine is the prototype phenothiazine.

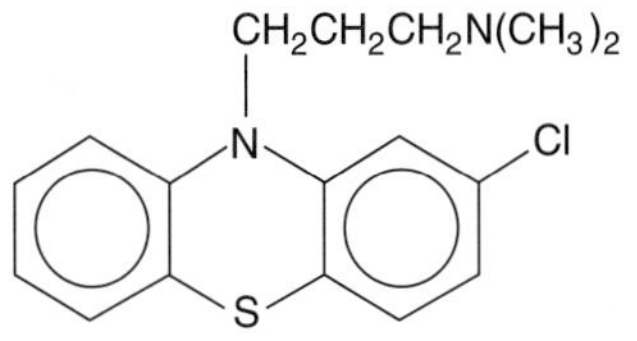

Uses

Phenothiazines are used to treat psychosis including schizophrenia; violent, agitated, disturbed behavior and mania. Other uses include treatment of pain, headache, hiccups, acute severe anxiety, idiopathic dystonia, withdrawal, taste disorders, leishmaniasis, alleviation of nausea and vomiting, and treatment of behavioral symptoms secondary to Alzheimer's disease and senile dementia.

Exposure Pathways

Phenothiazines are available in both injectable and oral dosage forms. The principal exposure pathway is intentional ingestion in adults or accidental ingestion in small children.

Toxicokinetics

Phenothiazines are readily but incompletely absorbed due to first-pass metabolism in the gut wall. Oral bioavailability ranges from 10 to 69%. Peak serum levels are reached at 2 or 3 hr. Phenothiazines are extensively metabolized in the liver through glucuronic acid conjugation, N-dealkylation, and sulfoxidation. Phenothiazines are widely distributed throughout the body, including the central nervous system (CNS). CNS levels may be up to 10 times greater than plasma levels. Phenothiazines are highly protein bound, 95–99% with a volume of distribution from 11 to 30 liters/kg, with a mean of 20 liters/kg. The main metabolites are excreted both in the urine and feces. Less than 1% is excreted in the urine unchanged. Elimination half-life ranges from 6 to 119 hr with an average of 18 hr.

Mechanism of Toxicity

Phenothiazines primarily block postsynaptic neurotransmission by binding to dopamine (D_1 and D_2), muscarinic, and serotonergic receptors. Phenothiazines also possess peripheral α-adrenergic receptor blockade and quinidine-like cardiac effects. Phenothiazines may also lower the seizure threshold.

Human Toxicity

Clinical signs of toxicity most frequently include sedation, coma, hypotension, extrapyramidal effects, and cardiac arrythmias. Anticholinergic effects including dry mouth, blurred vision, and tachycardia have been seen. Cardiac effects include mild hypotension and a prolonged Q-T interval. Quinidine-like effects have rarely resulted in sudden cardiac death. The most commonly reported dystonic reactions include akathisias, stiff neck, stiff or protruding tongue, and tremor. Neuroleptic malignant syndrome has been reported after therapeutic use and acute intoxication. Hypokalemia has also been noted. Seizures are rarely seen. The most common reported adverse reactions following therapeutic use include dry mouth, sedation, orthostatic hypotension, blurred vision, mydriasis, photosensitivity, anorexia, nausea, vomiting, constipation, diarrhea, and dyspepsia. Various hematologic changes have been reported. Clozapine has been linked to fatal agranulocytosis.

Clinical Management

All basic and advanced life-support measures should be implemented. Gastric decontamination should be performed. Phenothiazines readily bind to activated charcoal. Aggressive supportive care including airway management should be instituted when necessary. Hypotension usually responds to intravenous fluids and Trendelenburg's position. The vasopressor of choice is norepinephrine. Arrhythmias should be treated with lidocaine or phenytoin. Diazepam is the drug of choice for seizures; phenytoin is the preferred drug to prevent recurrence. Dystonic reactions respond well to intravenous benztropine or diphenhydramine. Oral therapy of diphenhydramine or benztropine should be continued for 2 days to prevent recurrence of the dystonic reaction. For patients suffering from neuroleptic malignant syndrome, dantrolene sodium and bromocriptine have been used in conjunction with cooling and other supportive measures. Hemodialysis and hemoperfusion have not been shown to be effective.

Animal Toxicity

Signs of toxicity reported in animals have included sedation, dullness, hypotension, respiratory depression, photosensitivity, weakness, anorexia, fever, icterus, colic, restlessness, seizures, anemia, and hemoglobinuria. Treatment consists of gastric decontamination and aggressive supportive care.

—Douglas J. Borys

Phenylmercuric Acetate

- CAS: 62-38-4
- SYNONYM: Acetoxyphenyl mercury
- CHEMICAL CLASS: Organomercurial
- CHEMICAL STRUCTURE:

C_6H_5—HgO—$COCH_3$

Uses

Phenylmercuric acetate is used as a seed dressing for the prevention of seed-borne diseases of vegetables, soybeans, cotton, peanuts, beets, and ornamental plants. It is sometimes used as a food preservative and antifungal agent. In paper, plastic, and fabric industries, this compound is also used as a preservative.

Exposure Pathways

Oral and dermal routes are the most common routes of exposure to phenylmercuric acetate.

Toxicokinetics

Phenylmercuric acetate is slowly absorbed through the skin; absorption is more efficient by the gastrointestinal tract. Relatively similar rates of absorption of phenylmercuric acetate and mercuric acetate were found in rat kidney slices. When absorption was studied in liver slices, however, the rate of absorption was found to be much higher (twice) for the organic form. Organic mercury has a greater affinity for the brain compared to inorganic mercury (probably because of its relative ease in crossing the blood–brain barrier).

Laboratory studies demonstrated that mercury from phenylmercuric acetate tends to distribute more in the liver and kidneys compared to inorganic mercury. A chronic study with phenylmercuric acetate and mercuric acetate showed greater (10–20 times) distribution of the phenyl derivative into these tissues. Organomercury compounds usually undergo cleavage of the carbon–mercury bond in the body, releasing ionic inorganic mercury.

Phenylmercuric acetate is mainly excreted through urine. The excretion of phenylmercuric acetate in humans was reported to exhibit two phases. The first phase showed a transient increase in urinary mercury concentration followed by a second slower phase.

Mechanism of Toxicity

Generally, mercury interferes with cellular enzymatic mechanisms by combining with sulfhydryl (-SH) groups of different enzymes and thereby produces nonspecific cell injury or death (see Mercury).

Human Toxicity

The principal manifestations of mercury salt poisoning are gastrointestinal, hepatic, and renal damage.

Acute

Ingestion of phenylmercuric acetate may cause metallic taste, thirst, severe abdominal pain, vomiting, and bloody diarrhea which may persist for several weeks. Acute renal failure characterized by decreased urine output was reported 1 day to 2 weeks after ingestion.

Chronic

Ingestion of phenylmercuric acetate over a prolonged period may cause skin disorders (urticaria and stomatitis), salivation, diarrhea, anemia, leukopenia, and hepatic and renal damage. Prolonged dermal exposure to phenylmercuric acetate may cause mercurialism.

Clinical Management

In case of acute poisoning, emergency measures should be taken by immediately removing the ingested poison using gastric lavage with tap water or using emesis or catharsis. Dimercaprol may be administered as an antidote for mercury poisoning with subsequent hemodialysis to accelerate the removal of the mercury–dimercaprol complex from the body. Penicillamine may also be administered as an antidote.

Animal Toxicity

The oral LD_{50} of phenylmercuric acetate in rats was found to be 60 mg/kg. In mice, the oral LD_{50} was 70 mg/kg. Dietary mercury (2 mg/kg/day for 2 years) in the form of phenylmercuric acetate did not affect rat growth, mortality, or organ weights. However, a dietary level of 160 ppm (8 mg/kg/day) of phenylmercuric acetate was found to retard the growth of rats and shorten their survival time. Histochemical changes in the rat kidney have been observed following a dietary level of 0.5 ppm of phenylmercuric acetate. Succinate dehydrogenase and alkaline and acid phosphatase activities in the renal epithelium were reported to be altered following intragastric administration of phenylmercuric acetate.

—*Tamal Kumar Chakraborti*

Related Topic

Metals

Phenylpropanolamine

- CAS: 14838-15-4
- SYNONYMS: PPA; *d,l*-norephedrine
- PHARMACEUTICAL CLASS: A synthetic sympathomimetic drug structurally related to ephedrine and amphetamine
- CHEMICAL STRUCTURE:

$$C_6H_5-\underset{OH}{CH}-\underset{NH_2}{CH}-CH_3 \cdot HCl$$

Uses

Phenylpropanolamine is used as a nasal decongestant and as an anorectic. It as approved by the U.S. FDA as an over-the-counter weight-loss product.

Exposure Pathway

Phenylpropanolamine is available in liquid and tablet oral dosage forms. Ingestion is the most common route of accidental and intentional exposure.

Toxicokinetics

Oral doses of phenylpropanolamine are rapidly and completely absorbed from the gastrointestinal tract, with maximal therapeutic effect in 1–3 hr. In overdose, the peak toxic reaction is usually seen within 2 or 3 hr following ingestion. Phenylpropanolamine is converted primarily to norephedrine. Small amounts of the drug are slowly metabolized in the liver to an active hydroxylated metabolite.

Phenylpropanolamine crosses the blood–brain barrier, resulting in central nervous system (CNS) effects. The brain-to-serum ratios are extremely close at 0.025 and 0.05 mmol per kilogram. The volume of distribution of phenylpropanolamine is 4.4 (±1.2) liters/kg. Phenylpropanolamine is eliminated 80–90% unchanged in the urine, along with the metabolite norephedrine. Phenylpropanolamine is a weak base with a pK_a of 9.4 and is eliminated more rapidly in acidic urine. Where the urine pH is normal (5.5–7.0), the plasma half-life of phenylpropanolamine is 5.6 hr (±1 hr).

Mechanism of Toxicity

The primary action of phenylpropanolamine is indirect α-adrenergic agonism, releasing norepinephrine at postganglionic sympathetic nerve terminals. Phenylpropanolamine also possesses direct α-adrenergic agonist properties and, to a lesser degree, β-adrenergic agonist activity. Hypertension results from α-adrenergic-mediated vasoconstriction of peripheral blood vessels.

Human Toxicity

Hypertension is the most common and most serious toxic effect of phenylpropanolamine. Hypertensive crisis, cerebral hemorrhage, and myocardial ischemia may result. Tachycardia is most often seen with phenylpropanolamine where it is combined with antihistamines in multisymptom products. Bradycardia (as a reflex response to hypertension) is more common when phenylpropanolamine is exclusively ingested. Concurrent substances that are prevalent in combination products and may contribute to the toxicological presentation of phenylpropanolamine exposures include analgesics, antihistamines, and antitussives. Consideration should be given to the alcohol component of liquid preparations. Caffeine may be added to phenylpropanolamine in illicit stimulant and weight-loss preparations. Phenylpropanolamine has a low therapeutic index and adverse effects can occur at doses two or three times the normal daily dose. The recommended adult daily dose is 75–150 mg. An amount over 10 mg/kg is toxic in children. Neurological symptoms include anxiety, confusion, headache, and altered mental status.

Clinical Management

Basic and advanced life-support measures should be instituted as indicated. Gastric decontamination may be performed depending on the patient's symptomatology and the history of the ingestion. Activated charcoal may be used to adsorb phenylpropanolamine. Careful monitoring of the heart and hemodynamic status should be performed. Antiarrhythmics and antihypertensive agents may be necessary in severe exposures. Management of poisoning with concurrent drugs ingested should be appropriate to the agent(s) involved. Laboratory analysis of the creatine phosphokinase and urinalysis should be performed.

Animal Toxicity

Following the ingestion of phenylpropanolamine, dogs and cats may exhibit hyperactivity, mydriasis, depression, vomiting, hyperthermia, disorientation, and bradycardia. Therapy is directed at prevention of absorption and control of tachyarrhythmias with lidocaine (dogs only) or procainamide (dogs only). Diazepam may be used for control of symptoms of CNS stimulation.

—*Carole Wezorek*

Phenytoin

- CAS: 57-41-0
- SYNONYMS: Diphenylhydantoin (DPH); 5,5-diphenylhydantoin, 5,5-diphenylimidazolidine-2,4-dione; Dilantin Infatabs; Fenitoina; Phenantoinum
  Phenytoin sodium (CAS: 630-93-3; 92% phenytoin)—diphenylhydantoin sodium; diphenin; phenytoinum natricum; soluble phenytoin; Dilantin; Epanutin; Diphenylan
- PHARMACEUTICAL CLASS: Hydantoin (a synthetic chemical that is structurally similar to barbituric acid)
- CHEMICAL STRUCTURE:

Uses

Phenytoin is used as an anticonvulsant and antidysrhythmic.

Exposure Pathways

Ingestion is the most common route of exposure. Phenytoin can also be administered intravenously.

Toxicokinetics

Oral absorption is dose dependent. Peak blood concentrations occur 2–4 hr after single 100-mg doses but may be delayed 4–12 hr after a loading dose (600 mg). Peak levels may not occur for 2–7 days after an oral overdose. The oral bioavailability of phenytoin averages 90% (range, 70–100%). Intramuscular absorption is unpredictable and erratic.

The major pathway of biotransformation is via hepatic hydroxylation to *p*-hydroxyphenytoin, which is subsequently conjugated to glucuronide. Minor metabolites include *m*-hydroxyphenytoin and 3,4-dihydrodihydroxyphenytoin. All metabolites are inactive. Phenytoin biotransformation is capacity limited, with linear (first-order) kinetics observed at low (therapeutic) doses, and zero-order (Michaelis–Menton) elimination observed at toxic and even high therapeutic doses. Phenytoin and its metabolites undergo enterohepatic recirculation prior to elimination.

The volume of distribution averages 0.5–0.8 liters/kg, and binding to plasma proteins is normally about 90%. Protein binding is altered in neonates and the elderly and under many conditions, including uremia, nephrotic syndrome, hypoalbuminemia, hyperbilirubinemia, and hepatic disease. Alterations in protein binding will result in variations in the amount of unbound (free) drug that is the active component. Thus, free phenytoin levels (therapeutic = 1–2 μg/ml) rather than total levels (therapeutic = 10–20 μg/ml) may correlate better with clinical efficacy and toxicity in the presence of these conditions. Phenytoin crosses the placenta and is excreted in breast milk.

Small amounts of phenytoin are excreted unchanged in the urine (2–4%) and feces (5%). Most is eliminated renally as inactive conjugated metabolites. The elimination half-life at linear doses averages 20–30 hr (12–20 hr in children) but may be as long as 60 hr and as high as 200 hr after overdose. The maximum rate of metabolism is estimated at 6 mg/kg/day.

Mechanism of Toxicity

Phenytoin possesses anticonvulsant activity without significant CNS depression. At various concentrations, phenytoin has been shown to inhibit inward Na^+ currents, outward K^+ currents, and Ca^{2+}-mediated action potentials. The ability to inhibit sodium channels is responsible for the antidysrhythmic action (class II-B) of phenytoin. Phenytoin can induce enzymes of the hepatic cytochrome P450 system.

Human Toxicity: Acute

Clinical effects after overdose are generally dose related and primarily involve the peripheral and central nervous systems; nystagmus (>20 μg/ml), ataxia (>30 μg/ml), and lethargy (>40 μg/ml) are most characteristic. Nausea, tremor, dysarthria, and confusion are also relatively common. Coma or significant cardiac dysrhythmias are unusual. Hypotension or dysrhythmias may be encountered with too rapid intravenous infusion. Paradoxical central nervous system (CNS) excitation has been reported, but the potential of phenytoin to actually cause seizures at very high serum concentrations is unclear. This phenomenon has typically occurred in patients with a preexisting seizure disorder on chronic phenytoin therapy.

Human Toxicity: Chronic

Chronic toxic effects are dose related and typically involve cerebellar and vestibular functions (nystagmus and ataxia). Nausea, dizziness, diplopia, behavioral changes, gingival hyperplasia, hirsutism, hyperglycemia, osteomalacia, pancytopenia, and skin eruptions are reported complications of chronic therapy. Hypersensitivity (idiosyncratic) reactions, including hepatic necrosis and Stevens–Johnson syndrome, can occur and are potentially fatal.

Phenytoin use during pregnancy has been associated with intrauterine growth retardation, mental retardation, craniofacial abnormalities, and digital hypoplasia (e.g., fetal hydantoin syndrome).

Clinical Management

The basis of treatment is the provision of supportive care. Hypotension should respond to intravenous fluid therapy. Seizures should be treated with intravenous doses of diazepam or lorazepam and discontinuation of phenytoin. Assessments of toxicity should be based on serum drug levels and not on the amount of drug ingested. Serum phenytoin concentrations should be determined in all symptomatic patients or patients with ingestions exceeding 20 mg/kg. Serial levels are needed to determine peak (highest measured) concentration. Serum levels of electrolytes, glucose, hepatic enzymes, blood urea nitrogen, and bilirubin should be determined in hospitalized patients. Activated charcoal is useful to prevent gastrointestinal absorption and to enhance elimination of absorbed drug (i.e., gastrointestinal dialysis). Multiple oral doses of charcoal are indicated to facilitate the lowering of toxic blood levels that possibly would require days to decline in conditions of zero-order metabolism. Other measures to enhance phenytoin elimination are not warranted. Continuous cardiac monitoring is not necessary in the absence of preexisting cardiac disease or massive overdose with hemodynamic compromise. Patients should be monitored until serum levels are (near) normal and they are neurologically competent. Death resulting from oral ingestion is rare.

Animal Toxicity

Toxicity in animals is expected to be similar to that in humans.

—*S. Rutherfoord Rose*

Phorbol Esters

Phorbol esters are a class of tumor promoters derived from or structurally related to phorbol (4,9,12-β-13, 20-pentahydrotz-1,6-tiglindiene-3-ol; CAS: 17673-25-5), the parent alcohol of the tumor-producing compounds in croton oil.

The concept of tumor promotion has had a long history but was principally derived from the early experimental research of Rous and Kidd, Berenblum, and Mottram. In these studies it was found that a single application of coal tar or a polycyclic hydrocarbon to the skin of rabbits or mice in subcarcinogenic amounts would initiate the process of skin carcinogenesis if followed by a promotional event.

Based on historical and voluminous subsequent research, operational criteria have been defined to describe the characteristic of a promoter in the mouse skin model. These criteria are as follows:

(1) That it should not be carcinogenic per se.

(2) That it should not increase tumor yield if administered before the initiating carcinogen.

(3) That when applied after an initiating, subcarcinogenic dose of the carcinogen, it should accelerate the rate of development of tumors and thus increase the total, time-related tumor incidence.

(4) That the yield of tumors produced should be dose related to the initiator, not to the promoter, providing the promoter is used in excess of the minimum amount required to promote all initiated cells.

(5) That unlike initiation, which can take place rapidly during a single exposure to the initiator and which is a permanent event, promotion requires long exposure to the promoter before the changes induced become irreversible.

These criteria have been the guidelines for the application of the concept of promotion to tumor induction in other organs, including liver, bladder, and colon, and have led to the following definition of tumor promotion as "the process by which an agent brings about the selective expansion of initiated cells which increase the probability of malignant transformation." From a mechanistic perspective this expansion of initiated cells is the result of altered gene expression induced by the presence of a promoting agent.

Such promotion can also be considered nongenotoxic or epigenetic carcinogenesis. The phorbol esters act as xenobiotic mitogens to cause these effects (as do phenobarbitol, DDT, and the peroxisomal proliferators).

The phorbol esters are the most widely studied skin tumor promoters. These compounds are derivatives of the tetracyclic diterpene phorbol, esterified in the 12 and 13 positions. The tumor-promoting activity of the phorbol esters appears to be related to a delicate hydrophobic–hydrophilic balance determined by positions 12-0, 13-0, and 20. TPA is the most potent of the phorbol esters series. The structure–activity relationship of phorbol esters, as well as those of other diterpene esters, has been reported in detail. Although the phorbol esters have been the most widely studied skin tumor promoters to date, many other chemical compounds have been shown to possess skin tumor-promoting properties.

Tumor-promoting agents produce substantial cellular changes when topically applied to mouse epidermis. Within a few hours after application of a single effective dose of the phorbol ester, TPA, to mouse skin, localized edema and erythema characteristic of inflammation and irritation are evident, and within 24 hr there is leukocytic infiltration of the dermis. At that time there is also a 5- to 10-fold increase in the percentage of darls cells (DCs) in the interfollicular epidermis. These DCs are characterized by their strong basophilia, dense chromatin, and large numbers of free ribosomes. They increase in number in TPA-induced hyperplasia to a greater extent than in hyperplasia induced by mezerin or more weakly promoting hyperplastic agents. These observations have led to the hypothesis that an increase in their number may be an important component of the promotion stage of skin carcinogenesis. Several investigators have reported the presence of both viable and nonviable DCs in promoter-treated epidermis. The importance of any or all of these types of DCs in the process of tumor promotion remains an open question at present.

Within 1 or 2 days after a single promoter treatment, stimulation of mitotic activity in the basal cell layer of the epidermis continues for several days and results in an increased number of nucleated cell layers. This is followed by a phase of increased keratinization of the upper layers of the epidermis. Without additional promoter treatments, all these responses to the promoter gradually subside and the epidermis regains its normal appearance within approximately 2 or 3 weeks of treatment. Repeated promoter treatment, however, prevents this decrease in response, and the skin appears to be in a chronic state of irritation and regenerative hyperplasia. In fact, repeated treatment with TPA leads to a potentiation of the hyperplasia response in species and mouse strains that are susceptible to skin tumor promotion by phorbol esters. Where adequately tested, all tumor promoters produce such a potentiated hyperplasia, although the magnitude and kinetics of this response can differ with each type of promoting agent. The ability to produce a potentiated hyperplasia after multiple treatments and the magnitude of this response appear to correlate most closely with the tumor-promoting ability of various compounds.

Further Reading

Hecker, E., Fusenig, N. E., Kunz, W., Marks, F., and Thielmann, H. W. (1982). *Cocarcinogenesis and Biological Effects of Tumor Promoters*. Raven Press, New York.

Marzulli, F. N., and Maibach, H. I. (1991). *Dermatotoxicology*, 4th ed. Hemisphere, New York.

—*Shayne C. Gad*

Related Topics

Carcinogenesis
DDT
Ocular and Dermal Studies
Peroxisome Proliferators
Polycyclic Aromatic Hydrocarbons
Skin
Toxicity Testing, Dermal

Phosgene

- CAS: 75-44-5
- SYNONYMS: Carbonyl chloride; chloroformyl chloride
- CHEMICAL CLASS: Haloform
- CHEMICAL STRUCTURE:

```
     O
     ‖
Cl—C—Cl
```

Uses

Phosgene is used in the production of war gases. It is also used in pesticide and herbicide production. It is a by-product of chloroform biotransformation.

Exposure Pathways

Inhalation and exposure to skin and mucous membranes are possible exposure routes.

Toxicokinetics

Phosgene is absorbed by the lungs and excreted via the liver and kidneys.

Mechanism of Toxicity

P450 cytochrome transform chloroform via a covalent bond to phosgene, a reactive metabolite. Metabolism via glutathione reduces phosgene to hydrogen chloride, carbon dioxide, along with mercapturic acid. Hydrogen chloride induces cell necrosis, decomposing a product of chlorinated hydrocarbons. Pulmonary edema is related to adenosine triphosphatase levels in the lungs.

Human Toxicity

Phosgene exposure is asymptomatic in the short term. Exposure may cause buildup of fluids in the lungs or pneumonia. High concentrations in the respiratory system can produce choking, chest constriction, pain in breathing, coughing, and blood in sputum. Exposure to eyes can be very irritating. Buildup of phosgene in the liver or kidneys may produce damage. The OSHA PEL for phosgene is 0.1 ppm.

Clinical Management

The exposed individual should be removed from exposure and given respiratory therapy. Cortisone or another steroid should also be given to mediate damage to tissue. Pulmonary edema should be treated, if necessary.

Animal Toxicity

In animals, phosgene exposure has resulted in liver or kidney damage, skin irritation, and respiratory damage. The inhalation LD_{50} is 1400 mg/m^3 in rats,

1800 mg/m^3 in mice, 4200 mg/m^3 in dogs, 600 mg/m^3 in monkeys, 1000 mg/m^3 in rabbits, and 1300 mg/m^3 in guinea pigs.

—*Shayne C. Gad*

Related Topics

Pesticides
Respiratory Tract
Sensory Organs

Phosphoric Acid

- CAS: 7664-38-2
- SYNONYMS: Orthophosphoric acid
- CHEMICAL CLASS: Inorganic acids; corrosive mineral acids
- CHEMICAL STRUCTURE:

$$(HO)_2P(=O)OH$$

Uses
Phosphoric acid is a component of detergents, fertilizers, food additives, gasoline additives, and water treatment products. It is also used in rustproofing, engraving, and metal coating.

Exposure Pathways
Dermal, ocular, and mucous membrane contact and ingestion are possible routes of exposure.

Toxicokinetics
Phosphoric acid is rapidly absorbed.

Mechanism of Toxicity
Corrosion and disruption of pH balance are the mechanisms of toxicity.

Human Toxicity
Exposure to high-concentrated solutions can irritate the skin and mucous membranes. The ACGIH TLV is 1 mg/m^3 of air. The estimated fatal dose in humans is 1 ml. Phosphoric acid is highly corrosive.

Clinical Management
Gastric lavage or emetics should be avoided. The exposed area should be washed with copious amounts of water and a neutralizer such as magnesium oxide, lime water, or aluminum hydroxide gel.

—*Jayne E. Ash and Shayne C. Gad*

Related Topics

Acids
Corrosives

Photoallergens

Introduction

Photoallergy is an acquired immunologically mediated reaction to a chemical initiated by the formation of photoproducts. A photoallergen is a chemical that leads to this response. The occurrence of a photoallergic response to a chemical is sporadic and highly dependent on the specific immune reactivity of the host. Photoallergic responses are thought to be cell-mediated hypersensitivity reactions involving two distinct mechanisms. In the first reaction type, light initiates the conversion of the hapten (synonymous with photosensitizer) to a complete allergen. Animal studies suggest that the photoreactive chemical in the skin absorbs light and is converted to a photoproduct that subsequently binds to tissue proteins producing a complete antigen.

$$\text{PS} \longrightarrow \underset{\text{(Hapten)}}{\text{Photoproduct}} + \text{Tissue Protein} \longrightarrow \underset{\text{(Antigen)}}{\text{Allergen}}$$

Halogenated salicylanilide photoproducts are believed to be formed in this fashion. In the second type of reaction, light absorbed by the photosensitizer results in its conversion to a photoproduct that is a more potent allergen than the parent compound.

PS (Weak Allergen) ⟶ Photoproduct (Strong Allergen)

The photoproduct of sulfanilamide is thought to be formed by this second pathway in which the parent sulfanilamide compound is converted by UV light to the potent allergic sensitizer *p*-hydroxyaminobenzene sulfonamide. Patients with this type of photoallergy have demonstrated an allergic reaction to sulfanilamide in the dark.

In contrast to phototoxicity, photoallergy represents a true type IV delayed hypersensitivity reaction. Hence, while phototoxic reactions can occur with the first exposure to the offending chemical, photoallergy requires prior sensitization. Induction and subsequent elicitation of reactions may result from topical or systemic exposure to the agent. If topical, the reactions are termed photocontact dermatitis, while systemic exposures are termed systemic photoallergy. In more situations, systemic photoallergy is the result of the administration of medications. Photocontact dermatitis was described over 50 years ago following the use of topical antibacterial agents. Thousands of cases were reported in the 1960s after halogenated salicylanilides were used in soaps as antibacterial additives. Tetrachlorosalicylanilide and tribromosalicylamide were quickly withdrawn from the market after numerous reports of photoallergy surfaced. Generally, the mechanisms of photocontact dermatitis and that of systemic photoallergy are the same as those described previously for allergic contact dermatitis. In the context of photocontact dermatitis, however, UV light is necessary to convert a potential photosensitizing chemical into a hapten that elicits an allergic response.

Testing for photoallergy is similar to patch testing for allergic contact dermatitis. Duplicate allergens are placed on the back under occlusion with stainless-steel chambers. Approximately 24 hr later, one set of patches is removed and irradiated with UVA. All patches are removed and clinical assessments of patch test sites are made 48 hr and then 1 week following placement. A reaction to an allergen solely on the irradiated side is deemed photocontact dermatitis. Reactions occurring simultaneously on the irradiated and unirradiated sides are consistent with an allergic contact dermatitis. There is disagreement about the likelihood of coexisting allergic contact and photocontact dermatitis to the same agent since a photopatch test may occasionally exhibit greater reactivity on the irradiated side compared to the unirradiated side. Table P-2 lists potential photoallergens used in photo-patch testing.

From a mechanistic standpoint, light-induced dermatopathologic changes can be divided into phototoxic and photoallergic categories. Phototoxic skin damage

TABLE P-2
Photoallergen Series for Photo-Patch Testing

p-Aminobenzoic acid
Bithionol (thiobis-dichlorophenol)
Butyl methoxydibenzolymethane
Chlorhexidine diacetate
Chlorpromazine hydrochloride
Cinoxate
Dichlorophen
4,5-Dibromosalicylanide
Diphenhydramine hydrochloride
Eusolex 8020 (1-(4-isopropylphenyl)-3-phenyl-1,2-propandione)
Eusolex 6300 (3-(4-methylbenzyliden)-camphor)
Fenticlor (thiobis-chlorophenol)
Hexachlorophene
Homosalate
Menthyl anthranilate
6-Methylcoumarin
Musk ambrette
Octyl dimethyl *p*-aminobenzoic acid
Octyl methoxycinnamate
Octyl salicylate
Oxybenzone
Petrolatum control
Promethazine
Sandalwood oil
Sulfanilamide
Sulisobenzone
Tetrachlorocarbanilide
Thiourea
Tribromosalicylanilide
Trichlorocarbanilide
Triclosan

results from the direct interaction of irradiation with subcellular targets, while photoallergic reactions pivot around immunomodulation of cutaneous photoreactivity. Both variants require initiation by exogenous light, but subsequent cytopathologic mechanisms may be substantially different.

With phototoxicity, light may originate directly from exogenous sources, such as the sun, artificial lighting, or photodynamic topical chemicals, or it may emanate from endogenous sources such as photodynamic drugs or chemicals following activation or excitation by percutaneous irradiation. Subcellular targets have not been completely characterized but may include the formation of thymine dimers, DNA–protein cross-links, or photodependent oxidations. Immunologic processes are not involved in this form of photosensitivity.

With photoallergic reactions, cytopathologic events are believed to be even more complex than with direct phototoxicity. Although many mechanistic features remain obscure, fundamental concepts include the photoactivation of endogenous or xenobiotic haptens so that they combine with cellular proteins and form a complete antigen. Subsequent immunologic reactions, especially cell-mediated hypersensitivity, complete the sensitivity process.

Although precise cytopathologic mechanisms have not been established for many photosensitivity reactions, clinical and pathological features have been extensively documented. The following outline describes key diagnostic findings that serve to differentiate photosensitivity reactions from other dermatologic phenomena.

Comparison with Contact Allergy

Photocontact allergic reactions are often compared with contact allergic reactions. Four pathogenetic mechanisms are present in both reaction types:

(1) Compounds with a low molecular weight can act as haptens.

(2) The antigen is produced by covalent binding of the hapten to skin components.

(3) The immunological reactions are T cell dependent.

(4) The histological pictures of contact and photocontact allergic reactions are similar.

Photoactivation of Molecules

The main difference between the two pathogenetic mechanisms is that in photoallergy light energy is necessary for the activation of the hapten or skin components to form covalent allergenic adducts. Besides photoactive exogenic or endogenic heteromolecules, the following skin components can be activated by photon energy: amino acids and proteins, blood components, lipoproteins, DNA, RNA, and so on. The reaction possibilities between hapten, light, and skin components can be classified in six different groups depending on the activated molecule:

(1) Through the absorbed light quantum the prohaptene is transformed into the haptene.

(2) Through the absorbed light quantum the active protein carrier is formed from the protein in the skin.

(3) The haptene formed by irradiation combines with a skin protein to form an antigen.

(4) The haptene combines with the protein changed by light to form an antigen.

(5) The haptene altered by light combines with the protein changed by light, thus forming an antigen.

(6) The haptene and light catalyze a chemical reaction on the protein which leads to an autoantigen.

Distinct photochemical processes are now known for molecular photoactivation. Most of the photoactive molecules have X electrons. If a molecule is activated by light, two different energy levels can be attained. The molecule can be activated from the ground state to the singlet energy level to the triplet energy level. In the case of the singlet-state level, an electron reaches a higher orbital while the original spin configuration is maintained. In the case of the triplet-state level, the electron in the higher orbital changes the spin configuration so that the two electrons in the different orbitals have parallel spin configurations.

The activated singlet-state molecules are short-lived and return to their ground state in time periods of 10^{-8} to maximal 10^{-6} sec. Fluorescence is one of the observed manifestations of the nascent energy. Triplet states are of longer duration, their lifetime can reach the range of 10^{-3} to 100 sec. Phosphorescence may be observed. Besides fluorescence and phosphorescence, nascent energy of activated molecules can also be released in the form of heat; electrical charges can be transferred to other molecules, and radicals can be formed or the molecule itself transformed.

In the case of photoallergic reactions, the formation of heteroadducts plays an important role. It comprises the combination of exogenous molecules with autologous tissue or cell components. This is the main process for the formation of the complete antigen. The formation of heteroadducts is also the most important factor in the treatment of psoriasis with 8-methoxypsoralen (8-MOP) and UV-A. The binding of 8-MOP to thymine molecules in the DNA is important not only for clinical treatment but also for possible late side effects (carcinogenicity).

An important complication of some of the chemicals inducing photoallergic responses is the development of persistent light reactions in which a marked sensitivity to light persists despite the apparent termination of exposure. Removal of the offending photoallergen in these cases does little to abate the condition and the action spectrum broadens to include the UVB as well as the UVA bands. As the phrase implies, this condition is long-lived and troublesome. This particular problem validates the importance of developing and utilizing screening tests for photoallergenicity to prevent exposure of a susceptible population of people to chemicals with this potential.

Clinical Findings

Usually, but not invariably, dermatologic lesions are restricted to light-exposed areas. Changes may vary from urticaria to papular and eczematous eruptions with subsequent exfoliation and lichenification. Microscopically, it is very difficult to distinguish photoallergic reactions from nummular eczema, atop dermatitis, eczematous drug eruptions, and, especially, allergic contact dermatitis.

Histopathologic Findings

Generally, microscopic findings do not provide an adequate basis for separating photoallergic reactions from the eczematous drug eruptions and allergic contact dermatitides previously discussed. Salient features include spongiosis with lymphocytic exocytosis, mild dermal edema, and mild to moderate dermal perivascular cuffing consisting of lymphocytes, histiocytes, and varying numbers of eosinophils. A feature that may distinguish photoallergy from contact allergy in human skin is that inflammatory cell infiltrations in light-induced allergic reactions may be both superficial and deep within the dermis, whereas with contact allergy they tend to be limited to the superficial dermis.

Assessment of Photosensitization

Photosensitivity reactions account for a very small percentage of the total number of undesirable effects from environmental chemicals. However, the increasing incidence and severe disability resulting from these types of skin changes suggest that additional photobiologic research efforts are needed, particularly when the photosensitivity response is of the persistent light reactor mechanism. Predictive testing is an obvious approach used to assess the photosensitizing potential of new chemicals entering the commercial market. These methods make it possible to identify and possibly minimize or eliminate exposures to those compounds demonstrating risk–benefit rations that are undesirable for the general population or especially sensitive individuals.

In vitro and *in vivo* methods with predictive value for estimating the photosensitizing potential of new compounds have developed rapidly to meet the demanding requirements of today's society. *In vitro* methods for assessing photosensitization are desirable because they are usually rapid and inexpensive and therefore allow screening of a large number of compounds. Many of these methods are not very specific, however, and will generate a greater percentage of false-positive results than *in vivo* tests using animal or human models. Complex *in vitro* test systems appear to be useful in identifying the site and mechanism of action in certain situations. Continued evolution of *in vitro* methodologies will add to the understanding of the photosensitization mechanism as better correlation is established with *in vivo* studies.

The first basic experimental work in photoallergy was done more than 50 years ago, when Epstein, in a straightforward and very perceptive study, demonstrated that sulfanilamide was both a phototoxin and a photoallergen. He and others had observed patients receiving sulfanilamide who developed a dermatitis in sun-exposed areas. Six naive subjects (one of whom was himself) were chosen and skin sites were injected intradermally with sulfanilamide (0.1 ml of a 1% saline solution). Then these areas were irradiated with ultraviolet light from a mercury arc lamp (UVA and UVB). In all six subjects, the procedure induced a mild erythema leading to hyperpigmentation at the injected sites; that is, a sulfanilamide-mediated phototoxic reaction. Repetition of the protocol (intradermal sulfanilamide and then UV irradiation) at a different site, some days later, caused a marked dermatitis in two of the six individuals. These two subjects had been photosensitized to sulfanilamide, and with further photo testing they continued to show an altered reactivity to sulfanilamide followed by UVR (but not to sulfanilamide alone); their photoallergy persisted. In later work, Epstein induced photoallergic contact dermatitis to chlorpromazine in human subjects, utilizing the topical application of chlorpromazine for photosensitization and photochallenge. Those results paralleled his findings with sulfanilamide: Chlorpromazine was both a phototoxin and a photoallergen. Biopsies of positive chlorpromazine photoallergic reaction sites showed a histopathological picture consistent with that of delayed-type hypersensitivity; that is, reactions similar to those of classical experimental allergic contact dermatitis in humans.

Over the ensuing years, a considerable number of compounds have been tested in humans for their possible photoallergenicity, and many of the larger dermatology units have photo testing sections for evaluating patients for possible photoallergy to materials with which they come into contact. Experimental work in humans sometimes followed the lead of clinical impressions, as was the case with chlorpromazine and tetrachlorosalysilanilide. Kaidbey and Kligman designed a prospective testing scheme in humans for evaluating possible photocontact allergens. Their method requires repeated photosensitizing exposures—that is, application of the test chemical to the skin—followed by ultraviolet light, for photosensitization; photochallenge is done 10–14 days after the last photosensitization at an untreated skin site. This routine, which is a variant of the "maximization" test in humans for classical contact allergens, has proven very useful for identifying the photoallergenicity of suspect materials.

Schwartz and Speck were the first to demonstrate photoallergy in an experimental animal, the guinea pig. Their initial investigation was with sulfanilamide and derivatives, and later experiments were with chlorpromazine. The common theme in tests is to photosensitize by the repeated successive application of prospective allergen, followed by UVR, to a clipped area (sometimes with the injection of complete Freund's adjuvant into the photosensitization site). Photochallenge is done at a different skin site some weeks later and reactions are evaluated by eye, as for classic allergic contact dermatitis in the guinea pig. The technique successfully identifies most known photocontact allergens, although in our experience and that of others, the substance bisphenol-A, by clinical report a photosensitizer of humans, does not photosensitize guinea pigs.

Test procedures designed to identify potentially photosensitizing chemicals evolved in the wake of the photosensitivity outbreak caused by the antimicrobial halogenated salicylanilides in the early 1960s. Photocontact allergy, although relatively uncommon, proved to be particularly troublesome. A minority of affected patients developed a persistent photodermatitis for many years despite avoidance of further contact with the offending chemical. While removal of the photosensitizing phenolic compounds from the marketplace reduced the incidence of photosensitivity, it quickly became apparent that other, chemically unrelated substances were also capable of inducing this adverse reaction. There was a clear need for a laboratory test to detect potentially photosensitizing agents.

Further Reading

Castel, S. W. (1991). Cutaneous photosensitization. In *Dermal and Ocular Toxicology* (D. W. Hobson, Ed.), pp. 193–220. CRC Press, Boca Raton, FL.

Maurer, T. (1983). *Contact and Photocontact Allergens.* Dekker, New York.

Marzulli, F. N., and Maibach, H. I. (1991). *Dermatotoxicology,* 4th ed. Hemisphere, New York.

—Shayne C. Gad

Related Topics

Ocular and Dermal Studies
Skin
Toxicity Testing, Dermal

Photochemical Oxidants

Introduction

Photochemical air pollution arises from a series of complex atmospheric reactions which result in a mixture of ozone, oxides of nitrogen, aldehydes, peroxyacetyl nitrates, and reactive hydrocarbons. If sulfur dioxide is present, sulfuric acid also may be formed because nitric acid vapor can be formed from nitrogen dioxide. From the point of view of the toxicology of photochemical air pollutants, the hydrocarbons as such are of less concern, though they may fall into the hazardous pollutant category (perhaps associated with cancer). The concentrations of these substances in ambient air generally do not reach levels high enough to produce other toxic effects. They are important, however, because they enter into the chemical reactions that lead to the formation of photochemical smog.

The oxidant of critical importance in the photochemical atmosphere is ozone (O_3). Several miles above the earth's surface there is sufficient shortwave ultraviolet (UV) light to directly split molecular O_2 to atomic O to combine with O_2 to form O_3. These UV wavelengths do not reach the earth's surface. In the troposphere, nitrogen dioxide efficiently absorbs longer wavelength UV light, which leads to the following simplified series of reactions:

$$NO_2 + h\nu \longrightarrow O + NO$$

$$O + O_2 \longrightarrow O_3$$

$$O_3 + NO \longrightarrow NO_2$$

This process is cyclic, with NO_2 regenerated by the reaction of the NO and O_3 formed. In the absence of hydrocarbons, this series of reactions would approach a steady state with no excess or buildup of O_3. The hydrocarbons, especially olefins and substituted aromatics, are attacked by the free atomic O, with NO to produce more NO_2. Thus, the balance of the reactions shown in Eqs. (1)–(3) is upset so that O_3 levels build up, particularly when the sun's intensity is greatest at midday, utilizing the NO_2 provided by morning commuters. These reactions are very complex and involve the formation of unstable intermediate free radicals that undergo a series of changes. Aldehydes are major products in these reactions. Formaldehyde and acrolein account for about 50 and 5%, respectively, of the total aldehyde in urban atmospheres. Peroxyacetyl nitrate (CH_3COONO_2), often referred to as PAN, and its homologs also arise in urban air, most likely from the reaction of the peroxyacyl radicals with NO_2.

Short-Term Exposures to Smog

The complexity of photochemical air pollution challenged toxicologists early on to ascertain its potential to affect human health adversely. Although ozone was quickly suspected as a primary toxicant because of its reactivity and abundance, a number of studies were undertaken with actual (outdoor-derived) smog or synthetic (photolyzed laboratory-prepared atmospheres) smog in an attempt to assess the potency of a more realistic pollution mix. When human subjects were exposed to actual photochemical air pollution (Los Angeles ambient air pumped into a laboratory exposure chamber), they experienced changes in lung function similar to those described in controlled clinical studies of ozone (i.e., reduction in spirometric lung volumes; see below), thus supporting the notion that ozone is of primary concern (see Ozone).

Acute animal studies utilized more easily controlled synthetic atmospheres (usually irradiated automobile exhaust) where the ozone target levels could be made to mimic high air pollution levels: approximately <0.5 ppm. Again, very much like ozone alone, just a few hours of exposure to irradiated exhaust resulted in deep lung damage, primarily within the alveolar or small airway epithelium. In some of these studies, early evidence of edema appeared in the interstitium, particularly in older animals. Additionally, similarly exposed mice were found to be more susceptible to bacterial challenge and lung pneumonias. With time after the termination of exposure, the end-airway lesions recovered and the susceptibility to infection waned, although some of the pathology in the distal lung persisted for more than 24 hr. While ozone appeared to be the prime toxicant in these studies, that was not always the case. When guinea pigs were exposed to irradiated automobile exhaust, airway resistance increased, indicating that a more soluble irritant probably was active, presumably reactive aldehydes. Thus, the array of effects of a complex atmosphere may be more diverse than would be predicted if it were assumed that ozone alone was responsible.

Chronic Exposures to Smog

Studies of both humans and animals exposed to smog have attempted to link chronic lung defects with photochemical air pollution. Cross-sectional and retrospective field studies have suggested an accelerated loss of lung function in people living in areas of high pollution relative to low pollution, but most of these studies have been imprecise because of confounding factors (meteorological factors, exposure measurement imprecision, and population variables). Recently, there has been a rejuvenation of interest in what are sometimes called sentinel studies, which allow a detailed study of animals exposed to the same highly polluted urban air to which people are exposed. This approach has had a troubled past, but newer studies have attempted to minimize or at least control for the problems of infection, animal care, and lack of control of the exposure atmosphere.

Synthetic smog studies in animals were undertaken to eliminate some of the concerns about ambient smog exposure. The most extensive effort to evaluate the potential long-term health effects of synthetic smog was undertaken at the Cincinnati U.S. EPA laboratory in the mid-1960s. Beagle dogs were exposed to synthetic atmospheres on a daily basis (16 hr) for 68 months, followed by a clean air recovery period of about 3 years. The lungs of exposed dogs then underwent extensive morphological examination to correlate physiological and morphological observations. While the study did not show time-related lung function changes, all exposure groups had abnormalities, most of which persisted or worsened over the 3-year recovery period in clean air. Enlargement of air spaces and loss of interalveolar septa in proximal acinar regions were most severe in dogs that were exposed to oxides of nitrogen, oxides of sulfur, or oxides of sulfur with irradiated exhaust. Oxidants such as ozone arising from the irradiated exhaust would be expected to act on the distal lung. These studies elucidated a morphological lesion that was degenerative and progressive in nature, not unlike that of chronic obstructive pulmonary disease, the condition most often noted in the epidemiological studies.

—*Shayne C. Gad*

Related Topics

Pollution, Air
Respiratory Tract

Phthalate Esters Plasticizers

- CAS: 117-82-8
- Representative Compounds: 1, 2-Benzenedicarboxylic acid; bis(2-methoxyethyl) ester
- Synonyms: Methyl glycol phthalate; phthalic acid; bis(2-methoxyethyl) ester
- Chemical Structure:

$$C_6H_4\left(\overset{O}{\overset{\|}{C}}-O-CH_2-CH_2-O-CH_3\right)_2$$

Uses

Phthalate esters are widely used in the production of plastics, such as containers used for storing and transporting blood and other substances.

Exposure Pathways

Dermal, intravenous, and inhalation routes of exposure are all possible.

Toxicokinetics

All phthalate esters are readily absorbed, but toxicokinetics vary based on the route of exposure. Once absorbed, they are quickly distributed to organs and other body tissues such as the liver (bile) or kidneys.

Mechanism of Toxicity

Phthalate esters metabolize quickly to a monoester but do not progress further. This monoester is toxic and can deregulate cellular activity by mimicking endogenous ligands.

Human Toxicity

The greatest risk of toxicity is through use of stored blood products. Central nervous system depression, lung damage, or kidney damage are possible effects. Phthalate esters may irritate eyes, skin, or mucous membranes.

Clinical Management

If ingested, gastric lavage should be performed and respiratory therapy administered, if needed. Treatment should be symptomatic.

Animal Toxicity

Phthalate esters are dose-related teratogens in rats and chicks. In mice, the intraperitoneal LD_{50} is 2.51 g/kg and the oral LD_{50} is 2–6.4 g/kg. In rats, the intraperitoneal LD_{50} is 3.7 g/kg and the oral LD_{50} is 4.4 g/kg.

—Jayne E. Ash and Shayne C. Gad

*Picloram**

- CAS: 1918-02-1
- SYNONYMS: 4-Amino-3,5,6-trichloro-2-pyridinecarboxylic acid; 3,5,6-trichloro-4-aminopicolinic acid; 4-amino-3,5,6-trichloro-2-picolinic acid
- CHEMICAL CLASS: Chlorinated pyridine herbicide

* Information Source: Hazardous Substance Data Bank, National Library of Medicine, Bethesda, MD, July 1996.

Uses

Picloram and its salts are systemic herbicides produced by chlorination of 2-methylpyridine followed by hydrolysis and reaction with ammonia. Most broadleaf crops, except crucifers, are sensitive; most grasses are resistant. Picloram is effective in controlling annual weeds, is used alone or in combination with 2,4-D against deep-rooted perennials on non-cropland, and is used typically as pellets or in combination with 2,4-D or 2,4,5-T for brush control.

Exposure Pathways

Picloram is either a colorless powder or crystalline solid having very low vapor pressure, making inhalation exposure unlikely unless the dust is inhaled. Exposure to picloram occurs mainly through its manufacture and its use as a herbicide in forests. Environmental exposures in humans occur when forest visitors or others not directly involved in spray operations come in contact with spray or sprayed foliage, inhale spray mist, eat plants or animals contaminated with the herbicide, or drink water containing the herbicide. A suggested no-adverse-effect level for drinking water is 1.05 mg/liter. The ACGIH TLV 8-hr TWA is 10 mg/m^3.

Toxicokinetics

The fate of picloram was defined in six healthy male volunteers following single po doses of 5.0 and 0.5 mg/kg and a dermal dose of 2.0 mg/kg. Picloram was administered orally as the sodium salt in grape juice. The dermal dose was applied to the volunteers backs as the free acid dissolved in ethanol. The data indicate that the compound was rapidly absorbed from the gastrointestinal tract and rapidly excreted unchanged in the urine. Over 90% of the oral dose was recovered as unchanged picloram in the urine excreted through 72 hr. Most of the dose ($\geqq$75%) was excreted within 6 hr. By comparison, picloram was slowly absorbed through the skin, and only a small fraction (0.2%) of the picloram applied to the skin was absorbed.

Picloram is not readily metabolized and is excreted unchanged in the urine and feces of Fischer 344 rats. Following a 10-mg/kg [^{14}C]picloram intravenous dose, the isotope was cleared as parent compound and excreted in the urine. Balance studies in rats indicated that 98.4% of the dose was recovered. Urinary excretion resulted in an 80–84% recovery, fecal excretion resulted in approximately 15% recovery; less than 0.5%

was recovered in the bile, and virtually no radioactivity was recovered as trapped $^{14}CO_2$ or as other volatile compounds. Studies with [^{14}C]picloram showed that 90% of the compound fed in the diet to dogs was excreted within 48 hr in the urine, with small amounts appearing in the feces.

Mechanism of Toxicity

Little is known about the mechanism of toxicity of picloram.

Human Toxicity

Picloram causes a mild skin irritation, although it is not a skin sensitizer in humans. Picloram is not likely to be absorbed readily through the skin. Contact with exposed eyes causes moderate irritation which heals readily; corneal injury is unlikely. Inhalation of contaminated dusts may be somewhat irritating but is not likely to cause illness. Possible nausea may result from ingestion of massive amounts. Because of a lack of information for humans and animals, picloram is not classifiable with regard to its carcinogenicity in humans.

Animal Toxicity

Signs of intoxication from acute oral administration include skin rashes, hair loss, tachycardia, diarrhea, and, in cases of very high exposure, seizures. No teratogenic or embryotoxic effects have been found in rats fed up to 1000 mg/kg on Gestational Days 6–15. Similar findings were noted in rabbits. A multigeneration study in which rats were exposed to picloram from gestation through reproductive cycles to levels as high as 3000 ppm diet produced no evidence of effects on fertility, gestation, viability of pups, lactation, or skeletal development. Pregnant rats receiving doses of 1000 mg/kg/day during organogenesis were normal, but there was a slight increase in embryo resorption. A dose of 2000 mg/kg/day was toxic to the mothers but did not induce malformations in the pups. Picloram administered orally at three dose levels (20, 200, and 2000 mg/kg body weight) introduced no cytogenic aberrations in bone marrow cells. B6C3F1 mice and Osborne–Mendel rats were fed picloram for 80 weeks. After treatment, mice were observed for 10 weeks. Upon death or sacrifice, major organs were examined. In rats there was a high incidence of follicular hyperplasia, C cell hyperplasia, and C cell adenoma of the thyroid. There was an increased incidence of hepatic neoplastic nodules considered to be benign in female and male rats. Both male and female rats showed lesions of the liver diagnosed as foci of cellular alteration. It was concluded that picloram was not carcinogenic in mice or male rats.

Lifetime daily exposure of rats and dogs to diets containing 150 mg/kg body weight doses of picloram resulted in no observable gross or microscopic signs of toxicity. Rat LD_{50} (oral) is given as 8200 mg/kg.

Picloram was not mutagenic in gene mutation assays in bacteria and yeast, with or without metabolic activation.

—R. A. Parent, T. R. Kline and R. E. Sharp

Related Topics

Pesticides
Pollution, Water

Picric Acid

- CAS: 88-89-1
- SYNONYMS: 2,4,6-Trinitrophenol piconitric acid; carbazotic acid; nitroxanthic acid
- CHEMICAL CLASS: Nitrogen-substituted phenols
- CHEMICAL STRUCTURE:

OH
O_2N O NO_2
NO_2

Uses

Picric acid is used in the production of explosives, matches, and electric batteries. It is also used in etching copper and manufacturing colored glass and as a textile mordant.

Exposure Pathways

Dermal contact, ingestion, and inhalation are possible routes of exposure.

Toxicokinetics

Picric acid is readily absorbed through the skin or through the respiratory tract.

Mechanism of Toxicity

Picric acid accelerates the body's metabolism.

Human Toxicity

Dermal exposure may cause an allergic reaction. It causes yellow staining of skin. Absorption into the skin or ingestion may cause nausea, vomiting, diarrhea, abdominal pain, olguria, anuria, staining of skin, pruritus, sudden acne, stupor, convulsions, and death. The ACGIH TLV is 0.1 mg/m^3.

Clinical Management

The victim should be removed from exposure. Gastric lavage with water should be performed. Activated charcoal is also recommended.

Animal Toxicity

In animals, picric acid is a dermal sensitizer and strong eye irritant. It also causes liver and kidney damage and produces central nervous system effects. It is a mutagen. The LD_{50} in rats is 200 mg/kg.

—*Jayne E. Ash and Shayne C. Gad*

Related Topic

Acids

Piperonyl Butoxide

- CAS: 51-03-6
- SYNONYMS: Alleviate; Butacide; Butocide; Butoxide; Pyrenone; 5-[[2-(2-butoxyetoxy)ethoxy]methyl]-6-propyl-1,3-benzodioxole
- CHEMICAI CLASS: Methylenedioxyphenyl insecticide synergist
- CHEMICAL STRUCTURE:

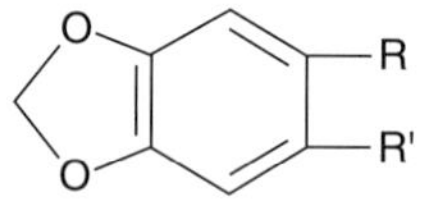

$$R-CH_2-(O-CH_2-CH_2)_2-O-(CH_2)_3-CH_3$$
$$R'-CH_2-CH_2-CH_3$$

Uses

Piperonyl butoxide is a synergist for pyrethrins, pyrethroids, and rotenone.

Exposure Pathways

Dermal exposure is the most common exposure pathway. Piperonyl butoxide is available as an aerosol, dust, emulsion, and solution.

Toxicokinetics

In experimental animals, piperonyl butoxide is poorly absorbed after oral and dermal exposure. The methylenedioxyphenyl moiety of piperonyl butoxide is cleaved by liver microsomal enzymes. The carbon atom of the methylene moiety is then hydrolyzed to a formate molecule which eventually forms carbon dioxide. The metabolites are conjugated with glucuronide or amino acid derivatives.

Mechanism of Toxicity

Piperonyl butoxide exerts toxicity by inhibiting mixed function oxidases. These enzymes are responsible for detoxifying pyrethrins and pyrethroids; their toxicity is therefore increased by piperonyl butoxide.

Human Toxicity: Acute

Piperonyl butoxide has a low incidence of acute toxicity. In one study, eight human volunteers given a single oral dose of 50 mg piperonyl butoxide did not show any signs of toxicity. Environmental exposures cause limited inhibition of microsomal enzymes. Laboratory findings indicate that piperonyl butoxide may cause various blood disorders (e.g., pancytopenia, thrombocytopenia, leukopenia, and polycythemia).

Human Toxicity: Chronic

Very little is known about the chronic effects of piperonyl butoxide.

Clinical Management

Basic life-support measures for respiratory and cardiovascular function should be utilized. Dermal decontamination should be accomplished by repeated washing with soap. Exposed eyes should be irrigated with copious amounts of room-temperature water for at least 15 min. Piperonyl butoxide may be mixed with other petroleum distillates; thus, emesis should be avoided. Activated charcoal or cathartics can be administered following oral exposure. The treatment is symptomatic. No antidote is available.

Animal Toxicity

Acute toxicity in laboratory animals following exposure to piperonyl butoxide is low (the oral LD_{50} in rats ranges from 6150 to 11,500 mg/kg). A single high dose of piperonyl butoxide can cause lacrimation, anorexia, unsteadiness, rough coat, irritation, coma, and death in rats. Repeated doses may also cause delayed onset of these same signs. Dogs also respond in the same way and may exhibit vomiting.

—Sushmita M. Chanda

Related Topics

Pesticides
Pyrethrin/Pyrethroids

Platinum (Pt)

- CAS: 7440-06-4
- SELECTED COMPOUNDS: *cis*-Dichlorodiammine platinum, DDP, cisplatin (CAS: 15662-27-1); *cis*-platinum chloride (CAS: 13454-96-1)
- CHEMICAL CLASS: Metals

Uses

Platinum and its alloys are used in jewelry, dentistry, the chemical industry, and the electrical industry. Most automobile catalytic converters contain platinum. Certain platinum compounds that have the *cis* configuration and can combine with DNA are useful therapeutic agents for many cancers that do not respond readily to conventional chemotherapy (especially testicular, ovarian, bladder, prostate, and thyroid cancers). Testicular cancer, which was once always fatal, now responds to platinum-containing drugs.

Exposure Pathways

Inhalation of industrial platinum compounds may be a problem. Platinum is usually a by-product of copper and nickel refining. Platinum and platinum-group metals (palladium, ruthenium, rhodium, and iridium) are also by-products of gold refining.

The general population is exposed to platinum by the dermal route, especially from jewelry. The oral route is not significant because absorption is very poor.

Toxicokinetics

Following inhalation, lung clearance of platinum metal is very slow. Approximately 1 week following ingestion of platinum-containing water, platinum is found in the kidneys and liver. Following injection of the cancer chemotherapeutic agent, *cis*-platinum, platinum is found mainly in the gonads. In autopsy specimens, platinum is found in adipose tissue.

The *cis*-platinum compounds can react with disulfides and amino groups and form adducts with some bases in nucleic acids. Serum creatinine levels correlate with *cis*-platinum doses.

Platinum compounds inhibit a few enzymes, including leucine aminopeptidase, and the hydrogenases of malate, liver alcohol, and lactate. Platinum compounds readily form a metallothionein.

Most platinum is excreted in the feces.

Human Toxicity

Inhalation of platinum dusts produces a pneumonitis characterized by coughing, wheezing, shortness of breath, and an asthma-like action. In some cases, cyanosis develops. The ACGIH TLV-TWA is 1 mg/m^3 for elemental platinum and 0.002 mg/m^3 for soluble salts as platinum.

Skin contact with various salts of platinum (especially the chlorides) can cause allergic dermatitis, characterized by eczematous patches. Type I hypersensitivity can be induced easily. Often the toxicity is not due to platinum itself but to its complexing with tissues.

Cisplatin produces a variety of serious side effects. It tends to deposit platinum in the corticomedullary area of the kidney and thus causes gastrointestinal upset (e.g., severe nausea and vomiting), nephrotoxicity (injuring both proximal and distal tubes), and blood changes (e.g., hypomagnesemia, leukopenia, and thrombocytopenia). Ototoxicity (e.g., tinnitus and hearing loss), peripheral neuropathy, and allergic reactions are also reported.

Clinical Management

Symptoms of platinum inhalation usually abate soon after terminating exposure. Dermal exposure should be treated by washing the affected area immediately after exposure. To prevent skin allergic responses to platinum, it is best to control platinum dusts in the environment.

The toxicity of the chemotherapeutic agent, cisplatin, can be reduced by prehydration using copious amounts of fluids.

Animal Toxicity

Cisplatin is an active mutagen in the Ames test. Administered subcutaneously, local tumors appear.

—*Arthur Furst and Shirley B. Radding*

Related Topics

Kidney
Metals

Poinsettia

- SYNONYMS: *Euphorbia pulcherrima;* Christmas star; Christmas flower; painted leaf; lobster plant; Mexican flame-leaf; star of Bethlehem; flower of nativity; Easter flower; pappagallo

Exposure Pathways

Ingestion and dermal contact are possible routes of exposure.

Mechanism of Toxicity

Diterpene esters are primary irritants to the gastrointestinal tract and dermal areas.

Human Toxicity

The amount of toxin found in the common greenhouse variety of poinsettia is minimal and very rarely causes symptoms. Irritation, whether dermal or oral, may be seen but not expected. The poinsettia, despite its unfavorable reputation, appears for the most part to be innocuous.

Clinical Management

For ingestion of plant material, treatment consists of dilution with cool liquids. Skin irritation may be treated with irrigation.

Animal Toxicity

Animals, particularly domestic animals, have shown gastrointestinal irritation progressing to diarrhea, hypersalivation, and weakness.

—*Rita Mrvos*

Poisoning Emergencies in Humans

Introduction

Over 2 million human poisoning exposures are reported by American poison centers each year. Estimates by the American Association of Poison Control Centers (AAPCC) fix the actual number of poisonings at approximately 5 million cases per year! The disparity in these data reflects the fact that a poison center is not contacted for advice each time a poisoning exposure occurs. However, the data illustrate that accidental and intentional poisoning in humans is a very common problem.

Despite the frequency of poisonings, the morbidity and mortality associated with these incidents can be minimized if medical intervention is aggressive, appropriate, and immediate. Morbidity and mortality can also be minimized if the lay and medical publics are aware of the most common poisons, how to treat exposures to those poisons, and, most important, how to prevent poisonings from occurring.

Toxicoepidemiology

Poisonings are among the most preventable public health problems. The reason being that the majority of exposures are accidental (86%) and occur in children under 6 years of age. However, poisoning exposures are not limited to children and occur during every decade of life (Fig. P-9).

The high incidence of pediatric exposures is a consequence of the patterns of growth and development in children as well as carelessness by caretakers and the lack of adult awareness about what constitutes a poison. Children aged 18–36 months are at the greatest risk due to excessive hand-to-mouth behavior. Their innate curiosity, which results in extensive exploration of their environment, is also a contributing factor. Combined with a general lack of awareness by adults about the fact that nearly everything is potentially hazardous (adding credence to a phrase attributed to Paracelsus: "the only thing that differentiates a poison from a remedy is the dose"), children are very prone to become victims of accidental poisonings. These incidents are largely preventable by recognizing the toxic potential of medications, household products, cosmetics, and botanicals and keeping them out of the reach of children.

Across all age groups, medications are involved in the preponderance of reported poisonings (Table P-3). Cleaning products are the leading cause of pediatric poisoning exposures, followed closely by analgesics, cosmetics, and plants. These agents result in the majority of exposures because they are commonly found in households where children reside. Contrary to popular belief, children do not usually seek out these substances in cupboards or medicine cabinets but suffer their exposure while the product is actively being used, usually by an adult. Approximately 80% of all pediatric poisoning exposures occur while a product is in use! Since medications are ubiquitous in today's society, it is not surprising that they are responsible for the majority of human poisonings. Various medications are also the leading cause of death due to poisoning.

Poisonings are associated with a relatively low mortality rate—only 0.03% of poisoned victims have fatal outcomes. Adults account for 95% of these fatalities and children account for only 5%. Most adult

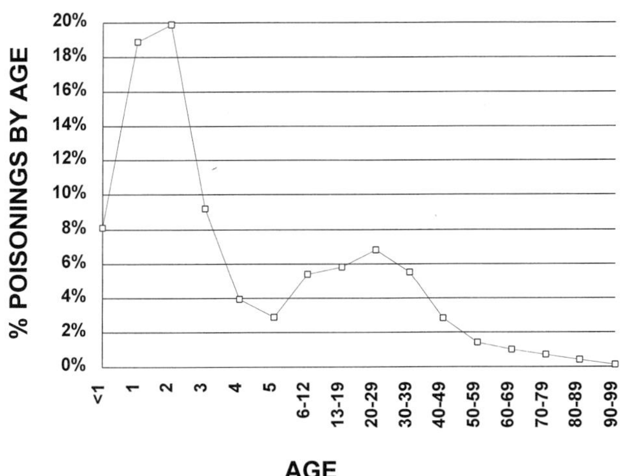

FIGURE P-9. Age distribution of poisoning exposures in humans (source: AAPCC annual reports, 1983-1992).

TABLE P-3
Poisoning Exposures vs Fatalities: Comparison of Exposure and Fatality Ranking

Poisoning exposures	*Fatality ranking*	*Poisoning fatalities*	*Common exposure ranking*
Cleaning products	10	Antidepressants	19
Analgesics	2	Analgesics	2
Cosmetics	28	Sedative/hypnotics	11
Plants	31	Street drugs	24
Cough/cold preps	17	Cardiovascular drugs	25
Hydrocarbons	11	Alcohols	14
Bites	27	Fumes	22
Topicals	24	Chemicals	10
Foreign bodies	39	Asthma medications	32
Chemicals	8	Cleaning products	1

Source: 1983–1992 AAPCC annual reports.

poisoning-related fatalities involve antidepressant agents or analgesics (Table P-3). Although the incidence of pediatric fatalities is low, they are tragic events that are largely preventable. Accidental ingestion of toxic amounts of iron accounts for most of the fatalities in children under 6 years of age. The other component of pediatric fatalities involves adolescent drug overdosage and substance abuse. Solvent inhalation alone accounts for approximately 30% of adolescent poisoning deaths.

Poison Prevention

Poison prevention education can reduce the number of accidental poisonings in children and adults alike. The severity of poisoning can also be reduced if people are educated about what to do if a poisoning exposure has occurred. This type of education, however, has little impact on individuals who intentionally expose themselves to potentially toxic substances for the purpose of self-harm.

The most important step in preventing and addressing poisonings is to know the telephone number of an AAPCC-certified regional poison center or your local poison center (Table P-4). Certified regional poison centers provide emergency poison and treatment information 24 hr per day, every day of the year. They are staffed by health professionals (nurses, pharmacists, and physicians) who are specialists in toxicology. A telephone call to the regional poison center may prevent an unnecessary trip to the emergency department or assist a health professional in the management of a challenging poisoning case. Regional poison centers can also provide poison prevention information; for example, guidance on how to "poison-proof" a home or guidance on poisonous versus nonpoisonous plants when planting a flower garden.

Since most accidental pediatric poisonings occur while products are in use, always attempt to store medications, cleaners, cosmetics, chemicals, and even plants out of the reach of children.

Child-resistant closures are not "child-proof." Consumer Product Safety Commission guidelines dictate that a limited number of children are permitted to open a child-resistant closure within a prescribed period of time. Therefore, despite the presence of a child-resistant closure on a container, the product should still be stored out of the reach of children. However, child-resistant closures should be used whenever possible.

TABLE P-4

American Association of Poison Control Centers Listing of Certified Regional Poison Centers (April 1997)

Alabama

Alabama Poison Center–Tuscaloosa
408-A Paul Bryant Drive
Tuscaloosa, AL 35401
Emergency phone: 800-462-0800 (AL only) or 205-345-0600

Regional Posion Control Center
The Children's Hospital of Alabama
1600-7th Ave. South
Birmingham, AL 35233-1711
Emergency phone: 800-292-6678 (AL only), 205-939-9201, or 205-933-4050

Arizona

Arizona Poison and Drug Information Center
Arizona Health Sciences Center; Rm. 1156
1501 N. Campbell Ave.
Tucson, AZ 85724
Emergency phone: 800-362-0101 (AZ only) or 520-626-6016

Samaritan Regional Poison Center
Good Samaritan Regional Medical Center
Ancillary-1
1111 E. McDowell Road
Phoenix, AZ 85006
Emergency phone: 602-253-3334

California

Central California Regional Poison Control Center
Valley Children's Hospital
3141 N. Millbrook, IN31
Fresno, CA 93703
Emergency phone: 800-346-5922 (central CA only) or 209-445-1222

San Diego Regional Poison Center
UCSD Medical Center
200 West Arbor Drive
San Diego, CA 92103-8925
Emergency phone: 800-876-4766 (in 619 area code only) or 619-543-6000

San Francisco Bay Area Regional Poison Control Center
San Francisco General Hospital
1001 Potrero Ave., Building 80, Room 230
San Francisco, CA 94110
Emergency phone: 800-523-2222

Santa Clara Valley Regional Poison Center
750 South Bascom Ave., Suite 310
San Jose, CA 95128
Emergency phone: 800-662-9886 (CA only) or 408-885-6000

University of California, Davis, Medical Center
Regional Poison Control Center
2315 Stockton Blvd.
Sacramento, CA 95817
Emergency phone: 800-342-9293 (northern CA only) or 916-734-3692

Colorado

Rocky Mountain Poison and Drug Center
8802 E. 9th Avenue
Denver, CO 80220-6800
Emergency phone: 303-629-1123

(*continues*)

*TABLE P-4 (*Continued)

Connecticut
Connecticut Regional Poison Center
University of Connecticut Health Center
263 Farmington Avenue
Farmington, CT 06030
Emergency phone: 800-343-2722 (CT only) or 203-679-3056

District of Columbia
National Capital Poison Center
3201 New Mexico Avenue NW, Suite 310
Washington, DC 20016
Emergency phone: 202-625-3333 or 202-362-8563 (TTY)

Florida
Florida Poison Information Center–Jacksonville
University Medical Center
University of Florida Health Science Center–Jacksonville
655 West 8th Street
Jacksonville, FL 32209
Emergency phone: 800-282-3171 (FL only) or 904-549-4480

The Florida Poison Information Center and Toxicology Resource Center
Tampa General Hospital
P.O. Box 1289
Tampa, FL 33601
Emergency phone: 800-282-3171 (FL only) or 813-253-4444 (Tampa)

Georgia
Georgia Poison Center
Grady Memorial Hospital
80 Butler Street SE
P.O. Box 26066
Atlanta, GA 30335-3801
Emergency phone: 800-282-5846 (GA only) or 404-616-9000

Indiana
Indiana Poison Center
Methodist Hospital of Indiana
1701 N. Senate Boulevard
P.O. Box 1367
Indianapolis, IN 46206-1367
Emergency phone: 800-382-9097 (IN only) or 317-929-2323

Kentucky
Kentucky Regional Poison Center of Kosair Children's Hospital
Medical Towers South, Suite 572
P.O. Box 35070
Louisville, KY 40232-5070
Emergency phone: 800-722-5725 (KY only) or 502-629-7275

Maryland
Maryland Poison Center
20 N. Pine St.
Baltimore, MD 21201
Emergency phone: 800-492-2414 (MD only) or 410-528-7701

National Capital Poison Center (DC suburbs only)
3201 New Mexico Avenue NW, Suite 310
Washington, DC 20016
Emergency phone: 202-625-3333 or 202-362-8563 (TTY)

Massachusetts
Massachusetts Poison Control System
300 Longwood Ave.
Boston, MA 02115
Emergency phone: 800-682-9211 or 617-232-2120

*TABLE P-4 (*Continued)

Michigan
Poison Control Center
Children's Hospital of Michigan
4160 John R, Suite 425
Detroit, MI 48201
Emergency phone: 800-764-7661 (800-POISON-1)

Minnesota
Hennepin Regional Poison Center
Hennepin County Medical Center
701 Park Ave.
Minneapolis, MN 55415
Emergency phone: 612-347-3141; Petline, 612-337-7387; TDD, 612-337-7474

Minnesota Regional Poison Center
8100 34th Avenue S.
P.O. Box 1309
Minneapolis, MN 55440-1309
Emergency phone: 612-221-2113

Missouri
Cardinal Glennon Children's Hospital
Regional Poison Center
1465 S. Grand Blvd.
St. Louis, MO 63104
Emergency phone: 800-366-8888 or 314-772-5200

Montana
Rocky Mountain Poison and Drug Center
8802 E. 9th Ave.
Denver, CO 80220-6800
Emergency phone: 303-629-1123

Nebraska
The Poison Center
8301 Dodge St.
Omaha, NE 68114
Emergency phone: 800-955-9119 (NE and WY) or 402-390-5555 (Omaha)

New Jersey
New Jersey Poison Information and Education System
201 Lyons Ave.
Newark, NJ 07112
Emergency phone: 800-764-7661 (800-POISON-1)

New Mexico
New Mexico Poison and Drug Information Center
University of New Mexico
Health Sciences Library, Room 125
Albuquerque, NM 87131-1076
Emergency phone: 800-432-6866 (NM only) or 505-843-2551

New York
Finger Lakes Regional Poison Center
University of Rochester Medical Center
601 Elmwood Avenue
Box 321, Room G-3275
Rochester, NY 14642
Emergency phone: 800-333-0542 or 716-275-5151

Hudson Valley Regional Poison Center
Phelps Memorial Hospital Center
701 North Broadway
North Tarrytown, NY 10591
Emergency phone: 800-336-6997 or 914-366-3030

(*continues*)

TABLE P-4 (Continued)

Long Island Regional Poison Control Center
Winthrop University Hospital
259 First Street
Mineola, NY 11501
Emergency phone: 516-542-2323, -2324, -2325, -3813

New York City Poison Control Center
New York City Department of Health
455 First Ave., Room 123
New York, NY 10016
Emergency phone: 212-340-4494, 212-P-O-I-S-O-N-S, or TTD 212-689-9014

North Carolina
Carolinas Poison Center
1000 Blythe Boulevard
P.O. Box 32861
Charlotte, NC 28232-2861
Emergency phone: 800-84-TOXIN (1-800-848-6946) or 704-355-4000

Ohio
Central Ohio Poison Center
700 Children's Drive
Columbus, OH 43205-2696
Emergency phone: 800-682-7625, 614-228-1323, 614-228-2272, TTY, 614-461-2021

Cincinnati Drug & Poison Information Center and Regional Poison Control System
P.O. Box 670144
Cincinnati, OH 45267-0144
Emergency phone: 800-872-5111 (OH only) or 513-558-5111

Oregon
Oregon Poison Center
Oregon Health Science University
3181 SW Sam Jackson Park Road, CB550
Portland, OR 97201
Emergency phone: 800-452-7165 (OR only) or 503-494-8968

Pennsylvania
Central Pennsylvania Poison Center
University Hospital
Milton S. Hershey Medical Center
Hershey, PA 17033
Emergency phone: 800-521-6110

The Poison Control Center
3600 Sciences Center, Suite 220
Philadelphia, PA 19104-2641
Emergency phone: 215-386-2100

Pittsburgh Poison Center
3705 Fifth Avenue
Pittsburgh, PA 15213
Emergency phone: 412-681-6669

Rhode Island
Rhode Island Poison Center
593 Eddy St.
Providence, RI 02903
Emergency phone: 401-277-5727

TABLE P-4 (Continued)

Texas
North Texas Poison Center
5201 Harry Hines Blvd.
P.O. Box 35926
Dallas, TX 75235
Emergency phone: 800-764-7661 (800-POISON-1)

Southeast Texas Poison Center
The University of Texas Medical Branch
301 University Avenue
Galveston, TX 77550-2780
Emergency phone: 800-764-7661 (800-POISON-1) or 409-747-1460

Utah
Utah Poison Control Center
410 Chipeta Way, Suite 230
Salt Lake City, UT 84108
Emergency phone: 800-456-7707 (UT only) or 801-581-2151

Virginia
Blue Ridge Poison Center
Box 67
Blue Ridge Hospital
Charlottesville, VA 22901
Emergency phone: 800-451-1428 or 804-924-5543

National Capital Poison Center (northern VA only)
3201 New Mexico Avenue NW, Suite 310
Washington, DC 20016
Emergency phone: 202-625-3333 or 202-362-8563 (TTY)

Washington
Washington Poison Center
155 NE 100th Street, Suite 400
Seattle, WA 98125
Emergency phone: 800-732-6985, 800-572-0638 (TDD only), 206-526-2121, 206-517-2394

West Virginia
West Virginia Poison Center
3110 MacCorkel Ave., SE
Charleston, WV 25304
Emergency phone: 800-642-3625 (WV only) or 304-348-4211

Wyoming
The Poison Center
8301 Dodge Street
Omaha, NE 68114
Emergency phone: 800-955-9119 (NE and WY) or 402-390-5555 (Omaha)

Some pediatric poisonings occur because adults place potentially toxic substances in food and beverage containers. For example, if motor oil is placed in a clear soft drink container, a curious child may perceive it to be the soft drink product and consume some of the contents. Never place chemicals in food or beverage containers or in unlabeled containers.

Children have a tendency to emulate adult behavior. Strive not to take medications in the presence of a child. Furthermore, never call medicine candy as an enticement to encourage a child to take their medication.

Most products are effective and safe if used properly. However, even good products can be potentially harmful if used improperly. To protect anyone who may be exposed to a product during use, always read and follow the directions for use and safety as indicated on product labels.

While there is an infinite litany of poison prevention techniques and tools, these guidelines provide the foundation for preventing most poisoning exposures. However, if a poisoning exposure does occur, always attempt to cease exposure to the poison, conduct life-support measures if necessary, and contact a regional poison center for further information. In some cases, gastric decontamination, the use of antidotes or pharmacologic antagonists, and basic or advanced life-support measures may be necessary.

Initial Basic Management of Human Poisoning

The practice of clinical toxicology is still very much a combination of art and science. Although knowledge about toxins has grown exponentially, there is still a considerable void of absolute knowledge about many toxins. Therefore, contrary to the false perceptions about the existence of antidotes, which abound in the lay literature, there are very few pharmacologic antagonists that can be used to reverse the adverse effects of toxins. Accordingly, good supportive care is the cornerstone of managing all poisoned patients. Immediate intervention utilizing the basic concepts of life support (airway, breathing, and circulation) limits the severity of many poisonings. The importance of establishing a patent airway and intravenous access cannot be overemphasized.

Airway Management

The evaluation and establishment of an airway should take precedence in the management of all poisoning exposures. Patients with a decreased level of consciousness should be viewed as candidates for endotracheal intubation. Patients who have been exposed to drugs or chemicals that produce respiratory depression may need intubation to secure an airway to maintain adequate ventilation. Combative patients who violently resist medical intervention may need to be paralyzed, and then intubated, to enable the nurse or physician to perform gastric decontamination or administer fluids or pharmacologic antagonists. Patients who are at risk of vomiting and the subsequent consequences of aspiration are candidates for aggressive airway management.

Intravenous Access

Intravenous access is extremely important in the prudent management of severely poisoned victims. Intravenous fluids may be necessary to maintain blood pressure and to rehydrate patients who have become volume depleted as a toxic consequence of the exposure. For example, salicylate toxicity may be associated with fluid losses from hyperventilation, fever, and vomiting. Electrolyte administration may be necessary to restore the proper electrolyte balance. Establishing intravenous access also creates a conduit for the administration of pharmacologic antagonists such as naloxone (for opioid poisoning) and flumazenil (for benzodiazepine overdosage) as well as pharmacotherapeutic agents like pressors and antiarrhythmics.

Pharmacologic Antagonists: "Antidotes"

The number of pharmacologic antagonists is quite limited. There are few agents that will rapidly reverse toxic effects and restore a patient to a previously healthy baseline state. Historically, administering some pharmacologic antagonists actually worsened patient outcome compared to merely employing basic supportive care. As an example, analeptic agents such as picrotoxin and nikethamide were used to reverse the central nervous system depressant effects of agents like barbiturates. The mortality rate that accompanied barbiturate overdosage and analeptic treatment actually exceeded the mortality rate associated with good supportive care. With the exception of *N*-acetylcysteine, naloxone, and the conventional coma drugs, there are few indications and little utilization of pharmacologic antagonists (see Table P-5 for the most commonly used antidotes).

Antidotes Used in Coma Management

The most common application of antidotal-type medications is in the empirical treatment of the comatose

TABLE P-5
The Most Commonly Used Antidotes

Antidote	*% of all antidote use*
N-acetylcysteine	37.0
Naloxone	34.6
Atropine	4.7
Deferoxamine	4.4
Antivenin	3.9
Ethanol	3.1
Hydroxocobalamin	2.4
Physostigmine	2.1
Pralidoxime	1.3
Digoxin immune Fab	1.3
Pyridoxine	1.0

Source: AAPCC annual reports 1983–1992.

patient. Unless there is an obvious reason for a decreased level of consciousness (e.g., disease state and trauma), comatose patients routinely receive glucose 50%, naloxone, and thiamine.

Glucose is administered to all patients with a decreased level of consciousness where an immediate cause is not ascertained or rapid determination of a patient's blood glucose is not possible. From a toxicologic perspective, this is most important if a patient overdosed accidentally or intentionally on insulin or an oral hypoglycemic agent. If a prolonged state of hypoglycemia (producing brain damage) or other pathologic conditions have not interfered, the intravenous administration of glucose should rapidly reverse the comatose state. Since the duration of action of the hypoglycemic agent may exceed that of glucose, a constant infusion or repeated boluses may be necessary. If intravenous access is not available, intramuscular administration of glucagon may reverse the hypoglycemia. Once consciousness is regained, supplementary oral feedings may help to maintain a normoglycemic state.

Thiamine is administered to comatose patients who receive glucose and may also be chronic alcoholics. Alcoholics are often compromised nutritionally and, therefore, thiamine deficient. Glucose administration further depletes thiamine stores, which may result in the development of Wernicke's encephalopathy.

The third drug in the coma drug panel is naloxone. It is used to reverse the effects of opioids, which produce profound central nervous and respiratory system depression (see Naloxone for more specific information). The empirical administration of naloxone is rarely effective because opioid overdosage is not the most common cause of toxin-induced coma. However, naloxone is inexpensive and little risk is associated with its use, making it one of the standard "coma drugs."

Specific Antidotes

As indicated previously, pharmacologic antagonists or antidotes are used with great specificity and little frequency. Most poisonings can be managed with aggressive supportive care. However, some antidotes may be life-saving. For example, the early use of *N*-acetylcysteine in an acetaminophen overdose patient can prevent the development of hepatotoxicity and even death. Naloxone can rapidly reverse the profound respiratory depression associated with opioid toxicity. Digoxin immune Fab can reverse the life-threatening events that accompany digitalis poisoning. However, there are not specific antidotes for most poisonings and clinical judgment and skills are the cornerstones of therapy.

N-Acetylcysteine

Acetaminophen overdosage, whether accidental or intentional, is the most common type of poisoning event reported to American poison centers. The incidence of poisoning exposures often parallels the availability of potential poisons. This is especially true for acetaminophen, which is the most common household analgesic. Most acetaminophen overdoses do not produce adverse effects because the majority are minor exposures in children. However, significant overdoses may need to be treated with *N*-acetylcysteine (NAC; Mucomyst) if the patient has a toxic serum acetaminophen concentration. NAC is thought to replace endogenous glutathione or serve as a glutathione surrogate. This is important since acetaminophen overdosage depletes glutathione, permitting the toxic metabolite to destroy hepatocytes. NAC is most effective if administered within 8 hr of the acetaminophen ingestion; however, it may still be effective 24 hr postingestion.

Only oral NAC therapy is approved in the United States. The patient receives a loading dose of 140 mg/kg NAC followed by an additional 17 doses of 70 mg/kg at 4-hr intervals. Intravenous NAC is used investigationally in the United States in one of two common regimens (24 or 48 hr) and in Europe as a 20-hr protocol. The 24-hr regimen consists of an intravenous loading dose of 150 mg/kg over 15 min followed by 50 mg/kg over 4 hr and 100 mg/kg over the ensuing 16 hr. In the 48-hr protocol, the intravenous loading dose is 140 mg/kg followed by doses of 70 mg/kg every 4 hr for an additional 12 doses. The European protocol involves the administration of 150 mg/kg followed by a dose of 50 mg/kg over 4 hr and then 100 mg/kg for 16 hr. Parenteral administration of NAC eliminates compliance problems associated with oral therapy (very bad taste and odor due to the sulfhydryl groups) and circumvents the problems associated with acetaminophen-induced vomiting. A poison center or clinical toxicologist should be consulted to assist in the selection of the most appropriate regimen—oral or intravenous.

Naloxone

Opioid poisoning from the abuse of morphine derivatives or synthetic narcotic agents may be reversed with the opioid antagonist naloxone (Narcan). Naloxone is commonly used in comatose patients as a therapeutic and diagnostic agent. The standard dosage regimen is to administer from 0.4 to 2.0 mg, preferably intravenously. Intramuscular administration is an alternative parenteral route, but if the patient is hemodynamically unstable, the naloxone may not be absorbed rapidly from the intramuscular injection site. The intravenous dose should be readministered at 2- or 3-min intervals until the desired endpoint is achieved—restoration of respiratory function and an improved level of consciousness. If the patient fails to respond to a dosage of 10 mg, additional increments can be administered if there is a high degree of suspicion that an opioid overdose is actually being treated or if a synthetic opioid is the suspected agent. Patients who have been exposed to synthetic opioids may not be as responsive to the antagonistic effects of naloxone due to the high affinity of the agent for opioid receptors. If the intravenous route of administration is not viable, alternative routes in addition to intramuscular injection are administration via the endotracheal tube in intubated patients as well as intralingual and sublingual injection. Intraosseous administration may be an alternative route in pediatric patients.

A patient may not respond to naloxone administration for a variety of reasons: insufficient dose of naloxone, the absence of an opioid exposure, a mixed overdose with other central nervous and respiratory system depressants (e.g., benzodiazepines and ethanol), or medical or traumatic reasons. Be cognizant that naloxone may produce the syndrome of opioid withdrawal. While it is unusual for withdrawal to be life-threatening, it is discomforting to the patient and may make treatment intervention more difficult.

Atropine

There are few indications for the use of atropine as an antidotal agent in the management of acute human poisonings. However, its antimuscarinic pharmacologic properties make it an important agent to treat toxicity caused by exposure to pesticides that inhibit acetylcholinesterase: carbamates and organophosphates. These pesticides produce cholinergic symptoms, which can be reversed with the aggressive use of atropine. The initial dose should be titrated to the desired effect and followed with doses that eliminate or reduce the severity of the cholinergic effects. It is not uncommon for individual atropine doses to be 2–4 mg administered over short intervals. The patient should be monitored carefully since repeated doses may be necessary within 5–60 min of the atropinizing dose. Organophosphates can irreversibly render red blood cell cholinesterase ineffective. Therefore, atropine administration may have to be prolonged (days to weeks) if the patient is not treated early with pralidoxime (which will cleave the organophosphate bond with red blood cell cholinesterase and reactivate the enzyme).

Deferoxamine

Iron overdosage is responsible for the majority of pediatric poisoning fatalities. While most accidental pediatric iron exposures do not even require gastrointestinal decontamination, a limited number of accidental exposures and many intentional exposures require aggressive therapy. The focus of treatment for iron poisoning is to address the life-threatening features, which include hypotension, bleeding, and shock. Severely toxic patients and those with high serum iron levels may benefit from the administration of deferoxamine (Desferal), an iron chelator. Deferoxamine chelates iron and converts it to a water-soluble complex, ferrioxamine, which is eliminated readily via the urine. In most patients with elevated free serum iron, the resultant ferrioxamine imparts a pink to orange-red hue to the urine (sometimes characterized as a vin rosé wine color). When serum iron concentrations are not readily available, the disappearance of the urine discoloration signals the clinician to terminate the deferoxamine therapy. Caution! On rare occasions, the characteristic urine discoloration has been reported to be absent even in patients suffering from severe iron poisoning with documented toxic serum iron levels.

The intravenous route is preferred over the intramuscular route for deferoxamine administration. Serious iron poisoning is often accompanied by profound hypotension, which would reduce deferoxamine bioavailability if it was administered intramuscularly. Pediatric and adult doses vary. A poison center or a clinical toxicologist should be consulted for specific recommendations. However, the traditional intravenous regimen is an initial dose of 1000 mg followed by 500 mg every 4 hr until the patient's clinical state has improved and the serum iron concentration has diminished to a nontoxic concentration. The only significant admonition that accompanies intravenous use is that the rate of administration should not exceed 15 mg/kg/hr. With either intravenous or intramuscular use, the maximum recommended daily dose is 6 g.

There is occasional reference to using deferoxamine as a gastric lavage fluid. However, there is no concrete evidence that this is efficacious; it may actually increase the body burden of iron through the absorption of ferrioxamine, and it is an expensive intervention.

Crotalidae Antivenin

There are a number of antivenins that find occasional use in clinical toxicology. North American coral snake (*Micrurus*) antivenin is available as is black widow spider (*Latrodectus*) antivenin. However, the most commonly used antivenin is polyvalent crotalidae antivenin, which is used to treat envenomation by a variety of North American pit vipers—namely, rattlesnakes (*Crotalus*), cottonmouths (*Agkistrodon*), water moccasins (*Massasauga* and *Sistrurus*), and copperheads. This antivenin is produced by injecting horses with the venom of two North American and two South American pit vipers. The horses develop immunity to the venoms and subsequently produce antibodies, which are harvested and prepared as a commercial product for human use.

Use of antivenin in the appropriate doses can control local swelling and serious systemic effects (e.g., neurologic effects and coagulopathies) that occur in patients who have been envenomated. However, the antivenin should not be used prophylactically since a significant number of snake bites are dry bites—no envenomation. Furthermore, because the antivenin is a horse serum derivative, it should not be administered until the snake bite victim has been skin tested to determine if the person is sensitive to horse serum. Even after skin testing, caution should prevail since there is a 10% incidence of false-negative skin tests. Serum sickness, although rarely serious, is a common manifestation of antivenin use and generally occurs several days after the conclusion of antivenin therapy.

There are numerous dosage regimens which vary with the degree of systemic toxicity and regional treatment preferences. Consultation with a poison center or a clinical toxicologist is advised for the most contemporary treatment recommendations. While the current antivenin is beneficial in selected patients, its nonspecific nature and the presence of foreign antibodies make it less than optimal therapy. Antibodies similar to digoxin immune Fab are being investigated and hold great promise for the future.

Ethanol

Ethanol is a common toxin that often complicates intentional poisonings by acting synergistically with substances such as benzodiazepines. However, ethanol is also an important antidote in the treatment of poisoning secondary to methanol and ethylene glycol, which are associated with significant morbidity and mortality. Neither ethylene glycol nor methanol are innately very toxic; however, their metabolic by-products produce profound toxicity. When ethanol and either ethylene glycol or methanol have been coingested, alcohol dehydrogenase will preferentially metabolize the ethanol substrate. As a result, neither methanol nor ethylene glycol will be metabolized to their toxic metabolites.

This metabolic inhibition can be accomplished by maintaining a serum ethanol level of approximately 100 mg/dl in the poisoned patient. To attain this serum ethanol level the patient should receive ethanol in a loading dose of 600–700 mg/kg followed by hourly doses of about 125 mg/kg (alcohol tolerance or intolerance may necessitate modification of the dose). The ethanol can be given orally, diluted (e.g., water and juice) to a concentration of 20–25%. Intravenous ethanol can be administered in the same doses, but the sterile ethanol solution for intravenous use should be given in a concentration of 5–10%. Hemodialysis is often employed to enhance the elimination of methanol and ethylene glycol; however, dialysis will also effectively remove ethanol. Therefore, the dose of ethanol must be approximately doubled during hemodialysis to maintain a serum ethanol level of 100 mg/dl.

In calculating the appropriate dose of ethanol, one must remember that ethanol percentages are not weight/volume relationships. For example 95% ethanol is not 95 g/dl (instead it is approximately 76 g/dl). The percentage ethanol must be multiplied by the specific gravity of ethanol to determine the grams of ethanol per deciliter of fluid. Therefore, 95% multiplied by ethanol's approximate specific gravity (0.80) yields 76 g/dl. If this consideration is not appreciated, the patient will be underdosed.

Hydroxocobalamin

The standard pharmacologic therapy for cyanide poisoning is to administer nitrites, to induce a state of methemoglobinemia (methemoglobin avidly binds cyanide), combined with sodium thiosulfate to further detoxify the cyanide. The toxicity of nitrites and the concern about producing methemoglobinemia in cyanide-poisoned fire victims, who may also suffer from carbon monoxide poisoning, has driven the development of other cyanide antidotes.

Hydroxocobalamin, although only investigational in the United States, is a safe and effective alternative. Also known as vitamin B_{12}, hydroxocobalamin combines with cyanide to produce another form of vitamin B_{12}, cyanocobalamin. Conventional hydroxocobalamin cannot be used since the recommended dose is 4 g, which would necessitate the injection of several liters of vitamin B_{12} as hydroxocobalamin. Investigationally and in Europe, hydroxocobalamin is available in a more concentrated form. As with the traditional therapy, hydroxocobalamin is coadministered with sodium thiosulfate.

Physostigmine

Once touted as the medication of choice to treat lethal tricyclic antidepressant overdoses, physostigmine (Antilirium) has very limited uses and has largely fallen into disfavor. Physostigmine is a cholinesterase inhibitor and finds its primary application in the treatment of severe anticholinergic poisoning. This type of severity is usually only observed following overdosage of belladonna alkaloids such as atropine or scopolamine and rarely occurs as a manifestation of antihistamine overdoses. Abuse of members of the *Datura* species (jimson weed—*D. stramonium*) may produce severe anticholinergic poisoning. When indicated, physostigmine is administered via SLOW (at least 2 or 3 min) intravenous injection, preferably in small incremental doses of 0.5 mg. Rapid injection or the administration of large doses may produce a cholinergic crisis or seizure activity.

Physostigmine has essentially no role in the treatment of tricyclic antidepressant overdoses. It was previously thought that antidepressant overdose toxicity was a consequence of parasympathetic stimulation. However, the life-threatening cardiovascular and central nervous system effects are not mediated by that mechanism, thereby eliminating the use of physostigmine.

Pralidoxime

Pralidoxime (Protopam), also commonly known as 2-PAM, is used to restore red blood cell cholinesterase activity in patients who have been poisoned by organophosphate insecticides or chemical warfare agents. Organophosphates bond with acetylcholinesterase and inactivate it. Atropine can reverse many of the muscarinic effects, but it cannot restore the red blood cell cholinesterase activity. Pralidoxime can sever those bonds and restore the compromised cholinesterase activity. It is especially effective if it is administered in the 24 hr postexposure and may have limited effectiveness up to 48 hr after the organophosphate exposure. Unlike atropine, pralidoxime will oppose the nicotinic effects induced by overexposure to organophosphates. Since carbamate insecticides do not produce permanent impairment of cholinesterase, only atropine, and not pralidoxime, is used in those exposures. The traditional dose of pralidoxime is 1 or 2 g infused in 100 ml of normal saline over a period of 15—30 min.

Digoxin Immune Fab

Digitalis glycoside poisoning is associated with relatively high morbidity and mortality. Until the advent of digoxin immune Fab (Digibind), the only intervention for these poisonings was supportive care and treatment of specific maladies, such as treatment of cardiac arrhythmias with antiarrhythmics. However, with digoxin immune Fab, patients suffering from digoxin and digitoxin poisoning, and even those with oleander (the botanical *Nerium oleander*) poisoning, have a much better prognosis.

The Fab fragments of antidigoxin antibodies are harvested from sheep and prepared for commercial use in humans. Unlike the snake antivenin extracted from horse serum, these specific antibody fragments are only rarely associated with any type of allergic response after administration.

The relative indications for digoxin immune Fab administration are limited to serious clinical toxicity manifest as life-threatening cardiac arrhythmias that are unresponsive to conventional intervention, hyperkalemia, digoxin overdosage in excess of 10 mg, and steady-state digoxin serum levels in excess of 10 ng/ml. A poison center or clinical toxicologist should be consulted for specific dosage recommendations. In the absence of serum concentration or exact overdose information, 10–20 vials are administered to adults. Digoxin immune Fab should not be used indiscriminately. It is extremely expensive—the acquisition cost of a course of therapy could easily exceed $10,000! More important, digoxin immune Fab will interfere with the inotropic effects of digoxin, which could produce a therapeutic dilemma for a patient dependent on those effects for hemodynamic performance.

Flumazenil

Benzodiazepines are involved in many intentional overdoses. While these overdoses are rarely fatal when a benzodiazepine is the sole ingestant, they often complicate overdoses with other central nervous system depressants (e.g., ethanol and sedatives) due to their synergistic activity. Flumazenil finds its greatest utility in the reversal of benzodiazepine-induced sedation from minor surgical procedures. In suspected benzodiazepine overdoses, 0.2 mg flumazenil should be administered intravenously over 30 sec. If no response occurs after an additional 30 sec, a second dose of 0.3 mg is recommended. Additional incremental doses of 0.5 mg may be administered at 1-min intervals until the desired response is noted or until a total of 3 mg has been administered. Flumazenil should not be administered injudiciously as a nonspecific coma-reversal drug (e.g., naloxone and dextrose) since it has the potential to precipitate withdrawal in benzodiazepine-dependent individuals (benzodiazepine withdrawal, unlike narcotic withdrawal, may be life-threatening). Furthermore, flumazenil is contraindicated in patients suffering from mixed benzodiazepine and cyclic antidepressant poisoning since it may unmask the seizurogenic potential of the antidepressants, which may otherwise be prevented by the benzodiazepines.

Pyridoxine

Previously thought to be contained, tuberculosis is reemerging in immunosuppressed populations. Isoniazid is among the agents used to treat patients who have converted to being positive in tuberculosis skin testing and to treat the active disease. In overdosage, isoniazid decreases the brain concentrations of γ-aminobutyric acid by inhibiting pyridoxal-5-phosphate activity, resulting in the development of severe seizure activity. The administration of pyridoxine (vitamin B_6) can prevent or actively treat the central nervous system toxicity associated with isoniazid poisoning. Pyridoxine is administered on a gram-for-gram basis with isoniazid (i.e., the amount of pyridoxine should equal the amount of isoniazid). If the ingested amount of isoniazid is unknown, the dose of pyridoxine should be 5 g administered intravenously. This dose can be repeated as needed.

There are numerous other antidotes, namely, those used to treat heavy metal poisoning and still others to reverse drug-induced hyperthermia or dystonic effects. While all these antidotal agents are important, they constitute just one aspect of patient management along with life-support measures and decontamination interventions.

Decontaminating the Poisoned Patient

If the absorption of a toxin can be prevented or the length of exposure to the toxin limited, the toxicity associated with exposure can be either limited or prevented. Therefore, it is essential to consider the use of decontamination techniques in all poisoned patients. Of course, not all poisoned patients are candidates for a decontamination procedure since there may be a significant amount of time between exposure to the poison and the ultimate treatment or there may be other extenuating circumstances that preclude the use of decontamination.

Since approximately 80% of all poisonings are ingestions, the most common type of decontamination performed is gastrointestinal decontamination using a variety of techniques including emesis, gastric lavage, activated charcoal, cathartics, and whole bowel irrigation. Early use of these techniques may eliminate the need to implement aggressive advanced life support and antidotes in poison victims. However, poisonings occur by all routes, including dermal and ocular routes, which necessitate external decontamination.

Dermal Decontamination

Dermal exposures represent the second most common route of poisoning exposure. These exposures are often associated with very low morbidity and merely require simple washing to remove the patient from further exposure to the potential toxin. Some dermal exposures may involve corrosive agents that can produce liquefaction or coagulation necrosis and extensive tissue damage. The general approach for most topical exposures is to remove any contaminated clothing and to remove the toxin from the skin by gently washing the region with mild hand soap and water (while being cautious not to expose contiguous areas of skin). An alternative, if soap is not available, is to irrigate the affected area with copious amounts of water for approximately 15 min. This commonsense approach will address the management of most dermal exposures.

If a corrosive exposure has occurred, the affected clothing should be removed immediately, and the affected area should be irrigated, as described previously, for a minimum of 15 min. If the skin is not damaged, it may be washed very cautiously and gently with mild hand soap and water to remove any additional corrosive residue. Do not attempt to neutralize acid and alkaline corrosives with the corresponding acid (e.g., vinegar) or base (e.g., baking soda). This may delay irrigation therapy and may worsen preexisting injury by producing an exothermic (heat-producing) injury.

Some toxins require unique decontamination methods. For example, hydrofluoric acid exposures should be treated by irrigating the affected area with copious amounts of water and then applying calcium gluconate gel topically. The calcium will bind and prevent the absorption of the fluoride ion. In a limited number of cases, water irrigation may not be advised. To further illustrate, patients exposed to elemental sodium or potassium (from an explosion resulting in these chemicals becoming imbedded in the skin) should not be exposed to water since this combination would produce the very caustic hydroxide (lye) salt of the chemical and result in even greater toxicity. An oil (olive or mineral) should be used to cover the imbedded chemicals prior to their removal through surgical debridement.

Ocular Decontamination

Ocular contamination by toxins as a common consequence of splash exposure can produce irritation and, occasionally, severe ocular damage. Since the eye is such a sensitive organ, the institution of ocular irrigation should not be delayed until a patient reaches an emergency care facility. Ocular irrigation should be performed as soon as possible by instillation of a gentle stream of lukewarm tap water into the affected eye(s); irrigation should continue for 15–30 min. The skin contiguous to the eye should be irrigated as well. In minor toxicity cases, this procedure can be conducted in the home with the understanding that referral to an emergency department may be necessary if irritation persists. In the emergency department, the patient should undergo ocular irrigation with sterile normal saline for a period of at least 1 hr. Some exposures to corrosives may necessitate prolonged ocular irrigation.

Inhalation Exposure

There is little that can be done to decontaminate the patient following inhalational exposures. Inhalation exposure to gases, solids, and liquids is common; however, unlike the gastrointestinal tract, skin, and eyes, there is little opportunity to decontaminate the lungs. Removing the patient from the toxic environment, palliative oxygen therapy, and good supportive care form the basis for treating inhalation exposures.

Gastrointestinal Decontamination

Emesis, gastric lavage, activated charcoal, cathartics, and whole bowel irrigation are the most common means of gastrointestinal decontamination. Emesis and gastric lavage have been revered as the cornerstones of gastric decontamination for decades. However, confidence in these modalities has diminished as the science of clinical toxicology has emerged. As experience and knowledge about specific toxins has grown, there is more confidence regarding the body's tolerance to toxins. Furthermore, considerable research has evaluated critically the effectiveness of gastric decontamination techniques and provided better direction regarding their use. The result is a trend away from the conventional measures of emesis and lavage and toward use of activated charcoal. Despite these decontamination revelations, there is still a limited role for most types of gastrointestinal decontamination in the management of the acute poisoning victim.

Emesis

The induction of emesis has been the decontamination choice when a potential poison has been ingested. Time-honored emetics have included apomorphine, egg whites, saltwater, copper sulfate, and household dishwashing liquid. However, their use is fraught with ineffectiveness and potential inherent toxicity.

Apomorphine is an effective emetic, but it must be given parenterally and it is not devoid of opioid effects. The potential toxicity associated with the therapeutic effects of apomorphine make it an unacceptable emetic for use in humans. The use of egg whites to induce emesis has no pharmacologic basis and may result in delaying the implementation of effective therapy. Salt water is not an effective emetic, and its use is accompanied by the risk of sodium chloride poisoning manifest as fluid and electrolyte abnormalities. Copper sulfate is an effective emetic with a very narrow therapeutic index. The potential toxicity associated with its use precludes it as a viable emetic. Dishwashing liquid (the mild hand dishwashing variety) is composed of surfactants, which are effective emetics. Due to the soapy nature of these products, patient compliance is difficult to achieve. Other liquid soaps, such as automatic dishwashing detergent and laundry detergents, can have irritant and even corrosive properties and should never be used for this purpose. Mild dishwashing detergent finds little utility as an emetic. The only acceptable emetic is syrup of ipecac.

Syrup of ipecac is an effective emetic that contains the alkaloids cephaline and emetine (derivatives of the plant *Cephaelis ipecacuanha*). Syrup of ipecac induces emesis via direct peripheral irritation of the stomach and secondarily by stimulating the vomiting center in the brain. Emesis will occur within 15–25 min following a recommended dose of 15–30 ml syrup of ipecac (children over 1 year of age, 15–30 ml; adolescents and adults, 30 ml) and 120–360 ml of water (water is the preferred beverage, but other liquids including soft drinks, juice, and even milk may be used if necessary). If vomiting does not occur within 30 min, a subsequent dose of 15–30 ml syrup of ipecac should be administered with additional water.

Utilizing these administration guidelines, syrup of ipecac-induced emesis is effective in >99% of patients. Based on marker drug studies, only 25–50% of the ingested toxin will be eliminated during the emetic process. The efficacy of syrup of ipecac is largely dependent on the amount of time between ingestion of the toxin and administration of ipecac. Syrup of ipecac may be effective if it is administered within the first 60 min after an ingestion. If there are delays between ingestion and treatment, emesis will still occur but the toxin may no longer reside in the stomach.

Syrup of ipecac has very limited indications. There are no data that demonstrate that ipecac reduces either morbidity or mortality. It finds its primary application as a pediatric remedy for home use. Most accidental poisoning exposures involving children are discovered within minutes of the ingestion. The administration of syrup of ipecac may help to remove a potentially toxic amount of a moderately toxic drug such as an analgesic or cold/cough preparation. If a child reaches an emergency department within a short time after an ingestion, ipecac-induced emesis may be effective. However, many adult cases involve intentional exposures with a significant delay between exposure and treatment, making emesis of little or no value.

If used properly, ipecac-induced emesis is well tolerated. Although a limited number of patients may have repeated episodes of emesis, the vomiting usually subsides within approximately 30 min. Complications are rare.

Emetine toxicity may occur as a consequence of syrup of ipecac abuse by individuals with eating disorders. With chronic use, emetine will accumulate and may produce neuromuscular and cardiovascular toxicity. Death has occurred from chronic ipecac abuse.

Syrup of ipecac-induced emesis should never be used in postictal patients or those with a decreased level of consciousness since aspiration may occur. Emesis is also contraindicated if rapidly acting and/or extremely toxic agents (e.g., tricyclic antidepressants and calcium channel blockers) have been ingested or if corrosive agents have been ingested. Emesis is relatively contraindicated following the ingestion of hydrocarbons since many are not absorbed and the aspiration of even a minuscule amount may produce severe aspiration pneumonitis. Contrary to popular opinion, neither pregnancy nor use in children less than 1 year of age are contraindications to emesis. However, in these cases the procedure should be performed in a health care facility.

Gastric Lavage

Until recently, gastric lavage had been thought to be the most effective means of gastric decontamination. The procedure consists of inserting a tube into the stomach and using suction to remove the stomach contents and any toxin(s) remaining in those contents. Contemporary experience and research confirms that gastric lavage is effective but that it has limitations similar to those of emesis—if there has been a significant delay (more than 60 min) between the ingestion and treatment, there will be little toxin in the stomach available for removal. In fact, like the other decontamination modalities, lavage has never been validated as having an effect on reducing the morbidity and mortality associated with poisonings.

Gastric lavage is a relatively safe procedure if performed properly. It is accomplished by orally introducing a large bore orogastric tube down the esophagus and into the stomach. The size of the tube will, in part, determine the efficacy of the procedure—a 34- to 40-French-diameter tube should be used in adults and a 24- to 28-French tube in children. Early literature described syrup of ipecac-induced emesis as being superior to gastric lavage; however, a careful review of the early research reveals that those conclusions were based on lavage that was performed inefficiently using small bore tubes and small fluid volumes. Ideally, patients should be placed in Trendelenburg's position on their left side. Patients should be intubated endotracheally if they have a decreased level of consciousness or if airway protection is necessary.

In adults, tap water may be used as the lavage fluid by instilling aliquots of approximately 300 ml per exchange via gravity flow lavage (Fig. P-10). After the instillation of 300 ml tap water, the inflow tube is clamped and the tube leading to the collection bag is opened to allow the fluid and gastric contents [and it is hoped, the toxin(s)] to flow, via gravity, into a collection bag. This procedure is repeated until the lavage returns are clear of gastric debris and a total of 10–20 liters has been instilled.

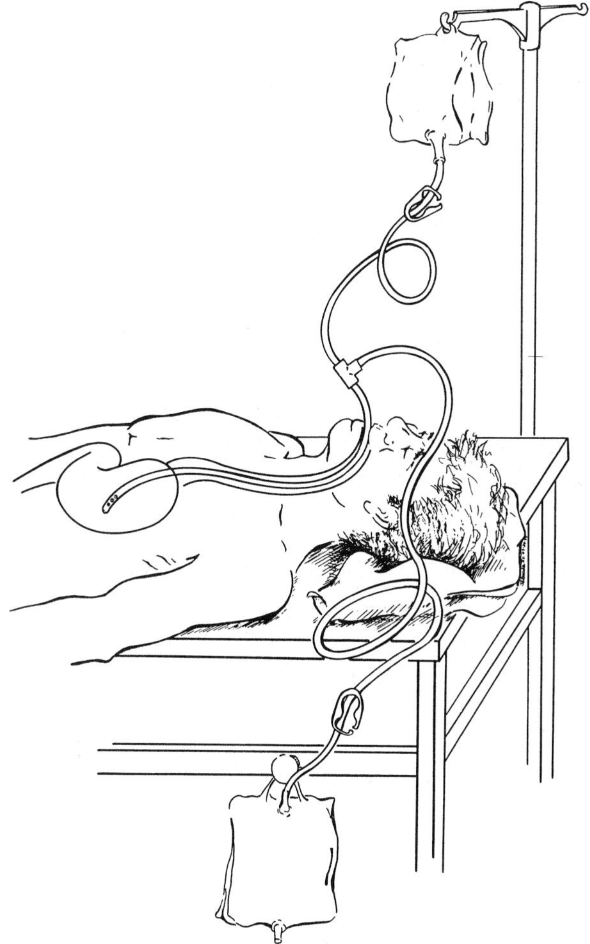

FIGURE P-10. Gravity flow lavage.

In young children, normal saline is used instead of tap water (to prevent electrolyte abnormalities) in aliquots of 10 ml/kg not to exceed 100–150 ml per aliquot. The procedure is repeated until the lavage returns are free of gastric debris and a total of 1–3 liters has been used.

The indications for gastric lavage are quite limited. It may be indicated in a comatose patient who has ingested an extremely toxic agent, a rapidly acting toxin, or an inordinately large amount of toxin within the previous 60 min. It may be more useful than the sole use of activated charcoal in these situations as well as in exposures in which activated charcoal does not effectively adsorb the toxin. Activated charcoal can be used early in gastric lavage to adsorb toxins that may be gastric-emptied during the lavage procedure. Furthermore, activated charcoal can serve as a marker to help determine when gastric lavage can be terminated. When the gross macroscopic evidence of activated charcoal is no longer obvious in the lavage returns, the procedure can be stopped.

Activated Charcoal

Prior to the 1980s, activated charcoal was relegated to the status of being an adjunct in the management of the poisoned patient. Contemporary research has demonstrated it to be as effective as, if not superior to, the traditional means of gastric decontamination (emesis and lavage). Activated charcoal is carbon that is produced from the combustion of petroleum products or wood pulp and "activated" when it is exposed to oxidizing gases, which have a cleaning action and also create a network of internal pores. The activation process gives the carbon (charcoal) its adsorptive properties and creates a massive surface area to adsorb toxins.

Activated charcoal effectively adsorbs toxins with a molecular weights ranging from 100 to 1000 Da. Therefore, it is capable of adsorbing most medications ingested in accidental and intentional overdoses. The most notable exceptions are low-molecular-weight compounds such as ethanol, methanol, ethylene glycol, lithium, iron, and heavy metals. However, the use of activated charcoal is never contraindicated solely based on the fact that one of the ingested toxins is not adsorbed.

Activated charcoal is available as a bulk powder for extemporaneous compounding, but most of the commercially available products for use in the poisoned patient are premixed aqueous slurries or sorbitol-containing mixtures. All of the products in the United States contain activated charcoal with a surface area of 950–2000 m^2/g. Activated charcoal tablets should never be used to treat poisonings since they do not have an adequate surface area to adsorb significant amounts of the toxin.

Activated charcoal can be administered orally or via the gastric lavage tube. The standard dose of activated charcoal for adults is 50–100 g; for children over 1 year, 25–50 g; and for children under 1 year, 1 or 2 g/kg. Since most products are aqueous slurries and not true suspensions, the containers should be agitated vigorously for at least 30 sec to resuspend the activated charcoal. The activated charcoal container should be rinsed repeatedly with water and the rinse water administered to the patient to ensure that the entire dose is delivered. Conscious patients can be offered the opportunity to drink the activated charcoal from a cup. Most aqueous activated charcoal products do not have any taste or odor; only the viscosity and gritty consistency of the product complicate drinking the activated charcoal. The addition of flavoring agents such as chocolate syrup and ice cream is not advised since they may compromise the adsorptive capacity of activated charcoal. However, the use of modest amounts may be necessary to enhance compliance in children. Noncompliant and comatose patients should receive the activated charcoal via a gastric lavage tube. The tube should be flushed with water to ensure administration of all of the charcoal.

Multiple-dose activated charcoal therapy has become a popular treatment to adsorb toxins that have a long residence time in the bowel (e.g., sustained-release pharmaceuticals) or to bind toxins that are enteroenterically or enterohepatically secreted into the gastrointestinal tract. Typically, 25–50 g of activated charcoal are administered every 2–6 hr to prevent the absorption of the toxin residing in the gastrointestinal tract. Sustained-release products are excellent candidates for multiple-dose therapy. Drugs such as phenobarbital and theophylline, which are secreted enteroenterically into the gastrointestinal tract, avail themselves to this form of gastrointestinal dialysis–the activated charcoal prevents reabsorption of the secreted drug and enhances gastrointestinal elimination. With theophylline and phenobarbital, this reduces the reliance on invasive extracorporeal elimination techniques such as hemodialysis. Some drugs undergo enterohepatic circulation; for example, digitoxin undergoes extensive biliary secretion. Multiple doses of activated charcoal can adsorb the digitoxin and prevent it from being reabsorbed to exert additional toxic manifestations.

Activated charcoal is finding greater applications and, in many situations, has replaced emesis and lavage as the primary form of gastric decontamination. There is often a substantial delay between a toxic ingestion and the ultimate treatment. In these situations, gastric emptying of the stomach contents [including the toxin(s)] has already occurred, making emesis and lavage of little value. Activated charcoal can be administered to adsorb any of the toxin still remaining in the stomach and, conceivably, to "catch up" with toxins in the small intestine. While this theory is in wide practice, it has never been validated. Potentially mild to moderately toxic exposures that are surrounded by an air of uncertainty as to the time of ingestion and the amount ingested, are cases in which the sole use of activated charcoal may be an option

Cathartics

Commercial activated charcoal preparations are also available in a sorbitol base. The sorbitol imparts a sweet taste to the product and also reduces the grittiness of activated charcoal by increasing the pharmaceutical elegance and viscosity of the product. Sorbitol is also a potent osmotic cathartic. The cathartic action is the primary reason for its presence in commercial products. Cathartics are sometimes used in conjunction with activated charcoal to enhance the gastrointestinal elimination of the activated charcoal:toxin complex from the bowel. The standard cathartic dose of sorbitol is 1.0–1.5 g/kg.

Since commercial products contain a fixed amount of sorbitol, it is possible to underdose a large individual and to grossly overdose an infant if they receive the commercial activated charcoal with sorbitol. In excess, sorbitol can produce significant fluid and electrolyte imbalance, which can complicate the management of a poisoned patient. Sorbitol is the most effective cathartic which has been used in the management of poisoning emergencies. However, the activated charcoal and sorbitol combination products should be avoided because the dose of sorbitol for the patient may be inappropriate. The combination products should never be used with each dose of activated charcoal during multiple-dose activated charcoal therapy.

Cathartics should not be used in the treatment of the poisoned patient. Their efficacy in reducing the morbidity and mortality associated with poisonings has not been demonstrated. Cathartics have the potential to produce fluid and electrolyte abnormalities.

Whole Bowel Irrigation

Whole bowel irrigation, long used for preoperative bowel preparation, is a relatively new intervention in clinical toxicology. The concept involves the administration of voluminous amounts of an iso-osmotic polyethylene glycol solution, which cleanses the bowel of toxins without being absorbed and without disturbing the delicate fluid and electrolyte balance of the body. The solution is administered orally at a rate of 0.5 (children) to 2.0 liters (adults) per hour. The solution is administered to an endpoint of either visible removal of the toxin from the bowel and clear rectal effuent or a total of 10 liters in adults.

Whole bowel irrigation has very limited indications. It may be effective in enhancing the elimination of poisons from the gastrointestinal tract that are incapable of being removed or detoxified in a safe alternative method. Heavy metals that are visualized on an abdominal X-ray may be removed using this technique. Patients who have ingested containers of illicit drugs (especially cocaine and heroin) to avoid prosecution ("body stuffers") or to smuggle them ("body packers") are excellent candidates for whole bowel irrigation. When large amounts of iron-containing dosage forms or sustained-release products are ingested, whole bowel irrigation may enhance their elimination and prevent absorption of the toxins. This elimination procedure does not lend itself to being convenient in patients who are comatose or critically ill. The endpoint of whole bowel irrigation has been estimated through clinical studies and the assumption cannot be made that all of the toxin has been totally eliminated from the gastrointestinal tract. Some of the toxin may have been absorbed and some may have been retained within the tract.

Alternative Means of Toxin Elimination

Gastric decontamination is the most commonly used means of eliminating a toxin from the gut. However, after absorption, most toxins are not secreted into the gastrointestinal tract and in rare circumstances other means of systemic elimination are employed.

Extracorporeal elimination of toxins is often considered but indicated rarely. Hemodialysis is available at many medical centers; however, there is a misconception that it is an effective modality to eliminate most toxins. To be removed effectively from the body by hemodialysis, a toxin should have high water solubility, low protein binding, a low molecular weight, and a small volume of distribution. Most substances do not meet that profile; only a limited number of common poisons are capable of being removed using hemodialysis (i.e., alcohols, lithium, theophylline, salicylates, and phenobarbital). Before embarking on a treatment regimen that includes a proposed option to dialyze a poisoned patient, a poison center or clinical toxicologist should be consulted.

The same admonition applies to the use of activated charcoal hemoperfusion where blood is percolated through a cartridge that contains activated charcoal. The concept is to have the toxins adsorbed by the activated charcoal. Many chemicals that are capable of being removed in this fashion have very low concentrations in the blood due to their fat solubility and large volume of distribution. Although these toxins may have an affinity to being adsorbed by activated charcoal, the small amount adsorbed is not sufficient to make a clinical difference in the patient. This procedure is not available in most hospitals.

Ion trapping is an intervention with considerable academic merit but without much clinical utility. It consists of manipulation of urinary pH (urinary acidification or alkalinization) to ionize a toxin and thus render it nonreabsorbable by the kidneys. Some drugs, such as salicylates and phenobarbital, appear to be vulnerable to enhanced elimination by altering the urinary pH. Clinically, however, the use of ion trapping followed by forced diuresis has never been demonstrated to have any impact on patient morbidity and mortality.

Further Reading

Bryson, P. D. (1989). *Comprehensive Review in Toxicology for Emergency Clinicians,* pp. 3–46. Taylor & Francis, Washington, DC.

Bowden, C. A., and Krenzelok, E. P. (1997). Clinical applications of commonly used contemporary antidotes. *Drug Exp.* **16**, 9–47.

Ellenhorn, M. J., and Barceloux, D. G. (1988). *Medical Toxicology: Diagnosis and Treatment of Human Poisoning*, pp. 54–85. Elsevier, New York.

Krenzelok, E. P., and Hall, A. H. (1996). In *Yearbook of Intensive Care and Emergency Medicine* (J.-L. Vincent, Ed.), pp. 780–790. Springer, Berlin.

Krenzelok, E. P., and Leikin, J. B. (1996). Approach to the poisoned patient. *Dis. Month* **42**, 509–608.

Litovitz, T. L., Smilkstein, M. Felberg, H., Klein-Schwartz, W., Berlin, R., and Morgan, J. L. (1997). 1996 Annual Report of the American Association of Poison Control Centers Toxic Surveillance System. *Am. J. Emerg. Med.* **15**, 447–500.

—Edward P. Krenzelok

Related Topics

American Association of Poison Control Centers
Carbamate Pesticides
Gastrointestinal System
Medical Surveillance
Organophosphate Pesticides
Sensory Organs
Skin

Pokeweed

- SYNONYMS: *Phytolacca americana; P. pecandra*; American nightshade; Indian polk; inkberry; pokeberry; red ink plant; red weed
- DESCRIPTION: Pokeweed is a tall, broad-leafed plant found in damp fields and wooded areas of southeastern Canada and the midwestern to eastern United States. The leaves and stalks are purplish. There are small greenish white to purplish flowers and dark berries in opposite clusters. The plant has a strong unpleasant odor. The large perennial root stalk can be up to 6 in. in diameter.

Uses

Pokeweed is used in pies, in tea, and as an herbal medicine. The young stems and sprouts are boiled and eaten after two changes of cooking water.

Exposure Pathways

Exposure to pokeweed is by ingestion and dermal contact.

Mechanism of Toxicity

The toxic activity of the plant is unclear. Pokeweed mitogen (PWM) noted in the plant fluids may initiate changes in the immune system that alter T and B lymphocytes. Pharmacology laboratories use PWM in experiments for its ability to penetrate cell membranes. The gastrointestinal irritant properties of phytolaccine enhance the absorption of triterpenoid glycosides (saponins), which may potentiate gastrointestinal toxicity.

Human Toxicity

Pokeweed contains phytolaccatoxin and related triterpenes. All plant parts are poisonous, especially the roots. Mature berries are relatively nontoxic, yet children have been poisoned by uncooked berries. Toxic exposures have occurred from eating uncooked leaves in salads or when the root is mistaken for horseradish, parsnip, or ginseng. Effects appear 2 or 3 hr after exposure. Symptoms include nausea, abdominal cramps, profuse sweating, and foamy diarrhea. Other effects include oral burning, a bitter taste in the mouth, dyspnea, weakness, tremors, and convulsions. Symptoms may last up to 48 hr. As few as 10 berries can result in toxic effects. Dermal exposures result in irritation, pain, and the sensation of heat.

Clinical Management

Symptoms usually resolve within 24 hr. In significant exposures, treatment should include gastric lavage or emesis, followed by activated charcoal. Late presentation cases will not benefit from emetics or cathartics. There is no antidote for exposure to pokeweed. Because cholinergic symptoms are prominent, treatment with atropine may be therapeutic.

—*Regina Wiechelt*

Pollution, Air

Types and Sources of Air Pollutants

Both man-made and natural sources contribute to the particles and gases which pollute our ambient environment. Episodic natural events, such as fires, wind erosion, and volcanic eruptions, produce considerable amounts of particulate matter and gases including mineral ash, pyrolysis products of combustion, carbon monoxide, and carbon dioxide. Although these "natural" particles and gases can have significant global effects such as short- and long-term alterations in weather conditions, little is known about the health effects resulting from inhalation of these materials. Obviously, little can be done to alter the contribution of pollutants from natural sources such as volcanic eruptions. A great deal more information is known regarding the generation, underlying chemistry, and adverse health effects of air pollutants from man-made (anthropogenic) sources. This continued interest in understanding the generation and health effects of man-made air pollutants stems largely from the fact that measures can be taken to control these pollutants and thus modify adverse health effects. Such control measures are often promulgated and regulated at the governmental level and are based on comparisons of the tangible (e.g., increased morbidity and mortality and financial) and intangible (e.g., quality of life) costs to society and the environment versus the cost of control measures.

Both stationary and mobile sources contribute to the particulate matter and gases that make up polluted urban and rural environments. Fossil fuel-powered electricity plants, heat generators, and waste incineration sites represent the major stationary point sources of pollution. Industrial processing plants such as smelters also produce a wide range of particulate matter and gases. Because these pollution sources are stationary, significant differences in both the quantity and the makeup of regional air pollution occur. For example, sulfur is present in fossil fuels (primarily in coal) used for heat production in the northeastern United States. The resulting acid components of ambient particles in the northeastern United States are thus primarily sulfates, whereas the acidic fraction of airborne particles in California is primarily nitrates.

A major portion of ambient air pollution results from gasoline- and diesel-powered automobiles and trucks. The mobile and ubiquitous nature of motor vehicles makes their pollution products widespread. While the presence of lead in automobile exhaust has been virtually eliminated, the contribution of motor vehicles to ambient concentrations of nitrogen oxides, hydrocarbons, and carbon monoxide in urban atmospheres is great. Indeed, transportation sources are responsible for 45% of the nitrogen oxides and 80% of the carbon monoxide emissions in the United States. Sunlight can drive a series of chemical reactions involving nitrogen oxides and hydrocarbons (a process known as photochemical oxidation) which result in secondary pollutants such as ozone. Though a secondary pollutant, ambient ground-level ozone is a major health concern for both urban and rural dwellers and produces agricultural crop losses and tree damage approaching several billions of dollars each year.

Regardless of the source of primary and secondary air pollutants, meteorological conditions play a significant role in the formation and transport of gases and particulate matter. One well-documented example occurs when sulfur dioxide released from industrial point sources in the northeastern United States forms acidic particles. These acidic precursors undergo long-range transport resulting in adverse effects due to acid rain in southern Canada. Thus, movement of masses of air can reduce ambient levels of pollutants in one region at the expense of air quality in another region. Meteorologic conditions also influence the creation of photochemical smog. Inversions occur when cooler air is trapped beneath a blanket of warm air, resulting in stagnant weather patterns. In southern California, the combination of inversions, sunlight, and motor vehicle emissions drives the photochemical reaction of trapped precursors and results in high ozone concentrations.

Regulation of Air Pollution

Reductions in ambient concentrations of some but certainly not all air pollutants has taken place over the past decade. In the United States, the U.S. EPA is the primary agency responsible for promulgating and regulating air pollution standards. National ambient air quality standards (NAAQS) have been established for six classes of outdoor pollutants: lead, carbon monoxide, ozone, nitrogen dioxide, sulfur dioxide, and particulate matter. These standards (Table P-6) are periodically reviewed and updated based on currently available data regarding adverse health effects. Bases on new evidence, the standards for ozone and particulate matter were recently changed. The ozone standard was amended to include an 8-hr average to reflect results of clinical studies which demonstrated cellular and biochemical pulmonary changes in exercising human subjects exposed to 0.10 ppm ozone for several hours. The particulate matter standard was also changed to include a standard for fine particles. Those metropolitan sites in which a particular pollution level exceeds the NAAQS are designated as nonattainment areas. Currently, more than half of the population in the United States lives in a nonattainment area for at least one regulated air pollutant. The Pollutant Standard Index, a more general ranking of air quality, is used for the daily reporting of air quality to the layperson via newspapers and telecasts in most major cities (Table P-7). It is noteworthy that five pollutants account for nearly 98% of the total mass of air pollution and that gaseous emissions make up the majority of air pollutants (Table P-8). These figures do not take into account fugitive dust emissions which are not inhalable (i.e., coarse dust

TABLE P-6
National Ambient Air Quality Standards (NAAQS)

Pollutant	*Primary standard*	*Type of average*	*Nonattainment population*[a]
Lead	1.5 $\mu g/m^3$	Maximum quarterly	5
Carbon monoxide	35 ppm (40 mg/m^3) 9 ppm (10 mg/m^3)	1 hr 8 hr	14
Ozone	0.08 ppm (157 $\mu g/m^3$)	Maximum daily 8 hr	45
Nitrogen dioxide	0.053 ppm (100 $\mu g/m^3$)	1 year	0
Sulfur dioxide	0.14 ppm (365$\mu g/m^3$) 0.03 ppm (80 $\mu g/m^3$)	1 year	0
PM_{10}	150 $\mu g/m^3$ 50 $\mu g/m^3$	24 hr 1 year	26
$PM_{2.5}$	50 $\mu g/m^3$ 15 $\mu g/m^3$	24 hr 1 year	Data not available

[a] Millions of persons living in counties with air quality levels not meeting the NAAQS in 1992. In 1992, the NAAQS for ozone was a maximum daily 1-hr concentration of 0.12 ppm.

TABLE P-7
Pollutant Standard Index Values

Index value descriptor[a]	*Air quality level*	*Health effect*
500	Significant harm	Hazardous
400	Emergency	Hazardous
300	Warning	Hazardous
200	Alert	Very unhealthful
100	NAAQS	Unhealthful
50	50% of NAAQS	Moderate
0	—	Good

[a]General health descriptor used in the lay press and media.

which is generated by wind erosion, farming, construction, and mining and quickly settles out due to its large size). Despite extensive legislation (two Clean Air Acts within the past 20 years) to set primary and secondary standards for the protection of human health and the environment, respectively, considerable numbers of air toxics are currently unregulated.

Control and reduction of ambient air pollutants in the United States has met with varying degrees of success. Unleaded gasoline now accounts for 99% of all gasoline sales. This change has virtually eliminated mobile sources as emitters of lead and reduced ambient lead levels by more than 75%. Likewise, stationary point sources of lead emissions, primarily industrial smelters, have dropped by more than 90% over the past two decades, although significant problems exist with individual smelters. Over the past decade, programs in reducing gaseous pollutants have been successful for carbon monoxide (8% decrease in total emissions) and sulfur dioxide (18% decrease). The reduction program for nitrogen dioxide has been partially successful. A slight increase in total nitrogen dioxide emissions occurred during a time period in which total motor vehicle miles in the United States increased substantially. A lack of major changes in ambient levels of nitrogen oxides and volatile organic compounds has resulted in only marginal success in reducing ambient levels of the secondary pollutant ozone. The long-term trend for ozone concentrations is downward, although meteorologic conditions appear to modify peak ozone levels monitored throughout the United States (high ozone levels have been measured during summers with hot, dry conditions and low levels measured during cool summers). In summary, legislative efforts have been successful in reducing ambient air pollution over the past two decades. Reduction of emissions from mobile sources such as motor vehicles has met with the greatest success, while reducing emissions from stationary point sources has often proven difficult as a result of conflicting interests of business, state and federal regulations, and enforcement agencies. While progress has been made in reducing ambient oxidant pollutants, it should be noted that a significant problem still exists and in the United States more than 140 million people lived in counties which exceeded the ozone standard in 1991.

TABLE P-8
Emission Estimates for the United States, 1995

Pollutant	*Total emissions*[a]	*10-Year trend*[b]
Carbon monoxide	92	15% decrease
Nitrogen dioxide	2	3% increase
Sulfur dioxide	18	9% decrease
Volatile organics	23	10% decrease
PM_{10}	43	12% decrease
$PM_{2.5}$	10	Not available
Lead	0.005	75% decrease

[a]Millions of short tons/year for 1995 except for $PM_{2.5}$, which is for 1990.

[b]Percentage change in estimated emissions between 1984 and 1994.

Health Effects of Air Pollution

There is mounting evidence that a number of air pollutants play a causal role in adverse health effects and that co-pollutants such as acid aerosols, ozone, and nitrogen oxides can have synergistic effects with each other. The major challenges for environmental health scientists are to identify the acute and long-term adverse health effects of ambient air pollution, pinpoint the relevant concentrations at which these effects occur, and determine sensitive subpopulations. This latter point is important in developing risk assessment paradigms as current federal legislation in the United States acknowledges the importance of protecting the health and welfare of all individuals.

In general, a great deal more is known about the acute effects of ambient air pollutants than is known about the chronic effects. The following discussion will outline the findings of epidemiologic, controlled clinical, and animal studies which have examined the adverse health effects of outdoor air pollutants. More detailed information can be found under Further Reading.

Ozone

Exposure to ozone in the ambient air is a major health concern in urban and rural communities throughout the United States. Current strategies to control the exposure of the general population to this highly reactive gas have been only marginally successful. Indeed, tens of millions of people reside in communities in which the ozone NAAQS has been exceeded.

Substantial evidence from epidemiological and controlled clinical studies suggests that acute ozone exposure at current ambient levels is associated with adverse respiratory effects in human subjects. The functional and symptomatic response of human subjects to inhaled ozone, however, appears to be highly variable. After performing moderate exercise during a single 6.6-hr exposure to 0.12 ppm ozone, the change in forced expiratory volume in 1 sec (FEV1) ranged from no decrement to −39% in healthy adult volunteers. The decrement in FEV1 and the increase in respiratory symptoms were dose dependent, with some volunteers responding to as little as 0.08 ppm ozone. Significant increases in the airway responsiveness to inhaled methacholine have also been observed after exposure to near-ambient ozone concentrations in laboratory studies. These functional effects are accompanied by an inflammatory response that occurs shortly after exposure and persists for at least 1 day. An influx of neutrophils and an increase in a number of mediators, including eicosanoids, neutrophil elastase, and cytokines, were measured in bronchoalveolar lavage fluid recovered from subjects exposed to near-ambient concentrations of ozone.

The adverse functional effects observed in controlled clinical studies are similar to those reported during exposure to ambient air. Decrements in lung function have been noted in a series of camp studies in which children were exposed to ambient ozone during normal outdoor play activity. Compared to controlled chamber studies, greater decrements in lung function were observed in the camp studies when the data were normalized for ozone concentration. A number of factors may explain the greater response in the camp studies, but the most likely reason is the simultaneous exposure to ambient copollutants such as acid aerosols. Epidemiologic studies have found strong correlations between respiratory symptoms, such as cough, throat irritation, and chest discomfort, and ambient ozone levels. Exacerbation of asthma, increases in hospital admissions for respiratory infections, and excess mortality have also been reported to be associated with oxidant air pollution episodes. Thus, a number of epidemiologic, field, and clinical studies provide evidence that adverse respiratory effects occur after acute exposure to ozone at or below the current NAAQS. Animal studies have corroborated these findings, although test animals in general appear to be less sensitive than human subjects to ozone.

Despite ample evidence for an acute response to ozone in human subjects, relatively little is known about the cumulative effects of acute injury and possible progression to adverse chronic lung dysfunction. Many studies have found that the functional decrements and symptoms observed after a single exposure to ozone lessen or are absent upon repeated exposure. The phenomenon of tolerance to the acute effects of ozone was described decades ago in animal studies. Clinical studies examining ozone-induced tolerance have clearly demonstrated that functional and inflammatory changes which are typically observed after the first day of exposure are attenuated by the second or third day of exposure for both normal and asthmatic subjects. Interestingly, the development of tolerance after repeated ozone exposure appears to occur for some functional parameters but not for others. For example, it has been observed in healthy adults that despite the rapid development of tolerance to decrements in FEV1 following repeated ozone exposure, ozone-induced increases in airway responsiveness to methylcholine were sustained throughout the five daily exposures. In addition, increases in markers of inflammation, such as an influx of neutrophils, are attenuated after five daily exposures. Markers of cell injury, however, do not appear to adapt as readily to repeated ozone exposure. These latter findings and similar results observed in animal studies suggest that although the respiratory tract is able to adapt to a major portion of the acute effects of ozone, long-term consequences may occur.

The few population-based and animal toxicology studies examining the chronic pulmonary effects of ozone suggest that ozone may be associated with long-term reductions in lung function and pathological changes. Animal studies using concentrations above the current NAAQS reveal that the centriacinar region of the airways and the nasal cavity are the most sensitive to pathological changes induced by chronic ozone. Epidemiologic studies have demonstrated that chronic exposure to ozone is associated with decrements in lung function and increases in the incidence and severity of asthma. The ability of these epidemiologic studies to establish cause and effect is hampered by confounding factors such as copollutants. Thus, the question whether chronic adverse health effects are clearly associated with ambient ozone exposure has not been answered at this time (see Ozone).

Sulfur Oxides

Significant and, on occasion, disastrous adverse health effects have accompanied acute air pollution episodes involving reducing-type pollutants. In the middle of this century, meteorologic inversion conditions resulted in high levels of particulate matter and sulfur dioxide in the Meuse Valley in Belgium, Donora in Pennsylvania, and London. Excess mortality accompanied each of these pollution episodes and has been attributed to the smoke and sulfur dioxide generated by fossil fuel combustion. A number of recent epidemiologic, clinical, and animal studies have confirmed that both particulate matter and sulfur oxides produce adverse health effects. These adverse effects have been observed during pollution episodes in which the gas and particle concentrations do not approach the magnitude of the three incidences mentioned previously. Delineating the relative contribution of particulate matter and sulfur oxides to these adverse effects is difficult because of the chemicophysical association of sulfur oxides and particles. This section is limited to the current state of knowledge on sulfur oxides and acid aerosol-related health effects. The following section will discuss particulate matter-related effects.

Sulfur dioxide is generated during the combustion of fossil fuels (primarily coal) containing traces of sulfur. Controlled laboratory studies using human subjects and test animals have demonstrated that sulfur dioxide can produce functional and pathological changes. These changes include increases in airway resistance and in mucus production. In general, the concentrations of sulfur dioxide necessary to produce these changes are greater than those encountered in the ambient environment. A notable exception is the bronchoconstrictive effect of sulfur dioxide on atopic and asthmatic subjects. Inhalation of 0.4 or 0.5 ppm sulfur dioxide in combination with moderate exercise causes substantial bronchoconstriction, shortness of breath, and cough in these sensitive individuals. Similar changes occur in normal (nonatopic) individuals only after exposure to at least a magnitude greater concentration of sulfur dioxide.

Despite the clear evidence of a subpopulation of individuals sensitive to near-ambient peak levels of sulfur dioxide, the two decade-old NAAQS for sulfur dioxide has not been changed nor has a short-term peak standard been instituted. A considerably greater amount of attention has been placed on the contribution of airborne particulates, particularly those associated with sulfur oxides, to adverse health effects. The carbon-, mineral-, and heavy metal-based particles produced during fossil fuel combustion and smelting promote the conversion of sulfur dioxide to sulfuric acid. Recognition of sulfur dioxide–particle interactions comes as a result of findings garnered from a number of animal studies and the characterization of sulfuric acid, ammonium sulfate, and ammonium bisulfate associated with atmospheric particles. The importance of the coexistence of sulfur oxides and particulate matter is reflected in the difficulty of epidemiology studies to separate the contribution of each pollutant to adverse health effects.

Epidemiological evidence from both Europe and North America suggests that acid aerosols formed by gas–particle interactions in the atmosphere play a major role in the adverse health effects seen during severe and moderate pollution episodes. The increases in mortality observed in London from 1958 to 1972 were more closely associated with acid aerosol concentrations than other pollutants such as smoke and sulfur dioxide. In the United States and Canada, cross-sectional analyses have demonstrated that ambient sulfate concentrations are better than indices of particulate concentrations as a predictor of excess mortality and hospital admissions due to air pollution. A prospective cohort study, known as the Six Cities Study, has found that increased mortality from cardiopulmonary deaths and lung cancer were strongly associated with sulfate and particulate concentrations. This same study has demonstrated that the incidence of bronchitis in children is correlated with ambient levels of acid aerosols. Similarly, in northern Europe, an acidic pollution episode in 1985 has been linked with significant excesses in respiratory mortality and morbidity and with persistent decrements in pulmonary function in children. In summary, a large body of evidence suggests that acid aerosols play a significant role in the adverse health effects attributed to air pollution.

Epidemiology studies are limited in their ability to establish direct cause and effect relationships. Many confounding factors such as smoking, occupational exposure, and copollutants such as ozone may contribute to observed effects and, for this reason, investigators have exposed human volunteers and animals to acid aerosols under controlled conditions.

Animal studies have demonstrated that exposure to near-ambient concentrations of sulfuric acid produces both conducting airway and alveolar changes, including increased airway resistance, airway hyperresponsiveness, and alterations in clearance mechanisms and macrophage function. Controlled human exposures to acid aerosols, however, have demonstrated few pulmonary effects at concentrations below 500–1000 $\mu g/m^3$. The adverse effects reported to occur after acute exposures to sulfuric acid aerosols have largely been observed in atopic subjects, are small in magnitude, and are readily reversible. Therefore, a research need has developed to explain the difference between the results of epidemiological studies and the paucity of data demonstrating adverse health effects in controlled human studies. One possible cause of this discrepancy is the type of acid aerosols used in the laboratory studies. Although pure sulfuric acid droplets are used almost exclusively in controlled exposures, ambient acid aerosols are chemically complex and are proposed to be composed of a core consisting of carbon, minerals, or heavy metals surrounded by acidic (sulfuric or nitric acid) surface material. Thus, knowing which chemical species is responsible for acid aerosol-induced adverse health effects is fundamental in developing proper control strategies for reducing air pollutants at their source.

Particulate Matter

Particulate emissions are by-products of fuel combustion, industrial processes, and motor vehicles and are believed to have a significant potential for causing adverse health effects. Carbonaceous material present in atmospheric aerosols is a combination of elemental carbon and organic and inorganic compounds. Particulate matter may also consist of fly ash, minerals, or road dust and contain traces of a number of heavy metals. Recent population-based studies have found that the association between adverse respiratory effects and particulate concentrations occurs in a number of regions throughout the United States. This association is strongest for PM_{10} and $PM_{2.5}$ indices (particulate matter less than 10 and 2.5 μm in diameter, respectively), but does occur for total suspended particulates. The observed adverse effects include increases in total mortality, mortality due to respiratory and cardiovascular causes, chronic bronchitis, and hospital visits and admissions for asthma. Elderly individuals and infants appear to comprise subpopulations that are most sensitive to the adverse health effects of PM_{10}.

Because the chemical makeup of particles varies greatly from region to region, the identification of the factor(s) responsible for the adverse health effects associated with PM_{10} is merely conjecture at this time. Few controlled human studies have used realistic particles and thus have contributed little to our understanding of particle-induced injury. Animal studies have been somewhat more productive and have demonstrated that particle-induced lung injury may be dependent on particle size, the presence of transition metals, and surface acid content. Effects of exposure to carbonaceous particles have been reported in studies investigating the toxicological significance of automotive diesel engine exhaust and fly ash. Long-term exposures to automotive diesel engine exhaust were found to cause focal fibrotic and proliferative lung disease accompanied by a progressive accumulation of soot in the lung and impaired alveolar clearance. Exposure of rats to high concentrations of diesel exhaust was also associated with an increase in lung cancer. Only minimal lung injury and irritant potency have been noted after repeated exposure of test animals to resuspended fly ash. Recent animal studies using freshly formed fly ash suggest that physical, chemical, and especially surface characteristics of the fly ash change substantially during the collection, storage, and resuspension processes. Using freshly generated fly ash, investigators have observed significant changes in lung function after acute exposure in guinea pigs. Thus, animal toxicology and controlled clinical studies have not yet provided clear answers to questions regarding the factor(s) responsible for the adverse health effects temporally associated with PM_{10} pollution episodes.

Nitrogen Oxides

Nitrogen oxide is produced in high-temperature combustion processes and is rapidly converted to nitrogen dioxide. Nitrogen dioxide is an irritant gas which produces oxidant lung injury similar to that produced by ozone. Nitrogen dioxide is far less potent than ozone and few functional or pathological changes have been observed in animals exposed to <0.5 ppm nitrogen dioxide. Pathological changes occur primarily in the terminal bronchioles and the alveolar region, although changes in mucociliary clearance have been observed during chronic exposures. Both long-term and short-term exposure to nitrogen dioxide can increase the susceptibility of animals to respiratory infection. Studied in a number of animal species, this effect includes increased mortality, decreased survival time, and impaired clearance of instilled pathogens. These findings reflect those obtained in epidemiologic studies which have found an increased incidence of respiratory infections in homes with gas appliances (see Indoor Air Pollution).

Nitrogen oxides other than nitrogen dioxide have been studied for possible adverse health effects. Chemical analysis of ambient aerosols collected in southern California has revealed that nitrates exhibit particularly high values compared to other parts of the United States. These aerosols are generally acidic in nature and are composed of nitric acid and nitrate salts that are formed through photochemical reactions with nitrogen dioxide and other oxides of nitrogen. These forms of nitrogen oxides contribute to acid aerosol formation in the ambient air and result from particle surface–gas interactions similar to those which have been described for sulfuric acid generation. Unique to the conditions of the coastal regions of California, acid fog forms from the interaction of nitrogen oxides and fog water droplets. A paucity of toxicologic and epidemiologic data does not allow a clear assessment of the health effects of either nitric acid-based particle.

Although research has clearly demonstrated a potential for nitrogen oxides, particularly nitrogen dioxide, to have serious health consequences, few exceedances of the NAAQS occur (see Table P-6). In general, health researchers are more concerned with (1) the key role nitrogen oxides play in the photochemical reactions which produce ozone and (2) the presence of nitrogen oxides indoors (both in occupational settings and in homes). Ambient concentrations of nitrogen oxides are generally lower than those found in grain silos and in homes using fossil fuel-consuming appliances.

Carbon Monoxide

Despite a nearly 40% increase in motor vehicle miles traveled over the period of 1983–1992, total emissions for carbon monoxide decreased by 25%. This dramatic change is attributed largely to controls initiated by the Federal Motor Vehicle Control Program. These figures do not reflect the additional decreases in carbon monoxide emissions which have resulted from the use of oxygenated fuels since 1992. Under the Clean Air Act of 1990, oxygenated fuels are required in all areas that do not meet the NAAQS standard for carbon monoxide during the winter months (when carbon monoxide levels are highest). Preliminary results of the oxygenated fuel program suggest that further decreases in carbon monoxide emissions will be achieved.

In general, ambient exposure to carbon monoxide is directly related to one's proximity to motor vehicle exhaust. Away from highways and industrial combustion processes, ambient carbon monoxide concentrations rarely exceed 1 ppm. Carbon monoxide levels can reach 3 or 4 ppm near roads and 5 ppm in the passenger compartment of automobiles. Heavier traffic conditions are typically associated with peak concentrations of 10–50 ppm. Even greater carbon monoxide concentrations can be encountered by workers in confined spaces such as tunnels. Significant exposures to carbon monoxide can also occur indoors (see Indoor Air Pollution). Levels as high as 10,000 ppm have been recorded in enclosed spaces in which a firefighter might enter. Operation of gasoline-powered equipment within a building can also result in significant carbon monoxide levels with ill-effects (e.g., Zamboni ice cleaners in skating rinks). Importantly, significant amounts of carbon monoxide are present in cigarette smoke. In nonsmoking human subjects, carboxyhemoglobin levels do not exceed 0.4% if environmental carbon monoxide levels are zero. Carboxyhemoglobin levels in cigarette smokers, however, can range from 5 to 10%.

Carbon monoxide is classified as a chemical asphyxiant. Its detrimental effects are mediated by its ability to combine with hemoglobin and other oxygen-carrying or -utilizing proteins. By binding avidly to hemoglobin and causing the formation of carboxyhemoglobin, the carrying capacity of hemoglobin for oxygen is reduced proportionately. One of the most sensitive measures of ill-effects after carbon monoxide inhalation is neurological testing. As little as 4% carboxyhemoglobin impairs neurologic function in repetitive tasks. In patients with preexisting angina or chronic pulmonary obstruction, increases in carboxyhemoglobin levels of only 2% were found to produce quicker onset of angina and dyspnea, respectively, during exercise. Reduced night and peripheral vision accompany carboxyhemoglobin levels of 10%. As levels exceed 10%, headaches may occur and at carboxyhemoglobin levels of 20–30%, nausea and weakness ensue. Decreases in mental function, collapse, and coma are evident as carboxyhemoglobin exceeds 35%.

Thus, carbon monoxide can produce a wide range of adverse effects. The concentration of carbon monoxide encountered in urban environments is relatively low and may have little effect on normal individuals. Several subpopulations, however, may be sensitive to current ambient exposure levels of carbon monoxide. These groups include individuals with chronic obstructive pulmonary disease, exertional angina, and cardiac arrhythmias. Fetuses may also be affected by carbon monoxide. Carbon monoxide binds more tightly to fetal hemoglobin and is cleared more slowly. Animal studies have demonstrated that maternal carbon monoxide exposure can reduce birth weight and increase neonatal mortality. Epidemiologic findings appear to confirm this effect of environmental carbon monoxide exposure on fetuses, although the confounding influences of smoking and indoor sources of carbon monoxide are hard to eliminate (see Carbon Monoxide).

Lead

Research on the health effects of chronic, low-level lead exposure is quite extensive and has been garnered from both epidemiologic and animal studies. The most critical of these adverse health effects have occurred in children and include deficits in physical and neurobehavioral development. In adults, small but consistent increases in blood pressure are significantly correlated with increases in blood lead concentrations. Acute, high-dose lead exposures result in more severe toxicological effects and these and other biological consequences of lead exposure are discussed in greater detail in the separate entry for Lead.

Exposure to lead can occur via a number of pathways including ingestion (drinking water, food, and soil) and inhalation. Although ingestion of lead contributes the majority of the average individual's body burden of lead, airborne lead has been estimated to be responsible for 7–40% of blood lead. The major sources of airborne lead are gasoline additives, metal smelters, and battery manufacturing/disposal. Total emissions for lead has decreased dramatically over the past two decades and has reduced ambient air concentrations by 89% nationwide (data from 1983 to 1992). The decrease in total emissions and ambient concentrations is a direct result of federal regulations issued by U.S. EPA requiring the removal of lead from gasoline. The dramatic decrease in lead emissions has been paralleled by an equally impressive decrease in average blood lead levels, making this one of the most successful federal intervention programs in the field of environmental health. Over a 4-year period (1976–1980), average blood levels decreased from approximately 15.5 to 9.5 μg/dl. Despite the improvement in nationwide airborne lead concentrations, industrial point source release is still a problem. As of 1992 and 1993, 13 areas in the United States were designated as nonattainment areas in regard to airborne lead and approximately 5 million people resided in counties that do not meet the NAAQS for lead.

Future Directions and Control Strategies

Improvements in air quality in the United States have occurred as a result of federal regulations promulgated by the Clean Air Acts of 1970 and 1990. While the decrease in emissions for some NAAQS pollutants has been impressive (e.g., lead and carbon monoxide), only minor changes have been documented for others (e.g., nitrogen and sulfur oxides and PM_{10}. Moreover, as of 1993, nonattainment regions have been identified for each of the NAAQS pollutants. Thus, it is important to acknowledge that a major air pollution problem still exists. The lack of significant improvement in various pollutant categories occurs as a result of several factors including economics, technological limitations, inability to identify proper control strategies, and politics. Reduction of pollutant emissions from point sources, in particular, has proven to be difficult to regulate and enforce.

The reported emissions for the air pollutants with NAAQS are only a portion of the total amount of toxic substances released by mobile and point sources. While regulations and controls set in place to reduce the release of particulate matter, volatile organics, and nitrogen oxides will also reduce the emissions of many air toxics, it is estimated that 1 million tons of air toxics are released in the United States each year. Air toxics are generally defined as hazardous air pollutants, other than the NAAQS pollutants, with the potential for causing increases in mortality or serious illnesses. The Clean Air Act Amendments of 1990 identify 189 substances requiring regulation. Regulation of these air toxics necessitates technology-based standards for reducing emissions and establishing an accidental release program. The top 10 air toxics, in terms of total emissions, are toluene, methanol, methyl ethyl ketone, xylene, chlorine, hydrochloric acid, carbon disulfide, and chlorinated alkanes and alkenes. Over a 9-year period (1987–1995), a sustained downward trend in total emissions of these air toxics was obtained. It must be emphasized that provisions in the Clean Air Act Amendments of 1990 focus on point sources of air toxics emissions rather than individual substances. Thus, key source categories have been identified and are to undergo prompt regulation for reducing hazardous emissions. Examples of key emissions sources for which regulations have been developed include chemical manufacturing plants (which emit as many as 150 of the 189 hazardous air toxics), coke oven batteries, dry cleaning facilities, ethylene oxide sterilization facilities, industrial cooling towers, and chromium electroplating operations.

Further Reading

Costa, D. L., and Amdur, M. O. (1996). Air pollutants. In *Casarett and Doull's Toxicology: The Basic Science of Poisons* (K. Klaassen, Ed.), pp. 857–882. Pergamon, Elmsford, NY.

Lippmann, M. (1993). Health effects of tropospheric ozone: Review of recent research findings and their implications to ambient air quality standards. *J. Expos. Anal. Environ. Epid.* 3, 103–129.

National Institute of Environmental Health Sciences (NIEHS) (1989). *Environmental Health Perspectives. Acid Aerosols,* Vol. 79, DHHS No. (NIH) 89-218. NIEHS, Washington, DC.

U.S. Environmental Protection Agency (1993). *National Air Quality and Emissions Trends Report,* EPA 454/R-93-031. U.S. EPA, Research Triangle Park, NC.

U.S. EPA. Air quality criteria documents for: (1) Ozone and related photochemical oxidants; (2) Particulate matter; (3) Lead; (4) Nitrogen oxides; (5) Sulfur oxides; and (6) Carbon monoxide. U.S. EPA, Research Triangle Park, NC.

World Health Organization and United Nations Environment Program (1992). *Urban Air Pollution in Megacities of the World.* Blackwell, Oxford, UK.

—Terry Gordon

Related Topics

Clean Air Act
Combustion Toxicology
Ecological Toxicology
Environmental Toxicology
Indoor Air Pollution
Photochemical Oxidants
Pollution, Water
Pollution, Soil
Respiratory Tract

Pollution Prevention Act

- AGENCY: U.S. EPA
- YEAR PASSED: 1990
- GROUPS REGULATED: Industrial manufacturers

Synopsis of Law

Rather than continue to spend millions of dollars annually to control the millions of tons of pollution each year, Congress decided to encourage industry to reduce source pollution through cost-effective changes in production, operation, and use of raw materials. Not only would these actions prevent pollution but they could also reduce the amount of raw materials used, limit liabilities of compliant industries, and reduce risks to workers as well as to the environment.

Prior to passage of the Pollution Prevention Act (PPA), control efforts within industry were reactive, focusing on treatment and disposal of waste. The act proposed a front-end approach to pollution control, reducing the amount of materials entering the production process. It also suggested technical support to business in order to adapt to source reduction praxis. The policy states,

> The Congress hereby declares it is to be the national policy of the United States that pollution should be prevented or reduced at the source whenever feasible; pollution that cannot be prevented should be recycled in an environmentally safe manner, whenever feasible; and disposal or other release into the environment

should be employed only as a last resort and should be conducted in an environmentally safe manner.

Under the PPA, U.S. EPA established an office responsible for creating standards to measure source reduction, ensuring that U.S. EPA policy is consistent with this initiative, and providing the public with such information. The act also established a Source Reduction Clearinghouse to promote industry efforts by providing information and workshops, helping set measurable goals, and establishing incentive and reward systems for efforts or innovations. Incentive systems included matching grants to states to establish their own source reduction programs.

PPA also included specific source reduction actions in conjunction with the businesses required to file an annual toxic chemical release form under the Superfund Amendments Reauthorization Act. The additional toxic chemical source reduction and recycling report documents the amount of the chemical entering the waste stream, the amount that is recycled, and efforts to reduce source use. In turn, U.S. EPA is required to report to Congress every 2 years with a detailed evaluation report of the source reduction program.

—Jayne E. Ash and Shayne C. Gad

Related Topics

Clean Air Act
Clean Water Act
Comprehensive Environmental Response, Compensation, and Liability Act
National Environmental Policy Act
Toxic Substances Control Act

Pollution, Soil

Introduction

Soil is the thin outer zone of the earth's crust that supports rooted plants and is the product of climate and living organisms acting on rock. A true soil is a mixture of air, water, mineral, and organic components. The relative mix of these components determines both the value of the soil for agricultural and other human uses. This relative mix also determines to a large extent how a chemical added to soil will be transported and/or transformed within the soil. Soils are characteristically heterogeneous. A trench dug into the soil zone typically reveals several horizontal layers having different colors and textures. These multiple layers are often divided into three major horizons: (1) the A horizon, which encompasses the root zone and contains a high concentration of organic matter; (2) the B horizon, which is unsaturated, is below the roots of most plants, and contains a much lower organic carbon content; and (3) the C horizon, which is the unsaturated zone of weathered parent rock consisting of bedrock, alluvial material, glacial material, and/or soil of an earlier geological period.

Soils are composed of three major phases—gases, liquids, and solids. The fraction by volume of soil that is gas varies with soil type and decreases with depth. The volume fraction of soil that is gas varies from a value of 10%, typical in clay soils, to 25%, typical in sandy soils. The soil solution is mostly water but includes dissolved minerals and nutrients. The volume fraction of soil that is liquid ranges from 10%, typical for sandy soils, to 40%, typical for clay soils. The solid phase makes up from 50 to 80% by volume of the soil composition and from 75 to 90% by mass of the soil. Soil solids include mineral (i.e. the parent rock) and organic components, including humic acids and decaying matter. The mineral component of soil is in the range of 70–90% by mass. The organic phase of soil is defined by the organic-carbon content of the soil. The organic-carbon content of soil ranges from much less than 1% by mass for desert and/or sandy soils to as much as 5% by mass for clay soils and even as high as 10% by mass for peat bogs.

Soils exist where the atmosphere, the hydrosphere, the geosphere, and the biosphere all converge. Thus, contaminants in soil can impact human health and the environment through a complex web of interactions. The following sections provide an introduction to three issues related to toxicology and soil: (1) the potential for soil contamination by chemical, biological, and radioactive contaminants; (2) the potential fate, including both transport and transformation processes, for contaminants in soil; and (3) the types of direct and indirect human and animal contacts with soil contaminants that can result in risks to human and ecological health.

Soil Contamination

Throughout the world, soils are contaminated to some extent from local, regional, and global pollution sources. Frequently, this contamination is the result of human and natural activities that lead to the direct application of contaminants to soil. However, soil contamination also results from the transfer by rain and dry deposition of contaminants from air; by the transfer of contaminants through the use of contaminated water for irrigating farms, gardens, or lawns; or by the soil itself through natural physical or biological agents that provide a source of contamination. Metal species and radionuclides released from combustion processes or from volcanoes and persistent organochlorine compounds are agents that can be carried globally in the atmosphere and result in low levels of soil contamination as a result of deposition from the atmosphere. Pesticide use and the disposal of radioactive, biological, and chemical wastes can lead to much higher but localized levels of soil contamination. Some sources of contamination, such local high concentrations of toxic elements, the natural production of radon in soils, and the replication of toxic organisms are not external but internal to the soil. In the following sections, sources of soil contamination are identified and discussed.

Direct Application of Contaminants to Soil

Direct releases to soil occur in the form of pesticide, herbicide, and fertilizer applications; burial or land farming of domestic and industrial wastes; applications of sewer sludge to agricultural lands; and chronic releases from motor vehicles, resulting from the wear of brakes and tires as well as oil leaks. In addition, accidental discharges to the soil from storage tanks and miscellaneous spills during the transport of toxic substances can also occur. Contaminant releases to soil are normally quantified in terms of mass per unit area per unit time. For example, pesticide applications to agricultural fields can range from under 1 kg/ha to over 20 kg/ha per year.

Deposition from the Atmosphere

Contaminants in the atmosphere can be transferred to soil either directly through dry deposition, wet deposition, and vapor partitioning or indirectly through deposition to plants, whose parts fall onto the soil. Dry deposition is the process by which particulate matter settles out of the atmosphere and onto soil and plant surfaces. Contaminants that are attached to these particles will be transferred to soil through this deposition process. Atmospheric contaminants on particles are also washed out of the air to soil with rain or snow in the wet deposition of the particles. Contaminants dissolved in the gas phase of air and not bound to particles can also be transferred to soil through a combination of wet deposition and chemical partitioning. Contaminants dissolved in air that are water soluble are easily washed out during rain and snow. This is wet deposition of a gas phase. In addition, contaminants that are water soluble can be transferred from air to soil through partitioning, which involves the diffusing of chemical from solution in air to solution in the soil water. Similarly, contaminants that are relatively insoluble in water but highly lipid soluble can be carried from air to soil through partitioning into the organic phases of soil. In this process, the contaminants diffuse from solution in air to solution in the organic phase of soil. Finally, contaminants in air can be transferred from air to vegetation surfaces by dry deposition, wet deposition, and by partitioning into the lipid and water phases of plants. When the plants decay, lose leaves, or are mowed; residual contamination is transferred to soil.

Use of Contaminated Water for Irrigation

The use of contaminated water supplies to irrigate farmlands, gardens, and lawns can result in the accumulation of persistent compounds in the irrigated soil. Organic contaminants with low water solubility, when introduced to the soil, will migrate to the organic carbon phase of the soil where they can be retained for relatively long periods. Some metal species can also accumulate and persist in soil if their soil chemistry favors the binding of these contaminants into the mineral phase.

Contaminant Sources Internal to the Soil

In some cases the source of soil contamination is the soil itself. For example, soils rich in toxic elements (e.g., arsenic, lead, mercury, and cadmium) provide their own source of contamination. In addition, soils rich in uranium and its radioactive decay product radium provide continuous long-term sources of the radioactive gas radon in soil. The radon can diffuse from soil into the air of buildings or into groundwater, with resulting radiation exposures to human and animal populations. Other possible sources of contamination internal to soil itself are biological organisms, which are either themselves health threatening or produce toxic chemicals.

TABLE P-9
Processes by Which Contaminants Are Transferred to and from Soils

Gains	*Losses*
Diffusion from air	Diffusion to air
Diffusion from root-zone soil	Diffusion to root-zone soil
Washout from air by rainfall	Advection to root-zone soil
Dry deposition of air particles	Soil solution runoff
Contaminant sources	Erosion (mineral runoff) to surface water
	Resuspension of soil particles
	Chemical/physical transformation

Transport and Transformation of Soil Contaminants

There are a number of competing processes that impact the fate of a contaminant found in soils. When a contaminant is added to or formed in a soil column, there are a number of mechanisms by which it can be transported out of the soil column to other parts of the environment or be transformed into some other chemical species. Therefore, once a contaminant has been identified in the soil column, one must also determine whether that substance will (1) remain or accumulate within the soil column; (2) be transported by dispersion or advection within the soil column; (3) be physically, chemically, or biologically transformed within the soil (i.e., by hydrolysis, oxidation, etc.); or (4) be transported to another part of the environment through cross-media transfer (e.g., volatilization, runoff, or groundwater infiltration). The purpose of this section is to provide an overview of the processes by which contaminants are transported in and out of soil layers (Table P-9) and to provide a summary of transformation processes.

Transport Processes in the Soil Column

In order to understand how chemical species are transported in soil, it is important to recognized that the soil column needs to be viewed as having a least three distinct reservoirs for contaminants. These reservoir are (1) the surface-soil layer, (2) the rooting zone, and (3) the deeper unsaturated zone. The nature of these soil components is described in the following sections.

The Ground-Surface-Soil Compartment

Studies of radioactive fallout in agricultural land-management units reveal that, in the absence of tilling, particles deposited from the atmosphere accumulate in and are resuspended from a thin ground- or surface-soil layer with a thickness in the range 0.1–1 cm. The ground-surface-soil layer is at the top of the A soil horizon. The ground-surface-soil layer has a lower water content and higher gas content than underlying layers. Contaminants in this surface-soil layer are more likely than deeper soil contaminants to be transported horizontally by mechanical runoff and soil-solution runoff to nearby surface waters. Surface-soil contaminants are susceptible to wind erosion, volatilization, photolysis, biodegradation, and transfer to plant surfaces by rainsplash. In contrast to contaminants in deeper soil, surface-soil contaminants are susceptible to chemical transformation by photolysis. Surface-soil contaminants are transferred to and from air by diffusion and resuspension/deposition and transferred to and from the rooting-zone soil by diffusion and leaching.

The Rooting-Zone Soil

Root-zone soil includes the A horizon below the surface layer. The roots of most plants are confined within the first meter of soil depth. In agricultural lands, the depth of plowing is 15–25 cm. In addition, the diffusion depth, which is the depth below which a contaminant is unlikely to escape by diffusion, is on the order of a meter or less for all but the most volatile contaminants. Soil-water content in the root zone is somewhat higher than that in surface soils. The presence of clay in this layer serves to retain water. Contaminants in root-zone soil are transported upward by diffusion, volatilization, root uptake, and capillary motion of water; transported downward by diffusion and leaching; and transformed chemically primarily by biodegradation or hydrolysis.

The Deeper Unsaturated Soil

The deeper unsaturated soil includes the soil layers below both the root zone and above the saturated zone, where all pore spaces are filled with water. This compartment can encompass both the B and the C soil horizons. The soil in this layer typically has a lower organic carbon content and lower porosity than the root-zone soil. Contaminants in this layer move downward to the groundwater zone primarily by capillary motion of water and leaching. Chemical transformation in this layer is primarily by biodegradation.

Transformation

The transformation of toxic substances in soil can have a profound effect on their potential for human exposure and accumulation by biota. Transformation processes in soil include physical processes such as radioactive decay; chemical processes such as photolysis, hydrolysis, and oxidation/reduction; and biological processes such as microbial transformations. All of these processes can significantly reduce the concentration of a substance or alter its structure in such a way as to enhance or diminish its toxicity.

Radioactive Decay

Radioactive elements are made up of atoms whose nuclei are unstable and give off atomic radiation as part of a process of attaining stability. The emission of radiation transforms radioactive atoms into another chemical element, which may be stable or may be radioactive such that it undergoes further decay.

Photolysis

Most organic contaminants are capable of undergoing photolytic decomposition. Such decompositions can be partial, resulting in the formation of stable by-products, or complete, resulting in the destruction of the compound. Although solar radiation at the earth's surface is attenuated by the atmosphere, it is generally sufficient to break bonds in many compounds. In soils, phototransformation impacts only those contaminants on the soil surface. However, in agricultural lands that are tilled, contaminants in the tilling horizon (approximately 20 cm) can be brought to the surface where phototransformation occurs. Phototransformations can result in relatively short half-lives (e.g., hours to days) for contaminants such as pesticides that are applied directly to crops or surface soils. Photolytic breakdown of pesticides can substantially reduce the concentrations of chemicals that are applied to crops and thereby diminish potential exposures to humans and animals that consume the crops.

Hydrolysis

Hydrolytic transformation of organic chemicals can be a significant destructive process for toxic compounds that are present in the aqueous phase of soils. Hydrolysis is most important for chemicals that have functional groups (e.g., amides, esters, carbamates, and organophosphates) that can be rapidly altered (e.g., minutes to days) in the presence of water. For amides and carbamates, hydrolytic cleavage yields aromatic and aliphatic amines with increased likelihood of toxic activity. Conversely, hydrolytic degradation of compounds that contain stable substituents (e.g., halogenated compounds such as carbon tetrachloride) can have half-lives of several thousand years. Because hydrolytic reactions are driven by the availability of hydrogen and hydroxide ions, the pH of the soil can have a dramatic influence on the rate of hydrolysis for any given compound. Hydrolytic transformations that are relatively slow at neutral pH can occur at rates that are several orders of magnitude greater under acidic or basic conditions.

Oxidation and Reduction

Many inorganic and organic chemicals can undergo oxidation or reduction reactions in soil. An indicator of a compound's ability to be oxidized or reduced is provided by a knowledge of its oxidation potential, which is the voltage at which it is transformed to its reduced state. A similar measure of a soil's ability to reduce a compound is provided by the redox potential, which is a measure of electron activity. Redox potentials are relatively high and positive in oxidized environments (e.g., surface waters) and low and negative in reduced environments (e.g., aquatic sediments and the subsurface soil layers). These environmental conditions are especially important for inorganic chemicals that are rarely present in their elemental form in the environment. Arsenic, for example, exists primarily in its oxidized form (arsenate) in the atmosphere and in surface waters and in its reduced form (arsenite) in sediments.

Microbial Transformation

Due to their broad range of enzymatic capabilities, microorganisms are capable of transforming many inorganic and organic compounds. Such transformations can result in the partial degradation of a compound (e.g., conversion of trinitrotoluene to dinitrotoluene), mineralization (i.e., complete transformation to carbon dioxide and water), or synthesis of a stable product (e.g., formation of methyl arsenicals from arsenate). While these processes generally result in the detoxification of the parent compound, toxic products may also be formed. For example, the microbial metabolism of aromatic amines can result in the formation of toxic byproducts.

Human Contact with Soil

Human contacts with soil can be multiple and complex. Table P-10 lists a matrix of potential human contacts with soils than can result in human uptake of soil contaminants through inhalation, ingestion, and dermal exposure routes. In the following sections, we consider what is known about some of these exposure pathways and how they might be assessed in a risk assessment or other health-effects study.

Direct Soil Ingestion

Both adults and children continuously ingest small amounts of soil through inadvertent hand-to-mouth activities. Children who spend a great deal of time outdoors have been observed to contact and ingest soil. Through activities such as gardening, outdoor labor, and cleaning, adults are also subject to inadvertent soil. ingestion. Some individuals have been observed to intentionally ingest rather large quantities of soil. The ingestion of nonfood substances such as soil is called pica. Geophagia is the intentional, chronic, and often addictive consumption of earth.

Several studies have been conducted to characterize soil ingestion by children. Some studies make use of measurements of soil levels on children's hands in combination with observations of hand-to-mouth activity to estimate soil uptake. Another approach to soil ingestion measurement makes use of tracer elements in feces. Both feces of children and soil in their play yard are analyzed for elements such as aluminum, silicon, and titanium—elements thought to be poorly absorbed in the gut. Assuming no non-soil sources of these elements, and based on fecal excretion rates, soil ingestion for each child is estimated on the basis of the mass of each tracer element in feces relative to that in soil. Hospitalized children who have little contact with soil are often used as control groups.

Transfer of Soil Contaminants to Vegetation and Food Products

Soil contaminants in both the rooting zone and the surface-soil layer can be transferred to edible parts of vegetation by a number of processes. Contaminants in the rooting zone are transferred to plants through root uptake. The partitioning of contaminants between soil and root tends to increase with increasing contaminant concentration since the root membrane on most plants

TABLE P-10
Matrix of Exposure Pathways That Link Humans with Contaminated Soils through Direct and Indirect Contact

Exposure route	*Exposure pathways linking contaminated soil with human contact*
Ingestion	Direct soil ingestion by humans
	Ingestion of fruits, vegetables, and grains contaminated by transfer from soil
	Ingestion of meat, milk, and eggs contaminated by transfer from soil to plants to animals
	Ingestion of meat, milk, and eggs contaminated through soil ingestion by animals
	Ingestion of groundwater contaminated by soil
Inhalation	Inhalation of soil vapors that migrate to indoor air
	Inhalation of soil particles transferred to indoor air
Dermal contact	Dermal contact with soil

restricts uptake to dissolved species. Contaminants in the rooting zone can be transferred to surface soil by plowing and tilling or by the activities of burrowing animals such as worms, ants, and rodents. Contaminants in surface soil can be transferred to edible plant parts through resuspension/deposition, rainsplash, and volatilization/partitioning. Resuspension/deposition is the process in which soil particles are blown by the wind up from the soil surface and then fall back onto the leaves of vegetation where the soil contaminants can be retained for some time on the leaf surfaces or absorbed by the plant into the leaf tissues and possibly transported to other parts of the plant. Rainsplash is a process in which the impact of falling raindrops onto the soil surface causes soil particles to be scattered into the air with impact onto plant surfaces. Volatilization/partitioning is a two-step process in which contaminants with a sufficiently high vapor pressure volatilize from the soil and then collect in the waxy surface or the water portion of leaves through a air/lipid or air/water exchange.

Contaminants in vegetation can be transferred to food products that are derived from the vegetation. The level of contamination of vegetative food products often depends on which part of a plant is being consumed. Translocation, which is the process by which a contaminant is transferred from one part of a plant to another, can result in significant differences in contaminant concentration between the total plant and the part of the plant being consumed, i.e., the fruit or seeds. In addition, ingestion of contaminated soil and the ingestion of soil-contaminated pasture or grains by food-producing animals can lead to the contamination of animal-based food products— that is, meat, milk, dairy products, and eggs.

Dermal Contact with Soil

Dermal exposure to contaminants in soil can occur during a variety of activities, such as construction work, gardening, and recreation outdoors. Adults who work outdoors in activities such as construction, farming, or gardening can have rather high soil loadings on their skin. Children playing outdoors also can have rather large soil loadings on their skin. Lipid-soluble chemicals have a strong tendency to move from a soil layer on the skin surface to the lipid-rich outer layer of human skin. However, the rate at which this transfer takes place is often very slow and could require hours or even days to reach an equilibrium state. Estimating doses that result from contact with a contaminated soil involves a number of difficult to measure parameters, including the contaminant concentration in soil, the soil-to-skin adherence factor, the chemical-specific absorption factor for the skin–soil system, the exposure frequency, and the exposure time. The exposure frequency expresses how often, i.e., days per year, an individual is involved in an activity that results in soil contact. The exposure time is a measure of how long, in hours, the soil is in contact with skin during an exposure activity.

Dose estimates for soil contact include a great deal of uncertainty. This uncertainty arises because we must deal with the transport of chemicals within the skin layer; the interaction of the soil layer on the skin with the skin surface; the dynamic conditions always involved in scenarios addressing interaction of the skin surface with chemicals, soil, air, and water; and addressing the level of protection provided by clothing.

Inhalation of Soil Particles Suspended as Dust

Soil contaminants that are bound to soil particles can be resuspended and inhaled along with the fine particles to which these contaminants are attached. The inhalation of suspended particles can take place both outdoors and inside buildings. In recent years there has been a recognition that fine and coarse particles in the indoor environment are attributable to both air and soil sources and enter the indoor environment by processes such as resuspension, deposition, and soil tracking. Soil tracking is the process by which soil particles are carried into the indoor environment by shoes and clothing of human occupants as well as on the feet and fur of pets.

Contaminant Vapor Transport into Buildings

The vapors of volatile contaminants, such as radon and volatile organic compounds, can be transport through diffusion from the soil pore spaces into buildings. Three principal factors are needed to define the ratio of contaminant concentration in indoor air to observed contaminant concentration in soil gas. These are (1) the distance between the contaminant source and the building foundation, (2) the permeability of the soil, and (3) the area of cracks in the foundation relative to the total area of the foundation.

Groundwater Contamination

Soil contaminants can be transformed by physical, chemical, and/or biological processes. Those that are not transformed can be carried to groundwater in areas of net recharge. Once contaminants move from soil into groundwater these contaminants can contact humans through a number of exposure pathways, such as direct water ingestion, dermal uptake in showers/baths, irrigation of crops, and the feeding of food-producing animals.

Summary

The purpose of this entry is to consider the nature of soils, how soils are contaminated by human activities, how these contaminants are transported and transformed in the soil column, and the types of human activities that could result in human exposure to soil contaminants. Soils are complex systems that exist at the interface among atmosphere, biosphere, hydrosphere, and lithosphere. A true soil includes gas, water, mineral, and organic components. Potential human contacts with soil can result in inhalation, ingestion, and dermal uptake of soil contaminants through both direct and indirect exposure pathways. The magnitude and persistence of exposure depends not only on the level of soil contamination but also on the physical and chemical properties of soil, the chemical properties of the contaminant, and the frequency and duration of human activities such as occupational and recreational activities or use of homegrown food, which result in direct and indirect soil contact. Toxicologists should be aware of the complex nature of soils, of the potential of soil contamination, and of types of direct and indirect contacts that human populations have with soil.

Further Reading

Allen, D. T., Cohen, Y., and Kaplan, I. R. (Eds.) (1989). *Intermedia Pollutant Transport: Modeling and Field Measurements*. Plenum, New York.

Bodek, I., Lyman, W. J., Reehl, W. F., and Rosenblatt, D. H. (1988). *Environmental Inorganic Chemistry Properties, Processes and Estimation Methods*. Pergamon, New York.

McKone, T. E., and Daniels, J. I. (1991). Estimating human exposure through multiple pathways from air, water, and soil. *Regul. Toxicol. Pharmacol.* **13**, 36–61.

National Research Council (1991). *Frontiers in Assessing Human Exposure to Environmental Toxicants*. National Academy Press, Washington, DC.

Paustenbach, D. J., Shu, H. P., and Murray, F. J. (1986). A critical examination of assumptions used in risk assessments of dioxin contaminated soil. *Regul. Toxicol. Pharmacol.* **6**, 284–307.

Thibodeaux, L. J. (1979). *Chemodynamics, Environmental Movement of Chemicals in Air, Water, and Soil*. Wiley, New York.

U.S. Environmental Protection Agency (1989). *Risk Assessment Guidance for Superfund. Volume I: Human Health Evaluation Manual (Part A)*, EPA/540/1-89/002. Office of Emergency and Remedial Response, Washington, DC.

Wauchope, R. D. (1978). The pesticide content of surface water draining from agricultural fields—A review. *J. Environ. Qual.* 7, 459–472.

—Thomas E. McKone

Related Topics

Carbamate Pesticides
Ecological Toxicology
Environmental Toxicology
Organochlorine
Organophosphates
Pesticides
Pollution, Air
Pollution, Water

Pollution, Water

Water is a major transporter of toxic chemicals in the environment. Our view of the hazards associated with water pollution varies considerably depending on how the water is to be used. Chemicals in water used for drinking or bathing result in direct exposure to humans and, if doses of chemical derived from these activities are sufficiently high, these exposures can lead to toxic effects. However, chemicals introduced into streams and lakes frequently result in exposures by less direct means, for example, by eating fish obtained from these waters. The nature of chemicals that are involved in exposure via drinking water and that of chemicals involved in exposure through food derived from contaminated water are frequently quite different. Generally, chemicals that are found in drinking water tend to have significant water solubility and low affinities for clay and organic matter found in soils. Those chemicals that are obtained in food derived from water are generally much less soluble in water and have very high solubility in fats. These properties account for their accumulation in fish tissues. Many of the chemicals which bioaccumulate are also poorly degraded in the environment. This further contributes to their accumulation. In many cases the impact of these latter chemicals on wildlife is more important than their effects on human health.

Chemicals are introduced into water in a variety of ways. In the past, the focus has been on industrial pollution. When industrial outfalls into bodies of water were less well controlled than they generally are today, these point sources were important. While it is important to recognize that point sources of chemicals can still be responsible for local problems in water quality, nonpoint sources of water pollution contribute much more to chemical contamination of water on a national basis. Chemical contamination of groundwater has occurred as the result of poor chemical disposal practices in the past. The types of chemicals that occur in these groundwaters are chemicals that are very mobile in soils. As with other point sources, the impact of these sites is local rather than national in scope. However, cleanup of groundwater is technically very difficult and expensive. Therefore, every effort must be made to prevent this type of contamination. While the actual impact on water used for drinking is apparently small when considered on a national basis compared to other types of water pollution, the problem of uncontrolled hazardous waste sites does occur in all regions of the country and produces a great deal of public concern. Non-point sources would include chemicals used in agriculture, such as fertilizers and various pesticides; fallout from products of incomplete combustion, such as the automobile; and chemicals that are washed into streams, rivers, and lakes by runoff of urban areas. Thus, the types and numbers of chemicals that can contaminate water from these sources are practically endless.

Chemicals are also deliberately added to water. In the treatment of wastewater, and more particularly in the treatment of drinking water, a variety of chemicals are added for purposes of disinfecting, clarifying, and preventing corrosion of pipes. Moreover, as water is distributed to consumers, the surfaces it contacts have the potential of contaminating the water. These surfaces may be the water mains and pipes in a municipal distribution system, or they may be the surface of a plastic bottle in which the water is purchased in a supermarket.

Because of the complex sources of chemicals in water, contaminants of water will be discussed as they are introduced into water; those introduced into ambient water, chemicals introduced during the treatment of water, and contaminants associated with the distribution of water.

Contaminants of Ambient Water

Natural Contaminants

It is important to recognize that the bulk of the chemicals found in water are of natural origin. Many of these chemicals are innocuous at even the highest concentrations that might be found in fresh water. Some are essential minerals and metals that are important to normal physiology of the body. These would include sodium, chloride, magnesium, calcium, bicarbonate, carbonate, sulfate, and iron. Occasionally, these materials are present at concentrations that will cause gastrointestinal disturbances (e.g. diarrhea induced by sulfates and nausea and vomiting due to copper).

Occasionally, water will come into contact with natural deposits of potentially hazardous chemicals. A relatively frequent contaminant of groundwaters in the western United States is arsenic. Usually the concentrations are below 100 μg/liter, but there are concerns that such concentrations may represent a cancer hazard. At higher doses, of course, arsenic is clearly toxic to a variety of organ systems. Less frequently, river water may erode deposits of asbestos. While asbestos is recognized as being carcinogenic when it is inhaled, there has been no convincing evidence that ingested asbestos presents such a hazard. This may be partially due to the small size of the asbestos fibers that are found in water. Fibers in excess of 5 μm appear to be most dangerous.

Surface waters (i.e., streams and lakes) or groundwater influenced by surface water also contain a complex mixture of organic chemicals. These may range from a fraction of a mg/liter up to 10's of mg/liter. Some of these chemicals are simple sugars, amino acids, and low-molecular-weight organic acids that are normal biological substrates. The bulk of these organic compounds, however, are humic substances. Humic substances consist of humic and fulvic acids which are polymers of small-molecular-weight products of biological decay that form over time. The size of the humic acid molecules can be quite large and they can involve very complex and individual structures. Fulvic acids are significantly smaller and tend to be more soluble. The properties of these substances vary considerably in different climates. They are responsible for the dark color seen in many standing waters. In themselves, these chemicals do not pose health hazards. However, they do serve as substrates for reactions with various oxidant chemicals used in the treatment of drinking water.

Agricultural Chemicals

Agricultural chemicals have a high probability of affecting water supplies if they have a significant water solubility, are not rapidly degraded, and have a low affinity for soils. Fortunately, most chemicals currently used in agriculture do not fit this category. However, the large volume used of certain chemicals that are mobile in soils does result in adverse impacts on both surface water and groundwater. The most widespread example of this is nitrates derived from the use of fertilizers. The concentrations of nitrate in surface waters frequently exceed drinking water standards during certain times of the year. A more pervasive problem, however, is the relatively widespread contamination of groundwaters by nitrate. These concentrations will remain high for years to come, even if practices introducing them into the groundwaters were stopped today.

Much of the public fear of agricultural products focuses on the use of various pesticides. Many of these compounds are highly toxic. Fortunately, those which are the most toxic and likely to contaminate water, the organophosphorus pesticides, are generally degraded in water. These chemicals would include parathion, methyl parathion, terbufos, and malathion. These chemicals have been found in water, but generally at low concentrations. On the other end of the spectra are the very water-insoluble compounds, such as DDT, chlordane, dieldrin, and lindane, that have high affinity for soils and will be found primarily in particulate matter in water. Paraquat is a very dangerous contact herbicide that appears to be very immobile in soils and has rarely, if ever, been found in ambient waters. Generally, these particulates are removed from water before it is used for human consumption and any chemical remaining in the water is at very low concentrations (<0.01 μg/liter). There are, however, a small number of pesticides, such as aldicarb (Temik) and diazinon, that are very mobile in soils and which can be significant contaminants of water. The other group of chemicals that are of some concern are low-molecular-weight halogenated compounds that are used as soil fumigants. These would include ethylene dibromide, dibromochloropropane, and 1,3-dichloropropene. The former two chemicals' use has recently been banned by the U.S. EPA. Herbicides such as atrazine, butylate, chloramben, DCPA (dacthal), MCPA, dicamba, metolachlor, metribuzin, picloram, prometon, pronamide, propachlor, propazine, simazine, and 2,4,5-T have also been detected in surface water and/or groundwater supplies. The latter compound is no longer in use in the United States because it was contaminated with low levels of a very toxic chemical, 2,3,7,8-tetrachlorodibenzodioxin.

Industrial Chemicals

Industrial contamination of water occurs as the result of directly introducing contaminated wastewaters into a body of water or lake or from improper disposal of chemicals to the land. The chemicals most frequently found in water from both of these activities are chemicals that are used in very high volume. However, the nature of surface water contamination is more likely to depend on the nature of the industry impacting a particular body of water. The soil surrounding a waste site frequently acts as an effective barrier to contamination to many chemicals found in hazardous waste sites.

Probably the most frequent contaminants of water from these two sources are spilled liquid fuels, such as gasoline, kerosene, and diesel oil, and low-molecular-weight solvents such as trichloroethylene, tetrachloroethylene, 1,1,1-trichloroethane (methyl chloroform), benzene, toluene, various xylene isomers, and aliphatic hydrocarbons. Other solvents may also be found in high concentrations in groundwaters where they have been disposed of in large quantities. These would include solvents no longer in common use such carbon tetrachloride or chloroform. The toxicology of these chemicals varies widely. Acutely and at very high doses most solvents depress the central nervous system (CNS). It is very unlikely that such concentrations would be achieved as a result of environmental contamination. Some of these chemicals have a high probability of producing liver or kidney damage as delayed effects or under conditions of more chronic exposure (e.g., carbon tetrachloride, chloroform, 1,1,2,2-tetrachloroethane, and 1,1,2-trichloroethane). Others present a specific hazards of producing delayed and cumulative nervous system deficits (e.g., methyl butyl ketone, *n*-hexane, trichloroethylene, and toluene). Again, these effects may be observed at levels of exposure encountered occupationally but would be rare from generalized environmental contamination. Generally, the major concern of concentrations found in the aquatic environment is with those chemicals that produce cancer (e.g., benzene, vinyl chloride, dichloromethane, trichloroethylene, tetrachloroethylene, and carbon tetrachloride). Among these chemicals, only benzene and vinyl chloride have induced cancer in humans. Estimates of the cancer risks that arise from environmental exposures to these chemicals are quite controversial.

Around military bases and weapons laboratories of the U.S. Department of Energy, there have been frequent incidents of groundwater contamination by explosives, specialized fuels, and radionuclides. Among the explosives identified in these circumstances are trinitrotoluene, HMX, and RDX. Radionuclides would include tritium, plutonium, and technetium.

Chemicals Introduced during Treatment of Drinking Water

Chemicals are used for a variety of purposes in the production of drinking water. Also, chemicals are added to water for a variety of purposes. Reservoirs are frequently treated with herbicides to prevent overgrowth of vegetation. Disinfectants are added as barriers to the spread of waterborne infectious disease. Other oxidants (potassium permanganate and chlorine dioxide) are utilized to remove unwanted color or to remove or prevent formation of chemicals that impart a bad taste or odor to the water. A variety of chemicals are utilized in the clarification of water. Alum and ferric chloride are utilized to aggregate particulate material in the water (i.e., coagulation). A variety of other polymeric chemicals are used to neutralize surface charge that prevents coagulation and settling of particulates and are referred to as coagulant aids. Lime is added to soften water and acids, bases, and buffers are added to adjust the pH and to control corrosion. It is impossible to catalog all the chemicals that are used in the treatment of water. For a more complete list, the interested reader is referred to the NSF International listing of chemicals that meet the NSF standards as drinking water additives (see Further Reading).

Disinfectants

In most of the world, disinfectants are reactive chemicals introduced into water to prevent the spread of waterborne infectious diseases. In situations in which sanitation is poor, the need for disinfection is very obvious. However, the large amounts of water that are needed in metropolitan areas inevitably means that microbial contaminants are introduced into some of the source water. Chemical disinfectants provide an economical and simple technology for controlling these contaminants. On the other hand, disinfectants vary in their toxicological properties. Therefore, it is important to establish that these chemicals can be used safely at effective concentrations. Chlorine presents no specific toxicological problems at effective concentrations. Monochloramine (i.e., chlorine + ammonia) is relatively safe at the concentrations that are used, but it is a much poorer disinfectant than chlorine. Ozone presents no particular toxicological threats because it is not sufficiently stable in water to reach the taps at which the water is consumed. However, this is also a disadvantage because there is no residual disinfectant to prevent outgrowth of microorganisms in the mains, service lines, and pipes that distribute the water. As a consequence, a second disinfectant is usually added after an initial treatment with ozone. Another chemical that has been proposed for use as a disinfectant is chlorine dioxide. This chemical is a very effective disinfectant, but it does produce thyroid disorders in experimental animals. Moreover, it degrades to two chemicals, chlorite and chlorate, that produce hemolytic anemia and methemoglobinemia. While it is probable that chlorine dioxide can be used safely in drinking water disinfection, there is less margin of safety with its use and the concentration needed for disinfection. Moreover, close attention must be paid to the amounts of chlorite and chlorate, which are inevitable by-products of this compound, that are produced in the distribution system and occur at the tap.

In 1974 it was discovered that the use of chlorine in the disinfection of water leads to the formation of a group of compounds referred to as the trihalomethanes. This group of compounds includes chloroform, bromodichloromethane, dibromochloromethane, and bromoform. The relative concentrations of the members of this class depend on the concentration of bromide in the water being disinfected. In recent studies, it has become clear that the trihalomethanes are only one class of by-product and that there are small concentrations of a wide variety of chemicals produced with chlorination. However, it should be recognized that all chemical disinfectants are reactive compounds and, as a consequence, all will produce unintended by-products as a result of their use.

Disinfectant by-products are produced by reaction of the disinfectant with other chemicals in the water. The bulk of these chemicals are of natural origin. Humic and fulvic acids are the most common organic chemicals present. These are formed by the natural decay of biological material and are in themselves harmless. As indicated previously, the bromide concentration in the water also influences the type of by-product that is formed. Chlorine and ozone oxidize bromide to hypobromous acid, which acts to add bromine to various chemicals. Under conditions of high pH (alkaline conditions) ozone can further react with hypobromite ion to produce bromate. Differences in pH also affect the levels of other chemicals that are produced. Acid pH results in the formation of a variety of mutagenic chemicals at very low concentrations when chlorine is utilized as the disinfectant, whereas high pH gives rise to higher concentrations of the trihalomethanes.

Epidemiological data suggest that chlorination of drinking water does increase the probability of developing bladder and cancer of the large intestine. The elevation of these cancers above background is relatively small. Consequently, the differences may be caused by other risk factors that were not identified. Animal studies do indicate that some of the chemicals that are produced with chlorination are capable of producing tumors, but the tumors have been more commonly found in the liver and kidney. Moreover, the actual risk predicted from the animal studies is much less than suggested by the epidemiological studies. These differences may indicate that the results of the epidemiology studies were not correct. However, many of the chemicals produced by chlorination have yet to be evaluated in experimental animals. This is a very important question because many of the by-products that have yet to be studied in experimental animals are also produced by other disinfectants such as ozone. The modifications that should be made in the use of disinfectants will not be clear until the toxicological effects of these compounds have been established.

The types of chemicals produced by disinfectants and some specific examples are provided in Table P-11. The reader should not be deceived by the fact that the list of by-products associated with chlorination is much longer than that of other disinfectants. This is the result of more thorough study, not necessarily an actual reflection of the numbers of by-products that are formed by each process.

Other Chemical Treatments of Water

An NSF International publication (NSF Listings, 1994) provides a complete list of products that have been approved for use as direct additives to drinking water by NSF's certification program. The number of specific products used is too large to summarize easily in limited space. Consequently, a partial list of the active ingredients that are representative of products used for specific purposes is provided in Table P-12.

Most chemicals that are direct additives to drinking water present little hazard to health. Many of these chemicals also have been used as food additives and have been subjected to appropriate levels of toxicological testing. Other additives, such as starch, are natural foodstuffs and would be generally regarded as safe, especially at the low concentrations that would be expected to reach the tap.

Polymeric chemicals are a somewhat special case. These are most frequently introduced as direct additives as coagulant aids. By virtue of their function, these polymers are almost quantitatively removed from the water during normal treatment. Even if applied inappropriately, these chemicals are of such high molecular weight that they would not be absorbed and are almost certainly not a threat to health if they have been properly tested. A potential difficulty with these chemicals

TABLE P-11
Classes of Disinfectant By-Products

Disinfectant	Inorganic	Organic: Halogenated	Organic: Nonhalogenated
Chlorine	Chlorate	Trihalomethanes Haloacetates Haloacetonitriles Haloaldehydes Haloketones Halofuranones Chloropicrin	Aldehydes Carboxylic acids
Monochloramine		Cyanogen chloride Others generally thought to be the same as chlorine, but of lower concentration	
Chlorine dioxide	Chlorite Chlorate	Not well characterized	
Ozone	Bromate Hydrogen peroxide	Bromomethanes Bromoacetates Bromoaldehydes Bromoketones Iodinated analogs	Aldehydes Carboxylic acids

TABLE P-12
Chemicals That Are Used as Direct Additives to Drinking Water

Chemical	*Purpose*
Alum (aluminum salts) Iron (iron salts) Cationic polymers Nonionic polymers Anionic polymers Starch	Coagulation and flocculation for removal of particulate
Phosphates Polyphosphates Orthophosphates	Antiscalants, corrosion control, and sequestering agents
Copper salts	Antifouling and algicides
Chlorine Calcium hypochlorite Sodium hypochlorite Ozone Chlorine dioxide Potassium permanganate Hydrogen peroxide	Oxidants (also disinfectants)
Calcium oxide (lime) Calcium hydroxide	Softening and pH adjustment
Potassium hydroxide Sodium hydroxide Hydrochloric acid Sodium bicarbonate	pH adjustment
Sodium flouride	Dietary supplement

is that they may contain varying amounts of the monomers used in their synthesis or other incompletely reacted material of lower molecular weight. Some of the monomeric compounds are quite toxic. Acrylamide is an example of one of these compounds that is neurotoxic, carcinogenic, and a reproductive toxin. Epichlorhydrin, vinyl chloride, and vinylidene chloride are additional examples of these chemicals. For this reason, the amount of unreacted monomer present in the product is closely regulated by certification agencies such as NSF International.

Chemicals Introduced during the Distribution of Water

Water used for human purposes is delivered in a variety of ways. It is placed in a container to be transported or it is forced by gravity into a system of mains, service lines, and pipes to deliver it to individual users. In both cases the water contacts a surface. Water is a very effective solvent and will invariably extract some chemicals from these surfaces. The surfaces that water contacts are metal, plastic, concrete, or a paint or other type of coating that is applied to the surface. In addition to pipes and containers, there are reservoirs and holding tanks in which similar problems are involved.

The chemicals leached from these surfaces depend on the corrosive properties of the particular water as well as the chemical nature of the surface. Hard water tends to deposit a mineral layer on the inside of pipes and on other surfaces that essentially limits the access of water to the surfaces. On the other hand, soft water, particularly at lower pHs, can actively dissolve toxic metals such as lead or cadmium from pipes or solder. Copper in pipes is also frequently leached from pipes at high concentrations when the water has corrosive properties. Asbestos-cement has been used widely in water mains. The extraction of the asbestos fibers from these surfaces is also very much increased at lower pH and with soft water. The use of lead pipe and solder in household pipes has pretty much been abandoned in the United States. However, alloys of lead are still utilized in many faucets and brass fixtures (e.g., submersible pumps). Rather high concentrations of lead can result if water stands in these fixtures overnight. As a result it is always wise to avoid using the water first drawn from the tap in the morning for human consumption. Low levels of lead exposure *in utero* or in the first few years of life have been associated with delayed CNS development in humans and experimental animals.

Plastic pipes are polymeric in nature (e.g., polyvinyl chloride). Within the pipe are traces of the monomers used in the manufacture of the pipe (e.g., vinyl chloride). In addition, there are a variety of other chemicals added during the manufacture of the pipe as lubricants to facilitate their manufacture or stabilizers to prevent the breakdown of the pipe. In Europe, lead has been used as the stabilizer of pipes, whereas various organic tin compounds have been utilized in the United States. Lead is widely recognized as being toxic. Inorganic tin has a very limited toxicity, but this is not the form of tin that is used. Some of the organic tin compounds are potent nervous system toxins (e.g., trimethyl or triethyl tin), while others appear to adversely affect the immune system (dioctyl tin). The forms of tin used in polyvinyl chloride pipe, however, are primarily monomethyl and dimethyl tin, which are much less active as neurotoxins than the trimethyl tin. There will be some extraction of all these chemicals from the pipe when it is first put into service. However, the concentrations that are found in the water decrease sharply with continued use of the pipe. This is only partially due to the depletion of the chemical from the pipe because many waters will form an impermeable barrier (e.g., calcium carbonate) on the interior of the pipe that minimize leaching from its surface.

Paints and coatings can be utilized on any surface in a distribution system all the way to the pipes in the consumer's home. However, most coatings are applied to storage tanks and water mains. In past years some rather dangerous coatings have been used. Coal tar paints were frequently utilized in the first several decades of this century. These paints contain very high concentrations of polycyclic aromatic hydrocarbons (PAHs). Generally this does not pose much of a problem because the solubility of these compounds in water is quite limited. This is particularly true of most of those which are carcinogenic. However, when the coating begins to degrade with age, it tends to come off the surface as small particles. These very small particles can contain very high concentrations of benzo(*a*)pyrene and other PAHs and have been shown to be carcinogenic when introduced into the stomach of mice. Fortunately, the coal tar paints have been largely replaced by asphalt paints which contain very much smaller concentrations of PAHs. However, many distribution systems throughout the country have mains which predate this conversion. Another suspect practice of the past was the use of red lead paint in water tanks. Fortunately, this product has also been abandoned.

Summary

The sources of water pollution are diverse. Some of this pollution occurs in the general environment and involves both point and nonpoint sources. Pollution of this kind can impact human health both directly, when the water is consumed for drinking purposes, and indirectly through accumulation of chemicals in foodstuffs derived from the water. The chemicals seen from these two sources have very different characteristics. Despite the fact that there is contamination of ambient water, most contamination of drinking water by chemicals occurs during its treatment and distribution. While there is no conclusive evidence that these sources of chemicals adversely affect health, it is important to keep this issue in mind in the development of new processes for treating drinking water and new materials for distributing drinking water.

Further Reading

Bull, R. J., and Kopfler, F. C. (1991). *Health Effects of Disinfectants and Disinfection By-Products.* American Water Works Association and AWWA Research Foundation, Denver, CO.

Department of Energy (DOE) (1992). *Chemical Contaminants on DOE Lands and Selection of Contaminant Mixtures for Subsurface Science Research,* DOE/ER-05471. U.S. DOE, Washington, DC.

NSF Listings (1994). *Drinking Water Additives—Health Effects.* NSF International. Ann Arbor, MI.

U.S. EPA (1989). *Drinking Water Health Advisory: Pesticides.* Lewis, Chelsea, MI.

—Richard J. Bull

Related Topics

Bioacummulation
Ecological Toxicology
Effluent Biomonitoring
Environmental Processes
Environmental Toxicology
Organophosphates
Pesticides
Polycyclic Aromatic Hydrocarbons
Polymers
Pollution, Air
Pollution, Soil

Polybrominated Biphenyls

- CAS: 59536-65-1
- Preferred Name: PBBs
- Synonyms: Polybromobiphenyls; Firemaster BP-6; Firemaster FF-1
- Chemical Class: Cyclic halogenated hydrocarbons. PBBs are bromine analogs of polychlorinated biphenyls (PCBs). As such, the toxicological properties of PBBs are essentially indistinguishable from those of structurally related PCBs and dibenzodioxins (see Polychlorinated Biphenyls).
- Chemical Structure:

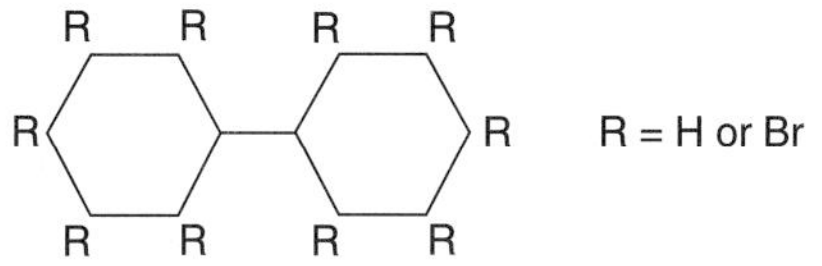

R = H or Br

Uses

PBBs are inert, stable chemicals used as plasticizers and fire retardants for textiles and electronic components. In 1973, in Michigan, PBBs were accidentally mixed in a high-protein supplement for dairy cows. This resulted in widespread contamination of animal feeds, domestic animals, animal products, and eventually humans.

Exposure Pathways

Historically, only workers manufacturing fire retardants were exposed to PBBs. However, following the accidental introduction of PBBs in the domestic animal food chain, humans and animals were extensively exposed to PBBs in their diet.

Toxicokinetics

In rodents, PBB dosing has been found to induce cytochrome P450.

Mechanism of Toxicity

PBBs have two target organs of toxicity: the liver and the skin. Liver damage can range from liver enlargement to scattered necrosis. Liver damage is manifested by its characteristic clinical symptoms that include nausea, vomiting, jaundice, weight loss, edema, and abdominal pain. Skin effects include chloracne, hyperpigmentation of the skin and nails. Neurological effects have also been documented in laboratory animals and are suspected in humans.

Human Toxicity

Epidemiological studies conducted following the Michigan incidence revealed no acute symptoms from the consumption of PBB contaminated food. For long-term exposure the only symptoms that were at least partially attributed to PBB consumption included chloracne, blurred vision, and fatigue. Just like PCBs, PBBs are capable of crossing the placental barrier and concentrate in breast milk. Infants born to and nursing from PBB-exposed mothers may uptake and accumulate PBBs. The half-life for PBBs in humans has been calculated to be 10.8 years.

Clinical Management

There is no specific treatment for PBB toxicity. Only supportive treatment is recommended.

Animal Toxicity

In a dairy cow herd that accidentally consumed Firemaster BP-6 in their diet, feed intake and milk production dropped to about half of normal levels. Initial symptoms noted in the herd included: hematomas, hoof and hair abnormalities, and weight loss. Subsequent experiments in ruminants revealed that approximately 45% of an oral PBB dose is excreted unchanged in the feces 7 days after dosing; 23% was excreted in the milk within 95 days postdosing.

In rodents, oral doses of PBB have been found to cause liver hypertrophy, fatty liver, and scattered necrosis. In addition, neurological effects of PBB poisoning have been demonstrated in rats. Specifically, offspring from rats fed PBBs at a dose of 2 mg/kg during gestation and lactation showed signs of neurological damage and growth retardation.

—Heriberto Robles

Polychlorinated Biphenyls

- CAS: 1336-36-3
- Preferred Name: PCBs
- Synonyms: Arochlor; chlorodiphenyls; clophen; fenchlor; kanechlor; phenochlor; pyralene
- Chemical Structure:

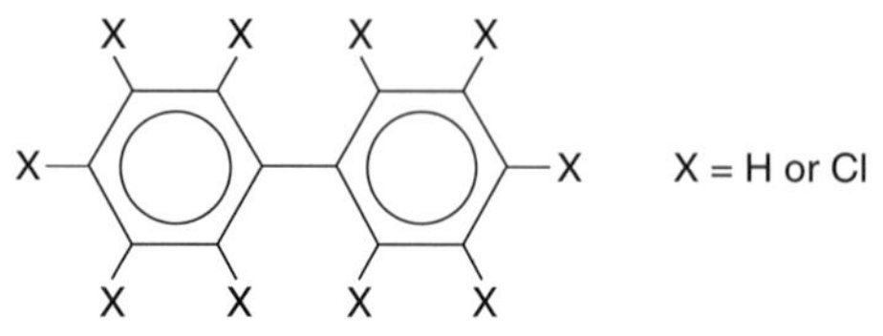

X X X X
X— biphenyl —X   X = H or Cl
X X X X

- Description: Polychlorinated biphenyls (PCBs) are mixtures of different congeners of chlorobiphenyl. The arochlors are characterized by four-digit numbers. The first two digits indicate that the mixture contains biphenyl (12), triphenyls (54), or both (25 and 44); the last two digits give the weight % of chlorine in the mixture. For example, Arochlor 1242 contains biphenyl with approximately 42% chlorine.

  Physical properties vary by product because of the varied composition. For example; Arochlor 1242 is a clear mobile liquid; Arochlor 1254 is a light yellow, viscous liquid, and Arochlor 1260 is a light yellow, soft sticky resin. PCBs are heat stable and resistant to biologic degradation as well as acids, bases, oxidation, and other chemical reactions.

Uses

PCBs were used in electrical capacitors, electrical transformers, vacuum pumps, and gas transmission tribunes. They were also formerly used as hydraulic fluids, plasticisers, adhesives, fire retardants, wax extenders, lubricants and cutting oils, inks, dedusting agents, etc. PCBs are no longer commercially produced in the United States.

Exposure Pathways

Most exposures are environmental or occupational with the delayed symptoms being the first indication that an intoxication has occurred.

Toxicokinetics

PCBs and polybromated biphenyls are absorbed by all routes. Dermal absorption varies depending on the compound, concentration, and species but is in the 15–56% range. PCBs are chemically inert and the more highly chlorinated compounds are resistant to metabolism. The liver is the primary site of metabolism and the primary mechanism is hydroxylation and conjugation with glucuronic acid and is inversely proportional to the chlorine content. PCBs are primarily distributed to the adipose tissues. During pregnancy, one-tenth of the maternal serum level can be found in cord blood and 107–119 times the serum level can be found in human milk. Excretion is variable depending on the species and is inversely related to the chlorine content. PCBs are excreted in breast milk.

Mechanism of Toxicity

The exact mechanism of action by which PCBs cause their toxicity is unclear. They are potent enzyme inducers and affect thiamine utilization.

Human Toxicity

PCBs have a low acute toxicity but they accumulate in the environment and in animal and human tissues; the potential for chronic or delayed toxicity is significant. The most dramatic case of PCB poisoning occurred in West Japan in 1968 (Yusho accident) when rice oil contaminated with PCBs poisoned more than 1600 people. Fatigue, headache, increased sweating of the palms, itching, visual disturbances, numbness of the extremities, subcutaneous facial edema, joint swelling and pain, cough, intermittent abdominal pain, and menstrual changes were noted. However, the symptoms may not be purely due to PCB toxicity since the oil also contained dibenzofurans and quaterphenyls which are known to be toxic. Fifteen cases of reproductive and fetotoxic human effects were observed in the Yusho epidemic. Decreased immunoglobulin levels were observed.

Acute

PCBs are mildly irritating to the eyes and skin. Facial edema, eye discharge, swollen eyelids, conjunctival hyperemia, and visual and hearing disturbances may result. Increases in diastolic and systolic blood pressure are possible. Neurobehavioral and psychomotor impairment have been seen after occupational exposure. Gastrointestinal disturbances and diarrhea have been noted. Clinical hepatitis has been seen in the Yusho epidemic. PCB exposure can cause elevation of serum triglycerides. Chloracne, which may occur from either dermal contact or systemic absorption, is a specific skin reaction associated with cyclic halogenated compounds and is characterized by distinct cystic, skin-colored lesions and comedones, both of which may become inflamed and infected. Edematous swelling of the limbs has been reported. Pruritis was observed in 14% of the exposed persons following exposure to combustion products of PCBs. Small elevation in urinary uroporphyrin levels and decreased coproporphyrin levels in a small number of humans accidentally exposed to PCBs have been reported.

Chronic

Long-term exposure to PCBs may cause embryo toxicity including fetal death, fetal resorption, cleft palate, dilated renal pelvis, and hypoplasia of the thymus. Males may be more susceptible to the teratogenic effects than females. It may cause reproductive and fetotoxic effects. Mammalian reproductive effects include changes in the estrus cycle, implantation failure, increased abortions, low birth-weight offspring, and decreased postnatal survival. PCBs are considered potential human carcinogens. A slight increase in melanoma of the skin in men occupationally exposed to PCBs has been reported. Renal adenocarcinoma in workers chronically exposed to PCBs has occurred.

The ACGIH TLV for chlorodiphenyl (42% chlorine) is 1 mg/m³ TWA. The ACGIH TLV for chlorodiphenyl (54% chlorine) is 0.5 mg/m³ TWA. ACGIH has not established a STEL for chlorodiphenyl.

The OSHA PEL for chlorodiphenyl (42% chlorine) is 1 mg/m³ PEL-TWA, with skin notation. The OSHA PEL for chlorodiphenyl (54% chlorine) is 0.5 mg/m³ PEL-TWA, with skin notation.

Clinical Management

Most exposures are environmental or occupational with the delayed symptoms being the first indication that an intoxication has occurred. There is no specific treatment, only supportive treatment. Emesis is of no use since ingestion of PCBs will not be recognized until long after emesis is of any value. Vomiting may cause aspiration. On ingestion, activated charcoal mixed with a saline cathartic or sorbitol may be used. On ocular exposure, the eyes should be flushed. On dermal exposure, multiple soap and water washings are necessary. On inhalation exposure, emergency airway support and 100% humidified supplemental oxygen with assisted ventilation may be needed. If a cough or difficulty in breathing develops, the victim should be evaluated for respiratory tract irritation, bronchitis, and pneumonitis.

Animal Toxicity

Liver damage is a consistent finding in animal studies. PCBs are carcinogenic in animals causing liver tumors in rats. In laboratory animals exposed orally or cutaneously to sublethal levels of various PCB mixtures, common findings are severe atrophy of 1° and 2° lymphoid organs, lower circulatory immunoglobulin levels, and decreased specific antibody responses following immunization with antigens. Both augmentation and suppression of cell-mediated immunity on exposure to PCBs has been reported.

—Swarupa G. Kulkarni and Harihara M. Mehendale

Related Topics

Bioaccumulation
Bioconcentration
Environmental Hormone Disruptors
Neurotoxicology: Central and Peripheral
Psychological Indices of Toxicity
Skin

Polycyclic Aromatic Amines

- CAS: 153-78-6
- Representative Compound: Fluoren-2-amine
- Synonyms: 2-Aminofluorine; fluorene
- Other Compounds: 3, 3′-Dichlorobenzidine
- Chemical Structure:

NH_2

Uses

Polycyclic aromatic amines occur naturally in coal tar. They are by-products of the coal refining process. They were used in the 1930s as an insecticide.

Exposure Pathways

Dermal contact, ingestion, and inhalation are possible routes of exposure.

Toxicokinetics

Polycyclic aromatic amines are readily absorbed into the body via the gastrointestinal tract, where metabolic activation takes place.

Mechanism of Toxicity

n-Hydroxy metabolites within the gastrointestinal tract transform fluoren-2-amine into a mutagen or carcinogen.

Human Toxicity

Carcinogenic properties are dependent on individual rates of acetylation. Persons who are slow acetylators are more susceptible to cancer, as are workers in industrialized countries. Nutrition is also implicated in the development.

Clinical Management

The victim should be removed from exposure.

Animal Toxicity

Fluoren-2-amine is a teratogen, mutagen, and carcinogen. It is tumorigenic in rats at 2420 mg (TD, oral). The oral LD_{50} in mice is 132 mg/kg.

—Jayne E. Ash and Shayne C. Gad

Polycyclic Aromatic Hydrocarbons

- Representative Compound: Pyrene (CAS: 129-00-0)
- Synonym: Benzo(*def*)phenanthrene
- Other Compounds: Benz(*a*)pyrene; 3-methylcholanthrene (see separate entries for these compounds)
- Chemical Structure:

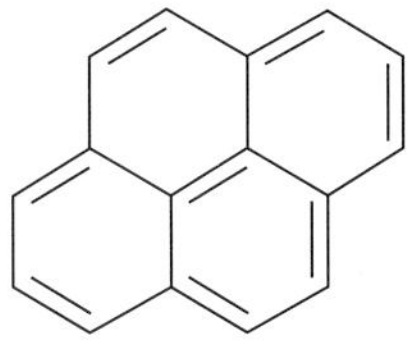

Uses

Pyrene is used in biochemical research. Polycyclic aromatic hydrocarbons occur naturally in coal tar, fossil fuel combustion, and forest fires.

Exposure Pathways

Dermal contact and inhalation are common exposure routes.

Mechanisms of Toxicity

Pyrene increases photosensitivity and suppresses the immune system. P450 metabolism releases carcinogenic and mutagenic potential.

Human Toxicity

Pyrene produces a carcinogenic effect from exposure to skin as well as a presence in bloodstream. It also produces immunodepression. The OSHA PEL for benzo(*a*)pyrene is 0.2 mg/m^3.

Clinical Management

The victim should be removed from exposure. Exposed skin and eyes should be thoroughly flushed with tepid water. Supportive therapy should be provided.

Animal Toxicity

In animals, pyrene is a mild dermal irritant, carcinogen, tumorigen, and primary irritant. The oral LD_{50} is 2.7 g/kg in rats and 800 mg/kg in mice.

—Shayne C. Gad and Jayne E. Ash

Related Topics

Absorption
Carcinogen–DNA Adduct Formation and DNA Repair
Respiratory Tract

Polyethylene Glycol

- Synonyms: α-Hydro-ω-hydroxypoly-(oxy-1,2-ethanediyl); macrogol; PEG; Carbowax; Jeffox; Nycolin; Pluracol E; Poly-G; Polyglycol E; Solbase
- Pharmaceutical Class: A distribution of liquid and solid polymers of varying molecular weights corresponding to an average number of oxyethylene groups

♦ CHEMICAL STRUCTURE:

$H(OCH_2-CH_2)_nOH$ where n = average number of oxyethylene groups

Uses

Polyethylene glycols are widely used in food, cosmetics, and topical pharmaceuticals (e.g., ointments and suppository base).

Exposure Pathways

Ingestion and skin contact are the most common routes of both accidental and intentional exposures.

Toxicokinetics

The absorption of orally administered polyethylene glycols is dependent on their molecular size. While 50–65% of liquid polyethylene glycols (molecular weight up to 600) are absorbed, only from 0 to 2% of solid polyethylene glycols (molecular weight, 1000–8000) are absorbed.

Polyethylene glycols are not appreciably metabolized. Ethylene glycol is not known to be a metabolite. The distribution of the higher members of polyethylene glycols within the body is extracellular, whereas the lower-molecular-weight members of the series diffuse intracellularly to a considerable extent.

Liquid polyethylene glycols are rapidly excreted in the urine, while the higher-molecular-weight members are mainly eliminated in the feces.

Mechanism of Toxicity

Many years of human experience in the workplace and in the use of consumer products containing polyethylene glycols have not shown any adverse health effects, except for administering high doses to sensitive or unhealthy persons. Nephrotoxicity associated with the topical treatment of burn patients with polyethylene glycols may reflect the sensitivity of the patients' kidneys rather than the direct toxic effects of polyethylene glycols.

Human Toxicity: Acute

There have not been any reports of acute toxic or irritative effects in humans exposed to polyethylene glycols. The lowest-molecular-weight members (200–300) have been observed to produce at most only a mild sensitization reaction in a very small percentage of individuals in skin patch testing studies.

Human Toxicity: Chronic

No epidemiological studies or case reports of ill effects in healthy humans attributable to chronic exposure to polyethylene glycols were found in the available literature.

Clinical Management

Animal toxicology and human experience have shown that polyethylene glycols are of very low acute toxicity and nonirritating. Emergency care is not anticipated. There is not a specific antidote for polyethylene glycols. Treatment of overexposure should be directed at the control of symptoms and the clinical condition of the patient.

Animal Toxicity

Polyethylene glycols have a very low level of acute toxicity to animals. They do not produce appreciable irritation to the rabbit skin and are only mildly irritating to the rabbit eyes. Subchronic feeding and drinking water studies in the rat and the dog revealed that polyethylene glycols have very low toxicity. Nephrotoxicity and hepatotoxicity have been observed in the monkey and the dog, respectively, after continuous infusion of high doses of polyethylene glycol. Carcinogenicity studies do not indicate any significant incidence of tumor production.

—Hon-Wing Leung

Polymers

Polymers are macromolecules formed by the chemical bonding of five or more identical units called monomers. In most cases the number of monomers is quite large (3500 for pure cellulose) and often is not precisely known. In synthetic polymers, this number can be controlled to a predetermined extent (e.g., by shortstopping agents). Combinations of two, three, or four monomers are called, respectively, dimers, trimers, and tetramers and are known collectively as oligomers. Such oligomers are not polymers.

A partial list of polymers by type includes the following:

I. Inorganic: siloxane, sulfur chains, black phosphorus, boron-nitrogen, silicones

II. Organic
 1. Natural
  a. Polysaccharides: starch, cellulose, pectin, seaweed gums (e.g., agar), vegetable gums (e.g., arabic)
  b. Polypeptides (proteins): casein, albumin, globulin, keratin, insulin, DNA
  c. Hydrocarbons: rubber and gutta percha (polyisoprene), also called elastomers
 2. Synthetic
  a. Thermoplastic polymers: nylon, polyvinyl chloride, polyethylene (linear), polystyrene, polypropylene, fluorocarbon resins, polyurethane, acrylate resins
  b. Thermosetting polymers: polyethylene (cross-linked) phenolics, alkyds, polyesters
 3. Semisynthetic cellulosics (rayon, methylcellulose, cellulose acetate) and modified starches (e.g., starch acetate)

For most devices, we are concerned only with the synthetic organic polymers. The principal class of natural polymers of concern is the elastomer class. The chief class of inorganic polymers of concern is the silicone class.

Polymers can be categorized in a number of ways. Homopolymers, for example, consist of only one repeating monomer unit. The most commonly encountered homopolymers are listed in Table P-13.

Copolymers are produced by the simultaneous polymerization of two or more dissimilar molecules. Examples include polyvinyl acetate, polyesters, and polyamides. Synthetic elastomers (such as SBR synthetic rubber, made from styrene and butadiene) are also copolymers. This pattern continues with the terpolymers (such as ABS), which consist of three different monomers.

The principal concerns with the biocompatability of polymers are additives, residual monomers, and contaminants that are leachable in the body. As shown in Table P-14, polymers themselves generally have very low toxicities. Partially as a reflection of their high molecular weights, true polymers themselves are not generally absorbed into the body, are not irritating, and are not sensitizers.

TABLE P-13
Commonly Used Homopolymers in Medical Devices

Polyacrylates
Polyamides
Polybutylene
Polychloroprene
Polyethylene
Polypropylene
Polysiloxanes
Polystyrene
Polysulfones
Polytetrafluoroethyene
Polyvinylchloride

Residual monomers, additives, and contaminants are a very different story. Each of these can be quite significant biologically.

Residual monomers are those remaining individual building-block units in homopolymers, copolymers, terpolymers, etc. that are not successfully incorporated into the plastic during the synthesis process. Technically, we should also include dimers, trimers, and other small-chain fragments that are left in the polymer mass but are not chemically bound to it. Many factors help determine how much residual monomer will be left in a polymer and how available such residuals are to a

TABLE P-14
Oral Lethalities of Common Polymers

Polymer	*Rat LD_{50} (g/kg body weight)*
Polyethylene	>8
Polypropylene	>8
Polychloroprene latex	>40
Chlorosulfonated polyethylene	>20
Polyvinyl acetate	>25
Polyacrylonitrile	>3
Polyacrylamide	>8.2
Aromatic polyamides	>7.5

TABLE P-15
Additives Used in Plastics

Plasticizers	UV absorbers
Lubricants	Blowing agents
Antioxidants	Fillers
Colorants	Release agents
Emulsifiers	Flame and fire retardants
Stabilizers	Accelerators
Curing agents	Antistatic agents

surrounding biological matrix. Moreover, some of the monomers are quite active biologically. When we test a plastic for biocompatibility, biologically available (leachable) residual monomers are a significant part of our concern. Examples of toxic monomers (and their principal toxicities) that can be found in polymers include the following:

- Acrylonitrile: human carcinogen (liver, brain)
- Vinyl chloride: human carcinogen (liver)
- Formaldehyde: animal carcinogen (nasal)
- Methylene dinaline: suspect human carcinogen

A wide variety of other chemical entities are specifically incorporated into plastics to achieve desired goals of structure, performance, and processing ease. A short list of the major categories of additives is provided in Table P-15.

Such additives can be quite significant biologically and may be very biologically available. An historical example is diethylhexylphthalate, a once widely used plasticizer that was found both to be an animal carcinogen and to migrate readily from plastic bags and tubing to the blood and intravenous solutions they contained.

The result of the additives and contaminants being in plastic is that a range of toxic materials may be leached from many plastics. A short list of some of the more significant toxic materials is provided in Table P-16.

TABLE P-16
Identified Toxic Materials in Polymers

Aluminum	Ketones and hydrocarbons
Acrylonitrile (monomer)	Lead
Arsenic	Mercaptobenzothiazole
Benzene	Methyl chloride (monomer)
Benzoic peroxide	Methylene chloride
Bisphenol A	Methylene dinaline
Cadmium	Nickel
Carbon tetrachloride	PAHs on carbon black
Dibutyl tin	Pyrene
Epoxy curing agents	Tin
Ethylene dichloride	Tricresyl phosphate
Ethylene oxide	Triphenyl phosphate
Formaldehyde	

Further Reading

Kroschwitz, J. I. (1990). *Concise Encyclopedia of Polymer Science and Engineering.* Wiley, New York.
Shefter, V. O. (1995). *Handbook of Toxic Properties of Monomers and Additives.* CRC Press, Boca Raton, FL.

—Shayne C. Gad

Related Topics

Combustion Toxicology
Pollution, Water

Population Density

The estimation of population densities is a major task in the generation of numerical endpoints in ecological toxicology. The populations of the species that make up a community interact with each other and with the chemical and physical characteristics of the site. When substances are introduced into a site that affect the ability of individuals to reproduce, to grow, and to compete, then there may be shifts in population abundance among the species in a community. Not all population shifts are due to chemical insult—all populations have naturally occurring fluctuations. When one begins to assess the biotic aspect of communities or ecosystems, it appears to be desirable to know which species are present, what is the abundance of each species, and what is the age–class distribution for each species. However, the assessment of the densities of populations (number of individuals per unit area) is a difficult and labor-intensive undertaking. Even the question of which species are present at a specific site can be overwhelming, especially if one wishes to be complete and include bacteria, fungi, algae, protozoans, mosses, invertebrates from nematodes through mollusks to arthropods, vascular plants, and the relatively few species of vertebrates from fish through mammals. The complexities of species identification by themselves have required that taxonomists specialize so that the detailed assessment of the species found at any one site would require engaging the services of many taxonomists. Consequently, surveys of species that are present at a site are biased in part by the available expertise in species identification. Furthermore, the number of species found is strongly influenced by the degree of effort; species with high population numbers are more easily detected than rare species. The physical and behavioral characteristics also exert a strong influence on whether individuals will be detected on a site. For instance, the conspicuous characteristics of a bald eagle result in a high probability of detection, even where it is relatively rare. On the other hand, the tiger salamander likes to hide under moist debris on the forest floor and come out to hunt at night, so the likelihood of detecting a tiger salamander is much lower. These kinds of biases need to be carefully considered, especially when the purpose of the survey is to demonstrate the presence or absence of a species in specific locations.

There are a number of methods for assessing population density, including direct counts, sample counts, and indices and signs of population abundance. The reliability of the information provided by these different methods differs significantly.

The Direct Count or Census

Direct counts are possible when the entire area to be enumerated is circumscribed and it is possible to count all individuals within the circumscribed area. Examples include the number of oak trees in a farmer's wood lot and the number of deer on a small island. As long as the population is enclosed and as long as there is no change in the population number during the count, the accuracy of the count depends solely on the precision of the count. This precision will vary with the counting method (e.g., ground survey vs aerial survey).

Sample Counts

These are counts on sample plots or along transects with defined dimensions. The population densities found on the representative sample areas are then extrapolated to larger areas. Sample plots and transects are particularly useful for the assessment of sessile organisms, such as plants or corrals. The distribution of individuals in an area has significant consequences for the sampling. Individuals may be randomly distributed across the area to be sampled. They may also be clumped (i.e., the individuals have a tendency to cluster because of mutual attraction), or they may be regularly distributed, which tends to occur during competition for territory (see Fig. P-11). The size of the sampling unit (size of the plot or width of the transect) relative to the cluster size will have a significant impact of the observed variability of the sample counts when populations are clumped.

Sample plots are often made with the help of simple shapes, such as circles, triangles, or squares, with known areas that can be conveniently carried into the field. Individuals within the sampling unit are then identified and counted. Transects are usually based on identifying and counting individuals along a strip on either side of a transect line.

$$\hat{D} = \frac{n \cdot CF}{2 \cdot w \cdot l}$$

where:
$\hat{D}$ = number of individuals per unit area
n = number of individuals found along the transect
CF = conversion factor:
if w and l are in feet, CF = 43,560 for acre, and 2.7878288×10^7 for mile^2;
if w and l are in meters, CF = 10,000 for hectare, and 10^6 for km^2;
w = width from centerline to the outer edge of the transect in feet or meters,
l = length of the transect in feet or meters.

where w is the width from centerline to the outer edge of the transect in feet or meters and l is the length of the transect in feet or meters.

There are many instances when one wishes to determine the population density of organisms that move and tend to flee from the observer. A basic assumption for any of these methods is that the individuals of the population are randomly distributed. In practice, animals are most frequently observed as they flee from the observer. This type of problem is complicated by the

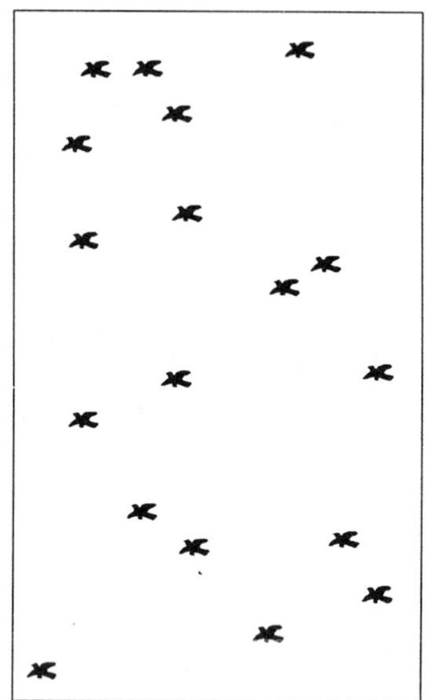
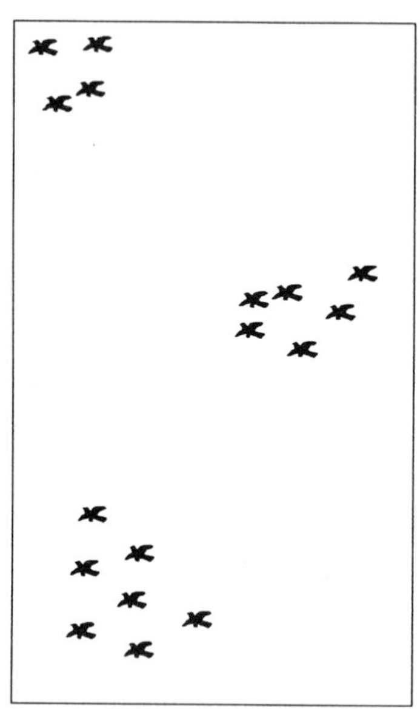
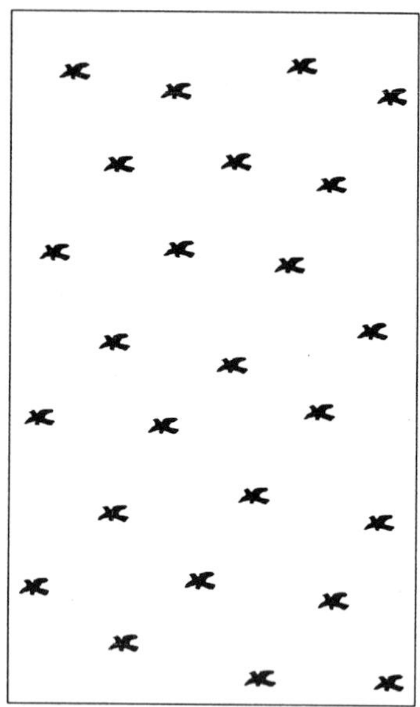

FIGURE P-11. Random, clumped, and regular distribution of individuals in an area.

fact that animals directly in the path of the advancing observer are more likely to flee than those some distance off the path. In addition, the ability to observe also tends to decrease with distance because of natural obstructions. A simple modification of the transect method can partially accommodate this by determining the distance (d) from the observer and the absolute angle (Θ) relative to the transect line where the animal is first observed. The previous equation is modified by using the average fleeing distance perpendicular to the transect line which is $w = d \times \sin\Theta$. However, because the arithmetic average of w falls by definition halfway between the centerline of the transect and the outer edge of the sampled strip, it needs to be modified to:

$$D = \frac{n \times CF}{d \times \sin\Theta \times l}$$

Even this modification can be improved by considering that the probability that an animal will become visible by fleeing is in part dependent on the angle of approach of the observer.

Capture–Recapture Methods

At their simplest, these methods are based on the recapture of previously marked animals and an analysis of their proportion in the population. The method is based on a simple ratio:

$$\frac{N}{M} = \frac{n}{m} \quad \textit{therefore} \quad N = \frac{M \times n}{m}$$

where:
N is the number of individuals in the population,
M is the number of individuals marked and released after initial capture,
n is the total number of animals caught at a subsequent time, and
m is the number of marked animals recaptured.

The method needs to satisfy a number of conditions in order to avoid biases:

1. The marking has no effect on the animal;
2. Marked animals mix completely with the animals that had not been captured.

3. The probability of recapture is the same as the probability of capture of any animal during the second catch effort.
4. The sampling time is discrete.
5. There is no immigration or emigration.
6. There are no births or deaths during the sampling interval.

As long as M and n are approximately equal, then the standard error (SE) can be estimated by

$$S.E. \approx \sqrt{\frac{M^2 \times n\,(n-m)}{m^3}}$$

More complex capture–recapture methods involve successive catch–mark–release operations on the same population in order to improve the robustness of the population estimate from a statistical point of view. However, such repeated trapping operations also increase the likelihood that individual animals become either trap shy or trap happy.

Nearest Neighbor Method

This method derives its population density estimates from measurements of the average distance ($\bar{r}$) between neighboring individuals. This method is very sensitive to the distribution pattern for the population. However, if a sufficient number of measurements of the distances between neighbors ($\bar{r}$) can be made, then it can be determined whether these are normally distributed. Furthermore, if the population density has been determined by an independent method, then the spacing characteristic (λ) can be used to identify distribution characteristics. The basic nearest neighbor relationship is:

$$D = \frac{CF}{\lambda x \bar{r}^2}$$

where:
D = number of individuals per unit area (population density);
CF = conversion factor, as above;
λ = spacing characteristic: $\lambda = 4$ for random spacing, $\lambda = 0.8666$ for uniform hexgonal spacing, $\lambda \gg 4$ for significant clumping;
$\bar{r}$ = average distance between nearest neighbors.

Indices and Signs

Often population densities may be arrived at indirectly through the use of indices. For example, a census of beaver lodges is much more easily accomplished than a direct count of the number of beaver in an area. If the average number of beaver per lodge can be established independently, then it is easy to calculate the estimated beaver population. Similar strategies are possible for muskrat houses and some territorial bird songs. Indices must be used with caution because the indirect approach to population numbers tends to introduce poorly defined biases and errors. Eventually the relationship between indicators of population density and the actual number of individuals becomes too tenuous to allow numerical estimates of population density. However, depending on the specific index used, it may still be possible to establish population trends.

The best established methods for the assessment of population trends are the catch per unit effort (CUE) methods used for the assessment of marine fisheries resources. These trend analyses are based on the use of standardized catching gear used for standardized periods over known locations. The basic assumption is that the catch is related to the population density and to the effort expended in making the catch (Bagenal, 1978). Counts of roadkills have also been used with variable success to establish trends for various mammalian populations. Studies of population trends for insects often employ traps using light, baits, or pheromones as attractants (Southwood, 1978).

It is not necessary that the animals actually be caught. The annual mail carrier pheasant survey along defined rural routes compares annual differences in sightings to gain insight into trends in pheasant populations. The annual Audubon Christmas bird count is also a type of CUE assessment without capture.

Finally, the occurrence of various signs, such as tracks, nests, scats, and evidence of feeding, can be used to establish indications of population density and trends, albeit with a fairly low degree of reliability.

Population Trends Based on Age Structure

The age structure of a population provides some indication of whether the population is increasing, level, or decreasing. This information needs to be used with much caution because the age structure is inherently due to the net reproductive rate, life span, and age-specific death rates; and these factors are due to interactions characteristic of the species and the particular environment. Within these limitations the relative abundance of young animals in relation to older animals provides a clue to the direction of abundance. Within the same species, the proportion of younger organisms in the population tends to be directly related to the rate of increase. Conversely, the population with a greater proportion of aged organisms tends to be decreasing.

Further Reading

Bagenal, T. (1978). *Methods for Assessment of Fish Production in Fresh Waters,* 3rd ed. Blackwell, Oxford, UK.

Bookhout, T. A. (Ed.) (1994). *Research and Management Techniques for Wildlife and Habitats.* The Wildlife Society, Bethesda, MD.

Southwood, T. R. E. (1978). *Ecological Methods,* 2nd ed. Chapman & Hall, London.

—*Rolf Hartung*

Related Topics

Biomarkers, Environmental
Ecological Toxicology
Ecological Toxicology, Experimental Methods
Environmental Processes
Environmental Toxicology
Risk assessment, Ecological

Potassium (K)

- CAS: 7440-09-7
- Selected Compounds: Potassium bromate, $KBrO_3$ (CAS: 7758-01-2); potassium chloride, KCl (CAS: 7447-40-7); potassium permanganate, $KMnO_4$ (CAS: 7722-64-7)
- Chemical Class: Metals

Uses

An essential element for humans, potassium is used in foods and as a salt substitute. It is an essential element for plants as well and is, therefore, a constituent of most fertilizers. Potassium and its compounds are used in specific medicinal preparations and used in cement and glass manufacturing. Potassium bromate is used in hair waving products. Potassium permanganate, a powerful oxidizing agent, is used in the photographic and chemical industries. A dilute solution is used for special dermatological applications.

Exposure Pathways

The primary exposure pathway is through ingestion of food; sources include milk, meat, and a variety of fruits. Many salt substitutes contain potassium chloride.

Toxicokinetics

Potassium salts are more than 90% absorbed, but blood levels are controlled by hemostatic mechanisms. Climate plays a role in potassium blood levels; people in warm climates have approximately 30% more potassium in their blood than people in very cold climates.

All tissues of the body contain potassium. It is found mainly in the muscle followed by the skeleton. Excretion of potassium via urine is also controlled by hemostatic mechanisms; the kidney regulates this so that there is not normally a major loss of this essential element. The amount of potassium excreted depends on the chloride ion concentration and the adrenal hormone secretion level.

Mechanism of Toxicity

Potassium is a cofactor and activates a large variety of enzymes, including glycerol dehydrogenase, pyruvate kinase, L-threonine dehydrase, and ATPase.

Human Toxicity

Excess intake of potassium, reduced renal excretion of potassium, or both can lead to hyperkalemia. The toxicity of excess potassium can be exacerbated by aldosterone antagonist drugs.

A word of caution: Periodically, a solution containing a relatively high concentration of a potassium salt is sold as a nutritional supplement. In light of the fact that ingestion of additional potassium can upset the sodium:potassium ratio, potassium supplements are only indicated on the advice of a physician. Unusually high intake of potassium can cause abnormal EKG readings (T-waves will be elevated and P-waves depressed). Ventricular fibrillation can result and lead to cardiac arrest. A large increase (about 18 g per day) may produce neuromuscular weakness or paralysis.

Potassium permanganate is a mucous membrane irritant. Taken internally, it can be corrosive to the stomach. It is poorly absorbed, but it can cause nervous system symptoms and increased methemoglobin levels.

Potassium perchlorate can induce aplastic anemia, which can be fatal.

Clinical Management

Intravenous injection of calcium gluconate can antagonize the cardiac effects of excess potassium. Also, intravenous injection of sodium bicarbonate and glucose will help diminish the effects of potassium hemodialysis overdose.

Animal Toxicity

Potassium is not associated with carcinogenic action. Moreover, there have not been any mutagenic or teratogenic effects attributed to this element.

—Arthur Furst and Shirley B. Radding

Related Topic

Metals

Primidone

- CAS: 125-33-7
- Synonyms: Primaclone; hexamidinum; 2-desoxyphenobarbital; 5-ethylperhydro-5-phenylpyrimidine-4,6-dione; Mysoline; Midone; Dilon; Mylepsin; Liskantin; Majsolin; Sertan
- Pharmaceutical Class: Desoxybarbiturate; a congener of phenobarbital
- Chemical Structure:

H
O N
CH
NH
O

Uses

An anticonvulsant, primidone is used in the treatment of generalized tonic–clonic seizures and partial focal seizures. It is often used in combination with phenytoin or carbamazepine.

Exposure Pathways

Ingestion is the route of exposure. Toxicity results from acute or chronic overdosage of tablets or oral suspension.

Toxicokinetics

Following therapeutic doses, primidone is usually well absorbed (bioavailability ranges from 70 to 95%) with peak plasma concentrations occurring in 3 or 4 hr. Primidone is converted by the liver to two metabolites: phenobarbital and phenylethylmalonamide (PEMA). Both metabolites are active and phenobarbital is thought to be primarily responsible for primidone's anticonvulsant activity. Phenobarbital appears in the blood 2–4 days after beginning primidone therapy. The volume of distribution averages 0.6 liters/kg, but there is a lot of interindividual variation (in all the kinetic parameters). Approximately 20% of primidone and PEMA is bound to plasma proteins, but the binding of phenobarbital is about 50%. Primidone crosses the placenta and is excreted in breast milk.

The majority of a dose is excreted in the urine as PEMA; about 15% is excreted as phenobarbital. The plasma elimination half-lives of primidone, PEMA, and phenobarbital are about 8–10, 24–36, and 100 hr, respectively. The metabolism of primidone is enhanced with chronic therapy, with a reduced half-life of 4–7 hr. An elimination half-life of 6.2 hr has been documented following overdose.

Mechanism of Toxicity

Primidone and PEMA appear to have weak anticonvulsant activity compared to that of phenobarbital. Both primidone and phenobarbital contribute to central nervous system (CNS) depression, probably through enhancement of GABA activity in the brain and resulting decreased neuronal excitability.

Human Toxicity: Acute

Acute intoxication resembles barbiturate toxicity. Clinical effects include dose-related CNS depression, nystagmus, ataxia, nausea and vomiting, dizziness, vertigo, and irritability. Doses in excess of 1500 mg (twice the maximum recommended daily dose) should be considered toxic. Less common are hypotension, hypothermia, and dermal bullae. Encephalopathy has been observed in an epileptic patient with high plasma levels and poor renal function. With plasma concentrations exceeding 80 μg/ml, primidone may precipitate and cause crystalluria. Plasma levels >10 μg/ml are associated with toxic effects. The therapeutic range is reportedly 5–10 μg/ml, but clinical effects correlate more closely with phenobarbital blood levels.

Human Toxicity: Chronic

With chronic exposure, side effects may include rash, thrombocytopenia, leukopenia, and a lupus-like disorder. Chronic therapy is likely to result in tolerance and withdrawal symptoms if primidone therapy is abruptly stopped.

Clinical Management

The most important aspect of treatment for acute overdose is provision of airway maintenance and ventilation. Hypotension and hypothermia should be corrected if present. Ipecac-induced emesis is probably unwise because of the potential for rapid absorption and CNS depression, but decontamination should be accomplished with oral activated charcoal. There are no antidotes. Analeptic drugs are not indicated. Patients with high plasma phenobarbital levels may be treated with multiple oral doses of activated charcoal and/or urinary alkalinization to enhance phenobarbital excretion. At therapeutic levels, hemodialysis has been shown to increase primidone clearance from 30 to 98 ml/min. Phenobarbital is also removed by hemodialysis. Primidone, PEMA, and phenobarbital can be removed by hemoperfusion. There is no evidence that extracorporeal drug removal has a beneficial clinical effect with respect to morbidity or mortality.

Animal Toxicity

Acute poisoning in animals may cause lethargy, incoordination, loss of reflexes, coma, or respiratory depression. Treatment is based on supportive care in consultation with a veterinarian.

—*S. Rutherfoord Rose*

Procainamide

- CAS: 51-06-9
- Synonyms: Procan SR; Pronestyl
- Pharmaceutical Class: Class IA antiarrhythmic
- Chemical Structure:

$NH_2-C_6H_4-CONHCH_2CH_2N(C_2H_5)_2 \cdot HCl$

Use

Procainamide is used in the management of ventricular arrhythmias.

Exposure Pathways

Ingestion is the most common route of both accidental and intentional exposures. Procainamide is available for parenteral administration and toxicity can occur via this route.

Toxicokinetics

Following oral administration, approximately 85% of procainamide is absorbed from the gastrointestinal tract within 1 or 2 hr. In overdose, absorption may be delayed especially if sustained-release preparations are involved. Procainamide is moderately distributed to tissue with a volume of distribution of approximately 2 liters/kg. Protein binding is minimal at 15–25%. Procainamide is metabolized to its active metabolite *n*-acetyl procainamide (NAPA). NAPA has a volume of distribution of approximately 1.5 liters/kg and is 10%

protein bound. Procainamide has an elimination half-life of approximately 3 hr; the half-life of NAPA is approximately 6 hr. Fifty percent of procainamide is eliminated unchanged in the urine.

Mechanism of Toxicity

Procainamide affects phase 0 depolarization of the cardiac action potential by decreasing rapid intracellular movement of sodium during this phase. The result is lengthening of the action potential as well as a decrease in its rate and amplitude. This is displayed on the electrocardiogram as a widening of the QRS complex. Procainamide may also affect phases 2–4 of the action potential. Effects on phase 2 result in a flattened plateau, whereas effects on phase 3 result in prolonged repolarization. These phase 3 effects are displayed as QTc prolongation on the electrocardiogram. Also, spontaneous depolarization is reduced in phase 4 resulting in a prolonged refractory period. Vasodilation associated with procainamide toxicity is due to interference with ganglionic transmission of catecholamine neurotransmitters. A reflex tachycardia may occur in response to this vasodilation. Also, procainamide may have weak anticholinergic effects that produce tachycardia. Negative inotropic effects, which are less prominent than those observed with other class IA antiarrhythmics, may occur in toxicity. The *n*-acetylprocainamide metabolite of procainamide has pharmacologic and toxicologic effects similar to those of the parent compound.

Human Toxicity

The primary toxicities observed with procainamide are cardiovascular in nature. Initially, a tachycardia may occur due to procainamide's anticholinergic properties or as a reflex response to vasodilation. Conduction disturbances are the most common cardiac toxicities that occur. On the EKG, these may be displayed as widening of the QRS and QTc prolongation. All types of heart block, functional rhythms, and asystole can occur. Procainamide can also cause ventricular tachycardia, ventricular fibrillation, and *Torsades de Pointes*. Severe hypotension due to decreases in cardiac output and/or vasodilation occurs in procainamide toxicity. The decreases in level of consciousness that occur in procainamide toxicity are secondary to the cardiovascular effects that occur. Seizure activity can occur in procainamide toxicity.

Clinical Management

Due to procainamide's potential for severe cardiovascular toxicity, advanced life-support may be required. Emergent intubation and ventilation may be necessary. Pulse oxymtry can be utilized at the bedside to assess respiratory status. Procainamide's proarrhythmic effects mandate a baseline 12-lead electrocardiogram as well as continuous EKG monitoring. Frequent monitoring of blood pressure should occur due to the hypotensive effects of procainamide. Invasive hemodynamic monitoring may be necessary to assess systemic vascular resistance, mean arterial pressure, and pulmonary capillary wedge pressure. Gastrointestinal decontamination can effectively decrease procainamide absorption. Due to procainamide's rapid absorption and potential for severe toxicity, syrup of ipecac-induced emesis is contraindicated. In recent substantial ingestions and/or in ingestions involving multiple substances, gastric lavage can be used to decontaminate the stomach. Activated charcoal adsorbs procainamide throughout the gastrointestinal tract. Whole bowel irrigation with a polyethylene glycol solution should be considered in ingestions involving sustained-release preparations. A transcutaneous or transvenous pacemaker should be placed to manage recalcitrant bradycardia and conduction disturbances. Isoproterenol has been suggested for treatment of hypotension, but it should be used with caution due to its vasodilatory properties. Ventricular arrhythmias can be treated with lidocaine, bretylium, and/or electrical therapy. If *Torsades de Pointes* occurs, magnesium sulfate should be administered. Isoproterenol can be administered in *Torsades* that does not respond to magnesium. Hypotension should be managed initially with fluid replacement. Volume repletion should not be overly aggressive due to decreases in cardiac output. If cardiac output is decreased, positive inotropic agents, such as sopamine, dobutamine, and amrinone, should be used. Vasodilation should be managed with vasopressors, such as dopamine, norepinephrine, and epinephrine. If seizures occur, benzodiazepines such as diazepam and lorazepam should be used initially. If seizures are refractory to the benzodiazepines, phenytoin and barbiturates should be considered. Due to their pharmacokinetic characteristics, moderate volume of distribution, and low protein binding, procainamide and NAPA can be removed via hemodialysis and hemoperfusion. Hemoperfusion is the preferred route of extracorporeal removal since clearance is greater. The clinical laboratory should be utilized in patient assessment. Both procainamide and NAPA serum concentrations should be obtained. Normal ranges for these are as follows: procainamide, 3–14 μg/ml; NAPA, 12–35 μg/ml. Measurement of electrolytes, renal function tests, and measurement of arterial blood gases should also be obtained.

—*Daniel J. Cobaugh*

Related Topics

Cardiovascular System
Gastrointestinal System

Prometryn

- CAS: 7287-19-6
- PREFERRED NAME: Prometryn(e)
- SYNONYMS: 2-Methylthio-4; 6-bis(isopropylamino)-*s*-triazine; G 34161
- CHEMICAL CLASS: Sulfur-substituted triazine pesticide
- CHEMICAL STRUCTURE:

MeS, NHPr-i, N, N, N, NHPr-i

Use
Prometryn is used as a herbicide.

Exposure Pathway
Ingestion is a possible route of exposure.

Toxicokinetics
Prometryn is excreted in urine or feces within 72 hr.

Mechanism of Toxicity
On ingestion, prometryn metabolizes, producing amine dealkylation and side chain oxidation. It affects the tricarboxylic acid cycle.

Human Toxicity
Prometryn has low acute toxicity. Symptoms include nausea or sore throat. The ACGIH TLV is 5 mg/m^3.

Clinical Management
Lavage and catharsis are recommended for ingestion. Oxygen therapy should be provided if needed.

Animal Toxicity
The LD_{50} in rats is 3750 mg/kg. The LD_{50} in bluegill sunfish is 10.0 ppm. The LD_{50} in rainbow trout is 2.5 ppm. Prometryn causes liver and kidney damage. Acute intoxication in rats produces ataxia, dyspnea, and convulsions. It causes point mutations in yeast. It is a mild eye and skin irritant.

—*Jayne E. Ash and Shayne C. Gad*

Related Topic

Pesticides

Propachlor

- CAS: 1918-16-7
- SYNONYMS: *N*-isopropyl-α-chloroacetanilide; Ramrod; Bexton
- CHEMICAL CLASS: Halogenated hydrocarbon pesticide
- CHEMICAL STRUCTURE:

i—Pr—N(Ph)—C(=O)—CH_2Cl

Use
Propachlor is used as a herbicide.

Exposure Pathways
Dermal contact, ocular contact, and ingestion are possible exposure routes.

Toxicokinetics

Approximately 50% is excreted as metabolites through urine or feces within 24 hr.

Mechanism of Toxicity

Propachlor inhibits production of cytochrome oxidase (brain and kidneys) and cholinesterase in the liver.

Human Toxicity

The ACGIH TLV is 100 mg/kg per day. Propachlor causes coma and convulsion and is irritating to the skin, gastrointestinal tract, and respiratory tract. It is a dermal sensitizer.

Clinical Management

Exposed skin should be washed with soap and water. Exposed eyes should be flushed with running water for 15 min. If a small amount has been ingested, an emetic (i.e., ipecac) should be given within the first hour. If the propachlor has been combined with a hydrocarbon, ipecac should not be used. Gastic lavage should be provided if a large amount has been ingested. If ingested more than 1 hr prior, activated charcoal or magnesium sulfate should be used.

Animal Toxicity

Propachlor is a mutagen. Death is preceded by weakness, salivation, tremors, and collapse. In rats, the oral LD_{50} is 710 mg/kg and the dermal LD_{50} is 2000 mg/kg. In mice, the oral LD_{50} is 392 mg/kg and the dermal LD_{50} is 380 mg/kg. In ducks, the oral LD_{50} is 512 mg/kg.

—Jayne E. Ash and Shayne C. Gad

Related Topics

Pesticides
Pollution, Water

Propane

- SYNONYMS: Dimethylmethane, propane (DOT, OSHA); propyl hydride, (UN1978, DOT); bottled gas
- CHEMICAL CLASS: Aliphatic hydrocarbon (C3)
- MOLECULAR FORMULA: C_3H_8
- DESCRIPTION: Propane is a colorless, odorless highly flammable/explosive gas that is heavier than air. It occurs in natural gas at concentrations ranging from 3 to 18%. It is emitted into the atmosphere from furnaces, automobile exhausts, and sources of natural gas; it is also found in trace amounts in human expired air. With sufficient oxygen, it is combusted to carbon dioxide and water, but carbon monoxide, a deadly gas, will be generated under leaner conditions.

Uses

Propane is used principally as a fuel source for homes and industries and as an aerosol propellant. It is also used in the synthesis of organic materials, in the manufacture of ethylene, as a refrigerant, and as an extractant.

Exposure Pathways

Because propane exists as a gas at normal temperature and pressure, exposure would occur by inhalation. Typical background concentrations detected at ground level in major U.S. cities range from 0.050 to 0.4 ppm. It is possible to spill liquid propane from a pressurized tank, causing frostbite upon skin contact due to rapid evaporation and loss of heat.

Mechanism of Toxicity

Propane is inert, and air concentrations up to 100,000 ppm (10%) will only produce slight dizziness in humans in a few minutes. Some sources classify propane as a simple anesthetic, although it can principally be classified as a simple asphyxiant, and concentrations that are high enough to displace oxygen would be expected to cause lightheadedness, loss of consciousness, and possibly death from asphyxiation.

Human Toxicity

Propane is not considered to be inherently toxic to humans. In high concentrations, it may have a narcotic effect, but at concentrations below 1000 ppm, propane will show no physiological effects in humans. OSHA classifies propane as a simple asphyxiant; it will cause chemical suffocation at concentrations that are high enough to displace oxygen. Currently, the U.S. FDA classifies propane as generally recognized as safe. Propane gas is also explosive and is, therefore, an explosion and/or fire hazard (the upper and lower explosive limits are 2.4 and 9.5% by volume, respectively). Industrially, propane is handled similarly to methane, and a threshold limit of 1000 ppm is suggested by both OSHA and ACGIH.

Clinical Management

Persons exposed to high concentrations of propane should vacate or be removed from the source of the gas and seek fresh air. Extreme care must be taken to keep areas of expected increased concentration free from ignition sources, such as sparks from static electricity. Explosion-proof apparatus should also be used in these areas.

Animal Toxicity

Propane has been shown to have adverse effects on the cardiovascular system in the primate, dog, cat, and mouse. Guinea pigs exposed to 2.2–5.5% of the gas showed sniffing and chewing movements. In dogs, 1% gas caused hemodynamic changes, whereas 3.3% showed decreases in aortic pressure, stroke volume, and cardiac output and an increase in pulmonary resistance. Ten percent propane in the mouse and 15% in the dog did not produce arrhythmia but did produce weak cardiac sensitization. Some microbes can utilize propane as an energy source, whereas others are inhibited by its presence.

—*Stephen Clough*

Related Topic

Neurotoxicology: Central and Peripheral

Propanil

- CAS: 709-98-8
- SYNONYMS: *N*-(3,4-dichlorophenyl)propanamide; Chem Rice; Drexel Prop-Job; DPA; Erban; FW-734, Herbax; Propanex; Propanilo; Riselect; Stam Supernox; Stampede 3E, Stam F-34; Sta M-4; Strel; Surcopur; Surpur; S10165 and Vertac; Bay 303130; a code designation FW-734
- CHEMICAL CLASS: Amide
- CHEMICAL STRUCTURE:

$NHCOC_2H_5$

Cl

Cl

Use

Propanil is a postemergence herbicide used primarily on rice and potatoes.

Exposure Pathways

Dermal exposure is most common but ocular and respiratory exposures also occur.

Toxicokinetics

Propanil shows little accumulation in mammalian tissues. No propanil was found in urine or milk after oral administration in a cow and only about 1% of the dose was recovered in the feces. Propanil was found to be stable in rumen fluid but rapidly metabolized by liver enzymes *in vitro*. Propanil is converted *in vitro* and *in vivo* to dichloroaniline (DCA) via amidases. Amidases capable of converting propanil to DCA are found in both plant and animal tissues.

Mechanism of Toxicity

Propanil acts as a nervous system depressant. Following metabolic conversion, DCA induces methemoglobinemia and can produce cyanosis. Propanil is also a chloracnegen, most likely because of contamination by tetrachlororazobenzene, a congener of dioxin.

Human Toxicity

The major forms of toxicity in humans from propanil exposure are irritation, chloracne, and methemoglobinemia. Because of the danger of chloracne, protective clothing is recommended at all times when propanil is handled. With high doses, nervous system depression can occur.

Clinical Management

Treatment is mainly symptomatic in nature, and any appropriate supportive therapy should be used.

Animal Toxicity

As with most herbicides, mammalian acute toxicity from propanil exposure is low (LD_{50} values >1 g/kg). Long-term reproductive studies indicated no propensity for reproductive toxicity. Inhibitors of liver amidases (e.g., tri-*ortho*-cresyl phosphate) can prevent the formation of DCA and methemoglobinemia from propanil exposure.

—Thuc Pham

Related Topic

Pesticides

Propargite

- CAS: 2312-35-8
- SYNONYMS: 2-[4-(1,1-Dimethylethyl)phenoxy]cyclohexyl 2-propynyl sulfite; BPPS; Omite; Comite
- CHEMICAL CLASS: Organic sulfite acaricide
- CHEMICAL STRUCTURE:

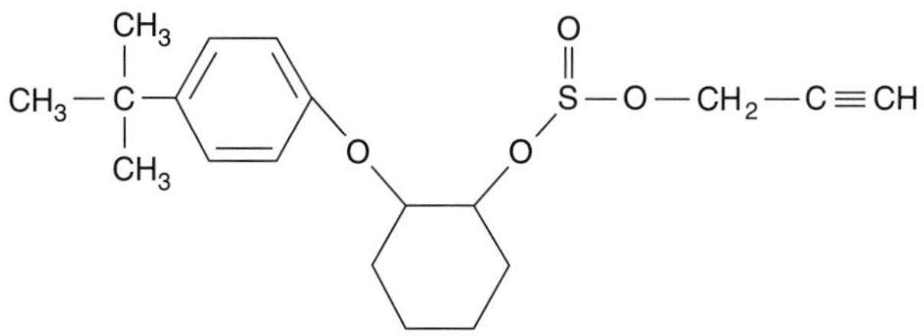

CH_3 — C(CH_3)(CH_3) — C$_6$H$_4$ — O — C$_6$H$_{10}$ — O — S(=O) — O — CH_2 — C≡CH

Use

Propargite is primarily used to control motile forms of mites.

Exposure Pathways

Dermal, oral, inhalation, and ocular exposures are all possible.

Toxicokinetics

Propargite can be absorbed from the gastrointestinal tract after oral administration. It undergoes hydroxylation at the sulfite ester. Metabolites of propargite are eliminated in both urine and feces.

Mechanism of Toxicity

The mechanism of toxicity of propargite is unclear. Propargite is, however, an inhibitor of monoamine oxidase and therefore can alter the metabolism of monoamines.

Human Toxicity

Dermatitis is the major form of toxicity following propargite exposure. Signs include erythema, burning, itching, exfoliation, and hyperpigmentation. Ocular exposure produces irritation. Changes in the chemical formulation have alleviated many of the acute irritant effects associated with propargite use.

Clinical Management

Treatment is symptomatic.

Animal Toxicity

Propargite exhibits low acute toxicity. The oral LD_{50} value in rats is about 1–4 g/kg, but it is somewhat lower with dermal exposure. Propargite was not mutagenic, tumorigenic, carcinogenic, or teratogenic in animal studies.

—Jing Liu

Related Topic

Pesticides

Propazine

- CAS: 139-40-2
- SYNONYMS: 2,4-bis(isopropylamino)-6-chloro-*s*-triazine; Gesamil; Milogard; G-30028

- Chemical Class: Chloro-substituted triazine
- Chemical Structure:

Cl, N, N, N, N—NHPri, NNPr-i

Use

Propazine is a herbicide.

Exposure Pathways

Dermal contact, inhalation, and ingestion are possible routes of exposure.

Toxicokinetics

Propazine is readily absorbed and metabolized by amine-dealkyation and side-chain oxidation. It is slowly excreted in urine and feces.

Mechanism of Toxicity

Propazine causes fatty degeneration. It also blocks metabolism of sugars and carbohydrates.

Human Toxicity

Propazine can cause dyspnea, muscle spasms, ataxia, anorexia, coma, convulsions, and liver and kidney damage. The ACGIH TLV is 5 mg/m^3.

Clinical Management

Affected areas should be flushed with water for 15 min. Contaminated clothing should be removed.

Animal Toxicity

The oral LD_{50} is 7700 mg/kg in rats and 5000 mg/kg in mice. Propazine causes skin irritation and blood and liver toxicity in rabbits. It is a mutagen.

—Jayne E. Ash and Shayne C. Gad

Related Topics

Pesticides
Pollution, Water

Propene

- CAS: 115-07-1
- Synonyms: Propylene; 1-propylene; methylethylene; liquid petroleum gas
- Chemical Class: Aliphatic alkene
- Molecular Formula: C_3H_6
- Chemical Structure:

H2C═CH—CH3

Uses

Propene is used as a chemical intermediate in the production of polypropylene, acrylonitrile, propylene oxide, isopropanol, and cumene. Refineries use much of their production of propene internally as a refinery heating gas and to produce alkylates in gasoline and to produce liquefied petroleum gas.

Exposure Pathway

Because propene is a gas, inhalation exposure is the primary route of entry.

Toxicokinetics

The toxicokinetics of propene has been studied in laboratory animals. In Sprague–Dawley rats, at steady state, 42% of inhaled propene is exhaled unchanged and is not absorbed into the bloodstream, with the remainder being metabolized and eliminated. Propene is metabolized to propene oxide, which reacts to form hemoglobin complexes at cysteine, histidine, and *N*-terminal valine. It is then further reacted to an alcohol and excreted.

Mechanism of Toxicity

Propene is classified as a simple asphyxiant and its toxicity is associated with the central nervous system effects associated with oxygen deprivation.

Human Toxicity

Propene is relatively nontoxic and has been investigated for use as an anesthetic. Its flammability and explosivity, however, has deemed this application as inappropriate. Exposure to a concentration of 6.4% for 2.25 min resulted in mild intoxication, a sensation of numbness, and an inability to concentrate. At 12.8% for 1 min, these same symptoms were more pronounced, with 24 and 33% for 3 min resulting in unconsciousness. Exposures from 40 to 75% for a few minutes caused reddening of the eyelids, flushing of the face, tearing, and coughing. This is consistent with the fact that liquefied propene may cause skin burns on direct contact. As with any asphyxiant, high exposures for sufficient time, resulting in oxygen deprivation, can result in death.

Clinical Management

Overexposure to propene is treated by simply moving the victim to fresh air. If skin or eye irritation has occurred, affected areas should be flushed with water for at least 15 min. Recovery is usually rapid and complete.

Animal Toxicity

Inhalation of high concentrations of propene by experimental animals results in anesthetic effects similar to those seen in humans. Anesthesia has been induced in cats after exposure to concentrations of propene at 20–31% without causing other signs of toxicity. At higher concentrations, from 40 to 80%, blood pressure decreased, pulse increased, and an unusual heartbeat was reported. Cardiac sensitization was reported following propene exposure in dogs. Subchronic propene exposure to rats and mice for 2–14 weeks at concentrations ranging from 625 to 10,000 ppm resulted in no reported toxicity. Male and female Sprague–Dawley rats were exposed to propene at concentrations of 200, 1,000, and 5,000 ppm for 7 hr/day, 5 days/week for 104 weeks, and male and female Swiss mice were exposed for 78 weeks. The mortality rate of the male rats increased slightly after exposures of 1000 and 5000 ppm and that of male mice after exposure to the highest dose. No evidence of other toxicity was observed. In another long-term study with exposures up to 10,000 ppm, 6 hr/day, 5 days/week for 103 weeks in rats and mice, nontumorigenic lesions were reported in the nasal cavity of male rats. The authors concluded that these effects were due to inflammatory changes from local irritation. No exposure-related changes in tumor incidence were reported.

—Patricia J. Beattie

Propionic Acid

- CAS: 79-09-4
- Preferred Name: Sodium propionate
- Synonym: Mycoban
- Chemical Class: Antifungal
- Chemical Structure:

$$HO-\overset{\overset{\displaystyle O}{\|}}{C}-CH_2-CH_3$$

Uses

Propionic acid is used as an antimold food preservative and as a skin fungicide.

Exposure Pathways

Dermal exposure, inhalation, and ingestion are possible routes of exposure.

Toxicokinetics

Propionic acid is rapidly absorbed through the skin. It is excreted primarily through expired air (77%) and urine and feces (7%). It is carried by blood to the liver, where it is metabolized and removed.

Mechanism of Toxicity

If sodium propionate is ingested or applied topically in an acid media, it becomes propionic acid. It oxidizes fatty acids, lowers pH values, and facilitates the citric acid cycle through interaction with coenzyme A. There has been evidence of heightened production of insulin in cows and sheep; the insulin later settles to an overall lower level.

Human Toxicity

Propionic acid produces burning or inflammation from contact with skin and mucous membranes. JECFA does not give an acceptable daily intake level. The ACGIH TLV is 10 ppm.

Clinical Management

The victim should be removed from exposure. Treatment is symptomatic.

Animal Toxicity

In animals, symptoms include polytropism. It also produces central nervous system, cardiovascular, respiratory, and blood effects.

—*Jayne E. Ash and Shayne C. Gad*

Related Topic

Acids

Proposition 65

- TITLE: Safe Drinking Water and Toxic Enforcement Act
- AGENCY: State of California
- YEAR PASSED: 1986
- GROUPS REGULATED: Those doing business in California (except as preempted by federal law)

Synopsis of Law

California's Safe Drinking Water and Toxic Enforcement Act requires the governor to revise and publish a list of chemicals known to the state to cause cancer or reproductive toxicity. This law is more familiarly known as Proposition 65. The administrative record of Proposition 65 in California clearly shows that several arguments and suggestions have been and are being repeatedly made regarding its reasonableness. If determinations of carcinogenicity or teratogenicity were made within the bounds of the published scientific and medical literature by nationally or internationally renowned experts in these highly specialized fields, the law might seem reasonable. If the determination took into account information supplied by national scientific, medical, and/or trade associations, the law might seem reasonable. If trace quantities of known carcinogens or teratogens in consumer products were suspect of their true biological risk to consumers, the law might seem reasonable.

Despite the previous arguments and suggestions, the California regulation relying on California state toxicologists and physicians retains its sovereignty in such determinations. Some useful and safe consumer products will be lost due to California's Proposition 65, making certain ingredients or trace contaminants unlawful in consumer products. More tellingly, the law may place a significant labeling and warning notice burden on retailers (such as grocery stores) and national manufacturers of products sold in California.

—*Shayne C. Gad*

Related Topics

Developmental Toxicology
State Regulation of Consumer Products
Toxicity Testing, Reproductive

Propoxur

- CAS: 114-26-1
- SYNONYMS: 2-Isopropoxyphenyl-*N*-methylcarbamate; Baygon; Blattanex; IMPC; Invisi-Gard, IPMC; Propogon; Sendra; Sendran; Suncide; Tendex; Tugon Fliegenkugel; Unden; Undene; BAY 39007; BAY 9010; BO 58 12315; ENT 25671; OMS33
- CHEMICAL CLASS: Carbamate pesticide
- CHEMICAL STRUCTURE:

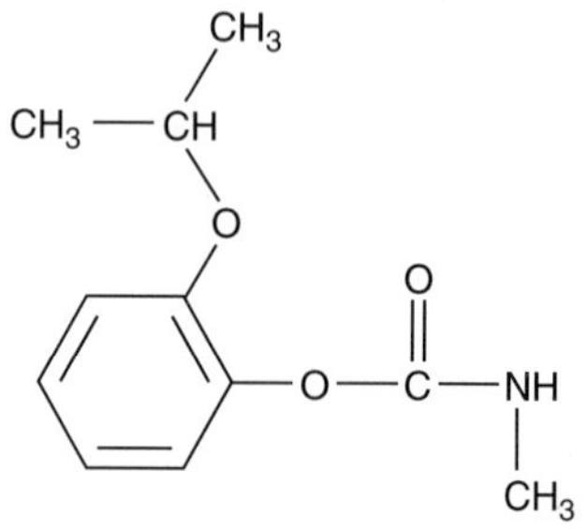

CH_3
CH_3—CH
O
O
O—C—NH
CH_3

Uses

The main uses of propoxur include control of household insect pests, domestic animal pests, and mosquitoes.

Exposure Pathways

Human exposure to propoxur has occurred through ingestion, dermal contact, and inhalation. The high vapor pressure of propoxur (which is advantageous for mosquito control) has been implicated in several cases of inhalation after recommended safety precautions were not observed.

Toxicokinetics

Dermal absorption in humans has been estimated to be approximately 16%; estimated absorption from the gastrointestinal tract in experimental studies with humans has been complicated due to propoxur-induced emesis. 2-Isopropoxyphenol is the major metabolite. The majority of the dose undergoes urinary excretion within 48 hr of exposure. In rats, both the parent compound and 2-isopropoxyphenol appear to be eliminated primarily in the urine as sulfate conjugates.

Mechanism of Toxicity

The mechanism of toxicity for propoxur is similar to that of aldicarb (see Aldicarb).

Human Toxicity: Acute

The acute effects of exposure are due to acetylcholinesterase inhibition and may include the typical symptoms of cholinergic overstimulation such as the SLUDGE syndrome (salivation, lacrimation, urination, diarrhea, gastrointestinal cramping, and emesis), respiratory depression, bronchospasms, increased bronchial secretions, pulmonary edema, blurred vision, miosis, headache, tremors, muscle fasiculations, convulsions, mental confusion, and coma. Respiratory failure is the cause of death.

Human Toxicity: Chronic

Currently, insufficient evidence exists to indicate any significant long-term health risk associated with propoxur exposure.

Clinical Management

Activated charcoal may be used to reduce absorption from the gastrointestinal tract. Syrup of ipecac-induced emesis may be used if the patient is conscious and alert. Emesis is contraindicated if the patient is, or may become, convulsive. For inhalation exposure, the patient should be removed from the exposure area and observed for signs of breathing difficulty. In cases of dermal exposure, contaminated clothing should be removed and disposed of. Any exposed areas of skin should be repeatedly washed with soap and water. For eye contact, the eyes should be flushed with generous amounts of lukewarm water for a minimum of 15 min.

Clinical management is basically symptomatic and supportive. Artificial ventilation with 100% humidified oxygen is necessary in cases of respiratory paralysis. An endotracheal tube may be required to maintain the airway. Erythrocytic acetylcholinesterase (AChE) levels, arterial blood gases, and cardiac function should be monitored. Because of the rapid reactivation of AChE, significant enzyme inhibition may not be seen unless blood samples are drawn and assayed within approximately 2 hr of the exposure. Atropine should be given to relieve the muscarinic (i.e., SLUDGE) symptoms. Convulsions may be treated with intravenous diazepam. Phenytoin may be used if the convulsions are recurrent. Pralidoxime is indicated in cases of mixed exposure to both carbamates and organophosphorus compounds but is contraindicated in cases of carbamate-only exposure.

Animal Toxicity

The acute oral LD_{50} in mice is 25 mg/kg.

Paul R. Harp

Related Topics

Carbamate Pesticides
Pesticides

Propoxyphene

- CAS: 469-62-5
- SYNONYMS: Dextropropoxyphene/*d*-propoxyphene (CAS: 1639-60-7); Propoxyphene hydrochloride; Propoxyphene napsylate; Darvon
- PHARMACEUTICAL CLASS: Opioid analgesic with local anesthetic activity; synthetic opioid

structurally related to methadone (see Methadone)

Use

Propoxyphene is used as a mild narcotic analgesic.

Exposure Pathways

All propoxyphene preparations are for oral use and ingestion is the most common route of exposure. Propoxyphene-containing pharmaceuticals are sometimes injected for abuse purposes.

Toxicokinetics

Propoxyphene is readily absorbed from the stomach and upper small intestine with measurable levels in 5 min. Peak plasma levels are seen in 1–2.5 hr following ingestion. The drug undergoes extensive first-pass metabolism at both the hepatic level and absorption sites in the gastrointestinal tract. It is primarily metabolized (90%) in the liver N-demethylation, leading to the formation of norpropoxyphene. Norpropoxyphene is then further metabolized in the liver to a number of inactive metabolites. Other metabolic pathways include aromatic hydroxylation and ester hydrolysis. Small amounts of dinorpropoxyphene have been detected in the plasma. Seven additional metabolites have been identified in the urine (propoxyphene metabolites: *p*-hydroxypropoxyphene and norpropoxyphene carbinol; norporpoxyphene metabolites: *p*-hydroxynorpropoxyphene, norpropoxyphene carbinol, and dinorpropoxyphene; dinorpropoxyphene metabolites: cyclic dinorpropoxyphene and dinorpropoxyphene carbinol).

It is highly protein bound (80%) and widely distributed to the liver, lungs, brain, kidneys, and fat. Concentrations in these tissues are approximately 10–40 times greater than in the blood. The volume of distribution is 12–26 liters/kg. Less than 10% is excreted unchanged in the urine. From 10 to 20% is excreted as norpropoxyphene. The α-phase (distribution) half-life of propoxyphene is approximately 5 hr. There is substantial individual variation in the elimination half-life of propoxyphene.

Mechanism of Toxicity

Propoxyphene produces excessive opioid receptor stimulation and local anesthetic activity.

Human Toxicity: Acute

Potentially lethal effects include coma, apnea, seizures, hypotension, arrhythmias, pulmonary edema, and cardiac arrest. Other characteristic effects include miosis, anxiety, restlessness, euphoria, nausea, and vomiting.

Human Toxicity: Chronic

Chronic toxicity may result in psychotic reactions with confusion, disorientation, and irrational behavior. Prolonged use has precipitated pressure point erythema, blisters, and skin necrosis.

Clinical Management

After life-support measures have been provided, gastric decontamination by gastric lavage and/or activated charcoal is recommended. Naloxone can be employed for respiratory depression and a decreased level of consciousness. Large doses may be needed. Chronic propoxyphene abusers may develop withdrawal symptoms after naloxone administration. Cardiac status should be monitored and treated as indicated.

Animal Toxicity

Central nervous system and cardiovascular effects in animals are similar to those seen in humans.

—*Regina M. Rogowski*

Prostaglandins

Prostaglandins are hormone-like substances derived from amino acids that mediate a wide range of physiological functions including metabolism, smooth muscle activity, and nerve transmission. They may occur endogenously or be produced for specific therapeutic purposes.

Endogenous production of prostaglandins is mediated by prostaglandin H synthase (PHS), a derivative of arachidonic acid. PHS is a peroxidase involved with biotransformation, adding a peroxide oxygen to the xenobiotic. Interaction with some substances, such as benzo(*a*)pyrene or aflatoxin B_1, may catalyze the release of tumorigenic metabolites. By oxidizing acetaminophen to *N*-acetyl-benzoquinoneimine, PHS may also contribute, along with P450 and glutathione, to the nephrotoxic effects of the drug.

PHS is suspected of contributing to bladder cancer in dogs by converting aromatic amines to reactive radicals through one-electron oxidation in the liver. This may imply that PHS could be a human carcinogen as well since dogs and humans have similar tumorigenic responses to aromatic amines. PHS peroxidation may also suppress bone marrow by binding to proteins and DNA in the marrow. The role of PHS in biotransformation is mediated by the availability of archidonic acid, which may be the key to controlling its toxic effect.

This particular use of aspirin suggests the use of prostaglandins to promote blood clotting. Prostaglandins have a number of therapeutic uses. They are used to prevent ulcers, reduce the potential size of myocardial infarctions, and treat glaucoma. Prostaglandins are also used to promote cervical or uterine contractions in pregnant women, either as a labor inducer or as an abortifacient (i.e., RU486).

Aside from endogenous production, prostaglandins can be absorbed into the body through ocular exposure, inhalation, ingestion, or injection. In the case of glaucoma treatment, a prostaglandin derivative (S-1033) is rapidly absorbed through the eyes and into the plasma with a half-life of 11 min at β-phase. On the other hand, E and F strains of progesterone are hemostable but rapidly metabolized by tissue-bound enzymes in the liver, kidneys, and lungs.

Since prostaglandins perform different functions throughout the body, there are various modes of toxicity as well. Prostaglandins contribute to platelet aggregation of blood clots and nonsteroidal antiinflammatory drugs (NSAIDs) such as aspirin or ibuprofen counteract that activity. Conversely, NSAIDs inhibit the production of and promote excretion of prostaglandins in the kidneys, which may lead to nephrotoxicity. Without the vasodilatory property, the kidneys fail to get needed blood. Misoprostol, or Cytotec, is a synthetic prostaglandin approved for the prevention of NSAID-induced ulcers.

Prostaglandins also regulate smooth muscle function in the lungs, heart, and uterus. This must be considered when administering it therapeutically or risk potentially toxic consequences. Asthmatics exposed to prostaglandin F2α (or Dinoprost) may experience bronchospasm, arrythmia, or hyperventilation. It may induce grand mal seizures in epileptics.

When used to induce labor, Dinoprost effects may include cervical laceration or rupture with retention of the placenta or hemorrhaging. It may affect the alimentary tract as well, causing nausea, vomiting, and diarrhea. In two cases, women died of cardiovascular collapse following a 40-mg dose of Dinoprost. The TD_{Lo} is 20 μg/kg.

Since prostaglandins are rapidly metabolized in the body, discontinued use and supportive therapy are usually the recommended treatments for a toxic response. In cases of placental retention, blood transfusions may be necessary.

—*Shayne C. Gad and Jayne E. Ash*

Prunus Species

- Species Names: *Prunus domestica* (common plum); *Prunus ceresidera* (myrobolan plum); *Prunus persica* (peach); *Prunus avium* or *P. cerasus* (cherry); *Prunus ameniaca* (apricot); *Prunus dulcis dulcis* (almond); *Prunus malus pumila* (apple)
- Description: Laurocerasus species includes a group of more than 400 trees and shrubs. They are often ornamental for their flowers, fruit, and nuts.
- Chemical Class: Cyanogenic glycosides exemplified by amygdalin

Exposure Pathway

Exposure is by ingestion of seeds, leaves, stems, roots, and fruit. Ingestion of seeds is the most common means of exposure.

Toxicokinetics

Amygdalin is erratically absorbed from most of the gastrointestinal tract but effectively absorbed from the duodenum. Amygdalin is metabolized to cyanide, which is converted to thiocyanate by an enzymatic reaction catalyzed by rhodanese, an enzyme that is widely distributed in tissue but has the highest concentration in the liver. Rhodanese can detoxify large amounts of cyanide but not rapidly enough to prevent fatalities (see Cyanide).

Mechanism of Toxicity

All plants contain high concentrations of cyanogenic glycoside. When seeds are crushed and the pulp is moistened, various enzymes catalyze the conversion of the glycosides to cyanide. The reaction takes place slowly in an acid pH, but an alkaline pH hastens the process. Slow hydrolysis explains the delay in symptom development after ingestion since time is needed to travel from the acidic stomach to the much more alkaline duodenum. Intestinal flora are also capable of hydrolyzing amygdalin to hydrocyanic acid. It forms a stable complex with ferric iron and cytochrome oxidase, inhibiting activity of the enzyme. Cells containing cytochrome oxidase are unable to utilize available oxygen and suffer hypoxia. The respiratory center ceases to function due to the cytotoxic effects of cyanide.

Human Toxicity

Cyanide poisoning due to the accidental ingestion of these plants is rare. Acute symptoms are the same as in cyanide poisoning and include difficulty breathing, dyspnea, muscular twitching, spasms, ataxia, seizures, coma, and death. The onset of symptoms may be very rapid with few premonitory signs. However, depending on a variety of factors, the signs and symptoms may be delayed. Respirations are usually rapid at first and then become slow and labored.

Clinical Management

If toxic amounts are ingested, the symptoms may have a rapid progression. Gastric lavage and/or activated charcoal may be effective to gastric decontaminate the patient. Oxygen (100%) should be administered to maintain an elevated PO_2. Clinically symptomatic patients may need the cyanide antidote kit, which contains amyl nitrite inhalant, sodium nitrite, and sodium thiosulfate. Diazepam may be used to control seizures. Methemoglobin levels should be monitored since the administered nitrites will produce some degree of methemoglobinemia. Acidosis should be treated with sodium bicarbonate. Although rarely used, hemodialysis may be effective by correcting resistant acidemia and thiosulfate–cyanide clearance.

Animal Toxicity

Studies show that large or small amounts of ingested plant material have not caused any problems in animals.

—Regina M. Rogowski

Pseudoephedrine

- CAS: 670-40-6
- Synonyms: Pseudoephedrine hydrochloride; pseudoephedrine sulfate; D-isoephedrine; isoephedrine; Sudafed
- Pharmaceutical Class: Pseudoephedrine is a stereo isomer of ephedrine, in the drug class of sympathiomimetics. It occurs naturally in plants of the genus *Ephedra*.
- Chemical Structure:

$$C_6H_5-CH(OH)-CH(NHCH_3)-CH_3 \cdot HCl$$

Use

Pseudoephedrine is used as an oral nasal decongestant.

Exposure Pathways

Accidental and intentional exposures to pseudoephedrine occur most often by the oral route and involve either the pure form or multisymptom cold preparations containing pseudoephedrine in combination with antihistamines, analgesics, and/or antitussive agents.

Toxicokinetics

Pseudoephedrine is well absorbed from the gastrointestinal tract. After oral administration of a 60-mg dose, nasal decongestion occurs within 30 min and persists for 4–6 hr. Extended release capsules may increase the duration of action to 12 hr. Pseudoephedrine is incompletely metabolized in the liver by N-demethylation to an inactive metabolite. Protein binding for pseudoephedrine is 20%. The volume of distribution is 2.1–3.3 liters/kg. Urinary excretion is the primary route of elimination for pseudoephedrine and metabolites. From 55 to 75% of the parent drug is excreted unchanged. A small amount is excreted as the active metabolite norpseudoephedrine. The half-life is 7 hr but may vary from 1.9 to 21 hr depending on the pH of the urine. The rate of urinary excretion is accelerated in acid urine and decreased in alkaline urine.

Mechanism of Toxicity

Pseudoephedrine is a weak base (pK_a 9.4) that stimulates both α- and β-adrenergic receptors, as well as the release of neuronal norepinephrine. β1 stimulation produces increased heart rate and blood pressure.

Human Toxicity

Hypertension and tachycardia are the primary toxic manifestations of pseudoephedrine overdose. An amount of more than three or four times the maximum daily dosage for adults or children may produce symptoms of β-adrenergic stimulation. In severe poisonings, cardiac arrhythmias and cerebral hemorrhage due to hypertensive crisis may occur. Anxiety, muscle tremor, and seizures may result from stimulation of the central nervous system (CNS). Hallucinations are a more common manifestation exhibited by children. Hypokalemia and hyperglycemia may be noted on laboratory examination. Acute renal failure and rhabdomyolysis have occurred in rare instances with large overdose.

Clinical Management

Basic and advanced life-support measures should be instituted as necessary. Appropriate gastric decontamination should be performed dependent on the patient's condition and symptomatology, amount of the ingested substance, and the history of the exposure. Activated charcoal may be used to adsorb pseudoephedrine. The cardiac and hemodynamic status should be carefully monitored. β-Adrenergic blocking agents and antiarrhythmic agents may be necessary to treat cardiac complications. Hypertension is generally transient, requiring only observation. Antihypertensive agents may be necessary in rare instances. Symptoms of CNS stimulation usually respond to a calm environment and supportive measures. Treatment of exposure to products in which pseudoephedrine is combined with antihistamines, antitussive agents, analgesics, and/or alcohol must include toxicological management of the concurrent drugs involved. Laboratory evaluation should include electrolytes, blood glucose, creatine phosphokinase, and urinalysis.

Animal Toxicity

Following the ingestion of a large dose of pseudoephedrine, dogs and cats may exhibit hyperactivity, mydriasis, depression, vomiting, hyperthermia, disorientation, bradycardia, and tachycardia. Therapy is directed at prevention of absorption and control of tachyarrhythmias with lidocaine (dogs only) or procainamide (dogs only). Diazepam may be used for control of symptoms of CNS stimulation.

—*Carole Wezorek*

Psychological Indices of Toxicity

The Emergence of Psychological Measures

Psychology is the science that strives to understand, to measure, and to modify our behavior: what we do, what we say, what we think, and what we feel. At its most basic level, behavior describes how we manipulate and respond to our environment. It is the ultimate output of the nervous system. Its domain ranges across the entire universe of human activities from simple reflexes to the creation of cosmological theories. Toxicology, however, at least in the formal sense, recognized the crucial role of behavioral neuroscience only recently. Perhaps behavior seemed somewhat exotic compared to the study and traditional endpoints of death and tissue damage. However, step back from the brink that these endpoints represent and toxicology swiftly becomes a more complex and subtle enterprise.

Behavior began to insinuate itself into toxicology in the late 1960s and early 1970s. It was not a total novice, though. It came with an impressive technology molded by the discipline of behavioral pharmacology, which had begun to emerge in the 1950s with the discovery of the tranquilizing drugs. These drugs, offering the prospect of chemotherapy for psychological disorders, needed a scientific support structure. Behavioral pharmacology provided the consummate scientific basis for appraising and discovering drugs designed to alter behavior. Neurochemistry blossomed at the same time, but only the patient's behavior, measured either in a clinical or in a laboratory setting, could be the arbiter of a successful search. The same technology transferred effortlessly to the study and measurement of adverse behavioral effects, the theme of the discipline of behavioral toxicology (see Behavioral Toxicology).

Acceptance of the notion that behavioral measures could yield evidence of toxicity also benefited from the insistence of Soviet scientists that central nervous system (CNS) function and behavior offered more sensitive and appropriate measures of toxicity than the criteria prevailing in the West. Because of its own scientific history, especially the influence of Pavlov, and its political doctrines, Soviet toxicology elevated the CNS to a dominant role. Soviet scientists maintained that their exposure standards, generally much lower than those prevailing in the West, derived from their reliance on indices of CNS function rather than detectable tissue damage. Although some of these claims proved scientifically equivocal, perhaps because they needed to comply with political doctrines, they aroused the interest and attention of Western scientists who then began to apply and develop a more sound behavioral technology.

Behavioral criteria had also been adopted by industrial hygienists to set exposure standards for inhaled materials. The short-term exposure limit prescribed by ACGIH singled out performance criteria, such as reduced work efficiency and impairment of self-rescue, as indications of excessive exposure. The courts also played a role. They had begun to accept complaints of defective psychological functioning as legitimate grounds for suits alleging excessive workplace exposure. Finally, the environmentalist movement, changing its focus from tangible pollution such as filthy waterways and mass kills of wildlife, began to recognize the possibility of subtle functional effects arising from prolonged low-level exposure to environmental chemicals. Reductions in IQ scores stemming from lead exposure prompted the elimination of lead from gasoline. Proposed links between environmental chemicals and neurodegenerative diseases such as Parkinson's disease and Alzheimer's disease further aroused the public's interest.

Data from both the laboratory and the field began to converge once behavior became a source of questions about adverse effects. Both information conduits offered evidence of widespread behavioral consequences of chemical exposure generally measurable only with the appropriate application of psychological assessment methods. Workplace surveys, for example, showed many more complaints of symptoms such as sleep disturbances, excitability, depression, irritability, restlessness, apathy, and nervousness in workers exposed to neurotoxicants than in unexposed workers. Animal experiments revealed deficits in critical functions such as learning, even in superficially healthy subjects. As the literature grew, the rationale for psychological testing became more solidly entrenched. No other approach seemed comparable in unmasking changes that typically would go undetected, nor did other indicators seem as responsive to early health effects.

Occupational Sources of Adverse Psychological Responses

Much of what we have learned about the detrimental psychological effects of exposure to chemicals has come from the workplace. One reason is that greater hazards were tolerated in the workplace than in the communal environment. Another is that research protocols could be more specific about the chemicals because they could be identified with designated industrial processes.

Metals

Heavy metals are acknowledged inducers of behavioral toxicity. Lead, mercury, and manganese, especially, are associated with unique syndromes. Other metals, such as aluminum, selenium, thallium, and tin, have also been implicated in adverse behavioral effects. Table P-17 lists some of the symptoms ascribed to metal toxicity. They range in severity from subjective complaints, such as fatigue and depression, to clear neurological deficits such as tremor. Manganese is especially intriguing. Most identified victims of manganese poisoning have been miners exposed by breathing dust containing the ore. The earliest indications of toxicity typically consist of psychological signs such as extreme emotional lability marked by abnormal laughter and crying. In the South American mining communities where manganese intoxication is endemic, the syndrome is known as "locura manganica," or manganese madness. Later, more direct neurological signs begin to loom. Some of these, such as abnormal gait and slowness of movement, are reminiscent of Parkinson's disease.

Other sources of manganese exposure, such as ferromanganese processing and ore-crushing plants, expose workers to much lower levels of inhaled manganese. Even in these workers, who give no indication of clinical deficits when examined by neurologists, psychological tests reveal an elevated incidence of fatigue, tinnitus, finger tremor, and increased irritability. Behavioral testing of animal subjects also unmasks subtle deficits at exposure levels too low to induce overt neurological signs. In monkeys trained to pull against a weight with a rowing motion, manganese treatment elicits long pauses between responses such as those that might be expected under conditions of fatigue. Such findings make many scientists wary of proposals to introduce manganese compounds as additives for gasoline. They fear that dispersal of manganese into the environment may create the same intractable health problems that followed the introduction of leaded gasoline.

Metallic (elemental) mercury, the mercury found in thermometers, can also generate a constellation of both behavioral and neurological signs. Mercury is extremely volatile so that it enters the body through inhalation. Mercury vapor readily passes from the lung into the blood and then penetrates into the brain, where, at high enough levels, it produces neurotoxicity. Such effects have been recognized for centuries. Bernardo Ramazzini, often called the father of occupational hygiene because of his celebrated work published in the eighteenth century, was keenly aware of mercury poisoning and its manifestations. His descriptions of the sufferings of Venetian mirror gilders and of workers in other occupations who came in contact with mercury are exquisitely detailed and vivid. High exposures to mercury were also experienced by mercury miners; even today, in the famed mercury mines of Almaden in Spain, miners work only a few hours each week to preclude mercury poisoning.

The cardinal neurological marker of mercury vapor intoxication is tremor. Workers in the hat industry frequently suffered from mercury poisoning. Mercury compounds helped convert the stiff, straight animal fur into a limp, flexible mat that could be shaped into a hat. Vapor escaped during the process, and, inhaled day after day by the workers, sometimes evoked tremor so severe that some found it difficult even to walk without support. A survey of hat factories conducted by the U.S. Public Health Service in 1940 found a clear relationship between workplace mercury levels and the severity and incidence of tremor. Eventually, the mercury compounds were replaced.

However, even in persons exposed to much lower ambient levels, abnormalities in the frequency components of the tremor can be detected with appropriate instrumentation and mathematical analysis. A technique introduced in 1973 involved having the worker insert a finger into a slot connected to a transducer that converted tremor into an electrical signal. The worker was instructed to maintain a pressure within limits signaled by a pair of lights. The tremor signal, fed directly into a digital computer, was then broken down into its frequency components. Unlike normal tremor, the mercury-induced tremor showed two peaks, at different frequencies, rather than one. This study of women exposed to mercury vapor in the course of calibrating pipettes was able to trace their recovery, after removal from the factory, by recording and analyzing the amplitude and frequency of the tremor. Another application of tremor measures, designed to guard against excessive exposure, was adopted in a study of chlor-alkali work-

TABLE P-17
Symptoms Ascribed to Metal Toxicity

Ansomia	Incoordination
Apetite loss	Irritability
Depression	Paresthesias
Disorientation	Polyneuritis
Dizziness	Somnolence
Fatigue	Tremor
Headache	Visual disturbances
Insomnia	Weakness

ers. Chlor-alkali processing plants convert brine into chlorine and caustic soda by electrolysis. Huge pools of elemental mercury serve as the electrodes in this process. Even with devices to restrict the emission of mercury vapor, enough may escape to induce incipient toxicity. In this application, the investigators monitored tremor by using these advanced signal processing techniques; one indication of excessive exposure was the appearance of two peaks in the frequency distribution of the tremor rather than a single peak, and this served as a criterion for transferring the worker to another part of the plant.

Tremor is often accompanied by a group of symptoms termed "erethism," a term derived from the Greek root for irritation or redness. The symptoms include hyperirritability, labile temperament, timidity and shyness, blushing easily, depression, insomnia, and fatigue. One description of erethism, from a report on women in a factory in which mercury was released in the production of motor components, is virtually a classic example. The worker complained of dizzy spells, weakness, fatigue, forgetfulness, grouchiness, and "a fluttery feeling like I was scared or floating in space."

Because the Mad Hatter in *Alice in Wonderland* exhibited some of the symptoms of erethism, he is sometimes held to be a model for the afflictions suffered by workers in the hat industry; whether Lewis Carrol intended such a parallel is still disputed, but the resemblances are uncanny. Even in the absence of identifiable symptoms, psychological testing has revealed what could be called nascent erethism in workers exposed to mercury vapor but showing no overt signs of toxicity. Tests of coordination and reaction time reveal differences between exposed and unexposed workers. Performance on elements of adult intelligence tests, such as the ability to repeat strings of digits, also shows differences.

A source of mercury other than the workplace has now assumed ascendancy in driving public unease. Recent publicity has indicted mercury amalgam dental fillings as a source of adverse health effects. Although it is true that chewing can release mercury vapor from amalgam fillings, the quantities are typically too small to produce elevations in blood or urine mercury levels that are hazardous to adults. Risks posed to the fetus and child are of greater concern but are characterized by a paucity of data.

Perhaps no other metal has aroused as much public discussion and attention as lead. It was one of the earliest metals exploited for practical uses; the word plumbing comes from the Latin word for lead. The Romans constructed cisterns and cooking utensils from lead. Lead pigments are found in glazes, even those that are used to decorate pottery; acidic foods leach the lead from the glaze. Lead permeates our current environment because of its presence in paint and in industrial products such as storage batteries and because of the lead added to gasoline.

Ancient physicians, such as Galen, were aware of lead's toxicity. Alice Hamilton, who founded the specialty of occupational medicine in the United States, termed lead the oldest of the industrial poisons except for carbon monoxide. In England, regulations designed to protect workers against the consequences of clinical lead poisoning, such as convulsions and coma, were prescribed in the nineteenth century. However, incipient lead poisoning remained a more formidable problem because the classical signs are absent. Instead, the symptoms tend to be vague; the workers may act sluggish, achy, and fatigued and be prone to errors on the job. Recent assessments of lead workers, undertaken with psychological tests, show adverse effects even in the absence of clinically overt problems. These take the form of reduced scores on tests of memory, vigilance, spatial relations, and coordination. Standardized inventories of affect and personality also show disturbances in exposed workers. Lead can also impair hearing; rises in the concentration of lead in blood, a marker of recent lead exposure, elevate hearing thresholds. The most destructive of lead's neurotoxic effects, however, is interference with brain development. This aspect will be addressed later.

Pesticides

Pesticides are another class of chemicals capable of damaging the nervous system and, even at low levels, produce deficits detectable by psychological testing. The organophosphorous insecticides, which are chemical relatives of the most potent nerve gases, are notorious poisons and, carelessly handled, as often happens in underdeveloped countries, can prove lethal. Parathion, diazinon, and malathion are representatives of this class and are widely used in the United States. Acute poisoning episodes produce signs such as eye irritation, headache, dizziness, nausea, and visual disturbances. These gross effects fade with time, usually in days or weeks. However, when farmworkers who had undergone an episode of acute poisoning were evaluated with psychological tests 1 year later, they showed persisting sequelae. Compared to controls, who were matched on age and education, they displayed lower scores on a widely used adult intelligence scale and on a test of coordination and higher scores on a battery of psychological tests designed to measure incipient neurological impairment. These results are consistent with those from similar studies and with experiments in monkeys showing enduring effects on the electrical activity of the brain.

Other studies demonstrate that effects of even rather modest exposures can be detected with psychological tests. In one example, even though they gave no indication of overt poisoning and seemed superficially healthy, farmworkers who had been exposed to organophosphorous insecticides displayed evidence of psychological disturbances on a test constructed to measure anxiety. They selected items indicating that they experienced more tension, more restlessness, more emotional instability, more nervousness, and more fitful sleep than a sample of unexposed workers.

The organochlorine insecticides such as DDT are also potent nervous system poisons. Like the organophosphorous compounds, they interfere with the nervous systems of insects, so it is no surprise that they exert similar effects in humans. At high doses, they cause convulsions. An epidemic of convulsions in an English town, in fact, was traced to flour inadvertently contaminated with an organochlorine insecticide. At lower doses, the effects are more subtle. One organochlorine insecticide, chlordecone, was responsible for an outbreak of poisoning in a Virginia factory. After workers began to complain of health problems to local physicians, public health officials began an investigation and confirmed that poor hygiene in the plant had exposed the employees to excessive amounts of the chemical. The most intriguing facet of this episode is that the earliest index of toxicity turned out to be complaints of excessive nervousness. Would even an alert plant physician be likely to consider chemical exposure as the source of such complaints? Wouldn't a more likely diagnosis be personal problems either at home or at the place of employment? Episodes such as this have led some observers to recommend that workers in comparable environments undergo periodic psychological assessments to detect adverse effects.

Solvents

Among the chemicals evoking the most attention from psychologists are the volatile organic solvents. Carbon disulfide, toluene, xylene, styrene, trichloroethylene, and methylene chloride are representative members of this class. They may have evoked such attention because they are demonstrably neurotoxic. Due to their volatility, they are inhaled. ACGIH exposure standards for solvents are based on this property. Because they are soluble in fatty tissues, they easily reach the brain. At high ambient levels, they produce narcosis; in fact, some have been used as surgical anesthetics. The question posed to investigators is whether low concentrations, even those meeting current workplace exposure standards, produce adverse effects.

Scandinavian investigators pioneered studies of chronically exposed workers. On the basis of their research, they posited what has been called the organic solvent syndrome, toxic encephalopathy, or painter's syndrome (because painters often work in an environment suffused with solvents). They asserted that chronic exposure in the workplace to volatile organic solvents produced permanent deficits reflected by diminished performance on psychological tests. They pointed to lower scores on tests of intelligence, memory, learning, and other cognitive functions and to elevated reaction times and personality changes. These claims were vigorously debated, with critics arguing that necessary controls, such as matching exposed and unexposed workers for education and drinking habits, were lacking. They also argued that the generous worker compensation regulations of some Scandinavian countries encouraged claims of solvent-induced impairment. Later investigations, with more rigorous controls, and in other countries, supported the original claims and have even expanded them to include an impaired sense of smell and deficits in color vision.

Solvents are ubiquitous in the workplace and are produced in the millions of kilograms annually. They also appear in many household products such as cleaners, glues, and paint thinners. Because so many workers are exposed to solvents, and because their use is so common in other settings, the U.S. EPA proposed that solvent manufacturers undertake a comprehensive evaluation of 10 solvents with high production volumes. They specified four components in the evaluation: functional observation battery, motor activity, neuropathology, and schedule-controlled operant behavior.

In the functional observation battery, rats or mice are exposed acutely and subchronically to a solvent. Technicians then make a number of systematic observations such as the response to prodding, orienting to a click, resistance to pulling, and other simple responses.

A numerical score, based on the individual components, is then calculated.

In evaluating motor activity, rats or mice are exposed acutely or subchronically and tested in a device that measures amount of movement. For example, the rat may be placed in a figure-eight maze equipped with photocells at the intersections. Motor activity is scored by the number of photobeams interrupted. Although motor activity can be influenced by many factors, it is especially responsive to chemicals acting on the CNS.

Neuropathology involves sacrificing rats or mice after subchronic exposure and inspecting for lesions in the brain.

Schedule-controlled operant behavior (see Behavioral Toxicology) has come to play a prominent role in behavioral toxicology because it provides a supple, flexible scheme for assessing the capacity for complex behavior. The U.S. EPA explained its choice of schedule-controlled operant behavior by focusing on its versatility:

> Solvents may have neurotoxic effects on memory, learning, and performance which can be permanent. These effects are less well understood. . . . The schedule-controlled operant behavior test has typically been required as a second tier test . . . it is proposed as a first-tier test . . . because of EPA's desire to obtain data on the effects of solvents on learning, memory, and performance.

The origins of this proposal from the U.S. EPA lie in the demonstrated efficacy of performance tests as measures of psychophysiological function and in their sensitivity to the effects of chemical exposures in the workplace. These tests come from two sources. One originated in the need to provide diagnostic guidance for psychologists evaluating clients or for personnel selection. Test design and construction comprise one of psychology's major specialties; its methods have evolved over at least eight decades. Psychometric techniques provide the basis for selection tools such as the Scholastic Achievement Test. The second was the experimental psychology laboratory, the site of fundamental research on all aspects of human performance including sensory function, motor function, and cognitive functions such as memory. Contributions from these two sources always overlapped and influenced one another, but they converged especially effectively to meet the growing interest in the measurement of performance stirred by evidence that such measures could uncover toxic effects that otherwise would remain concealed.

The demonstrated sensitivity of psychological test methods to solvent exposure led the World Health Organization (WHO) to call upon experts for the design of a test battery that could be applied even in underdeveloped countries lacking such a tradition. The basic WHO battery appears in Table P-18. More comprehensive batteries tend to be used in the advanced industrial countries, where psychologists have tried to exploit the potential of digital computers for test design, presentation, and analysis.

Psychological Measures of Impaired Development

Hardly any facet of psychology claims as much attention in toxicology as brain development. Teratology describes the discipline whose dominion is the study of congenital deformities, or birth defects. By analogy, some investigators appropriated the term to label a new area they called behavioral teratology. The label became accepted practice because it graphically described what these scientists viewed as a vital but previously neglected aspect of toxicology: the functional consequences, later in life, of exposure to neurotoxic agents during gestation or infancy. Although such functional consequences might include defects as severe as mental deficiency, most of the research in this area has taken the form of questions about less blatant outcomes. Learning disabilities, conduct disorders, slower than normal language acquisition, delayed motor development, and downward shifts in the distribution of IQ scores are among the outcomes reported in the scientific literature.

TABLE P-18
WHO Neurobehavioral Core Test Battery

Functional domain	*Core test*
Motor speed	Aiming; dot placing
Attention	Simple reaction time
Perceptual-motor	WAIS digit–symbol
Manual dexterity	Santa Ana test
Visual memory	Benton test
Auditory memory	WAIS digit span

In response to overwhelming public anxieties, regulatory agencies in Japan and the United Kingdom began to insist on behavioral teratology information for new drugs. The U.S. EPA has also been active in setting guidelines for developmental toxicity that also embrace potential behavioral effects. These guidelines prescribe a range of behavioral testing protocols ranging from simple locomotor activity to tests designed to measure learning and memory. The impetus for such protocols comes from the recognized vulnerability of the developing brain to neurotoxic chemicals. The fetal alcohol syndrome is one striking example. Three agents in particular have aroused the interest of toxicologists: lead, methylmercury, and the polychlorinated biphenyls.

Lead

Severe lead poisoning in children is now a much more infrequent event in the United States than even in the recent past. The current focus of attention is the impact of much lower exposure levels on how well children function. Twenty-five years ago, a blood lead concentration below 40 μg/dl was considered acceptable. By 1991, the CDC, weighing all the accumulated evidence, had concluded that levels exceeding 10 μg/dl gave cause for concern. The primary motive for this change stemmed from depressed scores on intelligence tests.

Attempts to construct a metric of intelligence have occupied the energies of many psychologists from the middle of the nineteenth century to the present. Definitions of intelligence continue to elicit intense debate. Intelligence testing of children, however, beyond doctrinal disagreements, has come to rest on a forthright principle: Measure the child against his or her peers. Intelligence tests vary widely in the items they choose for such comparisons but typically include an assessment of vocabulary, the ability to count and calculate, the ability to discern relationships among objects, and other markers of how well the child has mastered his or her environment. The components of a leading test, the Wechsler Intelligence Scale for Children-Revised, are listed in Table P-19. As in all psychological tests, items basically represent stimuli for the elicitation of behavior samples. They are not absolute measures of some fundamental property.

TABLE P-19
Components of the Wechsler Intelligence Scale for Children (Revised)

Verbal IQ	Performance IQ
Information	Picture completion
Vocabulary	Picture arrangement
Digit span	Block design
Arithmetic	Object assembly
Comprehension	Coding
Similarities	Mazes

From items such as those contained in the component subtests listed in Table P-19, a test score, equivalent to a test age, is derived. The IQ is computed as the quotient of the test age, based on the performance of a standardized population of children, divided by the child's chronological age. A child who is average for his or her age will yield an IQ of 100. An above-average child will obtain an IQ above 100. There is some dispute about the interpretation of an IQ based on a standardized population significantly different in ethnic background and socioeconomic status from the child being tested, so that exposure conditions and the child's other environmental circumstances should not be confounded.

IQ scores began their ascendancy in assessing the risks of childhood lead exposure as long ago as the 1950s, but poorly focused investigations, inadequate measures of exposure, and the then unrecognized scope of lead toxicity yielded little more than a stream of ambiguous studies. A pioneering report in 1979 by Herbert Needleman and colleagues marked the first of many well-designed studies showing significant IQ reductions in young children ascribable to quite modest increments of lead exposure. It adopted the then novel strategy of estimating cumulative exposure to lead by relying on baby teeth, which, like bone, store lead. The findings were so compelling that they stimulated additional investigations in many parts of the world that built further support for the lead and IQ relationship.

Subsequent investigations adopted an even more forceful strategy; they undertook prospective studies in which children with documented prenatal lead exposures were followed from birth. These studies demonstrated that even lead levels so low that they would have been considered insignificant just a few years earlier could reduce scores on IQ and analogous developmental tests.

Some critics charge that such findings possess little practical significance. They argue that a difference of a few IQ points exercises negligible influence on how well a child functions. However, such an argument neglects the implications for the population as a whole. Because of the way in which IQ scores are distributed, in a population of 100 million in which the mean IQ is 100, 2.3 million individuals will score above 130, the superior range. If the mean is shifted downward by five IQ points (5%), which the critics deem insignificant, the mean IQ becomes 95 and only 990,000 individuals will score above 130. Most observers would contend that such an impact on a society cannot be considered negligible. This perspective, gained from the results of psychological tests, made a key contribution to the CDC decision to designate a lead level of 10 μg/dl in blood as a level of concern.

Methylmercury

About 26 states now disseminate fish advisories for lakes and rivers based on methylmercury contamination. Methylmercury is an organic form of mercury and a potent nervous system poison. It is especially destructive to the developing brain. Although recognized as a poison for over 100 years, its impact on the fetal brain came to attention only in the 1950s, when the population of a small Japanese fishing village, Minamata, experienced widespread methylmercury poisoning. Fish and shellfish from Minamata bay had been contaminated by effluent from a factory that used mercury as a catalyst in the production of acetaldehyde. Many inhabitants died. Even more suffered permanent neurological damage. In addition, a much higher incidence of retarded brain development was observed in Minamata than elsewhere in Japan but the population was too small to yield a cogent answer.

The final evidence came in the form of an outbreak of methylmercury poisoning in Iraq. Because grain crops had been decimated by a severe drought in 1971, the Iraqi government ordered over 80,000 tons of seed grain from Mexico and the United States. The order specified that the grain be treated with a methylmercury fungicide, which ordinarily would dissipate into the soil after planting. Despite warnings, many farming communities in the Iraqi countryside, facing food shortages, baked the treated grain into bread. The result was a mass poisoning episode, in the winter of 1971–1972, that killed as many as 5000 people. It was the largest mass chemical disaster in history.

University of Rochester investigators, led by Dr. Thomas W. Clarkson, were called upon for assistance because of their research experience with mercury and with antidotes. They established a laboratory in Baghdad and began a project to survey the countryside. One phenomenon struck them with singular force. Offspring of mothers who had consumed large amounts of the tainted bread displayed evidence of brain damage. Some seemed afflicted with cerebral palsy. Some were prone to seizures. Others were late in speech and motor development. Because Clarkson and colleagues had discovered that growing hair took up methylmercury from the blood, hair became the ultimate measure of exposure. Because scalp hair grows about 1 cm (about one-half inch) per month, a 12-cm length of hair had engraved on it a year's history of methylmercury blood levels, which closely reflect consumption.

With this tool, the investigators were able to establish a relationship between maternal methylmercury exposure and indices of child development. Statistical analyses of the correlation between maternal hair levels and delayed walking, for example, suggested that even slightly elevated methylmercury consumption by a pregnant woman might pose a risk for fetal brain development.

The primary repository of methylmercury in the diet is fish. Natural sources of inorganic mercury, such as volcanoes, and human contributions from fossil fuel and waste combustion contribute to a global mercury cycle that deposits the mercury in waterways. Microorganisms in the bottom sediment convert the inorganic form into methylmercury, which ascends the food chain and concentrates in the predators at the apex of the food chain. Swordfish, shark, pike, snapper, and tuna are among these predatory species.

In New Zealand, comparisons among children whose mothers consumed different amount of fish during gestation indicated that higher consumption levels tended to depress scores on IQ and other psychological tests. Because a single study could not be definitive, other studies have been undertaken. Their results have now begun to appear and show little evidence of adverse outcomes. Studies of this kind must occupy several years, however, because some consequences of developmental damage, such as performance on certain components of IQ tests, cannot be assayed until the child is advanced enough to be tested. In the meantime, regulatory authorities have adopted a position of caution and advised against the consumption of certain species of fish from particular sites by pregnant women and young children.

Polychlorinated Biphenyls

The polychlorinated biphenyls (PCBs) are as ubiquitous in the environment as lead. They also share many properties in common with other organic halogen compounds such as the organochlorine insecticides and dioxins. Their health risks until recently have been dominated by potential carcinogenicity. Newer data sources now suggest that their most serious risks may stem from actions on the developing brain. Two poisoning episodes, one in Japan and one in Taiwan, yielded the first clues. In both instances, cooking oil had been contaminated by PCBs, which enjoyed wide use as insulating material for transformers. They are dissolved in a oil base, so contamination cannot easily be detected. Children born to mothers who had consumed the contaminated oil, besides showing skin darkening and other signs of PCB toxicity, also suffered from mental retardation. Suspicions that problems might lurk in lower levels of exposure stimulated studies equipped to measure more accurately the correlation between maternal PCB exposure and offspring development. The resulting data indicate to many scientists that current levels of tissue PCBs are disturbingly close to levels that represent a hazard to optimal brain development.

One origin of this altered point of view is a series of studies based on correlations between maternal intake of PCB-contaminated fish during pregnancy and the performance of the offspring on psychological tests. The higher the maternal PCB level (measured in blood samples or fat bioposies), the lower the IQ score. IQ scores of children whose mothers consumed Lake Michigan fish suffered a 6% (6 point) decline at 11 years of age. Additional psychological tests confirmed this relationship. Normal infants shown two pictures, one of which is familiar and one of which is novel, will tend to spend more time gazing at the novel picture. The degree of bias in the direction of novelty apparently correlates to a surprisingly degree with later IQ scores. Children later shown to be at risk for developmental retardation show little novelty bias. Maternal PCB levels are significant predictors of novelty bias; the higher the PCB level, the lower the degree of bias. These two psychological indices—IQ scores and visual recognition memory—established the PCBs, even at levels that produce no obvious indications of toxicity, as hazards to brain and behavioral development. The implications of these findings are disturbing because so many women maintain body burdens of PCBs uncomfortably close to the levels associated with lowered scores on psychological tests of developmental outcome. They are also disturbing because PCBs represent a class of chemicals, including the dioxins and DDT, that have been labeled endocrine disruptors and that have the potential to interfere with sexual differentiation of the brain, with immune system function, and with thyroid development.

Food Additives

An instructive instance of the changed perspectives that psychological measures may impose on toxicity evaluation and risk assessment emerged from claims that some foods and food additives might elicit behavioral disturbances in children. The claims were formulated by Dr. Ben Feingold, a pioneering pediatric allergist in the Kaiser-Permanente system in California. Feingold asserted that some of the children labeled as hyperactive, or suffering from what is currently called attention deficit disorder, actually were exhibiting adverse responses to certain dietary constituents. Among the additives, he singled out synthetic colors and flavors for elimination from diets because, in addition to reports in the allergy literature linking them to adverse reactions, they lacked nutritional value in any case.

The U.S. FDA does not require testing of food additives for neurobehavioral toxicity and Feingold's claims were based on clinical experience rather than on controlled clinical trials. His claims, however, generated sharp public interest, particularly on the part of agonizing parents, and provoked a series of clinical trials designed to test his hypothesis. Although the investigators adopted a wide variety of approaches, and most focused on food dyes for experimental convenience, the total published literature converges to the conclusion that, in principle, Feingold's claims were valid. The major disagreements stem from the estimated proportion of children at risk, which range from about 1 to 25%, and the scope of the dietary components evoking behavioral disturbances. Another source of disagreement arises from how risks are perceived. Some critics argue that a 1% prevalence of adverse responses to food dyes, for example, is not a reason to eliminate them from the food supply. At the same time, regulatory agencies such as the U.S. EPA strive to establish exposure levels to ensure cancer risks below one per million persons. An incidence of 1% is hardly trivial.

One of the experiments indicating the potential of food dyes to induce adverse behavioral responses was conducted by the author and coinvestigators with a sample of young California children. These children had been designated by their parents as responders. That is, their behavior had been seen to improve on a diet that eliminated food additives and some other foods. The parents enrolled in a study in which they provided daily behavioral observations of their child's response to a soft drink containing either a blend of food dyes or innocuous colorings such as caramel. The two drinks were not distinguishable. During the 11-week experimental period, the daily drink contained the blend of dyes on eight randomly assigned occasions.

Of the 22 enrolled children, 2 showed consistent responses to the blend of dyes. One of the children, a 34-month-old girl, gave highly elevated scores, after drinking the challenge drink, on the following items of a 10-item list: short attention span, acts as if driven by motor, runs away, throws and breaks things, and whines. She also showed elevated scores on a standardized rating scale of attention deficit disorder. Table P-20 shows the difference between the amount of U.S. FDA-approved food dyes evoking behavioral disturbances in sensitive children and the acceptable daily intakes based on the standard 2-year feeding study in rodents (a study required by the U.S. FDA). The differences between conventional assays, largely based on pathology, and those based on psychological measures are about 50- to 60-fold.

TABLE P-20
Food Dyes: Doses (mg/day) Eliciting Behavioral Responses vs FDA Acceptable Daily Intake

Color	*Behavior*[a]	*ADI*
Yellow 5	9.07	300
Yellow 6	10.70	300
Red 40	13.80	420
Red 3	0.57	150
Blue 1	0.80	200
Blue 2	0.15	37
Green 3	0.11	150

[a]Based on Weiss *et al.* (1980).

Psychological Measures of Enhanced Chemical Sensitivity

A new array of problems closely entwined with environmental toxicology is attached to labels such as sick building syndrome, multiple chemical sensitivity, chronic fatigue syndrome, and Gulf War syndrome. They have spawned a sizable literature and gripped public interest and anxieties. For all three labels, the primary clinical manifestations consist primarily of subjective complaints; conventional medical indices are lacking. Especially for multiple chemical sensitivity and sick building syndrome, the instigators are held to be toxic chemicals, but in most instances the offending agents lack clear identification.

Patients allegedly suffering from multiple chemical sensitivity complain of depression, excessive fatigue, sleep disorders, irritability, headaches, and symptoms, such as rhinitis, similar to those associated with allergies. Although immune system disorders are hypothesized as the most frequent underlying cause, compelling evidence in support of such a mechanism is lacking. Another puzzle is the emergence of such symptoms in response to chemical agents of widely divergent classes and, typically, at rather low concentrations. The vague, malleable contours of the syndrome and the absence of an identifiable etiology have engendered a countervailing skepticism about its validity on the part of many clinicians and scientists. The absence of sound investigational protocols and experiments, except for a sparse, scattered literature, has nourished such skepticism.

The sick building syndrome is another victim of sparse empirical support. The contemporary emphasis on energy efficiency has produced buildings notable for poor air quality manifested as inadequate ventilation coupled with contaminating agents ranging from infectious microorganisms to common allergens to volatile organic chemicals. Outbreaks of illness, attributed to such environmental conditions, have made their way into the biomedical literature and the popular media.

Like multiple chemical sensitivity patients, those asserted to be afflicted with the sick building syndrome exhibit a collection of largely subjective complaints: headaches, fatigue, and lightheadedness are among the symptoms. They are accompanied by complaints of persistent cough, chest tightness, wheezing, and eye and throat irritation. Although better documented than the multiple chemical sensitivity syndrome because the complaints often can be traced to a specific site, it too has often aroused suspicions of its validity. Some critics contend that most reports of widespread illness in particular buildings are more likely instances of suggestibility than of authentic illness. Others, citing unsuccessful attempts to relate variations in air quality to the quantity of complaints, also tend to belittle the syndrome as a disease entity.

U.S. EPA scientists are among the groups that have sought to view these two syndromes from an experimental perspective. The agency's unfortunate experience with its own building renovation program, which left a residue of sick building complaints, gave this effort a substantial impetus. They exposed healthy subjects to a mixture containing 22 volatile organic chemicals commonly detected in new or newly renovated buildings and asked the subjects to rate the intensity of various responses. During the 2.75-hr exposure periods, perceived odor intensity diminished and air quality ratings improved. Ratings of eye and throat irritation, headache, and dizziness either increased or remained stable. Such results indicate that odors alone, as suggested by some observers, do not trigger the symptoms of multiple chemical sensitivity or sick building syndrome. Concurrent assessments of neurobehavioral function found that subjects reported increased fatigue and confusion. At the same time, their performance on successive administrations of a battery of 13 psychological tests remained unimpaired, a finding the authors speculate may have been influenced by the tendency to improve with practice.

Chronic fatigue syndrome, although its reality is also debated, is more firmly established as a valid entity than the other two syndromes. The label is attached to patients who suffer prolonged feelings of fatigue, weakness, and even exhaustion. They report inability to concentrate, memory loss, depression, sleep disorders, and a variety of symptoms reminiscent of influenza. The prevailing view among those who accept the syndrome is that it reflects an immune system disorder, perhaps triggered by a viral infection, but its character and etiology remain equivocal.

When psychological testing of such patients has been undertaken, some are revealed to suffer reliable cognitive deficits. For example, they exhibit slowed reaction times, reduced accuracy in searching for target letters on a page of typed letters, impaired recall of a narrative, and lowered scores on various tests of memory. Such results are intriguing and perhaps significant. They are supported by data indicating that psychological test performance is impaired by experimentally induced viral or bacterial infections and that recovery of performance, despite recovery by clinical measures, may require a prolonged period. Another clue comes from animal experiments. In response to infections, the immune system releases substances called cytokines. Interleukins are members of this class. Interleukins also exert profound effects on behavior, and some scientists speculate that the nonspecific symptoms of infection, similar to the complaints vented by chronic fatigue syndrome patients, originate from the action of these and other cytokines.

Although these three syndromes are not intrinsically linked to the traditional domain of toxicology, they illustrate the role that psychological measures are increasingly assuming when adverse effects of environmental chemicals emerge as an issue. Clinical medicine prefers to deal with specific signs pointing to specific diseases. Environmental toxicants, however, far more often now than in the past, are being indicted as the sources responsible for diffuse aberrations of function such as conduct disorders, learning disabilities, memory and concentration difficulties, feelings of listlessness, fatigue, depression, and a galaxy of other disturbances beyond the catalog of accepted medical diagnoses. Psychological test methods, developed over a period of many decades, provide the tools for making the appropriate connections.

Further Reading

Annau, Z. (Ed.) (1986). *Neurobehavioral Toxicology.* Johns Hopkins Univ. Press, Baltimore, MD.

Environmental Neurotoxicology (1991). National Academy Press, Washington, DC.

Office of Technology Assessment, Congress of the United States (1990). *Neurotoxicology: Identifying and Controlling Poisons of the Nervous System*, OTA-BA-436. U.S. Government Printing Office, Washington, DC.

Russell, R. W., Flattau, P. E., and Pope, A. M. (Eds.) (1990). *Behavioral Measures of Neurotoxicity.* National Academy Press, Washington, DC.

Tilson, H. A., and Mitchell, C. L. (Eds.) (1992). *Neurotoxicology.* Raven Press, New York.

Weiss, B., and O'Donoghue, J. L. (Eds.) (1994). *Neurobehavioral Toxicity: Analysis and Interpretation.* Raven Press, New York.

—Bernard Weiss

Related Topics

Behavioral Toxicology
Food Additives
Indoor Air Pollution
Metals
Multiple Chemical Sensitivities
Neurotoxicology: Central and Peripheral
Pesticides
Short-Term Exposure Limit
Sick Building syndrome
Toxicity Testing, Behavioral

Pyrethrin/Pyrethroids

Extracts from pyrethrum flowers (*Chrysanthemum cineraraefolum* and *C. coccineum*) have been marketed as insecticidal agents since the early to mid-1800s. The pyrethrum flowers actually contain a mixture of six insecticidal esters broadly classified into one of two groups: Pyrethrin I and Pyrethrin II. Pyrethrin I, chrysanthemic acid esters, includes pyrethrin I, cinerin I, and jasmolin I. Pyrethrin II, pyrethric acid esters, includes pyrethrin II, cinerin II, and jasmolin II. Rapid knockdown of flying insects is a characteristic of the Pyrethrin II compounds but the Pyrethrin I compounds possess greater insecticidal activity.

Pyrethrum was commonly used in both domestic and agricultural applications until the more stable organochlorine compounds became available. When environmental persistence dictated replacement of the organochlorines, the pyrethrins and their more stable, more potent, synthetic derivatives, the pyrethroids, became widely used again. Pyrethroids are estimated to account for 25–30% of the current worldwide insecticide usage.

Pyrethroids are available in a variety of forms including emulsifiable concentrates, wettable powders, granules, and concentrates. Pyrethroids are often combined with synergists such as piperonyl butoxide (which inhibits enzymes involved in pyrethroid metabolism) or with other classes of pesticides such as organophosphates. Tank mixing of pyrethroids with other pesticides is also a common practice during application. Human ectoparasites can be treated with a cream containing 1% permethrin.

The pyrethroids are generally divided into one of two groups based on the presence of a cyano moiety group at the α-carbon position. Type I pyrethroids lack the cyano group; examples include allethrin, tetramethrin, kadethrin, resmethrin, phenothrin, and permethrin. Examples of type II compounds include cypermethrin, deltamethrin, fenpropanthrin, fenvalerate, flucythrinate, and fluvalinate. All pyrethroids share the same basic mechanism of action but the different types cause somewhat different symptoms.

Pyrethroids may be present as at least four different isomers and the sodium channel interactions are stereospecific with the 1*R* and 1*S cis* isomers binding differently than the 1*R* and 1*S trans* isomers. Additionally, only the 1*R* isomers are toxic to mammals, while the main action of the 1*S* isomers is to block effects of the 1*R* isomers. This stereospecificity, due to isomerism about the third carbon atom of the cyclopropane ring, accounts for the reported differences in toxicity of the pyrethroids available as isomeric mixtures. The R group of the type II pyrethroids has a cyano moiety providing an additional chiral carbon and a total of eight different isomeric forms (if the cyclopropane ring is present; a few pyrethroids do not have the ring structure). The cyano substitution also imparts specificity with only the α-S compounds affecting both mammals and insects.

Mechanisms of Toxicity

Pyrethroids have a selective high affinity for membrane sodium channels. Closing of the channel, which ends the action potential, is slowed resulting in a prolonged "tail" current and repetitive firing of presynaptic and accompanying postsynaptic cells following a single action potential. High enough doses/exposures can cause complete depolarization and blockade of nerve conduction. An interesting characteristic of pyrethroids is their selective affinity for active channels; closed or inactive channels are generally unaffected.

Other possible mechanisms of pyrethroid toxicity have been investigated. Inhibition of Ca^{2+}, Mg^{2+}-ATPase and the calcium-binding protein calmodulin have been observed with some pyrethroids. However, the increases in neurotransmitter release seen with the pyrethroids are thought to be due to increased sodium flux rather than increased intracellular calcium levels. The type II compounds have also been shown to interfere with the γ-aminobutyric acid-mediated chloride ionophore, but these effects occur only at doses higher than those required to affect sodium flux.

Several factors favor pyrethroid toxicity to insects rather than mammals. First, pyrethroids have a negative temperature coefficient. Mammals, because of their higher body temperature, are less susceptible. Also due to higher body temperatures, mammalian enzymes are more effective at detoxifying the pyrethroids.

Human Toxicity

Acute

Because of low absorption and rapid metabolism few systemic effects are usually seen in pyrethroid exposures. Extensive human dermal exposure causes temporary abnormal sensations including paresthesia, numbness, and tingling sensations. Mammalian systemic effects of the type I pyrethroids typically include hyperexcitation, enhanced startle response, tremors, and prostration. Type II motor symptoms in mammals are characterized by hyperactivity, incoordination, choreoathetosis, and convulsions. Human ingestion of type II pyrethroids has resulted in a variety of symptoms including nausea, vomiting, stomach pain, tenesmus, diarrhea, muscle fasiculations, coma, and death due to respiratory failure.

Chronic

Chronic effects in humans following pyrethroid exposure have not been reported.

Clinical Management

Oral exposures may be treated with syrup of ipecac-induced emesis, activated charcoal, or gastric lavage. Emesis is contraindicated in unconsciousness or convulsions. In cases of dermal exposure, contaminated clothing should be removed and disposed of. Any exposed areas of skin should be repeatedly washed with soap and water. Paresthesia may be treated with topical application of vitamin E. For eye contact, the eyes should be flushed with generous amounts of lukewarm water for a minimum of 15 min. Seizures can be treated with intravenous diazepam; phenytoin or phenobarbital may be helpful for uncontrollable or recurrent seizures. Atropine can be used to control excessive salivation. No specific antidotes for pyrethroid-induced neurotoxic effects have been approved for use in humans. Spontaneous recovery usually occurs with mild or moderate intoxication.

Animal Toxicity

Fish and crustaceans are extremely sensitive to pyrethroid compounds in laboratory settings. However, various factors (e.g., sediment binding) may reduce pyrethroid toxicity to these nontarget organisms in a natural environment.

Further Reading

Narahashi, T. (1996). Neuronal ion channels as the target sites of insecticides. *Pharmacol. Toxicol.* 79, 1–14.

—*Paul R. Harp*

Related Topics

Carboxylesterases
Neurotoxicology: Central and Peripheral

Pyridine

- CAS: 110-86-1
- SYNONYMS: Azabenzene; azine
- CHEMICAL CLASS: Heterocyclic nitrogen
- MOLECULAR FORMULA: C_5H_5N
- CHEMICAL STRUCTURE:

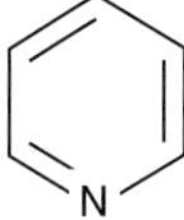

Uses

Pyridine is a solvent used in the synthesis of pharmaceuticals and other organic compounds.

Exposure Pathways

Inhalation, dermal contact, and ingestion are possible routes of exposure.

Toxicokinetics

Pyridine is absorbed from the gastrointestinal tract and skin and by inhalation. Part of it is excreted unchanged in the urine. Portions of a dose may be methylated at the N-position to form the urinary metabolite *N*-methylpyridinium hydroxide. Pyridine also may undergo oxygenation by liver microsomes (cytochrome P450) in the presence of NADPH and oxygen.

Human Toxicity

Despite widespread industrial use, reports of human injury as a result of pyridine are rare. Acute exposure to pyridine results in irritation to the skin, nose, and throat. Central nervous system (CNS) depression results in dizziness and lightheadedness. Exposure to high concentrations may result in coma and death. Contact with the eyes causes burning and leads to permanent damage. Ingestion of small amounts may produce narcotic effects including anorexia, nausea, fatigue, and mental depression. Larger quantities have resulted in systemic effects and death in 43 hr.

Chronic exposure at 6–16 ppm may result in severe liver damage and kidney injury. Permanent damage to the CNS may result in confusion and mental changes including headache, insomnia, and back pain. Chronic ingestion results in symptoms similar to inhalation. Chronic exposure causes liver and kidney damage.

Pyridine is an allergen and exposure may result in sensitization. It has no known carcinogenic effects.

Clinical Management

The victim should be removed from the source of exposure. For inhalation exposures, fresh air should be supplied. Artificial respiration should be provided if breathing has stopped; oxygen should be administered if available. Treatment should be symptomatic, noting narcotic effect of pyridine. Dermal exposure should be minimized by washing away all traces of the chemical with soap or mild detergent and large amounts of water. Symptoms of dermatitis should be treated.

For ingestion, if the victim is conscious and not convulsing, emesis should be induced with syrup of ipecac and water should be given. Vomiting should be encouraged with the head below the hips to reduce aspiration. Treatment should be repeated 20 min later if not initially effective. Activated charcoal may be administered. It should be noted that large doses can act as a heart poison.

Animal Toxicity

Dermal LD_{50}s include 1121 mg/kg for rabbits and 1 g/kg for guinea pigs. Oral LD_{50}s include 891 mg/kg for rats, 1500 mg/kg for mice, and 4 g/kg for guinea pigs. Intravenous LD_{50}s include 420 mg/kg for mice and 880 mg/kg for dogs. The LC_{Lo} (inhalation) in rats is 4000 ppm/4 hr.

—Kathryn Kehoe

Pyridoxine

- CAS: 65-23-6
- SYNONYMS: Vitamin B_6; pyridoxal; pyridoxamine; pyridoxin; 5-hydroxy-6-methyl-3,4-pyridinedimethanol
- PHARMACEUTICAL CLASS: Water-soluble vitamin
- MOLECULAR FORMULA: $C_6H_5NO_2$
- CHEMICAL STRUCTURE:

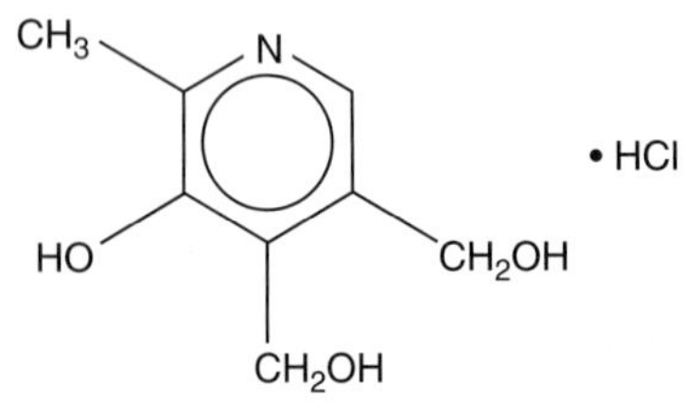

CH_3 N • HCl HO CH_2OH CH_2OH

Uses

Pyridoxine is a nutritional supplement used during deficiency states resulting from conditions such as severe diarrhea, malabsorption, congenital metabolic dysfunction, hyperthyroidism, renal and hepatic disease, congestive heart failure, alcoholism, and during pregnancy and lactation.

Exposure Pathways

Routes of exposure are oral, intravenous, and intramuscular. Dietary sources of pyridoxine include bananas, potatoes, eggs, lentils, legumes, cereals, chicken, liver, and kidneys. Cooking destroys some of the vitamins.

Toxicokinetics

Pyridoxine is readily absorbed from the gastrointestinal tract mainly in the jejunum. It is hepatically metabolized and stored mainly in the liver, muscle, and brain. Volume of distribution and protein binding are both low. The plasma half-life is 1.7 hr and the biological half-life is 15–20 days. Pyridoxine is excreted renally almost entirely as metabolites. Excess amounts of pyridoxine (beyond daily need) are excreted unchanged in the urine.

Mechanism of Toxicity

The exact mechanism of pyridoxine-induced neurotoxicity has not been established but may occur at the dorsal root ganglion.

Human Toxicity

Acute toxic effects are not expected but occasional allergic reactions have been reported. Chronic doses of ≧1 g pyridoxine per day for several months may cause severe sensory neuropathy, ataxia, incoordination of hands, weakness, and paresthesias. This most frequently occurs in women being treated for premenstrual syndrome. Seizures and ulcers have also been reported with extremely large doses given intravenously.

Clinical Management

Acute ingestions seldom require treatment. Chronic excessive use should be discontinued and any toxic effects treated symptomatically.

Animal Toxicity

Acute toxicity is not expected, and it would be unlikely for animals to be given chronic pyridoxine overdosage.

—Denise L. Kurta

Related Topic

Developmental Toxicology

Pyriminil

- CAS: 53558-25-1
- SYNONYMS: 1-(3-Pyridylmethyl-3-(4-nitrophenyl) urea; DLP-87; DLP-787; PNU; Pyrinuron; Vacor; RH-787
- CHEMICAL CLASS: Substituted urea
- CHEMICAL STRUCTURE:

O
NH—C—NH
CH_2
N
NO_2

Uses

Pyriminil was first introduced in 1975 as a rodenticide to control rats and house mice. It is especially effective against rodents resistant to anticoagulant poisons. Pyriminil was marketed for indoor use only in the form of a bait and tracking powder.

Exposure Pathways

Oral and dermal routes of exposure are possible.

Toxicokinetics

Pyriminil is absorbed from the gastrointestinal tract. Following absorption, pyriminil is distributed in the body and undergoes metabolism in the liver by the mixed function oxidase system. The hepatic metabolism of pyriminil is dependent on the 3-methylcholanthrene-inducible form of mixed function oxidase. Different metabolites have been identified in the urine of poisoned rats, dogs, and humans. These metabolites include pyriminilglucuronide, aminopyriminil, acetamidopyriminil, *p*-aminophenyl urea, *p*-acetamidophenyl urea, *p*-nitroaniline, *p*-phenylenediamine, *p*-acetamidoaniline, nicotinic acid, nicotinuric acid, and nicotinamide. Dogs develop tolerance to pyriminil, which may be partially attributed to enhanced hepatic detoxification and excretion.

Mechanism of Toxicity

Pyriminil acts as a nicotinamide antagonist and interferes in the synthesis of the coenzyme (NADH) and its phosphate (NADPH). It can also cause an insulin-deficient form of diabetes by acting as a direct pancreatic β-cell toxin similar to alloxan and streptozotocin.

Human Toxicity: Acute

The lowest acute toxic dose of pyriminil in humans was estimated at 5 mg/kg. Ingestion of one-half of one 39-g packet (2% pyriminil) of Vacor reportedly led to a fatality. A 7-year-old child was found dead one day after ingesting one packet of DLP-787 (2% Vacor). In another case, two of nine people died after ingestion of 39 g of Vacor; the remaining people developed chronic hypotension and permanent diabetes mellitus. Generally the symptoms of acute poisoning were characterized by rapid onset of insulin-dependent diabetes mellitus, severe orthostatic hypotension, autonomic dysfunction, autonomic neuropathy (dysphagia, impotence, urinary retention, constipation, or diarrhea), and peripheral neuropathy. Other symptoms included nausea, vomiting, abdominal cramp, diffuse myalgias, polyuria, polydipsia, dyspnea, malaise, and general weakness. Peripheral sensory and motor neuropathies are possible signs of pyriminil exposure. Neurological effects of pyriminil can occur within hours of ingestion and may persist for months.

Clinical Management

Because pyriminil can cause early onset seizures, induction of emesis is contraindicated. Gastric lavage may be useful if performed soon after ingestion. Activated charcoal/cathartic therapy may be adopted to retard the absorption of pyriminil from the gastrointestinal tract. According to U.S. FDA guidelines, 240 ml of diluent may be mixed with 30 g of charcoal. The usual charcoal dose is 30–100 g in adults and 15–30 g in children (1 or 2 g in infants).

Conventional anticonvulsants (e.g., diazepam, phenobarbital, and phenytoin) may be administered to treat pyriminil-induced seizures. Niacinamide has been demonstrated to be an effective antidote in pyriminil poisoning in rats but little information is available regarding its antidotal efficacy in humans. Insulin therapy could be instituted as a preventive measure for possible diabetes mellitus. Orthostatic hypotension due to pyriminil exposure may be treated with conventional mineralocorticoids.

Animal Toxicity

In rats, the LD_{50} is very low (about 5 mg/kg). Other species are markedly less sensitive (LD_{50} values from 0.5 to 4 g/kg). A horse was reported to show severe muscle fasciculations, sweating, dilated pupils, and tachycardia following ingestion of 0.25–0.5 kg of pyriminil. Other signs of toxicity in horses include colic, hindlimb weakness, ataxia, and persistent loss of appetite. Pyriminil intoxication in other animals causes gastrointestinal disorders (e.g., vomiting and abdominal cramp), visual problems, cardiovascular disorders, ataxia, tremor, and coma.

—Tamal Kumar Chakraborti

Related Topic

Pesticides